NEUROLOGIC INTERVENTIONS

for PHYSICAL THERAPY

NEUROLOGIC INTERVENTIONS for PHYSICAL THERAPY

Fourth Edition

SUZANNE "TINK" MARTIN, PT, PhD
Professor Emerita
Physical Therapy
University of Evansville
Evansville, Indiana

MARY KESSLER, PT, MHS
Dean
College of Education and Health Sciences
Associate Professor
Physical Therapy
University of Evansville
Evansville, Indiana

ELSEVIER

Elsevier
1600 John F. Kennedy Blvd.
Ste. 1800
Philadelphia, PA 19103-2899

NEUROLOGIC INTERVENTIONS FOR PHYSICAL THERAPY, FOURTH EDITION   ISBN: 978-0-323-66175-1

Notice

Practitioners and researchers must always rely on their own experience and knowledge in evaluating and using any information, methods, compounds, or experiments described herein. Because of rapid advances in the medical sciences, in particular, independent verification of diagnoses and drug dosages should be made. To the fullest extent of the law, no responsibility is assumed by Elsevier, authors, editors, or contributors for any injury and/or damage to persons or property as a matter of products liability, negligence, or otherwise, or from any use or operation of any methods, products, instructions, or ideas contained in the material herein.

Previous editions copyrighted 2016, 2007, and 2000.

ISBN 9780323661751

Content Strategist: Lauren Willis
Content Development Specialist: Sara Watkins
Publishing Services Manager: Deepthi Unni
Project Manager: Srividhya Vidhyashankar
Design Direction: Bridget Hoette

Printed in China

Last digit is the print number: 9   8   7   6   5   4

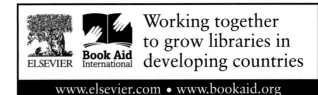

To my husband, *Terry*, who has always been there with love and support, and to my parents, *John* and *Sue Delker*, who were always supportive of my educational endeavors. Finally, to all the children, families, colleagues, and students who taught me what was important in life.

Tink Martin

To *Craig*, my husband, who continues to provide me with love, support, and encouragement to pursue this and all of my other professional goals, and to *Kyle* and *Kaitlyn*, who still like to see their photographs in print but more importantly were there to listen and encourage me to finish this edition. Thank you all from the bottom of my heart.

A final word of thanks to my parents, *John* and *Judy Oerter*, and my family who have always encouraged me to work hard and strive for excellence. You have always believed in me and my ability to succeed.

Mary Kessler

ACKNOWLEDGMENTS

I again want to acknowledge the dedication and hard work of my colleague, friend, and coauthor, Mary Kessler. Mary's focus on excellence is evident in the updated adult chapters, as well as in the introductory chapter. Special thanks to Dawn Welborn-Mabrey for her marvelous pediatric insights. A huge thank you to Dr. Beth Ennis for her contribution to the new chapter on autism. Thank you to the physical therapist assistant and doctor of physical therapy students at the University of Evansville. You are the reason this book happened in the first place and the reason it has evolved into its present form. Thank you to past contributors, Dr. Pam Ritzline, Mary Kay Solon, Dr. Donna Cech, and Terry Chambliss. I also want to acknowledge the work of those at Elsevier, Lauren Willis and Sara Watkins, for seeing us through the timely completion of the fourth edition.

Tink Martin

I must thank my good friend, mentor, colleague, and coauthor, Tink Martin. Without Tink, none of these editions would have been completed. She has continued to take care of many of the details, always keeping us focused on the end result. Tink's ongoing encouragement and support have been most appreciated.

A special thank you to all of the students at the University of Evansville. They are the reason that we originally started this project, and they have continued to encourage and motivate us to update and revise the text. Several individuals contributed significantly to the completion of this edition, including Dr. Tzurei Chen, Dr. Jason Pitt, Dr. Jordana Lockwich, Maghan Bretz, and Lauren Rennie. Additional thanks must be extended to all of the individuals who have assisted us in the past, including Dr. Catherine McGraw, Sara Snelling, Dr. Pam Ritzline, Mary Kay Solon, Janet Szczepanski, Terry Chambliss, Suzy Sims, Beth Jankauski, and Amanda Fisher. Every person mentioned has contributed to the overall excellence and success of this text.

Mary Kessler

We are pleased that the first three editions of *Neurologic Interventions for Physical Therapy* led to the request for a fourth edition. A new chapter on autism has been added to meet the needs of the clinicians working with this growing population, and the recognition that physical therapy has much to offer the children and families. We have updated references and maintained the developmental flow of the text. The role of neural plasticity and the understanding that motor development can enhance cognition and language are reinforced in the earlier chapters. Patient cases have been revised to assist students in problem solving and documentation. It has been one of the highlights of my professional career to contribute to the literature in our field.

Tink Martin

We are gratified by the very positive responses to the first three editions of the *Neurologic Interventions for Physical Therapy* text. In an effort to make a good reference even better, we have taken the advice of reviewers and our physical therapist and physical therapist assistant students to complete a fourth and final edition for the two of us. The sequence of chapters still reflects a developmental trend with motor development, handling, and positioning, and interventions for children coming before the content on adults. Chapters on specific pediatric disorders and neurologic conditions seen in adults remain, as well as introductory chapters on physical therapy practice and the role of the physical therapist assistant. The review of basic neuroanatomy structure and function and the chapter on proprioceptive neuromuscular facilitation have been revised and continue to provide foundational knowledge. The intervention components of each chapter have been enhanced to emphasize function and the use of current best evidence in the physical therapy care of these patients. Concepts related to neuroplasticity, the Core Outcome Measures, high intensity gait, and task-specific training are also included. All patient cases have been reworked again to reflect current practice and are formatted in a way to assist students with their documentation skills.

We continue to see that the text is used by students in both physical therapist assistant and doctor of physical therapy programs, and this certainly has broad appeal. However, as we indicated in our last preface, we continue to be committed to addressing the role of the physical therapist assistant in the treatment of children and adults with neurologic deficits. Additionally, the use of the textbook by physical therapy students should increase the understanding of and appreciation for the psychomotor and critical thinking skills needed by all members of the rehabilitation team to maximize the function of patients with neurologic deficits.

The Evolve site continues to be enhanced as we try to insert additional resources for faculty and students. The mark of sophistication of any society is how well it treats the young and old, the most vulnerable segments of the population. We hope in some small measure that our continuing efforts will make it easier to unravel the mystery of directing movement, guiding growth and development, and relearning lost functional skills to improve the quality of life for the people we serve.

Mary Kessler

LIST OF CONTRIBUTORS

Meghan Bretz
Director
St. Vincent Evansville & University of
    Evansville Physical Therapy Neurologic
    Residency
Rehabilitation
Ascension St. Vincent
Evansville, Indiana
Adjunct Faculty
Physical Therapy
University of Evansville
Evansville, Indiana

Tzurei Chen
Assistant Professor
Physical Therapy
Pacific University
Hillsboro, Oregon

Kevin Chui
Director and Professor
School of Physical Therapy and Athletic
    Training
Pacific University
Hillsboro, Oregon

Elizabeth Ennis
Associate Professor, Chair
Physical Therapy
Bellarmine University
Louisville, Kentucky
Coowner
All About Families, PLLC
Louisville, Kentucky

Mary Kessler
Dean
College of Education and Health Sciences
Associate Professor
Physical Therapy
University of Evansville
Evansville, Indiana

Jordana Lockwich
Assistant Professor
Physical Therapy
University of Evansville
Evansville, Indiana

Suzanne Martin
Professor Emerita
Physical Therapy
University of Evansville
Evansville, Indiana

Jason Pitt
Assistant Professor
Physical Therapy
University of Evansville
Evansville, Indiana

TABLE OF CONTENTS

The Roles of the Physical Therapist and Physical Therapist Assistant in Neurologic Rehabilitation

OBJECTIVES

After reading this chapter, the student will be able to:
1. Discuss the International Classification of Functioning, Disability, and Health and its relationship to physical therapy practice.

2. Explain the role of the physical therapist in patient/client management.
3. Describe the role of the physical therapist assistant in the treatment of adults and children with neurologic deficits.

INTRODUCTION

The practice of physical therapy in the United States continues to change to meet the increased demands placed on service provision by reimbursement entities and federal regulations. The profession has seen an increase in the number of physical therapist assistants (PTAs) providing physical therapy interventions for adults and children with neurologic deficits. PTAs are employed in outpatient clinics, inpatient rehabilitation centers, extended-care and pediatric facilities, school systems, and home health care agencies. Traditionally, the rehabilitation management of adults and children with neurologic deficits consisted of treatment derived from the knowledge of disease and interventions directed at the amelioration of patient signs, symptoms, and functional impairments. Physical therapists (PTs) and PTAs "help individuals maintain, restore, and improve movement, activity, and functioning, thereby enabling optimal performance and enhancing health, well-being, and quality of life" (APTA, 2014).

Physical therapy services are provided across the lifespan to children and adults "who have or may develop impairments, activity limitations, and participation restrictions" (APTA, 2014). These limitations develop as a consequence of various health conditions including those of the "musculoskeletal, neuromuscular, cardiovascular, pulmonary, and/or integumentary system" or the negative consequences of the interaction of personal and environmental factors on human performance (APTA, 2014).

Sociologist Saad Nagi developed a model of health status that has been used to describe the relationship between health and function (Nagi, 1991). The four components of the Nagi Disablement Model (*disease, impairments, functional limitations,* and *disability*) evolve as the individual loses health. *Disease* is defined as a pathologic state manifested by the presence of signs and symptoms that disrupt an individual's homeostasis or internal balance. *Impairments* are alterations in anatomic, physiologic, or psychological structures or functions. *Functional limitations* occur as a result of impairments and become evident when an individual is unable to perform everyday activities that are considered part of the person's daily routine. Examples of physical impairments include a loss of strength in the anterior tibialis muscle or a loss of 15 degrees of active shoulder flexion. These physical impairments may or may not limit the individual's ability to perform functional tasks. Inability to dorsiflex the ankle may prohibit the patient from achieving toe clearance and heel strike during ambulation, whereas a 15-degree limitation in shoulder range of motion may have little impact on a person's ability to perform self-care or dressing tasks.

According to the disablement model, a *disability* results when functional limitations become so great that the person is unable to meet age-specific expectations within the social or physical environment (Verbrugge and Jette, 1994). Society can erect physical and social barriers that interfere with a person's ability to perform expected life roles. The societal attitudes encountered by a person with a disability can result in the community's perception that the individual is handicapped. Fig. 1.1 depicts the Nagi classification system of health status.

The second edition of the *Guide to Physical Therapist Practice* incorporated the Nagi Disablement Model into its conceptual framework of physical therapy practice. The use of this model directed PTs to focus on the relationship between impairment and functional limitation and the patient's ability to perform everyday activities within the patient's home and community (APTA, 2003).

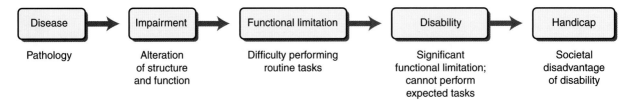

Fig. 1.1 Nagi classification system of health status.

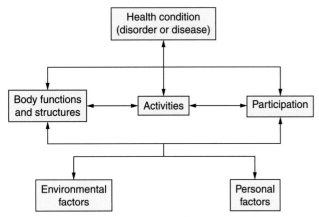

Fig. 1.2 Model of the International Classification of Functioning, Disability, and Health. (From Cech D, Martin S: *Functional movement development across the life span*, ed 3, St. Louis, 2012, Elsevier.)

The World Health Organization (WHO) developed the International Classification of Functioning, Disability, and Health (ICF), which was endorsed by the American Physical Therapy Association (APTA) in 2008. This system provides an updated frame of reference for physical therapy practice and standard language to describe health, function, and disability at both the individual and population level, and is incorporated into the third edition of the *Guide to Physical Therapist Practice*. Fig. 1.2 illustrates the ICF model. Health is much more than the absence of disease; rather, it is a condition of physical, mental, and social well-being that allows an individual to participate in functional activities and life situations (WHO, 2013; Cech and Martin, 2012). A biopsychosocial model of health is central to the ICF and defines a person's health status and functional capabilities by the interactions between one's biological, psychological, and social domains (Fig. 1.3). This conceptual framework recognizes that two

individuals with the same medical diagnosis might have very different functional outcomes and levels of participation based on environmental and personal factors.

The ICF also presents functioning and disability in the context of health and organizes the information into two distinct parts. Part 1 addresses the components of functioning and disability as they relate to the health condition. The health condition (disease or disorder) results from the impairments and alterations in an individual's body structures and functions (physiologic and anatomic processes). Activity limitations present as difficulties performing a task or action and encompass physical as well as cognitive and communication activities. Participation restrictions are deficits that an individual may experience when attempting to meet social roles and obligations within the environment. Functioning and disability are therefore viewed on a continuum in which functioning encompasses performance of activities and participation and disability implies activity limitations and restrictions in one's ability to participate in life situations such as employment, education, or relaxation (Centers for Disease Control and Prevention, 2017; WHO, 2013).

Part 2 of the ICF recognizes the contextual factors "external environmental factors (e.g., social attitudes, architectural characteristics, legal and social structures, and climate and terrain)" and internal personal factors (age, sex, social, and educational background, coping strategies, profession, life experiences, and other factors) that influence a person's response to the presence of a disability and the interaction of these factors on one's ability to participate in meaningful activities (APTA, 2014). Fig. 1.4 provides a diagram of the ICF Model of Functioning and Disability. All factors must be considered to determine the impact, both positive and negative, these factors have on function and participation (APTA, 2014; WHO, 2013).

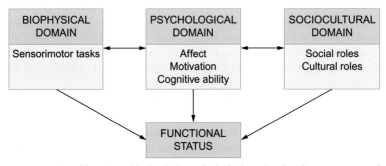

Fig. 1.3 The three domains of function—biophysical, psychological, sociocultural—must operate independently as well as interdependently for human beings to achieve their best possible functional status. (From Cech D, Martin S: *Functional movement development across the life span*, ed 3, St. Louis, 2012, Elsevier.)

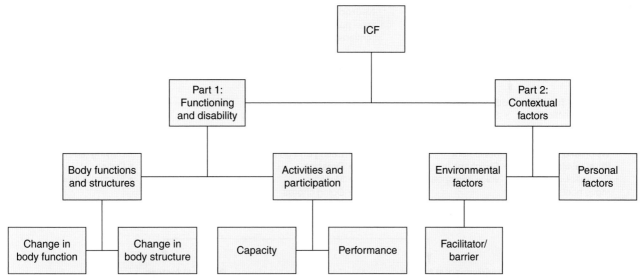

Fig. 1.4 Structure of the International Classification of Functioning, Disability, and Health (ICF) Model of Functioning and Disability. (Adapted from [http://www.apta.org], with permission of the American Physical Therapy Association. © 2019 American Physical Therapy Association. All rights reserved.)

The ICF emphasizes enablement rather than disability (Cech and Martin, 2012). In the ICF model, there is less focus on the cause of the medical condition and more emphasis directed to the impact that activity limitations and participation restrictions have on the individual. As individuals experience a decline in health, it is also possible that they may experience some level of disability. Thus the ICF "mainstreams the experience of disability and recognizes it as a universal human experience" (WHO, 2002).

An ICF for Children and Youth has been developed to provide greater detail for children from birth to age 18 years. This document addresses the "body functions and structures, activities, participation, and environments specific to infants, toddlers, children, and adolescents" and provides a framework for common language and documentation as it relates to health status and disability in children (APTA, 2014; WHO, 2007). Fig. 1.5 provides an example of the ICF applied to children with cerebral palsy, autism, and attention-deficit/hyperactivity disorder.

The third edition of the *Guide to Physical Therapist 3.0* recognizes the critical roles that PTs and PTAs play in providing "rehabilitation and habilitation, performance enhancement, and prevention and risk-reduction services" for patients and the overall population (APTA, 2014). Additionally, as professionals we play a critical role in developing standards for our practice and in recommending health care policy to ensure access, availability, and quality, patient-centered physical therapy care (APTA, 2014).

It is important that therapists continue to appreciate our role in optimizing patient function as various functional skills are needed in domestic, vocational, and community environments. Within the third edition of the *Guide to Physical Therapist Practice 3.0* (APTA, 2014), functioning is defined as "an umbrella term for body functions, body structures, activities and participation. Functioning is the positive

interaction between an individual with a health condition and that individual's environmental and personal factors" (APTA, 2014). Individuals often define themselves by what they are able to accomplish and how they are able to interact in the world (Cech and Martin, 2012). Function "comprises activities that an individual identifies as essential to support his or her physical, social, and psychological well-being and to create a personal sense of meaningful living" (APTA, 2014). *Function* is related to age-specific roles in a given social context and physical environment and is defined differently for a child of 6 months, an adolescent of 15 years, and a 65-year-old adult. Factors that contribute to an individual's *functional performance* include personal characteristics (age, race, sex, level of education), physical ability, sensorimotor skills, emotional status (depression, anxiety, self-awareness and self-esteem), and cognitive ability (intellect, motivation, concentration, and problem-solving skills). The environment in which the adult or child lives and works, such as one's home, school, or community, social supports, and the social and cultural expectations placed on the individual by the family, community, or society all impact performance of functional tasks and quality of life (APTA, 2014; Cech and Martin, 2012).

THE ROLE OF THE PHYSICAL THERAPIST IN PATIENT MANAGEMENT

As stated earlier, PTs are responsible for providing rehabilitation, habilitation, and services to maintain health and function, prevent functional decline, and in individuals who are healthy enhance performance (APTA, 2014). Ultimately, the PT is responsible for performing a review of the patient's history and systems, and for administering appropriate tests and measures to determine an individual's need for physical therapy services. If after the examination the PT concludes

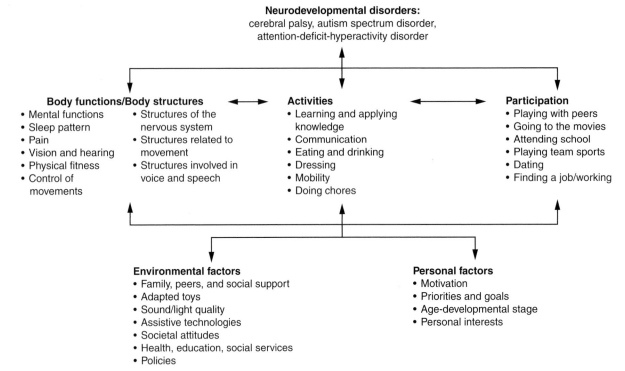

Neurodevelopmental disorders:
cerebral palsy, autism spectrum disorder,
attention-deficit-hyperactivity disorder

Body functions/Body structures
- Mental functions
- Sleep pattern
- Pain
- Vision and hearing
- Physical fitness
- Control of movements

- Structures of the nervous system
- Structures related to movement
- Structures involved in voice and speech

Activities
- Learning and applying knowledge
- Communication
- Eating and drinking
- Dressing
- Mobility
- Doing chores

Participation
- Playing with peers
- Going to the movies
- Attending school
- Playing team sports
- Dating
- Finding a job/working

Environmental factors
- Family, peers, and social support
- Adapted toys
- Sound/light quality
- Assistive technologies
- Societal attitudes
- Health, education, social services
- Policies

Personal factors
- Motivation
- Priorities and goals
- Age-developmental stage
- Personal interests

Fig. 1.5 The International Classification of Functioning, Disability, and Health biopsychosocial model applied to neurodevelopmental disorders. (From Schiariti V, Mahdi S, Bolte S: International Classification of Functioning, Disability, and Health Core Sets for cerebral palsy, autism spectrum disorder, and attention-deficit-hyperactivity disorder, *Dev Med Child Neurology* 60:933–941, 2018.)

that the patient will benefit from services, a plan of care is developed that identifies the goals, expected outcomes, and the interventions to be administered to achieve the desired patient outcomes (APTA, 2014). The PT may also determine that the patient is not appropriate for physical therapy services and will recommend referral or consultation to another health care provider.

The steps the PT utilizes in patient/client management are outlined in the third edition of the *Guide to Physical Therapist Practice*, and include *examination, evaluation, diagnosis, prognosis, interventions*, and *outcomes*. The PT integrates these elements to optimize the patient's health, function, or physical performance. Fig. 1.6 identifies the element of patient/client management. In the *examination*, the PT collects data through a review of the patient's history and a review of systems, and then administers appropriate tests and measures to determine the patient's need for services (APTA, 2014). The PT *evaluates* the data, interprets the patient's responses to tests and measures, and integrates that data with information obtained during the review of history and systems. Within the evaluation process, the therapist establishes a *physical therapy diagnosis* based on the patient's level of impairment and functional limitations. A *differential diagnosis* (a systematic process to classify patients into diagnostic categories) may be used. When PTs provide a differential diagnosis, they do so with consideration of the impact of the health condition on system function, especially the movement system, and take into consideration the entire person (APTA, 2014). Once the diagnosis is established,

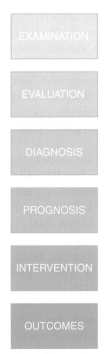

EXAMINATION

EVALUATION

DIAGNOSIS

PROGNOSIS

INTERVENTION

OUTCOMES

Fig. 1.6 The elements of patient/client management. (Adapted from [http://www.apta.org], with permission of the American Physical Therapy Association. © 2019 American Physical Therapy Association. All rights reserved.)

the PT develops a prognosis, which is the predicted level of functional improvement and an estimate to the amount of time needed to achieve those levels. As the PT determines the patient's prognosis, he or she must consider what the patient is capable of functionally, and what is likely to be habitual for the patient. Patient motivation is important to consider during this process. Therefore the PT must understand "the difference between what a person currently does and what the person potentially could do" as he or she makes a prognosis and develops realistic, achievable functional goals and outcomes (APTA, 2014). It is also important to note that the patient must be an active participant in this process and the PT must follow the decisions made by the patient as they relate to what constitutes meaningful function (APTA, 2014).

Intervention is the element of patient management in which the PT or the PTA interacts with the patient through the administration of "various interventions to produce changes in the [patient's] condition that are consistent with the diagnosis and prognosis" (APTA, 2014). Interventions are organized into nine categories: "patient or client instruction (used with every patient and client and in every practice setting); airway clearance techniques, assistive technology, biophysical agents; functional training in self-care and domestic, work, community, social, and civic life; integumentary repair and protection techniques; manual therapy techniques; motor function training; and therapeutic exercise" (APTA, 2014). The PT must prescribe the type and intensity of the interventions as well as the method, mode, duration, frequency, and progression. Reexamination of the patient may be necessary and includes performance of appropriate tests and measures to determine if the patient is progressing with treatment, if modifications in the techniques administered are needed, or if the episode of care is complete. "Outcomes are the actual results of implementing the plan of care that indicate the impact on functioning (body functions and structures, activities, and participation)" (APTA, 2014). The PT must determine the impact selected interventions have had on the following: disease or disorder, impairments, activity limitations, participation, risk reduction and prevention, health, wellness, fitness, societal resources, and patient satisfaction (APTA, 2014).

The development of the *plan of care* is the final step in the examination, diagnostic, and prognostic process. It is developed in collaboration with the patient, and if necessary other individuals who are involved in the patient's care. Goals should be developed to impact functioning (body functions and structures, activities, and participation) and should be objective, measurable, functionally oriented, time measurable, and meaningful to the patient. Goals may be written as short or long term depending on the practice setting. The plan of care must also discuss the patient's discharge from services, "conclusion of the episode of care" and follow-up visits or referrals needed (APTA, 2014). If a patient has not achieved his or her goals, a report of the patient's current status and rationale for discontinuation of services is provided.

Other aspects of patient/client management include coordination, "the working together of all parties involved with the patient," communication, and documentation of services provided (APTA, 2014). Documentation includes any and all entries into the patient's health record and should include the services provided and the patient's response to treatment administered. All documentation for physical therapy services should follow the APTA's Guidelines. (APTA, 2014).

Interventions are designed to produce changes in a patient's condition. The PT will select interventions based on information obtained in the examination and that are based on the patient's current condition and prognosis. Physical therapy interventions are designed to optimize patient function, emphasize patient education and instruction, and promote individual health, wellness, and fitness with the goal of preventing reoccurrence of the condition. Interventions are administered by the PT and when indicated by others involved in the patient's plan of care. PTAs may be "appropriately utilized in components of the intervention and in collection of selected examination and outcomes data" (APTA, 2018a). All other tasks remain the sole responsibility of the PT.

The guidelines for direction and supervision of PTAs follow those suggested by Dr. Nancy Watts in her 1971 article on task analysis and division of responsibility in physical therapy (Watts, 1971). This article was written to assist PTs with guidelines for delegating patient care activities to support personnel. Although the term *delegation* is not used today because of the implications of relinquishing patient care responsibilities to another practitioner, the principles of patient/client management, as defined by Watts, can be applied to the provision of present-day physical therapy services. PTs and PTAs unfamiliar with this article are encouraged to review it because the guidelines presented are still appropriate for today's clinicians and are referenced in APTA documents.

THE ROLE OF THE PHYSICAL THERAPIST ASSISTANT IN TREATING PATIENTS WITH NEUROLOGIC DEFICITS

There is little debate as to whether PTAs have a role in treating adults with neurologic deficits, as long as the individual needs of the patient are taken into consideration and the PTA follows the plan of care established by the PT. PTAs are the only health care providers who "assists a physical therapist in practice" (APTA, 2018a). The primary PT is still ultimately responsible for the patient, both legally and ethically, and is responsible for the actions of the PTA relative to patient management that can include the performance of selected interventions and the collection of certain examination and outcomes measures (APTA, 2018a). The APTA has identified the following responsibilities as those that must be performed exclusively by the PT (APTA, 2018a):

1. Interpretation of referrals when available
2. Initial examination, evaluation, diagnosis, and prognosis
3. Development or modification of the plan of care, which includes the goals and expected outcomes and is based on results of the initial examination

4. Determination of when the expertise and decision-making capabilities of the PT requires the PT to personally render services and when it is appropriate to utilize a PTA
5. Revision of the plan of care if indicated
6. Conclusion of a patient's episode of care
7. Responsibility for communication related to a "hand off"
8. Oversight of all documentation for services rendered

The APTA has stated that it is the responsibility of the PT to perform the examination, evaluation, diagnosis, prognosis, intervention, and outcomes. The entire evaluation, the creation of the patient's diagnosis and prognosis as well as components of the examination, intervention, and outcomes must be exclusively performed by the PT because of the need for continuous assessment and synthesis of information. Additionally, the APTA has identified selected interventions that are performed solely by the PT, which include "spinal and peripheral joint mobilization/manipulation and dry needling, which are components of manual therapy; and sharp selective debridement, which is a component of wound management" (APTA, 2018b). Any intervention that requires immediate and continuous examination and evaluation is to be performed by the PT (APTA, 2018b).

As stated earlier, PTAs may be utilized in administering interventions and in the collection of certain examination and outcomes. Before directing the PTA to perform specific components of the intervention, the PT must critically evaluate the patient's condition (*stability, acuity, criticality,* and *complexity*), he or she must also consider the practice setting in which the intervention is to be delivered, the type of intervention to be provided, and the predictability of the patient's probable outcome to the intervention (APTA, 2018a). The guidelines proposed follow those suggested by Dr. Watts (Watts, 1971).

In addition, the knowledge base of the PTA, his or her level of experience, training, and skill level must be considered when determining which tasks can be directed to the PTA. The APTA has developed two algorithms (PTA direction and PTA supervision; Figs. 1.7 and 1.8) to assist PTs with the steps that should be considered when a PT decides to direct certain aspects of a patient's care to a PTA and the subsequent supervision that must occur. Even though these algorithms exist, it is important to remember that communication between the PT and PTA must be ongoing to ensure the best possible outcomes for the patient. PTAs are also advised to become familiar with the Problem-Solving Algorithm Utilized by PTAs in Patient/Client Intervention (Fig. 1.9) as a guide for the clinical problem-solving skills a PTA should employ before and during patient interventions (APTA, 2007).

PTs and PTAs are advised to refer to APTA policy documents, their state practice acts, and the Commission on Accreditation in Physical Therapy Education guidelines for the most up-to-date information regarding interventions that are considered outside the scope of practice for the PTA. Practitioners are also encouraged to review individual state practice acts and payer requirements for supervision requirements as they relate to the PT/PTA relationship (Crosier, 2011).

State practice acts often describe the scope of practice and supervision requirements for PTAs. It is also important to note that levels of supervision are also described by the APTA. The APTA identifies three levels of supervision including: general supervision in which the PT is not required to be onsite but is available by telecommunications; direct supervision in which the PT is "physically present and immediately available for direction and supervision and has direct contact with the patient during each visit"; and direct personal supervision in which the PT or PTA is "immediately available to direct and supervise tasks that are related to patient management. The direction and supervision is continuous and telecommunications does not meet the requirement of direct personal supervision" (APTA, 2012). It is important to note that various policy documents define and mandate different levels of supervision (Crosier, 2010).

Unfortunately, in our current health care climate, there are times when the decision as to whether a patient should be treated by a PTA is determined by productivity concerns and the patient's payer source and not the patient's rehabilitation needs. An issue affecting some clinics and PTAs is the denial of payment by some insurance providers for services provided by a PTA. Consequently, decisions regarding the utilization of PTAs are sometimes determined by financial remuneration and not by the needs of the patient.

THE PHYSICAL THERAPIST ASSISTANT AS A MEMBER OF THE HEALTH CARE TEAM

The PTA functions as a member of the rehabilitation team in all treatment settings. Members of this team include the primary PT; the physician; speech, occupational, and recreation therapists; nursing personnel; the psychologist; case manager; and the social worker. However, the two most important members of this team are the patient and his or her family. In a rehabilitation setting, the PTA is expected to provide *interventions* to improve the patient's functional independence and participation in life situations. Relearning motor activities, such as bed mobility, transfers, ambulation skills, stair climbing, and wheelchair negotiation, if appropriate, are emphasized to enhance the patient's functional mobility. In addition, the PTA participates in patient and family education and is expected to provide input into the patient's discharge plan. Patient and family instruction include providing information, education, and the actual training of patients, families, significant others, or caregivers, and is a part of every patient's plan of care (APTA, 2014). As is the case in all team activities, open and honest communication and mutual respect among all team members is crucial to maximize the patient's participation and achievement of an optimal functional outcome.

Although PTAs work with adults who have had strokes, spinal cord injuries, and traumatic brain injuries, some PTs have viewed pediatrics as a specialty area of practice. This narrow perspective is held even though PTAs work with children in hospitals, outpatient clinics, schools, and community settings, including fitness centers and sports-training facilities.

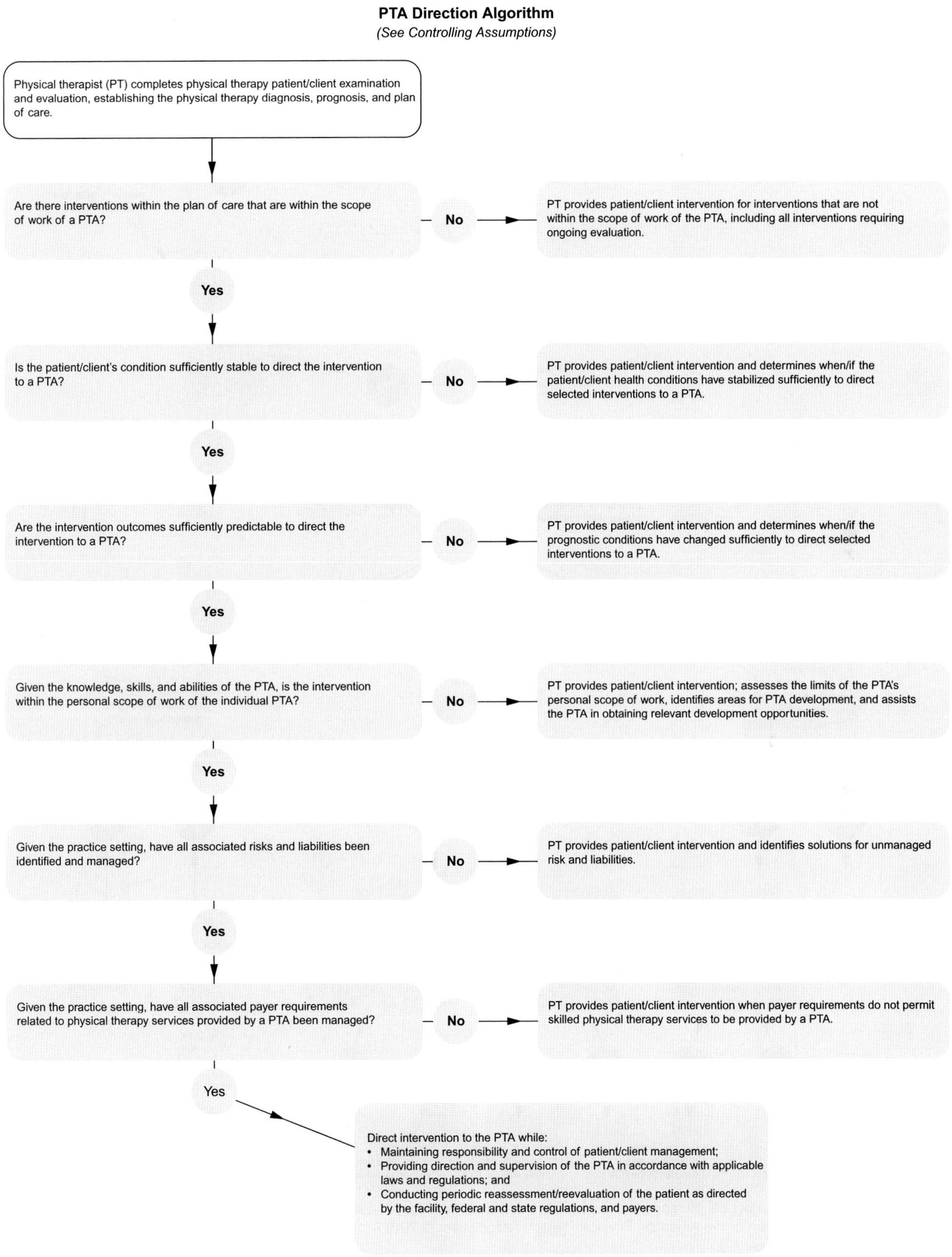

PTA Direction Algorithm
(See Controlling Assumptions)

Physical therapist (PT) completes physical therapy patient/client examination and evaluation, establishing the physical therapy diagnosis, prognosis, and plan of care.

Are there interventions within the plan of care that are within the scope of work of a PTA?

No → PT provides patient/client intervention for interventions that are not within the scope of work of the PTA, including all interventions requiring ongoing evaluation.

Yes

Is the patient/client's condition sufficiently stable to direct the intervention to a PTA?

No → PT provides patient/client intervention and determines when/if the patient/client health conditions have stabilized sufficiently to direct selected interventions to a PTA.

Yes

Are the intervention outcomes sufficiently predictable to direct the intervention to a PTA?

No → PT provides patient/client intervention and determines when/if the prognostic conditions have changed sufficiently to direct selected interventions to a PTA.

Yes

Given the knowledge, skills, and abilities of the PTA, is the intervention within the personal scope of work of the individual PTA?

No → PT provides patient/client intervention; assesses the limits of the PTA's personal scope of work, identifies areas for PTA development, and assists the PTA in obtaining relevant development opportunities.

Yes

Given the practice setting, have all associated risks and liabilities been identified and managed?

No → PT provides patient/client intervention and identifies solutions for unmanaged risk and liabilities.

Yes

Given the practice setting, have all associated payer requirements related to physical therapy services provided by a PTA been managed?

No → PT provides patient/client intervention when payer requirements do not permit skilled physical therapy services to be provided by a PTA.

Yes

Direct intervention to the PTA while:
• Maintaining responsibility and control of patient/client management;
• Providing direction and supervision of the PTA in accordance with applicable laws and regulations; and
• Conducting periodic reassessment/reevaluation of the patient as directed by the facility, federal and state regulations, and payers.

Fig. 1.7 Physical therapist assistant (PTA) direction algorithm. (Adapted from [http://www.apta.org], with permission of the American Physical Therapy Association. © 2019 American Physical Therapy Association. All rights reserved.)

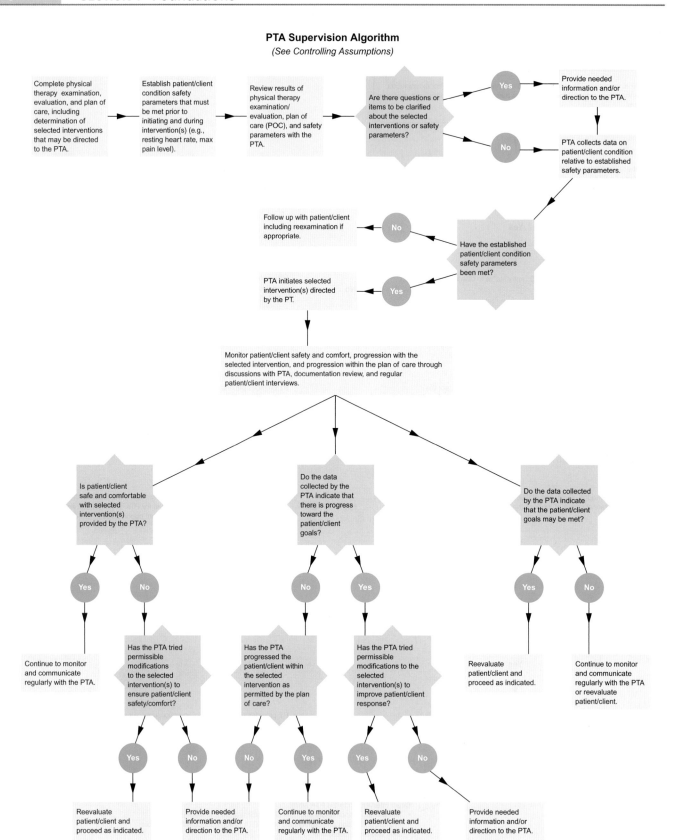

Fig. 1.8 Physical therapist assistant (PTA) supervision algorithm. (Adapted from [http://www.apta.org], with permission of the American Physical Therapy Association. © 2019 American Physical Therapy Association. All rights reserved.)

Problem-Solving Algorithm Utilized by PTAs in Patient/Client Intervention
(See Controlling Assumptions on previous page.)

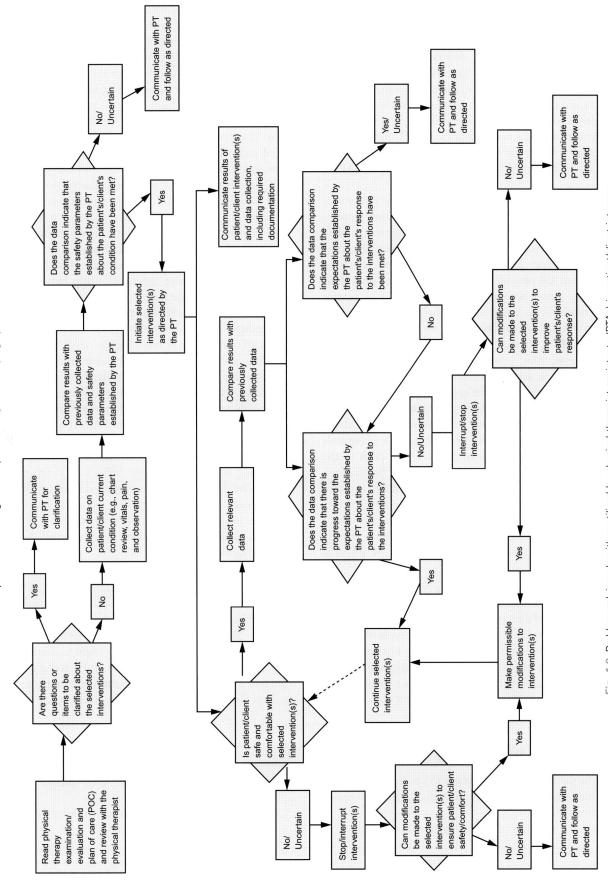

Fig. 1.9 Problem-solving algorithm utilized by physical therapist assistants (PTAs) in patient/client intervention. (Adapted from [http://www.apta.org], with permission of the American Physical Therapy Association. © 2019 American Physical Therapy Association. All rights reserved.)

Although some areas of pediatric physical therapy are specialized, many areas are well within the scope of practice of the generalist PT and PTA. The Academy of Pediatric Physical Therapy in their fact sheet state that "Physical therapist assistants may be involved with the delivery of physical therapy services under the direction and supervision of a licensed PT" (APPT, 2019). Additionally, the Academy states that "Physical therapists and physical therapist assistants must be graduates of accredited educational programs and comply with rules of state licensure and practice guidelines" (APPT, 2019). Practitioners may secure additional knowledge, certification, and credentials to recognize specialization in pediatrics (APPT, 2019).

The provision of pediatric services in school systems by PTAs is supported, however, because of supervision requirements it may be difficult for school systems to meet the PT/PTA supervision requirements. This can be especially problematic in rural areas where the number of providers may be limited. When it is possible to comply with supervision standards, many school settings find that the "PT/PTA service delivery model is an effective and efficient way to provide services for students, consistent with the need for cost containment" (APTA, 2014).

The rehabilitation team working with a child with a neurologic deficit usually consists of the child; his or her parents; the various physicians involved in the child's management, and other health care professionals, such as an audiologist and physical and occupational therapists; a speech language pathologist; and the child's classroom teacher. The PTA is expected to bring certain skills to the team and to the child, including knowledge of positioning, posture and lifting, use of adaptive equipment and assistive technology, management of abnormal muscle tone, knowledge of developmental activities that foster acquisition of functional motor skills and movement transitions, knowledge of family-centered care, and the role of physical therapy in an educational environment. Additionally, interpersonal communication and advocacy skills are beneficial as the PTA works with the child and the family, as well as others. Family teaching and instruction are expected within a family-centered approach to the delivery of various interventions embedded into the child's daily routine. Because the PTA may be providing services to the child in his or her home or school, the assistant may be the first to observe additional problems or be told of a parent's concern. These observations or concerns should be communicated immediately to the supervising PT. Because of the complexity of patients' problems and the interpersonal skill set needed to work with the pediatric population and their families, most clinics require prior work experience or residency training prior to employing a PT, or prior work experience or advanced proficiency for PTAs who wish to work in these practice settings (Clynch, 2012).

PTs and PTAs are valuable members of a patient's health care team. To optimize the relationship between the two and to maximize patient outcomes, each practitioner must understand the educational preparation and experiential background of the other. The preferred relationship between PTs and PTAs is one characterized by trust, understanding, mutual respect, effective communication, and an appreciation for individual similarities and differences (Clynch, 2012). This relationship involves direction, including determination of the tasks that can be directed to the PTA, supervision because the PT is responsible for supervising the assistant to whom tasks or interventions have been directed and accepted, communication, and the demonstration of ethical and legal behaviors. Positive benefits that can be derived from this preferred relationship include more clearly defined identities for both PTs and PTAs and a more unified, collaborative approach to the delivery of high-quality, cost-effective, patient-centered, physical therapy services.

CHAPTER SUMMARY

Changes in physical therapy practice have led to an increase in the number of PTAs, and greater variety in the types of patients treated by these clinicians. PTAs are actively involved in the treatment of adults and children with neurologic deficits. After a thorough examination and evaluation of the patient's status, the primary PT may determine that the patient's intervention or a portion of the intervention may be safely performed by an assistant. The PTA functions as a member of the patient's rehabilitation team, and works with the patient to maximize his or her ability to participate in meaningful activities. Improved function in the home, school, or community remains the primary goal of our physical therapy interventions.

REVIEW QUESTIONS

1. Discuss the ICF model as it relates to health and function.
2. List the factors that affect an individual's performance of functional activities.
3. Discuss the elements of patient/client management.
4. Identify the factors that the PT must consider before utilizing a PTA.
5. Discuss the roles of the PTA when working with adults or children with neurologic deficits.

REFERENCES

Academy of Pediatric Physical Therapy, American Physical Therapy Association: *Academy of pediatric physical therapy fact sheet, the ABCs of pediatric physical therapy*, Alexandria, VA, 2019, APTA. Available at: https://pediatricapta.org/includes/fact-sheets/pdfs/09 abcs of ped pt.pdf?v=1.1. Accessed May 4, 2019.

American Physical Therapy Association: *Guide to physical therapist practice 3.0*, Alexandria, VA, 2014, APTA. Available at: guidetoptpractice.apta.org. Accessed May 4, 2019.

American Physical Therapy Association: *Direction and supervision of the physical therapist assistant HOD P06-18-28- 35*, Alexandria, VA, 2018a, APTA. Available at: www.apta.org/uploadedFiles/APTAorg/About_Us/Policies/Practice/DirectionSupervisionPTA.pdf. Accessed January 4, 2019.

American Physical Therapy Association: *Guide to physical therapist practice*, ed 2, Alexandria, VA, 2003, APTA, pp 13–47, 679.

American Physical Therapy Association: *Interventions performed exclusively by physical therapists HOD P06-18-31-36*, Alexandria, VA, 2018b, APTA. Available at: www.apta.org/uploadedFiles/APTAorg/About_Us/Policies/Practice/ProceduralInterventions.pdf. Accessed May 4, 2019.

American Physical Therapy Association: *Levels of supervision HOD P06-00-15-26*, Alexandria, VA, 2012, APTA, Available at: www.apta.org/uploadedFiles/APTA/org/About_US/Policies/Terminology/Levels of Supervision.pdf. Accessed March 13, 2019.

American Physical Therapy Association Education Division: *A normative model of physical therapist professional education, version 2007*, Alexandria, VA, 2007, APTA, pp 84–85.

Cech D, Martin S: *Functional movement development across the life span*, ed 3, Philadelphia, 2012, Saunders, pp 1–13.

Centers for Disease Control and Prevention: *Disability and health overview, impairments, activity limitation and participation restrictions*, Atlanta, GA, 2017, CDC. Available at: www.cdc.gov/ncbddd/disabilityandhealth/disability.html. Accessed May 1, 2019.

Clynch HM: *The role of the physical therapist assistant: regulations and responsibilities*, Philadelphia, 2012, FA Davis, pp 23, 43–76.

Crosier J: PTA direction and supervision algorithms, *PTinMotion* 2010. Available at: www.apta.org/PTinMotion/2010/9/PTA supervisionalgorithmchart. Accessed January 7, 2014.

Crosier J: *The PT/PTA relationship: 4 things to know*, February 2011. Available at: www.apta.org/PTA/PatientCare/PTPTARelationship4ThingstoKnow. Accessed May 4, 2019.

Nagi SZ: Disability concepts revisited: implications for prevention. In Pope AM, Tarlox AR, editors: *Disability in America: toward a national agenda for prevention*, Washington, DC, 1991, National Academy Press, pp 309–327.

Section on Pediatrics American Physical Therapy Association: *School-based physical therapy: conflicts between Individuals with Disabilities Education Act (IDEA) and legal requirements of state practice acts and regulations*, Alexandria, VA, 2014, APTA. Available at: www.pediatricapta.org/includes/Fact-sheets?pdfs. Accessed May 4, 2019.

Verbrugge LM, Jette AM: The disablement process, *Soc Sci Med* 38:1–14, 1994.

Watts NT: Task analysis and division of responsibility in physical therapy, *Phys Ther* 51:23–35, 1971.

World Health Organization: *How to use the ICF: a practical manual for using the International Classification of Functioning, Disability and Health (ICF)*, Geneva, Switzerland, 2013, WHO.

World Health Organization: *International Classification of Functioning, Disability and Health: children and youth version*, Geneva, Switzerland, 2007, WHO.

World Health Organization: *International Classification of Functioning, Disability, and Health (ICF)*, World Health Organization. Available at: www.who.int/classifications/icf/en/. Accessed January 5, 2014.

World Health Organization: *Towards a common language for functioning, disability and health, ICF*, Geneva, Switzerland, 2002, WHO.

2

Neuroanatomy

Mary Kessler and Jason Pitt

OBJECTIVES

After reading this chapter, the student will be able to:
1. Differentiate between the central and peripheral nervous systems.
2. Identify significant structures within the nervous system.
3. Understand primary functions of structures within the nervous system.

4. Describe the vascular supply to the brain.
5. Discuss components of the cervical, brachial, and lumbosacral plexuses.

INTRODUCTION

The purpose of this chapter is to provide the student with a review of neuroanatomy. Basic structures within the nervous system are described and their functions discussed. This information is important to physical therapists and physical therapist assistants who treat patients with neurologic dysfunction because it assists clinicians with identifying clinical signs and symptoms. In addition, it allows the clinician to develop an appreciation of the patient's prognosis and potential functional outcome. It is, however, outside the scope of this text to provide a comprehensive discussion of neuroanatomy. The reader is encouraged to review neuroscience and neuroanatomy texts for a more in-depth discussion of these concepts.

OVERVIEW OF THE NERVOUS SYSTEM

Individuals are able to perceive sensory experiences, to initiate movement, and to perform cognitive tasks as a result of a functioning nervous system. To function properly, nervous systems have to solve two very different problems. On the one hand, nervous systems must be able to reliably communicate with the rest of the body to accurately convey sensory and motor signals. However, nervous systems must also be flexible enough to change over time to learn and solve problems. Our nervous system is able to balance reliability and flexibility through several divisions of labor.

The nervous system is divided into two parts: the flexible *central nervous system* (CNS) and the reliable *peripheral nervous system* (PNS). The CNS is the site of information integration and is composed of the *brain* and *spinal cord*. The PNS is designed to provide robust communication between the CNS and body and comprises all of the components outside the

cranium and spine. Physiologically, the PNS is divided into the *somatic nervous system* and the *autonomic nervous system* (ANS). The ANS is further subdivided into sympathetic and parasympathetic components. Fig. 2.1 illustrates the major components of the CNS. Before we discuss the functions of these nervous system divisions, we will review the cellular makeup of nervous tissue and the specializations that allow for rapid communication.

CELLULAR COMPONENTS OF THE NERVOUS SYSTEM

The nervous system is a highly organized communication system comprising more than 100 billion nerve cells. *Nerve cells* allow us to properly navigate our world by communicating with sensory and motor structures throughout the body. For example, sensations, such as touch, proprioception, pain, and temperature, are transmitted from the periphery as *electrochemical impulses* to the CNS through sensory tracts. Once information is processed within the CNS, it is relayed as new electrochemical impulses to peripheral structures through motor tracts. A *tract* is a group of nerve fibers that are similar in origin, destination, and function. In this section, we will review the basic types of nerve cells and how they participate in the electrochemical signaling of tracts.

Types of Nerve Cells

There are two basic types of nerve cells: neurons and neuroglia. *Neurons* are specialized for communication through their ability to generate rapid electrochemical signals. *Neuroglia* are diverse support cells that facilitate neuron function and survival. Although it is increasingly clear that neuroglia can also play an active role in electrochemical signaling, this

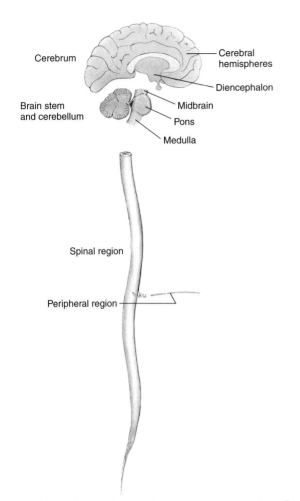

Cerebrum

Cerebral
hemispheres

Diencephalon

Brain stem
and cerebellum

Midbrain

Pons

Medulla

Spinal region

Peripheral region

Fig. 2.1 Lateral view of the regions of the nervous system. Regions are listed on the left, and subdivisions are listed on the right. (From Lundy-Ekman L: *Neuroscience: fundamentals for rehabilitation,* ed 4, St. Louis, 2013, Elsevier.)

topic is beyond the scope of this chapter (Halassa et al., 2007).

Neurons are sometimes divided into the three following categories: (1) afferent neurons, (2) interneurons, and (3) efferent neurons. Afferent neurons project toward a given structure (i.e., they arrive), efferent neurons project away from a given structure (i.e., they exit), and interneurons relay signals between two neurons. Although these may sound like clear divisions, a single neuron can actually be all three types. For example, all neurons in the cortex are interneurons. Interneurons in layer five of the cortex that make up the corticospinal tract project their axons to the spinal cord, acting as cortical efferents and spinal afferents. To avoid this confusion, we suggest you use the following function categories: (1) *motor neurons,* which convey output from the CNS to the muscles, and (2) *sensory neurons,* which detect environmental or bodily stimuli and relay it to the CNS. All other neurons should simply be called neurons (or interneurons, if you prefer). It should be noted that there is no strict naming convention for neurons. In fact, the same layer five cortical neurons mentioned earlier that make up the corticospinal

tract are called upper motor neurons, even though they do not innervate muscles.

Neuroglia are nonneuronal supporting cells that provide critical services for neurons. Different types of neuroglia (astrocytes, oligodendrocytes, microglia, and ependymal cells) have been identified in the CNS. Fig. 2.2 depicts the types of neuroglia. *Astrocytes* are responsible for maintaining the capillary endothelium and as such provide a vascular link to neurons. Additionally, astrocytes contribute to the metabolism of the CNS, regulate extracellular concentrations of ions and neurotransmitters, and proliferate after an injury to create a glial scar (Fitzgerald et al., 2012). *Oligodendrocytes* wrap myelin sheaths around axons, forming the white matter of the CNS. Nonmyelinating oligodendrocytes (*satellite oligodendrocytes*) associate with the cell bodies of neurons and appear to regulate ion concentrations, similar to astrocytes. *Microglia* are known as the phagocytes of the CNS. They engulf and digest pathogens and assist with nervous system repair after injury. *Ependymal cells,* which line the ventricular system, produce and circulate cerebrospinal fluid (Fitzgerald et al., 2012).

Neuroglia in the PNS fulfill similar functions as in the CNS. *Satellite cells* buffer extracellular ion concentrations around neuronal cell bodies. The major neuroglial cell of the PNS is the *Schwann cell,* which is further divided into different functional classes. Myelinating Schwann cells ensheath axons in myelin, similar to oligodendrocytes. Nonmyelinating Schwann cells outnumber myelinating Schwann cells ~4:1 and have similar functions to astrocytes, as they contact vasculature and participate in ion buffering. Terminal Schwann cells help maintain the neuromuscular junction (Ko and Robitaille, 2015).

Neuron Structures

As depicted in Fig. 2.3, a typical neuron consists of dendrites, a cell body, and an axon. *Dendrites* are responsible for transducing extracellular physical or chemical input into an intracellular signal. Most commonly, a dendrite produces electrical currents, which are transferred to the cell body for processing. Neurons have variable morphologies, differing in size, number of dendrites, and degree of dendrite branching (Fig. 2.4). Neurons with no true dendrite are *unipolar* or *pseudounipolar,* neurons with a single dendrite are *bipolar,* and neurons with multiple dendrites are called *multipolar.* The number and arrangement of dendrites is related to the function of the neuron. For example, somatosensory neurons are pseudounipolar, allowing for linear communication of sensory stimuli. However, multipolar Purkinje cells in the cerebellum have elaborate dendrites, allowing them to integrate a large number of inputs and allow for motor learning. As mentioned earlier, nervous system function requires both reliable and flexible signaling.

The *cell body* or *soma* is composed of a nucleus and a number of different cellular organelles. The cell body is responsible for synthesizing proteins and supporting functional activities of the neuron, such as transmitting electrochemical impulses and repairing cells. The fact that the cell body is responsible

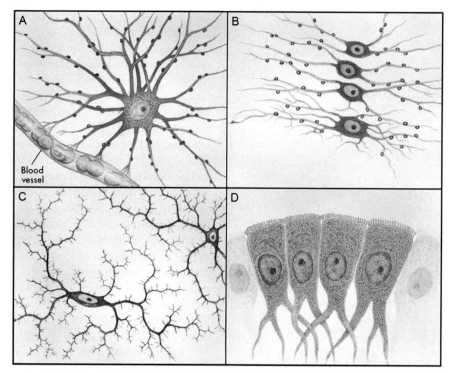

Fig. 2.2 The four types of neuroglia cells: **(A)** astrocytes, **(B)** oligodendrocytes, **(C)** microglia, and **(D)** ependymal cells. (From Copstead LEC, Banasik JL: *Pathophysiology: biological and behavioral perspectives*, ed 2, Philadelphia, 2000, WB Saunders.)

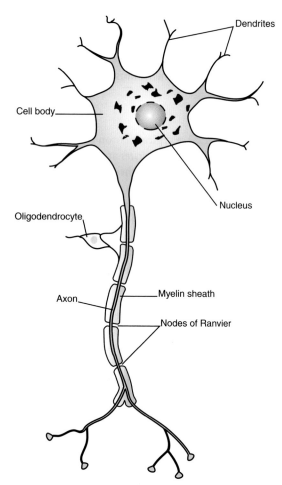

Fig. 2.3 Diagram of a neuron.

for protein synthesis explains why axons degrade distally to the site of injury—they are unable to produce protein and survive. Cell bodies of neurons with similar functions are often grouped together to form *nuclei* in the CNS and *ganglia* in the PNS.

The *axon* is the message-sending component of neurons. Axons extend from the cell body and contact target cells that can include muscle cells, glands, or other neurons. Neurons communicate with target cells by conducting electrical signals called *action potentials* down their axon. Action potentials stimulate the release of chemical signals called *neurotransmitters* that bind to receptors on target cells to elicit a response. All nerve signaling pathways involve this alternating pattern of electrical signaling within neurons, and chemical signaling between a neuron and a target cell.

Electrical Conduction Within Neurons

Electrical signaling occurs through the movement of ions across the membrane. Ions can only cross the membrane through proteins called *ion channels*. In some axons, electrical conduction is facilitated by *myelin*, a lipid/protein that encases and insulates the axon.

Myelin in the CNS and PNS have some important distinctions. Myelin produced by oligodendrocytes in the CNS is more compact, which is an advantage because space is limited by the skull. Myelin produced by Schwann cells in the PNS is less compact, providing additional protection for peripheral nerves. PNS myelin also allows for axon regrowth, whereas CNS myelin appears to prevent axon regrowth

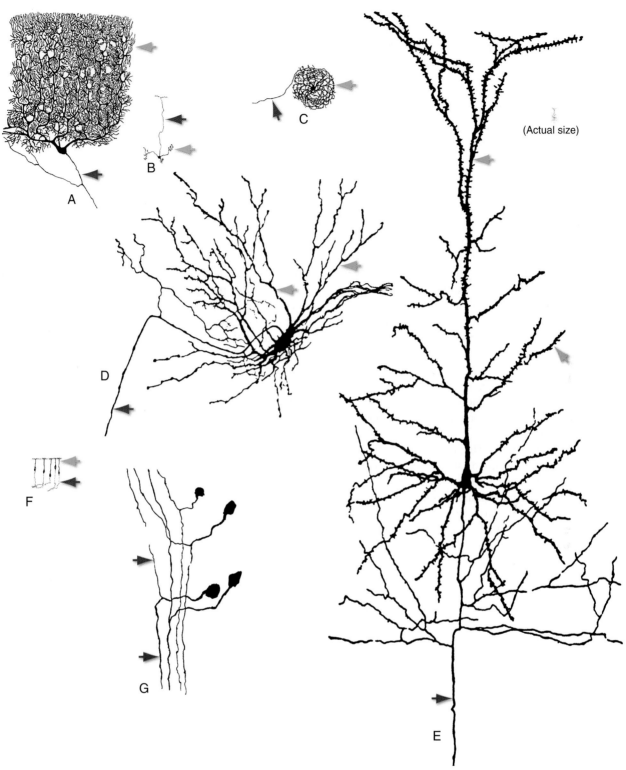

(Actual size)

Fig. 2.4 Morphologies of different types of neurons. All neurons are drawn to roughly the same scale to illustrate the diversity of cell size. Drawings are based on Golgi stains. The dendrites and axons are labeled with green and blue arrows, respectively. All neurons have a single axon but can vary in terms of dendrite number and branching. Multipolar neurons **(A-E)** have multiple dendrites emerging from their cell body. Bipolar neurons **(F)** have a single dendrite. Unipolar and pseudounipolar neurons **(G)** have no true dendrites. **(A)** Purkinje cell from the cerebellar cortex; **(B)** granule cell from the cerebellar cortex; **(C)** projection neuron from the inferior olivary nucleus; **(D)** spinal cord motor neuron; **(E)** large pyramidal neuron from the cerebral cortex (the inset shows the actual size); **(F)** olfactory receptor neurons; **(G)** dorsal root ganglion cells. (From Vanderah T, Gould DJ: *Nolte's the human brain e-book: an introduction to its functional anatomy, Philadelphia*, 2015, Elsevier Health Sciences, Fig. 1.4, p. 5.)

TABLE 2.1   Conduction Velocities in Different Axon Types

Group Name	Diameter (μm)	Myelinated	Conduction Velocity (m/s)	Information Transmitted
Group I (Aα)	13–20	Yes	70–120	Motor signals
Group II (Aβ)	6–12	Yes	40–70	Touch sensation
Group III (Aδ)	1–5	Yes	12–36	First pain
Group IV (C)	0.2–1.5	No	0.5–2	Second pain

following injury. This difference in myelin may explain the limited recovery in spinal cord injuries compared with peripheral nerve injuries.

Myelin increases the efficiency of action potential conduction down the axon in two important ways: (1) increased conduction velocity, and (2) decreased metabolic expenditure. Myelinated axons conduct action potentials more rapidly than unmyelinated axons (Table 2.1). Myelination increases conduction velocity by insulating the axon. Myelinated regions of the axon are devoid of ion channels, which prevents electrical charge from leaking out of the axon. The myelin sheath also prevents the charge within the axon from being stored at the membrane, allowing it to more rapidly flow within the axon. As a result of this, there is a noticeable delay (approximately 0.5 to 1 second) of our perception of tactile sensation conveyed by myelinated fibers, and painful sensation conveyed by unmyelinated fibers.

The myelin sheath surrounding the axon is not continuous; it contains interruptions or spaces within the myelin called the *nodes of Ranvier* (or, more simply, nodes). Nodes are only 2 μm in length and contain ion channels that restore the action potential as it travels along the axon. However, myelinated regions (or *internodes*) each span 0.3 to 2 mm in length and are devoid of ion channels. The lack of ion channels in internodes causes action potentials to "leap" from node to node in a process called *saltatory conduction* (*saltare* means "to leap" in Latin). Saltatory conduction is much faster than active conduction that takes place in unmyelinated axons, which contain ion channels along their entire length (Fig. 2.5).

The second advantage of myelin arises from the fact that over 99% of the axon length is myelinated, and thus ion impermeable. Myelinated axons conduct far fewer ions across the membrane than unmyelinated axons. Because of this, myelinated axons have fewer ions to pump back across the membrane, which reduces the adenosine triphosphate (ATP) cost of each action potential. The importance of this concept is illustrated by demyelinating states. For example, multiple sclerosis is a neurodegenerative disorder caused by the autoimmune destruction of oligodendrocytes. Early on, the loss of myelin impairs action potential conduction. Over time, demyelinated neurons must continue to spend higher amounts of ATP for each action potential. The production of additional ATP leads to the production of free radicals, which damage macromolecules and are generally toxic to cells. Thus myelination helps keep neurons alive.

Synapses

The site of contact between the axon and its target cell is called a *synapse*. Synapses are the site at which electrical signals within the axon (i.e., action potentials) are translated into a chemical signal that creates some effect on the target cell. These chemical messages are called *neurotransmitters*. After neurotransmitters are released from the axon, they diffuse across the 20 nm space between the axon and the target cell. This space is called the *synaptic cleft*. After crossing the synaptic cleft, neurotransmitters bind to *receptors* and create some change in the function of the target cell. Neurotransmitter receptors may cause long-lived changes in cell function by altering gene expression in the target cell. More commonly, neurotransmitter receptors are ion channels that create fast electrical events to cause some short-term effect. For example, motor neurons cause muscles to contract, whereas interneurons alter the electrical activity of a neighboring neuron, perhaps stimulating an action potential and another round of neurotransmitter release.

Neurotransmitters

Neurotransmitters are chemicals that are released from neurons to communicate with target cells. An in-depth discussion of neurotransmitters is beyond the scope of this text. We will, however, discuss some common neurotransmitters because of their relationship to CNS disease. Furthermore, many of the pharmacologic interventions available to patients with CNS pathology act by facilitating or inhibiting neurotransmitter activity.

Common neurotransmitters include acetylcholine, glutamate, γ-aminobutyric acid, dopamine, serotonin, and norepinephrine. Acetylcholine conveys information in the PNS and is the neurotransmitter used by lower motor neurons that synapse onto skeletal muscle fibers (Lundy-Ekman, 2018). Acetylcholine also plays a role in regulating heart rate and other autonomic functions. Glutamate is an excitatory neurotransmitter used widely throughout the CNS. Excessive glutamate release is thought to contribute to neuron destruction after an injury to the CNS—this is discussed further in the last section of this chapter. γ-Aminobutyric acid is the major inhibitory neurotransmitter of the brain, and glycine is the major inhibitory neurotransmitter of the spinal cord. Dopamine influences motor activity, motivation, general arousal, and cognition. Serotonin plays a role in "mood, behavior, and inhibits pain" (Dvorak and Mansfield, 2013). Norepinephrine is used by the sympathetic nervous systems and produces the

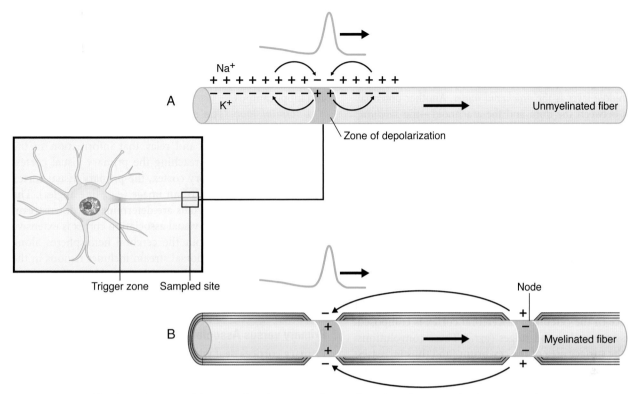

Fig. 2.5 Action potential propagation along axons. Current flow along the axons of active neurons. At rest, neurons have a negative charge at their membrane (represented as "−" signs and a light pink color inside the axon). As the action potential moves down the axon, it creates areas of positive charge (represented as "+" signs and a darker pink color inside the axon). Unmyelinated axons **(A)** move ions across the membrane along the entire length of the axon. Myelinated axons **(B)** only move ions across the membrane at nodes, allowing for more rapid saltatory conduction. (From Mtui E, Gruener G, Dockery P: *Fitzgerald's clinical neuroanatomy and neuroscience e-book*, Philadelphia, 2015, Elsevier Health Sciences, Fig. 7.12, p. 83.)

"fight-or-flight response" to stress (Fitzgerald et al., 2012; Lundy-Ekman, 2018).

ANATOMIC COMPONENTS OF THE CENTRAL NERVOUS SYSTEM

The CNS comprises the brain and spinal cord. The brain consists of the cerebrum, the thalamic complex, the brainstem, and the cerebellum. We will cover each of these major divisions of the CNS from top to bottom. Before we cover the CNS, we must first discuss the protective structures that house it.

Supportive and Protective Structures

The CNS is protected by a number of different structures and substances to minimize the possibility of injury (Fig. 2.6). First, the brain and spinal cord are surrounded by bony skull and vertebral column, which provide mechanical protection against injury. Immediately below the skull and within the vertebrae, we find three layers of membranes called the *meninges*, which provide additional protection.

The outermost layer is the *dura mater*. The dura is a thick, fibrous connective tissue membrane that adheres to the skull. The dural covering has two distinct projections: the falx cerebri, which separates the cerebral hemispheres, and the tentorium cerebelli, which provides a separation between the posterior

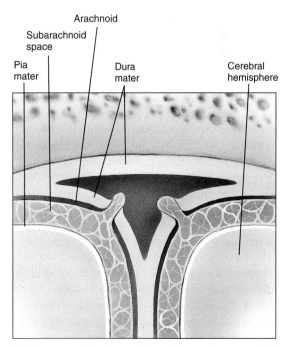

Fig. 2.6 Coronal section through the skull, meninges, and cerebral hemispheres. The section shows the midline structures near the top of the skull. The three layers of meninges, the superior sagittal sinus, and arachnoid granulations are indicated. (From Lundy-Ekman L: *Neuroscience: fundamentals for rehabilitation*, ed 4, St. Louis, 2013, Elsevier.)

cerebral hemispheres and the cerebellum. The area between the dura mater and the skull is a potential space known as the *epidural space*. The epidural space is called a potential space because it only exists in the case of injury. Assuming we don't have any cranial bleeding, the epidural space should not be visible. The next or middle layer is the *arachnoid mater*. Another potential space lies between the dura and the arachnoid—the *subdural space*. Below the arachnoid mater, we find our first bona fide space: the *subarachnoid space*, which contains the cerebral arteries. The subarachnoid space is filled with cerebrospinal fluid, which allows it to act as a cushion for the CNS. The third layer is the *pia mater*. This is the innermost layer and adheres to the brain and spinal cord. The pia mater is delicate and fairly permeable compared with the other layers. For the most part, the meninges are continuous with the connective tissues found in peripheral nerves. The dura mater forms the epineurium and the arachnoid mater forms the perineurium.

The Cerebral Cortex

The surface of the cerebrum or cerebral cortex is composed of depressions *(sulci)* and ridges *(gyri)*. These convolutions increase the surface area of the cerebrum (and thus increases the number of cortical neurons) without requiring an increase in the size of the brain. The outer surface of the cerebrum is composed of gray matter approximately 2 to 4 mm thick, whereas the inner surface is composed of white matter fiber tracts (Fitzgerald et al., 2012).

Lobes of the Cerebrum

The cerebrum is divided into four lobes—frontal, parietal, temporal, and occipital—each having unique functions, as shown in Fig. 2.7, *A*. The hemispheres of the brain, although apparent mirror images of one another, have specialized functions as well. This sidedness of brain function is called hemispheric specialization or lateralization.

Frontal lobe. The *frontal lobe* contains the *primary motor cortex* (PMC). The frontal lobe is responsible for voluntary control of complex motor activities. In addition to its motor responsibilities, the frontal lobe also exhibits a strong influence over cognitive functions, including judgment, attention, awareness, abstract thinking, mood, and aggression. The principal motor region responsible for speech (the Broca area) is located within the frontal lobe, near the primary motor regions that control the lips, tongue, and larynx.

Parietal lobe. The *parietal lobe* contains the primary somatosensory cortex. Incoming sensory information is processed within this lobe and meaning is provided to the stimuli. Perception is the process of attaching meaning to sensory information and requires interaction between the brain, body, and the individual's environment (Lundy-Ekman, 2018). Much of our perceptual learning requires a functioning parietal lobe. Specific body regions are assigned locations within the parietal lobe for this interpretation. This mapping is known as the sensory homunculus (Fig. 2.7, *B*).

Temporal lobe. The *temporal lobe* contains the primary auditory cortex. The primary auditory cortex decodes pitch and volume of sounds. The meaning of sounds is distinguished in other cortical regions. One particularly important region is the Wernicke area, which ascribes meaning to particular sounds (i.e., words). The temporal lobe is also involved in declarative memory function (i.e., factual memories), as it houses important memory-relevant structures such as the amygdala and hippocampus.

Occipital lobe. The *occipital lobe* contains the primary visual cortex. The eyes take in visual signals concerning objects in the visual field and relay that information to the thalamus before finally reaching the primary visual cortex. Like the primary auditory cortex, the primary visual cortex distinguishes fine details of an image (e.g., line angles). The meaning of these fine details are determined in downstream association regions. The visual association cortex is extensive and is located throughout the cerebral hemispheres along two main streams. The dorsal stream includes regions in the parietal lobes and determines object location. The ventral stream includes regions in the temporal lobes and determines object identity.

Primary versus Association Cortex

Primary cortices deal with granular details, whereas association cortices create meaning from these details. For example, neurons in the primary visual cortex are responsive to very specific visual stimuli, such as the angle of a line, whereas visual association cortices will construct objects (e.g., an octagon) and ascribe meaning to these objects (e.g., a stop sign). An excellent example of an association cortex for the physical therapist is the *parietoinsular vestibular cortex*. The parietoinsular vestibular cortex constructs our sense of balance based on input from the somatosensory cortex (*What is our body position?*), visual cortex (*Is anything around us moving?*), and vestibular system (*Is our body moving?*). Association areas are responsible for all higher-order functions of the CNS, including personality, intelligence, memory, and consciousness. Fig. 2.7, *C* depicts association areas within the cerebral hemispheres.

Motor Areas of the Cerebral Cortex

The PMC, located in the frontal lobe, is primarily responsible for contralateral voluntary control of the upper and lower extremity and facial movements. Thus a greater proportion of the total surface area of this region is devoted to neurons that control these body parts. It is important to understand that although neurons in the PMC do control specific body parts, they do not map to specific muscles. Instead, PMC neurons are organized around movements, whereas lower motor neurons in the spinal cord are organized around muscles. Other motor areas include the *premotor area* and *supplementary motor area* (SMA). Both of these regions project directly to the spinal cord and to the PMC. The premotor area is involved in well-patterned, bilateral movements and appears to direct our movements based more on external cues (i.e., sensory information). The SMA is involved with eye control and appears to create sequences of movements based more on internal cues (i.e., learned information).

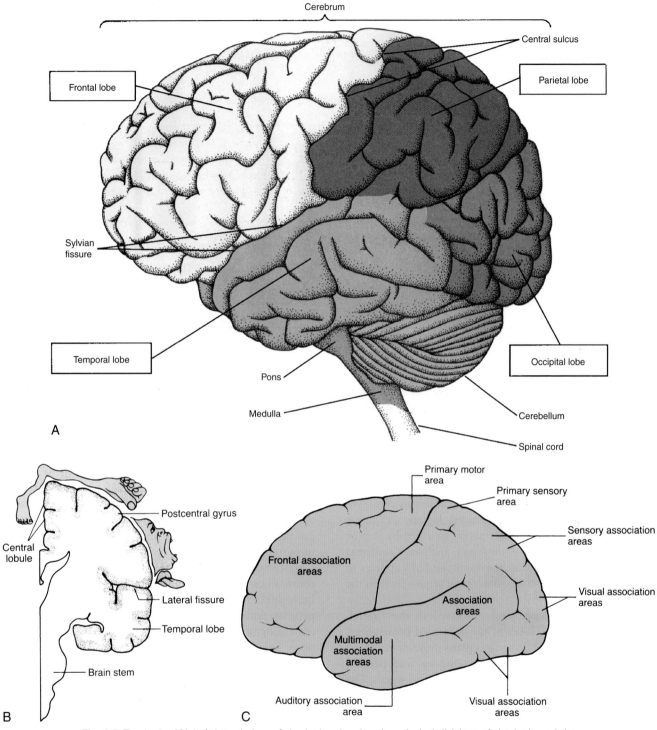

Fig. 2.7 The brain. **(A)** Left lateral view of the brain, showing the principal divisions of the brain and the four major lobes of the cerebrum. **(B)** Sensory homunculus. **(C)** Primary and association sensory and motor areas of the brain. (A, from Guyton AC: *Basic neuroscience: anatomy and physiology*, ed 2, Philadelphia, 1991, WB Saunders; B and C, from Cech D, Martin S: *Functional movement development across the life span*, ed 3, St. Louis, 2012, Elsevier.)

Hemispheric Specialization

The cerebrum can be further divided into the right and left *cerebral hemispheres*. Gross anatomic differences have been demonstrated within the hemispheres. The hemisphere that is responsible for language is considered the dominant hemisphere. Approximately 95% of the population, including all right-handed individuals, are left-hemisphere dominant. Even in individuals who are left-hand dominant, the left hemisphere is the primary speech center in about 50% of these people (Geschwind and Levitsky, 1968; Gilman and Newman, 2003; Guyton, 1991). Table 2.2 lists primary functions of both the dominant and nondominant cerebral

TABLE 2.2 Behaviors Attributed to the Dominant and Nondominant Brain Hemispheres

Behavior	Dominant Hemisphere	Nondominant Hemisphere
Cognition/intellect	Processing information in a sequential, linear manner Observing and analyzing details	Processing information in a simultaneous, holistic, or gestalt manner Grasping overall organization or pattern
Perception/cognition	Processing and producing language, processing verbal cues and instructions	Processing nonverbal stimuli (environmental sounds, visual cues, speech intonation, complex shapes, and designs) Visual-spatial perception Drawing inferences, synthesizing information
Academic skills	Reading: sound-symbol relationships, word recognition, reading comprehension Performing mathematical calculations	Mathematical reasoning and judgment Alignment of numerals in calculations
Motor and task performance	Planning and sequencing movements Performing movements and gestures to command	Sustaining a movement or posture, consistency in movement performance
Behavior and emotions	Organization, expressing positive emotions	Ability to self-correct, judgment, awareness of disability, and safety concerns Expressing negative emotions and perceiving emotion

Modified from O'Sullivan SB: Stroke. In O'Sullivan SB, Schmitz TJ, editors: *Physical rehabilitation assessment and treatment,* ed 4, Philadelphia, 2001, FA Davis; O'Sullivan SB: Stroke. In O'Sullivan SB, Schmitz TJ, Fulk GD, editors: *Physical rehabilitation,* ed 6, Philadelphia, 2014, FA Davis.

hemispheres. Damage to either hemisphere can lead to sensory and motor impairments. Language deficits (e.g., aphasia) are suggestive of damage to the dominant hemisphere, whereas deficits in spatial awareness (e.g., hemineglect) are suggestive of damage to the nondominant hemisphere.

Dominant hemisphere functions. The dominant hemisphere has been described as the verbal or analytic side of the brain. The dominant hemisphere allows for the processing of information in a sequential, organized, logical, and linear manner. The processing of information in a step-by-step or detailed fashion allows for thorough analysis. Consistent with this "stepwise" function, the dominant SMA appears to play a greater role in planning movement sequences than the nondominant SMA.

Language is produced and processed in the frontal, temporal, and parietal lobes of the dominant hemisphere. In the frontal lobes, the Broca area plans movements of the mouth to produce speech. In the temporal and parietal lobes, the Wernicke area attributes meaning to words. The Broca area and Wernicke area work together during speech production, and damage to either one causes severe language deficits. Additional regions in the parietal lobe play a role in recognizing written words. Common impairments seen in patients with dominant hemispheric injury include an inability to plan motor tasks (apraxia); difficulty in initiating, sequencing, and processing a task; difficulty in producing or comprehending speech; and perseveration of speech or motor behaviors (Deutsch and O'Sullivan, 2019).

Nondominant hemisphere functions. The nondominant cerebral hemisphere is responsible for an individual's nonverbal and artistic abilities. The nondominant side of the brain allows individuals to process information in a complete or holistic fashion without specifically reviewing all the details. The individual is able to grasp or comprehend general concepts. Consistent with this "big picture" function, the nondominant SMA is more active during bilateral movements than unilateral movements.

The principal function of the nondominant hemisphere is to determine spatial relationships. For example, the nondominant hemisphere is involved in hand-eye coordination, determining the location of objects, and perceiving one's position in space. The nondominant hemisphere plays an important role in nonverbal communication, as the area that corresponds to the Broca area is responsible for nonverbal communication, including gestures and adjustments of the individual's tone of voice. Deficits that can be observed in patients with nondominant hemisphere damage include poor judgment and safety awareness, unrealistic expectations, denial of disability or deficits, disturbances in body image, irritability, and lethargy.

Hemispheric connections. Even though the two hemispheres of the brain have discrete functional capabilities, they perform many of the same actions. Communication between the two hemispheres is constant, so individuals can be analytic and yet still grasp broad general concepts. It is possible for the right hand to know what the left hand is doing and vice versa. The *corpus callosum* is a large group of axons that connect the right and left cerebral hemispheres and allow communication between the two cortices.

Subcortical Structures

Subcortical structures lie deep within the brain and include the internal capsule, the basal ganglia, and the limbic system. These structures are briefly discussed because of their significance to motor function.

Internal Capsule

The *internal capsule* contains the major projection fibers that run to and from the cerebral cortex (Fig. 2.8). The internal capsule can be broken down into three different regions. The anterior limb connects the frontal cerebral cortex to the thalamus and pons. The genu contains cortical motor fibers that project to brainstem motor nuclei. The posterior limb contains motor fibers from the frontal cortex that form the corticospinal tract and sensory fibers projecting from the thalamus to the parietal cortex. The posterior limb also contains visual and auditory fibers projecting from the thalamus to the occipital and temporal lobes, respectively. A lesion within the internal capsule typically causes contralateral loss of voluntary movement and conscious somatosensation, whereas visual and auditory deficits occur rarely.

Basal Ganglia

Another group of nuclei located at the base of the cerebrum comprises the *basal ganglia*. The basal ganglia form a subcortical structure made up of the caudate nucleus, putamen, globus pallidus, substantia nigra, and subthalamic nuclei. The globus pallidus and putamen form the lentiform nucleus, and the caudate and putamen are known as the striatum. The basal ganglia project to motor regions of the thalamus to regulate posture and muscle tone, as well as volitional and automatic movements. In addition to their role in motor control, the basal ganglia are also involved in cognitive functions. Of particular importance is reward or drive, which involves dopamine input to the ventral striatum (i.e., the nucleus accumbens). In short, actions that increase dopamine input to the ventral striatum are more likely to be repeated in the future.

The most common condition that results from dysfunction within the basal ganglia is Parkinson disease. Parkinson disease is caused by the loss of *dopamine neurons* in the substantia nigra. Dopamine input to the dorsal striatum stimulates the basal ganglia to initiate planned movements. Therefore the loss of dopamine input to the basal ganglia interferes with movement initiation. This explains many of the motor symptoms of Parkinson disease, including bradykinesia (slowed movement), hypokinesia (reduced movement amplitude), akinesia (a lack of movement), rigidity, and postural instability. The resting tremor that occurs early on in Parkinson disease is likely caused by network dysfunction in the basal ganglia, although a detailed explanation of this is beyond the scope of this chapter.

Limbic System

The *limbic system* is a group of deep brain structures that are involved in memory and emotion. The brain structures included in the limbic system have changed over the years as we discover new regions involved in memory and emotion. Thus the limbic system is a functional classification, rather than anatomic. Currently, major components of the limbic system include thalamic and hypothalamic nuclei, mammillary bodies, basal forebrain, anterior cingulate cortex, insula,

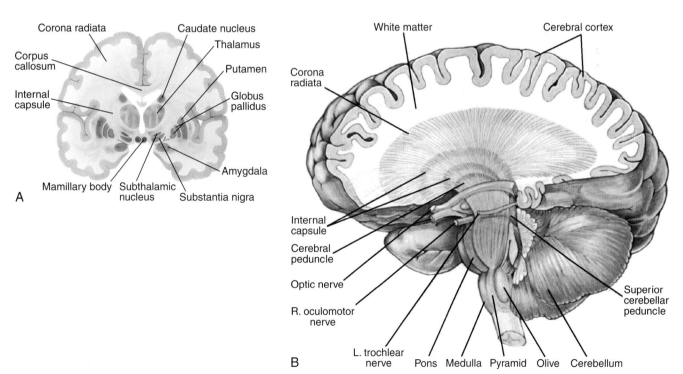

Fig. 2.8 The cerebrum. **(A)** Diencephalon and cerebral hemispheres. Coronal section. **(B)** A deep dissection of the cerebrum showing the radiating nerve fibers, the corona radiata, that conduct signals in both directions between the cerebral cortex and the lower portions of the central nervous system. (A, from Lundy-Ekman L: *Neuroscience: fundamentals for rehabilitation,* ed 4, St. Louis, 2013, WB Elsevier; B, from Guyton AC: *Basic neuroscience: anatomy and physiology,* ed 2, Philadelphia, 1991, WB Saunders.)

nucleus accumbens, amygdala, hippocampus, and entorhinal cortex. Based on this collection of brain regions, the limbic system appears to control memory, pain, pleasure, rage, affection, sexual interest, fear, and sorrow.

The overlap between emotion and memory has important functional significance. Emotionally salient events are far more memorable because of the increased activation of the limbic system. In this way, our emotions can prime memory circuits to facilitate memory encoding. Unfortunately, this robust memory encoding for emotionally charged events can lead to maladaptive states, such as phobias or posttraumatic stress disorder.

Thalamic Complex

The thalamic complex is situated deep within the cerebrum and is composed of the thalamus, epithalamus, subthalamus, and hypothalamus. The *thalamus* is the area where the major sensory tracts (dorsal columns and lateral spinothalamic) and the visual and auditory pathways synapse. The thalamus consists of a large collection of nuclei and synapses that are reciprocally connected with sensory and motor regions of the cortex. In this way, the thalamus serves as a central relay station for sensory impulses, and channels them to appropriate primary and association areas of the cortex for interpretation. Motor output from the basal ganglia and cerebellum converge at the thalamus, where they are transmitted to the cortex to influence motor output.

The *hypothalamus* is a group of nuclei that lie at the base of the brain, underneath the thalamus. The hypothalamus regulates homeostasis, which is the maintenance of a balanced internal environment. This structure is primarily involved in automatic functions, including the regulation of hunger, thirst, digestion, body temperature, blood pressure,

sexual activity, and sleep-wake cycles. The hypothalamus is responsible for integrating the functions of both the endocrine system and the ANS through its regulation of the pituitary gland and its release of hormones.

Brainstem

The *brainstem* is located between the thalamus and the spinal cord and is divided into three sections (Fig. 2.9). Moving cephalocaudally, the three areas are the midbrain, pons, and medulla. Each of the different areas is responsible for specific functions. The *midbrain* connects the diencephalon to the pons and acts as a relay station for tracts passing between the cerebrum and the spinal cord or cerebellum. The midbrain also houses reflex centers for visual, auditory, and tactile responses. The *pons* contains bundles of axons that travel between the cerebellum and the rest of the CNS and functions with the medulla to regulate breathing rate, chewing, and swallowing. It also contains reflex centers that assist with orientation of the head in response to visual and auditory stimulation. Cranial nerve nuclei can also be found within the pons, specifically cranial nerves V through VIII, which carry motor and sensory information to and from the face. The *medulla* is an extension of the spinal cord and contains the fiber tracts that run through the spinal cord. Motor and sensory nuclei for the neck and mouth region are located within the medulla, as well as the control centers for heart rate and respiration. Reflex centers for vomiting, sneezing, and swallowing are also located within the medulla.

The *reticular formation* is a collection of relay nuclei within the brainstem that extends vertically throughout its length. The system projects to the cortex and thalamus to maintain and adjust an individual's level of arousal, including sleep-wake cycles. In addition, the reticular formation

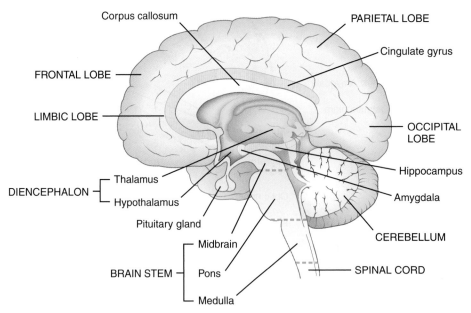

Fig. 2.9 Schematic midsagittal view of the brain shows the relationship between the cerebral cortex, cerebellum, spinal cord, and brainstem, and the subcortical structures important to functional movement. (From Cech D, Martin S: *Functional movement development across the life span,* ed 3, St. Louis, 2012, Elsevier.)

facilitates the voluntary and autonomic motor responses necessary for certain self-regulating, homeostatic functions, and is involved in the modulation of muscle tone throughout the body.

Cerebellum

The *cerebellum* controls balance and complex muscular movements. Lying below the occipital lobes and posterior to the brainstem, the cerebellum fills the posterior fossa of the cranium. The cerebellum consists of two symmetric *hemispheres* and a midline *vermis*. The cerebellum is organized such that the vermis controls the trunk and central regions of the body and assists in balance and posture, whereas the hemispheres control the limbs and allows us to smoothly execute complex, multijoint movements. Smooth movement requires precise regulation of the initiation, timing, sequencing, and force generation of agonist and antagonist muscle groups. Damage to the cerebellum is characterized by gait instability, intention tremor, uncoordinated movements, slurred speech, and difficulty with smooth eye movements.

The cerebellum is a major site of motor learning, allowing us to execute complex movements with little thought. When we first learn movements (e.g., walking), the movements are driven largely by the cortex, and thus require great concentration. Over time, the cerebellum acquires the patterns necessary to complete movements, unloading the task from the cortex and allowing us to perform the task with little to no conscious effort. In addition to learning the movements we want to execute the cerebellum also learns to carry out anticipatory movements that appropriately shift our balance during voluntary movements. For example, immediately before we lift a weight, the cerebellum initiates anticipatory muscle contractions in our postural muscles to keep us upright during the lift.

Spinal Cord

The *spinal cord* is a direct continuation of the brainstem, specifically the medulla (Fig. 2.10). The spinal cord extends approximately to the level of the intervertebral disc between the first two lumbar vertebrae. At approximately the vertebral L1 level, the spinal cord becomes a cone-shaped structure called the *conus medullaris*. Below this level, the spinal cord becomes a mass of spinal nerve roots called the *cauda equina*. The cauda equina consists of the nerve roots for spinal nerves L2 through S5. A thin filament, the *filum terminale*, extends from the caudal end of the spinal cord and attaches to the coccyx.

The spinal cord has two enlargements—one that extends from the third cervical segment to the second thoracic segment and another that extends from the first lumbar to the third sacral segment (Fig. 2.11). These enlargements accommodate the great number of neurons needed to innervate the upper and lower extremities located in these regions. These spinal enlargements give rise to the cervical, brachial, and lumbosacral nerve plexuses discussed later in this chapter.

The spinal cord has two primary functions: coordination of movement patterns and communication of sensory

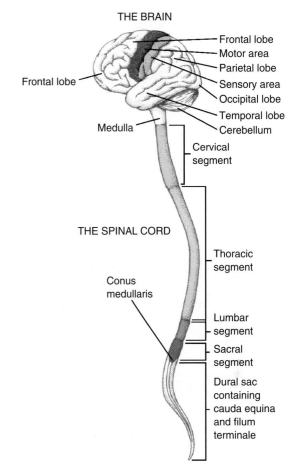

Fig. 2.10 The principal anatomic parts of the nervous system. (From Guyton AC: *Basic neuroscience: anatomy and physiology,* ed 2, Philadelphia, 1991, WB Saunders.)

information. The motor and sensory tracts are discussed in the next section. Briefly, motor tracts from upper motor neurons stimulate lower motor neurons in the spinal cord, which initiate muscle contraction. Sensory tracts arise from neurons in the *dorsal root ganglia* that extend their axons into the skin, muscles, and joints. Some sensory tracts synapse locally in the spinal cord, whereas others project directly to the brainstem before reaching the thalamus and cortex. The spinal cord contains local circuits that link sensory and motor pathways to allow for the execution of subconscious reflexes, including withdrawal and stretch reflexes.

MAJOR TRACTS OF THE CENTRAL NERVOUS SYSTEM

Gray Matter and White Matter

Gray matter refers to areas that contain large numbers of nerve cell bodies and dendrites. Collectively, these cell bodies give the region its grayish coloration. Gray matter covers the entire surface of the cerebrum and is called the cerebral cortex. The cortex is estimated to contain 50 billion neurons—approximately 500 billion neuroglial cells and a significant capillary network (Fitzgerald et al., 2012). Gray matter is also

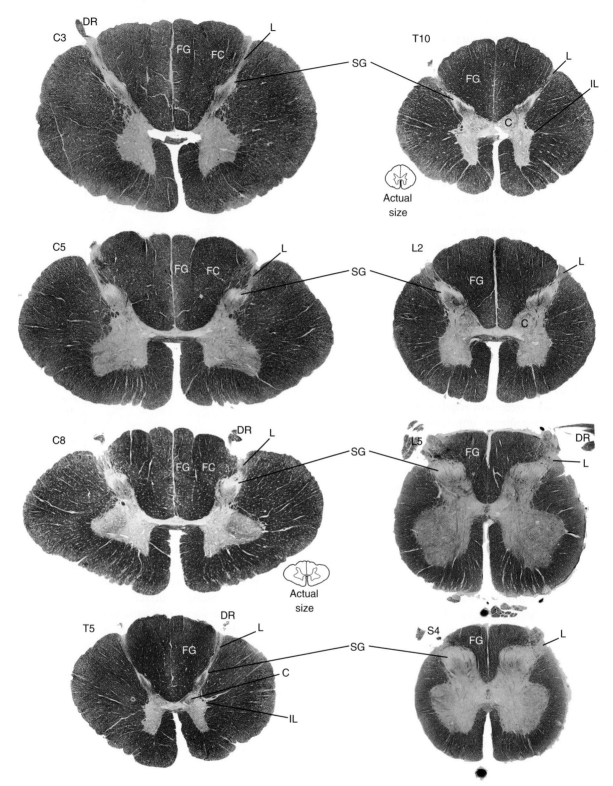

Fig. 2.11 Cross-section of the spinal cord at different levels. Fiber stained sections of the spinal cord are shown. The gray matter (lighter purple) is found within the surrounding white matter tracts (dark purple). Higher levels of the spinal cord contain a greater number of fiber tracts, and thus have more white matter. Regions of the spinal cord that innervate limbs (e.g., C5, C8, L5, and S4) contain a greater number of motor neurons, and thus have expanded anterior horns. Thoracic and lumbar spinal segments (T1–L2) contain preganglionic sympathetic neurons that are visible as the intermediolateral cell column. *C*, Clarke nucleus; *DR*, dorsal root; *FC*, fasciculus cuneatus; *FG*, fasciculus gracilis; *IL*, intermediolateral cell column; *L*, Lissauer tract; *SG*, substantia gelatinosa. (From Vanderah T, Gould DJ: *Nolte's the human brain e-book: an introduction to its functional anatomy*, Philadelphia, 2015, Elsevier Health Sciences, Fig. 10.8, p. 242.)

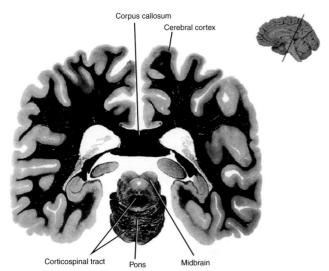

Corpus callosum
Cerebral cortex

Corticospinal tract   Pons   Midbrain

Fig. 2.12 Cross-section of cerebrum and brainstem. Fiber stained cross-sections of the brain are shown. In the cerebrum, the gray matter (tan) surrounds the fiber tracts (black). In the brain stem, the gray matter and white matter are intermixed. Cerebral cortex (not labeled), corpus callosum (1), midbrain (not labeled), pons (below 8), corticospinal tract (8 and fibers below 8). (From Vanderah T, Gould DJ: *Nolte's the human brain e-book: an introduction to its functional anatomy*, Philadelphia, 2015, Elsevier Health Sciences, Fig. 25.10, p. 650.)

present deep within the spinal cord and is discussed in more detail later in this chapter.

Areas of the nervous system with a high concentration of myelin appear white because of the fat content within the myelin. Consequently, *white matter* is composed of axons and associated glia. White matter is found in the brain and spinal cord, although its location relative to gray matter varies (Figs. 2.11 and 2.12). In the brain, gray matter of the cerebral cortex surrounds the white matter that comprises axons projecting to and from the cortex. As these myelinated fiber tracts project down the spinal cord, they weave their way through the deep nuclei and brainstem. At the level of the spinal cord, myelinated fibers surround the central gray matter.

Internal Anatomy of the Spinal Cord

The internal anatomy of the spinal cord can be visualized in cross-sections and is viewed as two distinct areas. Fig. 2.13, *A* illustrates the internal anatomy of the spinal cord. The center of the spinal cord, the gray matter, is distinguished by its H-shaped or butterfly-shaped pattern. The gray matter contains cell bodies of motor and sensory neurons, as well as interneurons that link motor and sensory neurons to create spinal circuits. The ventral or *anterior horns* house the lower motor neurons, whereas the dorsal or *posterior horns* house sensory neurons (Fig. 2.13, *B*). Sensory neurons in the posterior horns receive input from the primary sensory neurons that innervate the body. These primary sensory neurons are housed in the dorsal root ganglia, which lie immediately outside the spinal cord, but still within the vertebral column. The

lateral horns are present at the T1 to L2 levels and contain cell bodies of preganglionic sympathetic neurons.

The periphery of the spinal cord is composed of white matter. The white matter is composed of sensory (ascending) and motor (descending) fiber tracts. These fiber tracts carry impulses between the spinal cord and brain. In addition, these fiber tracts cross over from one side of the body to the other at various points within the spinal cord and brain. The point at which fiber tracts cross the midline, or *decussate*, varies between tracts, but this crossing occurs once for all of the major tracts involving the cerebral cortex. This explains why the left side of our brain controls the right side of our bodies (this is called *contralateral innervation*).

Major Afferent (Sensory) Tracts

Two primary ascending sensory tracts are present in the white matter of the spinal cord. The dorsal or *posterior columns* carry information about position sense (proprioception), vibration, two-point discrimination, and deep touch. Fig. 2.14 shows the location of this tract. The fibers of the dorsal columns synapse in the medulla. Fibers from these medullary neurons form the *medial lemniscus*, which crosses the midline and projects to the thalamus. Thalamic neurons project to the cortex to create conscious perceptions of somatosensory information.

The *spinothalamic tract* transmits pain and temperature sensations (Fig. 2.14). Fibers from this tract enter the spinal cord, synapse in the posterior horn, and cross within three spinal segments. The spinothalamic tract ultimately terminates in the thalamus. As mentioned earlier, thalamic neurons project to the cortex to create (1) awareness of the location of pain, and (2) the negative affect associated with pain. The spinothalamic tract is a part of a larger collection of fibers called the *anterolateral tract*, which conveys crude touch and nociceptive input to brainstem nuclei to carry out reflexive responses to painful stimuli.

Although the posterior column-medial lemniscus pathway and the spinothalamic tract convey different types of information, they are quite similar. Both contain three neurons. The first neuron is housed in the dorsal root ganglia. The second neuron projects its axon across the midline. The third neuron projects from the thalamus to the cortex. These two tracts are summarized in Fig. 2.15 and Table 2.3.

Major Efferent (Motor) Tract

The *corticospinal tract* is the primary motor pathway and controls skilled movements of the extremities. This tract originates from *upper motor neurons* in the frontal lobes (including primary motor, premotor, supplementary motor, and even sensory cortices), descends through the internal capsule, decussates at the medullospinal junction, and projects downward with anterior and lateral regions of the spinal cord to finally synapse on *lower motor neurons* in the anterior horns. Thus the corticospinal tract is a fairly straightforward two neuron circuit in which upper motor neurons stimulate lower motor neurons, which then stimulate individual muscles to cause contraction and carry out movements.

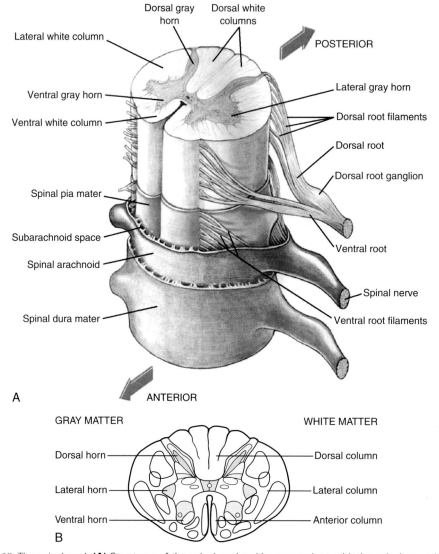

Fig. 2.13 The spinal cord. **(A)** Structures of the spinal cord and its connections with the spinal nerve by way of the dorsal and ventral spinal roots. Note also the coverings of the spinal cord, the meninges. **(B)** Cross-section of the spinal cord. The central gray matter is divided into horns and a commissure. The white matter is divided into columns. (A, from Guyton AC: *Basic neuroscience: anatomy and physiology,* ed 2, Philadelphia, 1991, WB Saunders.)

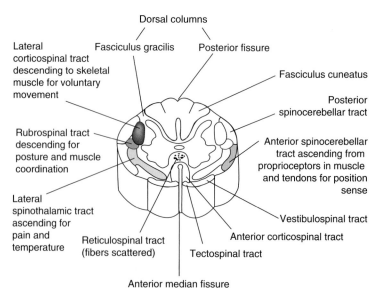

Fig. 2.14 Cross-section of the spinal cord showing tracts. (From Gould BE: *Pathophysiology for the health-related professions,* Philadelphia, 1997, WB Saunders.)

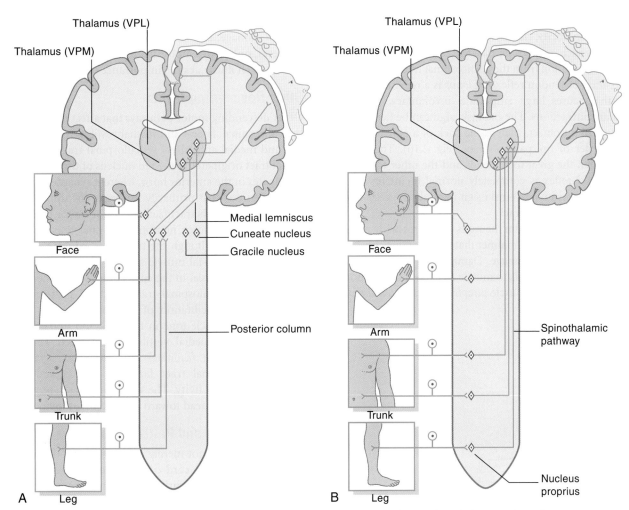

Fig. 2.15 Ascending tracts of the spinal cord that reach the cortex. Summaries of the posterior column-medial lemniscus pathway (*PCML*, **A)** and the spinothalamic tract (*ST*, **B)** are shown. With the exception of the face, all first-order sensory neurons are located in the dorsal root ganglia. First-order sensory neurons for the face are found in the trigeminal ganglion. Second-order sensory neurons in the medulla (PCML) and spinal cord (ST) cross the midline. Third-order neurons in the thalamus project to the cortex to create conscious perceptions. *VPL*, ventral posterolateral nucleus; *VPM*, ventral posteromedial nucleus. (From Mtui E, Gruener G, Dockery P, *Fitzgerald's clinical neuroanatomy and neuroscience e-book*, Philadelphia, 2015, Elsevier Health Sciences, Fig. 15.7, p. 164.)

TABLE 2.3	Location of Neurons in the Major Sensory Tracts of the Spinal Cord	
	Posterior Column-Medial Lemniscus	**Spinothalamic Tract**
Primary neuron	Ipsilateral dorsal root ganglion	Ipsilateral dorsal root ganglion
Secondary neuron	Ipsilateral *medulla*, crosses midline within *medulla*	Ipsilateral *dorsal horn of spinal cord*, crosses midline within *three spinal segments*
Tertiary neuron	Contralateral thalamus: ventral posterior lateral nucleus	Contralateral thalamus: ventral posterior lateral nucleus, *dorsomedial nucleus, and interstitial nuclei*

NOTE: To facilitate studying, common features of the two pathways are underlined and distinct features are italicized.

To carry out movements, the corticospinal tract has to stimulate lower motor neurons as well as inhibit spinal reflexes. As we will see later in this chapter, spinal reflexes exist to prevent involuntary movements. The basic logic of the stretch reflex is to contract any muscle that is stretched to prevent any overt change in muscle length. Thus to produce a change in muscle length, the corticospinal tract inhibits spinal reflexes through a variety of mechanisms (one is discussed later).

The clinical significance of reflex inhibition by the corticospinal tract cannot be overstressed. Besides muscle weakness and/or paralysis, common indicators of corticospinal tract damage are *spasticity*, *clonus*, and the reemergence of primitive reflexes such as the *Babinski sign*. Spasticity is caused by the loss of inhibition from the corticospinal tract and leads to *hyperreflexia* of tendon reflexes. *Clonus* is a repetitive stretch reflex that causes large amplitude, involuntary, rhythmic muscular contractions. The Babinski sign can be detected by running a blunt object, such as the back of a pen, along the lateral border of the patient's foot (Fig. 2.16). The sign is present when the great toe extends and the other toes splay. The Babinski reflex is completely normal in infants up to 2 years old. A positive Babinski sign in adults suggests damage to the corticospinal tract.

Damage to lower motor neurons interferes with muscle strength and reflexes in a manner that is distinguishable from upper motor neuron damage. Damage to both upper and lower motor neurons leads to muscle weakness. Lower motor damage leads to severe muscle *atrophy*, muscle *fasciculations*,

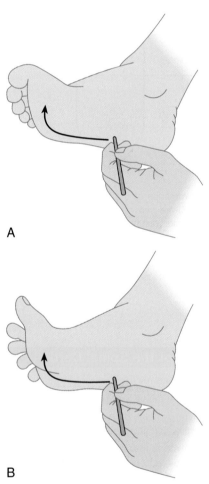

A

B

Fig. 2.16 Babinski sign. **(A)** Normal. Stroking from the heel to the ball of the foot along the lateral sole, then across the ball of the foot, normally causes the toes to flex. **(B)** Developmental or pathologic. Babinski sign in response to the same stimulus. In people with corticospinal tract lesions, or in infants younger than 7 months old, the great toe extends. Although the other toes may fan out, as shown, movement of the toes other than the great toe is not required for the Babinski sign. (From Lundy-Ekman L: *Neuroscience: fundamentals for rehabilitation*, ed 4, St. Louis, 2013, Elsevier.)

and *hyporeflexia*. Muscle atrophy can occur with upper motor neuron damage, and stress can cause muscle fasciculations. However, only lower motor neuron damage leads to hyporeflexia, which illustrates the importance of reflex testing.

Other Descending Tracts

Other descending motor pathways that affect muscle tone are the rubrospinal, lateral and medial vestibulospinal, tectospinal, and medial and lateral reticulospinal tracts. The rubrospinal tract originates in the red nucleus of the midbrain and terminates in the anterior horn, where it synapses with lower motor neurons that primarily innervate the upper extremities. Fibers from this tract facilitate flexor motor neurons and inhibit extensor motor neurons. Proximal muscles are primarily affected, although the tract does exhibit some influence over more distal muscle groups. The rubrospinal tract has been said to assist in the correction of movement errors. The lateral vestibulospinal tract assists in postural adjustments through facilitation of proximal extensor muscles. Regulation of muscle tone in the neck and upper back is a function of the medial vestibulospinal tract. The medial reticulospinal tract facilitates limb extensors, whereas the lateral reticulospinal tract facilitates flexors and inhibits extensor muscle activity. The tectospinal tract provides for orientation of the head toward a sound or a moving object.

Spinal Reflexes and Pattern Generators

The spinal cord is not merely a relay between the brain and the PNS. The spinal cord contains neural circuits that are capable of generating fairly complex movements in the absence of input from the cerebrum. For example, decerebrate cats (which have connections with their cerebrum severed) are still capable of walking and running on a treadmill, so long as their body weight is supported. These movements are carried out by spinal circuits called *central pattern generators*, which are responsible for coordinating alternating, bilateral movements and spinal reflexes.

Lower motor neurons send out axons through the ventral or anterior spinal root; these axons eventually become peripheral nerves and innervate muscle fibers. There are two types of lower motor neurons: alpha lower motor neurons (αLMNs) and gamma lower motor neurons (γLMNs). αLMNs stimulate *extrafusal muscle fibers* and cause forceful muscle contraction. γLMNs stimulate *intrafusal muscle fibers* and control muscle tone by regulating the excitability of sensory organs in the muscle called *muscle spindles*. Muscle spindles are sensory organs that are less than 1 cm long and distributed throughout skeletal muscles. Muscle spindles are stimulated by muscle stretch and provide sensory feedback regarding muscle length.

Muscle spindles keep muscle length constant by providing excitatory input to αLMNs that innervate the stretched muscle. This is the basis of the stretch reflex. If a muscle is involuntarily stretched, perhaps because of a tap on a tendon, the muscle stretch stimulates muscle spindles. Stretched muscle spindles then stimulate muscle contraction by activating two types of neurons: (1) the αLMNs that innervate the stretched muscle, and (2) inhibitory interneurons that ensure the antagonist αLMNs remain silent. Let us consider the patellar reflex. A tap on the patellar tendon stretches the quadriceps and stimulates muscle spindles. Stretched muscle spindles stimulate αLMNs that innervate the quadriceps and inhibit (via an interneuron) αLMNs that innervate the hamstrings, which causes contraction of the quadriceps.

An important note about stretch or deep tendon reflexes is that their activation and subsequent motor response can occur without higher cortical influence. The sensory input entering the spinal cord does not have to be transmitted to the cortex for interpretation. This has clinical implications because it means that a patient with a cervical spinal cord injury can continue to exhibit lower extremity deep tendon reflexes despite lower extremity paralysis.

How does the corticospinal tract override the stretch reflex to carry out voluntary movements? It all comes down to γLMNs. Muscle spindles are flanked by intrafusal muscle fibers. When intrafusal muscle fibers contract following input from γLMNs, the muscle spindle is elongated. The lengthening of the muscle spindle by γLMNs offsets the shortening of the muscle spindle that occurs when αLMNs stimulate muscle contraction via extrafusal muscle fibers. Thus the activity of both αLMNs and γLMNs is required in order for movements to take place. The αLMN stimulates muscle contraction, whereas the γLMN prevents spinal reflexes from interfering with muscle contraction.

PERIPHERAL NERVOUS SYSTEM

The PNS consists of the nerves leading to and from the CNS, including the cranial nerves exiting the brainstem and the spinal roots exiting the spinal cord, many of which combine to form peripheral nerves. These nerves connect the CNS functionally with the rest of the body through sensory and motor impulses. Fig. 2.17 provides a schematic representation of the PNS and its transition to the CNS.

The PNS is divided into two primary components: the somatic (body) nervous system and the ANS. The somatic or voluntary nervous system is concerned with conscious reactions to external stimulation. This system is under

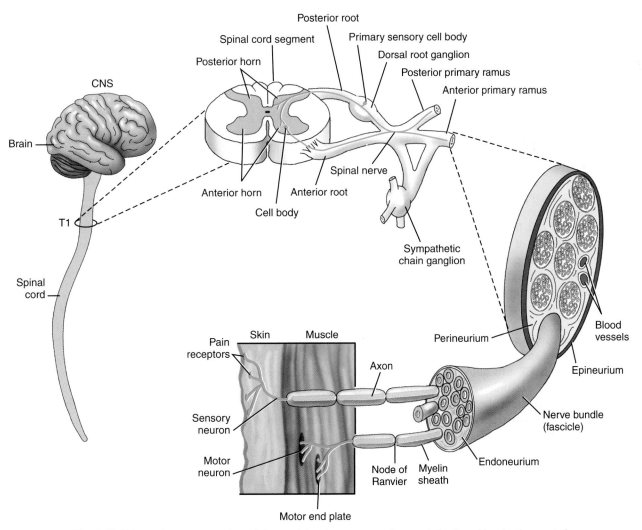

Fig. 2.17 Schematic representation of the peripheral nervous system and the transition to the central nervous system.

TABLE 2.4 Cranial Nerves

Number	Name	Related Function	Connection to Brain
I	Olfactory	Smell	Inferior frontal lobe
II	Optic	Vision	Diencephalon
III	Oculomotor	Moves eye up, down, medially; raises upper eyelid; constricts pupil; adjusts the shape of the lens of the eye	Midbrain (anterior)
IV	Trochlear	Moves eye medially and down	Midbrain (posterior)
V	Trigeminal	Facial sensation, chewing, sensation from temporomandibular joint	Pons (lateral)
VI	Abducens	Abducts eye	Between pons and medulla
VII	Facial	Facial expression, closes eye, tears, salivation, taste	Between pons and medulla
VIII	Vestibulocochlear	Sensation of head position relative to gravity and head movement; hearing	Between pons and medulla
IX	Glossopharyngeal	Swallowing, salivation, taste	Medulla
X	Vagus	Regulates viscera, swallowing, speech, taste	Medulla
XI	Accessory	Elevates shoulders, turns head	Spinal cord and medulla
XII	Hypoglossal	Moves tongue	Medulla

From Lundy-Ekman L: *Neuroscience: fundamentals for rehabilitation,* ed 4, St. Louis, 2013, Elsevier.)

conscious control and is responsible for skeletal muscle contraction by way of the nine cranial nerves with motor function and 31 pairs of spinal nerves. By contrast, the ANS is an involuntary system that innervates glands, smooth (visceral) muscle, and the myocardium. The primary function of the ANS is to maintain *homeostasis,* an optimal internal environment. Specific functions include the regulation of digestion, circulation, and cardiac muscle contraction.

Somatic Nervous System

Within the PNS are 12 pairs of cranial nerves, 31 pairs of spinal nerves, and the ganglia or cell bodies associated with the cranial and spinal nerves. The cranial nerves are located in the brainstem and can be sensory or motor nerves, or mixed. Primary functions of the cranial nerves include eye movement, smell, sensation perceived by the face and tongue, auditory and vestibular functions, and innervation of the sternocleidomastoid and trapezius muscles. See Table 2.4 for a more detailed list of cranial nerves and their major functions.

The spinal nerves consist of 8 cervical, 12 thoracic, 5 lumbar, and 5 sacral nerves and 1 coccygeal nerve. Cervical spinal nerves C1 through C7 exit above the corresponding vertebrae. Because there are only seven cervical vertebrae, the C8 spinal nerve exits above the T1 vertebra. From that point on, each succeeding spinal nerve exits below its respective vertebra. Fig. 2.18 shows the distribution and innervation of the peripheral nerves. Spinal nerves, consisting of sensory (posterior or dorsal root) and motor (anterior or ventral root) components, exit the *intervertebral foramen.* Once through the foramen, the spinal nerve divides into two primary rami. This division represents the beginning of the PNS. The dorsal or posterior rami innervate the paravertebral muscles, the posterior aspects of the vertebrae, and

the overlying skin. The ventral or anterior primary rami innervate the intercostal muscles, the muscles and skin in the extremities, and the anterior and lateral trunk. The region of skin innervated by sensory afferent fibers from an individual spinal nerve is called a *dermatome.* The group of muscles innervated by a spinal nerve is called a *myotome.* Because dermatomes and myotomes are consistent between different people, they are useful clinical tools for localizing areas of damage to the nervous system.

The 12 pairs of thoracic nerves do not join with other nerves and maintain their segmental relationship. However, the anterior primary rami of the other spinal nerves join together to form local networks known as the cervical, brachial, and lumbosacral plexuses (Guyton, 1991). The reader is given only a brief description of these nerve plexuses because a detailed description of these structures is beyond the scope of this text.

Cervical Plexus

The cervical plexus is composed of the C1 through C4 spinal nerves. These nerves primarily innervate the deep muscles of the neck, the superficial anterior neck muscles, the levator scapulae, and portions of the trapezius and sternocleidomastoid. The phrenic nerve, one of the specific nerves within the cervical plexus, is formed from branches of C3 through C5. This nerve innervates the diaphragm, the primary muscle of ventilation, and is the only motor and main sensory nerve for this muscle (Guyton, 1991). Fig. 2.19 identifies components of the cervical plexus.

Brachial Plexus

The anterior primary rami of C5 through T1 form the brachial plexus. The plexus divides and comes together several times, providing muscles with motor and sensory innervation from more than one spinal nerve root level.

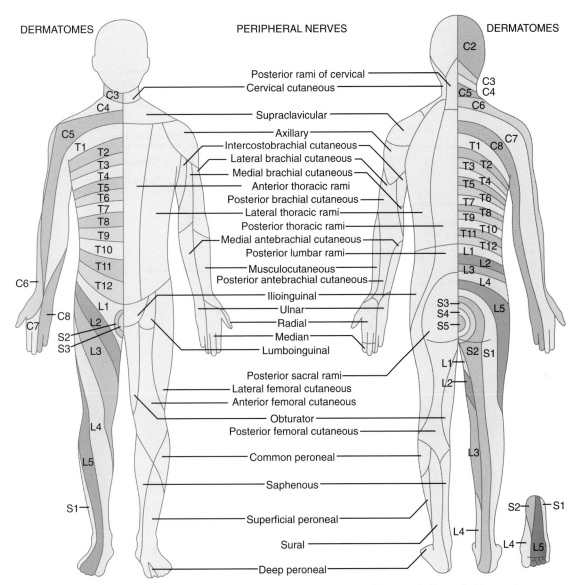

DERMATOMES PERIPHERAL NERVES DERMATOMES

Posterior rami of cervical
Cervical cutaneous
Supraclavicular
Axillary
Intercostobrachial cutaneous
Lateral brachial cutaneous
Medial brachial cutaneous
Anterior thoracic rami
Posterior brachial cutaneous
Lateral thoracic rami
Posterior thoracic rami
Medial antebrachial cutaneous
Posterior lumbar rami
Musculocutaneous
Posterior antebrachial cutaneous
Ilioinguinal
Ulnar
Radial
Median
Lumboinguinal
Posterior sacral rami
Lateral femoral cutaneous
Anterior femoral cutaneous
Obturator
Posterior femoral cutaneous
Common peroneal
Saphenous
Superficial peroneal
Sural
Deep peroneal

Fig. 2.18 Dermatomes and cutaneous distribution of peripheral nerves. (From Lundy-Ekman L: *Neuroscience: fundamentals for rehabilitation*, ed 3, Philadelphia, 2007, WB Saunders.)

The five primary nerves of the brachial plexus are the musculocutaneous, axillary, radial, median, and ulnar nerves. Fig. 2.20 depicts the constituency of the brachial plexus. These five peripheral nerves innervate the majority of the upper extremity musculature, with the exception of the medial pectoral nerve (C8), which innervates the pectoralis muscles; the subscapular nerve (C5 and C6), which innervates the subscapularis; and the thoracodorsal nerve (C7), which supplies the latissimus dorsi muscle (Guyton, 1991).

The musculocutaneous nerve innervates the forearm flexors. The elbow, wrist, and finger extensors are innervated by the radial nerve. The median nerve supplies the forearm pronators and the wrist and finger flexors, and it allows thumb abduction and opposition. The ulnar nerve assists the median nerve with wrist and finger flexion, abducts and adducts the fingers, and allows for opposition of the fifth finger (Guyton, 1991).

Lumbosacral Plexus

Although some authors discuss the lumbar and sacral plexuses separately, they are discussed here as one unit because together they innervate lower extremity musculature. The anterior primary rami of L1 through S3 form the lumbosacral plexus. This plexus innervates the muscles of the thigh, lower leg, and foot. This plexus does not undergo the same separation and reuniting as does the brachial plexus. The lumbosacral plexus has eight roots, which eventually form six primary peripheral nerves: obturator, femoral, superior gluteal, inferior gluteal, common peroneal, and tibial. The sciatic nerve, which is frequently discussed in physical therapy practice, is actually composed of the common peroneal and tibial nerves encased in a sheath. This nerve innervates the hamstrings and causes hip extension and knee flexion. The sciatic nerve separates into its components just above the knee (Guyton, 1991). The lumbosacral plexus is shown in Figs. 2.21 and 2.22.

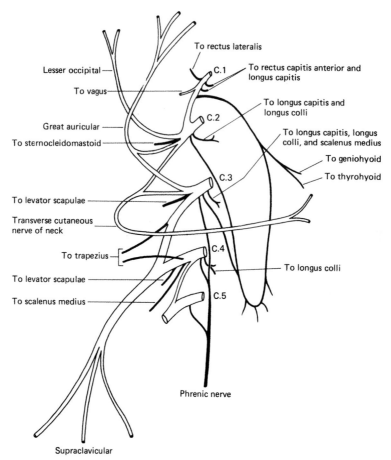

Fig. 2.19 The cervical plexus and its branches. (From Guyton AC: *Basic neuroscience: anatomy and physiology,* ed 2, Philadelphia, 1991, WB Saunders.)

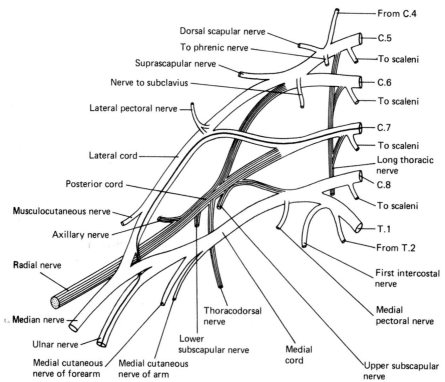

Fig. 2.20 The brachial plexus and its branches. (From Guyton AC: *Basic neuroscience: anatomy and physiology,* ed 2, Philadelphia, 1991, WB Saunders.)

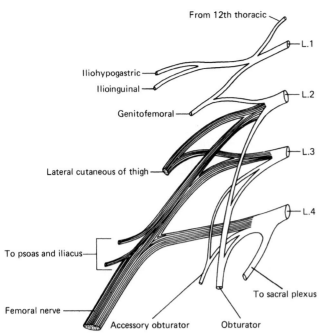

Fig. 2.21 The lumbar plexus and its branches, especially the femoral nerve. (From Guyton AC: *Basic neuroscience: anatomy and physiology*, ed 2, Philadelphia, 1991, WB Saunders.)

Autonomic Nervous System

The ANS innervates smooth muscle, cardiac muscle, and glands to regulate "circulation, respiration, digestion, metabolism, secretions, body temperature, and reproduction" (Lundy-Ekman, 2018). The ANS is divided into the sympathetic and parasympathetic divisions. Both the sympathetic and parasympathetic divisions innervate internal organs, using a two-neuron pathway comprising (1) a preganglionic neuron, and (2) a postganglionic neuron that provides the connection from the CNS to the autonomic effector organs. Cell bodies of the preganglionic neurons are located within the brainstem or spinal cord. The myelinated axons exit the CNS and synapse on the neurons in the peripheral ganglia, where they release acetylcholine to stimulate a postganglionic neuron. Postganglionic neurons project unmyelinated axons to target cells of the effector organ, where they release either acetylcholine (parasympathetic) or norepinephrine (sympathetic) (Lundy-Ekman, 2018). Fig 2.23 provides a schematic representation of this organization, whereas Fig. 2.24 shows the influence of the sympathetic and parasympathetic divisions on effector organs.

The preganglionic sympathetic fibers of the ANS arise from the thoracic and lumbar portions of the spinal cord.

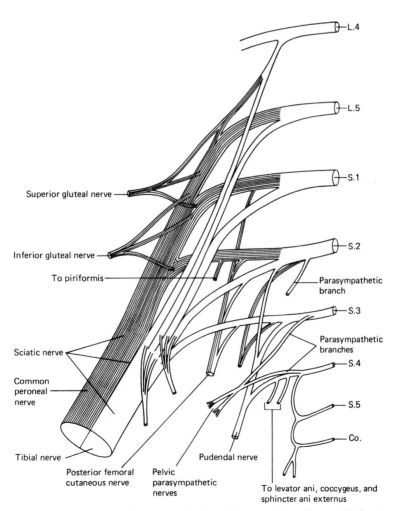

Fig. 2.22 The sacral plexus and its branches, especially the sciatic nerve. (From Guyton AC: *Basic neuroscience: anatomy and physiology*, ed 2, Philadelphia, 1991, WB Saunders.)

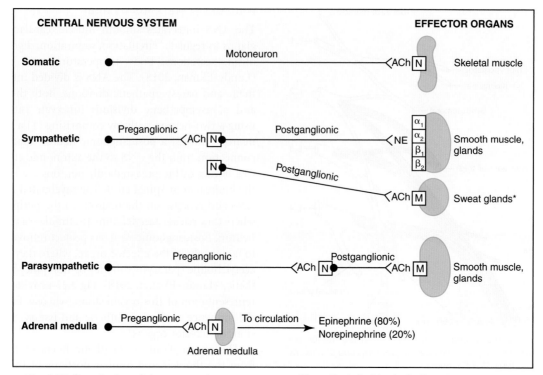

Fig. 2.23 Organization of the autonomic nervous system. (From Cech D, Martin S: *Functional movement development across the life span,* ed 3, St. Louis, 2012, Elsevier.)

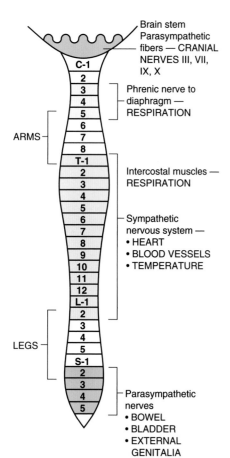

Fig. 2.24 Functional areas of the spinal cord. (From Gould BE: *Pathophysiology for the health-related professions,* Philadelphia, 1997, WB Saunders.)

Axons of preganglionic neurons terminate in either the sympathetic chain or the prevertebral ganglia located in the abdomen. The sympathetic division of the ANS facilitates energy expenditure, allowing the individual to respond in stressful situations. As such, the sympathetic nervous system is often referred to as the *"fight-or-flight response."* Sympathetic responses help the individual prepare to cope with the stimulus by maintaining an optimal blood supply. Activation of the sympathetic system stimulates smooth muscle in the blood vessels to contract, thereby causing vasoconstriction. Norepinephrine, also known as noradrenaline, is the major neurotransmitter responsible for this action. Consequently, heart rate and blood pressure are increased as the body prepares for a fight or to flee a dangerous situation. Blood flow to muscles is increased as it is diverted from the gastrointestinal tract.

The preganglionic parasympathetic fibers of the ANS arise from the brainstem—specifically cranial nerves III (oculomotor), VII (facial), IX (glossopharyngeal), and X (vagus)—and from lower sacral segments of the spinal cord. Parasympathetic postganglionic neurons are located in plexuses nearby or within target tissues. The parasympathetic division of the ANS assists in energy storage by slowing heart rate and facilitating blood flow to the digestive system, rather than the skeletal muscles. As such, the parasympathetic division is often referred to as the *"rest-and-digest response."* The vagus nerve is a major component of the parasympathetic ANS, innervating the myocardium and the smooth muscles of the lungs and digestive tract. Activation of the vagus nerve can produce the following effects: bradycardia, decreased force of cardiac muscle contraction, bronchoconstriction, increased mucus production, increased peristalsis, and increased glandular secretions. Efferent activation of the sacral components results in emptying of the bowel and bladder and arousal of sexual organs. These functions are accomplished by the release of acetylcholine, which dilates arterioles in smooth muscles. Figs. 2.25 and 2.26 show the influence of the sympathetic and parasympathetic divisions on effector organs.

Both branches of the ANS function automatically to control homeostatic functions (e.g., blood flow). Thus autoregulation is achieved by integrating information from both

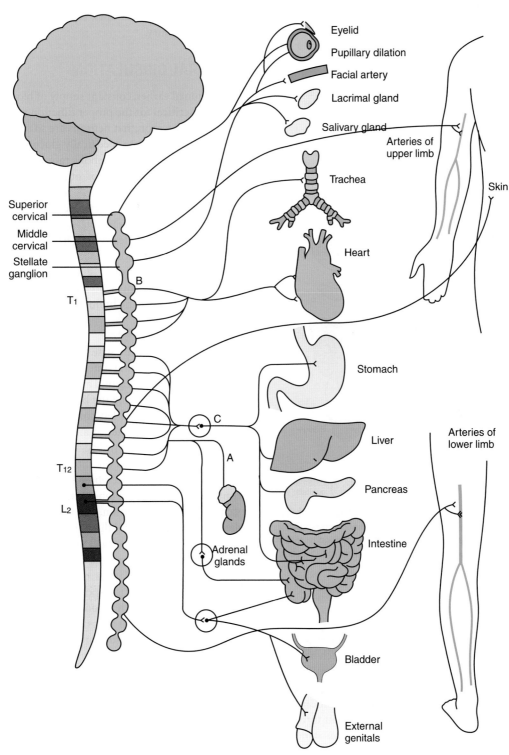

Fig. 2.25 Efferents from the spinal cord to sympathetic effector organs. **(A)** Direct, one-neuron connections to the adrenal medulla. **(B)** Two-neuron pathways to the periphery and thoracic viscera, with synapses in paravertebral ganglia. **(C)** Two-neuron pathways to the abdominal and pelvic organs, with synapses in outlying ganglia. Note that all sympathetic presynaptic neurons originate in the thoracic cord and the lumbar cord. (From Lundy-Ekman L: *Neuroscience: fundamentals for rehabilitation*, ed 4, St. Louis, 2013, Elsevier.)

internal carotid artery. When blood pressure drops, these pressure-sensitive afferents stimulate the sympathetic nervous system to increase blood pressure. When blood pressure increases, the parasympathetic nervous system is stimulated. A malfunctioning baroreflex leads to conditions such as postural hypotension, in which patients experience dramatic drops in blood pressure when standing, potentially leading to fainting and injury.

CEREBRAL CIRCULATION

As mentioned earlier, constant supply of blood to the brain is absolutely critical for the proper function and survival of our neurons. The reason that neurons are so sensitive to changes in blood flow (or more specifically glucose and oxygen flow) is because of their high metabolic rate. Even though the brain accounts for a mere ~2% of our body mass, it consumes ~25% of our glucose and ~20% of our oxygen (Erbsloh et al., 1958). Although a few seconds of disrupted blood flow can lead to lightheadedness, a few minutes of hypoxia can lead to neuron death and irreversible brain damage. Knowledge of cerebrovascular anatomy is the basis for understanding the clinical manifestations, diagnosis, and management of patients who have sustained cerebrovascular accidents and traumatic brain injuries.

Anterior Circulation

All arteries to the brain arise from the aortic arch. The first major arteries ascending anteriorly and laterally within the neck are the common carotid arteries. The carotid arteries are responsible for supplying the bulk of the cerebrum with circulation. The right and left common carotid arteries bifurcate just behind the posterior angle of the jaw to become the external and internal carotids. The external carotid arteries supply the face, whereas the internal carotids enter the cranium and supply the cerebral hemispheres, including the frontal lobe, the parietal lobe, and parts of the temporal and occipital lobes. In addition, the internal carotid artery supplies the optic nerves and the retina of the eyes. At the base of the brain, each of the internal carotids bifurcate into the right and left anterior and middle cerebral arteries. The middle cerebral artery is the largest of the cerebral arteries and is most often occluded. It is responsible for supplying the lateral surface of the brain with blood and also the deep portions of the frontal and parietal lobes. The anterior cerebral artery supplies the superior border of the frontal and parietal lobes. Both the middle cerebral artery and the anterior cerebral artery make up what is called the anterior circulation to the brain. Figs. 2.27 and 2.28 depict the cerebral circulation.

Posterior Circulation

The posterior circulation is composed of the two vertebral arteries, which are branches of the subclavian. The vertebral arteries supply blood to the brainstem and cerebellum. The vertebral arteries leave the base of the neck and ascend posteriorly to enter the skull through the foramen magnum. The two vertebral arteries supply the medulla and upper spinal

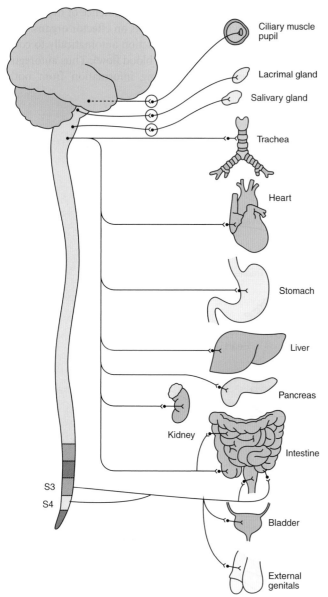

Fig. 2.26 Parasympathetic outflow through cranial nerves III, VII, IX, and X and S2–S4. Note that all parasympathetic preganglionic neurons originate in the brainstem or the sacral spinal cord. (From Lundy-Ekman L: *Neuroscience: fundamentals for rehabilitation,* ed 4, St. Louis, 2013, Elsevier.)

peripheral afferents with input from higher-level structures in the CNS. The region most closely associated with this control is the hypothalamus, which regulates functions such as feeding behaviors, digestion, heart rate, and respiration. Let us consider how the ANS controls blood flow based on peripheral and central input. Blood, like everything else on earth, is subject to gravitational pull and inertia. When you turn upside down, blood rushes to your head. When you stand up from a sitting position, blood is pulled out of your head to some degree. You may have felt light-headed when you "stood up too quickly" at some point in your life. The ANS prevents massive fluctuations in cerebral blood flow via the *baroreflex.* In the baroreflex, afferent neurons sense blood pressure in the

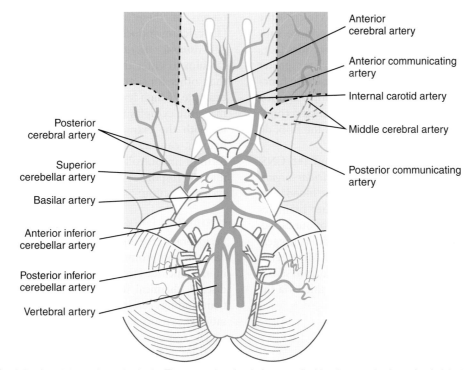

Fig. 2.27 Arterial supply to the brain. The posterior circulation supplied by the vertebral arteries is labeled on the left. The anterior circulation, supplied by the internal carotids, is labeled on the right. The watershed area, supplied by small anastomoses at the ends of the large cerebral arteries, is indicated by dotted lines. (From Lundy-Ekman L: *Neuroscience: fundamentals for rehabilitation*, ed 4, St. Louis, 2013, Elsevier.)

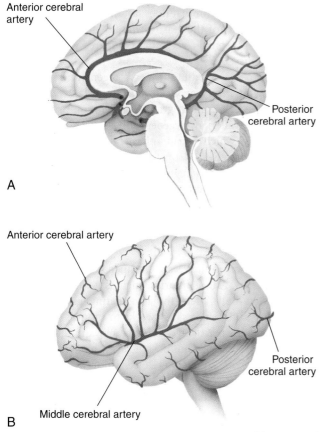

Fig. 2.28 Arterial supply to the medial **(A)** and lateral **(B)** portions of the cerebral hemispheres. (From Lundy-Ekman L: *Neuroscience: fundamentals for rehabilitation,* ed 2, St. Louis, 2002, Elsevier.)

cord and fuse to form the basilar artery. The basilar artery supplies the pons, cerebellum, and then divides into the right and left posterior cerebral arteries. The posterior cerebral artery connects to the carotid system via the posterior communicating artery. Both of these arteries supply the structures of the midbrain. The posterior cerebral artery then continues to supply the occipital and temporal lobes.

The anterior and posterior communicating arteries, which are branches of the carotid, are interconnected at the base of the brain and form the circle of Willis. This connection of blood vessels provides a protective mechanism to the structures within the brain. Because of the circle of Willis, failure or occlusion of one cerebral artery does not critically decrease blood flow to that region. Consequently, the occlusion can be circumvented or bypassed to meet the nutritional and metabolic needs of cerebral tissue.

Blood–Brain Barrier

Our blood contains a host of nutrients, metabolites, wastes, and toxins. Some of these are great for nerve cells (e.g., glucose and O_2). Others may be toxic to neurons (e.g., glutamate or pesticides from food). The entry of bloodborne substances into the CNS is restricted by the *blood–brain barrier* (BBB). The BBB is a collection of *tight junctions* and specific *transporter proteins* that control what is able to move from the blood into the nervous system. Tight junctions form a continuous intercellular barrier between neighboring cells that prevents diffusion between cells. Nonpolar substances, such as O_2 and CO_2 can freely cross the BBB. However, any water-soluble substances in the blood must rely on specific transporter proteins to cross the BBB. A variety of transporter proteins exist to move substance ranging from ions to glucose to entire peptides (e.g., insulin). Water-soluble substances without a transporter protein are unable to enter the CNS and affect neuron function. This explains why first-generation antihistamines, which can cross the BBB, make us drowsy, whereas second-generation antihistamines, which cannot cross the BBB, do not make us drowsy.

The BBB is not uniformly tight throughout the CNS. Certain areas of the CNS called *circumventricular organs* have a "leaky" BBB to allow them to sample the blood. Circumventricular organs communicate with other brain regions to adjust our behavior based on the state of our blood. For example, the area postrema, within the medulla, triggers vomiting when toxins are detected in the blood. More pertinent to our everyday lives, the subfornical organ senses blood osmolarity and triggers the sensation of thirst via the hypothalamus.

REACTION TO INJURY

What happens when the CNS or the PNS is injured? The CNS and the PNS are prone to different types of injury, and each system reacts differently. Within the CNS, artery obstruction causes cell and tissue death within minutes because of a lack of glucose and oxygen. Within about 2 minutes, neurons deplete their ATP stores, which prevents them from maintaining the negative charge across their membrane. This change in electrical activity leads to two key events: (1) the uncontrolled accumulation of calcium within the neuron, and (2) the uncontrolled release of neurotransmitters, particularly glutamate. Both of these events influence one another and can lead to neuron loss through a process called *excitotoxicity*.

Excitotoxicity

Briefly, excitotoxicity occurs when intracellular calcium levels rise sufficiently to create pores within mitochondrial membranes. These pores allow for the leakage of mitochondrial components into the cytoplasm, which initiate cell death through a process called *apoptosis*. Although a detailed discussion of apoptosis is beyond the scope of this book, you should appreciate that in apoptosis, the cell cuts itself up and degenerates in an orderly fashion. When neurons run out of ATP and lose their negative charge, calcium channels in the membrane open and allow calcium to rush into the neuron. Thus when an area of the brain is deprived of blood flow, the neurons accumulate calcium and die off via apoptosis.

Under typical circumstances, calcium is not toxic to neurons and plays an important role in neuron function. For example, calcium triggers the release of neurotransmitters. That means that when neurons run out of ATP and begin to accumulate intracellular calcium, they also release neurotransmitters uncontrollably. Excessive release of the excitatory neurotransmitter glutamate places the postsynaptic

targets of these neurons at risk by two mechanisms: (1) calcium-induced apoptosis as discussed earlier, and (2) *osmotic necrosis*. Many glutamate receptors allow calcium to enter the cell. Although calcium is more toxic than other ions, any ion can be toxic due to osmosis. For example, if high levels of sodium move into a neuron, they make the cytoplasm hyperosmotic. To reestablish isotonicity with the extracellular fluid, water will rush into the neuron, causing it to swell and eventually rupture. This form of uncontrolled cell death can then trigger an inflammatory response that can further compromise nervous system function.

Peripheral Nerve Injuries

Peripheral nerve injuries often result from means other than vascular compromise. Common causes of peripheral nerve injuries include stretching, laceration, compression, traction, disease, chemical toxicity, and nutritional deficiencies. Patient findings can include paresthesia (pins and needles sensations), sensory loss, and muscle weakness.

The response of a peripheral nerve to the injury is different from that in the CNS. The CNS is only permissive to axon regrowth during development. After birth, axon growth in the CNS is heavily restricted, likely as a means of preserving the intricate patterns of connectivity established during development. Axon growth in the CNS is restricted by the myelin produced by oligodendrocytes. Schwann cells produce a different type of myelin that does not hinder axon regrowth. This explains part of the reason why functional recovery is poor following a spinal cord injury compared with a peripheral nerve injury.

Schwann cells contribute to nerve regeneration in many ways. Following injury, axons degenerate distal to the site of injury—this is called anterograde degeneration or *Wallerian degeneration*. Wallerian degeneration is accomplished by Schwann cells, which recruit phagocytes and even act as phagocytes themselves to some degree (Fig. 2.29). Once the debris is cleared, axon regrowth is stimulated by trophic factors from Schwann cells. Axons crawl along Schwann cells to find their postsynaptic targets and restore function. This is a slow process, with axons growing only about 1 mm per day, depending on the size of the nerve fiber (Dvorak and Mansfield, 2013).

Peripheral nerve injuries are classified based on the severity of the injury. Minor injuries, such as gentle nerve compression, that only affect the myelinating glia are called *neurapraxia*. Recovery is slow (weeks to months) and complete owing to the regrowth of injured Schwann cells. Injuries that cause axon damage but do not sever the nerve itself are called *axonotmesis*. Recovery is slower (months to years) but still likely owing to the preserved axon sheath, which contains Schwann cells and guidance cues that help the axon regrow to its appropriate target. The most severe injuries are called *neurotmesis*, and they involve crushing or severing of the nerve. Functional recovery is the least likely in this case, as regenerating axons do not have a clear path back to their original targets.

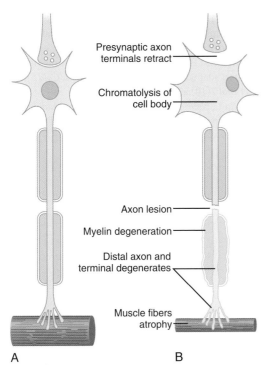

Fig. 2.29 Wallerian degeneration. **(A)** Normal synapses before an axon is severed. **(B)** Degeneration following severance of an axon. Degeneration following axonal injury involves several changes: (1) the axon terminal degenerates; (2) myelin breaks down and forms debris; and (3) the cell body undergoes metabolic changes. Subsequently, (4) presynaptic terminals retract from the dying cell body, and (5) postsynaptic cells degenerate. (From Lundy-Ekman L: *Neuroscience: fundamentals for rehabilitation*, ed 4, St. Louis, 2013, Elsevier.)

Labels in figure:
Presynaptic axon terminals retract
Chromatolysis of cell body
Axon lesion
Myelin degeneration
Distal axon and terminal degenerates
Muscle fibers atrophy
A   B

Neural Plasticity

For many years, it was thought that brain injuries were permanent and that there was little opportunity for repair. This viewpoint is no longer considered accurate as our understanding of *neural plasticity* has evolved. Neural plasticity is the brain's ability to adapt and for neurons "to alter their structure and function in response to a variety of internal and external pressures, including behavioral training" (Kleim and Jones, 2008). For example, areas of the cortex can modify the parts of the body with which they correspond. This has been widely studied using amputations, in which the removal of a limb or digit causes the cortical regions to respond to different neighboring body parts.

Neural plasticity occurs throughout our CNS through at least two distinct mechanisms, which we will mention briefly. First, changes in the strength of existing synaptic connections can modify neural networks and allow brain regions to become more or less responsive to other parts of the brain or body. This likely accounts for our associative learning. Second, the sprouting of new axons can allow neurons to create new connections with denervated body parts. This occurs more readily outside the CNS and appears to occur at the neuromuscular junction throughout aging as lower motor neurons die off. As clinicians, we must design treatment sessions that will maximize CNS recovery to provide our patients with the best functional outcome and quality of life possible. Examples of specific treatment interventions that potentially maximize neural plasticity will be presented throughout the rest of the book.

CHAPTER SUMMARY

An understanding of the structures and functions of the nervous system is necessary for physical therapists and physical therapist assistants. This knowledge assists practitioners in working with patients with neuromuscular dysfunction because it allows the therapist to have a better appreciation of the patient's pathologic condition, deficits, and potential capabilities. In addition, an understanding of neuroanatomy is helpful when educating patients and their families regarding the patient's condition and possible prognosis.

REVIEW QUESTIONS

1. Describe the major components of the nervous system.
2. What is the function of the white matter?
3. What are some of the primary functions of the parietal lobe?
4. What is Broca aphasia?
5. Discuss the primary function of the thalamus.
6. What is the primary function of the corticospinal tract?
7. What is an anterior horn cell? Where are these cells located?
8. Discuss the components of the PNS.
9. Where is the most common site of cerebral infarction?
10. What are some clinical signs of an upper motor neuron injury?

REFERENCES

Deutsch JE, O'Sullivan SB: Stroke. In O'Sullivan SB, Schmitz TJ, Fulk GD, editors: *Physical rehabilitation*, ed 7, Philadelphia, 2019, FA Davis, pp 592–661.

Dvorak L, Mansfield PJ: *Essentials of neuroanatomy for rehabilitation*, Boston, 2013, Pearson, pp 50–74, 141–143.

Erbsloh F, Bernsmeier A, Hillesheim H: The glucose consumption of the brain & its dependence on the liver, *Arch Psychiatr Nervenkr Z Gesamte Neurol Psychiatr* 196(6):611, 1958.

Fitzgerald MJT, Gruener G, Mtui E: *Clinical neuroanatomy and neuroscience*, St. Louis, 2012, Elsevier, pp 78, 97–110, 299.

Geschwind N, Levitsky W: Human brain: Left-right asymmetries in temporal speech regions, *Science* 161:186–187, 1968.

Gilman S, Newman SW: *Manter and Gatz's essentials of clinical neuroanatomy and neurophysiology*, ed 10, Philadelphia, 2003, FA Davis, pp 1–11, 61–63, 147–154, 190–203.

Guyton AC: *Basic neuroscience: anatomy and physiology*, ed 2, Philadelphia, 1991, WB Saunders, pp 1–24, 39–54, 244–245.

Halassa MM, Fellin T, Haydon PG: The tripartite synapse: roles for gliotransmission in health and disease, *Trends Mol Med* 13(2):54–63, 2007.

Kleim JA, Jones TA: Principles of experience-dependent neural plasticity: implications for rehabilitation after brain damage, *J Speech Lang Hear Res* 51:S225–S239, 2008.

Ko CP, Robitaille R: Perisynaptic Schwann cells at the neuromuscular synapse: adaptable, multitasking glial cells, *Cold Spring Harb Perspect Biol* 7(10):a020503, 2015.

Lundy-Ekman L: *Neuroscience: fundamentals for rehabilitation*, ed 5, St. Louis, 2018, Elsevier, pp 121–136, 170–184, 503.

Motor Control and Motor Learning

OBJECTIVES

After reading this chapter, the student will be able to:

1. Define motor development, motor control, motor learning, and neural plasticity.
2. Understand the relationship among motor control, motor learning, and motor development.
3. Differentiate models of motor control and motor learning.
4. Understand the development of postural control and balance.
5. Discuss the role of experience and feedback in motor control and motor learning.
6. Relate motor control, motor learning, and neural plasticity principles to therapeutic intervention.

INTRODUCTION

Motor abilities and skills are acquired during the process of motor development through motor control and motor learning. Once a basic pattern of movement is established, it can be varied to suit the purpose of the task or the environmental situation in which the task takes place. Early motor development displays a fairly predictable sequence of skill acquisition through childhood. However, the ways in which these motor abilities are used functionally are highly variable. Individuals rarely perform a movement exactly the same way every time. Variability must be part of any model used to explain how posture and movement are controlled.

Any movement system must be able to adapt to the changing demands of the individual mover and the environment in which the movement takes place. The individual mover must be able to learn from prior movement experiences. Different theories of motor control emphasize different developmental aspects of posture and movement. Development of postural control and balance is embedded in the development of motor control. Understanding the relationship among motor control, motor learning, and motor development provides a valuable framework to understand the treatment of individuals with neurologic dysfunction at any age.

Motor development is a product as well as a process. The products of motor development are the skills of the developmental sequence and the kinesiologic components of movement, such as head and trunk control, necessary for these motor abilities. These products are discussed in Chapter 4. The process of motor development is the way in which those abilities emerge. The process and the product are affected by many factors, such as time (age), maturation (genes), adaptation (physical constraints), and learning. Motor development is the result of the interaction of the innate or built-in species blueprint for posture and movement and the person's experiences with movement afforded by the environment. Sensory input is needed for the mover to learn about moving and the results of moving. Sensory input contributes to perceptual development because perception is the act of attaching meaning to sensation. Motor development is the combination of the nature of the mover and the nurture of the environment. Part of the genetic blueprint for movement is the means to control posture and movement. Motor development, motor control, and motor learning contribute to an ongoing process of change throughout the lifespan of every person who moves.

MOTOR CONTROL

Motor control, the ability to maintain and change posture and movement, is the result of a complex set of neurologic and mechanical processes. Those processes include motor, cognitive, and perceptual development. Motor control begins with the control of self-generated movements and proceeds to the control of movements in relationship to changing demands of the task and the environment. Control of self-movement largely results from the development of the neuromotor systems. As the nervous and muscular systems mature, movement emerges. The perceptual consequences of self-generated movements drive motor development (Anderson et al., 2014). Motor control allows the nervous system to direct what muscles should be used, in what order, and how quickly, to solve a movement problem. The infant's first movement problem relates to overcoming the effects of gravity. A second, but related, problem is how to move a larger head as compared with a smaller body to establish head control. Later, movement problems are related to controlling the interaction between stability and mobility of the head, trunk, and limbs. Control of task-specific movements, such as stringing beads or riding a tricycle, depends on cognitive and perceptual abilities. The task to be carried out by the person within the environment dictates the type of movement solution that will be needed.

Because the motor abilities of a person change over time, the motor solutions to a given motor problem may also change. The

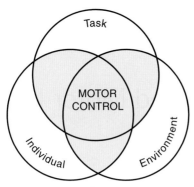

Fig. 3.1 Movement emerges from an interaction between the individual, the task, and the environment. (From Shumway-Cook A, Woollacott MH: *Motor control: theory and practical applications*, ed 4, Baltimore, 2012, Williams & Wilkins.)

individual's motivation to move may also change over time and may affect the intricacy of the movement solution. An infant encountering a set of stairs sees a toy on the top stair. She creeps up the stairs but then has to figure out how to get down. She can cry for help, bump down on her buttocks, creep down backward, or even attempt creeping down forward. A toddler faced with the same dilemma may walk up the same set of stairs one step at a time holding onto a railing, and descend sitting holding the toy, or may be holding the toy with one hand and the railing with the other and descend the same way she came up the stairs. An older child will walk up and down without holding on, and an even older child may run up those same stairs. The relationship among the task, the individual, and the environment is depicted graphically in Fig. 3.1. All three components must be considered when thinking about motor control.

Motor Control Time Frame

Motor control happens not in the space of days or weeks, as is seen in motor development, but in fractions of seconds. Fig. 3.2 illustrates a comparison of time frames

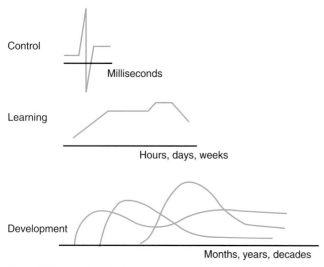

Fig. 3.2 Time scales of interest from a motor control, motor learning, and motor development perspective. (From Cech D, Martin S, editors: *Functional movement development across the life span*, ed 3, St. Louis, 2012, Elsevier.)

associated with motor control, motor learning, and motor development. Motor control occurs because of physiologic processes that happen at cellular, tissue, and organ levels. Physiologic processes have to happen quickly to produce timely and efficient movement. What good does it do if you extend an outstretched arm after falling down? Extending your arm in a protective response has to be quick enough to be useful, that is, to break the fall. People with neurologic dysfunction may exhibit the correct movement pattern, but they have impaired timing, producing the movement too slowly to be functional, or they have impaired sequencing of muscle activation, producing a muscle contraction at the wrong time. Both of these problems, impaired timing and impaired sequencing, are examples of deficits in motor control.

Role of Sensation in Motor Control

Sensory information plays an important role in motor control. Initially, sensation cues reflexive movements in which few cognitive or perceptual abilities are needed. A sensory stimulus produces a reflexive motor response. Touching the lip of a newborn produces head turning, whereas stroking a newborn's outstretched leg produces withdrawal. Sensation is an ever-present cue for motor behavior in the seemingly reflex-dominated infant. As voluntary movement emerges during motor development, sensation provides feedback accuracy for hand placement during reaching and later for creeping. Sensation from weight bearing reinforces maintenance of developmental postures, such as the prone on elbows position and the hands and knees position. Sensory information is crucial to the mover when interacting with objects and maneuvering within an environment. Fig. 3.3 depicts how sensation provides the necessary feedback for the body to know whether a task, such as reaching or walking, was performed and how well it was accomplished. Sensory experience contributes to development of postural control and motor skill acquisition.

Role of Feedback

Feedback is a very crucial feature of motor control. *Feedback* is defined as sensory or perceptual information received as a result of movement. There is intrinsic feedback, or feedback produced by the movement. Sensory feedback can be used to detect errors in movement. Feedback and error signals are important for two reasons. First, feedback provides a means to understand the process of self-control. Reflexes are initiated and controlled by sensory stimuli from the environment surrounding the individual. Motor behavior generated from feedback is initiated as a result of an error signal produced by a process within the individual. The highest level of many motor hierarchies is a volitional, or self-control function, but there has been very little explanation of how it works.

Second, feedback also provides the fundamental process for learning new motor skills. Intrinsic feedback comes from any sensory source inside the body, such as from proprioceptors, or outside the body when the person sees that the target was not hit or the ball was hit out of bounds

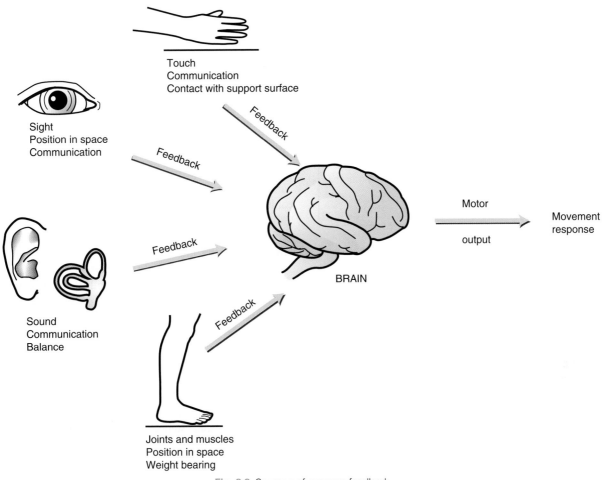

Fig. 3.3 Sources of sensory feedback.

(Schmidt and Wrisberg, 2013). Extrinsic feedback is extra or augmented sensory information given to the mover by some external source (Schmidt and Wrisberg, 2013). A therapist or coach may provide enhanced feedback on the person's motor performance. For this reason, feedback is a common element in motor control and motor learning theories.

Theories of Motor Control

Early theories of motor control were first presented in the 1800 with Sherrington and others proposing a reflex/hierarchical model to explain the production of movement. This model was based on varying levels of the nervous system being responsible for development of postural control and balance. A relationship exists between the maturation of the developing brain and the emergence of motor behaviors seen in infancy. One of the ways in which nervous system maturation has been routinely gauged is by the assessment of reflexes. The reflex is seen as the basic unit of movement in this motor control model. A reflex is the pairing of a sensory stimulus with a motor response, as shown in Fig. 3.4. Some reflexes are simple and others are complex. An example of a simple infantile reflex is the flexor withdrawal. A touch or noxious stimulus applied to the bottom of the foot produces lower extremity withdrawal. These reflexes are also referred to as primitive reflexes because

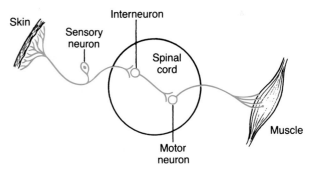

Fig. 3.4 Three-neuron nervous system. (Redrawn from Romero-Sierra C: *Neuroanatomy: a conceptual approach*, New York, 1986, Churchill Livingstone.)

they occur early in the lifespan of the infant, not because they are not sophisticated. Another example is the palmar grasp. Primitive reflexes are listed in Table 3.1.

Tonic reflexes are associated with the brain stem of the central nervous system. These reflexes produce changes in muscle tone and posture. Examples of tonic reflexes exhibited by infants are the tonic labyrinthine reflex and the asymmetric tonic neck reflex. In the latter, when the infant's head is turned to the right, the infant's right arm extends and the left

TABLE 3.1	Primitive Reflexes	
Reflex	**Age at Onset**	**Integration**
Suck-swallow	28 weeks' gestation	2–5 months
Rooting	28 weeks' gestation	3 months
Flexor withdrawal	28 weeks' gestation	1–2 months
Crossed extension	28 weeks' gestation	1–2 months
Moro	28 weeks' gestation	4–6 months
Plantar grasp	28 weeks' gestation	9 months
Positive support	35 weeks' gestation	1–2 months
Asymmetric tonic neck	Birth	4–6 months
Palmar grasp	Birth	9 months
Symmetric tonic neck	4–6 months	8–12 months

From Cech D, Martin S, editors: *Functional movement development across the life span*, ed 3, St. Louis, 2012, Elsevier, p. 54.

arm flexes. The tonic labyrinthine reflex produces increased extensor tone when the infant is supine and increased flexor tone in the prone position. In this model, most infantile reflexes (sucking and rooting) and tonic reflexes are integrated by 4 to 6 months. Exceptions do exist. Integration is the mechanism by which less mature responses are incorporated into voluntary movement.

Nervous system maturation is seen as the ultimate determinant of the acquisition of postural control in the reflex/hierarchical model. Righting reactions utilize sensory information to orient the head in space and the body relative to the head and the support surface. Equilibrium reactions are complex postural responses that respond to slow balance disturbances. They continue to be present even in adulthood. These reactive postural responses involve the head and trunk and provide the body with an automatic way to respond to movement of the center of gravity within and outside the body's base of support. Extremity movements in response to quick displacements of the center of gravity out of the base of support are called protective reactions. These are also considered postural reactions and serve as a back-up system should the righting or equilibrium reaction fail to compensate for a loss of balance. A more complete description of these reactive postural responses is given as part of the development of postural control from a hierarchical perspective.

Development of Motor Control

Development of motor control can be described by the relationship of mobility and stability of body postures (Sullivan et al., 1982) and by the acquisition of automatic postural responses (Cech and Martin, 2012). Initial random movements (mobility) are followed by maintenance of a posture (stability), movement within a posture (controlled mobility), and finally, movement from one posture to another posture (skill). The sequence of acquiring motor control is seen in key developmental postures in Fig. 3.5. With acquisition of each new posture comes the development of control within that posture. For example, weight shifting in the prone position precedes rolling from prone to supine; rocking on hands and knees precedes creeping; and cruising, or lateral weight shifting in standing, precedes walking. The actual motor accomplishments of rolling, reaching, creeping, cruising, and walking are skills in which mobility is combined with stability, and the distal parts of the body (i.e., the extremities) are free to move. The infant develops motor and postural control in the following order: mobility, stability, controlled mobility, and skill.

Stages of Motor Control

Stage one. Stage one is mobility, when movement is initiated. The infant exhibits random movements within an available range of motion for the first 3 months of development. Movements during this stage are erratic. They lack purpose and are often reflex-based. Random limb movements are made when the infant's head and trunk are supported in the supine position. Mobility is present before stability. In adults, mobility refers to the availability of range of motion to assume a posture and the presence of sufficient motor unit activity to initiate a movement.

Stage two. Stage two is stability, the ability to maintain a steady position in a weight-bearing, antigravity posture. It is also called static postural control. Developmentally, stability is further divided into tonic holding and co-contraction. Tonic holding occurs at the end of the shortened range of movement and usually involves isometric movements of antigravity postural extensors (Stengel et al., 1984). Tonic holding is most evident when the child maintains the pivot prone position (prone extension), as seen in Fig. 3.5. Postural holding of the head begins asymmetrically in prone, followed by holding the head in midline, and progresses to holding the head up past 90 degrees from the support surface. In the supine position, the head is turned to one side or the other; then it is held in midline; and finally, it is held in midline with a chin tuck while the infant is being pulled to sit at 4 months (Fig. 3.6).

Co-contraction is the simultaneous static contraction of antagonistic muscles around a joint to provide stability in a midline position or in weight bearing. Various groups of muscles, especially those used for postural fixation, allow the developing infant to hold such postures as prone extension, prone on elbows and hands, all fours, and a semisquat. Co-contraction patterns are shown in Fig. 3.5. Once the initial relationship between mobility and stability is established in prone and later in all fours and standing, a change occurs to allow mobility to be superimposed on the already established stability.

Stage three. Controlled mobility is mobility superimposed on previously developed postural stability by moving within a posture. Proximal mobility is combined with distal stability. This controlled mobility, the third stage of motor control, occurs when the limbs are weight bearing and the body moves such as in weight shifting on all fours or in standing. The trunk performs controlled mobility when it is parallel to the support surface or when the line of gravity is perpendicular to the trunk. In prone and all-fours positions, the limbs and the trunk are performing controlled mobility when shifting weight.

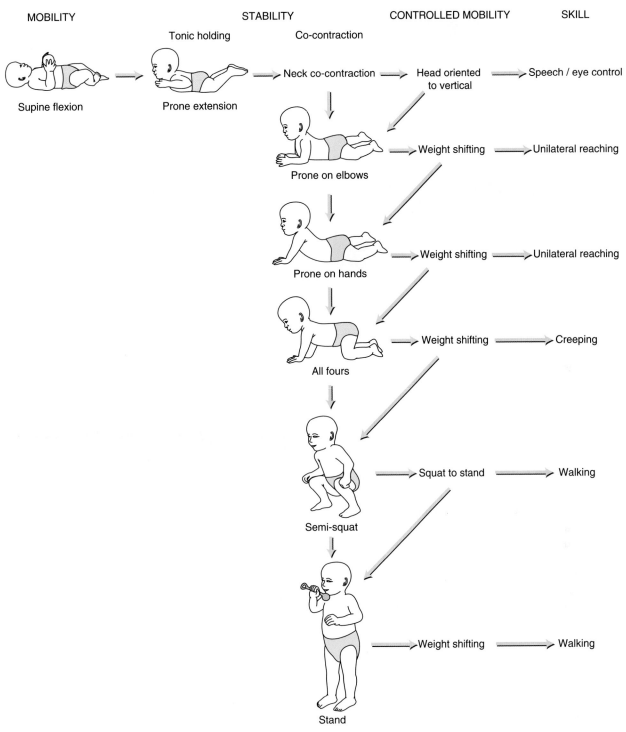

Fig. 3.5 Key postures and sequence of development.

The infant's first attempts at weight shifts in the prone position happen accidentally with little control. As the infant tries to reproduce the movement and practices various movement combinations, the movement becomes more controlled. Another example of controlled mobility is demonstrated by an infant in a prone on-elbows position who sees a toy. If the infant attempts to reach for the toy with both hands, which she typically does before reaching with one hand, the infant is likely to fall on her face. If she perseveres and learns to shift weight onto one elbow, she has a better chance of obtaining the toy. Weight bearing, weight shifting, and co-contraction of muscles around the shoulder are crucial to the development of shoulder girdle stability. Proximal shoulder stability supports upper extremity function for skilled distal manipulation. If this stability is not present, distal performance may be impaired. Controlled mobility is also referred to as dynamic postural control.

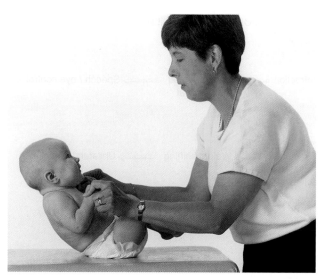

Fig. 3.6 Chin tuck when pulled to sit.

Stage four. Skill, the most mature type of movement, is usually mastered after controlled mobility within a posture. For example, after weight shifting within a posture, such as in a hands-and-knees position, the infant frees the opposite arm and leg to creep reciprocally. Creeping is a skilled movement. Other skill patterns are also depicted in Fig. 3.5. Skill patterns of movement occur when mobility is superimposed on stability in non–weight bearing; proximal segments stabilize while distal segments are free for movement. The trunk does skilled work when it is upright or parallel to the force of gravity. In standing, only the lower extremities are using controlled mobility when weight shifting occurs. If the swing leg moves, it performs skilled work while the stance limb performs controlled mobility. When an infant creeps or walks, the limbs that are in motion are using skill, and those in contact with the support surface are using controlled mobility. Creeping and walking are considered skilled movements. Skilled movements involve manipulation and exploration of the environment.

Development of Reactive Postural Control

Postural control develops in a cephalocaudal direction in keeping with Gesell's developmental principles, which are discussed in Chapter 4. Postural control is demonstrated by the ability to maintain the alignment of the body—specifically, the alignment of body parts relative to each other and the external environment. The infant learns to use a group of automatic postural responses to attain and maintain an upright erect posture. These postural responses are continuously used when balance is lost in an effort to regain equilibrium.

The sequence of development of postural reactions entails righting reactions, followed by protective reactions, and then equilibrium reactions. In the infant, head righting reactions develop first and are followed by the development of trunk righting reactions. Protective reactions of the extremities emerge next in an effort to safeguard balance in higher postures, such as sitting. Finally, equilibrium reactions develop in all postures, beginning in prone. Traditionally, posture and movement develop together in a cephalocaudal direction, so balance is achieved in different positions relative to gravity. Head control is followed by trunk control; control of the head on the body and in space comes before sitting and standing balance.

Righting reactions. Righting reactions are responsible for orienting the head in space and keeping the eyes and mouth horizontal. This normal alignment is maintained in an upright vertical position and when the body is tilted or rotated. Righting reactions involve head-and-trunk movements to maintain or regain orientation or alignment. Some righting reactions begin at birth, but most are evident between 4 and 6 months of age, as listed in Table 3.2. Gravity and change of head or body position provide cues for the most frequently used righting reactions. Vision cues an optical righting reaction, gravity cues the labyrinthine righting reaction, and touch of the support surface to the abdomen cues the body-on-the-head reaction. These three head-righting reactions assist the infant in developing head control.

Head turning can produce neck-on-body righting, in which the body follows the head movement. If either the upper or lower trunk is turned, a body-on-body righting reaction is elicited. Either neck-on-body righting or body-on-body righting can produce log rolling or segmental rolling.

TABLE 3.2 **Righting and Equilibrium Reactions**		
Reaction	**Age at Onset**	**Integration**
Head righting		
Neck (immature)	34 weeks' gestation	4–6 months
Labyrinthine	Birth–2 months	Persists
Optical	Birth–2 months	Persists
Neck (mature)	4–6 months	5 years
Trunk righting		
Body (immature)	34 weeks' gestation	4–6 months
Body (mature)	4–6 months	5 years
Landau	3–4 months	1–2 years
Protective		
Downward lower extremity	4 months	Persists
Forward upper extremity	6–7 months	Persists
Sideways upper extremity	7–8 months	Persists
Backward upper extremity	9 months	Persists
Stepping lower extremity	15–17 months	Persists
Equilibrium		
Prone	6 months	Persists
Supine	7–8 months	Persists
Sitting	7–8 months	Persists
Quadruped	9–12 months	Persists
Standing	12–24 months	Persists

From Cech D, Martin S, editors: *Functional movement development across the life span*, ed 3, St. Louis, 2012, Elsevier, p. 269.

Log rolling is the immature righting response seen in the first 3 months of life; the mature response emerges around 4 months of age. The purpose of righting reactions is to maintain the correct orientation of the head and body in relation to the ground. Head and trunk righting reactions occur when weight is shifted within a base of support; the amount of displacement determines the degree of response. For example, in the prone position, slow weight shifting to the right produces a lateral bend or righting of the head and trunk to the left. If the displacement is too fast, a different type of response may be seen—a protective response. Slower displacements are more likely to elicit head and trunk righting. These can occur in any posture and in response to anterior, posterior, or lateral weight shifts.

Righting reactions have their maximal influence on posture and movement between 10 and 12 months of age, although they are said to continue to be present until the child is 5 years old. Righting reactions are no longer considered to be present if the child can come to standing from a supine position without using trunk rotation. The presence of trunk rotation indicates a righting of the body around the long axis. Another explanation for the change in motor behavior could be that the child of 5 years has sufficient abdominal strength to perform the sagittal plane movement of rising straight forward and attaining standing without using trunk rotation.

Protective reactions. Protective reactions are extremity movements that occur in response to rapid displacement of the body by diagonal or horizontal forces. They have a predictable but invariant developmental sequence, which can be found in Table 3.2. By extending one or both extremities, the individual prepares for a fall or prepares to catch herself. A 4-month-old infant's lower extremities extend and abduct when the infant is held upright in vertical and quickly lowered toward the supporting surface. At 6 months, the upper extremities show forward protective extension, followed by sideways and backward extension. Protective stepping in the lower extremities is evident around 3 months of walking experience (Roncesvalles et al., 2000). Protective reactions of the upper extremities should not be confused with the ability of the infant to prop on extended arms, a movement that can be self-initiated by pushing up from prone or by being placed in the position by a caregiver. Because an infant must be able to bear weight on extended arms to exhibit protective extension, training an infant to prop on extended arms or to push up from prone can be useful treatment intervention.

Equilibrium reactions. Equilibrium reactions, the most advanced postural reactions, are the last to develop. These reactions allow the body as a whole to adapt to slow changes in the relationship of the center of mass with the base of support. By incorporating the already learned head-and-trunk righting reactions, the equilibrium reactions add extremity responses to flexion, extension, or lateral head-and-trunk movements to regain equilibrium. In lateral weight shifts, the trunk may rotate in the opposite direction of the weight shift to further attempt to maintain the body's center of mass within the base of support. The trunk rotation is evident only during lateral displacements. Equilibrium reactions can occur if the body moves relative to the support surface, as in leaning sideways, or if the support surface moves, as when one is on a tilt board. In the latter case, these movements are called tilt reactions. The three expected responses to a lateral displacement of the center of mass toward the periphery of the base of support in standing are as follows: (1) lateral head and trunk righting occurs away from the weight shift; (2) the arm and leg are opposite the direction of the weight shift abduct; and (3) trunk rotation away from the weight shift may occur. If the last response does not happen, the other two responses can provide only a brief postponement of the inevitable fall. At the point at which the center of gravity leaves the base of support, protective extension of the arms may occur, or a protective step or stagger may reestablish a stable base. Thus, the order in which the reactions are acquired developmentally differs from the order in which they are used for balance.

Equilibrium reactions also have a set developmental sequence and timetable (see Table 3.2). Because prone is a position from which to learn to move against gravity, equilibrium reactions are typically seen first in prone, then supine, sitting, all fours, and last in standing. The infant is always working on more than one postural level at a time so equilibrium reactions in a lower posture mature after the infant has acquired the ability to move in a higher posture. For example, sitting equilibrium matures after the infant is creeping.

Motor Program Model of Motor Control

Motor program theory was developed to directly challenge the notion that all movements are generated through chaining or reflexes because even slow movements occur too fast for sensory input to influence them (Gordon, 1987). The implication is that for efficient movement to occur in a timely manner, an internal representation of movement actions must be available to the mover. "Motor programs are associated with a set of muscle commands specified at the time of action production, which do not require sensory input" (Wing et al., 1996). Schmidt (1988) expanded motor program theory to include the notion of a generalized motor program or an abstract *neural representation* of an action, distributed among different systems. Being able to mentally represent an action is part of developing motor control (Gabbard, 2009).

The term motor program may also refer to a specific neural circuit called a central pattern generator (CPG), which is capable of producing a motor pattern, such as walking. CPGs exist in the human spinal cord. Stepping pattern generators (SPGs) are located in each leg that controls stepping movements at the hip and the knee (Yang et al., 2005). Postural control of the head and trunk and voluntary control of the ankle are also required for walking. Sensory feedback adjusts timing and reinforces muscle activation (Knikou, 2010).

Systems Models of Motor Control

A systems model of motor control is currently used to describe the relationship of various brain and spinal centers working together to control posture and movement. In a systems model, the neural control of posture and movement is *distributed*, that is, which areas of the nervous system that control posture or movement depend on the complexity of the task to be performed. Because the nervous system has the ability to self-organize, it is feasible that several parts of the nervous system are engaged in resolving movement problems; therefore, solutions are typically unique to the context and goal of the task at hand (Thelen, 1995). The advantage of a systems model is that it can account for the flexibility and adaptability of motor behavior in a variety of environmental conditions.

A second characteristic of a systems model is that body systems other than the nervous system are involved in the control of movement. The most obvious other system to be involved is the musculoskeletal system. The body is a mechanical system. Muscles have viscoelastic properties. Physiologic maturation occurs in all body systems involved in movement production: muscular, skeletal, nervous, cardiovascular, and pulmonary. For example, if the contractile properties of muscle are not mature, certain types of movements may not be possible. If muscular strength of the legs is not sufficient, ambulation may be delayed. Muscle strength, posture, and perceptual abilities exhibit developmental trajectories, which can affect the rate of motor development by affecting the process of motor control.

Feedback is a third fundamental characteristic of the systems models of motor control. To control movements, the individual needs to know whether the movement has been successful. In a closed-loop model of motor control, sensory information is used as feedback to the nervous system to provide assistance with the next action. A person engages in closed-loop feedback when playing a video game that requires guiding a figure across the screen. This type of feedback provides self-control of movement. A loop is formed from the sensory information that is generated as part of the movement and is fed back to the brain. This sensory information influences future motor actions. Errors that can be corrected with practice are detected, and performance can be improved. This type of feedback is shown in Fig. 3.7.

By contrast, in an open-loop model of motor control, movement is cued either by a central structure, such as a motor program, or by sensory information from the periphery. The movement is performed without feedback. When a baseball pitcher throws a favorite pitch, the movement is too quick to allow feedback. Errors are detected after the fact. An example of action spurred by external sensory information is what happens when a fire alarm sounds. The person hears the alarm and moves before thinking about moving. This type of feedback model is also depicted in Fig. 3.7 and is thought to be the way in which fast movements are controlled. Another

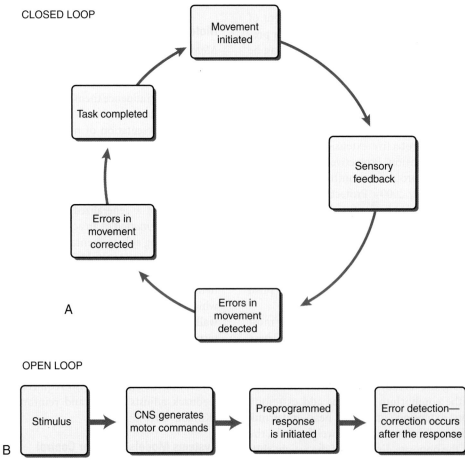

Fig. 3.7 (A, B) Models of feedback. (Redrawn from Montgomery, PC, Connolly BH: *Motor control and physical therapy: theoretical framework and practical application*, Hixson, 1991, Chattanooga Group.)

way to think of the difference between closed-loop and open-loop motor controls can be exemplified by someone who learns to play a piano piece. The piece is played slowly while the student is learning and receiving feedback, but once it is learned, the student can sit down and play it through quickly, from beginning to end.

Components of the postural control system. In the systems models, both posture and movement are considered systems that represent the interaction of other biologic and mechanical systems and movement components. The relationship between posture and movement is also called postural control. As such, posture implies a readiness to move, an ability not only to react to threats to balance but also to anticipate postural needs to support a motor plan. A motor plan or program is a plan to move, usually stored in memory. Seven components have been identified as part of a postural control system, as depicted in Fig. 3.8. These are limits of stability, sensory organization, eye-head stabilization, the musculoskeletal system, motor coordination, predictive central set, and environmental adaptation. Postural control like motor control is a complex and ongoing process.

Limits of stability. Limits of stability are the boundaries of the base of support (BOS) of any given posture. As long as the center of mass (COM) is within the base of support, the person is stable. An infant's BOS is constantly changing relative to the body's size and amount of contact the body has with the supporting surface. Supine and prone are more stable postures by virtue of having so much of the body in contact with the support surface. However, in sitting or standing, the size of the BOS depends on the position of the lower extremities and on whether the upper extremities are in contact with the supporting surface. In standing, the area in which the person can move within the limits of stability or base of support is called the cone of stability, as shown in Fig. 3.9. The central nervous system perceives the body's limits of stability through various sensory cues.

Keeping the body's COM within the BOS constitutes balance. During quiet stance, as the body sways, the limits of stability depend on the interaction of the position and velocity of movement of the COM. We are more likely to lose

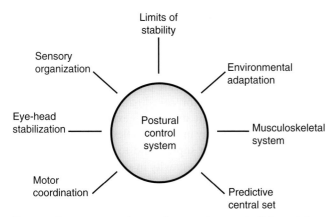

Fig. 3.8 Components of normal postural control. (Adapted from [http://www.apta.org], with permission of the American Physical Therapy Association. © 2019 American Physical Therapy Association. All rights reserved.)

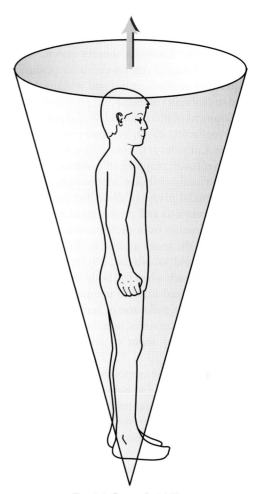

Fig. 3.9 Cone of stability.

balance if the velocity of the COM is high and at the limits of the BOS. The body perceives changes in the COM in a posture by detecting amplitude of center of pressure (COP) motion. The COP is the point of application of the ground reaction force. In standing, there would be a COP under each foot. You can feel how the COP changes as you shift weight forward and back while standing.

Sensory organization. The visual, vestibular, and somatosensory systems provide the body with information about movement and cue postural responses. Maturation of the sensory systems and their relative contribution to balance have been extensively studied with some conflicting findings. Some of these conflicts may be related to the way balance is studied, whether static or dynamic balance is assessed, and to the maturation of sensorimotor control. Regardless of these differences, sensory input appears to be needed for the development of postural control.

Vision is very important for the development of head control. Newborns are sensitive to the flow of visual information and can even make postural adjustments in response to this information (Jouen et al., 2000). Input from the visual system is mapped to neck movement initially and then to trunk movement as head and trunk control is established. The production of spatial maps of the position of various body parts appears to be linked to muscular action. The linking of posture at the neck to vision occurs before somatosensation is mapped to neck muscles (Shumway-Cook and Woollacott, 2017). Vision is the dominant sensory system for the first 3 years of life and infants rely on vision for postural control in the acquisition of head control and walking. Visual input is also used to calibrate vestibular and proprioceptive systems in the development of internal models of posture (Shumway-Cook and Woollacott, 2017). Vestibular information is also mapped to neck muscles at the same time as somatosensation is mapped. Eventually, mapping of combinations of sensory input, such as visual-vestibular information, is done (Jouen, 1984). This bimodal mapping allows for comparisons to be made between previous and present postures. The mapping of sensory information from each individual sense proceeds from the neck to the trunk and on to the lower extremities (Shumway-Cook and Woollacott, 2017). Information from vision acts as feedback when the body moves and as an anticipatory cue in a feed-forward manner before movement. As the child learns to make use of somatosensory information from the lower extremities, somatosensory input emerges as the primary sensory input on which postural response decisions are made.

Somatosensation is the combined input from touch and proprioception. Adults use somatosensation as their primary source for making a postural response. When there is a sensory conflict, the vestibular system acts as a tiebreaker in making the postural response decision. If somatosensation says you are moving and vision says you are not, the vestibular input should be able to resolve the conflict to maintain balance. However, vestibular function relative to standing postural control does not reach adult levels even at the age of 15 according to Hirabayashi and Iwasaki (1995).

Eye-head stabilization. The head carries two of the most influential sensory receptors for posture and balance: the eyes and labyrinths. These two sensory systems provide ongoing sensory input about the movement of the surroundings and head, respectively. The eyes and labyrinths provide orientation of the head in space. The eyes must be able to maintain a stable visual image even when the head is moving, and the eyes have to be able to move with the head as the body moves. The labyrinths relay information about head movement to ocular nuclei and about position, allowing the mover to differentiate between *egocentric* (head relative to the body) and *allocentric* (head relative to objects in the environment) motion. Lateral flexion of the head is an egocentric motion. The movement of the head in space while walking or riding in an elevator is an example of exocentric motion.

The head stabilization in space strategy (HSSS) involves an anticipatory stabilization of the head in space before body movement. A child first displays this strategy at 3 years of age while walking on level ground (Assaiante and Amblard, 1993). By maintaining the angular position of the head with regard to the spatial environment, vestibular inputs can be better interpreted. The HSSS matures between the ages of 7 and 8 years (Assaiante and Amblard, 1995; Assaiante, 1998). Anticipatory control of the head during locomotion is a steering process whereby the gaze leads the locomotor trajectory or walking path (Belmonti et al, 2016). This anticipatory control matures in early adolescence (Belmonti et al, 2013). Head orientation in adults is used to anticipate walking direction and orientation of lower body segments (Grasso et al., 1996). Older adults have been shown to adopt the HSS strategy when faced with distorted or incongruent somatosensory and visual information (DiFabio and Emasithi, 1997).

Musculoskeletal system. The body is a mechanically linked structure that supports posture and provides a postural response. The viscoelastic properties of the muscles, joints, tendons, and ligaments can act as inherent constraints to posture and movement. The flexibility of body segments, such as the neck, thorax, pelvis, hip, knee, and ankle, contributes to attaining and maintaining a posture or making a postural response. Each body segment has mass and grows at a different rate. Each way in which a joint can move represents a degree of freedom. Because the body has so many individual joints and muscles with many possible ways in which to move, certain muscles work together synergistically to control the degrees of freedom.

Normal muscle tone is needed to sustain a posture and to support normal movement. Muscle tone has been defined as the resting tension in the muscle (Lundy-Ekman, 2018) and the stiffness in the muscle as it resists being lengthened (Basmajian and DeLuca, 1985). Muscle tone is determined by assessing the resistance felt during passive movement of a limb. Resistance is caused mainly by the viscoelastic properties of the muscle. On activating the stretch reflex, the muscle proprioceptors, the muscle spindles, and Golgi tendon organs contribute to muscle tone or stiffness. The background level of activity in antigravity muscles during stance is described as postural tone by Shumway-Cook and Woollacott (2017). Others also describe patterns of muscular tension in groups of muscles as postural tone. Together, the viscoelastic properties of muscle, the spindles, Golgi tendon organs, and descending motor tracts regulate muscle tone.

Motor coordination. *Motor coordination* is the ability to coordinate muscle activation in a sequence that preserves posture. The use of muscle synergies in postural reactions and sway strategies in standing are examples of this coordination and are described in the upcoming section on neural control. Determination of the muscles to be used in a synergy is based on the task to be done and the environment in which the task takes place.

Strength and muscle tone are prerequisites for movement against gravity and motor coordination. Head-and-trunk control require sufficient strength to extend the head, neck, and trunk against gravity in prone; to flex the head, neck, and trunk against gravity in supine; and to flex the head, neck, and trunk laterally against gravity in side-lying.

Predictive central set. Predictive central set is that component of postural control that can best be described as postural readiness. Sensation and cognition are used as anticipatory cues before movement as a means of establishing a state of postural readiness. This readiness or postural set must be present to support movement. Think of how difficult it is to move in the morning when waking up; the body is not posturally ready to move. Contrast this state of postural unpreparedness with an Olympic competitor who is so focused on the motor task at hand that every muscle has been put on alert, ready to act at a moment's notice. Predictive central set is critical to postural control. Mature motor control is characterized by the ability of the body, through the postural set, to anticipate what movement is to come, such as when you tense your arm muscles before picking up a heavy weight. Anticipatory preparation is an example of feed-forward processing, in which sensory information is sent ahead to prepare for the movement to follow, in contrast to feedback, in which sensation from a movement is sent back to the nervous system for comparison and error detection. Many adult patients with neurologic deficits lack this anticipatory preparation, so postural preparedness is often a beginning point for treatment. Children with neurologic deficits may never have experienced using sensation in this manner.

Environmental adaptation. Our posture and movement adapt to the environment in which the movement takes place in much the same way as we change our stance if riding on a moving bus and have nothing stable to grasp. Infants have to adapt to moving in a gravity-controlled environment after being in utero. The body's sensory systems provide input that allows the generation of a movement pattern that dynamically adapts to current conditions. In a systems model, this movement pattern is not limited to the typical postural reactions. With development of postural networks, anticipatory postural control develops and is used to preserve posture. Adaptive postural control allows changes to be made to movement performance in response to internally or externally perceived needs. Anticipatory postural control develops in parallel with reactive postural control in sitting and standing.

Nashner's model of postural control in standing. Nashner (1990) formulated a model for the control of standing balance over the course of some 20 years. His model describes three common sway strategies seen in quiet steady-state standing: the ankle strategy, the hip strategy, and the stepping strategy. An adult in a quiet standing position sways about the ankles. This strategy depends on having a solid surface in contact with the feet and intact visual, vestibular, and somatosensory systems. If the person sways backward, the anterior tibialis fires to bring the person forward; if the person sways forward, the gastrocnemius fires to bring the person back to midline.

A second sway strategy, called the hip strategy, is usually activated when the base of support is narrow, as when standing crosswise on a balance beam. The ankle strategy is not effective in this situation because the entire foot is not in contact with the support surface. In the hip strategy, muscles are activated in a proximal-to-distal sequence, that is, muscles around the hip are activated to maintain balance before the muscles at the ankles.

The last sway strategy is that of stepping. If the speed and strength of the balance disturbance are sufficient, the individual may take a step to prevent loss of balance or a fall. This stepping

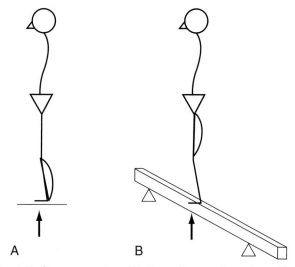

Fig. 3.10 Sway strategies. **(A)** Postural sway about the ankle in quiet standing. **(B)** Postural sway about the hip in standing on a balance beam. (Modified from Cech D, Martin S, editors: *Functional movement development across the life span*, ed 3, St. Louis, 2012, Elsevier, p. 271.)

response is the same as a lower extremity protective reaction. The ankle and the hip strategies are shown in Fig. 3.10.

The visual, vestibular, and somatosensory systems previously discussed provide the body with information about movement and cue appropriate postural responses in standing. For the first 3 years of life, the visual system appears to be the dominant sensory system for posture and balance. Vision is used both as feedback as the body moves and as feedforward to anticipate that movement will occur. Children as young as 18 months demonstrate an ankle strategy when quiet standing balance is disturbed (Forssberg and Nashner, 1982). However, the time it takes for them to respond is longer than in adults. Results of studies of 4- to 6-year-old children's responses to disturbances of standing balance were highly variable, almost as if balance was worse in this age group when compared with younger children. Sometimes the children demonstrated an ankle strategy, and sometimes they demonstrated a hip strategy (Shumway-Cook and Woollacott, 1985). It was originally postulated that children did not have adult-like responses until 10 years of age.

Postural sway in standing on a moveable platform under normal vestibular and somatosensory conditions is greater for children 4 to 6 years of age than for children 7 to 10 years of age (Shumway-Cook and Woollacott, 1985). By 7 to 10 years of age, an adult sway strategy is demonstrated wherein the child is thought to depend primarily on somatosensory information. Vestibular information is also being used, but the system is not yet mature. Interestingly, children with visual impairments are not able to minimize postural sway to the same extent as children who are not visually impaired (Portfors-Yeomans and Riach, 1995). This may be related to the child's inability to use either somatosensory or vestibular information fully during this age period.

Research supports that there is a transition period around 7 to 8 years that can be explained by the use of the HSSS

(Rival et al., 2005). By 7 years of age, children are able to make effective use of HSSS that depends on dynamic vestibular cues (Assaiante and Amblard, 1995). However, the transition to adult postural responses in standing is not complete by 12 years of age. Children at 12 to 14 years of age are still not able to handle misleading visual information to make appropriate adult balance responses (Ferber-Viart et al., 2007). These researchers found that, although the somatosensory inputs and scores in the 6- to 14-year-old subjects were as good as the young adults studied, their sensory organization was different. They concluded that children prefer visual input to vestibular input for determining balance responses and that vestibular information is the least effective for postural control.

ISSUES RELATED TO MOTOR CONTROL

Top Down or Distributed Control

The issue of where the control of movement resides has always been at the heart of the discussion of motor control. Remember that motor control occurs in milliseconds as compared with the time it takes to learn a movement or to develop a new motor skill. The reflex/hierarchical model was predicated on the cortex being the controller of movement. However, if there is no cortex, movement is still possible. The cortex can initiate movement, but it is not the only neural structure able to do so. From studying pathology involving the basal ganglia, it is known that movement initiation is slowed in people with Parkinson disease. Other neural structures that can initiate or control movement include the basal ganglia, the cerebellum, and the spinal cord. The spinal cord can produce rudimentary reciprocal movement from activation of central pattern generators. The reflexive withdrawal and extension of the limbs has been modified to produce cyclical patterns of movement that help locomotion be automatic, but is modifiable by higher centers of the brain. Lastly, the cerebellum is involved in movement coordination and timing of movements. The fact that more than one structure within the nervous system can affect and control movement lends credence for a distributed control of movement.

No one location of control exists in the systems view of movement; movement emerges from the combined need of the mover, the task, and the environment. The structures, pathways, and processes needed to produce the movement most efficiently are discovered as in finding the best way to get the task done. The structures, pathways, or processes that are continually used get better at the task and become the preferred way of performing that particular task. Developmentally, only certain structures, pathways, or processes are available early in development so that movements become refined and control improves with age. Movement control improves because of maturation of both the nervous system and musculoskeletal systems.

Degrees of Freedom

The mechanical definition of *degrees of freedom* is "the number of planes of motion possible at a single joint"

(Kelso, 1982). The degrees of freedom of a system have been defined as all of the independent movement elements of a control system and the number of ways each element can act (Schmidt and Wrisberg, 2013). There are multiple levels of redundancy within the CNS. Bernstein (1967) suggested that a key function of the CNS was to control this redundancy by minimizing the degrees of freedom or the number of independent movement elements that are used. For example, muscles can fire in different ways to control particular movement patterns or joint motions. In addition, many different kinematic or movement patterns can be executed to accomplish one specific outcome or action. During the early stages of learning novel tasks, the body may produce very simple movements, often "linking together two or more degrees of freedom" (Gordon, 1987), limiting the amount of joint motion by holding some joints stiffly via muscle co-contraction. As an action or task is learned, we first hold our joints stiffly through muscle co-contraction and then, as we learn the task, we decrease co-contraction and allow the joint to move freely. This increases the degrees of freedom around the joint (Vereijken et al., 1992). This concept is further discussed later in the chapter.

Certainly an increase in joint stiffness used to minimize degrees of freedom at the early stages of skill acquisition may not hold true for all types of tasks. In fact, different skills require different patterns of muscle activation. For example, Spencer and Thelen (1997) reported that muscle coactivity increases with the learning of a fast vertical reaching movement. They proposed that high-velocity movements actually result in the need for muscle coactivity to counteract unwanted rotational forces. However, during the execution of complex multijoint tasks, such as walking and rising from sitting to standing, muscle co-contraction is clearly undesirable and may in fact negatively affect the smoothness and efficiency of the movements. The resolution of the degrees of freedom problem varies depending on the characteristics of the learner as well as on the components of the task and environment. Despite the various interpretations of Bernstein's original hypothesis (1967), the resolution of the degrees of freedom problem continues to form the underlying basis for a systems theory of motor control.

Age-Related Changes in Postural and Motor Control

Variability in postural control is seen during infancy. Variability is needed for the development of functional movement. Furthermore, being able to vary and adapt one's posture makes exploration of the surrounding environment easier and affords opportunities for perception and action. An infant who lacks postural and movement variability is at risk for movement dysfunction. Dusing and Harbourne (2010) have suggested that lack of complex postural control may be an early indicator of developmental problems. Conversely, adding complexity to posture and movement variability may provide an impetus for functional changes in motor function.

Infants learn to move by moving. Utilization of sensory information during infancy reinforces development of the motor system (Dusing, 2016). Postural control supports movement and provides strategies on which to scaffold motor actions, such as reaching, grasping, crawling, and walking. Postural control and reaching are coordinated by 4 to 6 months of age (de Graaf-Peters et al., 2007). Optimal postural complexity allows the learner to select a strategy based on the perceptual information. Early movements are characterized by large amounts of postural variability. Adaptation of movement is not evident initially. but develops with experience (Hadders-Algra, 2010). Variability in postural control is evident when an infant scales the postural responses of the head to the surrounding visual information (Bertenthal et al., 1997). The ability to use visual information for postural responses improves from 5 to 9 months of age.

Balance Strategies in Sitting

Infants develop directionally specific postural responses before being able to sit (Hadders-Algra, 2008). These responses appear to be innate and are guided by an internal representation of the limits of stability, such as orientation of the vertical axis and relationship of COM to BOS. Control of the trunk develops segmentally in a top-down manner between 3 and 9 months (Saavedra et al, 2012). Saavedra identified four stages of sitting in her study: (1) no control; (2) attempts to initiate upright; (3) partial control with a large range of sway; and (4) functional control minimal sway. Head control improved as the infant developed control over successive trunk segments. The Segmental Assessment of Trunk Control (SATCo) was developed based on these findings. It has been recommended as an outcome measure for adults and children with cerebral palsy (Saether et al., 2013).

Most studies of the development of anticipatory postural control have been conducted in the sitting position using reaching as the task. Postural activity in the trunk was measured while an infant reached from a seated posture (Riach and Hayes, 1990). Trunk muscles were activated before muscles used for reaching in 6- to 8-month-old infants (van der Fits and Hadders-Algra, 1998). Rachwani et al. (2015) in a longitudinal study found that 4-month-old infants demonstrated twice as many compensatory postural responses than anticipatory ones. Anticipatory control of sitting increases from 2 to 11 years of age, but is still variable and incomplete when compared with adults (van der Heide et al., 2003). Older children demonstrate more refined scaling of postural responses. In other words, children become better at matching the amount of postural preparation needed for a specific task. Less postural activation is needed when picking up a light object when compared with picking up a heavy object.

Strategies in Standing

Reactive postural responses and anticipatory postural responses develop in tandem between the age of 1 and 10 years as the child learns to make use of feed-forward control (Chen et al., 2008). Infants' sitting posture is disturbed when they learn to walk (Chen et al., 2007). Young children tend to quickly make fast corrections to try and maintain standing balance. Around 8 or 9 years they demonstrate more accurate control and smaller corrections (Riach and Starkes, 1994). Postural control matures between 10 and 12 years. Spontaneous sway with eyes open reaches adult levels between 9 and 12 and with eyes closed between 12 and 15 years (Taguchi and Tada, 1988).

Older adults have more spontaneous sway than younger individuals (Maki and McIlroy, 1996; Sturnieks et al., 2008). The increase in sway is thought to be a compensation for the effects of gravity. However, the older adult may use increased sway to provide ongoing sensory information to postural control mechanisms in the CNS. Altering the sensory conditions provides a challenge to both young and older adults. With eyes closed, older adults stand more asymmetrically than younger adults. Older adults have been found to use a stiffening response of co-contracting muscles around the ankles joints rather than switching to using other sensory cues when vision is eliminated in quiet standing (Benjuya et al., 2004). Increased sway in a medial lateral direction is most predictive of falls in older adults (Maki et al., 1994). Stepping response may be more of a real-life response to external perturbations even if the position of the COM does not exceed the BOS (Rogers et al., 1996; Maki and McIlroy, 1997).

The model of motor control that best explains changes in posture and movement seen across the lifespan depends on the age and experience of the mover, the physical demands of the task to be carried out, and the environment in which the task is to be performed. The way in which a 2-year-old child may choose to solve the movement problem of how to reach the cookie jar in the middle of the kitchen table will be different from the solution devised by a 12-year-old child. As the infant grows, the movement solutions become more varied, and that, in itself, may reflect the self-organizing properties of the systems of the body involved in posture and movement. Posture has multiple roles in preparing, executing, and evaluating any movement task. Posture should be thought of as preparation for movement. Once anticipatory postural control is present, the postural system can anticipate postural needs prior to a task. A person would not think of starting to learn to in-line skate from a seated position. The person would have to stand with the skates on and try to balance while standing before taking off on the skates. The person's body tries to anticipate the posture that will be needed before the movement. Therefore, with patients who have movement dysfunction, the clinician must prepare them to move before movement is initiated.

When learning in-line skating, the person continually tries to maintain an upright posture. Postural control maintains alignment while the person moves forward. If the person loses balance and falls, posture is reactive. When falling, an automatic postural response comes from the nervous system; arms are extended in protection. Stunt performers have learned to avoid injury by landing on slightly bent arms, then tucking and rolling. Through the use of prior experience and knowledge of present conditions, the end result is modified and a full-blown protective response is generated. In many instances, automatic postural responses must be unlearned to learn and perfect fundamental motor skills. Think of a broad jumper who is airborne and moving forward in a crouch position. To prevent falling backward, the jumper must keep his arms forward and counteract the natural tendency to reach back.

MOTOR LEARNING

Across the lifespan, individuals are faced with new motor challenges and must learn to perform new motor skills. An infant must learn how to hold up her head, roll over, sit, crawl, and eventually walk. Each skill takes time to master and occurs only after the infant has practiced each skill in several different ways and in multiple environments. The young child then masters running, climbing on furniture, walking up stairs, jumping, and playing ball. The school-age child takes these tasks further to specifically kick a soccer ball into a net, throw a ball into a basketball hoop, or ride a bike or skateboard. As teens and adults learn new sports, they refine their skills, becoming more efficient at turning while on snow skis or pitching a baseball into the strike zone with more speed. Adults also learn to perform tasks related to their occupation efficiently. These tasks vary widely from one occupation to another and may include efficient computer keyboarding, climbing up a ladder, or lifting boxes. Older adults may need to modify their motor skill performance to accommodate for changes in strength and flexibility. For example, the older adult golfer may change her stance during a swing or learn to use a heavier golf club to maximize the distance of her drive. Injury or illness often requires an individual to relearn how to sit up, walk, put on a shirt, or get into or out of a car. The method each individual uses to learn new movements demonstrates the process of motor learning. Motor learning examines how an individual learns or modifies a motor task. As discussed in the section on motor control, the characteristics of the task, the learner, and the environment will have an impact on the learning and performance of the skill. With motor learning, general principles apply to individuals of any age, but variations have been found in the motor learning methods used by children, adults, and older adults.

Definition and Time Frame

Motor learning is defined as the process that brings about a permanent change in motor performance as a result of practice or experience (Schmidt and Wrisberg, 2013). The time frame of motor learning falls between the milliseconds involved in motor control and the years involved in motor development. Hours, days, and weeks of practice are part of motor development. It takes an infant the better part of a year to overcome gravity and learn to walk. The perfection of some skills takes years; ask anyone trying to improve a batting average or a soccer kick. Even though motor development, motor control, and motor learning take place within different time frames, these time frames do not exclude one or the other processes from taking place. In fact, it is possible that

because these processes do have different time bases for action, they may be mutually compatible.

THEORIES OF MOTOR LEARNING

Two theories of motor learning have generated a great deal of study about how we control and acquire motor skills. Both theories use programs to explain how movements are controlled and learned; they are Adams' closed-loop theory of motor learning (Adams, 1971) and Schmidt's schema theory (Schmidt, 1975). The two theories differ in the amount of emphasis placed on open-loop processes that can occur without the benefit of ongoing feedback (Schmidt and Lee, 2011). Schmidt incorporated many of Adams' original ideas when formulating his schema theory in an attempt to explain the acquisition of both slow and fast movements. Intrinsic and extrinsic feedbacks, as defined earlier in this chapter, are both important factors in these two theories.

Adams' Closed-Loop Theory

The name of Adams' theory emphasized the crucial role of feedback. The concept of a closed loop of motor control is one in which sensory information is funneled back to the central nervous system for processing and control of motor behavior. The sensory feedback is used to produce accurate movements.

The basic premise of Adams' theory is that movements are performed by comparing an ongoing movement with an internal reference of correctness that is developed during practice. This internal reference is termed as *perceptual trace*, which represents the feedback one would receive if the task were performed correctly. A perceptual trace is formed as the learner repeatedly performs an action. Through ongoing comparison of the feedback with the perceptual trace, a limb may be brought into the desired position. To learn the task, it would be necessary to practice the exact skill repeatedly to strengthen the correct perceptual trace. The quality of performance is directly related to the quality of the perceptual trace. The trace is made up of a set of intrinsic feedback signals that arise from the learner. Intrinsic feedback here means the sensory information that is generated through performance; for example, the kinesthetic feel of the movement. As a new movement is learned, correct outcomes reinforce development of the most effective, correct perceptual trace, although perceptual traces that lead to incorrect outcomes are discarded. The perceptual trace becomes stronger with repetition and more accurate in representing the correct performance as a result of feedback.

With further study limitations of the closed-loop theory of motor learning have been identified. One limitation is that the theory does not explain how movements can be explained when sensory information is not available. The theory also does not explain how individuals can often perform novel tasks successfully, without the benefit of repeated practice and perceptual trace. The ability of the brain to store individual perceptual traces for each possible movement has also been questioned, considering the memory storage capacity of the brain (Schmidt, 1975).

Schmidt's Schema Theory

Schmidt's schema theory was developed in direct response to Adams' closed-loop theory and its limitations. Schema theory is concerned with how movements that can be carried out without feedback are learned, and it relies on an open-loop control element—the motor program–to foster learning. The *motor program* for a movement reflects the general rules to complete the movement successfully. These general rules, or schema, can then be used to produce the movement in a variety of conditions or settings. For example, the general rules for walking can be applied to walking on tile, on grass, on an icy sidewalk, or going up a hill. The motor program provides the spatial and temporal information about muscle activation needed to complete the movement (Schmidt and Lee, 2011). The motor program is composed of the schema, or abstract memory, of rules related to skilled actions.

According to schema theory, when a person produces a movement, four kinds of information are stored in short-term memory.

1. The initial conditions under which the performance took place (e.g., the position of the body, the kind of surface on which the individual carried out the action, or the shapes and weights of any objects that were used to carry out the task)
2. The parameters assigned to the motor program (e.g., the force or speed that was specified at the time of initiation of the program)
3. The outcome of the performance
4. The sensory consequences of the movement (e.g., how it felt to perform the movement, the sounds that were made as a result of the action, or the visual effect of the performance)

These four kinds of information are analyzed to gain insight into the relationships among them and to form two types of schema: the recall schema and the recognition schema.

The *recall schema* is used to select a method to complete a motor task. It is an abstract representation of the relationship among the initial conditions surrounding performance, parameters that were specified within the motor program, and the outcome of the performance. The learner, through the analysis of parameters that were specified in the motor program and the outcome, begins to understand the relationship between these two factors. For example, the learner may come to understand how far a wheelchair travels when varying amounts of force are generated to push the chair on a gravel pathway. The learner stores this schema and uses it the next time the wheelchair is moved on a gravel path.

The *recognition schema* helps assess how well a motor behavior has been performed. It represents the relationship among the initial conditions, the outcome of the performance, and the sensory consequences that are perceived by the learner. Because it is formed in a manner similar to that of the recall schema, once it is established, the recognition schema is used to produce an estimate of the sensory consequences of the action that will be used to adjust and evaluate the motor performance of a given motor task.

In motor learning, the motor behavior is assessed through use of the recognition schema. If errors are identified, they are used to refine the recall schema. Recall and recognition schemas are continually revised and updated as skilled movement is learned. Limitations of the schema theory have also been identified. One limitation is that the formation of general motor programs is not explained. Another question has arisen from inconsistent results in studies of effectiveness of variable practice on learning new motor skills, especially with adult subjects.

STAGES OF MOTOR LEARNING

It is generally possible to tell when a person is learning a new skill. The person's performance lacks the graceful, efficient movement of someone who has perfected the skill. For example, when adults learn to snow ski, they typically hold their bodies stiffly, with knees straight and arms at their side. Over time, as they become more comfortable with skiing, they will bend and straighten their knees as they turn. Finally, when watching the experienced skier, the body fluidly rotates and flexes or extends as she maneuvers down a steep slope or completes a slalom race. The stages associated with mastery of a skill have been described and clearly differentiated between the early stages of motor learning and the later stages of motor learning. Two models of motor learning stages are described below and in Table 3.3.

TABLE 3.3 **Stages of Motor Learning**			
Model	**Stage 1**	**Stage 2**	**Stage 3**
Fitts' stages of motor learning	Cognitive stage Actively think about goal Think about conditions	Associative stage Refine performance Error correction	Autonomous stage Automatic performance Consistent, efficient performance
"Neo-Bernsteinian" model of motor learning	Novice stage Decreased number of degrees of freedom	Advanced stage Release of some degrees of freedom	Expert stage Uses all degrees of freedom for fluid, efficient movement
General characteristics	Stiff looking Inconsistent performance Errors Slow, nonfluid movement	More fluid movement Fewer errors Improved consistency Improved efficiency	Automatic Fluid Consistent Efficient Error correction

From Cech D, Martin S, editors: *Functional movement development across the life span*, ed 3, St. Louis, 2012, Elsevier, p. 77.

In the early stages of motor learning, individuals have to think about the skill they are performing and may even "talk" their way through the skill. For example, when learning how to turn when snow skiing, the novice skier may tell herself to bend the knees upon initiating the turn, then straighten the knees through the turn, and then bend the knees again as the turn is completed. The skier might even be observed to say the words "bend, straighten, bend" or "down, up, down" as she turns. Early in the motor learning process, movements tend to be stiff and inefficient. The new learner may not always be able to complete the skill successfully or might hesitate, making the timing movements within the skill inaccurate.

In the later stages of motor learning, the individual may not need to think about the skill. For example, the skier will automatically go through the appropriate motions with the appropriate timing as she makes a turn down a steep slope. Likewise, the baseball player steps up to the plate and does not think too much about how he will hit the ball. The batter will swing at a ball that comes into the strike zone automatically. If either the experienced skier or batter makes an error, he or she will self-assess their performance and try to correct the error next time.

Fitts' Stages

In analyzing acquisition of new motor skills, Fitts (1964) described three stages of motor learning. The first stage is the cognitive phase, in which the learner consciously has to consider the goal of the task to be completed and recognize the features of the environment to which the movement must conform (Gentile, 1987). In a task such as walking across a crowded room, the surface of the floor and the location and size of the people within the room are considered regulatory features. If the floor is slippery, a person's walking pattern is different than if the floor is carpeted. Background features, such as lighting or noise, may also affect task performance. During this initial cognitive phase of learning, an individual tries a variety of strategies to achieve the movement goal. Through this trial-and-error approach, effective strategies are built upon and ineffective strategies are discarded.

At the next stage of learning, the *associative phase*, the learner has developed the general movement pattern necessary to perform the task and is ready to refine and improve the performance of the skill. The learner makes subtle adjustments to adjust errors and to adapt the skill to varying environmental demands of the task. For example, a young baseball player may learn that he can more efficiently and consistently hit the ball if he chokes up on the bat. During this phase, the focus of the learner switches from "what to do" to "how to do the movement" (Schmidt, 1988).

In the final stage of learning, the *autonomous phase*, the skill becomes more "automatic" because the learner does not need to focus all of her attention on the motor skill. She is able to attend to other components of the task, such as scanning for subtle environmental obstacles. At this phase, the learner is better able to adapt to changes in features in the environment. The young baseball player will be relatively

successful at hitting the ball even when using different bats or if a cheering crowd is present.

"Neo-Bernsteinian" Model

This model of staging motor learning considers the learner's ability to master multiple degrees of freedom as she learns a new skill (Bernstein, 1967; Vereijken et al., 1992). Within this model, the initial stage of motor learning, the *novice stage*, is when the learner reduces the degrees of freedom that need to be controlled during the task. The learner will "fix" some joints so that motion does not take place and the degree of freedom is constrained at that joint. For example, think of the new snow skier who holds her knees stiffly extended while bending at the trunk to try to turn. The resultant movement is stiff-looking and not always effective. For example, if the slope of the hill is too steep or if the skier tries to turn on an icy patch, the movement may not be effective. The second stage in this model, the *advanced stage*, is seen when the learner allows more joints to participate in the task, in essence releasing some of the degrees of freedom. Coordination is improved as agonist and antagonist muscles around the joint can work together to produce the movement, rather than co-contracting as they did to "fix" the joint in earlier movement attempts. The third stage of this model, the *expert stage*, is when all degrees of freedom necessary to perform a task in an efficient, coordinated manner are released. Within this stage, the learner can begin to adjust performance to improve the efficiency of the movement by adjusting the speed of the movement. Considering the skier, the expert may appreciate that by increasing the speed of descent, a turn may be easier to initiate.

Effects of Practice

Motor learning theorists have also studied the effects of practice on learning a motor task and whether different types of practice make initial learning easier. Practice is a key component of motor learning. Some types of practice make initial learning easier but make transferring that learning to another task more difficult. The more closely the practice environment resembles the actual environment where the task will take place, the better the transfer of learning will be. This is known as task-specific practice. Therefore, if you are going to teach a person to walk in the physical therapy gym, this learning may not transfer to walking at home, where the floor is carpeted. Many facilities use an Easy Street (a mock or mini home, work, and community environment) to help simulate actual conditions the patient may encounter at home. Of course, providing therapy in the home is an excellent opportunity for motor learning.

Massed versus Distributed Practice

The difference between massed and distributed practice schedules is related to the proportion of rest time and practice time during the session. In massed practice, greater practice time than rest time occurs in the session. The amount of rest time between practice attempts is less than the amount of time spent practicing. In distributed practice conditions, the amount of rest time is longer than the time spent practicing. Constraint-induced therapy can be considered a modified form of massed practice in which learned nonuse is overcome by shaping or reinforcing (Taub et al., 1993). Shaping incorporates the motor learning concept of part practice as a task is learned in small steps, which are individually mastered. Successive approximation of the completed task is made until the individual is able to perform the whole task. In an individual with hemiplegia, the uninvolved arm or hand is constrained, thereby necessitating use of the involved (hemiplegic) upper extremity in functional tasks.

Random versus Blocked Practice

Another consideration in structuring a practice session is the order in which tasks are practiced. *Blocked practice* occurs when the same task is repeated several times in a row. One task is practiced several times before a second task is practiced. *Random practice* occurs when a variety of tasks is practiced in a random order, with any one skill rarely practiced two times in a row. *Mixed practice* sessions may also be useful in some situations in which episodes of both random and blocked practice are incorporated into the practice session.

Constant practice occurs when an individual practices one variation of a movement skill several times in a row. An example would be repeatedly practicing standing up from a wheelchair or throwing a basketball into a hoop. *Variable practice* occurs when the learner practices several variations of a motor skill during a practice session. For example, a patient in rehabilitation may practice standing up from the wheelchair, standing up from the bed, standing up from the toilet, and standing up from the floor. A child might practice throwing a ball into a hoop, throwing a ball at a target on the wall, throwing a ball underhand, throwing a ball overhand, or throwing a ball to a partner all within the same session. Variable practice training is useful in helping the learner generalize a motor skill over a wide variety of environmental settings and conditions. Learning is thought to be enhanced by the variable practice because the strength of the general motor program rules, specific to the new task, would be increased. This mechanism is also considered as a way that an individual can attempt a novel task because the person can incorporate rules developed for previous motor tasks to solve the novel motor task.

Whole versus Part Task Training

A task can be practiced as a complete action (*whole task practice*) or broken up into its component parts (*part practice*). Continuous tasks, such as walking, running, or stair climbing, are more effectively learned as a whole task practice. It has been demonstrated that if walking is broken down into part practice of a component, such as weight shifting forward over the foot, the learner demonstrates improvements in weight-shifting behavior but does not generalize this improvement into the walking sequence (Winstein et al., 1989).

Skills that can be broken down into discrete parts may be most effectively taught using part practice training. For example, a patient learning how to transfer out of a wheelchair

independently might first be taught how to lock the brakes on the chair, then how to scoot forward in the chair. After these parts of the task are mastered, the patient might learn to properly place his feet, lean forward over the feet, and finally stand. Similarly, when learning a dressing task, a child might first be taught to pull a shirt over her head then push in each arm. Once these components are completed, the focus might be on learning how to fasten buttons or a zipper.

Open and Closed Tasks

Movement results when an interaction exists among the mover, the task, and the environment. We have discussed the mover and the environment, but the task to be learned can be classified as either open or closed. Open tasks are those done in environments that change over time, such as playing softball, walking on different uneven surfaces, or driving a car. Closed tasks are skills that have set parameters and stay the same, such as walking on carpet, holding an object, or reaching for a target. These tasks appear to be processed differently. Which type involves more perceptual information? Open tasks require the mover constantly to update movements and to pay attention to incoming information about the softball, movement of traffic, or the support surface. Would a person have fewer motor problems with open or closed tasks? Closed tasks with set parameters pose fewer problems. Remember that open and closed tasks are different from open-loop and closed-loop processing used for motor control or motor learning.

OPTIMAL Theory

The OPTIMAL theory of motor learning is so named because it stands for optimizing performance through intrinsic motivation and attention for learning (Wulf and Lewthwaite, 2016). These researchers present a different perspective on motor learning. They propose that because motor behavior is embedded in a culture, motor behavior has a social context. Their theory assumes that attention and motivation (social-cognitive and affective) influence motor learning behavior. The literature on the effect of motivation and attention on motor learning has shown that a focus on positive expectations will enhance motor learning; providing the learner autonomy, such as allowing choices of task, practice, or environment can positively influence learning; and lastly that an external focus of attention on the intended movement effect rather than on body movements improves motor learning. Children's motor skill learning is influenced by their conceptions of ability (Drews et al., 2013). The theory has been applied when working with children with autism, children with intellectual disability, adults with Parkinson disease, and older adults with balance issues (Reis, 2018; Chiviacowsky et al., 2013; Chiviacowsky et al., 2012; Chiviacowsky et al., 2010). "Implications of the OPTIMAL theory for optimizing motor performance and learning in applied and clinical contexts involve finding the right approaches to boosting or supporting positive motivation and directing attention to effective external foci" (Wulf and Lewthwaite, 2016). Furthermore, the proponents of the theory think that when we as clinicians fail to provide ways to enhance learners' expectations, or support the mover's need for autonomy or induce an internal focus of attention there are negative learning outcomes.

Constraints to Motor Development, Motor Control, and Motor Learning

Our movements are constrained or limited by the biomechanical properties of our bones, joints, and muscles. No matter how sophisticated the neural message is or how motivated the person is, if the part of the body involved in the movement is limited in strength or range, the movement may occur incorrectly or not at all. If the control directions are misinterpreted, the intended movement may not occur. A person is only as good a mover as the weakest part of the entire movement system. For some, that weakest part is a specific system, such as the muscular or nervous system; for others, it is a function of a system, such as cognition.

Development of motor control and the acquisition of motor abilities occur while both the muscular and skeletal systems are growing and the nervous system is maturing. Changes in all the body's physical systems provide a constant challenge to the development of motor control. Thelen and Fisher (1982) showed that some changes in motor behavior, such as an infant's inability to step reflexively after a certain age, probably occur because the infant's legs become too heavy to move, not because some reflex is no longer exhibited by the nervous system. We have already discussed that the difficulty an infant encounters in learning to control the head during infancy can be attributed to the head's size being proportionately too big for the body. With growth, the body catches up to the head. As a linked system, the skeleton has to be controlled by the tension in the muscles and the amount of force generated by those muscles. Learning which muscles work well together and in what order is a monumental task.

Adolescence is another time of rapidly changing body relationships. As children become adolescents, movement coordination can be disrupted because of rapid and uneven changes in body dimensions. The most coordinated 10- or 12-year-old can turn into a gawky, gangly, and uncoordinated 14- or 16-year-old. The teenager makes major adjustments in motor control during the adolescent growth spurt.

Age-Related Changes in Motor Learning

Children learn differently than adults. Children practice, practice, practice. For example, when learning to walk, an infant covers a distance equal to 29 football fields daily (Adolph et al., 2003). A typical 14-month-old takes more than 2,000 steps per hour (Adolph, 2008). These two examples lend support to using block practice to learn and retain a new skill. Infants demonstrate inherent variability in task performance. Learning in one posture such as standing does not generalize to other actions such as going down a ramp, which is performed in the same upright postures under different conditions (Adolph, 2007; Berger et al., 2007). Adolph's work supports the dynamic systems theory that developing a level of skill in one position does not automatically transfer to another posture. Knowing how to crawl on a slope does not carry over to walking on a slope. The infant constantly needs to be problem solving in order to meet the challenges of the task and environment.

As young children are learning new gross motor tasks, blocked practice appears to lead to better transfer and performance of the skill. Del Rey et al. (1983) had typically developing children (approximately 8 years old) practice a timing task at different speeds in either a blocked or random order and then tested them on a transfer test with the new coordination pattern. The researchers found that blocked practice led to better performance on the transfer task than did random practice. In Frisbee throwing experiments, accuracy in throwing the Frisbee at a target was improved by blocked practice in children, although adults improved accuracy the most with random practice (Pinto-Zipp and Gentile, 1995; Jarus and Goverover, 1999). The contextual interference provided by random practice schedules does not appear to help children learn new motor skills (Perez et al., 2005).

Although most of the literature on children supports a blocked or mixed schedule for learning whole body tasks, some researchers have found that typically developing children may learn skilled or sport-specific skills if a variable practice schedule is used (Vera et al., 2008; Douvis, 2005; Granda and Montilla, 2003). This variable practice schedule combines blocked and random practice elements and allows the child to benefit from practicing the new skill with elements of contextual interference. Vera et al. (2008) found that 9-year-old children performed the skill of kicking a soccer ball best by following blocked or combined practice, but only children in a combined practice situation improved in dribbling the soccer ball. Similarly, Douvis (2005) examined the impact of variable practice on learning the tennis forehand drive in children and adolescents. Adolescents did better than children on the task, reflecting the influence of age and development, but both age groups did the best with variable practice. The variable practice sessions allowed the tennis players to use the forehand drive in a manner that more resembled the actual game of tennis, where a player may use a forehand drive, then a backhand drive.

Older adults' motor learning is affected by aging. In general older adults demonstrate deficits in sequential learning, learning new technology, and effortful bimanual coordination patterns. Some of these deficits may be age-related declines in force production, sensory capacity, or speed of sensory processing, and issues with divided attention. The good news is that older adults can improve motor performance with practice. Older adults perform tasks they are learning more slowly and with greater errors when compared with younger adults, but they do benefit equally, as compared with younger adults, from practice schedules conducive to motor learning.

Neural Plasticity

Neural plasticity is the ability of the nervous system to change. Although it has always been hypothesized that the nervous system could adapt throughout life, ample evidence now indicates that the adult brain maintains the ability for reorganization or plasticity (Doyon and Benali, 2005; Bruel-Jungerman et al., 2007). Traditionally, it was thought that plasticity was limited to the developing nervous system. Activity-dependent changes in neural circuitry usually occur during a restricted time in development or critical period, when the organism is sensitive to the effects of experience. *Critical periods* are times when neurons compete for synaptic sites. The concept of plasticity includes the ability of the nervous system to make structural changes in response to internal and external demands. Learning and motor behavior appear to modulate neurogenesis throughout life.

Experience is critical to development. In the course of typical prenatal and postnatal development, the infant is expected to be exposed to sufficient environmental stimuli (visual, vestibular, and auditory) at appropriate times to complete the development of these sensory systems. If the infant is not exposed to the proper quality and quantity of input within a critical time period, development of these systems will not proceed normally. Neural plasticity also allows the nervous system to incorporate other types of information from environmental experiences that are relatively unpredictable and idiosyncratic. These experiences are unique to the individual and depend on the context in which development occurs, such as the physical, social, and cultural environment. Lebeer (1998) refers to this as *ecological plasticity*, whereas the term *activity-dependent plasticity* is used by Johnston (2009). Climate, social expectations, and child-rearing practices can alter movement experiences. What each child learns depends on the unique physical challenges encountered. Motor learning as part of motor development is an example of *activity-dependent* neural plasticity. Experiences of infants in different cultures may result in alterations in the acquisition of motor abilities. Similarly, not every child experiences the exact same words, but every child does learn language. *Activity-dependent* plasticity is what drives changes in synapses or neuronal circuits as a result of experience or learning.

Recovery following injury to the nervous system occurs in one of two ways. One is a result of spontaneous recovery and the other way is function induced. For a more in-depth discussion of injury-induced plasticity and recovery of function, see Shumway-Cook and Woollacott (2017). Function-induced recovery is also known as use-dependent cortical reorganization. Regardless of the terminology, change results from activity that produces cortical reorganization, just as early experience drives motor and sensory development. Experience can drive recovery of function. Kleim and Jones (2008) summarized the research to date on activity-dependent neural plasticity and recommended 10 principles for neurorehabilitation. These are listed in Table 3.4 and are congruent with the principles of motor learning involving repetition and task-specific practice.

Interventions Based on Motor Control, Motor Learning, and Neural Plasticity Principles

Evidence-based practice is the integration of clinical expertise, the best available evidence, and patient characteristics (Sackett et al., 2000). Previous interventions have focused on

TABLE 3.4   Principles of Experience-Dependent Plasticity

Principle	Description
Use it or lose it	Lack of activity of certain brain functions can lead to functional loss.
Use it and improve it	Training a specific brain function can lead to improvement in that function.
Specificity	The training experience must be specific to the expected change.
Repetition	Active repetition is needed to induce change.
Intensity	Training must be of a sufficient intensity to induce change.
Salience	The stimulus used to produce a response must be appropriate.
Age	Plasticity is more likely to occur in the young brain versus the older brain.
Time	Timing of intervention may help or hinder recovery.
Transference	Training on one task may positively affect another similar task.
Interference	Plasticity in response to one experience can interfere with the acquisition of other behaviors.

(Adapted from Kleim JA, Jones TA: Principles of experience-dependent neural plasticity: implications for rehabilitation after brain damage, *J Speech Lang Hear Res* 51:S225–S239, 2008.)

the impairments seen in individuals with neurologic dysfunction. Evidence is lacking to support that changing impairments changes function. The adoption of the International Classification of Functioning, Disability, and Health (ICF) by the American Physical Therapy Association (APTA) has shifted emphasis toward interventions that focus on preventing or minimizing activity limitations and eliminating participation restrictions encountered by those children and adults with neurologic deficits. Embracing the ICF necessitates a broader, more functionally based view of interventions and the impact of those interventions on the quality of life of the individual. Interventions must be relevant to the individual, whether a child or an adult. Interventions must be evaluated as to the outcomes they produce. The Academy of Neurologic Physical Therapy has recommended the use of specific outcome measures for adults with neurologic dysfunction undergoing rehabilitation (Moore et al., 2018). Both Academies of Neurologic and Pediatric Physical Therapy are working to codify a movement systems nomenclature for describing movement problems in adults and children with movement dysfunction. This will certainly have an impact on evaluation, treatment planning, and rehabilitation.

Treatment planning must encompass the task, the environment, and the mover. The therapist planning interventions has to make them interesting and engaging. The motor activities selected must be engaging and meaningful to the person. The therapist selects the task to be performed and the environment as well as determines the type of practice and when feedback is given. The "just right challenge" is a concept that is often utilized in pediatric physical therapy practice. Devices can be used; for example a body weight support harness can be used to assist locomotion training or a wearable garment may be used to assist reaching. Active participation is required for motor learning.

The physical therapist's and physical therapist assistant's view of motor control and motor learning influence the choice of approach to therapy with children and adults with neuromotor deficits. Given that the prevailing view of motor control and motor learning is a systems view, all body systems must be taken into consideration when planning an intervention. Size and level of maturity of the body systems involved in movement must be considered. The age appropriateness of tasks relative to the mover's cognitive ability to understand the task should also be considered. Some interventions used in treating children with neurodevelopmental disorders focus only on developing reactive postural reactions. Although children need to be safe within any posture that they are placed in or attain on their own, children also need to learn adaptive postural responses. Adaptive responses are learned within the context of reaching and grasping, locomotion, and play activities. Movement experiences should be as close to reality as possible. Therapists will need to educate parents to provide opportunities for motor learning by adapting the physical and play environment. Increasing the infant or child's participation is of the utmost importance during therapy and at home. Activity-based approaches can maximize physical function and foster social, emotional, and cognitive development by providing movement challenges and repetitive training.

Enriched environments have been found to promote optimal brain injury recovery in infants at high risk for cerebral palsy by taking advantage of neuroplasticity (Morgan et al., 2013). The following interventions are recommended to promote motor, cognitive, and communication skills in children with cerebral palsy: Learning Games Curriculum (Palmer et al., 1988) and Goals-Activity-Motor Enrichment (GAME) (Morgan, et al., 2016). These programs take advantage of using sensorimotor experiences to further drive motor and cognitive development.

Constraint-induced movement therapy (CIMT) involves both constraint of the noninvolved upper extremity of an individual with hemiplegia and repetitive practice of skilled activities or functional tasks. Principles of forced use of an upper extremity that might be ignored has been extremely effective in adults and children with hemiplegia (Taub et al., 1993; Charles et al., 2001; 2006). Lin (2007) found that patients with chronic stroke had improved motor control strategies during goal-directed tasks after CIMT. The Hand-Arm Bimanual Intervention (HABIT) program is an example of an effective CIMT program for children with hemiplegic cerebral palsy (Charles and Gordon, 2006; Gordon et al., 2007). A systematic review by Huang et al. (2009) found that CIMT increases upper extremity use in children. Despite a recent systematic review and meta-analysis of CIMT in adults post stroke, best

dosage and optimal time to start the intervention is lacking (Etoom et al., 2016). The mass practice in CIMT is thought to induce cortical reorganization and mapping, which increases efficiency of task performance in the hemiplegic upper extremity (Taub et al., 2004; Nudo et al., 1996). These findings reflect the influence of CIMT on activity-dependent neural plasticity. (See Chapters 6 and 11 for further discussion.)

Use of body weight support treadmill training (BWTT) as a form of gait practice does not require the person to have postural control of the trunk before attempting to walk. Task-specific practice has been shown to have a positive effect on outcomes in adults with hemiplegia, incomplete spinal cord injuries, and in children with Down syndrome and cerebral palsy. BWTT has been studied extensively and has been found to be safe for patients post stroke (Moseley et al., 2017). In a recent Cochrane review, Mehrholz et al. (2017) found that BWTT significantly increased both gait and walking velocity during rehabilitation. The authors concluded that treadmill training, with or without body weight support, may improve gait speed and endurance after a stroke in patients who could walk, but not in dependent walkers. The authors encouraged future research focus on duration, frequency, and intensity of training.

Treadmill training is also used with patients who have incomplete spinal cord injuries. In this case, the lower extremities are maximally loaded for weight bearing while using a body weight support system and manual cues. Evidence from studies shows an increase in endurance, gait speed, balance, and independence (Behrman and Harkema, 2000; Dobkin et al., 2006; Field-Fote and Roach, 2011; and Harkema et al., 2012). A recovery model has been developed for rehabilitation of individuals with incomplete spinal cord injury (Behrman et al, 2017).

Treadmill training has been successfully used as an intervention for children with spinal cord injury (Behrman et al., 2014). Young children with Down syndrome who participated in treadmill training walked earlier than the control group (Ulrich et al., 2001). When comparing intensity of training, the higher intensity group walked earlier than the lower intensity group (Ulrich et al., 2008). Positive results are reported in children with cerebral palsy. In those children at Gross Motor Function Classification Scale level III and IV, there was a significant increase in gait speed motor performance (Willoughby et al., 2010).

How a therapy session is designed depends on the type of motor control theory espoused. Theories guide clinicians' thinking about what may be the reason the patient has a problem moving and about what interventions may remediate the problem. Therapists who embrace a systems approach may have the patient perform a functional task in an appropriate setting, rather than just practice a component of the movement thought to be needed for that task. Rather than having the child practice postural responses on a ball, the assistant has the child sit on a bench and take off her shoes and socks prior to playing a game involving repeated balance challenges.

Therapists who use a systems approach in treatment may be more concerned about the amount of practice and the schedule for when feedback is given than about the degree or normality of tone in the trunk or extremity used to perform the movement. Intensive gait is an example of intense practice that pushes the individual post stroke to work hard enough to drive recovery of the ability to walk. Treadmill training with a harness, overground walking, and stair climbing are used to produce activity-dependent change. Using this systems approach, an assistant would keep track of the person's rate of perceived exertion, heart rate, and time on task. Intensity matters and is thought to be the catalyst for neural changes post stroke. Knowledge of results is important for learning motor tasks. The goal of every therapeutic intervention, regardless of its theoretic basis, is to teach the patient how to produce functional movements in the clinic, at home, and in the community.

Another promising area of rehabilitation which utilizes neural plasticity involves those interventions that promote activity-dependent plasticity by associating the patient's motor intent with artificially generated movement and afferent activity using electrical stimulation. Ethier et al. (2015) reviewed research that showed that coordinating electrical stimulation with the patient's own efforts via brain machine interface or brain-computer interface (BCI) could enhance neurorehabilitation and promote functional recovery. An example of paired stimulation would be using transcranial magnetic stimulation along with peripheral nerve stimulation, such as functional electrical stimulation (FES) of the peroneal nerve during the swing phase of gait. Biasiucci et al. (2018), in a recent study, showed that pairing brain-actuated stimulation (BCI) with FES resulted in lasting arm motor recovery after stroke.

Interventions must be developmentally appropriate regardless of the age of the person. Although it may not be appropriate to have an 80-year-old creeping on the floor or mat table, it may be an ideal activity for an infant. All of us learn movement skills better within the context of a functional activity. Play provides a perfect functional setting for an infant and child to learn how to move (Dusing et al., 2018). The physical therapist assistant working with an extremely young child should strive for the most functional skills possible for the child's age, realizing that the amount and extent of the neurologic damage incurred may determine what movements are possible. Remember that it is also during play that a child learns valuable cause-and-effect lessons when observing how her actions result in moving herself or moving an object. Movement through the environment is an important part of learning spatial concepts.

Motor learning must always occur within the context of function. It would not be an appropriate context for learning about walking to teach a child to walk on a movable surface, for example, because this task is typically performed on a nonmovable surface. The way a task is first learned is usually the way it is remembered best. When stressed or in an unsafe situation, we often revert to this way of moving. For example, on many occasions a daughter of a friend is observed to go up and down the long staircase in her parents' home, foot over foot without using a railing. When her motor skills were filmed in a studio in which the only stairs available were ones that had no back, the same child reverted to stepping up with one foot and bringing the other foot up to the same step (marking time) to ascend and descend. She perceived the stairs to be less safe and chose a less risky way to move. Infants and young children should be given every opportunity to learn to move correctly from the start. This is one of the major reasons for intervening early when an infant exhibits motor dysfunction. Motor learning requires practice and feedback. Remember what had to be done to learn to ride a bicycle without training wheels. Many times, through trial and error, you tried to get to the end of the block. After falls and scrapes, you finally mastered the task, and even though you may not have ridden a bike in a while, you still remember how. That memory of the movement is the result of motor learning.

Assessing functional movement status is a routine part of the physical therapist's examination and evaluation. Functional status may provide cues for planning interventions within the context of the functional task to be achieved. Use of core outcome measures is critical to documenting change in the patient with neurologic conditions. When the physical therapist reexamines and reevaluates a patient with movement dysfunction, the physical therapist assistant can participate by gathering objective data about the number of times the person can perform an activity, what types of cues (verbal, tactile, pressure) result in better or worse performance, and whether the task can be successfully performed in more than one setting, such as the physical therapy gym or the patient's dining room. Additionally, the physical therapist assistant may comment on the consistency of the patient's motor behavior in the patient documentation.

CHAPTER SUMMARY

Motor control is ever-present. It directs posture and movement. Without motor control, no motor development or motor learning could occur. Motor learning provides a mechanism for the body to attain new skills regardless of the age of the individual. Motor learning requires feedback in the form of sensory information about whether the movement occurred and how successful it was. Practice and experience play major roles in motor learning. Motor development is the age-related process of change in motor behavior. Motor development is made up of the tasks acquired and learned during the process of moving. Neural plasticity is the ability of the nervous system to adapt to experience whether during the developmental process or as part of relearning actions limited by a neurologic insult. A neurologic deficit can affect an individual's ability to engage in age-appropriate motor tasks (motor development), to learn or relearn motor skills (motor learning), or to perform functional movements with sufficient efficiency to be effective (motor control). Purposeful movement requires that all three processes be used continually and contingently across the lifespan.

REVIEW QUESTIONS

1. Define and give examples of motor control, motor learning, and neural plasticity.
2. How do sensation, perception, and sensory organization contribute to motor control and motor learning?
3. How does posture influence motor development, motor control, and motor learning?
4. How is a postural response determined when visual and somatosensory input conflict?
5. When in the lifespan can "adult" sway strategies be consistently demonstrated?
6. How much attention to a task is needed in the various phases of motor learning?
7. Give an example of an open task and of a closed task.
8. Which type of feedback loop is used to learn movement? To perform a fast movement?
9. How much and what type of practice are needed for motor learning in a child? In an adult?
10. How do the principles of neuroplasticity relate to the principles of motor learning?

REFERENCES

Adams JA: A closed-loop theory of motor learning, *J Motor Behav* 3:110–150, 1971.

Adolph KE: Learning to move, *Curr Dir Psychol Sci* 17:213–218, 2008.

Adolph KE, Berger SE: Learning and development in infant locomotion, *Prog Brain Res* 164:237–255, 2007.

Adolph KE, Vereijken B, Shrout PE: What changes in infant walking and why, *Child Dev* 74:475–497, 2003.

Anderson DI, Campos JJ, Rivera M, et al.: The consequences of independent locomotion for brain and psychological development. In Shephard RB, editor: *Cerebral palsy in infancy*, London, UK, 2014, Churchill Livingstone, pp 199–224.

Assaiante C: Development of locomotor balance control in healthy children, *Neurosci Biobehav Rev* 22:527–532, 1998.

Assaiante C, Amblard B: Ontogenesis of head stabilization in space during locomotion in children: influence of visual cues, *Exp Brain Res* 93:499–515, 1993.

Assaiante C, Amblard B: An ontogenetic model of the sensorimotor organization of balance control in humans, *Hum Move Sci* 14:13–43, 1995.

Basmajian JV, DeLuca CJ: *Muscles alive: their function revealed by electromyography*, ed 5, Baltimore, 1985, Williams & Wilkins.

Behrman AL, Ardolino EA, Harkema SJ: Activity-based therapy: From basic science to clinical application for recovery after spinal cord injury, *J Neurol Phys Ther* 41(Suppl 3):S39–S45, 2017. doi:10.1097/NPT.0000000000000184.

Behrman AL, Harkema SJ: Locomotor training after human spinal cord injury: a series of case studies, *Phys Ther* 80:688–700, 2000.

Behrman A, Trimble SA, Fox EJ, Howland DR: Rehabilitation and recovery in children with severe SCI. Presented at CSM Feb 6, 2014, Las Vegas.

Belmonti V, Cioni G, Berthoz A: Anticipatory control and spatial cognition in locomotion and navigation through typical development and in cerebral palsy, *Dev Med Child Neurol* 58(Suppl 4):22–27, 2016.

Belmonti V, Cioni G, Berthoz A: Development of anticipatory orienting strategies and trajectory formation in goal-oriented locomotion, *Exp Brain Res* 227:131–147, 2013.

Benjuya N, Melzer I, Kaplanski J: Aging-induced shift from reliance on sensory input to muscle co-contraction during balanced standing, *J Gerontol A Biol Sci Med Sci* 59:166–171, 2004.

Berger SE, Theuring C, Adolph KE: How and when infants learn to climb stairs, *Infant Behav Dev* 30:36–49, 2007.

Bernstein N: *The coordination and regulation of movements*, Oxford, UK, 1967, Pergamon.

Bertenthal B, Rose JL, Bai DL: Perception-action coupling in the development of visual control of posture, *J Exp Psychol Hum Percept Perform* 23:1631–1643, 1997.

Biasiucci A, Leeb R, Iturrate I, et al.: Brain-actuated functional electrical stimulation elicits lasting arm motor recovery after stroke, *Nat Commun* 9(1):2421, 2018. doi:10.1038/s41467-018-04673-z.

Bruel-Jungerman E, Rampon C, Laroche S: Adult hippocampal neurogenesis, synaptic plasticity and memory: facts and hypotheses, *Rev Neurosci* 18:93–114, 2007.

Cech D, Martin S, editors: *Functional movement development across the life span*, ed 3, St. Louis, 2012, Elsevier.

Charles J, Gordon AM: Development of hand-arm bimanual intensive training (HABIT) for improving bimanual coordination in children with hemiplegic cerebral palsy, *Dev Med Child Neurol* 48:931–936, 2006.

Charles J, Lavinder G, Gordon AM: Effects of constraint-induced therapy on hand function in children with hemiplegic cerebral palsy, *Pediatr Phys Ther* 13:68–76, 2001.

Charles JR, Wolf SL, Schneider JA, Gordon AM: Efficacy of a child-friendly form of constraint-induced movement therapy in hemiplegic cerebral palsy: a randomized control trial, *Dev Med Child Neurol* 48:635–642, 2006.

Chen LC, Metcalfe SJ, Chang TY, Jeka JJ, Clark JE: The development of infant upright posture: sway less or sway differently? *Exp Brain Res* 186:293–303, 2008.

Chen LC, Metcalfe SJ, Jeka JJ, Clark JE: Two steps forward and one back: learning to walk affects infants' sitting posture, *Infant Behav Dev* 30:16–25, 2007.

Chiviacowsky S, Wulf G, Avila L: An external focus of attention enhances motor learning in children with intellectual disabilities, *J Intellect Disabil Res* 57:627–634, 2013.

Chiviacowsky S, Wulf G, Lewthwaite R, Campos T: Motor learning benefits of self-controlled practice in persons with Parkinson's disease, *Gait Posture* 35:601–605, 2012.

Chiviacowsky S, Wulf G, Wally R: An external focus of attention enhances balance learning in older adults, *Gait Posture* 32:572–575, 2010.

de Graaf-Peters VB, Bakker H, van Eykern LA, et al.: Postural adjustments and reaching in 4- and 6-month-old infants: an EMG and kinematical study, *Exp Brain Res* 181(4):647–656, 2007.

Del Rey P, Whitehurst M, Wughalter E, et al.: Contextual interference and experience in acquisition and transfer, *Percept Mot Skills* 57:241–242, 1983.

DiFabio RP, Emasithi A: Aging and the mechanisms underlying head and postural control during voluntary action, *Phys Ther* 77:458–475, 1997.

Dobkin B, Apple D, Barbeau H, et al.: Weight-supported treadmill vs overground training for walking after acute incomplete SCI, *Neurology* 66:484–493, 2006.

Douvis SJ: Variable practice in learning the forehand drive in tennis, *Percept Mot Skills* 101:531–545, 2005.

Doyon J, Benali H: Reorganization and plasticity in the adult brain during learning of motor skills, *Curr Opin Neurobiol* 15:161–167, 2005.

Drews R, Chiviacowsky S, Wulf G: Children's motor skill learning is influenced by their conceptions of ability, *J Mot Learn Dev* 2:38–44, 2013.

Dusing SC: Postural variability and sensorimotor development in infancy, *Dev Med Child Neurol* 58(Suppl 4):17–21, 2016.

Dusing SC, Harbourne RT: Variability in postural control during infancy: implications for development, assessment, and intervention, *Phys Ther* 90:1838–1849, 2010.

Dusing SC, Tripathi T, Marcinowski EC, et al.: Supporting play exploration and early developmental intervention versus usual care to enhance development outcomes during the transition from the neonatal intensive care unit to home: a pilot randomized controlled trial, *BMC Pediatrics* 18:46, 2018. doi:10.1186/s12887-018-1011–014.

Ethier C, Gallego JA, Miller LE: Brain-controlled neuromuscular stimulation to drive neural plasticity and functional recovery, *Curr Opin Neurobiol* 33:95–102, 2015.

Etoom M, et al.: Constraint-induced movement therapy as a rehabilitation intervention for upper extremity in stroke patients: systematic review and meta-analysis, *Int J Res* 39(3):197–210, 2016.

Ferber-Viart C, Ionescu E, Morlet T, Froehlich P, Dubreauil C: Balance in healthy individuals assessed with Equitest: maturation and normative data for children and young adults, *Int J Pediatr Otorhinolaryngol* 71:1041–1046, 2007.

Field-Fote EC, Roach KE: Influence of a locomotor training approach on walking speed and distance in people with chronic spinal cord injury: a randomized clinical trial, *Phys Ther* 91(1):48–60, 2011.

Fitts PM: Categories of human learning. In Melton AW, editor: *Perceptual motor skills learning*, New York, 1964, Academic Press, pp 243–285.

Forssberg H, Nashner L: Ontogenetic development of postural control in man: adaptation to altered support and visual conditions during stance, *J Neurosci* 2:545–552, 1982.

Gabbard C: Studying action representation in children via motor imagery, *Brain Cogn* 71(3):234–239, 2009.

Gentile AM: Skill acquisition: action, movement, and neuromotor processes. In Carr JA, Shepherd RB, Gordon J, Gentile AM, Held JM, editors: *Movement science: foundations for physical therapy in rehabilitation*, Rockville, MD, 1987, Aspen, pp 93–154.

Gordon AM, Schneider JA, Chinnan A, Charles JR: Efficacy of a hand-arm bimanual intensive therapy (HABIT) in children with hemiplegic cerebral palsy: a randomized control trial, *Dev Med Child Neurol* 49:830–838, 2007.

Gordon J: Assumptions underlying physical therapy intervention. In Carr JA, Shephard RB, editors: *Movement science: foundations for physical therapy in rehabilitation*, Rockville, MD, 1987, Aspen, pp 1–30.

Granda VJ, Montilla MM: Practice schedule and acquisition, retention, and transfer of a throwing task in 6-year-old children, *Percept Mot Skills* 96:1015–1024, 2003.

Grasso R, Glasauer S, Takei Y, Berthoz A: The predictive brain: anticipatory control of head direction for the steering of locomotion, *NeuroReport* 7:1170–1174, 1996.

Hadders-Algra M: Development of postural control. In Hadders-Algra M, Carlberg EB, editors: *Postural control: a key issue in developmental disorders*, London, 2008, Mac Keith Press, pp 22–73.

Hadders-Algra M: Variation and variability: key words in human motor development, *Phys Ther* 90:1823–1837, 2010.

Hadders-Algra M, Brogren E, Forssberg H: Ontogeny of postural adjustments during sitting in infancy: variation, selection and modulation, *J Physiol* 493:287–288, 1996.

Harkema SJ, Schmidt-Read M, Lorenz DJ, et al.: Balance and ambulation improvements in individuals with chronic incomplete spinal cord injury using locomotor training-based rehabilitation, *Arch Phys Med Rehabil* 93(9):1508–1517, 2012.

Hirabayashi S, Iwasaki Y: Developmental perspective of sensory organization on postural control, *Brain Dev* 17:111–113, 1995.

Huang HH, Fetter L, Hale J, McBride A: Bound for success: a systematic review of constraint-induced movement therapy in children with cerebral palsy supports improved arm and hand use, *Phys Ther* 89:1126–1141, 2009.

Jarus T, Goverover Y: Effects of contextual interference and age on acquisition, retention, and transfer of motor skill, *Percept Mot Skills* 88:437–447, 1999.

Johnston MV: Plasticity in the developing brain: implications for rehabilitation, *Dev Disabil Res Rev* 15(2):94–101, 2009.

Jouen F: Visual-vestibular interactions in infancy, *Infant Behav Dev* 7:135–145, 1984.

Jouen F, Lepecq JC, Gapenne O, Bertenthal BI: Optic flow sensitivity in neonates, *Infant Behav Dev* 23:271–284, 2000.

Kelso JAS: *Human motor behavior*, Hillsdale, NJ, 1982, Erlbaum Associates.

Kleim JA, Jones TA: Principles of experience-dependent neural plasticity: implications for rehabilitation after brain damage, *J Speech Lang Hear Res* 51:S225–S239, 2008.

Knikou M: Neural control of locomotion and training-induced plasticity after spinal and cerebral lesions, *Clin Neurophysiol* 121:1655–1668, 2010.

Lebeer J: How much brain does a mind need? Scientific, clinical, and educational implication of ecological plasticity, *Dev Med Child Neurol* 40:352–357, 1998.

Lin KC: Effects of modified constraint-induced movement therapy on reach-to-grasp movements and functional performance after chronic stroke: a randomized controlled study, *Clin Rehabil* 21:1075–1086, 2007.

Lundy-Ekman L: *Neuroscience: fundamentals for rehabilitation*, ed 5, St. Louis, 2018, Elsevier.

Maki BE, McIlroy WE: Postural control in the older adult, *Clin Geriatr Med* 12:635–658, 1996.

Maki BE, McIlroy WE: The role of limb movements in maintaining upright stance: the "change-in-support" strategy, *Phys Ther* 77:488–507, 1997.

Maki BE, Holliday PJ, Topper AK: A prospective study of postural balance and risk of falling in an ambulatory and independent elderly population, *J Gerontol* 49:M72–M84, 1994.

Mehrholz J, Thomas S, Elsner B: Treadmill training and body weight support for walking after stroke, *Cochrane Database Syst Rev* 8:CD002840, 2017. doi:10.1002/14651858.CD002840.pub4.

Moore JL, et al.: A core set of outcome measures for adults with neurologic conditions undergoing rehabilitation: a clinical practice guideline, *J Neurol Phys Ther* 42(3):174–220, 2018. doi:10.1097/NPT.0000000000000229.

Morgan C, Novak I, Badawi N: Enriched environments and motor outcomes in cerebral palsy: systematic review and meta-analysis, *Pediatrics* 132:e735–e746, 2013. doi:10.1542/peds.2012–3985.

Morgan C, Novak I, Dale RC, et al.: Single blind randomized controlled trial of GAME (Goals-Activity-Motor Enrichment) in infants at high risk of cerebral palsy, *Res Dev Disabil* 55:256–267, 2016.

Moseley AM, Stark A, Cameron ID, Pollock A: Treadmill training and body weight support for walking after stroke, *Cochrane Database Syst Rev* 8:CD002840, 2017. doi:10.002/14651858.CD002840.pub4.

Nashner LM: Sensory, neuromuscular, and biomechanical contributions to human balance. In Duncan P, editor: *Balance: proceedings of the APTA forum*, Alexandria, VA, 1990, American Physical Therapy Association, pp 5–12.

Nudo RJ, Wise BM, SiFuentes F, et al.: Neural substrates for the effects of rehabilitation training on motor recovery following ischemic infarct, *Science* 272:1791–1794, 1996.

Palmer FB, Shapiro BK, Wachtel RC, et al.: The effects of physical therapy on cerebral palsy: a controlled trial in infants with spastic diplegia, *N Eng J Med* 318(13):803–808, 1988.

Perez CR, Meira CM, Tani G: Does the contextual interference effect last over extended transfer trials? *Percept Mot Skills* 10:58–60, 2005.

Pinto-Zipp G, Gentile AM: Practice schedules in motor learning: children vs adults, *Soc Neurosci Abstr* 21:1620, 1995.

Portfors-Yeomans CV, Riach CL: Frequency characteristics of postural control of children with and without visual impairment, *Dev Med Child Neurol* 37:456–463, 1995.

Rachwani J, Santamaria V, Saavedra SL, et al.: The development of trunk control and its relation to reaching in infancy: a longitudinal study, *Front Hum Neurosci* 9:94, 2015. doi:10.3389/fnhum.2015.00094.

Reis E: Physical therapy for people with autism, *PTinMOTIONmag*, July 2018. Available at: https://www.apta.org/PTinMotion/2018/7/Feature/Autism/.

Riach CL, Hayes KC: Anticipatory control in children, *J Mot Behav* 22:25–26, 1990.

Riach CL, Starkes JL: Velocity of center of pressure excursions as an indicator of postural control systems in children, *Gait Posture* 2:167–172, 1994.

Rival C, Ceyte H, Olivier I: Development changes of static standing balance in children, *Neurosci Lett* 376:133–136, 2005.

Rogers MW, Hain TC, Hanke TA, Janssen I: Stimulus parameters and inertial load: effects on the incidence of protective stepping responses in healthy human subjects, *Arch Phys Med Rehabil* 77:363–368, 1996.

Roncesvalles NC, Woollacott MH, Jensen JL: Development of compensatory stepping skills in children, *J Mot Behav* 32:100–111, 2000.

Saavedra S, van Donkelaar P, Woollacott MH: Learning about gravity: segmental assessment of upright control as infants develop independent sitting, *J Neurophysiol* 18:2215–2229, 2012.

Sackett DL, Straus SE, Richardson WS, Rosenberg W: *Evidence-based medicine: how to practice and teach EBM*, New York, 2000, Churchill Livingstone.

Saether R, Helbostad JL, Ripagen II, Vik T: Clinical tools to assess balance in children and adults with cerebral palsy: a systematic review, *Dev Med Child Neurol* 55:988–999, 2013.

Schmidt RA: A schema theory of discrete motor skill learning, *Psychol Rev* 82:225–260, 1975.

Schmidt R: *Motor control and learning*, Champaign, IL, 1988, Human Kinetics.

Schmidt RA, Lee TD: *Motor control and learning: a behavioral emphasis*, ed 5, Champaign, IL, 2011, Human Kinetics.

Schmidt RA, Wrisberg CA: *Motor learning and performance*, ed 5, Champaign, IL, 2013, Human Kinetics.

Shumway-Cook A, Woollacott M: The growth of stability: postural control from a developmental perspective, *J Motor Behav* 17:131–147, 1985.

Shumway-Cook A, Woollacott M: *Motor control: translating research into clinical practice*, ed 5, Philadelphia, 2017, Wolters Kluwer.

Spencer JP, Thelen E: A multimuscle state analysis of adult motor learning, *Exp Brain Res* 128:505–516, 1997.

Stengel TJ, Attermeier SM, Bly L, et al.: Evaluation of sensorimotor dysfunction. In Campbell SK, editor: *Pediatric neurologic physical therapy*, New York, 1984, Churchill Livingstone, pp 13–87.

Sturnieks DL, St George R, Lord SR: Balance disorders in the elderly, *Clin Neurophysiol* 38:467–478, 2008.

Sullivan PE, Markos PD, Minor MA: *An integrated approach to therapeutic exercise: theory and clinical application*, Reston, VA, 1982, Reston Publishing.

Taguchi K, Tada C: Change in body sway with growth of children. In Amblard B, Berthoz A, Clarac F, editors: *Posture and gait: development, adaptation and modulation*, Amsterdam, The Netherlands, 1988, Elsevier, pp 59–65.

Taub E, Miller NE, Novack TA, et al.: Technique to improve chronic motor deficit after stroke, *Arch Phys Med Rehabil* 74:347–354, 1993.

Taub E, Ramey SL, DeLuca S, et al.: Efficacy of constraint-induced movement therapy for children with cerebral palsy with asymmetric motor impairment, *Pediatrics* 113:305–312, 2004.

Thelen E: Rhythmical stereotypies in infants, *Anim Behav* 27:699–715, 1979.

Thelen E: Motor development. A new synthesis, *Am Psychol* 50:79–95, 1995.

Thelen E, Fisher DM: Newborn stepping: an explanation for a "disappearing" reflex, *Dev Psychobiol* 16:29–46, 1982.

Ulrich DA, Lloyd MC, Tiernan CW, Looper JE, Angulo-Barroso RM: Effects of intensity of treadmill training on developmental outcomes and stepping in infants with Down syndrome: a randomized trial, *Phys Ther* 88:114–122, 2008.

Ulrich DA, Ulrich BD, Angulo-Kinzler RM, Yun J: Treadmill training of infants with Down syndrome: evidence-based developmental outcomes, *Pediatrics* 108:E84, 2001.

van der Fits IB, Hadders-Algra M: The development of postural response patterns during reaching in healthy infants, *Neurosci Biobehav Rev* 22(4):521–526, 1998.

van der Heide JC, Otten B, van Eykern LA, Hadders-Algra M: Development of postural adjustments during reaching in sitting children, *Exp Brain Res* 151(1):32–45, 2003.

Vera JG, Alvarez JC, Medina MM: Effects of different practice conditions on acquisition, retention, and transfer of soccer skills by 9-year-old school children, *Percept Mot Skills* 106(2):447–460, 2008.

Vereijken B, van Emmerik REA, Whiting HTA, Newell KM: Freezing degrees of freedom in skill acquisition, *J Mot Behav* 24:133–142, 1992.

Willoughby KL, Dodd KJ, Shields N, Foley S: Efficacy of partial body weight-supported treadmill training compared with overground walking practice for children with cerebral palsy: a randomized controlled trial, *Arch Phys Med Rehabil* 91:333–339, 2010.

Wing AM, Haggard P, Flanagan J: *Hand and brain: the neurophysiology and psychology of hand movements*, New York, 1996, Academic Press.

Winstein CJ, Gardner ER, McNeal DR, et al.: Standing balance training: effect on balance and locomotion in hemiparetic adults, *Arch Phys Med Rehabil* 70:755–762, 1989.

Wolpert DM, Ghahramani Z, Jordan MI: Are arm trajectories planned in kinematic or dynamic coordinate? An adaptation study, *Exp Brain Res* 103:460–470, 1995.

Wulf G, Lewthwaite R: Optimizing performance through intrinsic motivation and attention for learning: the OPTIMAL theory of motor learning, *Psychon Bull Rev* 23:1382–1414, 2016.

Yang JF, Lamont EV, Pang MY: Split-belt treadmill stepping in infants suggests autonomous pattern generators for the left and right leg in humans, *J Neurosci* 25:6869–6876, 2005.

Motor Development

OBJECTIVES

After reading this chapter, the student will be able to:

1. Define the lifespan concept of development.
2. Understand the relationship between cognitive and motor development.
3. Discuss the major theories of motor development.
4. Identify important motor accomplishments of the first 5 years of life.
5. Describe the acquisition and refinement of fundamental movement patterns during childhood.
6. Describe age-related changes in functional movement patterns across the lifespan.
7. Describe how age-related systems' changes affect posture, balance, and gait in older adults.

INTRODUCTION

The Lifespan Concept

Normal developmental change is typically presumed to occur in a positive direction; that is, abilities are gained with the passage of time. Aging for the infant and child means being able to do more. The older infant can sit alone, and the older child can run. With increasing age, a teenager can jump higher and throw farther than an elementary school-age child. Developmental change can also occur in a negative direction. Speed and accuracy of movement decline after maturity. When one looks at the ages of the gold medal winners in the last Olympics, it is apparent that motor performance peaks in early adolescence and early adulthood. Older adults perform motor activities more slowly and take longer to learn new motor skills. Traditional views of motor development are based on the positive changes that lead to maturity and the negative changes that occur after maturity.

A true lifespan perspective of motor development includes all motor changes occurring as part of the continuous process of life. This continuous process is not a linear one but rather is a circular process. Some even describe motor development as a spiral process. Motor development does not occur in isolation of other developmental domains, such as the psychological domain or the sociocultural domain. Fig. 4.1 depicts the relationship of an individual's mind and body developing within the sociocultural environment. Movement develops within three domains: biological, psychological, and sociological.

A Lifespan Approach

The concept of lifespan development is not new. Baltes (1987) originally identified five characteristics to use when assessing a theory for its lifespan perspective. The following are criteria that must be met to be considered a lifelong perspective:

- Lifelong
- Multidimensional
- Plastic
- Embedded in history
- Multicausal

Baltes et al. (2006) reinforced the idea that development is NOT complete at maturity; it is a lifelong occurrence. The multidimensional quality of lifespan theory provides a complete framework for ontogenesis (development). Culture and the knowledge gained from all domains have a significant impact on a person's life course. Biological plasticity is accompanied by cultural competence so that a gain/loss dynamic occurs during development. There are no gains without losses and no loss without gains. In essence, this is the adaptive capacity of the person. Context, the original fifth criterion, has been replaced by multicausal meaning that one can arrive at the same destination by different means or by a combination of means. Lifespan development is not constrained to travel a single course or developmental trajectory. There is variability.

No one period of life can be understood without looking at its relationship to what came before and what lies ahead. History affects development in three ways as seen in Fig. 4.2. The normative age-graded influence is seen in those developmental tasks described by Havinghurst (1972) for each period of development. Age-graded physical, psychological, and sociological milestones would fall into this category. Walking at 12 months and obtaining a driver's license at 16 years of age are examples of physical age-graded tasks. Understanding simple concepts, such as round objects always roll, and getting along with same-age peers in adolescence are examples from the psychological and social domains. Moreover, normative history-graded influences come from the effect of when a person is born. Each of us is part of a birth cohort or group. Some of us are Baby Boomers, Millennials, or Generation Z. All people in an age cohort share the same history of events, such as the terrorist attack of 9/11, Hurricane Katrina, and the Boston Marathon bombing.

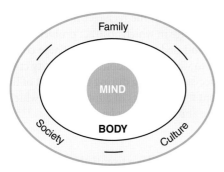

Fig. 4.1 Depiction of the relationship of an individual's psychological (mind) and physical (body) self within the sociocultural environment. (From Cech D, Martin S: *Functional movement development across the life span*, ed 3, Philadelphia, 2012, WB Saunders, p. 17.)

TABLE 4.1 Developmental Time Periods (Changes to Older Adulthood)	
Period	**Time Span**
Infancy	Birth to 2 years
Childhood	2–10 years (females)
	2–12 years (males)
Adolescence	10–18 years (females)
	12–20 years (males)
Early adulthood	18/20–40 years
Middle adulthood	40–70 years
Older adulthood	70 years to death

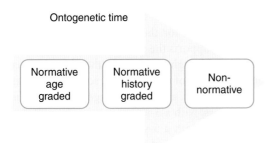

Fig. 4.2 Three major biocultural influences on lifespan development. (From Cech D, Martin S: *Functional movement development across the life span*, ed 3, Philadelphia, 2012, WB Saunders, p. 17.)

When you were born makes a difference in expectations and behaviors; these historical events shape the life of the cohort. The last history-related influence comes from things that happen to a person that have no norms or no expectations, such as winning the lottery, losing a parent, or having a child with a developmental disability. These are part of your own unique personal history. Lifespan development provides a holistic framework in which aging is a lifelong process of growing up and growing old. Biopsychosocial development is enriched when viewed from a lifespan perspective.

Lifespan View of Motor Development

The concept of motor development has been broadened to encompass any change in movement abilities that occurs across the span of life, so changes in the way a person moves after childhood are included. Motor development continues to elicit change, from conception to death. Think of the classic riddle of the pharaohs: what creeps in the morning and walks on two legs in the afternoon and on three in the evening? The answer is a human in various stages, as an infant who creeps, a toddler who walks alone throughout adulthood, and an older adult who walks with a cane at the end of life.

DEVELOPMENTAL PERIODS

Age is the most useful way to measure change in development because it is a universally recognized marker of biological, psychological, and social progression. Infants become children,

then adolescents, and finally adults at certain ages. Aging is a developmental phenomenon. Stages of cognitive development are associated with age, as are societal expectations regarding the ability of an individual to accept certain roles and functions. Defining these time periods gives everyone a common language when talking about motor development and allows comparison across developmental domains (biological, psychological, and sociological). Everyone knows that a 3-year-old child is not an adult, but when does childhood stop and adolescence begin? When does an adult become an older adult? A list of commonly defined time periods that are used throughout the text is found in Table 4.1.

Infancy

Infancy, the first period of development, spans the initial 2 years of life following birth. During this time, the infant establishes trust with caregivers and learns to be autonomous. This is an example of Erikson's first two stages of development to establish personality (Erikson, 1968). His eight stages are described in Table 4.2. The world is full of sensory experiences that can be sampled and used to learn about actions and the infant's own movement system. The infant uses sensory information to cue movement and uses movement to explore and learn about the environment. Therefore, a home must be baby-proofed to protect an extremely curious and mobile infant or toddler.

Childhood

Childhood begins at 2 years and continues until adolescence. Childhood fosters the initiative to plan and execute movement strategies and to solve daily problems. The child is extremely aware of the surrounding environment, at least one dimension at a time. During this time, she begins to use symbols, such as language, or uses objects to represent things that can be thought of but are not physically present. The blanket draped over a table becomes a fort, or pillows become chairs for a tea party. Thinking is *preoperational*, with reasoning centered on the self. Self-regulation is learned with help from parents regarding appropriate play behavior and toileting. Self-image begins to be established during this time. By 3 to 5 years of age, the preschooler has mastered many tasks, such as sharing, taking turns, and repeating the plot of a story. Childhood

TABLE 4.2   Erikson's Eight Stages of Development

Lifespan Period	Stage	Characteristics
Infancy	Trust versus mistrust	Self-trust, attachment
Late infancy	Autonomy versus shame or doubt	Independence, self-control
Childhood (pre-school)	Initiative versus guilt	Initiation of own activity
School age	Industry versus inferiority	Working on projects for recognition
Adolescence	Identity versus role confusion	Sense of self: physically, socially, sexually
Early adulthood	Intimacy versus isolation	Relationship with significant other
Middle adulthood	Generativity versus stagnation	Guiding the next generation
Late adulthood	Ego integrity versus despair	Sense of wholeness, vitality, wisdom

Adapted from Erikson E: *Identity: youth and crisis.* ©1968 by W.W. Norton & Company. Used by permission of W.W. Norton & Company.

encompasses Erikson's next two stages (see Table 4.2). The school-age child continues to work industriously for recognition on school projects or a special school fund-raising assignment. Now the child is able to classify objects according to certain characteristics, such as round, square, color, and texture. This furtherance of thinking abilities is called *concrete operations*. The student can experiment with which container holds more water (the tall, thin one or the short, fat one) or which string is longer. Confidence in one's abilities strengthens an already established positive self-image.

Adolescence

Adolescence covers the period right before, during, and after puberty, encompassing different age spans for boys and girls because of the time difference in the onset of puberty. Puberty and, therefore, adolescence begins at age 10 for girls and age 12 for boys. Adolescence is 8 years in length regardless of when it begins. Because of the age difference in the onset of adolescence, girls may exhibit more advanced social emotional behavior than their male counterparts. In a classroom of 13-year-olds, many girls are completing puberty, whereas most boys are just entering it.

Adolescence is a time of change. The identity of the individual is forged, and the values by which the person will live life are embraced. This is Erikson's fifth stage (see Table 4.2). Physical and social-emotional changes abound. A sense of the physical, psychological, social, and sexual self is usually achieved. The end result of a successful adolescence is the ability to know who one is, where one is going, and how one is going to get there. The pursuit of a career or vocation assists the teenager in moving away from the egocentrism of childhood. Cognitively, the teenager has moved into the *formal operations stage* in which abstract problems can be solved by inductive and deductive reasoning. These cognitive abilities help one to weather the adolescent identity crisis. Practicing logical decision making during this period of life prepares the adolescent for the rigors of adulthood, in which decisions become more and more complex.

Adulthood

As a concept, adulthood is a twentieth-century phenomenon. Adulthood is the longest time period of human life and the one about which the least is known. Adulthood is achieved by 20 years of age biologically, but psychologically it may be marked by as much as a 5-year transition period from late adolescence (17 years) to early adulthood (22 years). Levinson (1986) called this period the *early adulthood transition* because it takes time for the adolescent to mature into an adult. Research supports the existence of this and other transition periods. Although most of adulthood has been considered one long period of development, some researchers, such as Levinson, identify age-related stages. *Middle adulthood* begins at 40 years, with a 5-year transition from early adulthood, and it ends with a 5-year transition into *older adulthood* (age 60). Erikson's last three stages span the entirety of adulthood (see Table 4.2).

Arnett (2000, 2004, 2007) proposed a theory of emerging adulthood. The period between adolescence and the beginning of adulthood is seen as beginning at age 18 and ending at age 25. The characteristics seen during this time are: (1) a feeling of being in-between, (2) instability, (3) identity exploration, (4) self-focus, and (5) possibility. Arnett suggests that the forging of the person's identity occurs during this time period as opposed to adolescence as espoused by Erikson. Since the 60s there has been a trend to spend a longer time in education, thus delaying taking on adult roles until after graduation (Arnett et al., 2014; Arnett and Padilla-Walker, 2015).

George Vaillant (2002), a psychiatrist and director of the Harvard study of adult development, inserted two new stages into Erikson's original eight stages: career consolidation and keeper of the meaning. Career consolidation comes between Erikson's stages of intimacy and generativity. In the career consolidation stage, a person chooses a career. It begins between 20 and 40 years of age when young adults become focused on assuming a social identity within the work world. This is an extension of the person's personal identity forged in earlier stages. Vaillant (2002) identified four criteria that transform a "job" or "hobby" into a "career." They are competence, commitment, contentment, and compensation. Another stage will be discussed later in this section.

What makes a person an adult? Is there a magic age or task to be attained that indicates when a person is an adult? Legally, you are an adult at 18. However, many 18-year-olds more than likely would consider themselves as emerging adults. Regardless of the socioeconomic group a person belongs to, four criteria for adulthood continue to resound in the literature (Arnett and Padilla-Walker, 2015). To be an adult, one must accept responsibility for one's actions, make independent decisions, be more considerate of others, and be financially independent. Accepting responsibility and showing empathy for others are marks of maturity (Haddad et al., 2019).

Keeper of meaning is the additional stage Vaillant (2002) interjected between Erikson's generativity and integrity stages. It comes near the end of generativity so the person is in late middle adulthood. The role of the keeper of meaning is to preserve one's culture rather than care for successive generations. The focus is on conservation as well as preservation of society's institutions. The person in this stage guides groups and preserves traditions. Think of the interest older adults often have in genealogy as an example of this stage in development.

Family Systems

The concept of family is very broad, with families having many different structures and lifestyles. Single-parent families have increased tremendously over the past decades. Regardless of structure, family function is affected by each member of the family. This can be thought of as family dynamics or in Bronfenbrenner's (1979) ecological model as a system of interacting elements. The ecological model is seen in Fig. 4.3. Each parent affects the other, the child or children, and in turn, the child or children affect the parent. The family as a system is embedded in larger social systems, such as the extended family, neighborhood, and school and religious

organizations. All of these systems can influence the family. Recognizing the dynamics within a family is very important when establishing a therapeutic relationship. Family-centered intervention is a lifespan approach (Chiarello, 2013). Families have a life cycle in which stages and transitions have been identified. However, the reader is referred to McGoldrick et al. (2016) for an expanded and updated discussion of family.

Older Adulthood

We are aging from the moment we are born. Much is known about aging but medical research is ongoing. The major theory of aging continues to be the *free radical theory* (Mitteldorf and Fahy, 2018). It is also known as the *oxidative damage hypothesis*. Oxidative damage accumulates in the large molecules of our body, such as DNA, RNA, protein, carbohydrates, and lipids. The nervous and muscular systems are particularly susceptible to oxidative damage caused by the tissues' high metabolic rate. Systemic inflammation, increased risk of disease with advancing age, and metabolic dysregulation (increased insulin resistance) add to elimination of healthy cells (Raz and Daugherty, 2018). Age-related systems' decline can in some ways be offset by good nutrition, hydration, and exercise. The National Institute on Aging https://www.nia.nih.gov/ provides excellent science-based information on health and aging, including cognitive health, exercise and physical activity, and healthy eating.

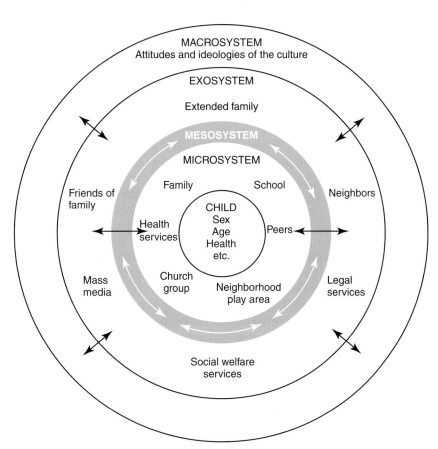

Fig. 4.3 Bronfenbrenner's ecological model is one of the few comprehensive frameworks for understanding the role of the environment in the child's development. (From Cech D, Martin S: *Functional movement development across the life span,* ed 3, 2012, WB Saunders, p. 26; Figure 2.7.)

Successful aging is possible if the older adult stays engaged mentally and physically to the best of the individual's ability. Three components of successful aging based on longitudinal studies by the MacArthur Foundation are avoiding disease and disability; having a high cognitive and physical functional capacity; and being actively engaged in life. Maximizing physical activity and participation should include all of the following types of exercises: endurance, strength, flexibility, and balance. Physical activity/exercise in a group has social value as well as physical value to safeguard health and add longevity and quality of life.

The following sections contain psychological theories that reflect the role movement may play in the development of motivation, intelligence, and perception. All of these psychologists present important information that may be helpful to you when you work with people of different ages. A lifespan perspective can assist in an understanding of motor development by acknowledging and taking into consideration the level of cognitive development the person has attained or is likely to attain.

MASLOW

Maslow (1954) identified the needs of the individual and how those needs change in relation to a person's social and psychological development. Rather than describing stages, Maslow developed a hierarchy in which each higher level depends on mastering the one before it. The last level mastered is not forgotten or lost but is built on by the next. Maslow stressed that an individual must first meet basic physiological needs to survive; then and only then can the individual meet the needs of the others. The individual fulfills *physiological needs, safety needs, needs for loving and belonging, needs for esteem*, and finally *self-actualization*. Maslow's theory is visually depicted in Fig. 4.4. A self-actualized person is self-assured, autonomous, and independent; is oriented to solving problems; and is not self-absorbed.

SELF-DETERMINATION THEORY

Self-determination is another theory of motivation which identifies three basic human needs: autonomy, competence, and relatedness (Deci and Ryan, 2000, 2008). Self-determination is the term used in the literature to describe someone who makes her own decisions. Competence is the need to master tasks important to the person. Relatedness is the need to be close and affectionate with others. Adolescents and young adults were found to make healthier life choices if they exhibited autonomous motivation and competence (Ryan et al., 2008). This theory can be used to assess youth with special health care needs (SHCN) readiness to transition from pediatric to adult-oriented health care. Only 40% of adolescents with SHCN meet core outcomes for transition (McManus et al., 2013). Intrinsic motivation has also been linked to increased attention and learning (Di Dominico and Ryan, 2017).

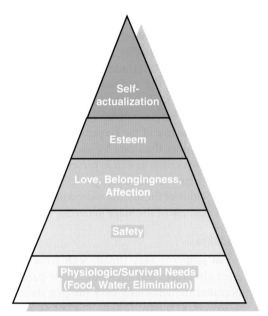

Fig. 4.4 Maslow's hierarchy. (From Cech D, Martin S, editors: *Functional movement development across the life span*, ed 3, Philadelphia, 2012, WB Saunders.)

DEVELOPMENTAL COGNITIVE THEORY: PIAGET

Piaget (1952) developed a theory of intelligence based on the behavioral responses of his children. He designated the first 2 years of life the *sensorimotor stage of intelligence*. During this stage, the infant learns to understand the world by associating sensory experiences with physical actions. Piaget called these associations *schemas*. The infant develops schemas for looking, eating, and reaching, to name just a few. From 2 to 7 years is the *preoperational stage of intelligence* during which the child is able to represent the world by symbols, such as words and objects. The increased use of language is the beginning of symbolic thought. During the next stage called *concrete operations*, logical thought occurs. Between 7 and 11 years of age, children can mentally reverse information. For example, if they learned that 6 plus 4 equals 10, then 4 plus 6 would also equal 10. The last stage is that of *formal operations*, which Piaget thought began at 12 years of age. Although research has not completely supported the specific chronologic years to which Piaget attributed these stages, the stages do occur in this order. The stage of formal operations begins in adolescence, which, according to our time periods, begins at 10 years in girls and at 12 years in boys. Piaget's stages are related to developmental age in Table 4.3.

Piaget studied the development of intelligence up to adolescence, when *abstract thought* becomes possible. Because abstract thought is the highest level of cognition, he did not continue to look at what happened to intelligence after maturity. Because Piaget's theory does not cover the entire lifespan, it does not represent a lifespan approach to intellectual development. However, Piaget does offer useful information about how an infant can and should interact with the

TABLE 4.3 Piaget's Stages of Cognitive Development

Lifespan Period	Stage	Characteristics
Infancy	Sensorimotor	Pairing of sensory and motor reflexes leads to purposeful activity
Preschool	Preoperational	Unidimensional awareness of environment Begins use of symbols
School age	Concrete operational	Solves problems with real objects Classification, conservation
Pubescence	Formal operational	Solves abstract problems Induction, deduction

Data from Piaget J: *Origins of intelligence*, New York, 1952, International University Press.

environment during the first 2 years of life. These first 2 years are critical to the development of intelligence. Regardless of the age of the child, the cognitive level must always be taken into account when one plans therapeutic intervention.

PERCEPTUAL-COGNITIVE THEORY

Perception has been linked to cognition from the beginning of the field of psychology. Piaget linked sensation to movement as an initial step in the development of intelligence. Eleanor Gibson championed the perceptual-cognitive theory of cognition. She pioneered the view that perception has the ability to detect order and structure, not just to organize sensory information. Her research and those that followed her focus on how perception guides action (Pick and Gibson, 1992).

The goal of perception is action (Gibson, 1979). Perception of the surrounding environment, which includes objects and people, serves the functional purpose to bring about contact and interaction. The objects afford the opportunity to act; in acting, the object and action are changed. This is the concept of *affordance* (Gibson, 1982). Affordance goes beyond adaptation and integration because both the object and perceiver are changed in the encounter. A jungle gym may afford a seat for one child or a place to hang upside down for another child. Perception is the means by which the child comes in contact with the world and adapts to it. The ecological view of perceptual development does not require the child to construct actions with objects as did Piaget's model. Gibson's concept of environmental affordance highlights the ecological perspective of cognition. The quality of the learning environment and the affordances available to the learner can have an impact on the development of cognitive abilities.

GROUNDED COGNITION

Grounded cognition is a concept in which cognition is embedded in the environment and the body (Barsalou, 2010). It has also been described as embodied cognition in which

intelligence develops from the interaction of the child within the environment as a result of sensorimotor experiences. This theory is similar to the perception-action theory in which the child makes use of perceptual motor experiences to develop cognition in a learning to learn paradigm. Perception and action are both required to build the brain. There appears to be a strong connection between what our bodies do and what we know about what our bodies do. Researchers have called for therapists to recognize that the development of object interaction, sitting and reaching, and locomotion are models of grounded cognition (Lobo et al., 2013).

THEORY OF MIND

Theory of mind is a concept whereby children learn to understand human behavior. It is a process that is supported by development of family interaction, pretend play, language, and executive function. Development of theory of mind begins in infancy with the development of joint attention. Usually an adult and an infant will mutually attend to the same object or action. When children learn to pretend play around 2 years of age they show that they can substitute one object for another. Pretend play requires that a child be able to have a mental representation of and object in the mind. As the child gets older he builds on the pretense and is able to separate things from the thoughts about them (Astington and Barriault, 2001). Theory of mind develops within the first 5 years of life. Three-year-olds are aware of others' wants, feelings, and perceptions and preschoolers understand the role of mental states when pretending (Ganea et al., 2004). It appears that the same symbolic phenomenon that underpins pretend play also underpins theory of mind. Understanding the mental world seems to be critically important for learning from others (Carlson et al., 2013)

MOTOR LEARNING COGNITIVE THEORY

Movement is also a way of exerting control over the environment. Remember the old sayings: "mind over matter" and "I think I can." Learning to control the environment begins with controlling one's own body. Gravity is a force to be reckoned with in the typical newborn. What worked in utero does not translate to the postpartum world. Postural control is learned by moving and integrating sensory information to reinforce posture. Learning to learn to move takes lots of practice. The first stage of motor learning according to Fitts (1964) does involve cognition. (See the previous chapter for the stages of motor learning.) To interact with objects and people within the environment, the child must be oriented within space. We learn spatial relationships by first orienting to our own bodies, then using ourselves as a reference point to map our movements within the environment. Physical educators and coaches have used the ability of the athlete to know where he or she is on the playing field or the court to better anticipate the athlete's own or the ball's movement.

Motor Imagery

Motor control is needed for motor learning, for the execution of motor programs, and for acquisition of motor skills. The areas of the brain involved in idea formation can be active in triggering movement. Movement is affected by the ability of the mind to understand the rules of moving. Children around the age of 5 begin to develop the ability to imagine motion or mentally represent action (Gabbard, 2009). This is termed motor imagery. Motor imagery is functionally equivalent to motor planning. A positive association exists between motor abilities in children and their motor imagery (Gabbard et al., 2012). Problems with motor imagery are associated with motor control problems seen in children with cerebral palsy (Craje et al., 2010). Spruijt et al. (2015) reviewed the literature on motor imagery and concluded motor imagery training could be a beneficial addition to pediatric rehabilitation in children at 5 years. Children continue to show improvements in this ability even into adolescence (Molina et al., 2008; Choudhury et al., 2007).

The role of mentally visualizing movement as a way to improve motor performance is well documented in the literature (Wang and Morgan, 1992). Sports psychologists have extensively studied cognitive behavioral strategies, including motivation, and recognize how powerful these strategies can be in improving motor performance (Meyers et al., 1996; Frank and Schack, 2017). We have all had experience with trying to learn a motor skill that we were interested in as opposed to one in which we had no interest. Think of the look on an infant's face as she attempts that first step; one little distraction and down she goes. Think also of how hard you may have to concentrate to master in-line skating; would you dare to think of other things while careening down a sidewalk for the first time?

MASTERY MOTIVATION

Motivation to move comes from intellectual curiosity. Typically developing children are innately curious about the movement potential of their bodies. Infants become visually aware of their own movement. This optically produced awareness is called visual proprioception (Gibson, 1966; Gibson, 1979). Locomotion affords toddlers more exploration of the environment, which supports psychological development (Anderson et al., 2014; Gibson and Pick, 2000). Mastery motivation is the multifaceted psychological force that encourages the child to master a more challenging task (Wang et al., 2013). The task could be playing with toys, playing with other children, or learning to ride a bike. Children move to be involved in some sports-related activities, such as tee-ball or soccer. Adolescents often define themselves by their level of performance on the playing field, so a large part of their identity is connected to their athletic prowess. Adults may routinely participate in sports-related activities as part of their leisure time. One hopes that activity is part of a commitment to fitness developed early in life.

SOCIAL COGNITIVE LEARNING

Lev Vygotsky, a Russian psychologist, thought that cognitive development could take place only as a result of social interaction (Vygotsky, 1986). The child partners with an adult who assists the child's learning. The adult provides the tools of the particular culture, such as alphabetical and numbering schemes, and its concepts about distance and time. He called that support given by the other person *scaffolding*. Anyone who has watched a building being erected can grasp this concept. In this instance, the support is given for learning and problem solving. Unlike Piaget, who thought children became little scientists on their own, Vygotsky thought that the nature of cognitive development could only be understood within a cultural and social context. The *zone of proximal development* is the area of performance or level of performance that a child can demonstrate when assisted that is not possible when left to work on her own. This zone is the potential for growth in cognitive abilities that is made possible by the assistance of a skilled adult or peer. Vygotsky thought that children could not make significant progress alone. He and Piaget both appreciated the role of play in cognitive development (Vygotsky, 1966; Piaget, 1951). (See Chapter 5 for a discussion of play development.)

INFLUENCE OF COGNITION ON MOTOR DEVELOPMENT

Motor development, motor control, and motor learning are influenced to varying degrees by a person's intellectual ability. Impairments in cognitive ability can affect an individual's ability to learn to move and adapt movement to tasks in varying environments. A child with intellectual disability may not have the ability to learn movement skills at the same rate as a child of average intelligence. The rate of developmental change in a child with an intellectual disability is decreased in all domains: biological, psychological, and sociological. Thus, acquisition of motor skills is often as delayed as the acquisition of other knowledge. Just as cognition can affect motor development, the motor system can affect cognition. Diamond (2000), Piek et al. (2008), and Pitcher et al. (2011) linked motor development and subsequent cognitive ability. The close interrelation of the prefrontal cortex and the cerebellum parallels the protracted development of the motor system. Motor experience can have an impact on cognition. Motor development of children between birth and 4 years predicted cognitive performance at school age (Piek et al., 2008). The most negative outcomes of being born premature and having a low birth weight are impaired motor, cognitive, and language development (Lebarton and Iverson, 2016; Leisman et al., 2016). Marrus and a team of investigators (2018) described neural networks of early motor development. They suggest that changes in the developing networks explain the emergence of gross motor abilities in toddlers. Motor learning requires cognitive operations, such as object permanence, means/end, and joint attention.

Object Permanence/Means End

The child must perceive the world and the objects in the world as being real. This is the concept of object permanence. The classic experiment to see if the child has object permanence is to partially cover a ball with a cloth and see if the child will recognize the object as being present when only part of it is visible. Once object permanence is present, the child may be enticed to engage in object exploration. Object play is associated with the emergence of words (Lifter and Bloom, 1989). A concept from Piaget in which the child uses an object or person to perform an action on another object is called means-end. An example of means-end is using a stick to bring an object closer so it can be grasped. Means end is an example of early cause and effect learning.

Joint Attention

The ability to jointly attend supports cognitive and motor learning. Joint attention occurs when two individuals, usually a parent and child, attend to the same object or event. Attention is necessary for motor learning and socialization. Without joint attention, the parent would not be able to engage the child socially or to have an opportunity to scaffold behavior. Joint attention affords an opportunity to create a zone of proximal development. Children with autism have poor joint attention. (See Chapter 9 for more information on children with autism.) Joint attention is related to language development and motor imitation (Dalton et al., 2017).

THEORIES OF MOTOR DEVELOPMENT

The two major theories of motor development are the dynamic systems theory and the neuronal group selection theory. These theories best reflect the state of our current knowledge about motor development. According to dynamic systems theory (DST) movement emerges from the interaction of multiple body systems (Thelen and Smith, 1994). DST incorporates the developmental biomechanical aspects of the mover, along with the developmental status of the mover's nervous system, the environmental context in which the movement occurs, and the task to be accomplished by the movement. The acquisition of postural control and balance are driven by the requirement of the specific task demands and the demands of gravity. Movement abilities associated with the developmental sequence are the result of selective motor control, which organizes movements into efficient patterns. DST is both a theory of motor control and of motor development. The brain and the neuromotor systems must interact to meet the developmental demands of the mover.

Growth, maturation, and adaptation of all body systems contribute to the acquisition of movement, not just the nervous system. Movement emerges from the interaction of all body systems, the task at hand, and the environment in which it takes place. To acquire motor skills, the mover has to control the number of planes of motion possible at a single joint and then multiple joints. This is the degrees of freedom problem discussed in Chapter 3. Bernstein thought that the new or novice mover minimized the number of independent movement elements used until control was developed. The new walker is a great example of controlling degrees of freedom. The upper trunk is kept in extension by placing the arms in high guard while the lower trunk is kept stable by anteriorly tilting the pelvis. The infant is left with only having to pick up each leg at a time as if stepping in place. A little forward momentum is used to propel the new walker.

Neuronal group selection theory proposes that motor skills result from the interaction of developing body dynamics and the structure or functions of the brain. The brain's structures are changed by how the body is used (moved). The brain's growing neural networks are sculpted to match efficient movement solutions. Three requirements must be met for neuronal selection to be effective in a motor system. First, a basic repertoire of movement must be present. Second, sensory information has to be available to identify and select adaptive forms of movement, and third, there must be a way to strengthen the preferred movement responses.

The infant is genetically endowed with spontaneously generated motor behaviors. Fig. 4.5 illustrates rudimentary neural networks that produce initial motor behaviors. This example

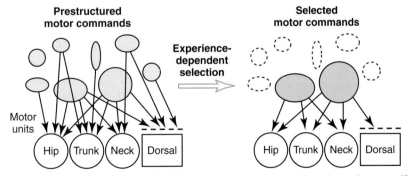

Fig. 4.5 A developmental process according to the neuronal group selection theory is exemplified by the development of postural muscle activation patterns in sitting infants. Before independent sitting, the infant exhibits a large variation of muscle activation patterns in response to external perturbations, including a backward body sway. Various postural muscles on the ventral side of the body are contracted in different combinations, sometimes together with inhibition of the dorsal muscles. Among the large repertoire of response patterns are those later used by adults. With increasing age, the variability decreases and fewer patterns are elicited. Finally, only the complete adult muscle activation patterns remain. If balance is trained during the process, the selection is accelerated. (Redrawn from Forssberg H: Neural control of human motor development, *Curr Opin Neurobiol* 9:676–682, 1999.)

involves activation of postural muscles in sitting infants. As the infant's multiple sensory systems provide perception, the strength of synaptic connections between brain circuits varies with selection of some networks that predispose one action over another. Environmental and task demands become part of the neural ensemble for producing movements. Spatial maps are formed and mature neural networks emerge as a product of use and sensory feedback. The maps that develop via the process of neuronal selection are preferred pathways. They become preferred because they are the ones that are used more often. Neurons that fire together wire together. Large amounts of the nervous system are interconnected in order to organize perception, cognition, emotion, and movement.

The theory of neuronal group selection supports a dynamic systems theory of motor control/motor development. According to neuronal group selection, the brain and nervous system are guided during development by a genetic blueprint and initial activity, which establishes rudimentary neuronal circuits. These early neuronal circuits are examples of self-organization. The use of certain circuits over others reinforces synaptic efficacy and strengthens those circuits. This is the selectivity that comes from exploring different ways of moving. Lastly, maps are developed that provide the organization of patterns of spontaneous movement in response to mover and task demands. The linking of these early perception-action categories is the cornerstone of development (Edelman, 1987). Other body systems, such as the skeletal, muscular, cardiovascular, and pulmonary, develop and interact with the nervous system so that the most efficient movement pattern is chosen for the mover. According to this theory, there are no motor programs. The brain is not thought of as a computer and movement is not hardwired. This theory supports the idea that neural plasticity may be a constant feature across the lifespan. Neural plasticity is the ability to adapt structures in the nervous system to support desired functions. Neurons that fire together wire together. Movement variability has always been considered a hallmark of normal movement. Integration of multiple systems allows for a variety of movement strategies to be used to perform a functional task. In other words, think of how many different ways a person can reach for an object or how many different ways it is possible for a person to move across a room.

DEVELOPMENTAL CONCEPTS

The concepts about human development are presented to help organize information on motor development. There is a sequence to early motor development; however, the sequence exhibits variability. The age of acquisition of specific motor skills is used to diagnosis delayed motor performance.

Epigenesis

Motor development is *epigenetic. Epigenesis* is a theory of development that states that a human being grows and develops from a simple organism to a more complex one through progressive differentiation. *Epigenesis* is the process by which the environmental influences alter genetic expression.

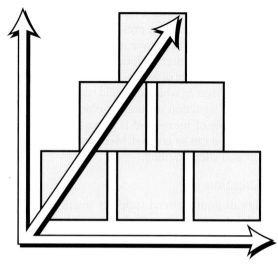

Fig. 4.6 Epigenetic development.

Epigenesis recognizes the role of the biological, psychological, and sociological environments that support and change the genetics of the person. An example from the plant world is the description of how a simple, round seed becomes a beautiful marigold. Motor development generally occurs in an orderly sequence, based on what has come before; not like a tower of blocks, built one on top of the other, but like a pyramid, with a foundation on which the next layer overlaps the preceding one. This pyramid allows for growth and change to occur in more than one direction at the same time (Fig. 4.6).

DEVELOPMENTAL SEQUENCE

The developmental sequence is generally recognized to consist of the development of head control, rolling, sitting, creeping, and walking (Gesell, 1940). The sequence of acquisition of motor skills has previously been known as *motor milestones*. The rate of change in acquiring each skill may vary from child to child within a family, among families, and among families of different cultures. Sequences may overlap as the child works on several levels of skills at the same time. For example, a child can be perfecting rolling while learning to balance in sitting. The lower-level skill does not need to be perfect before the child goes on to try something new. Some children even bypass a motor skill, such as creeping, and go on to another higher-level skill, such as walking, without doing any harm developmentally.

Cephalocaudal Development

Gesell (1974) recognized that development of postural control proceeded from cephalic to caudal and proximal to distal during postnatal development. Head control in infants begins with neck movements and is followed by development of trunk control. Postnatal postural development mirrors what happens in the embryo when the primitive spinal cord closes. Closure occurs first in the cervical area and then progresses in two directions at once, toward the head and the tail of the embryo. The infant develops head and neck and then trunk

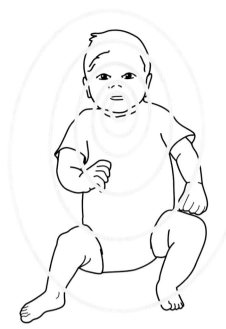

Fig. 4.7 Infant and spiral development.

control. Overlap exists between the development of head-and-trunk control; think of a spiral beginning around the mouth and spreading outward in all directions encompassing more and more of the body (Fig. 4.7). Development of postural control of the head and neck can be a rate-limiting factor in early motor development. If control of the head and neck is not mastered, subsequent motor development will be delayed.

Proximal to Distal Development

As a linked structure, the axis or midline of the body must provide a stable base for head, eye, and extremity movements to occur with any degree of control. The trunk is the stable base for head movement above and for limb movements distally. Imagine what would happen if you could not maintain an erect sitting posture without the use of your arms and you tried to use your arms to catch a ball thrown to you. You would have to use your arms for support, and if you tried to catch the ball, you would probably fall. Or imagine not being able to hold your head up. What chance would you have of being able to follow a moving object with your eyes? Early in development, the infant works to establish midline neck control by lifting the head from the prone position, then establishes midline trunk control by extending the spine against gravity, followed by establishing proximal shoulder and pelvic girdle stability through weight bearing. In some positions, the infant uses the external environment to support the head and trunk to move the arms and legs. Reaching with the upper extremities is possible early in development but only with external trunk support, as when placed in an infant seat in which the trunk is supported.

Dissociation/Fractionation

Development proceeds from *mass movements* to *specific movements* or from simple movements to complex movements.

This concept can be interpreted in several different ways. *Mass* can refer to the whole body, and *specific* can refer to smaller parts of the body. For example, when an infant moves, the entire body moves; movement is not isolated to a specific body part. The infant learns to move the body as one unit, as in log rolling, before she is able to move separate parts. The ability to separate movement in one body part from movement in another body part is called *dissociation*. Mature movements are characterized by *dissociation*, and typical motor development provides many examples. When an infant learns to turn her head in all directions without trunk movement, the head is said to be dissociated from the trunk. Reaching with one arm from a prone on elbows position is an example of dissociation of limb movement from the trunk. While the infant creeps on hands and knees, her limb movements are dissociated from trunk movement. Additionally, when the upper trunk rotates in one direction and the lower trunk rotates in the opposite direction during creeping (counter-rotation), the upper trunk is dissociated from the lower trunk and vice versa. Fractionation is another term sometimes used to describe how movement is broken down or fractionated into component parts. For example, babies go from having a mass grasp with all fingers moving into or away from the palm to being able to isolate or fractionate movement so that only one finger is isolated as a pointer.

Stability/Instability

Periods of stability and instability of motor actions have been observed by many people who have studied development. Gesell et al. (1974) described cyclic changes in motor control of children over the course of early development. Periods of equilibrium were balanced by periods of disequilibrium. Head control, which appeared to be fairly good at one age, was seen to lessen at an older age, only to recover as the infant developed further. At each stage of development, abilities emerge, merge, regress, or are replaced. During periods of disequilibrium, movement patterns regress to what was present at an earlier time, but after a while, new patterns emerge with newfound control. At other times, motor abilities learned in one context, such as control of the head in the prone position, may need to be relearned when the postural context is changed; for example, when the child is placed in a sitting position. Some patterns of movement appear at different periods, depending on need. One of the better examples of a reappearance of a pattern of movement is seen in the use of scapular adduction. Initially, this pattern of movement is used by the infant to reinforce upper trunk extension in the prone position. Later in development, the toddler uses the pattern again to maintain upper trunk extension as she begins to walk. This use in walking is described as a high-guard position of the arms.

Variation and Variability

Motor development can be described as occurring in two phases of variability. During the initial phase of variability, motor patterns are extremely variable as the mover explores

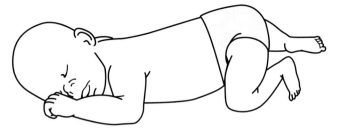

Fig. 4.8 Physiologic flexion in a newborn.

all kinds of possible movement combinations. The sensory information generated by these movements continues to shape the nervous system's development as shown in Fig. 4.5. Self-produced sensorimotor experience plays a pivotal role in motor development (Hadders-Algra, 2010; Dusing, 2016). All basic motor functions are thought to reach a beginning stage of secondary variability around 18 months of age. These basic motor functions include posture and locomotion as well as reaching and grasping. Variation and variability have always been considered hallmarks of typical motor development. Children who move in stereotypical ways or appear stuck in a restricted pattern of movement have been deemed to be at risk. Assessment of variability in postural control during infancy is now being used to identify motor problems (Novak et al., 2017).

Biomechanical Considerations in Motor Development

Some movements are easier to perform at certain times during development. Factors affecting movement include the biomechanics of the situation, muscle strength, level of neuromuscular maturation, and postural control. Full-term babies are born with predominant flexor muscle tone (*physiologic flexion*). The limbs and trunk naturally assume a flexed position (Fig. 4.8). As development progresses active movement toward extension occurs if the infant spends time in a prone position. Babies have a C-shaped spine at birth. Exposure to head lifting in prone develops the secondary cervical curve. Without exposure to the prone position in the form of *tummy time*, the ability of the infant to lift and turn the head is diminished. The risk of plagiocephaly or a misshapen head is increased, because in supine, the infant tends to assume an asymmetric head posture. The neck muscles are not strong enough to maintain the head in midline while in supine. *Tummy time* is essential to encourage lifting and turning of the head to strengthen the neck muscles bilaterally.

DEVELOPMENTAL PROCESSES

Motor development is a result of three processes: growth, maturation, and adaptation.

Growth

Growth is any increase in dimension or proportion. Examples of ways that growth is typically measured include size, height, weight, and head circumference. Infants' and children's growth is routinely tracked at the pediatrician's office by use of growth charts (Fig. 4.9). Growth is an important parameter of change during development because some changes in motor performance can be linked to changes in body size. Typically, the taller a child grows, the farther she can throw a ball. Strength gains with age have been linked to increases in a child's height and weight. Failure to grow or discrepancies between two growth measures can be an early indicator of a developmental problem.

Maturation

Maturation is the result of physical changes caused by pre-programmed internal body processes. Maturational changes are those that are genetically guided, such as myelination of nerve fibers, the appearance of primary and secondary bone growth centers (ossification centers), increasing complexity of internal organs, and the appearance of secondary sexual characteristics. Some growth changes, such as those that occur at the ends of long bones (*epiphyses*), occur as a result of maturation; when the bone growth centers (under genetic control) are active, length increases. After these centers close, growth is stopped, and no more change in length is possible.

Adaptation

Adaptation is the process by which environmental influences guide growth and development. Adaptation occurs when physical changes are the result of external stimulation. An infant adapts to being exposed to a contagion, such as chickenpox, by developing antibodies. The skeleton is remodeled during development in response to weight bearing and muscular forces (*Wolfe's law*) exerted on it during functional activities. As muscles pull on bone, the skeleton adapts to maintain the appropriate musculotendinous relationships with the bony skeleton for efficient movement. This same adaptability can cause skeletal problems if musculotendinous forces are abnormal (unbalanced) or misaligned and may thus produce a deformity.

MOTOR SKILLS

The attainment of typical motor abilities and the ages at which these skills can be expected to occur can be found in Tables 4.4 and 4.5. Remember there are wide variations in time frames during which motor skills are typically achieved.

Head Control

An infant should exhibit good head control by 4 months of age. The infant should be able to keep the head in line with the body (ear in line with the acromion) when he or she is pulled to sit from the supine position (Fig. 4.10). When the infant is held upright in a vertical position and is tilted in any direction, the head should tilt in the opposite direction. A 4-month-old infant, when placed in a prone position, should be able to lift the head up against gravity past 45 degrees (Fig. 4.11). The infant acquires an additional component of antigravity head control, the ability to flex the head from supine position, at 5 months.

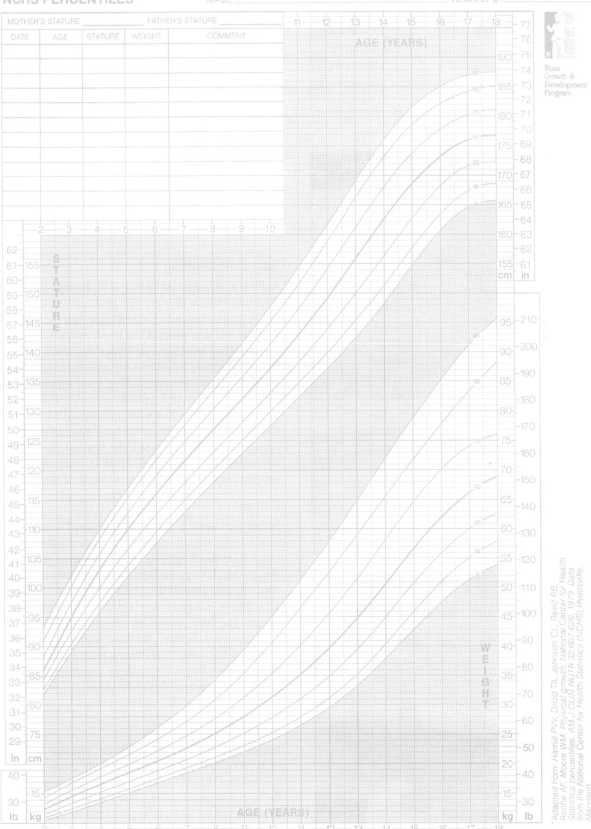

Fig. 4.9 Growth chart. (Used with permission of Ross Products Division, Abbott Laboratories Inc., Columbus, OH 43216. From NCHS Growth Charts, Ross Products Division, Abbott Laboratories Inc.)

TABLE 4.4   Infant Motor Skills

Motor Skill	Age
Head control (no head lag when pulled to sit)	4 months
Roll segmentally supine to prone	6–8 months
Sit alone steadily	6–8 months
Creep reciprocally, pulls to stand	8–9 months
Cruising	10–11 months
Walk alone	12 months

TABLE 4.5   Reach, Grasp, and Release Progression

Motor Action/Skill	Age
Visual regard of objects	0–2 months
Swipes at objects	1–3 months
Visually directed reaching	3.5–4.5 months
Reaching from prone on elbow	6 months
Retains objects placed in hand	4 months
Palmar grasp	6 months
Radial-palmar grasp	7 months
Scissors grasp	8 months
Radial-digital grasp	9 months
Inferior pincer	10–12 months
Superior pincer	12 months
Three-jaw chuck	12 months
Involuntary release	1–4 months
Transfers at midline	4 months
Transfers across body	7 months
Voluntary release	7–10 months
Releases a block into small container	12 months
Releases pellet into small container	15 months

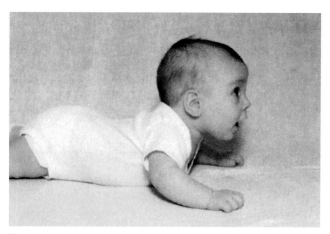

Fig. 4.11 **Head Lifting in Prone.** A 4-month-old infant lifts and maintains head past 45 degrees in prone. (From Wong DL: *Whaley and Wong's essentials of pediatric nursing*, ed 5, St. Louis, 1997, Mosby.)

Segmental Rolling

Rolling is an acquired motor skill. Infants log roll (at 4 to 6 months) before they are able to demonstrate segmental rotation (at 6 to 8 months). When log rolling the head and trunk move as one unit without any trunk rotation. Segmental rolling or rolling with separate upper and lower trunk rotation should be accomplished by 6 to 8 months of age. Rolling from prone to supine precedes rolling from supine to prone, because extensor control typically precedes flexor control. The prone position provides some mechanical advantage because the infant's arms are under the body and can push against the support surface. If the head, the heaviest part of the infant, moves laterally, gravity will assist in bringing it toward the support surface and will cause a change of position.

Sitting

Sitting represents a change in functional orientation for the infant. Previously the norm for achieving independent sitting was 8 months of age (Fig. 4.12). However, according to the World Health Organization (WHO) (2006) the mean age at which infants around the world now sit is 6.1 months (SD of 1.1). *Sitting independently* is defined as sitting alone when placed. The back should be straight, without any kyphosis (forward trunk flexion). No hand support is needed. The infant does not have to assume a sitting position, but is expected to free hands for reaching and manipulating objects/people. Independent sitting develops over several months as postural control of the trunk improves.

Creeping and Cruising

Babies may first crawl on their tummy, but according to WHO (2006), infants reciprocally creep on all fours at 8.5 months (SD 1.7) (see Fig. 4.13). *Reciprocal* means that the opposite arm and leg move together and leave the other opposite pair of limbs to support the weight of the body. By 10 to 11 months of age, most infants are pulling up to stand and are cruising around furniture. *Cruising* is walking sideways while being supported by hands or tummy on a surface

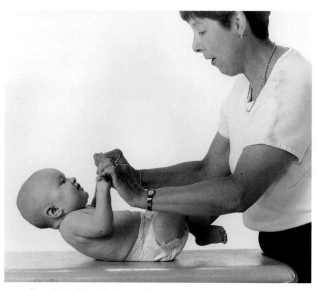

Fig. 4.10 Head in line with the body when pulled to sit.

(Fig. 4.14). The coffee table and couch are perfect for this activity because they are usually the correct height to provide sufficient support to the infant (Fig. 4.14). Some infants skip crawling on the belly and go into creeping on hands and knees. Other infants skip both forms of prone movement and pull to stand and begin to walk.

Walking

The last major gross motor milestone is walking (Fig. 4.15). The new walker assumes a wide base of support, with legs abducted and externally rotated; exhibits lumbar lordosis; and holds the arms in high guard with scapular adduction. The traditional age range for this skill has been 12 to 18 months; however, an infant as young as 7 months may demonstrate this ability. Children demonstrate great variability in achieving this milestone. The most important motor skills to acquire are probably head control and sitting, because if an infant is unable to achieve control of the head and trunk, control of extremity movements will be difficult if not impossible. WHO (2006) gives an average age of 12.1 months (SD 1.8) for children to accomplish independent movement in upright. There are ethnic differences in the typical age of walking. African-American children have been found to walk earlier (10.9 months) (Capute et al., 1985), whereas some Caucasian children walk as late as 15.5 months (Bayley, 2005). It is acceptable for a child to be ahead of typical

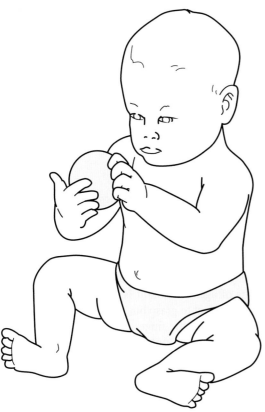

Fig. 4.12 Sitting independently.

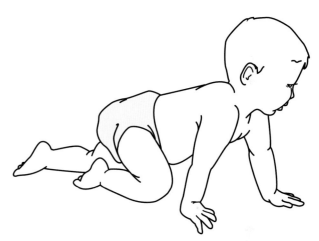

Fig. 4.13 Reciprocal creeping.

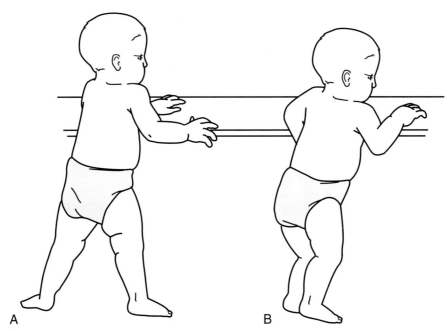

Fig. 4.14 **A** and **B,** Cruising around furniture.

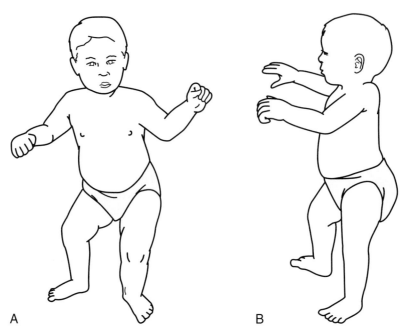

Fig. 4.15 **A** and **B,** Early walking: wide stance, pronated feet, arms in high guard, "potbelly," and lordotic back.

developmental guidelines; however, delays in achieving these milestones are cause for concern.

Reach, Grasp, and Release

Reaching patterns influence the ability of the hand to grasp objects. Reaching patterns depend on the position of the shoulder. Take a moment to try the following reaching pattern. Elevate your scapula and internally rotate your shoulder before reaching for the pencil on your desk. Do not compensate with forearm supination, but allow your forearm to move naturally into pronation. Although it is possible for you to obtain the pencil using this reaching pattern, it would be much easier to reach with the scapula depressed and the shoulder externally rotated. Reaching is an upper arm phenomenon. The position of the shoulder can dictate which side of the hand is visible. *Prehension* is the act of grasping. To prehend or grasp an object, one must reach for it.

Vision is used to entice the infant to reach, but is not initially used to guide the reach. Development of reach, grasp, and release is presented in Table 4.5.

Hand Regard

The infant first recognizes the hands at 2 months of age, when they enter the field of vision (Fig. 4.16). The asymmetric tonic neck reflex, triggered by head turning, allows the arm on the face side of the infant to extend and therefore is in a perfect place to be seen or regarded. Because of the predominance of physiologic flexor tone in the newborn, the hands are initially loosely fisted. The infant can visually regard other objects, especially if presented to the peripheral vision.

Reflexive and Palmar Grasp

The first type of grasp seen in the infant is *reflexive,* meaning it happens in response to a stimulus, in this case, touch. In a newborn, touch to the palm of the hand once it opens, especially on the ulnar side, produces a reflexive palmar grasp. Reflexive grasp is replaced by a voluntary palmar grasp by 6 months of age. The infant is no longer compelled by the touch of an object to grasp but may grasp voluntarily. *Palmar grasp* involves just the fingers coming into the palm of the hand; the thumb does not participate.

Voluntary Grasp

Once grasp is voluntary at 6 months, a progressive change occurs in the form of the grasp. At 7 months, the thumb begins to adduct, and this allows for a radial-palmar grasp. The radial side of the hand is used along with the thumb to pick up small objects, such as 1-inch cubes. Radial palmar grasp is replaced by radial-digital grasp as the thumbs begin to oppose (Figs. 4.17 and 4.18) Objects can then be grasped by the ends of the fingers, rather than having to be brought into the palm of the hand. The next two types of grasp involve the thumb and index finger only and

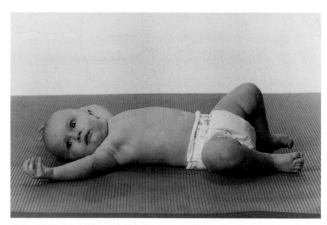

Fig. 4.16 Hand regard aided by an asymmetric tonic neck reflex.

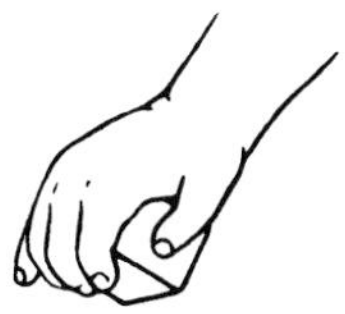

Fig. 4.17 Age 7 months: radial palmar grasp (thumb adduction begins); mouthing of objects. (From Cech D, Martin S, editors: *Functional movement development across the life span*, ed 3, Philadelphia, 2012, WB Saunders.)

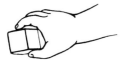

Fig. 4.18 Age 9 months: radial digital grasp (beginning opposition). (From Cech D, Martin S, editors: *Functional movement development across the life span*, ed 3, Philadelphia, 2012, WB Saunders.)

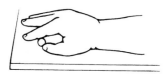

Fig. 4.19 Age 9 to 12 months: inferior pincer grasp (isolated index pointing). (From Cech D, Martin S, editors: *Functional movement development across the life span*, ed 3, Philadelphia, 2012, WB Saunders.)

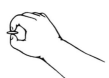

Fig. 4.20 Age 1 year: superior pincer grasp (tip to tip). (From Cech D, Martin S, editors: *Functional movement development across the life span*, ed 3, Philadelphia, 2012, WB Saunders.)

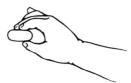

Fig. 4.21 Age 1 year: three-jaw chuck grasp (wrist extended with ulnar deviation); maturing release. (From Cech D, Martin S, editors: *Functional movement development across the life span*, ed 3, Philadelphia, 2012, WB Saunders.)

are called *pincer grasps*. In the inferior pincer grasp, the thumb is on the lateral side of the index finger, as if you were to pinch someone (Fig. 4.19). In the superior pincer grasp, the thumb and index finger are tip to tip, as in picking up a raisin or a piece of lint (Fig. 4.20). An inferior pincer grasp is seen between 9 and 12 months of age, and a superior pincer grasp is evident by 1 year. Another type of grasp that may be seen in a 1-year-old infant is called a *three-jaw chuck grasp* (Fig. 4.21). The wrist is extended, and the middle and index fingers and the thumb are used to grasp blocks and containers.

Release

As voluntary control of the wrist, finger, and thumb extensors develops, the infant is able to demonstrate the ability to release a grasped object (Duff, 2012). Transferring objects from hand to hand is possible at 5 to 6 months because one hand can be stabilized by the other. True voluntary release is seen around 7 to 9 months and is usually assisted by the infant's being externally stabilized by another person's hand or by the tray of a highchair. Mature control is exhibited by the infant's release of an object into a container without any external support (12 months) or by putting a pellet into a bottle (15 months). Release continues to be refined and accuracy improved with ball throwing in childhood.

TYPICAL MOTOR DEVELOPMENT

The important stages of motor development in the first year of life are those associated with even months 4, 6, 8, 10, and 12 (Table 4.6). Typical motor behavior of a 4-month-old infant is characterized by head control, support on arms and hands, and midline orientation. Symmetric extension and abduction of the limbs against gravity and the ability to extend the trunk against gravity characterize the 6-month-old infant. An infant 6 to 8 months old demonstrates controlled rotation around the long axis of the trunk that allows for segmental rolling,

TABLE 4.6 Important Stages of Development	
Age	Stage
1–2 months	Internal body processes stabilize Basic biological rhythms are established Spontaneous grasp and release are established
3–4 months	Forearm support develops Head control is established Midline orientation is present
4–5 months	Antigravity control of extensors and flexors begins Bottom lifting is present
6 months	Strong extension-abduction of limbs is present Complete trunk extension is present Pivots on tummy Sits alone Spontaneous trunk rotation begins
7–8 months	Trunk control develops along with sitting balance
8–10 months	Movement progression is seen in crawling, creeping, pulling to stand, and cruising
11–12 months	Independent ambulation occurs May move in and out of full squat
16–17 months	Carries or pulls an object while walking Walks sideways and backward
20–22 months	Easily squats and recovers toy
24 months	Arm swing is present during ambulation Heel strike is present during ambulation

counter-rotation of the trunk in crawling, and creeping. The 6-month-old may sit alone and play with an object. This milestone is being reached earlier than previously reported. Arm support may be needed until the child shows more dynamic control of the trunk and can make postural adjustments to lifting the limbs. A 10-month-old balances in standing, and a 12-month-old walks independently. Although the even months are important because they mark the attainment of these skills, the other months are crucial because they prepare the infant for the achievement of the control necessary to attain these milestones.

Infant

Birth to 3 Months

Newborns assume a flexed posture regardless of their position because physiologic flexor tone dominates at birth. Initially, the newborn is unable to lift the head from a prone position. The newborn's legs are flexed under the pelvis and prevent contact of the pelvis with the supporting surface. If you put yourself into that position and try to lift your head, even as an adult, you will immediately recognize that the biomechanics of the situation are against you. With your hips in the air, your weight is shifted forward, thus making it more difficult to lift your head even though you have more muscular strength and control than a newborn. Although you are strong enough to overcome this mechanical disadvantage, the infant is not. The infant must wait for gravity to help lower the pelvis to the support surface and for the neck muscles to strengthen to be able to lift the head when in the prone position. The infant will be able to lift the head first unilaterally (Fig. 4.22), then bilaterally.

Over the next several months, neck and spinal extension develop and allow the infant to lift the head to one side, to lift and turn the head, and then to lift and hold the head in the midline. As the pelvis lowers to the support surface, neck and trunk extensors become stronger. Extension proceeds from the neck down the back in a cephalocaudal direction, so the infant is able to raise the head up higher and higher in the prone position. By 3 months of age, the infant can lift the head to 45 degrees from the supporting surface. Spinal extension also allows the infant to bring the arms from under the body into a position to support herself on the forearms (see Fig. 4.23). This position also makes it easier to extend the trunk. Weight bearing through the arms and shoulders provides greater sensory awareness to those structures and allows the infant to view the hands while in a prone position.

When in the supine position, the infant exhibits random arm and leg movements. The limbs remain flexed, and they never extend completely. In supine, the head is kept to one side or the other because the neck muscles are not yet strong enough to maintain a midline position. If you wish to make eye contact, approach the infant from the side because asymmetry is present. An asymmetric tonic neck reflex may be seen when the baby turns the head to one side (Fig. 4.24). The arm on the side to which the head is turned may extend and may allow the infant to see the hand while the other arm, closer to the skull, is flexed. This "fencing" position does not dominate the infant's posture, but it may provide the beginning of the functional connection between the eyes and the hand that is necessary for visually guided reaching. Initially, the baby's hands are normally fisted, but in the first month, they open. By 2 to 3 months, eyes and hands are sufficiently linked to allow for reaching, grasping, and shaking a rattle. As the eyes begin to track ever-widening distances, the infant will watch the hands explore the body.

When an infant is pulled to sit from a supine position before the age of 4 months, the head lags behind the body. Postural control of the head has not been established. The baby lacks sufficient strength in the neck muscles to overcome the force of gravity. Primitive rolling may be seen as the infant turns the head strongly to one side. The body may

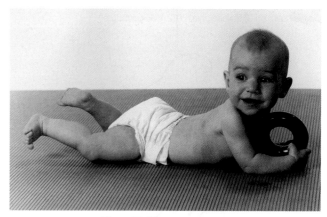

Fig. 4.23 Prone on elbows.

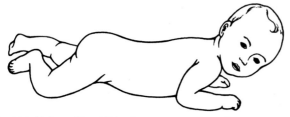

Fig. 4.22 Unilateral head lifting in a newborn. (From Cech D, Martin S, editors: *Functional movement development across the life span*, ed 3, Philadelphia, 2012, WB Saunders.)

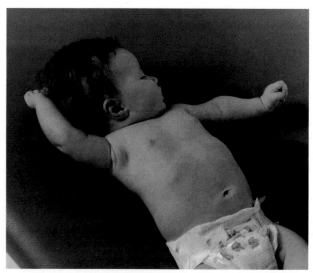

Fig. 4.24 Asymmetric tonic neck reflex in an infant.

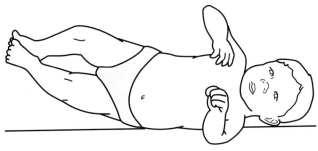

Fig. 4.25 Primitive rolling without rotation.

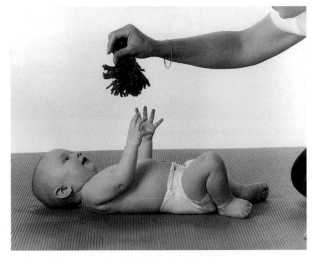

Fig. 4.26 Midline head position in supine.

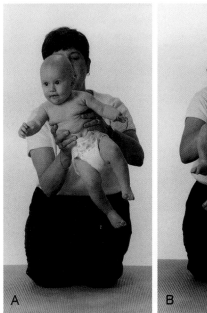 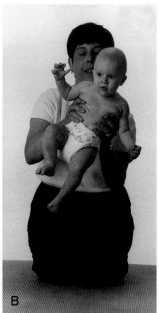

Fig. 4.27 **A** and **B,** Head control while held upright in vertical and tilted. The head remains either in midline or tilts as a compensation.

rotate as a unit in the same direction as the head moves. The baby can turn to the side or may turn all the way over from supine to prone or from prone to supine (Fig. 4.25. This turning as a unit is the result of a primitive neck righting reflex. A complete discussion of reflexes and reactions is presented following this section. In this stage of primitive rolling, separation of upper and lower trunk segments around the long axis of the body is missing.

Four Months

Four months is a critical time in motor development because posture and movement change from asymmetric to more symmetric. The infant is now able to lift the head in midline past 90 degrees in the prone position. When the infant is pulled to sit from a supine position, the head is in line with the body. Midline orientation of the head is present when the infant is at rest in the supine position (Fig. 4.26). The infant is able to bring her hands together in the midline and to watch them. In fact, the first time the baby gets both hands to the midline and realizes that her hands, to this point only viewed wiggling in the periphery, are part of her body, a real "aha" occurs. Initially, this discovery may result in hours of midline hand play. The infant can now bring objects to the mouth with both hands. Bimanual hand play is seen in all possible developmental positions. The hallmark motor behaviors of the 4-month-old infant are head control and midline orientation.

Head control in the 4-month-old infant is characterized by being able to lift the head past 90 degrees in the prone

position, to keep the head in line with the body when the infant is pulled to sit (see Fig. 4.10), to maintain the head in midline with the trunk when the infant is held upright in the vertical position and is tilted in any direction (Fig. 4.27). Midline orientation refers to the infant's ability to bring the limbs to the midline of the body, as well as to maintain a symmetric posture regardless of position. When held in supported sitting, the infant attempts to assist in trunk control. The positions in which the infant can independently move are still limited to supine and prone at this age. Lower extremity movements begin to produce pelvic movements. Pelvic mobility begins in the supine position when, from a hook-lying position, the infant produces anterior pelvic tilts by pushing on her legs and increasing hip extension, as in bridging (Bly, 1983). Active hip flexion in supine produces posterior tilting. Random pushing of the lower extremities against the support surface provides further practice of pelvic mobility that will be used later in development, especially in gait.

Five Months

Even though head control as defined earlier is considered to be achieved by 4 months of age, lifting the head against gravity from a supine position (*antigravity neck flexion*) is not achieved until 5 months of age. Antigravity neck flexion may first be noted by the caregiver when putting the child down in the crib for a nap. The infant works to keep the head from falling backward as she is lowered toward the supporting surface. This is also the time when infants look as though they are trying to get out of their car or infant seat by straining to bring the head forward. When the infant is pulled to sit from a supine position, the head now leads the movement with a chin tuck. The head is in front of the body. In fact, the infant often uses forward trunk flexion to reinforce neck flexion and to lift the legs to counterbalance the pulling force (Fig. 4.28).

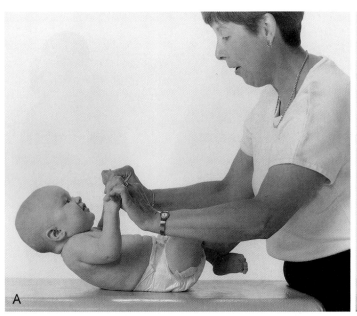
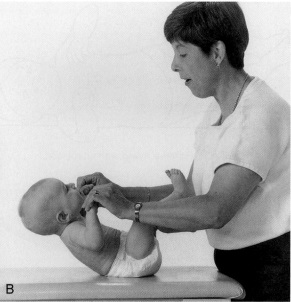

Fig. 4.28 **A,** Use of trunk flexion to reinforce neck flexion as the head leads during a pull-to-sit maneuver.
B, Use of leg elevation to counterbalance neck flexion during a pull-to-sit maneuver.

From a froglike position, the infant is able to lift her bottom off the support surface and to bring her feet into her visual field. This "bottom lifting" allows her to play with her feet and even to put them into her mouth for sensory awareness (Fig. 4.29). This play provides lengthening for the hamstrings and prepares the baby for long sitting. The lower abdominals also have a chance to work while the trunk is supported. Reciprocal kicking is also seen at this time.

As extension develops in the prone position, the infant may occasionally demonstrate a "swimming" posture (Fig. 4.30). In this position, most of the weight is on the tummy, and the arms and legs are able to be stretched out and held up off the floor or mattress. This posture is a further manifestation of extensor control against gravity. The infant plays between this swimming posture and a prone on elbows or prone on

extended arms posture (Fig. 4.31). The infant makes subtle weight shifts while in the prone on elbows position and may attempt reaching. Movements at this stage show *dissociation* of head and limbs.

A 5-month-old infant cannot sit alone, but may be supported at the low back. The typically developing infant can sit in the corner of a couch or on the floor if propped on extended arms. A 5-month-old infant placed in sitting demonstrates directionally appropriate activation of postural muscles in response to movement of the support surface (Hadders-Algra et al., 1996). The 5-month-old may be able to sit for short periods of time as she tries to reach for objects frequently falling and learning (Harbourne et al., 2013). She may stabilize one arm and attempt to reach with the other.

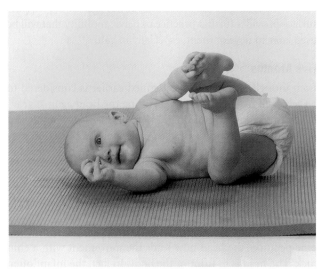

Fig. 4.29 Bottom lifting.

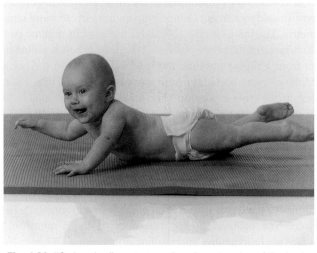

Fig. 4.30 "Swimming" posture, antigravity extension of the body.

Six Months

A 6-month-old infant becomes mobile in the prone position by pivoting in a circle (Fig. 4.32). The infant is also able to shift weight onto one extended arm and to reach forward with the other hand to grasp an object. The reaching movement is counterbalanced by a lateral weight shift of the trunk that produces lateral head and trunk bending away from the side of the weight shift (Fig. 4.33). This lateral bending in response to a weight shift is called a *righting reaction*. Righting reactions of the head and trunk are more thoroughly discussed in the next section. Maximal extension of the head and trunk is possible in the prone position along with extension and abduction of the limbs away from the body. This extended posture is called the *Landau reflex* and represents total body righting against gravity. It is mature when the infant can demonstrate hip extension when held away from the support surface, supported only under the tummy. The infant appears to be flying (Fig. 4.34). This final stage in the development of extension can occur only if the hips are relatively adducted. Too much hip abduction puts the gluteus maximus at a biomechanical disadvantage

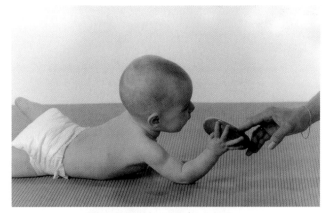

Fig. 4.33 Lateral righting reaction.

and makes it more difficult to execute hip extension. Excessive abduction is often seen in children with low muscle tone and increased range of motion, such as in Down syndrome. These children have difficulty performing antigravity hip extension.

Segmental rolling is now present and becomes the preferred mobility pattern when rolling, first from prone to supine, which is less challenging, and then from supine to prone. Antigravity flexion control is needed to roll from supine to prone. The movement usually begins with flexion of some body part, depending on the infant and the circumstances. Regardless of the body part used, segmental rotation is essential for developing transitional control (Fig. 4.35). *Transitional movements* are those that allow change of position, such as moving from prone to sitting, from the four-point position to kneeling, and from sitting to standing. Only a few movement transitions take place without segmental trunk rotation, such as moving from the four-point position to kneeling and from sitting to standing. Individuals with movement dysfunction often have problems making the transition smoothly and efficiently from one position to another. The quality of movement affects the individual's ability to perform transitional movements.

The 6-month-old infant can sit up if placed in sitting. A 6-month-old cannot purposefully move into sitting from a prone position but may incidentally push herself backward along the floor. Coincidentally, while pushing, her abdomen may be lifted off the support surface, allowing the pelvis to move over the hips, with the end result of sitting between the feet. Sitting between the feet is called *W sitting* and should be avoided in infants with developmental movement problems, because it can make it difficult to learn to use trunk muscles for balance. The posture provides positional stability, but it does not require active use of the trunk muscles. Concern also exists about the abnormal stress this position places on growing joints. In typically developing children, there is less concern because these children move in and out of the position more easily, rather than remaining in it for long periods of time.

Having developed trunk extension in the prone position, the infant can sit with a relatively straight back with the

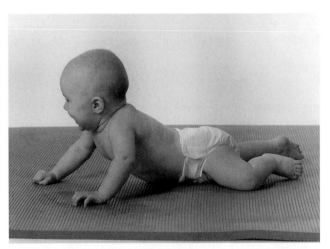

Fig. 4.31 Prone on extended arms.

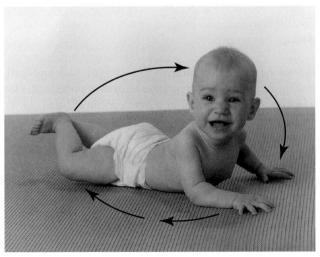

Fig. 4.32 Pivoting in prone.

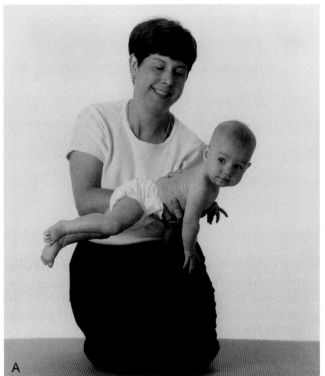

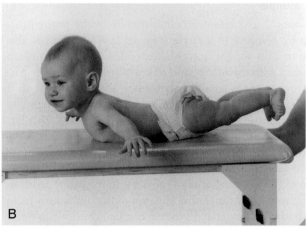

Fig. 4.34 **A,** Eliciting a Landau reflex. **B,** Spontaneous Landau reflex.

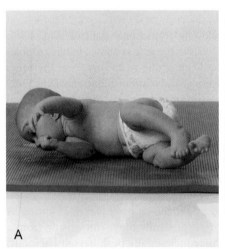

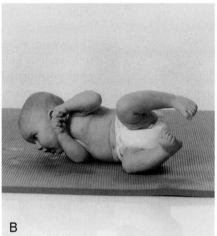

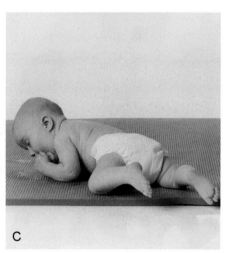

Fig. 4.35 **A–C,** Segmental rolling from supine to prone.

exception of the lumbar spine (Fig. 4.36). Both hands can be freed to explore objects and to engage in more sophisticated play. When balance is lost during sitting, the infant extends the arms for protection while falling forward. In successive months, this same upper extremity protective response will be seen in additional directions, such as laterally and backward. Different types of sitting postures, such as ring sitting, wide abducted sitting, and long sitting, provide the infant with different amounts of support.

The pull-to-sit maneuver with a 6-month-old often causes the infant to pull all the way up to standing (Fig. 4.37). The infant will most likely reach forward for the caregiver's hands as part of the task. A 6-month-old likes to bear weight on the feet

and will bounce in this position if she is held. Back-and-forth rocking and bouncing in a position seem to be prerequisites for achieving postural control in a new posture (Thelen, 1979). Repetition of rhythmic upper extremity activities is also seen in the banging and shaking of objects during this period. Reaching becomes less dependent on visual cues as the infant uses other senses to become more aware of body relationships. The infant may hear a noise and may reach unilaterally toward the toy that made the sound (Duff, 2012).

Although complete elbow extension is lacking, the 6-month-old's arm movements are maturing such that a mid–pronation-supination reaching pattern is seen. A position halfway between supination and pronation is considered neutral. Pronated reaching is the least mature reaching pattern and is seen early in development. Supinated reaching is the most mature pattern because it allows the hand to be visually oriented toward the thumb side, thereby increasing grasp precision (Fig. 4.38). Reaching patterns originate from the shoulder because early in upper extremity development, the arm functions as a whole unit. Reaching patterns are different from grasping patterns, which involve movements of the fingers.

Seven Months

Trunk control improves in sitting and allows the infant to free one or both hands for playing with objects and become independent in sitting. Fig. 4.39 shows examples of sitting postures in typically developing infants with and without hand support. The infant can narrow her base of support in sitting by adducting the lower extremities as the trunk begins to be able to compensate for small losses of balance. Dynamic stability develops from muscular work of the trunk. An active trunk supports dynamic balance and complements the positional stability derived from the size and configuration of the base of support. Lateral protective reactions begin to emerge in sitting at this time (Fig. 4.40). Unilateral reach is displayed by the 7-month-old infant (Fig. 4.41), as is an ability to transfer objects from hand to hand.

Sitting is a functional and favorite position of the infant. Because the infant's back is straight, the hands are free to play with objects or extend and abduct to catch the infant if a loss of balance occurs, as happens less frequently at this age. Upper trunk rotation is demonstrated during play in sitting as the child reaches in all directions for toys (see Fig. 4.39, C). If a toy is out of reach, the infant can prop on one arm and reach across the body to extend the reach using trunk

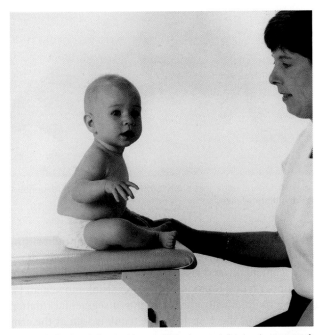

Fig. 4.36 Early sitting with a relatively straight back except for forward flexion in the lumbar spine.

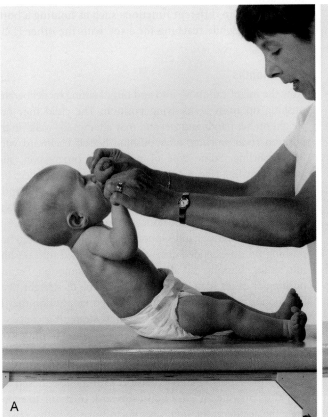
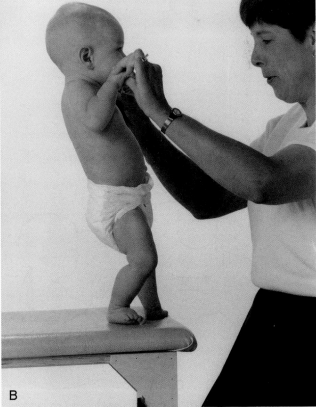

A   B

Fig. 4.37 **A** and **B,** Pull-to-sit maneuver becomes pull-to-stand.

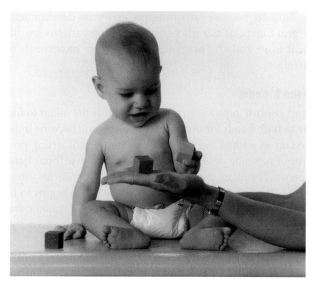

Fig. 4.38 Supinated reaching.

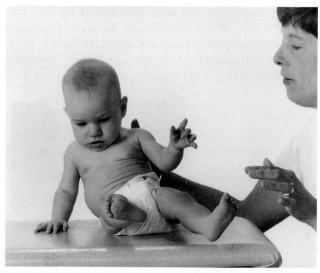

Fig. 4.40 Lateral upper extremity protective reaction in response to loss of sitting balance.

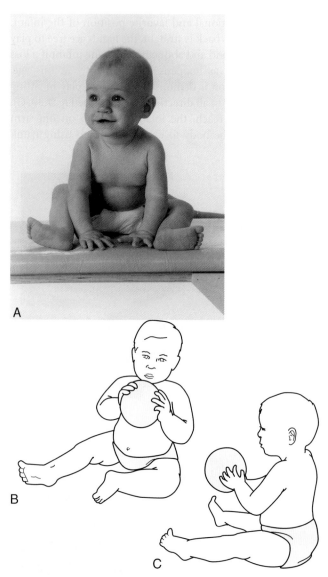

Fig. 4.39 Sitting postures. **A,** Ring sitting propped forward on hands. **B,** Half-long sitting. **C,** Long sitting.

rotation and reverse the rotation to return to upright sitting. With increased control of trunk rotation, the body moves more segmentally and less as a whole. This trend of dissociating upper trunk rotation from lower trunk movement began at 6 months with the beginning of segmental rotation. Dissociation of the arms from the trunk is seen as the arms move across the midline of the body. More external rotation is evident at the shoulder (turning the entire arm from palm down, to neutral, to palm up) and allows supinated reaching to be achieved. By 8 to 10 months, the infant's two hands are able to perform different functions such as holding a bottle in one hand while reaching for a toy with the other (Duff, 2012).

Eight Months

Now the infant can move into and out of sitting by deliberately pushing up from a side-lying position. The child may bear weight on her hands and feet and may attempt to "walk" in this position *(bear walking)* after pushing herself backward while belly crawling. Some type of prewalking progression, such as belly crawling (Fig. 4.42), creeping on hands and knees (see Fig. 4.13), or sitting and hitching, is usually present by 8 months. Hitching in a sitting position is an alternative way for some children to move across the floor. The infant scoots on her bottom with or without hand support. We have already noted how pushing up on extended arms can be continued into pushing into sitting. Pushing can also be used for locomotion. Because pushing is easier than pulling, the first type of straight plane locomotion achieved by the infant in a prone position may be backward propulsion. Pulling is seen as strength increases in the upper back and shoulders. All this upper extremity work in a prone position is accompanied by random leg movements. These random leg movements may accidentally cause the legs to be pushed into extension with the toes flexed and may thus provide an extra boost forward. In trying to reproduce the accident, the infant begins to learn to belly crawl or creep forward.

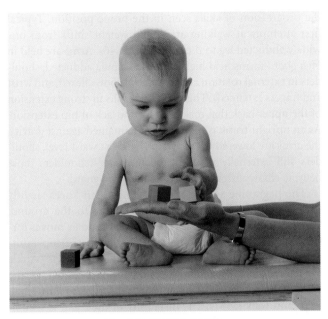

Fig. 4.41 Unilateral reach.

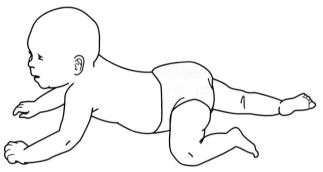

Fig. 4.42 Belly crawling.

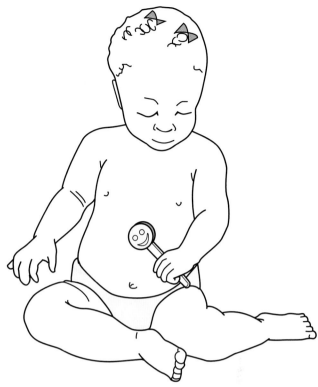

Fig. 4.43 Side sitting.

Nine Months

A 9-month-old is constantly changing positions, moving in and out of sitting (including side sitting) (Fig. 4.43) and into the four-point position. As the infant experiments more and more with the four-point position, she rhythmically rocks back and forth and alternately puts her weight on her arms and legs. In this endeavor, the infant is aided by a new capacity for hip extension and flexion, other examples of the ability to dissociate movements of the pelvis from movements of the trunk. The hands-and-knees position, or quadruped position, is a less supported position requiring greater balance and trunk control. As trunk stability increases, simultaneous movement of an opposite arm and leg is possible while the infant maintains weight on the remaining two extremities. This form of reciprocal locomotion is called *creeping*. Creeping is often the primary means of locomotion for several months, even after the infant starts pulling to stand and cruising around furniture. Creeping provides fast and stable travel for the infant and allows for exploration of the environment. A very small percentage (4.3%) of infants do not creep according to the WHO (2006).

Reciprocal movements used in creeping require counter-rotation of trunk segments; the shoulders rotate in one direction while the pelvis rotates in the opposite direction. Counter-rotation is an important element of erect forward progression (walking), which comes later. Other major components needed for successful creeping are extension of the head, neck, back, and arms, and dissociation of arm and leg movements from the trunk. Extremity dissociation depends on the stability of the shoulder and pelvic girdles, respectively, and on their ability to control rotation in opposite directions. Children practice creeping about 5 hours a day and can cover the distance of two football fields (Adolph, 2003).

When playing in the quadruped position, the infant may reach out to the crib rail or furniture and may pull up to a kneeling position. Balance is maintained by holding on with the arms rather than by fully bearing the weight through the hips. The infant at this age does not have the control necessary to balance in a kneeling or half-kneeling (one foot forward) position. Even though kneeling and half-kneeling are used as transitions to pull to stand, only after learning to walk is such control possible for the toddler. Pulling to stand is a rapid movement transition with little time spent in either true knee standing or half-kneeling. Early standing consists of leaning against a support surface, such as the coffee table or couch, so the hands can be free to play. Legs tend to be abducted for a wider base of support, much like the struts of a tower. Knee position may vary between flexion and extension, and toes alternately claw the floor and flare upward in an attempt to assist balance. These foot responses are considered equilibrium reactions of the feet (Fig. 4.44).

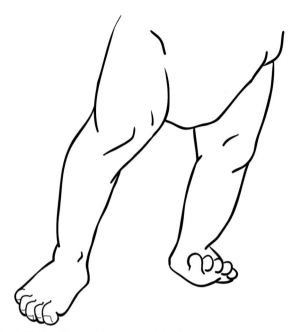

Fig. 4.44 **Equilibrium Reactions of the Feet.** Baby learns balance in standing by delicate movements of the feet: "fanning" and "clawing." (Redrawn by permission of the publisher from Connor FP, Williamson GG, Siepp JM, editors: *Program guide for infants and toddlers with neuromotor and other developmental disabilities,* New York, Teachers College, Columbia University, p. 117. All rights reserved.)

Once the infant has achieved an upright posture at furniture, she practices weight shifting by moving from side to side. While in upright standing and before cruising begins in earnest, the infant practices dissociating arm and leg movements from the trunk by reaching out or backward with an arm while the leg is swung in the opposite direction. When side-to-side weight shift progresses to actual movement sideways, the baby is cruising. Cruising is done around furniture and between close pieces of furniture. This sideways "walking" is done with arm support and may be a means of working the hip abductors to ensure a level pelvis when forward ambulation is attempted. These maneuvers always make us think of a ballet dancer warming up at the barre before dancing. In this case, the infant is warming up, practicing counter-rotation in a newly acquired posture, upright, before attempting to walk (Fig. 4.45). Over the next several months, the infant will develop better pelvic-and-hip control to perfect upright standing before attempting independent ambulation.

Toddler

Twelve Months

The infant becomes a toddler at 1 year. Most infants attempt forward locomotion by this age. The caregiver has probably already been holding the infant's hands and encouraging walking, if not placing the infant in a walker. Use of walkers continues to raise safety issues from pediatricians. The American Academy of Pediatrics (AAP) reaffirmed their policy statement on injuries associated with walker use (AAP, 2012). Also, too early use of walkers does not allow the infant to develop sufficient upper body and trunk strength needed for

the progression of skills seen in the prone position. Typical first attempts at walking are lateral weight shifts from one widely abducted leg to the other (Fig. 4.46). Arms are held in *high guard* (arms held high with the scapula adducted, shoulders in external rotation and abducted, elbows flexed, and wrist and fingers extended). This position results in strong extension of the upper back that makes up for the lack of hip extension. As an upright trunk is more easily maintained against gravity, the arms are lowered to *midguard* (hands at waist level, shoulders still externally rotated), to *low guard* (shoulders more neutral, elbows extended), and finally to no guard.

The beginning walker keeps her hips and knees slightly flexed to bring the center of mass closer to the ground. Weight shifts are from side to side as the toddler moves forward by total lower extremity flexion, with the hip joints remaining externally rotated during the gait cycle. Ankle movements are minimal, with the foot pronated as the whole foot contacts the ground. Toddlers take many small steps and walk slowly. The instability of their gait is seen in the short amount of time they spend in single-limb stance. As trunk stability improves, the legs come farther under the pelvis. As the hips and knees become more extended, the feet develop the plantar flexion needed for the push-off phase of the gait cycle.

Sixteen to Eighteen Months

By 16 to 17 months, the toddler is so much at ease with walking that a toy can be carried or pulled at the same time. With help, the toddler goes up and down the stairs, one step at a time. Without help, the toddler creeps up the stairs and may creep or scoot down on her buttocks. Most children will be able to walk sideways and backward at this age if they started walking at 12 months or earlier. The typically developing toddler comes to stand from a supine position by rolling to prone, pushing up on hands and knees or hands and feet, assuming a squat, and rising to standing (Fig. 4.47).

Most toddlers exhibit a reciprocal arm swing and heel strike by 18 months of age, with other adult gait characteristics manifested later. They walk well and demonstrate a "running-like" walk. Although the toddler may still occasionally fall or trip over objects in her path because eye-foot coordination is not completely developed, the decline in falls appears to be the result of improved balance reactions in standing and the ability to monitor trunk and lower extremity movements kinesthetically and visually. The first signs of jumping appear as a stepping off "jump" from a low object, such as the bottom step of a set of stairs. Children are ready for this first step-down jump after being able to walk down a step while they hold the hand of an adult (Wickstrom, 1983). Momentary balance on one foot is also possible.

Two Years

The 2-year-old's gait becomes faster, arms swing reciprocally; steps are bigger and time spent in single-limb stance increases. Many additional motor skills emerge during this year. A 2-year-old can go up and down stairs one step at a time, jump off a step with a two-foot take-off, kick a large ball, and throw

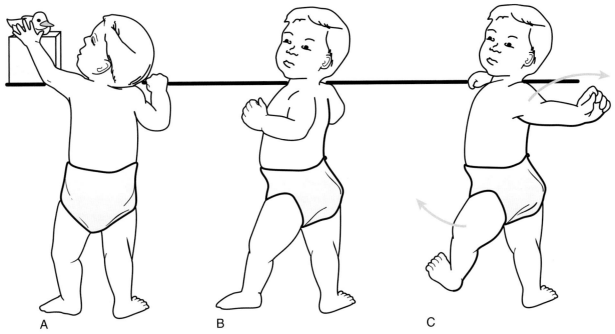

Fig. 4.45 **Cruising Maneuvers. A,** Cruising sideways, reaching out. **B,** Standing, rotating upper trunk backward. **C,** Standing, reaching out backward, elaborating with swinging movements of the same-side leg, thus producing counterrotation. (Redrawn by permission of the publisher from Connor FP, Williamson GG, Siepp JM, editors: *Program guide for infants and toddlers with neuromotor and other developmental disabilities,* New York, Teachers College, Columbia University, p. 121. All rights reserved.)

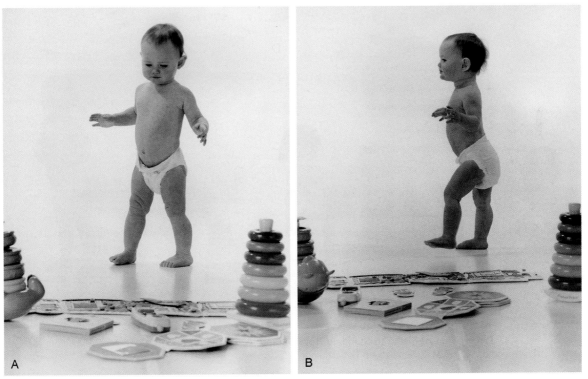

Fig. 4.46 **A** and **B,** Independent walking.

a small one. Stair climbing and kicking indicate improved stability during shifting of body weight from one leg to the other. Stepping over low objects is also part of the child's movement capabilities within the environment. True running, characterized by a "flight" phase when both feet are off the ground, emerges at the same time. Quickly starting to run and stopping from a run are still difficult, and directional changes by making a turn require a large area. As the child first attempts to jump off the ground, one foot leaves the ground, followed by the other foot, as if the child were stepping in air.

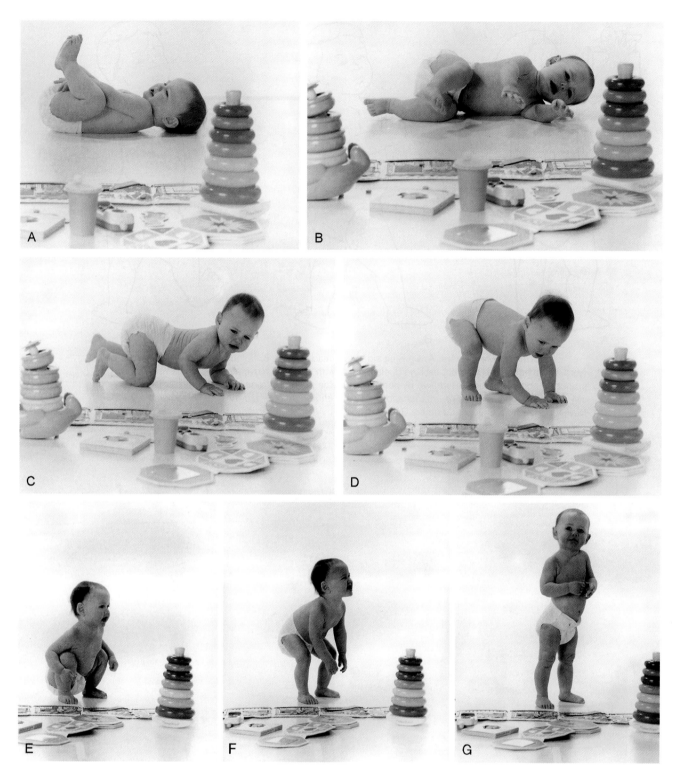

Fig. 4.47 Progression of Rising to Standing from Supine. **A,** Supine. **B,** Rolling. **C,** Four-point position. **D,** Plantigrade. **E,** Squat. **F,** Semi-squat. **G,** Standing.

Fundamental Movement Patterns (Three to Six Years)

Three Years

Fundamental motor patterns, such as hopping, galloping, and skipping, develop from 3 to 6 years of age. Wickstrom (1983) also includes running, jumping, throwing, catching, and striking in this category. Other reciprocal actions mastered by age 3 are pedaling a tricycle and climbing a jungle gym or ladder. Locomotion can be started and stopped based on the demands from the environment or from a task such as playing dodge ball on a crowded playground. A 3-year-old child can make sharp turns while running and can balance on toes and heels in standing. Standing with one foot in front of the other, known as tandem standing, is possible, as is standing on one foot for at least 3 seconds. A reciprocal gait is now used to ascend stairs with the child placing one foot on each step in alternating fashion but marking time (one step at a time) when descending.

Jumping begins with a step-down jump at 18 months and progresses to jumping up off the floor with two feet at the same time at age 2. Jumps can start with a one-foot or two-foot take-off. The two-foot take-off and land is more mature. Jumps can involve running then jumping as in a running broad jump or jumping from standing still, as in a standing broad jump. Jumping has many forms and is part of play or game activities. Jumping ability increases with age.

Hopping on one foot is a special type of jump requiring balance on one foot and the ability to push off the loaded foot. It does not require a maximal effort. "Repeated vertical jumps from 2 feet can be done before true hopping can occur" (Wickstrom, 1983) (see Fig. 4.48). Neither type of jump is seen at an early age. Hopping one or two times on the preferred foot may also be accomplished by 3½ years when there is the ability to stand on one foot and balance long enough to push off on the loaded foot. A 4-year-old child should be able to hop on one foot four to six times. Improved hopping ability is seen when the child learns to use the nonstance leg to help propel the body forward. Before that time, all the work is done by pushing off with the support foot. A similar pattern is seen in arm use; at first, the arms are inactive; later, they are used opposite the action of the moving leg. Gender differences for hopping are documented in the literature, with girls performing better than boys (Wickstrom, 1983). This may be related to the fact that girls appear to have better balance than boys in childhood.

Four Years

Rhythmic relaxed galloping is possible for a 4-year-old child. Galloping consists of a walk on the lead leg followed by a running step on the rear leg. Galloping is an asymmetric gait. A good way to visualize galloping is to think of a child riding a stick horse. Toddlers have been documented to gallop as early as 20 months after learning to walk (Whitall, 1989), but the movement is stiff with arms held in high guard as in beginning walking. A 4-year-old has better static and dynamic balance as evidenced by the ability to stand on either foot for a longer period of time (4 to 6 seconds) than a 3-year-old. Now she can descend stairs with alternating feet.

Four-year-olds can catch a small ball with outstretched arms if it is thrown to them, and they can throw a ball overhand from some distance. Throwing begins with an accidental letting go of an object at about 18 months of age. From 2 to 4 years of age, throwing is extremely variable, with underhand and overhand throwing observed. Gender differences are seen. A child of 2½ years can throw a large or small ball 5 feet. The ball is not thrown more than 10 feet until the child is more than 4 years of age. The distance a child is able to propel an object has been related to a child's height, as seen in Fig. 4.49 (Cratty, 1979). Development of more mature throwing is related to using the force of the body and a combination of leg and shoulder movements to improve performance.

"Although throwing and catching have a close functional relationship, throwing is learned a lot more quickly than catching" (Wickstrom, 1977). Catching ability depends on many variables, the least of which is ball size, speed, arm position of the catcher, skill of the thrower, and age-related sensory and perceptual factors. Some of these perceptual factors involve the use of visual cues, depth perception, eye-hand coordination, and the amount of experience the catcher has had with playing with balls. Closing the eyes when an object is thrown toward one is a fear response common in children (Wickstrom, 1977) and has to be overcome to learn to catch or strike an object.

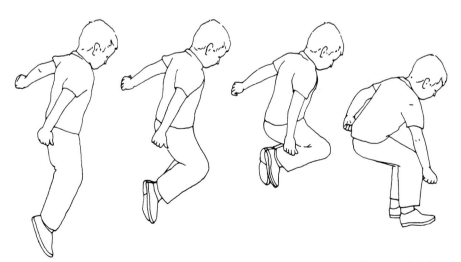

Fig. 4.48 **Vertical Jump.** Immature form in the vertical jump showing "winging" arm action, incomplete extension, quick flexion of the legs, and slight forward jump. (From Wickstrom RL: *Fundamental motor patterns*, ed 3, Philadelphia, 1983, Lea & Febiger.)

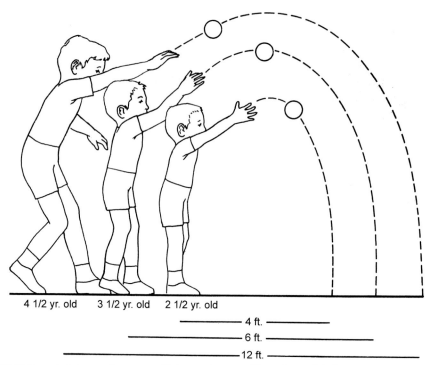

4 1/2 yr. old   3 1/2 yr. old   2 1/2 yr. old

——————— 4 ft. ———————
—————————— 6 ft. ——————————
————————————— 12 ft. —————————————

Fig. 4.49 Throwing distances increase with increasing age. (From Cratty BJ: *Perceptual and motor development in infants and children*, ed 2, Englewood Cliffs, NJ, 1979, Prentice Hall. Reprinted by permission of Pearson Education, Inc., New York.)

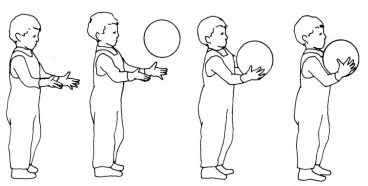

Fig. 4.50 **Immature Catching.** A 33-month-old boy extends his arms before the ball is tossed. He waits for the ball without moving, responds after the ball has touched his hands, and then gently traps the ball against his chest. It is essentially a robot-like performance. (From Wickstrom RL: *Fundamental motor patterns*, ed 3, Philadelphia, 1983, Lea & Febiger.)

Precatching requires the child to interact with a rolling ball. Such interaction typically occurs while the child sits with legs outstretched and tries to trap the ball with legs or hands. Children learn about time and spatial relationships of moving objects first from a seated position and later in standing when chasing after a rolling or bouncing ball. The child tries to stop, intercept, and otherwise control her movements and to anticipate the movement of the object in space. Next, the child attempts to "catch" an object moving through the air. Before reaching age 3, most children must have their arms prepositioned to have any chance of catching a ball thrown to them. Most of the time, the thrower, who is an adult, bounces the ball to the child, so the burden is on the thrower to calculate where the ball must bounce to land in the child's outstretched arms. Figs. 4.50 and 4.51 show two immature catchers, one 33 months old and the other 48 months old. As catching matures, the hands are used more, with less dependence on the arms and body. The 4-year-old still has maturing to do in perfecting the skill of catching.

Striking is the act of swinging and hitting an object. Developmentally, the earliest form of striking is for the child to use arm extension to hit something with her hand. When a child holds an implement, such as a stick or a bat, she continues to use this form of movement, which results in striking down the object. A 2- to 4-year-old demonstrates this immature striking behavior. Common patterns of striking are overhand, sidearm, and underhand. Without any special help, the child will progress slowly to striking more horizontally. Mature form of striking is

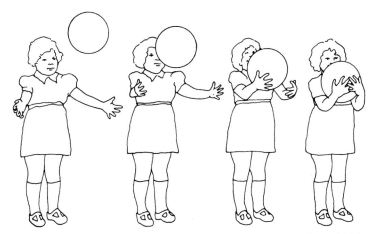

Fig. 4.51 A 4-year-old girl waits for the ball with arms straight and hands spread. Her initial response to the ball is a clapping motion. When one hands contacts the ball, she grasps at it and gains control by clutching it against her chest. (From Wickstrom RL: *Fundamental motor patterns*, ed 3, Philadelphia, 1983, Lea & Febiger.)

usually not demonstrated until at least 6 years of age (Malina et al., 2004). As the child progresses from striking down to a more horizontal striking (sidearm), more and more trunk rotation is seen as the child's swing matures (Roberton and Halverson, 1977). A mature pattern of striking consists of taking a step, turning away, and then swinging (step-turn-swing) (Wickstrom, 1983).

Kicking is a special type of striking and one in which the arms play no direct role. Children most frequently kick a ball in spontaneous play and in organized games. A 2-year-old is able to kick a ball on the ground. A child of 5 years is expected to kick a ball rolled toward her 12 feet in the air, and a child of 6 years is expected to run and kick a rolling ball up to 4 feet (Folio and Fewell, 2000). Gesell (1940) expected a 5-year-old to kick a soccer ball up to 8 to 11½ feet and a 6-year-old to be able to kick a ball up to 10 to 18 feet. Measuring performance in kicking is difficult before the age of 4 years. Annual improvements begin to be seen at the age of 5 years (Gesell, 1940). Kicking requires good static balance on the stance foot and counterbalancing the force of the kick with arm positioning.

Five Years

At 5 years of age, a child can stand on either foot for 8 to 10 seconds, walk forward on a balance beam, hop 8 to 10 times on one foot, make a 2- to 3-foot standing broad jump, and skip on alternating feet. Skipping requires bilateral coordination. At this age, the child can change directions and stop quickly while running. She can ride a bike, roller-skate, and hit a target with a ball from 5 feet away.

Six Years

A 6-year-old child is well-coordinated and can stand on one foot for more than 10 seconds, with eyes open or eyes closed. This ability is important to note because it indicates that vision can be ignored and balance can be maintained. A 6-year-old can throw and catch a small ball from 10 feet away. A first grader can walk on a balance beam on the floor, forward, backward, and sideways without stepping off. She continues to enjoy and use alternate forms of locomotion, such as

riding a bicycle or roller-skating. Patterns of movement learned in game-playing form the basis for later sports skills. Throughout the process of changing motor activities and skills, the nervous, muscular, and skeletal systems are maturing, and the body is growing in height and weight. Power develops slowly in children because strength and speed within a specific movement pattern are required.

Fundamental motor skills demonstrate changes in form over time. Between 6 and 10 years of age, a child masters the adult forms of running, throwing, and catching. Fig. 4.52 depicts when 60% of children were able to demonstrate a certain developmental level for the listed fundamental motor skills. Stage 1 is an immature form of the movement, and stage 4 or 5 represents the mature form of the same movement. A marked gender difference is apparent in overhand throwing. It is not uncommon to see young children demonstrate a mature pattern of movement at one age and a less mature pattern at a later age. Regression of patterns is possible when the child is attempting to combine skills. For example, a child who can throw overhand while standing may revert to underhand throwing when running. Alterations between mature and immature movement is in line with Gesell's concept of reciprocal interweaving. Individual variation in motor development is considerable during childhood. Even though 60% of children have achieved the fundamental motor skills as listed in Fig. 4.52, 40% of the children have not achieved them by the ages given.

1.1 Gait

Most children begin walking at the end of the first year of life but it takes years for a child to exhibit mature gait characteristics. Factors associated with the achievement of upright gait are sufficient extensor muscle strength, dynamic balance, and postural control of the head within the limits of stability of the base of support. A new walker's movement is judged by how long she has been walking, not by the age at the onset of the skill. After about 5 months of walking practice, the infant is able to exhibit an inverted pendulum mechanism that makes walking more efficient (Ivanenko et al., 2007). With

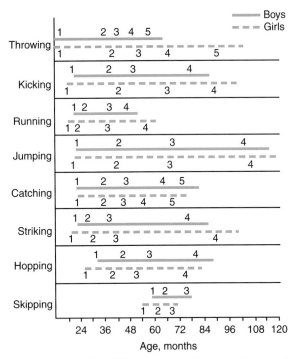

Fig. 4.52 Ages at which 60% of boys and girls were able to perform at specific developmental levels for several fundamental motor skills. Stage 1 is immature; stage 4 or 5 is mature. (Reprinted by permission from Seefledt V, Haubenstricker J: Patterns, phases, or stages: an analytical model for the study of developmental movement. In Kelso JAS, Clark JE, editors: *The development of movement control and coordination*, 1982, p. 314.)

practice, the duration of single limb support increases and the period of double limb support declines. Arm swing and heel strike are present by 2 years of age (Sutherland et al., 1988). Out-toeing has been reduced and pelvic rotation and a double knee-lock pattern are present. This pattern refers to the two periods of knee extension in gait, one just before heel strike and another as the body moves over the foot during the stance phase. In between, at the moment of heel strike, the knee is flexed to help absorb the impact of the body's weight. Cadence decreases as stride length increases.

Gait velocity almost doubles between 1 and 7 years, and the pelvic span-to-ankle spread span ratio increases. The latter gait laboratory measurement indicates that the base of support narrows over time. Rapid changes in temporal and spatial gait parameters occur during the first 4 years of life with slower changes continuing until 7 years when gait is considered mature by motion standards. Experience and practice play a significant role in gait development.

Age-Related Differences in Movement Patterns beyond Childhood

Many developmentalists have chosen to look only at the earliest ages of life when motor abilities and skills are being acquired. The belief that mature motor behavior is achieved by childhood led researchers to overlook the possibility that movement could change as a result of factors other than

nervous system maturation. Although the nervous system is generally thought to be mature by the age of 10 years, changes in movement patterns do occur in adolescence and adulthood.

Research shows a developmental order of movement patterns across childhood and adolescence with trends toward increasing symmetry with increasing age (Sabourin, 1989; VanSant, 1988a). VanSant (1988b) identified three common ways in which adults came to stand. These are shown in Fig. 4.53. The most common pattern was to use upper extremity reach, symmetric push, forward head, neck and trunk flexion, and a symmetric squat (see Fig. 4.53, A). The second most common way was identical to the first pattern up to an asymmetric squat (see Fig. 4.53, B). The next most common way involved an asymmetric push and reach, followed by a half-kneel (see Fig. 4.53, C). In a separate study of adults in their 20s through 40s, a trend was seen toward increasing asymmetry with age (Ford-Smith and VanSant, 1993). Adults in their 40s were more likely to demonstrate the asymmetric patterns of movement seen in young children (VanSant, 1991). The asymmetry of movement in the older adult may reflect less trunk rotation resulting from stiffening of joints or lessening of muscle strength, factors that make it more difficult to come straight forward to sitting from a supine position.

Thomas et al. (1998) studied movement from a supine position to standing in older adults using VanSant's descriptive approach. In a group of community-dwelling elders with a mean age of 74.6 years, the 70- and 80-year-old adults were more likely to use asymmetric patterns of movement in the upper extremity and trunk regions, whereas those younger than 70 showed more symmetric patterns in the same body regions. Furthermore, researchers found a shorter time to rise was related to a younger age, greater knee extension strength, and greater hip and ankle range of motion (flexion and dorsiflexion, respectively). However, older adults who maintain their strength and flexibility rise to standing faster and more symmetrically than do those who are less strong and flexible.

Although the structures of the body are mature at the end of puberty, changes in movement patterns continue throughout a person's entire life. Mature movement patterns have always been associated with efficiency and symmetry. Early in motor development, patterns of movement appear to be more homogenous and follow a fairly prescribed developmental sequence. As a person matures, movement patterns become more symmetric. With aging, movement patterns become more asymmetric. Because an older adult may exhibit different ways of moving from supine to standing than a younger person, treatment interventions should be taught that match the individual's usual patterns of movement.

POSTURE, BALANCE, AND GAIT CHANGES WITH AGING

Posture

The ability to maintain an erect aligned posture declines with advanced age. Fig. 4.54 shows the difference in posture

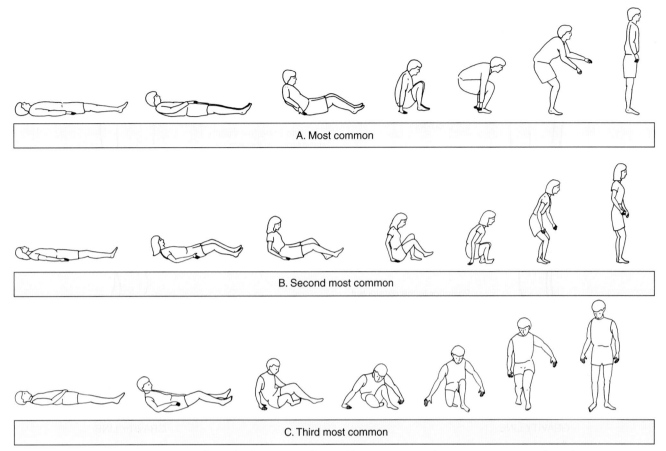

Fig. 4.53 Most common form of rising to a standing position: upper extremity component, symmetric push; axial component, symmetric; lower extremity component, symmetric squat. (Reprinted from VanSant AF: Rising from a supine position to erect stance: Description of adult movement and a developmental hypothesis, *Phys Ther* 68:185–192, 1988. With permission of the APTA.)

anticipated with typical aging. The secondary curves developed in infancy begin to be modified. The cervical curve decreases. The lumbar curve usually flattens. Being sedentary can accentuate age-related postural changes. The older adult who sits all day may be at greater risk for a flattened low back. The thoracic spine becomes more kyphotic. Aging alters the properties and relative amount of connective tissue in the interior of the intervertebral disc (Zhao et al., 2007). The discs lose water, and initially, flexible connective tissue stiffens, causing older adults to lose spinal flexibility. The strength of the muscles declines with age and could contribute to a decline in the maintenance of postural alignment in the older adult.

Balance

Older adults can have major problems with balance and falling. One-third of community dwelling older adults fall (Hopewell et al., 2018). Whether a person's ability to balance always declines with age is still undecided. Sensory information from the three sensory systems (visual, vestibular, and somatosensory) responsible for posture and balance undergo age-related changes. These changes can impair the older adult's ability to respond quickly to changes within the internal and external environments. Fall risk from environmental factors includes but is not limited to stairs, slippery surfaces,

and poor lighting. Intrinsic factors include physiologic changes in sensory receptors, especially vision, musculoskeletal weakness, gait difficulties, and psychosocial issues such as depression or dementia. The most evidence-supported measures of fall risk are the Berg Balance, Timed Up and Go, and five times sit to stand (Lussardi et al., 2017).

A decline in structural integrity of these sensory receptors decreases the quality and quantity of the information relayed. The actual number of receptors also decreases. Awareness of vibration, especially in the ankles, is lessened in the elderly and has been related to an increase in postural sway during quiet stance. The visual system is less able to pick up contours and depth cues because of a decline in contrast sensitivity. Age-related declines in visual acuity, depth significantly affect an older person's ability to detect threats to balance. Removal of visual information during balance testing in the elderly has been shown to increase postural sway (Lord et al., 1991). Scovil et al. (2008) found that stored visuospatial information from the environment is needed for planning and executing a stepping reaction. Muscular responses needed to react to a perturbation of balance may be lacking along with inaccurate sequencing, timing, or an inability to adapt to a change in environment or task demand (anticipatory balance).

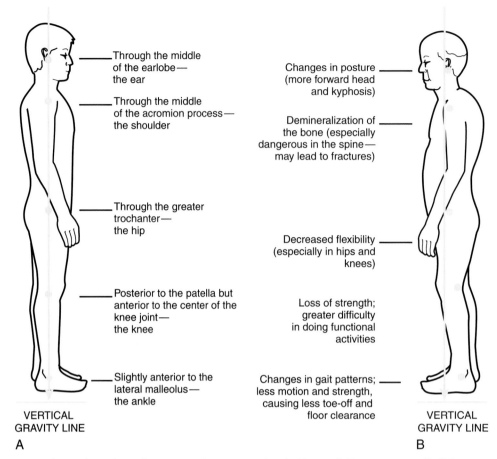

Through the middle
of the earlobe—
the ear

Through the middle
of the acromion process—
the shoulder

Through the greater
trochanter—
the hip

Posterior to the patella but
anterior to the center of the
knee joint—
the knee

Slightly anterior to the
lateral malleolus—
the ankle

VERTICAL
GRAVITY LINE

A

Changes in posture
(more forward head
and kyphosis)

Demineralization of
the bone (especially
dangerous in the spine—
may lead to fractures)

Decreased flexibility
(especially in hips and
knees)

Loss of strength;
greater difficulty
in doing functional
activities

Changes in gait patterns;
less motion and strength,
causing less toe-off and
floor clearance

VERTICAL
GRAVITY LINE

B

Fig. 4.54 Comparison of standing posture: changes associated with age. **A,** Younger person. **B,** Older person. (Modified from Lewis C, editor: *Aging: the health care challenge*, ed 2, Philadelphia, 1990, FA Davis.)

The sway that typically occurs during quiet standing is increased in older adults compared with younger adults (Maki and McIlroy, 1996; Sturnieks et al., 2008). Larger sway in older adults has been correlated with lower extremity strength and changes in sensory function, but no cause-and-effect relationship has been elucidated. It has been suggested that some older adults increase sway to increase sensory input to the lower extremities while able to stay within their limits of stability. Older individuals rely on vision more than somatosensation and respond to loss of visual input by standing more asymmetrically or swaying even more. Researchers found a difference in functional stability limits between community and noncommunity-dwelling older adults based on their performance on the Functional Reach (Rosa et al., 2019). All aspects of balance—steady-state, functional limits of stability, reactive, and anticipatory—are impacted by typical aging and by neuromotor disorders (Shumway-Cook and Woollacott, 2017).

Gait in the Older Adult

Numerous changes in gait can be expected to occur in an older population. Generally, the older adult is more cautious while walking. Cadence and velocity are decreased, as is stride length. Stride width increases to provide a wider base of support for better balance. Increasing the base of support and taking shorter steps means that an older adult spends more time in double limb support than a young adult. Walking velocity slows as stride length decreases, and double-support time increases. Double-support time reflects how much time is spent with both feet on the ground. Step initiation is delayed with a prolongation of the time it takes to transfer weight to the forward foot. Older adults shift more weight toward the support limb than younger adults, which represents a conservative strategy. Older adults have problems coordinating postural responses to leg movements (Hanke and Martin, 2012). Gait speed below 1.0 m/s is a strong indicator for falls (Kyrdalen et al., 2019).

Age-related changes in gait can create difficulties in other aspects of functional movement, such as stepping over objects and going up and down stairs. Chen et al. (1991) found that healthy older adults had more difficulty than healthy young adults in stepping over obstacles of increasing heights. In a recent systematic review, Galna et al. (2009) found that older adults adopt a conservative obstacle-crossing strategy, which involves greater hip flexion during swing phase for both the lead and trail limbs. When constrained by performing crossing an obstacle under timed conditions, the older adults were at greater risk for contacting the objects. Harley et al. (2009) found that under dual task conditions, increased cognitive demands lead to compromised safety and more variability in foot placement when stepping over obstacles.

Variability in gait when approaching obstacles is another indicator of fall risk (Pieruccini-Faria and Montero-Odasso, 2018). Stair climbing requires a period of single-limb stance while the swing leg is lifted up to the next step. Given the changes in gait with age already described, it is no surprise that older adults go up and down stairs more slowly. Challenging gait conditions have been used to predict a 1-year decline in gait speed in older adults who had normal gait speeds at initial testing (Brach et al., 2011).

Implications for Treatment

Age-related losses of range of motion, strength, and balance can be compounded in the older adult by a lack of habitual physical activity and can be intensified in the presence of neurologic deficits resulting from a stroke, spinal cord injury, or traumatic brain injury. The good news is that the decline in muscular strength and endurance can be partially reversed with an appropriate amount of resistive and endurance exercise. Precautions must always be considered in light of other preexisting conditions that would require modification of therapeutic intervention. The physical therapist is responsible for accurately documenting the patient's present level of abilities, recognizing mitigating circumstances, and planning appropriate therapeutic interventions. The therapist should instruct the physical therapist assistant in how the patient's exercise response should be monitored during treatment. If this information is not provided, the physical therapist assistant should request the information before treatment is initiated.

When the patient with a neurologic insult also has pulmonary or cardiac conditions, the physical therapist assistant should monitor the patient's vital signs during exercise. Decline in cardiopulmonary reserve capacity resulting from age can be compounded by a loss of fitness and loss of conditioning. A person who is in the hospital may be extremely deconditioned or become deconditioned. As the patient is being mobilized and acclimated to the upright position in preparation for discharge, the decline in physiologic reserve can affect the patient's ability to perform normal activities of daily living. Walking can require up to 40% of the oxygen taken in by an individual. Therefore, an older person may need to slow down the speed of walking depending on how much oxygen taken in is available. Measurements of heart rate, blood pressure, and respiratory rate are important, providing the supervising therapist with information about the patient's response to exercise. More specific monitoring of oxygen saturation, rate of perceived exertion, level of dyspnea (shortness of breath), or angina may be indicated by the supervising physical therapist, but further discussion of these methods is beyond the scope of this text. The complexity and acuity of the patient's condition may warrant limiting the involvement of the physical therapist assistant.

CHAPTER SUMMARY

Age and age-related changes in different body systems significantly alter the functional movement expectations for any given individual. Movement emerges from the interaction among the body systems in response to task demands within a changing biopsychosocial environment. Functional tasks are defined by the age and social and psychological expectations of the individual. An infant's function is to overcome gravity and learn to move into the upright position. The toddler explores the world in the upright position and adds fundamental movement patterns of running, hopping, and skipping during childhood. Manipulation of objects is continually refined from finger feeding cereal to learning to write. Exploring the environment provides sensory information that informs and predisposes the child to acquire cognitive and linguistic skills. Self-care skills are mastered by the time a child enters school. Sport skills build on the fundamental movement patterns and are important in childhood and adolescence. Work and leisure skills become important during late adolescence and adulthood. Older adulthood presents movement challenges for gait and balance that can be countered by exercise. Every period of the life span has different functional movement expectations that are driven by the mover, the task, and the social, physical and psychological environments.

REVIEW QUESTIONS

1. What are the criteria used to identify a developmental theory as being lifespan in approach?
2. What theorist described a pyramid of needs that the individual strives to fulfill?
3. What is an example of a directional concept of development?
4. What three processes guide motor development?
5. When does a child typically achieve gross- and fine-motor milestones?
6. What are the typical postures and movements of a 4-month-old and a 6-month-old?
7. What motor abilities constitute fundamental motor patterns?
8. Why do motor patterns continue to change throughout the lifespan?
9. What role does decreased activity play in an older adult's posture?
10. What gait changes can have an impact on functional abilities in older adults?

REFERENCES

Adolph K: Advances in research on infant motor development. Paper presented at APTA Combined Sections Meeting 2003, Tampa, FL.

American Academy of Pediatrics. Committee on Injury and Poison Prevention: Injuries associated with infant walkers, *Pediatrics* 129:e561, 2012.

Anderson DI, Campos JJ, Rivera M, et al.: The consequences of independent locomotion for brain and psychological development. In Shepherd RB, editor: *Cerebral palsy in infancy*, New York, 2014, Churchill Livingstone, pp 199–224.

Arnett JJ: Emerging adulthood: a theory of development from the late teens through the twenties, *Am Psychol* 55:469–480, 2000.

Arnett JJ: *Emerging adulthood: the winding road from the late teens through the twenties*, New York, 2004, Oxford University Press.

Arnett JJ: Suffering, selfish, slackers? Myths and reality about emerging adults, *J Youth Adolesc* 36:23–29, 2007.

Arnett JJ, Padilla-Walker LM: Brief report: Danish emerging adults' conceptions of adulthood, *J Adolesc* 38:39–44, 2015.

Arnett JJ, Zukauskiene R, Sugimura K: The new life stage of emerging adulthood at ages 18-29 years: implications for mental health, *Lancet Psychiatry* 1(7):569–576, 2014.

Astington JW, Barriault T: Children's theory of mind: how young children come to understand that people have thoughts and feelings, *Infants Young Child*, 13:1–12, 2001.

Baltes PB: Theoretical propositions of lifespan developmental psychology: on the dynamics between growth and decline, *Dev Psychol* 23:611–626, 1987.

Baltes PB, Lindenburger U, Staudinger UM: Lifespan theory in developmental psychology. In Damon W, Lerner RM, editors: *Handbook of child psychology*, ed 6, New York, 2006, Wiley & Sons, pp 569–664.

Barsalou LW: Grounded cognition: past, present, and future, *Top Cogn Sci* 2:716–724, 2010.

Bayley N: *Bayley scales of infant and toddler development*, ed 3, San Antonio, TX, 2005, Pearson.

Bly L: *Components of normal movement during the first year of life and abnormal development*, Chicago, 1983, Neurodevelopmental Treatment Association.

Brach JS, Perera S, VanSwearingen JM, Hiles ES, Wert DM, Studenski SA: Challenging gait conditions predict 1-year decline in gait speed in older adults with apparently normal gait, *Phys Ther* 91:1857–1864, 2011.

Bronfenbrenner U: *The ecology of human development. Experiments by nature and design*, Cambridge, MA, 1979, Harvard University Press.

Capute AJ, Shapiro BK, Palmer FB, et al. Normal gross motor development the influences of race, sex, and socio-economic status, *Dev Med Child Neurol* 27:635–643, 1985.

Carlson SM, Koenig MA, Harms MB: Theory of mind, *WIREs Cogn Sci* 4:391–402, 2013.

Chen HC, Ashton-Miller JA, Alexander NB, et al.: Stepping over obstacles gait patterns of healthy young and old adults, *J Gerontol* 46:M196–M203, 1991.

Chiarello LA: Family-centered care. In Effgen SK, editor: *Meeting the physical therapy needs of children*, ed 2, Philadelphia, 2013, FA Davis, pp 153–180.

Choudhury S, Charman T, Bird V, Blakemore S: Development of action representation during adolescence, *Neuropsychologia* 45:255–262, 2007.

Crajé C, van Elk M, Beeren M, et al.: Compromised motor planning and motor imagery in right hemiparetic cerebral palsy, *Res Dev Disabil* 31:1313–1322, 2010.

Cratty BJ: *Perceptual and motor development in infants and children*, ed 2, Englewood Cliffs, NJ, 1979, Prentice Hall.

Dalton JC, Crais ER, Vellman SL: Joint attention and oromotor abilities in young children with and without autism spectrum disorder, *J Commun Disord* 69:27–43, 2017.

Deci EL, Ryan RM: The "what" and "why" of goal pursuits: human needs and the self-determination of behavior, *Psychol Inq* 11:227–268, 2000.

Deci EL, Ryan RM: Self-determination theory: a macrotheory of human motivation, development and health, *Can Psychol* 49(3):182–185, 2008.

Diamond A: Close interrelation of motor development and cognitive development and of the cerebellum and the prefrontal cortex, *Child Dev* 71:44–56, 2000.

Di Dominico SI, Ryan RM: The emerging neuroscience of intrinsic motivation: a new frontier in self-determination research, *Front Hum Neurosci* 11:145, 2017. doi:10.3389/fnhum.2017.00145. eCollection 2017.

Duff SV: Prehension. In Cech D, Martin S, editors: *Functional movement development across the lifespan*, ed 3, Philadelphia, 2012, WB Saunders, pp 309–334.

Dusing SC: Postural variability and sensorimotor development in infancy, *Dev Med Child Neurol* 58(Suppl 4):17–21, 2016.

Dusing SC, Harbourne RT: Variability in postural control during infancy: implications for development, assessment, and intervention, *Phys Ther* 90:1838–1849, 2010.

Edelman GM: *Neural Darwinism*, New York, 1987, Basic Books.

Eishima K: The analysis of sucking behaviour in newborn infants, *Early Hum Dev* 27:163–173, 1991.

Erikson EH: *Identity, youth, and crisis*, New York, 1968, W.W. Norton.

Fitts PM: Categories of human learning. In Melton AW, editor: *Perceptual motor skills learning*, New York, 1964, pp 243–285.

Folio M, Fewell R: *Peabody developmental motor scales*, ed 2, Austin, TX, 2000, Pro-Ed.

Ford-Smith CD, VanSant AF: Age differences in movement patterns used to rise from a bed in the third through fifth decades of age, *Phys Ther* 73:300–307, 1993.

Frank C, Schack T: The representation of motor (inter)action, states of action, and learning: three perspectives on motor learning by way of imagery and execution, *Front Psychol* 8:678, 2017. doi:10.3389/fpsyg.2017.00678.

Gabbard C: Studying action representation in children via motor imagery, *Brain Cog* 71:234–239, 2009.

Gabbard C, Cacola P, Bobbio T: The ability to mentally represent action is associated with low motor ability in children: a preliminary investigation, *Child Care Health Dev* 38:390–393, 2012.

Galna B, Peters A, Murphy AT, Morris ME: Obstacle crossing deficits in older adults: a systematic review, *Gait Posture* 30:270–275, 2009.

Ganea PA, Lillard AS, Turkheimer E: Preschooler's understanding of the role of mental states and action in pretense, *J Cogn Dev* 5(2):213–238, 2004.

Gesell A: *The first five years of life*, New York, 1940, Harper & Brothers.

Gesell A, Ames LB, et al. *Infant and child in the culture of today*, rev, New York, 1974, Harper & Row.

Gibson JJ: *The senses as perceptual systems*, Boston, 1966, Houghton-Mifflin.

Gibson EJ: *The ecological approach to visual perception*, Boston, 1979, Houghton-Mifflin.

Gibson EJ: The concept of affordance in development: the renaissance of functionalism. In Collins WA, editor: *Minnesota symposium on child psychology*, vol 15, Hillsdale, NJ, 1982, Erlbaum.

Gibson EJ, Pick AD: *An ecological approach to perceptual learning and development*, New York, 2000, Oxford University Press.

Haddad AM, Purtillo RB, Doherty RF: *Health professional and patient interaction*, ed 9, St. Louis, 2019, Elsevier.

Hadders-Algra M: Variation and variability: key words in human motor development, *Phys Ther* 90:1823–1837, 2010.

Hadders-Algra M, Brogren E, Forssberg H: Ontogeny of postural adjustments during sitting in infancy: variation, selection, and modulation, *J Physiol* 493:273–288, 1996.

Hanke T, Martin S: Posture and balance. In Cech D, Martin S, editors: *Functional movement across the life span*, ed 3, St. Louis, 2012, Elsevier, pp 263–287.

Harbourne RT, Lobo MA, Karst GM, Galloway JC: Sit happens: does sitting development perturb reaching development or vice versa? *Infant Behav Dev* 36(3):438–450, 2013.

Harley C, Wilkie RM, Wann JP: Stepping over obstacles: attention demands and aging, *Gait Posture* 29:428–432, 2009.

Havinghurst RJ: *Developmental tasks and education*, ed 3, New York, 1972, David McKay.

Hopewell S, et al.: Multifactorial and multiple component interventions for preventing falls in older people living in the community, *Cochrane Database Syst Rev* 7:CD012221, 2018. doi:10.1002/14651858.CD01221.pub2.

Ivanenko YP, Dominici N, Lacquaniti F: Development of independent walking in toddlers, *Exerc Sport Sci Rev* 35:67–73, 2007.

Kyrdalen IL, Thingstad P, Sandrik L, Ormstad H: Associations between gait speed and well-known fall risk factors among community-dwelling older adults, *Physiother Res Int* 24(1):e1743, 2019. doi:10.1002/pri.1743.

Lebarton ES, Iverson JM: Associations between gross motor and communicative development in at-risk infants, *Infant Behav Dev* 44:59–67, 2016.

Leisman G, Moustafa A, Shafir T: Thinking, walking, talking: integratory motor and cognitive brain function, *Front Public Health* 4:94, 2016.

Levinson DJ: A conception of adult development, *Am Psychol* 41:3–13, 1986.

Lifter K, Bloom L: Object knowledge and the emergence of language, *Infant Behav Dev* 12: 395–423, 1989.

Lobo MA, Harbourne RT, Dusing SC, McCoy SW: Grounding early intervention: physical therapy cannot be about motor skills anymore, *Phys Ther* 93:94–103, 2013.

Lord SR, Clark RD, Webster IW: Visual acuity and contrast sensitivity in relation to falls in an elderly population, *Age Ageing* 20:175–181, 1991.

Lusardi MM, et al.: Determining risk of falls in community dwelling older adults: a systematic review and meta-analysis using posttest probability, *J Geriatr Phys Ther* 40:1–36, 2017.

Maki BE, McIlroy WE: Postural control in the older adult, *Clin Geriatr Med* 12:635–658, 1996.

Malina RM, Bouchard C, Bar-Or O: *Growth, maturation, and physical activity*, ed 2, Champaign, IL, 2004, Human Kinetics Books.

Marrus N, et al.: Walking, gross motor development, and brain functional connectivity in infants and toddlers, *Cereb Cortex* 28:750–763, 2018.

Maslow A: *Motivation and personality*, New York, 1954, Harper & Row.

McGoldrick M, Garcia Preto N, Carter BA: *The expanded family life cycle: individual, family, and social perspectives*, ed 5, New York, 2016, Pearson.

McManus MA, Pollack LR, Cooley WC, et al.: Current status of transition preparation among youth with special needs in the United States, *Pediatrics* 131:1090–1097, 2013.

Meyers AW, Whelan JP, Murphy SM: Cognitive behavioral strategies in athletic performance enhancement, *Prog Behav Modif* 30:137–164, 1996.

Mitteldorf J, Fahy GM: Questioning the inevitability of aging, *Proc Natl Acad Sci U S A* 115(4):E558, 2018. doi:10.1073/pnas.1720331115. Epub 2018.

Molina M, Tijus C, Jouen F: The emergence of motor imagery in children, *J Exp Child Psychol* 99:196–209, 2008.

Novak I, et al.: Early and accurate diagnosis and early intervention in cerebral palsy: advances in diagnosis and treatment, *JAMA Pediatr* 171(9):897–907, 2017.

Piaget J: *Play, dreams, and imitation in childhood*, London, 1951, Heinemann.

Piaget J: *Origins of intelligence*, New York, 1952, International University Press.

Pick HL, Gibson EL: Learning to perceive and perceiving to learn, *Dev Psychol* 28:787–794, 1992.

Piek JP, Dawson L, Smith LM, Gasson N: The role of early and fine and gross motor development on later motor and cognitive ability, *Hum Mov Sci* 27:668–681, 2008.

Pieruccini-Faria F, Montero-Odasso M: Obstacle negotiation, gait variability, and risk of falling: results from the "Gait and Brain Study," *J Gerontol A Biol Sci Med Sci* 2018. doi:10.1093/gerona/gly254. [Epub ahead of print].

Pitcher JB, Schneider LA, Drysdale JL, et al. Motor system development of the preterm and low birthweight infant, *Clin Perinatol* 38:605–625, 2011.

Raz N, Daugherty AM: Pathways to brain aging and their modifiers: free-radical-induced energetic and neural decline in senescence (friends) model—a mini-review, *Gerontology* 64:49–57, 2018.

Roberton M, Halverson L: The developing child: his changing movement. In Logsdon BJ, editor: *Physical education for children: a focus on the teaching process*, Philadelphia, 1977, Lea & Febiger.

Rosa MV, Parracini MR, Ricci NA: Usefulness, assessment and normative data of the Functional Reach Test in older adults: a systematic review and meta-analysis, *Arch Gerontol Geriatr Suppl* 81:149–170, 2019.

Ryan RM, Patrick H, Deci EL, et al.: Facilitating health behavior change and its maintenance: interventions based on self-determination theory, *Eur Psychol* 10:2–5, 2008.

Sabourin P: *Rising from supine to standing: a study of adolescents*, unpublished masters' thesis, 1989, Virginia Commonwealth University.

Scovil CY, Zettel JL, Maki BDE: Stepping to recover balance in complex environments: is online visual control of the foot motion necessary or sufficient? *Neurosci Lett* 445:108–112, 2008.

Shumway-Cook A, Woollacott M: *Motor control: translating research into clinical practice*, ed 5, Philadelphia, 2017, Wolters Kluwer.

Spruijt S, van der Kamp J, Steenbergen B: Current insights in the development of children's motor imagery ability, *Front Psychol* 6:787, 2015. doi:10.3389/fpsyg.2015.00787.

Sturnieks DL, St George R, Lord SR: Balance disorders in the elderly, *Clin Neurophysiol* 38:467–478, 2008.

Sutherland DH, Olshen RA, Biden EN, Wyatt MP: *The development of mature walking*, London, 1988, MacKeith Press.

Thelen E: Rhythmical stereotypies in infants, *Anim Behav* 27:699–715, 1979.

Thelen E, Smith LB: *A dynamic systems approach to the development of cognition and action*, Cambridge, MA, 1994, MIT Press.

Thomas RL, Williams AK, Lundy-Ekman L: Supine to stand in elderly persons: relationship to age, activity level, strength, and range of motion, *Issues Aging* 21:9–18, 1998.

Vaillant GE: *Aging well*, New York, 2002, Little Brown.

VanSant AF: Age differences in movement patterns used by children to rise from a supine position to erect stance, *Phys Ther* 68:1130–1138, 1988a.

VanSant AF: Rising from a supine position to erect stance: description of adult movement and a developmental hypothesis, *Phys Ther* 68:185–192, 1988b.

VanSant AF: Lifespan motor development. In Lister MJ, editor: *Contemporary management of motor control problems: proceedings of the II STEP Conference*, Alexandria, VA, 1991, American Physical Therapy Association, pp 77–84.

Vygotsky L: Play and its role in the mental development of the child, *Sov Psychol* 12:62–76, 1966.

Vygotsky L: *Thought and language*, MIT Press (Kozulin A, translator) Cambridge, MA, 1986.

Wang PJ, Morgan GA, Hwang AW, Liao HF: Individualized behavioral assessments and maternal ratings of mastery motivation in mental age-matched toddlers with and without motor delay, *Phys Ther* 93:79–87, 2013.

Wang Y, Morgan WP: The effect of imagery perspectives on the psychophysiological responses to imagined exercise, *Behav Brain Res* 52:1667–1674, 1992.

Whitall J: A developmental study of the inter-limb coordination in running and galloping, *J Motor Behav* 21:409–428, 1989.

Wickstrom RL: *Fundamental movement patterns*, ed 2, Philadelphia, 1977, Lea & Febiger.

Wickstrom RL: *Fundamental movement patterns*, ed 3, Philadelphia, 1983, Lea & Febiger.

World Health Organization (WHO): Motor development study: windows of achievement for six gross motor milestones, *Acta Paediatr Suppl* 450:86–95, 2006.

Zhao CQ, Wang LM, Jiang LS, et al.: The cell biology of the intervertebral disc aging and degeneration, *Ageing Res Rev* 6(3):247–261, 2007.

Positioning and Handling to Foster Motor Function

After reading this chapter, the student will be able to:

1. Understand the importance of using positioning and handling as interventions when treating children with neurodevelopmental disorders.
2. Describe the use of positioning and handling as interventions to improve function in children with neurodevelopmental disorders.
3. List handling tips that can be used when treating children with neurodevelopmental disorders.
4. Describe transitional movements used in treating children with neurodevelopmental disorders.
5. List the goals for use of adaptive equipment with children who have neurodevelopmental disorders.
6. Describe how play can be used therapeutically with children who have neurodevelopmental disorders.

INTRODUCTION

The purpose of this chapter is to detail some of the most frequent positioning and handling used as interventions when working with children who have neurodevelopmental disorders. Basic interventions such as positioning are used for many reasons: (1) to meet general patient goals such as improving head or trunk control; (2) to accommodate a lack of muscular support; (3) to provide proper postural alignment; (4) to manage muscle tone and extensibility; and (5) to afford an opportunity for self-generated movement. Handling techniques can be used to improve the child's performance of functional tasks, such as sitting, walking, and reaching, by promoting postural alignment prior to and during movement. Other specific sensory interventions, such as tapping a muscle belly, tactile cuing, or pressure, are tailored to specific impairments the child may have. Impairments include such things as difficulty in recruiting a muscle contraction for movement initiation, lack of pelvic control for midline positioning, or inability to control certain body segments during changes of position. The ultimate goal of any type of therapeutic intervention is functional movement. Positioning and handling can also be used to foster age appropriate play in children with neurodevelopmental disorders.

CHILDREN WITH NEURODEVELOPMENTAL DISORDERS

Children with neurodevelopmental disorders may exhibit delays in motor development and impairments in muscle tone, sensation, range of motion, strength, and coordination. These children are at risk for musculoskeletal deformities and contractures and often have or are susceptible to develop activity limitations in performing functional activities. Activity limitations in transfers, locomotion, manipulation, and participation restrictions in self-care and play may result from impairments. The reader is referred to Table 1.5 which depicts the ICF bio-psychosocial model as applied to neurodevelopmental disorders. What remains unclear is whether changing impairments changes function. Some or all of these impairments may be evident in any child with neurodevelopmental disorders. The activity limitations may be related to the impairments documented by the physical therapist during an initial examination and evaluation, such as deficits in strength, range of motion, and coordination. A lack of postural responses, balance, and motor milestone acquisition can be expected, given the specific pathologic features of the neurodevelopmental disorder.

Children with motor disabilities, such as seen in children with autism, cerebral palsy, Down syndrome, and myelomeningocele, demonstrate delays in play (Barton, 2015; Martin, 2014; Pfeifer et al., 2011). Children with disabilities play less well, often demonstrating lower levels of age-expected play (Jennings et al., 1988). Children with autism lack the ability to pretend and do not demonstrate pretend play (Charman and Baron-Cohen, 1997; Jarrold, 2003). In fact, the lack of pretend play in a young child is part of the diagnostic process for autism (Rutherford et al., 2007). Specific neurodevelopmental disorders are presented in more depth in Chapters 6, 7, 8, and 9.

GENERAL PHYSICAL THERAPY GOALS

The guiding goal of therapeutic intervention in working with children with neurodevelopmental disorders is to improve function. The physical therapist and physical therapist assistant team must strive to provide interventions designed to make the child as independent as possible within the parameters of the child's diagnosis. Specific movement goals may vary depending on the type of neurodevelopmental disorder. Children with low tone and joint hypermobility need to be stabilized, whereas children with increased tone and limited joint range need mobility. Joint and muscle extensibility may be limited or excessive. Children must be able to move from one position to another with selective motor control. Movement from one position to another is called *transitional movement*. Important movement transitions to be mastered include moving from supine position to prone; moving from supine or prone position to a sitting position; and moving from sitting position to standing position. Additional transitional movements usually acquired during normal development are moving from prone position to four-point position, followed by moving to kneeling, half-kneeling, and finally standing.

Movement is needed to engage in play and self-care, including self-feeding. Certain positions (such as sitting) are more amenable to engaging the child in play, although playing in side-lying or prone may be possible if the child has sufficient head control and ability to bear weight on one upper extremity while reaching with the other arm. Play should not only be used as a medium for therapy but as a goal in and of itself. Children with neurodevelopmental disorders often need assistance to interact with the caregiver and to explore the environment. Lobo et al. (2013) promote using early perceptual-motor behaviors to facilitate global development. All therapists and assistants, regardless of discipline, should use activity-focused interventions to promote participation (Fig. 5.1). Objects and their placement within the environment drive motor behavior. Acquisition of motor skills, especially sitting and locomotion, supports environmental exploration and perceptual motor development. Play is certainly an early perceptual-motor behavior and play is fun, therefore play is one of the hallmarks of participation in the life of a child (Rosenbaum and Gorter, 2011). Play is also a vehicle for developmental change that reinforces motor behavior. Play also affords opportunities for social, emotional, and cognitive linguistic development. Our interventions have to go beyond movement into the larger realm of social play and cognition (Lobo et al., 2013).

Children who exhibit excessive and extraneous movement, such as children with athetoid or ataxic cerebral palsy, need practice in maintaining stable postures against gravity because their natural tendency is to be moving all the time. Children with fluctuating muscle tone find it difficult to stabilize or maintain a posture and often cannot perform small weight shifts from the midline without falling. The ability to control transfer of weight within a posture is the beginning of selective motor control. With controlled weight transfer comes the ability to change positions safely or free the arms to play, feed, or dress. Regardless of the type of movement experience needed, all children with neuromuscular difficulties need to be able to function in as many postures as possible. Some postures are more functional than others, and may provide therapeutic benefits and afford possibilities for participation.

FUNCTION RELATED TO POSTURE

Posture provides a base for movement and function. Impairment of postural control, either in attaining or in maintaining a posture, can produce activity limitations. If an infant cannot maintain postural control in sitting without hand support, then the ability to play with toys is limited. Think of posture as a pyramid, with supine and prone positions at the base, followed by sitting, and erect standing at the apex (Fig. 5.2). As the child gains control, the base of support

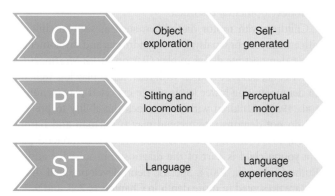

Fig. 5.1 How therapies support play and cognition.

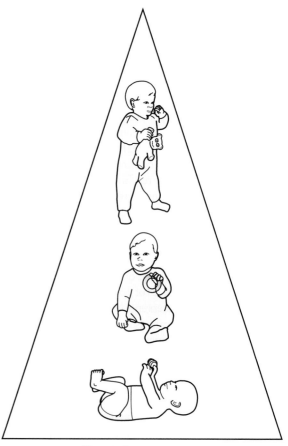

Fig. 5.2 Posture pyramid.

becomes smaller. Children with inadequate balance or postural control often widen their base of support to compensate for a lack of stability. A child with decreased postural muscle activity may be able to sit without arm support to play if the legs are straight and widely abducted (abducted long sitting). When the base of support is narrowed by bringing the legs together (long sitting), the child wobbles and may even fall over. The sitting posture, not the child's trunk musculature, was providing the stability.

Supine and Prone

Supine and prone are the lowest postural levels in which a child can function. The supine position is defined as being flat on the back on the support surface. Motor function at this level can involve rolling, reaching with upper extremities, looking, or propelling the body by pushing off flexed lower extremities. The prone position includes lying flat on the tummy with the head turned to one side or lifted, prone on elbows, or prone on extended arms. Mobility in the prone position is possible by means of rolling or crawling on the tummy. Many children push themselves backward when they are prone before they are able to pull themselves forward. Children with weak or uncoordinated lower extremities commonly perform a "commando crawl" using only the arms to pull along the support surface. This is also called "drag crawling" if the lower extremities do not assist in producing the movement, but are dragged along by the pull of the arms.

Sitting

Sitting, the next highest posture, affords the child the opportunity to move the extremities while the head and trunk are in a more upright position. In sitting, the child is appropriately oriented to the world, eyes oriented vertically and mouth horizontally. Typically developing children are sitting around 6 months of age. The muscles of the neck and trunk are in the same orientation with gravity, and it is actually easier to maintain head-and-trunk alignment in this position as compared with being in prone or supine, where the force of gravity must be constantly overcome. Sitting upright affords the child the chance to learn to be mobile in a wheelchair or to use the upper extremities for feeding, self-care, and play. Functional use of the upper extremities requires trunk control, whether that comes from postural muscle control or from a seating system. Alternative mobility patterns available to a child who is seated include scooting or hitching along the floor on the buttocks, with or without hand support.

Quadruped

Quadruped, as a developmental posture, allows creeping to emerge sometime between independent sitting and erect standing. In typically developing children, quadruped, or the four-point position as it may be called, provides quick mobility in a modified prone position before the child has mastered moving in an upright position. Quadruped is considered a dependent and flexed posture; therefore, it has been omitted from the pyramid posture. The child is dependent because the child's head is not always correctly oriented to the world, and with only a few exceptions, the limbs are flexed. It can be difficult for a child to learn to creep reciprocally, so this posture is often omitted as a therapeutic goal. A small number of infants never creep before walking (World Health Organization, 2006).

The quadruped position can provide excellent opportunities for the child to bear weight through the shoulders and hips and thereby promote proximal stability at these joints. Such weight-bearing opportunities are essential to preparing for the proximal joint control needed for making the transition from one posture to another. Although the quadruped position does make unique contributions to the development of trunk control, because the trunk must work maximally against gravity, other activities can be used to work the trunk muscles without requiring the upper extremities to be fully weight bearing and the hips and knees flexed. Deviating from the developmental sequence may be necessary in therapy because of a child's inability to function in quadruped or because of an increased potential for the child to develop contractures from overusing this posture.

Standing

The last and highest level of function is upright standing, in which ambulation may be possible. Most typically developing infants attain an upright standing position by pulling up on furniture at around 9 months of age. Supported standing programs have routinely been used in pediatric physical therapy practice. Evidence supports that standing can increase bone mineral density and range of motion, decrease spasticity, and improve hip stability (Paleg et al., 2013). For children not able to attain or maintain upright on their own, a supported standing program can be beneficial and a first step toward active participation in the environment.

By 12 months of age, most children are walking independently. Ambulation significantly increases the ability of toddlers to explore their surroundings. Ask the parent of an infant who has just begun to walk how much more challenging it is to keep up with and safeguard the child's explorations. Attainment of the ability to walk is one of our most frequent therapeutic goals. Being able to move around within our society in an upright standing position is a huge sign that one is "normal." For some parents who are dealing with the realization that their child is not exhibiting typical motor skills, the goal of walking may represent an even bigger achievement, or the final thing the child cannot do. We have worked with parents who have stated that they would rather have their child walk than talk. The most frequently asked questions you will hear when working with very young children are "Will my child walk?" and "When will my child walk?" These are difficult questions. The ambulation potential of children with specific neurologic deficit is addressed in the following chapters. The assistant should consult with the supervising therapist before answering inquiries related to patient prognosis.

PHYSICAL THERAPY INTERVENTION

Developmental intervention consists of positioning and handling, including guided movements and planned environmental experiences that allow the infant and young child to enjoy the feeling of typical movement. By modifying the environment or the task the child is afforded the opportunity to generate movement. These movement experiences must occur within the framework of the infant's or child's role within the family and in the natural environment—the home, and later, the school. An infant's social role is to interact with caregivers and the environment to learn about herself and the world. Piaget called the first 2 years of life the sensorimotor period for that reason. Intelligence (cognition) begins with associations the infant makes between the self and the people and objects within the environment. These associations are formed by and through movement of the body and objects within the environment.

Our intent is to enable the physical therapist and physical therapist assistant to see multiple uses of certain interventions in the context of an understanding of the overall nature of developmental intervention. Initially, when you work with an infant with neurodevelopmental issues, the child may have a diagnosis of only being "at risk" for developmental delay or cerebral palsy. The family may not have been given a specific developmental diagnosis. The therapist and physician may have discussed only the child's tight or loose muscles and problems with head control. One of the most important ways to help family members of an "at risk" child is to show them ways to position and handle (hold and move) the child to make it easier for the child and family to interact. Certain positions may support the infant's head better, thus enabling feeding, eye movement, and looking at the caregiver. Other positions may make diapering easier. Flexing the infant's head, trunk, and limbs while she is being carried is usually indicated because this handling method approximates the typical posture of a young infant and provides a feeling of security for both the child and the caregiver.

Research on the variability of postural control in infants and the effect of enhanced handling and positioning reinforces the need to teach/coach the caregiver how to provide meaningful sensorimotor experiences from the beginning. Lobo and Galloway (2012) documented advances in motor development from a 3-week program of enhanced handling and positioning taught to caregivers. These experiences consisted of encouraging pushing up in prone, positioning in supported sitting, and standing to promote head control. The caregiver was asked to engage the infant in face-to-face interaction without objects for 15 minutes every day. Short- and long-term advancements were reported. These finding support the use of small and varied movements to build prospective postural control. Infants need to try multiple strategies of moving to develop postural control (Dusing and Harbourne, 2010). A child's position was found to affect results of cognitive testing in a case report by O'Grady and Dusing (2016).

Daily Routines

Many handling and positioning techniques can be incorporated into the routine daily care of the child. Picking a child up and putting her down can be used to provide new movement experiences that the child may not be able to initiate on her own. Optimal positioning for bathing, eating, and playing is in an upright sitting position, provided the child has sufficient head control. As the infant develops head control (4 months) and trunk control, a more upright position can be fostered. If the child is unable to sit with slight support at 6 months, the appropriate developmental time, it may be necessary to use an assistive device, such as a feeder seat or a corner chair, to provide head or trunk support to allow the child to experience a more upright orientation to the world.

An upright orientation is also important in developing the child's interest and engaging her socially. Think of how you would automatically position a baby to interact. More than likely, you would pick him or her up and bring the baby's face toward you. An older child may need only minimal assistance to maintain sitting to perform activities of daily living, as in sitting on a bench to dress or sitting in a chair with arms to feed herself or to color in a book. Some children require only the support at the lower back to encourage and maintain an upright trunk, as seen in Fig. 5.3. Being able to sit at the table with the family includes the child in everyday occurrences, such as eating breakfast or reviewing homework. Upright positioning with or without assistive devices provides the appropriate orientation to interact socially while the child plays or performs activities of daily living (Fig. 5.4).

Home Program

Positioning and handling should be part of every home program. When positioning and handling are seen as part of the

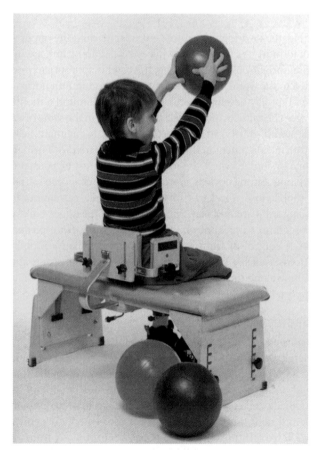

Fig. 5.3 Child sitting on a bench with pelvic support. (Courtesy Kaye Products, Inc., Hillsborough, NC.)

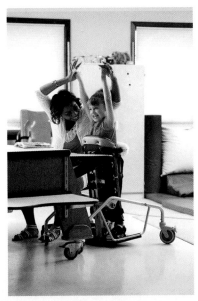

Fig. 5.4 Upright positioning fosters social interaction. (Courtesy Rifton Equipment, Rifton, NY.)

daily routine, parents are more likely to do these activities with the child. By recognizing all the demands placed on parents' time, you need to make realistic requests of them. Remember, a parent's time is limited. Stretching can be incorporated into bath time or diaper changes. In addition, by suggesting a variety of therapeutic play positions that can be incorporated into the daily routine of the child, you may make it unnecessary for the caregiver to have to spend as much time stretching specific muscles. Pictures are wonderful reminders. Providing a snapshot of how you want the child to sit can provide a gentle reminder to all family members, especially those who are unable to attend a therapy session. If the child is supposed to use a certain adaptive device, such as a corner chair, sometime during the day, help the caregiver to determine the best time and place to use the device. Good planning ensures carryover.

POSITIONING AND HANDLING INTERVENTIONS

Positioning for Function

One of the fundamental skills a physical therapist assistant learns is how to position a patient. The principles of positioning include alignment, comfort, and support. Additional considerations include prevention of deformity and readiness to move. When positioning the patient's body or body part, the alignment of the body part or the body as a whole must be considered. In the majority of cases, the alignment of a body part is considered along with the reason for the positioning. For example, the position of an upper extremity in relation to the upper trunk is normally at the side; however, when the patient cannot move the arm, it may be better positioned away from the body to prevent tightness of muscles around the shoulder. The patient's comfort is also important

to consider because, as we have all experienced, no matter how "good" the position is for us, if it is uncomfortable, we will change to another position. Underlying the rules governing how to position a person in proper body alignment is the need to prevent any potential deformity, such as tight heel cords, hip dislocation, or spinal curvature.

Positioning for support may also be thought of as positioning for stability. Children and adults often assume certain positions or postures because they feel safe. For example, the person who has hemiplegic involvement usually orients or shifts weight over the noninvolved side of the body because of better sensory awareness, muscular control, and balance. Although this positioning may be stable, it can lead to potential muscle shortening on the involved side that can impair functional movement. Other examples of postures that provide positional stability include W sitting, wide abducted sitting, and propped sitting on extended arms (Fig. 5.5). All these positions have a wide base of support that provides inherent stability. W sitting is not desirable because the child does not have to use trunk muscles for postural support; the stability of the trunk comes from the position. Asymmetric sitting or sitting with weight shifted more to one side may cause the trunk to develop muscle imbalance. Common examples of asymmetry are seen in children with hemiplegic cerebral palsy who, even in symmetric sitting postures such as short or long sitting, do so with their weight shifted away from the involved side.

In working with individuals with neurologic deficit, the clinician often must determine safe and stable postures that can be used for activities of daily living. The child who uses W sitting because the position leaves the hands free to play needs to be given an alternative sitting position that affords the same opportunities for play. Alternatives to W sitting may include some type of adaptive seating, such as a corner chair or a floor sitter (Fig. 5.6). A simple solution may be to have the child sit on a chair at a table to play, rather than sitting on the floor.

The last consideration for positioning is the idea that a position provides a posture from which movement occurs. This concept may be unfamiliar to those who are used to working with adults. Adults have a greater motivation to move because of prior experience. Children, on the other hand, may not have experienced movement and may even be afraid to move because they cannot do so with control. Safety is of paramount importance in the application of this concept. A child should be able to be safe in a posture; that is, be able to maintain the posture and demonstrate a protective response if she falls out of the posture. Often, a child can maintain sitting only if she is propped on one or both upper extremities. If the child cannot maintain a posture even when propped, some type of assistance is required to ensure safety while she is in the position. The assistance can be in the form of a device or a person. Proper alignment of the trunk must always be provided to prevent unwanted spinal curvatures, which can hamper independent sitting and respiratory function.

Any position in which you place a child should allow the child the opportunity to shift weight within the posture for pressure relief. The next movement possibility that should be

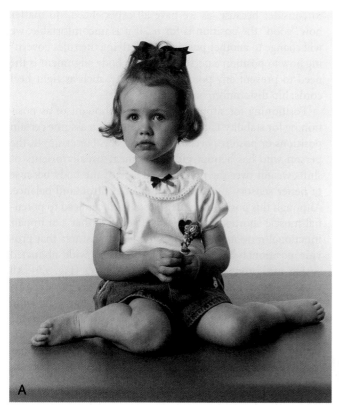

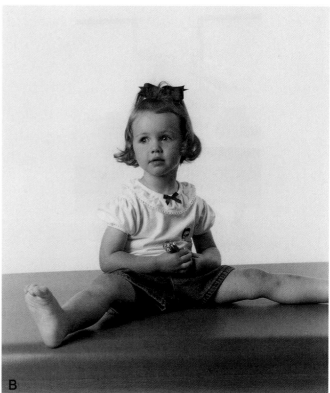

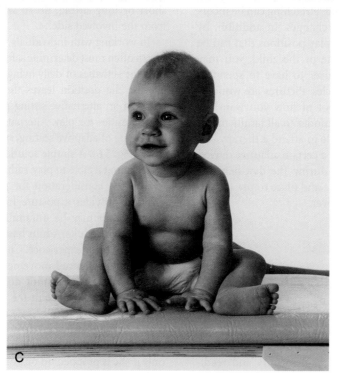

Fig. 5.5 **Sitting Postures. (A)** W sitting, which is to be avoided. **(B)** Wide abducted long sitting. **(C)** Propped sitting with legs abducted.

provided the child is to move from the initial posture to another posture. Many patients, regardless of age and for many reasons, have difficulty in making the transition from one position to another. We often forget this principle of positioning because we are more concerned about the child's safety

within a posture than about how the position may affect mobility. When we work with children, we must take into account both mobility and stability to select therapeutic positions that encourage static and dynamic balance. *Dynamic postures* are ones in which controlled mobility can be exhibited; that is,

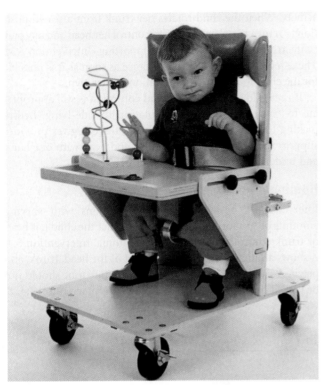

Fig. 5.6 Corner chair with head support. (Courtesy Kaye Products, Inc., Hillsborough, NC.)

shifting weight so the center of gravity stays within the base of support. In typical development, the child rocks or shifts weight in a hands-and-knees position for long periods before making the transition to creeping. The ability to shift weight with control within a posture indicates preparation and readiness to move out of that posture into another posture. Dynamic balance is also exhibited when the child moves from the four-point position to a side-sitting position. The center of gravity moves diagonally over one hip and down until a new base of support is created by sitting.

The type of activity the child is expected to perform in a particular posture must also be considered when a position is chosen. For example, how an infant or child is positioned for feeding by a caregiver may vary considerably from the position used for self-feeding or for playing on the floor. A child's position must be changed often during the day, so teaching the parent or caregiver only one position rarely suffices. For example, modifications of sitting positions may be required for bathing, feeding, dressing, playing, and toileting, depending on the degree of assistance the child requires with each of these activities. Other positions may be employed to accomplish therapeutic goals related to head control, trunk control, or extremity usage.

The job or occupation of infants and children is merely to play. Although play may appear to be a simple task, it is a constant therapeutic challenge to help parents identify ways to allow their child to participate fully in the world. More broadly, a child's job is interacting with people and objects within the environment and learning how things work. Usually, one of a child's first tasks is to learn the rules of moving, a difficult task when the child has a developmental disability. A child should be encouraged to participate in playful learning. Rosenbaum and Gorter (2011) incorporated "F-words" into the already existing concepts from the International classification of Functioning, Disability, and Health (ICF) model of childhood disability. Function has already been identified as pivotal to a child's participation in life. The other words, suggested by Rosenbaum and Gorter (2011), are family, fitness, fun, and future. These concepts will be highlighted throughout the remainder of the chapter.

Handling at Home

Parents and caregivers should be taught the easiest ways to move the child from one position to another. For example, Intervention 5.1 shows how to assist an infant with head

---

INTERVENTION 5.1   Prone to Sitting

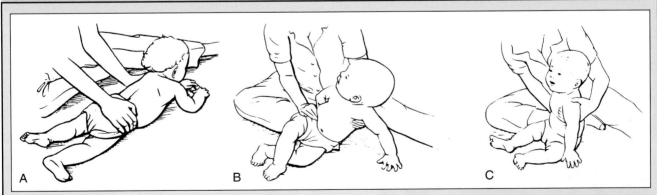

Moving a child with head control from prone into sitting.
A. Place one hand under the arm next to you and the other hand on the child's opposite hip.
B. Initiate rotation of the hip, and assist as needed under the shoulder. Allow the child to push up if she is able to.
C. Perform the activity slowly to allow the child to help and support the trunk if necessary in sitting.

control to move from prone into a sitting position for dressing or feeding. Most children benefit from being picked up while they are in a flexed position and then placed or assisted into sitting. Caregivers are taught how to encourage the infant or child to assist as much as possible during any movement. If the child has head control but decreased trunk control, encouraging the child to turn to the side and push up on an elbow or extended arm will result in sitting (Intervention 5.2). Manual assistance can be given when and where needed; the goal is self-initiated movement if possible. Movement transitions are a major part of a home program. For example, the caregiver can incorporate practicing coming to sit from a supine or prone position and alternate which side of the body the child rolls toward during the maneuver. In this manner, transitions become part of the child's daily routine, not an extra burden on the caregiver. Although it may seem easier for the caregiver to move the child, it is far more beneficial for the caregiver to encourage the child's participation in the activity. When the child rotates her trunk from a seated position to return to prone, she has to control her head and any part of the trunk the caregiver is not supporting (Intervention 5.3). The caregiver should reduce assistance as soon as it is possible for the child to initiate trunk rotation on her own.

If the child does not have head control, it is still appropriate to try to promote trunk rotation to side-lying. Before picking the child up from side-lying, the caregiver provides support under the child's shoulders and head with one hand and under the knees with the other hand.

Holding and Carrying Positions

Intervention 5.4 depicts carrying positions with varying amounts of support, depending on whether the child has head or trunk control, hypertonia, or hypotonia. Intervention 5.4, *A* shows an infant cradled for support of the head, trunk, and pelvis. A child with increased lower extremity tone should not be picked up under the arms, as shown in Intervention 5.4, *B*.

INTERVENTION 5.2   Supine to Side-lying to Sitting

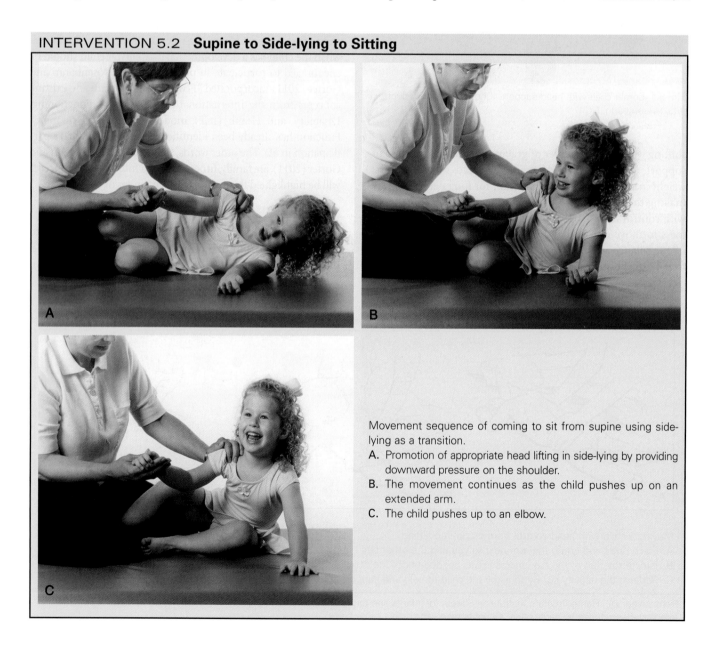

Movement sequence of coming to sit from supine using side-lying as a transition.
A. Promotion of appropriate head lifting in side-lying by providing downward pressure on the shoulder.
B. The movement continues as the child pushes up on an extended arm.
C. The child pushes up to an elbow.

INTERVENTION 5.3 Sitting to Prone

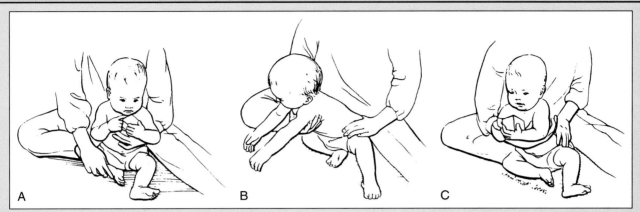

Moving a child with head control from sitting to prone.
A. With the child sitting, bend the knee of the side toward which the child will rotate.
B. Initiate the movement by rotating the child's upper trunk.
C. Complete the rotation by guiding the hip to follow until the child is prone.

(From Jaeger DL: Home Program Instruction Sheets for Infants and Young Children. ©1987 Therapy Skill Builders, a Harcourt Health Sciences Company. Reproduced by permission. All rights reserved.)

The legs stiffen into extension and may even cross or "scissor." This way of picking up an infant should also be avoided in the presence of low tone because the child's shoulder girdle stability may not be sufficient for the caregiver to hold the infant safely. Intervention 5.4, *C* and *E* demonstrates correct ways to hold a child with increased tone. The child's lower extremities are flexed, with the trunk and legs supported. Trunk rotation is encouraged. By having the child straddle the caregiver's hip, as in Intervention 5.4, *E*, the child's hip adductors are stretched, and the upper trunk, which is rotated outward, is dissociated from the lower trunk. The caregiver must remember to carry the child on opposite hips during the day, to avoid promoting asymmetric trunk rotation. The child with low tone needs to be gathered close to you to be given a sense of stability (see Intervention 5.4, *D*). Many infants and children with developmental delay find prone an uncomfortable position, but may tolerate being carried in the prone position because of the contact with the caregiver and the movement stimulation (see Intervention 5.4, *F*).

Holding an infant in the prone position over the caregiver's lap can provide vestibular system input to reinforce midline orientation or lifting of the head. Infants with head control and some trunk control can be held on the caregiver's lap while they straddle the caregiver's knee, to abduct their tight lower extremities.

Handling Techniques for Movement

Because children with disabilities do have similar problems, grouping possible treatment interventions together is easier based on the position and goal of the intervention, such as positioning in prone to encourage head control. The intervention should be matched to the child's problem, and one should always keep in mind the overall functional goal. Depending on the severity of neuromotor involvement of the child, lower-level developmental milestones may be the highest goal possible. For example, in a child with spastic quadriplegic cerebral palsy (Gross Motor Function Measure [GMFCS] level V) therapeutic goals may consist of the development of head control and the prevention of contractures, whereas in a child with quadriplegia and classification at GMFCS level IV, independent sitting and wheelchair mobility may be the goals of intervention. See Chapter 6 for a description of GMFCS levels of motor function.

Use of Manual Contacts

When you are promoting a child's head or trunk control using manual contact at the shoulder girdle, placing your hands under the child's axillae while facing her can serve in mobilizing the scapulae and lifting the extremities away from the body. Your fingers should be spread out in such a way to control both the scapulae and the upper arms. By controlling the scapulae in this way, you can promote movement of the child's head, trunk, arms, and legs but prevent the arms from pulling down and back, as may be the child's typical movement pattern. If you do not need to control the child's upper extremities, your hands can be placed over the child's shoulders to cover the clavicles, the scapulae, and the heads of the humeri. This second strategy can also promote alignment and therefore can increase stability and is especially useful in the treatment of a child with too much movement, as in athetoid cerebral palsy. Varying amounts of pressure can be given through the shoulders and can be combined with movement in different directions to provide a stabilizing influence.

INTERVENTION 5.4   Carrying Positions

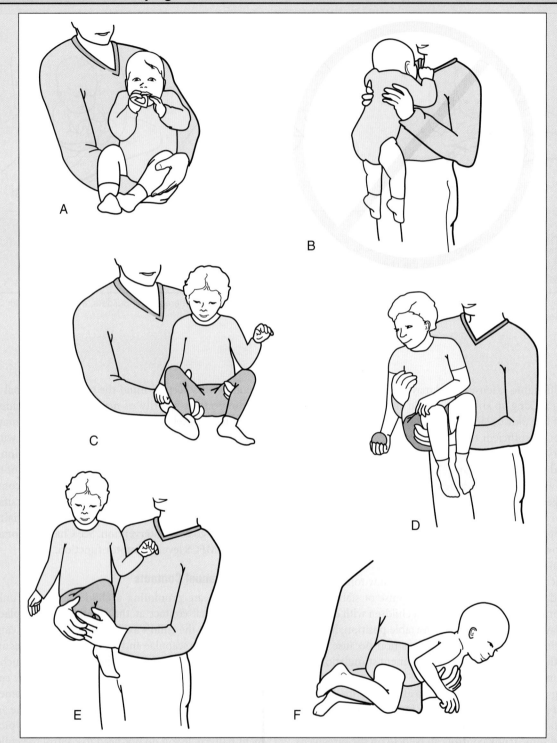

A. Place the child in a curled-up position with shoulders forward and hips flexed. Place your arm behind the child's head, not behind the neck.

B. INCORRECT: Avoid lifting the child under her arms without supporting the legs. The child with hypertonicity may "scissor" (cross) the legs. The child with hypotonicity may slip through your hands.

C. CORRECT: Bend the child's legs before picking her up. Give sufficient support to the trunk and legs while allowing trunk rotation.

D. Hold the child with low tone close, to provide a feeling of stability.

E. Have the child straddle your hips to separate tight legs. Be sure the child's trunk is rotated forward and both her arms are free.

F. Prone position.

Wherever your hands are on the child, the child is not in control; you are, so the child must be given practice controlling the body parts used to guide movement. For example, if you are using the child's shoulders to guide movement, the child needs to learn to control movement at the shoulder. As the child exhibits more proximal control, your manual contacts can be moved more distally to the elbow or hand. Stability can be facilitated by positioning the limbs in a weight-bearing or loaded position. If the child lacks sufficient control, pediatric air or fabric splints can be used to control the limb position, thus enabling the child to bear weight on an extended knee or to keep the weight-bearing elbow straight while reaching with the other arm (Fig. 5.7).

Handling Tips

The following should be considered when you physically handle a child with neuromotor deficit.

1. Allow the child to do as much of the movement as possible. You will need to go more slowly than you may think. For example, when bringing a child into a sitting position from supine, roll the child slowly to one side and give the child time to push up onto her hand, even if she can only do this part of the way, such as up to an elbow. In addition, try to entice the child to roll to the side before attempting to have her come to sit. Using a toy to encourage reaching to roll can also be used. The effects of gravity can be reduced by using an elevated surface, such as a wedge, under the head and upper trunk to make it easier to move into side-lying before coming to sit.

2. When carrying a child, encourage as much head and trunk control as the child can demonstrate. Carry the child in such a way that head and trunk muscles are used to maintain the head and trunk upright against gravity while you are moving. This allows the child to look around and see where you are going.

3. When trying to move the limbs of a child with spasticity, do not pull against the tightness. Do move slowly and rhythmically, starting proximally at the child's shoulders and pelvis. The position of the proximal joints can influence the position of the entire extremity. Changing the position of the proximal joint may also reduce tone throughout the extremity.

4. Many children with severe involvement and those with athetosis show an increased sensitivity to touch, sound, and light. These children startle easily and may withdraw from contact to their hands, feet, and mouth. Encourage the child to keep her head in the midline of the body and the hands in sight. Weight bearing on hands and feet is an important activity for these children because it provides some stability.

5. Children with low postural tone can be handled more vigorously unless there is a seizure precaution, but they tire more easily and require more frequent rest periods. Avoid placing children in a supine position to play because they need to work against gravity in the prone position to develop their extensor muscles. Their extensors are so weak that the extremities assume a "frog" position of abduction when these children are supine. Strengthening of abdominal muscles can be done with the child in a semi-reclined supine position. Encourage arm use and visual learning. By engaging visual tracking, the child may learn to use the eyes to encourage head and trunk movement. Infant seats are appropriate for the young child with low tone who needs head support, but an adapted corner chair is better for the older child.

6. When encouraging movements from proximal joints, remember that wherever your hands are, the child will not be in control. If you control the shoulders, the child has to control the head and trunk, that is, above and below where you are handling. Keep this in mind anytime you are guiding

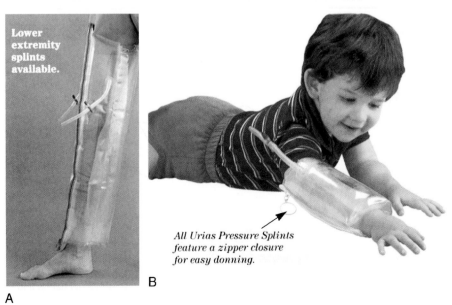

A   B

Fig. 5.7 (**A** and **B**) Use of pediatric air splints for knee control in standing and elbow control in prone reaching. (Courtesy Arden Medical, Ltd.)

movement. If you want the child to control a body part or joint, you should not be holding on to that area.

7. Ultimately, the goal is for the child to initiate and guide her own movements. Use of manual cues (handling) should be decreased as the child gains more motor control. If the child exhibits movement only while you are guiding the movement but is not able to assist in making the same movements on her own, you must question whether motor learning is actually taking place. The child must *actively participate* in movement to learn to move. For movement to have meaning, it must have a **goal,** such as object exploration or locomotion. Function is the bottom line for engagement, not necessarily "perfect" movement. Very few of us are ballerinas.

Use of Sensory Input to Promote Positioning and Handling

Touch

An infant begins to define the edges of her own body by touch. Touch is also the first way in which an infant finds food and experiences self-calming when upset. Infant massage is a way to help parents feel comfortable about touching their infant. The infant can be guided to touch the body as a prelude to self-calming (Intervention 5.5). Positioning the infant in side-lying often makes it easier for her to touch her body and to see her hands and feet (an important factor). Awareness of the body's midline is an essential perceptual ability. If asymmetry in movement or sensation exists, then every effort must be made to equalize the child's awareness of both sides of the body when the child is being moved or positioned. Additional tactile input can be given to that side of the body in the form of touch or weight bearing. The presence of asymmetry in sensation and movement can contribute to arm and leg length differences. Shortening of trunk muscles can occur because of

lack of equal weight bearing through the pelvis in sitting or as compensation for unilateral muscular paralysis. Trunk muscle imbalance can also lead to scoliosis.

Touch and movement play important roles in developing body and movement awareness and in balance. Children with hypersensitivity to touch may need to be desensitized. Usually, gentle but firm pressure is better tolerated than light touch when a child is overly sensitive. Light touch produces withdrawal of an extremity or turning away of the face in children who exhibit tactile defensiveness (Lane, 2002). Most typically developing children like soft textures before rough ones, but children who appear to misperceive tactile input may actually tolerate coarse textures, such as terry cloth, better than soft textures.

General guidelines for the use of tactile stimulation with children with tactile defensiveness have been outlined by Koomar and Bundy (2002). These include the following: (1) having the child administer the stimulation; (2) using firm pressure but realizing that light touch can be used if the child is indeed perceiving light touch as deep pressure; (3) applying touch to the arms and legs before the face; (4) applying the stimulation in the direction of hair growth; (5) providing a quiet, enclosed area for the stimulation to take place; (6) substituting proprioception for tactile stimulation or combining deep pressure with proprioception. Textured mitts, paintbrushes, sponges, and vibrators provide different types of tactile stimulation. Theoretically, deep touch or pressure to the extremities has a central inhibitory effect that is more general, even though this touch is applied to a specific body part (Ayres, 1972). The expected outcome is that the child will have an increased tolerance to touch, be able to concentrate better, and exhibit better organized behavior. If handling the child is to be an effective part of intervention, the infant or child must be able to tolerate touch.

INTERVENTION 5.5 **Teaching Self-Calming**

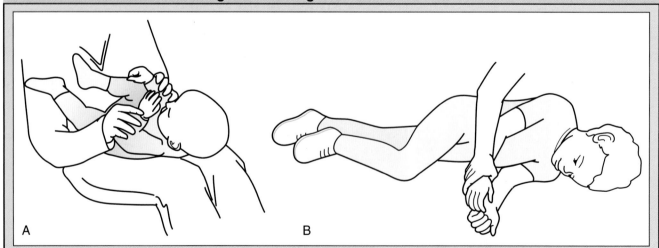

Using touch to self-calm in supported supine and side-lying positions.
A. The infant can be guided to touch the body as a prelude to self-calming.
B. Positioning the child in side-lying often makes it easier for him to touch his body and to see his hands and feet—important points of reference.

A child who is defensive about touch to the face usually also has increased sensitivity to touch inside the mouth. Such children may have difficulty in eating textured foods. Oral motor therapy is a specialized area of practice that requires additional education. A physical, occupational, or speech therapist may be trained to provide this type of care. The physical therapist assistant may be taught specific interventions by the therapist that are only applicable to a particular child in a specific setting. However, those interventions are beyond the scope of this book and are only referred to in general terms.

Vestibular System

The three semicircular canals of the vestibular system are fluid-filled. Each set of canals responds to movement in different planes. Cartwheels, somersaults, and spinning produce movement in different canals. Linear movement (movement in line with the body orientation) can improve head lifting when the child is in prone or supine position. Swinging a child in a hammock in a prone or supine position produces such linear movement and encourages head lifting (Fig. 5.8). Movement stimulation often works to alert a child affected by lethargy or one with low muscle tone because the vestibular system has a strong influence on postural tone and balance. The vestibular system causes a response when the flow of fluid in the semicircular canals changes direction. However, constant movement results in the child's habituation or becoming used to the movement and does not produce a response. Rapid, quick movement, as in sitting on a movable surface, can alert the child. Fast, jerky movement facilitates an increase in tone if the child's resting tone is low. Slow, rhythmic movement decreases high tone. Vestibular is a very powerful sensory system and the child's responses to it should be monitored and thoroughly documented.

Approximation

Application of compression through joints in weight bearing is *approximation*. Rocking on hands and knees and bouncing on a ball in sitting are examples of activities that provide approximation. Additional compression can be given manually through the body parts into the weight-bearing surface. Joints may also be approximated by manually applying constant pressure through the long axis of aligned body parts. Intermittent compression can also be used. Both constant pressure and intermittent pressure provide proprioceptive cues to alert postural muscles to support the body, as in sitting and bouncing on a trampoline. The speed of the compressive force and the give of the support surface provide differing amounts of joint approximation. The direction of movement can be varied while the child is rocking on hands and knees. Compression through the length of the spine is achieved from just sitting, as a result of gravity, but this compression can be increased by bouncing. Axial compression or pressure through the head and neck must be used cautiously in children with Down syndrome because of the 15% incidence of atlantoaxial instability in this population (Tassone and Duey-Holtz, 2008). External compression can also be given through the shoulders into the spine while the child is sitting, or through the shoulders or hips when the child is in a four-point position (Intervention 5.6). The child's body parts must always be aligned prior to receiving manual compression, with compression graded to the tolerance of the child. Less compression is better in most instances. Use of approximation is illustrated in the following example involving a young girl with athetoid cerebral palsy. When the clinician placed a hand lightly but firmly on the girl's head as she was attempting to maintain a standing position, the child was more stable within the posture. She was then asked to assume various ballet positions with her feet, to help her learn to adjust to different-sized bases of support and still maintain her balance. During the next treatment session, the girl initiated the stabilization by placing the therapist's hand on her head. Gradually, external stabilization from the therapist's hand was able to be withdrawn.

Intermittent or sustained pressure can also be used to prepare a limb or the trunk to accept weight prior to loading the limb as in gait or laterally shifting weight onto the trunk. Prior to weight bearing on a limb, such as in propped sitting, the arm can be prepared to accept the weight by applying pressure from the heel of the hand into the shoulder with the elbow straight but not locked (Intervention 5.7). This is best done with the arm in about 45 degrees of external rotation. Think of the typical position of the arm when it is extended to catch yourself. The technique of using sustained pressure for the trunk is done by applying firm pressure along the side of the trunk on which the weight will be shifted (Intervention 5.8). The pressure is applied along one side of the trunk from the middle of the trunk out toward the hip and shoulder prior to assisting the child to turn onto that side. This intervention can be used as preparation for rolling or coming to sit through side-lying. A modification of this intervention is used prior to or as you initiate a lateral weight shift to assist trunk elongation.

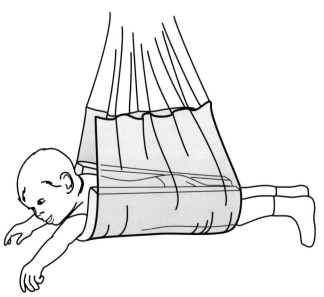

Fig. 5.8 Child in a hammock.

INTERVENTION 5.6   Compression of Proximal Joints

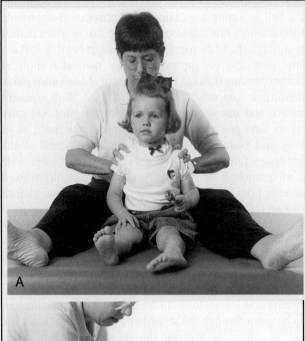

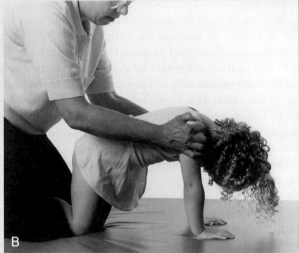

A. Manual approximation through the shoulders in sitting.
B. Manual approximation through the shoulders in the four-point position.

Vision

Visual images entice a child to explore the environment. Vision also provides important information for the development of head control and balance. Visual fixation is the ability to look with both eyes for a sustained time. To encourage looking, find out whether the child prefers faces or objects. In infants, begin with black and white objects or a stylized picture of a face and then add colors such as red and yellow to try to attract the child's attention. You will have the best success if you approach the infant from the periphery because the child's head will most likely be turned to the side. Next, encourage tracking of objects to the midline and then past the midline. Before infants can maintain the head in the midline, they can track from the periphery toward the midline,

INTERVENTION 5.7   Preparation for Upper Extremity Weight Bearing

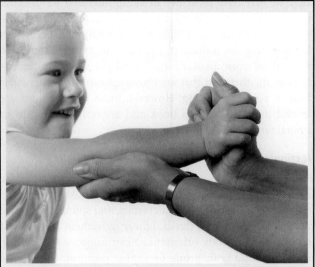

Application of pressure through the heel of the hand to approximate the joints of the upper extremity.

then through ever-widening arcs. Directional tracking ability then progresses horizontally, vertically, diagonally, and rotationally (clockwise and counterclockwise).

If the child has difficulty using both eyes together or if the eyes cross or turn out, alert the supervising physical therapist, who may suggest that the child see an optometrist or an ophthalmologist. Children who have eye problems corrected early in life may find it easier to develop head control and the ability to reach for objects. Children with permanent visual impairments must rely on auditory signals within the environment to entice them to move. Just as you would use a toy to help a child track visually, use a rattle or other noisemaker to encourage head turning, reaching, and rolling toward the sound. The child has to be able to localize or determine where the sound is coming from before these types of activities are appropriate. Children with visual impairments generally achieve motor milestones later than typically developing children.

Hearing

Although hearing does not specifically play a role in the development of posture and movement, if the acoustic nerve responsible for hearing is damaged, then the vestibular nerve that accompanies it may also be impaired. Impairment of the vestibular nerve or any part of the vestibular system may cause balance deficits because information from head movement is not translated into cues for postural responses. In addition, the close coordination of eye and head movements may be compromised. When working with preschoolers with hearing impairment, clinicians have often found that these children have balance problems. Studies have shown that both static and dynamic balance are impaired in this population and produce motor deficits, especially gait disturbances (Melos, 2017; de

INTERVENTION 5.8   Preparation for Weight Acceptance

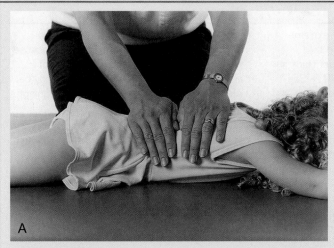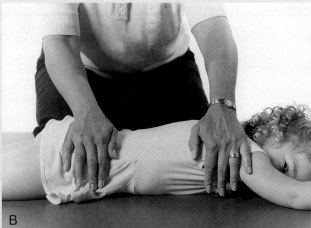

Firm stroking of the trunk in preparation for weight acceptance.
A. Beginning hand position.
B. Ending hand position.

Sousa et al., 2012; Livingstone and McPhillips, 2011). Auditory cues can be used to encourage movement and, in the visually impaired, may provide an alternative way to direct or guide movement.

PREPARATION FOR MOVEMENT

Postural Readiness

Postural readiness is the usual preparation for movement. It is defined as the ability of the muscles to exhibit sufficient resting tone to support movement. Sufficient resting tone is evident by the child's ability to sustain appropriate postural alignment of the body before, during, and after performing a movement task. In children with neurologic deficit, some positions can be advantageous for movement, whereas others may promote abnormally strong tonic reflexes (Table 5.1). A child in the supine position may be dominated by the effect of the tonic labyrinthine reflex, which causes increased extensor tone, and thus decreases the possibility that the child will be able to roll to prone or come to sit easily. If the tone is too high or too low, or if the body is not appropriately aligned, movement will be more difficult, less efficient, and less likely to be successful.

Postural Alignment

Alignment of the trunk is required prior to trying to elicit movement. When you slump in your chair before trying to come to a stand, your posture is not prepared to support efficient movement. When the pelvis is either too anteriorly or too posteriorly tilted, the trunk is not positioned to respond with appropriate righting reactions to any weight shift. Recognizing that the patient is lying or sitting asymmetrically should cue repositioning in appropriate alignment. To promote

weight bearing on the hands or feet, one must pay attention to how limbs are positioned. Excessive rotation of a limb may provide mechanical locking into a posture, rather than afford the child's muscles an opportunity to maintain the position. Examples of excessive rotation can be seen in the elbows of a child with low tone who attempts to maintain a hands-and-knees position or whose knees are hyperextended in standing. Advantages and disadvantages of different positions are discussed in Chapter 6 as they relate to the effects of exaggerated tonic reflexes, which are most often evident in children with spastic or dystonic cerebral palsy.

Manual Contacts

Manual contacts at proximal joints are used to guide movement or to reinforce a posture. The shoulders and hips are most commonly used, either separately or together, to guide movement from one posture to another. Choosing manual contacts is part of movement preparation. The more proximal the manual contacts, the more you control the child's movements. Moving contacts more distally to the elbow or knee or to the hands and feet requires that the child take more control. A description of the use of these manual contacts is given in the section of this chapter on positioning and handling.

Rotation

Slow, rhythmic movement of the trunk and extremities is often helpful in decreasing muscle stiffness (Intervention 5.9). Some children are unable to attempt any change in position without this preparation. When using slow, rhythmic movements, one should begin at proximal joints. For example, if tightness in the upper extremities is evident, then slow, alternating pressure can be applied to the anterior chest wall, followed by manual protraction of the scapula and depression

TABLE 5.1   Advantages and Disadvantages of Different Positions

Position	Advantages	Disadvantages
Supine	Can begin early weight bearing through the lower extremities when the knees are bent and feet are flat on the support surface. Positioning of the head and upper trunk in forward flexion can decrease the effect of the STLR. Can facilitate use of the upper extremity in play or object exploration. Lower extremities can be positioned in flexion over a roll, ball, or bolster.	Effect of STLR can be strong and not easily overcome. Supine can be disorienting because it is associated with sleeping. The level of arousal is lowest in this position, so it may be more difficult to engage the child in meaningful activity.
Side-lying	Excellent for dampening the effect of most tonic reflexes because of the neutral position of the head; achieving protraction of the shoulder and pelvis; separating the upper and lower trunk; achieving trunk elongation on the down side; separating the right and left sides of the body; and promoting trunk stability by dissociating the upper and lower trunk. Excellent position to promote functional movements, such as rolling and coming to sit, or as a transition from sitting to supine or prone.	It may be more difficult to maintain the position without external support or a special device, such as a side lyer. Shortening of the upper trunk muscles may occur if the child is always positioned on the same side.
Prone	Promotes weight bearing through the upper extremities (prone on elbows or extended arms); stretches the hip and knee flexors and facilitates the development of active extension of the neck and upper trunk. In young or very developmentally disabled children, it may facilitate development of head control and may promote eye-hand relationships. With the addition of a movable surface, upper extremity protective reactions may be elicited.	Flexor posturing may increase because of the influence of the PTLR. Breathing may be more difficult for some children secondary to inhibition of the diaphragm, although ventilation may be better. Prone is not recommended for young children as a sleeping posture because of its relationship with an increased incidence of sudden infant death syndrome.
Sitting	Promotes active head and trunk control; can provide weight bearing through the upper and lower extremities; frees the arms for play; and may help normalize visual and vestibular input as well as aid in feeding. The extended trunk is dissociated from flexed lower extremities. Excellent position to facilitate head and trunk righting reactions, trunk equilibrium reactions, and upper extremity protective extension. One or both upper extremities can be dissociated from the trunk. Side sitting promotes trunk elongation and rotation.	Sitting is a flexed posture. A child may be unable to maintain trunk extension because of a lack of strength or too much flexor tone. Optimal seating at 90-90-90 may be difficult to achieve and may require external support. Some floor-sitting postures, such as cross-sitting and W sitting, promote muscle tightness and may predispose to lower extremity contractures.
Quadruped	Weight bearing through all four extremities with the trunk working against gravity. Provides an excellent opportunity for dissociation and reciprocal movements of the extremities and as a transition to side sitting if trunk rotation is possible.	The flexed posture is difficult to maintain because of the influence of the STNR, which can encourage bunny hopping as a form of locomotion. When trunk rotation is lacking, children often end up W sitting.
Kneeling	Kneeling is a dissociated posture; the trunk and hips are extended while the knees are flexed. Provides a stretch to the hip flexors. Hip and pelvic control can be developed in this position, which can be a transition posture to and from side sitting or to half-kneeling and standing.	Kneeling can be difficult to control, and children often demonstrate an inability to extend at the hips completely because of the influence of the STNR.
Standing	Provides weight bearing through the lower extremities and a stretch to the hip and knee flexors and ankle plantar flexors; can promote active head and trunk control and may normalize visual input.	A significant amount of external support may be required; may not be a long-term option for the child.

PTLR, Prone tonic labyrinthine reflex; *STLR*, supine tonic labyrinthine reflex; *STNR*, symmetric tonic neck reflex.
Modified from Lemkuhl LD, Krawczyk L: Physical therapy management of the minimally-responsive patient following traumatic brain injury: coma stimulation, *Neurol Rep* 17:10–17, 1993.

INTERVENTION 5.9 **Trunk Rotation**

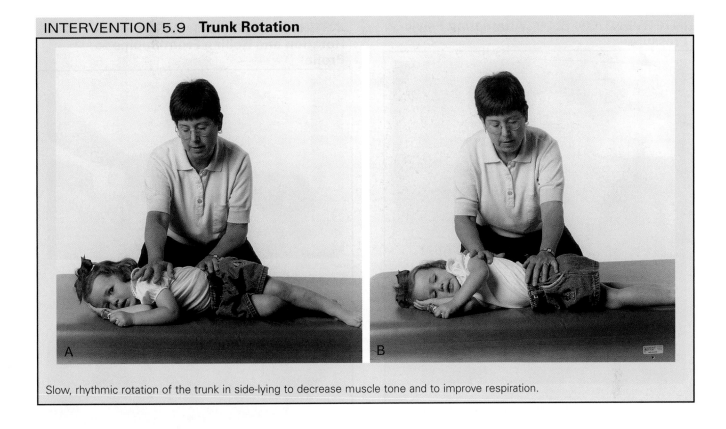

Slow, rhythmic rotation of the trunk in side-lying to decrease muscle tone and to improve respiration.

of the shoulder, which is usually elevated. The child's extremity is slowly and rhythmically externally rotated as the arm is abducted away from the body and elevated. The abduction and elevation of the arm allow for some trunk lengthening, which can be helpful prior to rolling or shifting weight in sitting or standing. Always starting at proximal joints provides a better chance for success. Various hand grasps can be used when moving the upper extremity. A handshake grasp is commonly used, as is grasping the thumb and thenar eminence (Fig. 5.9). Extending the carpometacarpal joint of the thumb also decreases tone in the extremity. Be careful to avoid pressure in the palm of the hand if the child still has a palmar grasp reflex. Do not attempt to free a thumb that is trapped in

a closed hand without first trying to alter the position of the entire upper extremity.

When a child has increased tone in the lower extremity muscles, begin with alternating pressure on the pelvis (anterior superior iliac spine), first on one side and then the other (Intervention 5.10). As you continue to rock the child's pelvis slowly and gently, externally rotate the hip at the proximal thigh. As the tone decreases, lift the child's legs into flexion because bending the hips and knees can significantly reduce the bias toward extension. With the child's knees bent, continue slow, rhythmic rotation of one or both legs and place the legs into hook lying. Pressure can be given from the knees into the hips and into the feet to reinforce this flexed position. The more the hips and knees are flexed, the less extension is possible, so in cases of extreme increased tone, the knees can be brought to the chest with continued slow rotation of the bent knees across the trunk. By positioning the child's head and upper body into more flexion in the supine position, you may also flex the child's lower extremities more easily. A wedge, bolster, or pillows can be used to support the child's upper body in the supine position. The caregiver should avoid positioning the child supine without ensuring that the child has a flexed head and upper body, because the legs may be too stiff in extension as a result of the supine tonic labyrinthine reflex. Lower trunk rotation initiated with one or both of the child's lower extremities can also be used as a preparatory activity prior to changing position, such as rolling from supine to prone (Intervention 5.11). If the child's hips and knees are too severely flexed and adducted, gently rocking the child's pelvis by moving the legs into abduction

Fig. 5.9 Handshake grasp.

INTERVENTION 5.10 Alternating Pelvic Pressure

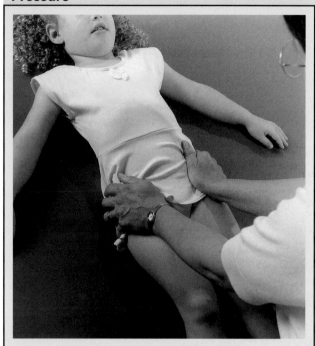

Alternating pressure with manual contact on the pelvis can be used to decrease muscle tone and to facilitate pelvic and lower extremity motion.

INTERVENTION 5.11 Lower Trunk Rotation and Rolling From Supine to Prone

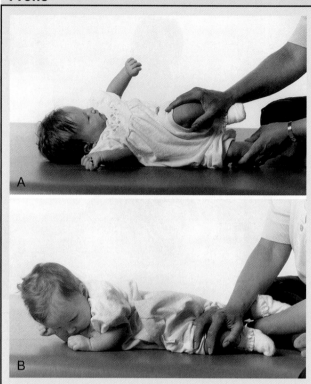

Lower trunk rotation initiated by flexing one leg over the other and facilitating rolling from supine to prone.

by means of some outward pressure on the inside of the knees and downward pressure from the knees into the hips may allow you to slowly extend and abduct the child's legs (Intervention 5.12). When generalized increased tone exists, as in a child with quadriplegic cerebral palsy, slow rocking while the child is prone over a ball may sufficiently reduce tone to allow initiation of movement transitions, such as rolling to the side or head lifting in prone (Intervention 5.13).

INTERVENTIONS TO FOSTER HEAD AND TRUNK CONTROL

The following positioning and handling interventions can be applied to children with a variety of disorders. They are arranged developmentally, because children need to acquire some degree of head control before they are able to control the trunk in an upright posture. Both head and trunk control are necessary components for sitting and standing.

Head Control

Several different ways of encouraging head control through positioning in prone, in supine, and while being held upright in supported sitting are presented here. The interventions can be used to promote development of head control in children who do not exhibit appropriate control. Many interventions can be used during therapy or as part of a home program. The decision about which interventions to use should be

INTERVENTION 5.12 Lower Trunk Rotation and Pelvic Rocking

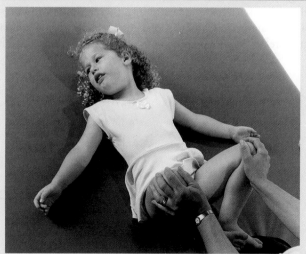

Lower trunk rotation and pelvic rocking to aid in abducting the lower extremities in the presence of increased adductor muscle tone.

INTERVENTION 5.13   Use of the Ball for Tone Reduction and Head Lifting

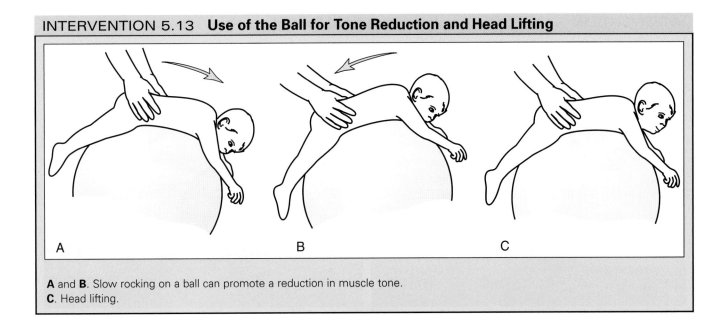

A   B   C

A and **B**. Slow rocking on a ball can promote a reduction in muscle tone.
C. Head lifting.

---

based on a thorough examination by the physical therapist and the therapeutic goals outlined in the child's plan of care.

Positioning to Encourage Head Control

Prone over a bolster, wedge, or half-roll. Prone is usually the first position in which the newborn experiences head lifting; therefore, it is one of the first positions used to encourage development of head control. When an infant is placed over a small roll or bolster, the child's chest is lifted off the support surface, and this maneuver takes some weight off the head. In this position, the infant's forearms can be positioned in front of the roll, to add further biomechanical advantage to lifting the head. The child's elbows should be positioned under the shoulders to provide weight-bearing input for a support response from the shoulder girdle muscles. A visual and auditory stimulus, such as a mirror, brightly colored toy, or noisemaker, can be used to encourage the child to lift the head. Lifting is followed by holding the head up for a few seconds, first in any position, then in the midline. A wedge may also be used to support the infant's entire body and to keep the arms forward. The advantage of a half-roll is that because the roll does not move, the child is less likely to "roll" off it. It may be easier to obtain forearm support when the child is positioned over a half-roll or a wedge of the same height as the length of the child's upper arm (Intervention 5.14, *A*).

Supine on a wedge or half-roll. Antigravity flexion of the neck is necessary for balanced control of the head. Although most children exhibit this ability at around 5 months of age, children with disabilities may find development of antigravity flexion more of a challenge than cervical extension, especially children with underlying extensor tone. Preparatory positioning in a supine position on a wedge or half-roll puts the child in a less difficult position against gravity to attempt head lifting (Intervention 5.14, *B*). The child should be encouraged to keep the head in the midline while he is positioned in supine.

A midline position can be encouraged by using a rolled towel arch or by providing a visual focus. Toys or objects can be attached to a rod or frame, as in a mobile, and placed in front of the child to encourage reaching with the arms. If a child cannot demonstrate any forward head movement, increasing the degree of incline so the child is closer to upright than to supine may be beneficial. This can also be accomplished by using an infant seat or a feeder seat with a Velcro base that allows for different degrees of inclination (Intervention 5.14, *C*).

Interventions to Encourage Head Control

Modified pull-to-sit maneuver. The beginning position is supine. The hardest part of the range for the child's head to move through in the pull-to-sit maneuver is the initial part in which the force of gravity is directly perpendicular to the head (Fig. 5.10). The infant or child has to have enough strength to initiate the movement. Children with disabilities may have extreme head lag during the pull-to-sit transition. Therefore, the maneuver is modified to make it easier for the child to succeed. The assistant provides support at the child's shoulders and rotates the child toward herself and begins to move the child toward sitting on a diagonal (Intervention 5.15). The assistant may need to wait for the child to bring the head and upper body forward into sitting. The child may be able to help with only the last part of the maneuver as the vertical position is approached. If the child tries to reinforce the movement with shoulder elevation, the assistant's index fingers can depress the child's shoulders and thus can avoid this substitution. Improvement in head control can be measured by the child's ability to maintain the head in midline in various postures, by exhibiting neck-righting reactions, or by assisting in the maneuver earlier during the range. As the child's head control improves, less trunk rotation is used to encourage the neck muscles to work against gravity as much

INTERVENTION 5.14   Positions to Encourage Head Control

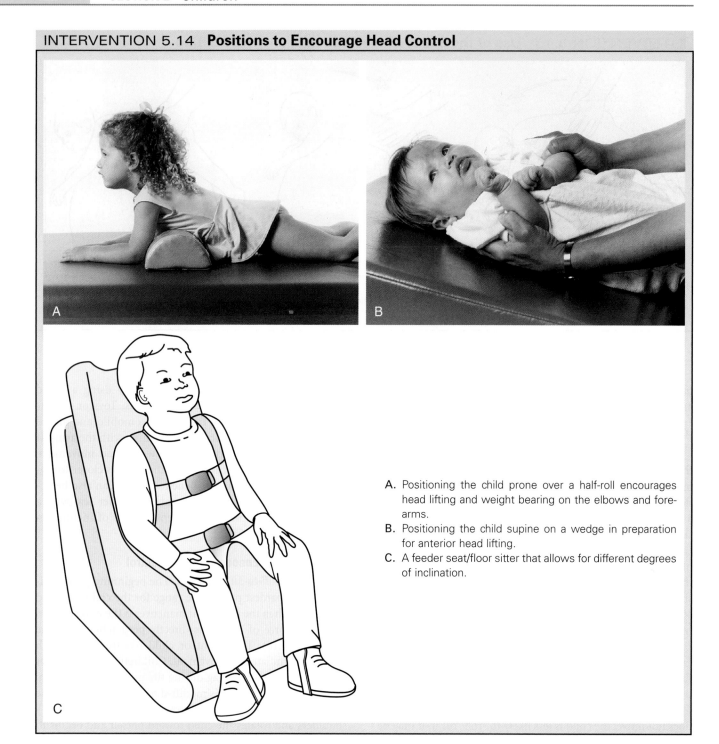

A. Positioning the child prone over a half-roll encourages head lifting and weight bearing on the elbows and forearms.
B. Positioning the child supine on a wedge in preparation for anterior head lifting.
C. A feeder seat/floor sitter that allows for different degrees of inclination.

as possible. More distal contacts, such as the elbows and finally the hands, can be used to initiate the pull-to-sit maneuver (see Intervention 5.2). These distal manual contacts are not recommended if the child has too much joint laxity.

Upright in supported sitting. In the child's relation to gravity, support in the upright sitting position (Box 5.1) is probably an easier position in which to maintain head control, because the orientation of the head is in line with the force of gravity. The head position and the force of gravity are parallel (see Fig. 5.10), whereas when a child is in supine or prone

position, the force of gravity is perpendicular to the position of the head at the beginning of head lifting. This relationship makes it more difficult to lift the head from either the supine or prone position than to maintain the head when either is held upright in vertical or held upright in supported sitting. This is why a newborn has total head lag as one tries to pull the baby to sit, but once the infant is sitting, the head appears to sit more stably on the shoulders. A child who is in supine or prone position uses only neck flexors or extensors to lift the head. In the upright position, a balance of flexors and

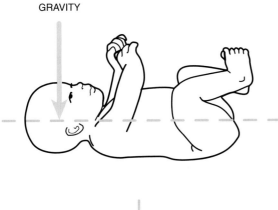

GRAVITY

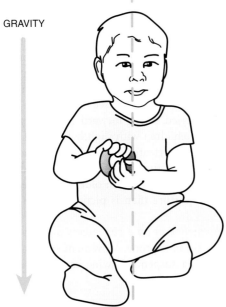

GRAVITY

Fig. 5.10 Relationship of gravity with the head in supported supine and supported sitting positions.

extensors is needed to maintain the head position. The only difference between being held upright in the vertical position and being held upright in supported sitting is that the trunk is supported in the latter position and thus provides some proprioceptive input by approximation of the spine and pelvis. Manual contacts under or around the shoulders are used to support the head (Fig. 5.11). Establishing eye contact with the child also assists head stability because it provides a stable visual input to orient the child to the upright position. To encourage head control further, the child can be placed in supported sitting in an infant seat or a feeder seat as a static position, but care should be taken to ensure the infant's safety in such a seat. Never leave a child unattended in an infant seat or other seating device without a seat belt and/or shoulder harness to keep the child from falling forward, and never place such a device on a table unless the child is constantly supervised.

Weight shifting from supported upright sitting. The beginning position is with the child seated on the lap of the assistant or caregiver and supported under the arms or around the shoulders. Support should be firm to provide some upper trunk stability without causing any discomfort to the child. Because the child's head is inherently stable in this position, small weight shifts from the midline challenge the infant to

---

BOX 5.1 Progression of Supported Sitting

1. Sitting in the corner of a sofa
2. Sitting in a corner chair or a beanbag
3. Side sitting with one arm propped over a bolster or half-roll
4. Sitting with arms forward and supported on an object, such as a pillow or a ball
5. Sitting in a high chair

INTERVENTION 5.15 Modified Pull-to-Sit Maneuver

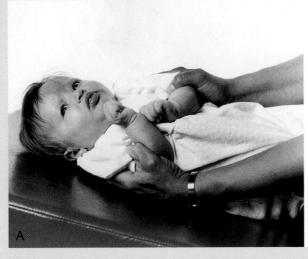
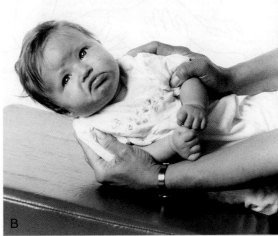

A   B

A. Position the child on an inclined surface supine in preparation for anterior head lifting.
B. Provide support at the child's shoulder, rotate the child toward yourself, and begin to move the child toward sitting on a diagonal.

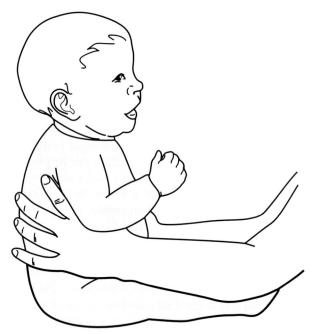

Fig. 5.11 Early head control in supported sitting.

Carrying in prone. The child's beginning position is prone. Because prone is the position from which head lifting is the easiest, when a child is in the prone position with support along the midline of the trunk, this positioning may encourage head lifting, as shown in Intervention 5.4, *F*. The movement produced by the person who is carrying the child may also stimulate head lifting because of the vestibular system's effect on postural muscles. Another prone position for carrying can be used in the case of a child with flexor spasticity (Intervention 5.16, *A*). One of the caregiver's forearms is placed under the child's shoulders to keep the arms forward, while the other forearm is placed between the child's thighs to keep one hip straight. Some lower trunk rotation is achieved as the pelvis is turned from the weight of the dangling leg.

Carrying in upright. The beginning position is upright. To encourage use of the neck muscles in the development of head control, the child can be carried while in an upright position. The back of the child's head and trunk can be supported against the caregiver's chest (see Intervention 5.16, *B*). The child can be carried, facing forward, in a snuggler or a backpack. For those children with slightly less head control, the caregiver can support around the back of the child's shoulders and head in the crook of an elevated elbow, as shown in Intervention 5.4, *A*. An older child needs to be in a more upright posture than is pictured, with the head supported.

Prone in a hammock or on a suspended platform swing. The beginning position is prone. Movement stimulation using a hammock or a suspended swing can give vestibular

maintain the head in the midline. If possible, just visually engaging the child may be enough to assist the child in maintaining head position or righting the head as weight is shifted. As the child becomes able to accept challenges, larger displacements may be given.

INTERVENTION 5.16   **Carrying Positions to Encourage Head Control**

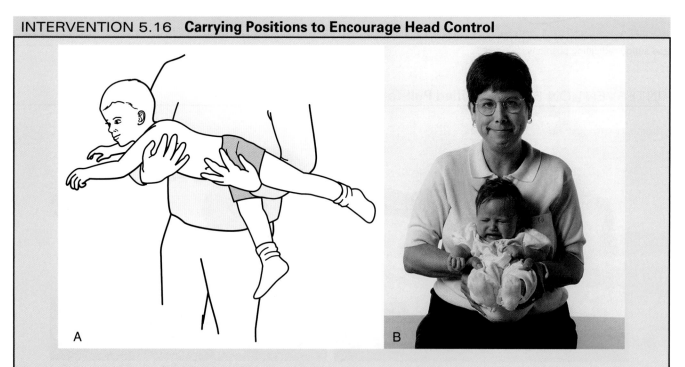

A. In the case of a child with flexor spasticity, the caregiver can place one forearm under the child's shoulders to keep his arms forward and place the other forearm between his thigh, while keeping one hip straight.

B. When the child is carried in the upright position, the back of the child's head is supported against the caregiver's chest.

input to facilitate head control when the child is in a prone position. When using a mesh hammock, you should place pillows in the hammock and put the child on top of the pillows. The child's head should be supported when the child is not able to lift it from the midline (see Fig. 5.8). As head control improves, support can gradually be withdrawn from the head. When vestibular stimulation is used, the change in direction of movement is detected, not the continuous rhythm, so be sure to vary the amount and intensity of the stimulation. Always watch for signs of overstimulation, such as flushing of the face, sweating, nausea, or vomiting. Vestibular stimulation may be used with children who are prone to seizures. However, you must be careful to avoid visual stimulation if the child's seizures are brought on by visual input. The child can be blindfolded or wear a baseball cap pulled down over the eyes to avoid visual stimulation.

Trunk Control

Positioning for Independent Sitting

As stated previously, sitting is the position of function for the upper extremities, because self-care activities, such as feeding, dressing, and bathing, require use of an upper extremity, as does playing with objects. Positioning for independent sitting may be more crucial to the child's overall level of function than standing, especially if the child's ambulation potential is questionable. Independent sitting can be attained in many ways. Propped sitting can be independent, but it will not be functional unless one or both hands can be freed to perform meaningful activities. Progression of sitting based on degree of difficulty is found in Box 5.2.

Sitting propped forward on both arms. The beginning position is sitting, with the child bearing weight on extended arms. Various sitting postures can be used, such as abducted long sitting, ring sitting, or tailor sitting. The child must be able to sustain some weight on the arms. Preparatory activities can include forward protective extension or pushing up from prone on elbows. Gentle approximation through the shoulders into the hands can reinforce the posture. Weight bearing encourages a supporting response from the muscles of the shoulder girdle and the upper extremities to maintain the position.

Sitting propped forward on one arm. The beginning position is sitting, as described in the previous paragraph. When bilateral propping is possible, weight shifting in the position

can encourage unloading one extremity for reaching or pointing and can allow for propping on one arm.

Sitting propped laterally on one arm. If the child cannot support all her weight on one arm laterally, then part of the child's weight can be borne by a bolster placed between the child's side and the supporting arm (Fig. 5.12). Greater weight acceptance can be practiced by having the child reach with the other hand in the direction of the supporting hand. When the location of the object to be reached is varied, weight is shifted and the child may even attempt to change sitting postures.

Sitting without hand support. Progressing from support on one hand to no hand support can be encouraged by having the child shift weight away from the propped hand and then have her attempt to reach with the propped hand. A progression of propping on objects and eventually on the child's body can be used to center the weight over the sitting base. Engaging the child in clapping hands or batting a balloon may also afford opportunities to free the propping hand. Short sitting with the feet supported can also be used as a way to progress from sitting with hand support to using one hand to using no hands for support.

Side sitting propped on one arm. Side sitting is a more difficult sitting posture in which to play because trunk rotation is required to maintain the posture to have both hands free for play. Some children are able to attain and maintain the posture only if they prop on one arm, a position that allows only one hand free for play and so negates any bimanual or two-handed activities. Again, the use of a bolster can make it easier to maintain the propped side-sitting posture. Asymmetric side sitting can be used to promote weight bearing on a hip on which the child may avoid bearing weight, as in hemiplegia. The lower extremities are asymmetrically positioned. The lower leg is externally rotated and abducted while the upper leg is internally rotated and adducted.

Side sitting with no hand support. Achievement of independent side sitting can be encouraged in much the same way as described in the previous paragraph.

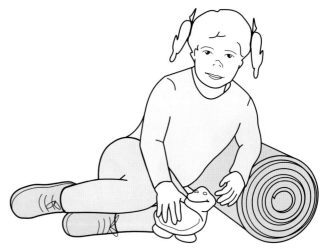

Fig. 5.12 Sitting propped laterally on one arm over a bolster.

BOX 5.2	**Progression of Sitting Postures Based on Degree of Difficulty**

1. Sitting propped forward on both arms
2. Sitting propped forward on one arm
3. Sitting propped laterally on both arms
4. Sitting propped laterally on one arm
5. Sitting without hand support
6. Side sitting with hand support
7. Side sitting with no hand support

Movement Transitions that Encourage Trunk Rotation and Trunk Control

Once a child is relatively stable within a posture, the child needs to begin work on developing dynamic control. One of the first things to work on is shifting weight within postures in all directions, especially those directions used in making the transition or moving from one posture to another. The following are general descriptions of movement transitions commonly used in functional activities. These transitions can be used during therapy and can also be an important part of any home program.

Rolling from supine to prone using the lower extremity. The beginning position is supine. Intervention 5.17 shows this transition. Using your right hand, grasp the child's right lower leg above the ankle and gently bring the child's knee toward the chest. Continue to move the child's leg over the body to initiate a rolling motion until the child is side-lying or prone. Alternate the side toward which you turn the child. Initially, infants roll as a log or as one complete unit. As they mature, they rotate or roll segmentally. If the lower extremity is used as the initiation point of the movement, the pelvis and lower trunk will rotate before the upper trunk and shoulders. As the child does more of the movement, you will need to do less and less until, eventually, the child can be enticed to roll using a sound or visual cue or by reaching with an arm.

Coming to sit from supine. The beginning position is supine. Position yourself to one side of the child. Reach across the child's body and grasp the hand farthest away from you. Bring the child's arm across the body so the child has turned to the side and is pushing up with the other arm. Stabilize the child's lower extremities so the rotation occurs in the trunk and is separate from leg rotation.

Coming to sit from prone. The beginning position is prone. Elongate the side toward which you are going to roll the child. Facilitate the roll to side-lying and proceed as follows in coming to sit from side-lying as described in the next paragraph.

Coming to sit from side-lying. The beginning position is with the child lying on one side, facing away from you with the head to the right. The child's lower extremities should be flexed. If lower extremity separation is desirable, the child's lower leg should be flexed and the top leg allowed to remain straight. Apply gentle pressure on the uppermost part of the child's shoulder in a downward and lateral direction. The child's head should right laterally, and the child should prop on the downside elbow. If the child experiences difficulty in moving to propping on one elbow, use one hand to assist the downward arm into the correct position. Your upper hand can now move to the child's top hip to direct the weight shift diagonally back over the flexed hip while your lower hand assists the child to push up on the downward arm. Part of this movement progression is shown in Intervention 5.2.

INTERVENTION 5.17   Rolling From Supine to Prone

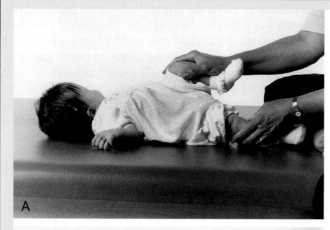

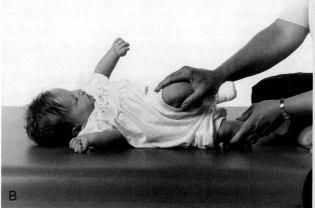

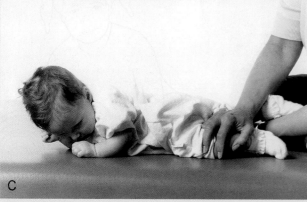

Movement sequence of rolling supine to prone.
- **B** and **A**. With the right hand, grasp the child's left lower leg above the ankle and gently bring her knee toward the chest.
- **B** and **C**. Continue to move the child's leg over the body to initiate a rolling motion until the child is in the side-lying or prone position.

The child's movements can be halted anywhere during the progression to improve control within a specific range or to encourage a particular component of the movement. The child ends up sitting with or without hand support, or the support arm can be placed over a bolster or half-roll if more support is needed to maintain the end position. The child's sitting position can range from long abducted sitting, propping forward on one or both extended arms, to half-ring sitting with or without propping. These positions can be maintained without propping if the child is able to maintain them.

Sitting to prone. This transition is used to return to the floor after playing in sitting. It can be viewed as the reverse of coming to sit from side-lying. In other words, the child laterally shifts weight to one side, first onto an extended arm and then to an elbow. Finally, the child turns over the arm and into the prone position. Some children with Down syndrome widely abduct their legs to lower themselves to prone. They lean forward onto outstretched arms as they continue to swing their legs farther out and behind their bodies. Children with hemiplegic involvement tend to move or to make the transition from sitting to prone position by moving over the noninvolved side of the body. They need to be encouraged to shift weight toward and move over the involved side and to put as much weight as possible on the involved upper extremity. Children with bilateral involvement need to practice moving to both sides.

Prone to four-point. The beginning position is prone. The easiest way to facilitate movement from prone to four-point is to use a combination of cues at the shoulders then the hips, as shown in Intervention 5.18. First, reach over the upper back of the child and lift gently. The child's arms should be flexed beside the upper body at the beginning of the movement. By lifting the shoulders, the child may bring the forearms under the body in a prone on elbows or puppy position. Continue to lift until the child is able to push up on extended arms. Weight bearing on extended arms is a prerequisite for assuming a hands-and-knees position. If the child requires assistance to maintain arms extended, a caregiver can support the child at the elbows, or pediatric air splints can be used. Next, lift the hips up and bring them back toward the feet, just far enough to achieve a four-point position. If the child needs extra support under the abdomen, a bolster, a small stool, or pillows can be used to help sustain the posture. Remember, four-point may just be a transitional position used by the child to go into kneeling or sitting. Not all developmentally normal children learn to creep on hands and knees. Depending on the predominant type of muscle tone, creeping may be too difficult to achieve for some children who demonstrate mostly flexor tone in the prone position. Children with developmental delays and minimal abnormal postural tone can be taught to creep.

Four-point to side sitting. The beginning position is four-point. Once the child can maintain a hands-and-knees position, work on moving to side sitting to either side. This transition works on control of trunk lowering while the child is in a rotated position. Dissociation of lower trunk movements from upper trunk movements can also be practiced. A prerequisite is for the child to be able to control or tolerate diagonal weight shifts without falling. So many times, children can shift weight anteriorly and posteriorly, but not diagonally. If diagonal weight shifting is not possible, the child will often end up sitting on the heels or between the feet. The latter position can have a significant effect on the development of lower extremity bones and joints. The degree to which the child performs side sitting can be determined by whether the child is directed to go all the way from four-point to side sitting on the support surface, or by whether the movement is shortened to end with the child side sitting on pillows or a low stool. If movement to one side is more difficult, movement toward the other side should be practiced first.

Four-point to kneeling. The beginning position is four-point. Kneeling is accomplished from a four-point position by a backward weight shift followed by hip extension with the rest of the child's body extending over the hips (see Intervention 5.18, *E*). Some children with cerebral palsy try to initiate this movement by using head extension. The extension should begin at the hips and should progress cephalad (toward the head). A child can be assisted in achieving an upright or tall-kneeling position by placement of extended arms on benches of increasing height to aid in shifting weight toward the hips. In this way, the child can practice hip extension in smaller ranges before having to move through the entire range.

Kneeling to Side Sitting. The beginning position is kneeling. Kneeling is an extended position because the child's back must be kept erect with the hips extended. Kneeling is also a dissociated posture because while the hips are extended, the knees are flexed and the ankles are passively plantar flexed to extend the base of support and to provide a longer lever arm. Lowering from kneeling requires eccentric control of the quadriceps. If this lowering occurs downward in a straight plane, the child will end up sitting on his feet. If the trunk rotates, the lowering can proceed to allow the child to achieve a side-sitting position.

Kneeling to Half-Kneeling. The beginning position is kneeling. The transition to half-kneeling is one of the most difficult to accomplish. Typically developing children often use upper limb support to attain this position. To move from kneeling to half-kneeling, the child must unweight one lower extremity. This is usually done by performing a lateral weight shift. The trunk on the side of the weight shift should lengthen or elongate while the opposite side of the trunk shortens in a righting reaction. The trunk must rotate away from the side of the body toward which the weight is shifted to assist the nonweighted lower extremity's movement (Intervention 5.19). The nonweighted leg is brought forward, and the foot is placed on the support surface. The resulting position is a dissociated one in which the forward leg is flexed at all joints, while the loaded limb is flexed at the knee and is extended at the hip and ankle (plantar flexed).

Coming to stand. The beginning position is sitting. Coming to stand is probably one of the most functional movement transitions. Clinicians spend a great deal of time working with people of all ages on this movement transition. Children initially have to roll over to prone, move into a hands-and-knees

INTERVENTION 5.18   Promoting Progression From Prone to Kneeling

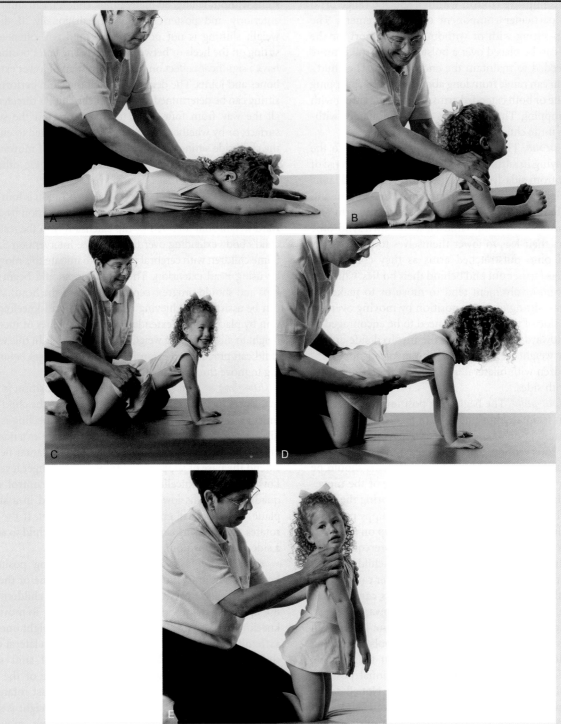

Facilitating the progression of movement from prone to prone on elbows to quadruped position using the shoulders and hips as key points of control.

- **C** and **A**. Before beginning, the child's arms should be flexed beside the upper body. Reach over the upper back of the child and lift her shoulders gently.
- **C** and **B**. As her shoulders are lifted, the child may bring her forearms under the body in a prone on elbows or puppy position. Continue to lift until the child is able to push up on extended arms.
- **C** and **C**. Next, lift the child's hips up and bring them back toward her feet, just far enough to achieve a four-point position.
- **C** and **D**. Promoting movement from quadruped to kneeling using the shoulders. The child extends her head before her hips. Use of the hips as a key point may allow for more complete extension of the hips before the head is extended.

INTERVENTION 5.19   Kneeling to Half-Kneeling

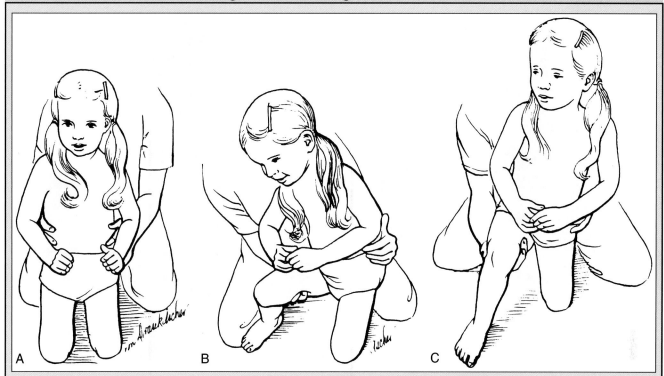

A. Kneel behind the child and place your hands on the child's hips.
B. Shift the child's weight laterally, but do not let the child fall to the opposite side, as is depicted. The child's trunk should elongate on the weight-bearing side; with some trunk rotation, the child may be able to bring the opposite leg forward.
C. If the child is unable to bring the opposite leg forward, assist as depicted.

position, creep over to a person or object, and pull up to stand through half-kneeling. The next progression in the developmental sequence adds moving into a squat from hands-and-knees and pulling the rest of the way up on someone or something. Finally, the 18-month-old can usually come to stand from a squat without assistance (Fig. 5.13). As the abdominal muscles become stronger, the child in supine turns partially to the side, pushes with one arm to sitting, then goes to a squat and on up to standing. The most mature pattern is to come straight up from supine, to sitting with no trunk rotation, to assuming a squat, and then coming to stand. From prone, the most mature progression is to push up to a four-point position, to kneeling and half-kneeling, and then to standing. Independent half-kneeling is a difficult position because of the configuration of the base of support and the number of body parts that are dissociated from each other.

ADAPTIVE EQUIPMENT FOR POSITIONING AND MOBILITY

Decisions regarding adaptive equipment for positioning and mobility should be made based on input from the team working with the infant or child. Adaptive equipment can include bolsters, wedges, walkers, and wheeled mobility devices. The decision about what equipment to use, however, is ultimately up to the parents. Barriers to the use of adaptive equipment may include, but are not limited to, architectural, financial, cosmetic, and behavioral constraints. Sometimes, children do not like the equipment the therapist thinks is most therapeutic. Any piece of equipment should be used on a trial basis before being purchased. Regarding wheelchair selection, a team approach is advocated. Members of the assistive technology team may include the physical therapist, the occupational therapist, the speech therapist, the classroom teacher, the rehabilitation engineer, and the vendor of durable medical equipment. The child and family are also part of the team because they are the ones who will use the equipment. The physical therapist assistant may assist the physical therapist in gathering information regarding the need for a wheelchair or piece of adaptive equipment, as well as providing feedback on how well the child is able to use the device. Positioning and mobility are only two of 10 areas covered under assistive technology. For more information on assistive technology, refer to O'Shea and Bonfiglio (2017).

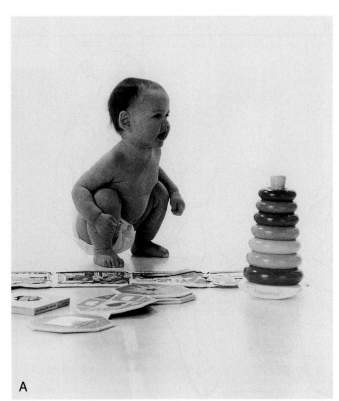
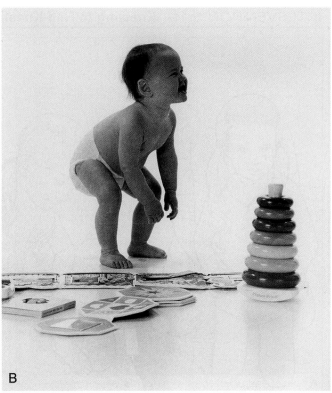
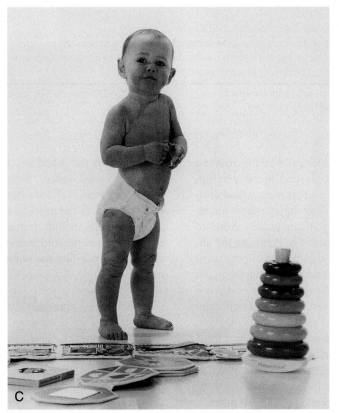

Fig. 5.13 (**A-C**) Coming to stand from a squat requires good lower extremity strength and balance.

Theoretically, the 90-90-90 rule for sitting alignment is a good place to begin; this would mean that the feet, knees, and hips are flexed to approximately 90 degrees. This degree of flexion allows weight to be taken on the back of the thighs, as well as the ischial tuberosities of the pelvis. An erect trunk and pelvic alignment is crucial for optimal head control and arm and hand function. For most children a seat to back angle of 90 degrees is most practical. However, if the child sits with a posterior pelvic tilt, an anterior tilt of the seat may provide trunk extension. In this example the seat-to-back angle is increased or open. If the child has difficulty keeping a seat because of increased extensor tone or spasms, raising the front edge of the seat can provide a better seated position by decreasing the seat-to-back angle. Using an anteriorly tilted seated surface has been reported to improve hand function in children with cerebral palsy, but the evidence is inconclusive (Costigan and Light, 2011). Presently, a neural pelvic position appears to be recommended clinically (O'Shea and Bonfiglio, 2017).

If the person cannot maintain the normal spinal curves while in sitting, consider providing lumbar support. The seat should be deep enough to support most of the thigh, but avoid pressure on the structures behind the knee. Other potential problems, such as neck extension, scapular retraction, and lordosis of the lumbar spine, can occur if the child is not able to keep the trunk extended for long periods of time. In such cases, the child may feel as though he is falling forward. Lateral trunk supports are indicated to control asymmetries in the trunk that may lead to scoliosis. Seating systems can improve social participation, mobility, speech and communication, and pulmonary function (Costigan and Light, 2011; Walls and Rosen, 2008).

Goals for Adaptive Equipment

Goals for adaptive equipment are listed in Box 5.3. Many of these goals reflect what is expected from positioning because adaptive equipment is used to reinforce appropriate postures. For example, positioning should give a child a stable postural base by providing postural alignment needed for functional movement. Changing the alignment of the trunk can have a positive effect on the child's ability to reach. Supported sitting may counteract the deforming forces of gravity, especially in a child with poor trunk control who cannot maintain an erect trunk posture. Simply supporting the child's feet takes much of the strain off trying to keep weight on the pelvis in a chair that is too high. When at all possible, the child's sitting posture with adaptive equipment should approximate that of a developmentally typical child's by maintaining all spinal curves. Ease of use by the caregiver and comfort level of the child will ensure that a piece of adaptive equipment is used, not stored in a closet.

What follows is a general discussion of considerations for positioning in supine and prone, sitting, side-lying, and standing.

BOX 5.3 Goals for Use of Adaptive Equipment

- Support best available postural alignment.
- Facilitate functional mobility.
- Provide mobility and encourage exploration.
- Increase opportunities for social and educational interactions.
- Improve participation in the classroom and at home.
- Improve physiologic functions.
- Increase comfort.

Supine and Prone Posture Positioning

Positioning the child prone over a half-roll, bolster, or wedge is often used to encourage head lifting, as well as weight bearing on forearms, elbows, and even extended arms. These positions are seen in Intervention 5.20. Supine positioning can be used to encourage symmetry of the child's head position and reaching forward in space. Wedges and half-rolls can be used to support the child's head and upper trunk in more flexion. Rolls can be placed under the knees, which also encourages flexion.

Sitting Posture Positioning

Many sitting postures are available for the typically developing child who moves and changes position easily. However, the child with a disability may have fewer positions from which to choose, depending on the amount of joint range, muscle extensibility, and head and trunk control required in each position. Children normally experiment with many different sitting postures, although some of these positions are more difficult to attain and maintain. Sitting on the floor with the legs extended is called long sitting. Long sitting requires adequate hamstring length (see Fig. 5.14, *A*) and is often difficult for children with cerebral palsy, who tend to sit on the sacrum with the pelvis posteriorly tilted (Fig. 5.15). During ring sitting on the floor, the soles of the feet are touching, the knees are abducted, and the hips are externally rotated such that the legs form a ring. Ring sitting is a comfortable sitting alternative because it provides a wider base of support; however, the hamstrings can and do shorten if this sitting posture is used exclusively (see Fig. 5.13, *B*). Tailor sitting, or cross-legged floor sitting, also takes some strain off the hamstrings and allows some children to sit on their ischial tuberosities for the first time (see Fig. 5.13, *C*). Again, the hamstrings will shorten if this sitting posture is the only one used by the child. The use of tailor sitting must be carefully evaluated in the presence of increased lower extremity muscle tone, especially in the hamstring and gastrocnemius-soleus muscles. In addition, in many of these sitting positions, the child's feet are passively allowed to plantar flex and invert, thereby encouraging tightening of the heel cords. If independent sitting is not possible, then adaptive seating should be considered.

The most difficult position to move into and out of appears to be side sitting. Side sitting is a rotated posture and requires internal rotation of one lower extremity and external rotation of the other lower extremity (Fig. 5.16, *A*). Because of the flexed lower extremities, the lower trunk is rotated in one direction—a maneuver necessitating that the upper trunk be rotated in the opposite direction. A child may have to prop on one arm to maintain side sitting if trunk rotation is insufficient (Fig. 5.16, *B*). Some children can side sit to one side but not to the other because of lower extremity range-of-motion limitations. In side sitting, the trunk on the weight-bearing side lengthens to keep the center of gravity within the base of support. Children with hemiplegia may not be able to side sit on the involved side because of an inability to elongate or rotate the trunk. They may be able to side sit only if they are propped

INTERVENTION 5.20   Encouraging Head Lifting and Upper Extremity Weight Bearing Using Prone Supports

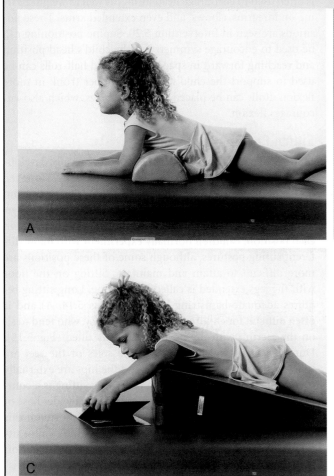

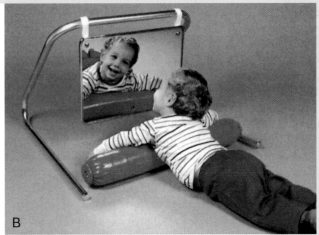

A. Positioning the child prone over a half-roll encourages head lifting and weight bearing on elbows and forearms.
B. Positioning the child prone over a bolster encourages head lifting and shoulder control.
C. Positioning the child prone over a wedge promotes upper extremity weight bearing and function.

on the involved arm, a maneuver that is often impossible. Because weight bearing on the involved side is a general goal with any person with hemiplegia, side sitting is a good position to work toward with these children (Intervention 5.21). Actively working into side sitting from a four-point or tall-kneeling position can be therapeutically beneficial because so many movement transitions involve controlled trunk rotation. Advantages of using the four-point position to practice this transition are that some of the weight is taken by the arms and less control is demanded of the lower extremities. As trunk control improves, you can assist the child in moving from tall kneeling on the knees to heel sitting and finally from tall kneeling to side sitting to either side. From tall kneeling, the base of support is still larger than in standing, and the arms can be used for support, if needed.

Children with disabilities often have one preferred way to sit, and that sitting position can be detrimental to lower extremity development and the acquisition of trunk control. For example, W sitting puts the hips into extreme internal rotation and anteriorly tilts the pelvis, thereby causing the spine to be extended (see Fig. 5.5, A). In this position, the tibias are subjected to torsional factors that, if sustained, can produce permanent structural changes. Children with low postural tone may accidentally discover this position by pushing themselves back between their knees. Once these children "discover" that they no longer need to use their hands for support, it becomes difficult to prevent them from using this posture. Children with increased tone in the hip adductor group also use this position frequently because they lack sufficient trunk rotation to move into side sitting from prone. Behavior modification has been typically used to attempt to change a child's habit of W sitting. Some children respond to verbal requests of "sit pretty," but often the parent is worn out from constantly trying to have the child correct the posture. As with most habits, if the child can be prevented from ever discovering W sitting, that is optimal. Otherwise, substitute another sitting alternative for the potentially deforming position. For example, if the only way the child

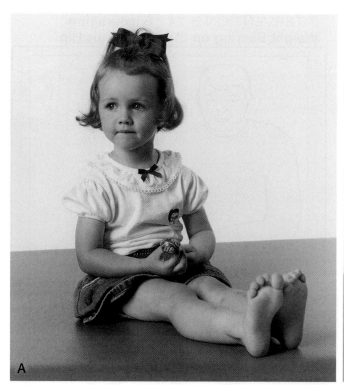

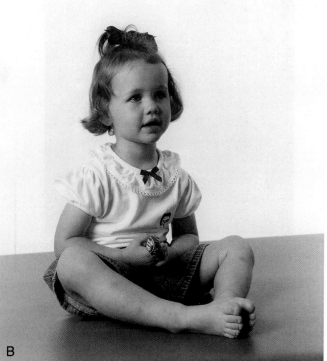

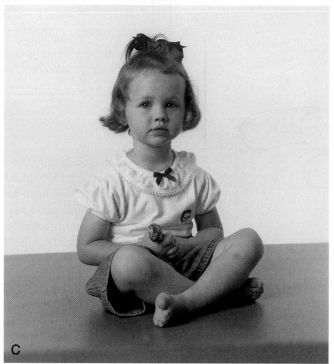

Fig. 5.14 Sitting Postures. **(A)** Long sitting. **(B)** Ring sitting. **(C)** Tailor sitting.

can independently sit on the floor is by W sitting, place the child in a corner chair or other positioning device that requires a different lower extremity position.

Adaptive Seating

Many positions can be used to facilitate movement, but the best position for activities of daily living is upright sitting.

How that posture is maintained may necessitate caregiver assistance or adaptive equipment for positioning. In sitting, the child can more easily view the world and can become more interested in interacting with people and objects within the environment. Ideally, the position should allow the child as much independence as possible while maintaining safety. Adaptive seating may be required to meet both these criteria.

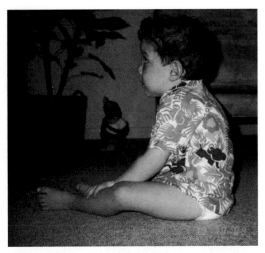

Fig. 5.15 **Sacral Sitting.** (From Burns YR, MacDonald J: *Physiotherapy and the growing child*, London, WB Saunders Company Ltd., 1996.)

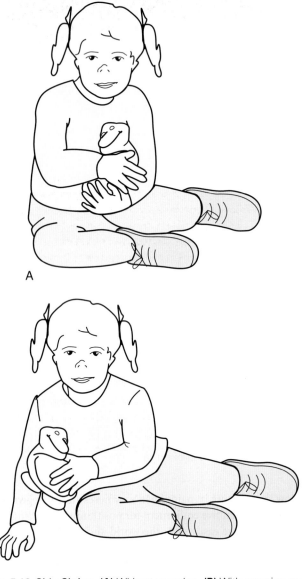

A

B

Fig. 5.16 **Side Sitting. (A)** Without propping. **(B)** With propping on one arm for support.

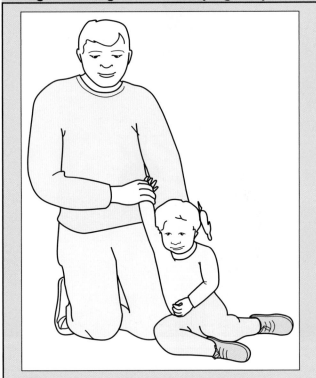

INTERVENTION 5.21   Encouraging Weight Bearing on the Hemiplegic Hip

Place the child in side sitting on the hemiplegic side. Elevation of the hemiplegic arm promotes trunk and external rotation elongation.

Some examples of seating devices are shown in Fig. 5.17. The easier it is to use a piece of adaptive equipment, the more likely the caregiver will be to use it with the child.

Children without good head control often do not have sufficient trunk control for sitting. Stabilizing the trunk alone may improve the child's ability to maintain the head in midline. Additionally, the child's arms can be brought forward and supported on a lap tray. If the child has poor head control, then some means to support the head will have to be incorporated into the seating device (see Fig. 5.6). When sitting a child with poor head and trunk control, the child's back must be protected from the forces of gravity, which accentuate a forward-flexed spine. Although children need to be exposed to gravity while they are in an upright sitting position to develop trunk control, postural deviation can quickly occur if muscular control is not sufficient.

Children with low tone often demonstrate flared ribs (Fig. 5.18) as a result of an absence of sufficient trunk muscle development to anchor the rib cage for breath support. Children with trunk muscle paralysis secondary to myelomeningocele may require an orthotic device to support the trunk during sitting. Although the orthosis can assist in preventing the development of scoliosis, it may not totally prevent its development

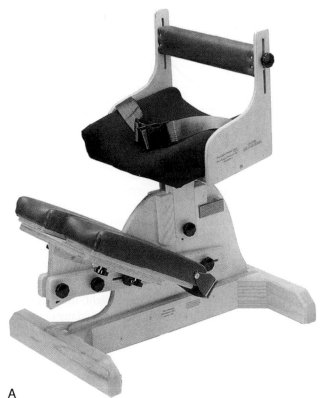

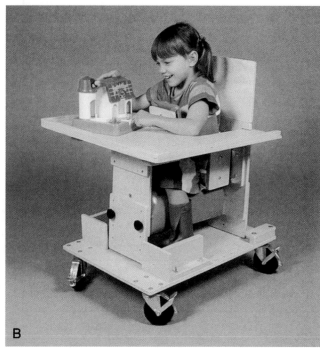

Fig. 5.17 **Adaptive Seating Devices. (A)** Posture chair. **(B)** Bolster chair. (A, Courtesy ©TherAdapt Products, Inc., Ludington, MI. B, Courtesy Kaye Products, Inc., Hillsborough, NC.)

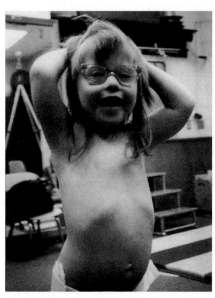

Fig. 5.18 **Rib Flare.** (From Moerchen VA: Respiration and motor development: a systems perspective. *Neurol Rep* 18:9, 1994. Reprinted from the Neurology Report with the permission of the Neurology Section, APTA.)

because of the inherent muscle imbalance. The orthosis may or may not be initially attached to lower extremity bracing.

Adaptive seating is widely used for children with disabilities despite the fact that there is limited research supporting its effectiveness. In the most recent systematic review of effectiveness of adaptive seating for children with cerebral palsy, the authors concluded there was limited high-quality research available (Chung et al., 2008). Despite that finding, some positive effects on participation, play, and family life have been documented (Rigby et al., 2009; Ryan et al., 2009). A bolster chair is depicted in Fig. 5.17, *B*. Sitting on a chair with an anteriorly inclined seat, such as seen in Fig. 5.17, *A*, was found to improve trunk extension (Miedaner, 1990; Sochaniwskyz et al., 1991). Others (Dilger and Ling, 1986) found that sitting a child with cerebral palsy on a posteriorly inclined wedge decreased her kyphosis (Intervention 5.22). The evidence is not conclusive for whether seat bases should be anteriorly or posteriorly inclined (Chung et al., 2008; Costigan and Light, 2011). Seating requirements must be individually assessed, depending on the therapeutic goals. A child may benefit from several different types of seating, depending on the positioning requirements of the task being performed.

Adjustable-height benches are excellent therapeutic tools because they can easily grow with the child throughout the preschool years. They can be used in assisting children with making the transition from sitting to standing, as well as in providing a stable sitting base for dressing and playing. The height of the bench is important to consider, relative to the amount of trunk control demanded from the child. Depending on the child's need for pelvic support, a bench allows the child to use trunk muscles to maintain an upright

INTERVENTION 5.22 Facilitating Trunk Extension

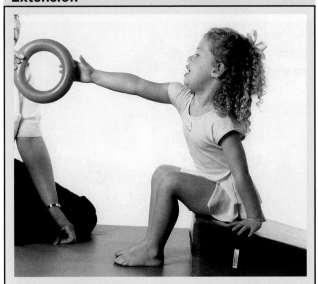

Sitting on a posteriorly inclined wedge may facilitate trunk extension.

INTERVENTION 5.23 Using a Side-Lyer

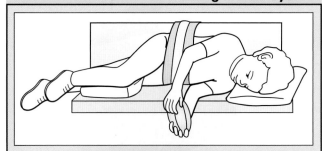

Use of a side-lyer ensures that a child experiences a side-lying position and may promote hand regard, midline play, or orientation. Positioning in side lying is excellent for dampening the effects of most tonic reflexes.

trunk posture during play or to practice head and trunk postural responses when weight shifts occur during dressing or playing. Additional pelvic support can be added to some therapeutic benches, as seen in Fig. 5.3. The bench can be used to pull up on and to encourage cruising.

Side-Lying Position

Side-lying is frequently used to orient a child's body around the midline, particularly in cases of severe involvement or when the child's posture is asymmetric when the child is placed either prone or supine. In a child with less severe involvement, side-lying can be used to assist the child to develop control of flexors and extensors on the same side of the body. Side-lying is often a good sleeping posture because the caregiver can alternate the side the child sleeps on every night. For sleeping, a long body pillow can be placed along the child's back to maintain side-lying, with one end of the pillow brought between the legs to separate them and the other end under the neck or head to maintain midline orientation. Lower extremities should be flexed if the child tends to be in a more extended posture. For classroom use, a commercial side lyer or a rolled-up blanket (Intervention 5.23) may be used to promote hand regard, midline play, or orientation.

Positioning in Standing

Positioning in standing is often indicated for its positive physiologic benefits, including growth of the long bones of the lower extremities. Standing can also encourage alerting behavior, peer interaction, and upper extremity usage for play and self-care. The upper extremities can be weight bearing or free to move because they are no longer needed to support the child's posture. The upright orientation can afford the child perceptual opportunities. Many devices can be used to promote an upright standing posture, including prone and supine standers, vertical standers, standing frames, and standing boxes. Standing programs can have beneficial effects on bone mineral density, hip development, range of motion, and spasticity (Paleg et al., 2014).

A standing device is indicated for children who are nonambulatory, minimally ambulatory, or who are not active in standing, as long as there are no contraindications. For hip health, standing should be introduced to children between 9 and 10 months of age. A posture management program should include a passive component using a prone/supine or vertical standing device and a dynamic component in which the stander moves, vibrates, changes from sit to stand, or is propelled by the user (Paleg et al., 2013) (Fig. 5.19).

Prone standers support the anterior chest, hips, and anterior surface of the lower extremities. The angle of the stander determines how much weight is borne by the lower extremities and feet. When the angle is slightly less than 90 degrees, weight is optimal through the lower extremities and feet. If the child exhibits neck hyperextension or a high-guard position of the arms when in the prone stander, its continued use needs to be reevaluated by the supervising physical therapist. Use of a prone stander is indicated if the goal is physiologic weight bearing or hands-free standing.

Supine standers are an alternative to prone standers for some children. A supine stander is similar to a tilt table, so the degree of tilt determines the amount of weight borne by the lower extremities and feet. For children who exhibit too much extension in response to placement in a prone stander, a supine stander may be a good alternative. However, postural compensations develop in some children with the use of a supine stander. These compensations include kyphosis from trying to overcome the posterior tilt of the body. Asymmetric neck postures or a Moro response may be accentuated, because the supine stander perpetuates supine positioning. Use of a supine stander in these situations may be contraindicated.

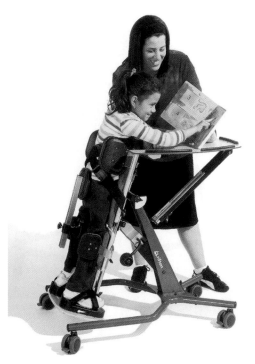

Fig. 5.19 Prone stander with table attachment. (Courtesy Rifton Equipment, Rifton, NY.)

Vertical standers support the child's lower extremities in hip and knee extension and allow for complete weight bearing. The child's hands are free for upper extremity tasks, such as writing at a blackboard (Intervention 5.24). The child controls the trunk. The need to function within different environments must be considered when one chooses adaptive equipment for standing. In a classroom, the use of a stander is often an alternative to sitting, and because the device is adjustable, more than one child may be able to benefit from its use. Continual monitoring of a child's response to any type of stander should be part of the physical therapist's periodic reexamination of the child. The physical therapist assistant should note changes in posture and abilities of any child using any piece of adaptive equipment.

Dosage for standing programs has recently been presented by Paleg et al. (2013, 2014) and are in Table 5.2.

Positioning in upright standing is important for mobility, specifically ambulation. Orthotic support devices and walkers are routinely used with young children with myelodysplasia. Ambulation aids can also be important to children with cerebral palsy who do not initially have the balance to walk independently. Two different types of walkers are most frequently used in children with a motor deficit. The standard walker is used in front of the child, and the reverse posture control

INTERVENTION 5.24 Vertical Standers

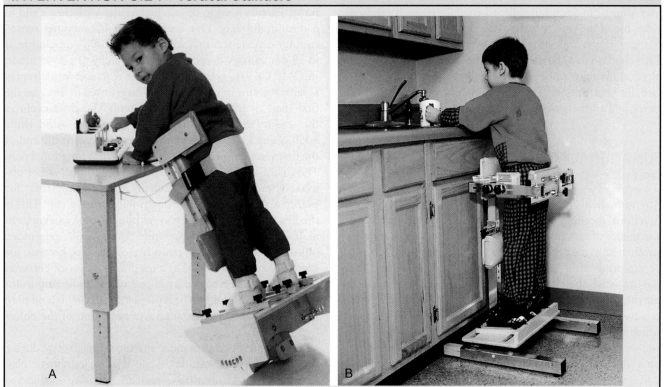

Vertical standers support the child's lower extremities in hip and knee extension and allow for varying amounts of weight bearing, depending on the degree of inclination. The child's hands are free for upper extremity tasks, such as writing at a blackboard, playing with toys (**A**), or working in the kitchen (**B**).

(Courtesy Kaye Products, Hillsborough, NC.)

TABLE 5.2 Recommended Optimal Dosages for Pediatric Supported Standing Programs		
Outcome	**Dosage**	**Level of Evidence**
Bone mineral density	60–90 minutes/day	Levels 2–4
Hip biomechanics	60 minutes/day in 30° to 60° of total bilateral hip abduction	Levels 2–5
Range of motion	45–60 minutes/day	Level 2
Spasticity	30–45 minutes/day	Level 2

From Paleg G, Smith B, Glickman L: Evidence-based clinical recommendations for dosing of pediatric supported standing programs. Presented at the APTA Combined Sections Meeting, February 4, 2014, Las Vegas, NV.

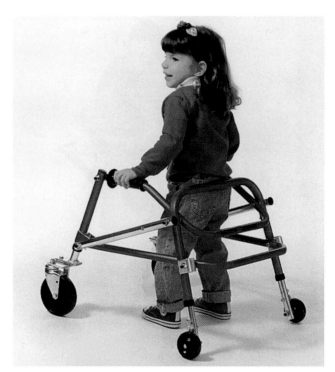

Fig. 5.20 **Reverse Posture Walker.** (Courtesy Kaye Products, Inc., Hillsborough, NC.)

walker is used behind the child. These walkers can have two wheels in the front. The traditional walker is then called a rollator. Difficulties with the standard walker include a forward trunk lean. The child's line of gravity ends up being anterior to the feet, with the hips in flexion. When the child pushes a reverse walker forward, the bar of the walker contacts the child's gluteal muscles and gives a cue to extend the hips. Because the walker is behind the child, the walker cannot move too far ahead of the child. The reverse walker can have two or four wheels. In studies conducted in children with cerebral palsy, use of the reverse walker (Fig. 5.20) resulted in positive changes in gait and upright posture (Levangie et al., 1989). Each child needs to be evaluated on an individual basis by the physical therapist to determine the appropriate assistive device for ambulation. The device should provide stability, safety, and an energy-efficient gait pattern.

FUNCTIONAL MOVEMENT IN THE CONTEXT OF THE CHILD'S WORLD

Any movement that is guided by the clinician should have functional meaning. This meaning could be derived as part of a sequence of movement, as a transition from one posture to another, or as part of achieving a task such as touching a toy or exploring an object. Play is a child's occupation and the way in which the child most frequently learns the rules of moving. Physical therapy incorporates play as a means to achieve therapeutic goals. Structuring the environment in which the treatment session occurs and planning which toys you want the child to play with are all part of therapy. Setting up a situation that challenges the child to move in new ways is motivating to most children. Some suggestions from Linder (2008) for toys and strategies to use with children of different ages can be found in Table 5.3.

Play can and should be a therapy goal for any young child with a motor deficit. Play fosters language and cognition in young children in addition to providing motivation to move. Parents need to be coached to play with their child in a meaningful way. Play encourages self-generated sensorimotor experiences that will support a child's development in all domains. A developmental hierarchy of play is found in Table 5.4. Play gets more complex with age. Initially, play is sensorimotor in nature, a term Piaget used to describe the first stage of intellectual development. The child explores the sensory and motor aspects of his or her world while establishing a social bond with the caregivers. At the end of the first year, sensorimotor play evolves into functional play. The infant begins to understand the functional use of objects. The child plays functionally with realistic toys; for example, combing her hair or drinking from a cup. This is the beginning of pretend play, although some categorize it as functional play with pretense. As the child gets older, objects are used to represent other objects not present, for example, a banana is used as a telephone or a stick becomes a magic wand. Pretend play is one of the most important forms of play, because in order to demonstrate pretend play, the child has to have a mental representation of the object in mind.

Pretend play becomes more and more imaginative during preschool years and can be described as sociodramatic play. Children who demonstrate pretend play are considered socially competent (Howes and Matheson, 1992). Increasing the complexity of play in children with neurodevelopmental disorders should be a goal in any physical therapy plan of care. Additionally, two other forms of play are seen during the

TABLE 5.3 **Appropriate Toys and Intervention Strategies for Working With Children**		
Age	**Toys**	**Intervention Strategies**

Infants	Rattles, plastic keys
	Stuffed animals
	Mobiles
	Busy box
	Blocks
	Mirror
	Push toys, ride-on toys
	Plastic cups, dishes
		Smiling, cooing, tickling while face to face
		Present interesting toys
		Play peek-a-boo; play "So big!"
		Dangle toys that make noise when contacted
		Push, poke, pull, turn
		Encourage reaching, changing positions by moving
		   toys; demonstrate banging objects together, progress
		   to knocking down
		Tummy time
		Demonstrate making things "go"
		Pretend to drink and eat; take turns

Toddlers	Stackable or nesting toys,
	   blocks
	Farm set, toy animals
	Grocery cart, pretend food
	Dolls
	Dump truck
	Water toys
	Pop-up toys
	Push toys, ride-on toys
	Books
		Demonstrate stacking; use different size containers
		   to put things in
		Set up enticing environments and stories
		Pretend to pour and feed the baby doll
		Encourage the child to include the doll in multistep
		   routines such as going to bed
		Pretend to fill and empty a dump truck
		Include in bath time
		Making things "go"
		Demonstrate making things "go"
		Read and describe, turn pages

Preschoolers	Balls, plastic bats, blocks
	Pillows, blankets, cardboard
	   boxes
	Obstacle course
	Play dough, clay
	Sand box
	Books
	Puzzles, peg board, string
	   beads
	Building toys, such as blocks
	Dress-up clothes, costumes
	Musical toys, instruments
	Playground equipment
		Gross motor play, rough housing
		Build a fort, play house
		Seek and find objects, spatial concepts of over,
		   under, around, and through
		Manipulate shapes
		Encourage digging, pouring, finding buried objects
		Encourage the child to tell the story
		Encourage and assist as needed
		Construct real or imaginary things
		Create scenarios for child or encourage the child to
		   create scripts and then follow her lead
		Incorporate music and dance into play with instruments
		   and costumes
		Kickball or "duck, duck, goose"

School-age	Playground equipment Bicycles Balls, nets, bats, goals Dolls and action figures Beads to string Blocks Magic sets Board games Roller skates, ice skates Building sets Computer games	Imaginative games (pirates, ballet dancers, gymnastics) Ride around neighborhood, go on a treasure hunt Encourage peer play and sports Develop scripts as a basis for play Start with large and move to smaller beads Copy design Create illusions Give child sense of success Physical play, endurance Constructive play Use adaptive switches if needed

From Linder T: *Transdisciplinary play-based intervention*, ed 2, Baltimore, 2008, Brooks.

TABLE 5.4   Play Development

Age	Type of Play	Purpose/Child Actions
0–6 months 6–12 months	Sensorimotor play: social and exploratory play Sensorimotor play→functional play	Establish attachment with caregivers Explore the world Learn cause and effect
12–24 months	Functional/relational play Pretend play emerges	Learn functional use of objects and to orient play toward peers Play functionally with realistic toys Pretend one object can symbolically represent another object
2–5 years	Pretend play Constructive play Physical play	Pretend dolls and animals are real Develop scripts as a basis for play Draw and do puzzles Engage in rough and tumble play, jumping, chasing, swinging, sliding
6–10 years	Games with rules	Problem solving, think abstractly Negotiate rules Play games with friends

BOX 5.4   Principles to Support Play Complexity

1. Provide opportunities for many kinds of play
   - Take into consideration cultural differences regarding floor play or messy play.
   - Example: Locate areas of the home (inside or outside) that would support the child's play.
   - Example: Demonstrate how to play with common every-day objects.
2. Increase the play level
   - The parent or caregiver can demonstrate a higher level of play by modeling.
   - Plan play dates with a child who plays at a higher level of play; the child will provide the modeling.
   - Example: Change the child's activity of putting blocks into a cup to pretending to pour something from the cup or drinking from the cup. The parent could pretend to take a bite of the block as if it were a piece of cake.
3. Add materials
   - Add a new object once a child is repeating actions in order to expand the child's routine.
   - Example: Give a cloth to a child playing with a doll to entice the child to cover the doll with the cloth, or to use the cloth as a burp cloth.
4. Add language
   - Add sounds, words, and/or rhythms to the play to enrich the context and encourage attention.

- Describing what is happening increases the child's vocabulary.
- Example: The child is moving a toy bus across the floor and the parent makes appropriate sounds or asks what sounds the bus would make. Sing The Wheels on the Bus.
5. Add actions
   - Add an action once a child repeats an action in order to expand the child's routine.
   - Example: The child pretends to put on a hat; expand that action to then pretending to go for a walk in the park or ask what would the child need to put on or take with her if it were raining?
6. Add ideas
   - Present novel ideas to the child that build on what the child is already thinking.
   - Example: Suggest making a card for the teacher and providing the child with paper, markers, and/or glitters to combine on her own.
   - Example: Provide the child with various hats or a dress-up box that might trigger scenarios like being a fireman, postman, cowboy, or a chef.

(Modified from Linder T: *Transdisciplinary play-based intervention*, ed 2, Baltimore, 2008 Brooks.)

preschool years—constructive and physical play. Constructive play involves drawing, doing puzzles, and constructing things out of blocks, cardboard boxes, or any other material at hand. Physical play is very important during this time as physical play develops fundamental motor skills that are prerequisites for games and sports. The last stage of play involves games with rules. Physical play is to be encouraged to provide a foundation for a lifetime of fitness as well as fun. Linder identified six principles for supporting appropriate complexity of play that can be used with children at all levels (Box 5.4).

CHAPTER SUMMARY

Children with neurologic impairments, regardless of the cause of the deficits, need to move and play. Part of any parent's role is to foster the child's movement exploration of the world. To be a good explorer, the child has to come in contact with objects and people of the world. By teaching the family how to assist the child to move and play, the clinician can encourage full participation in life. By supporting areas of the child's body that the child cannot support, functional movement of other body parts, such as eyes, hands, and feet, can be engaged in object exploration. The adage that if the individual cannot get to the world, the world should be brought to the individual, is true. The greatest challenge for physical therapists and physical therapist assistants who work with children with neurodevelopmental disorders may be to determine how to bring the world to a child with limited head or trunk control or limited mobility. Therapists need to foster function, family, fun, friends, and fitness as measures of participation in life (Rosenbaum and Gorter, 2011). There is never just one answer, but rather many possibilities to the challenges presented by these children. The typical developmental sequence has always been a good source of ideas for positioning and handling. Additional ideas can come from the child's play interests and curiosity and the imagination of the therapist and the family.

REVIEW QUESTIONS

1. What two activities should always be part of any therapeutic intervention?
2. What are the purposes of positioning?
3. What sensory inputs help to develop body and movement awareness?
4. Identify two of the most important handling tips.
5. How can play complexity be expanded in therapy?
6. Give three reasons to use adaptive equipment.
7. What are the two most functional postures (positions to move from)?
8. What are the disadvantages of using a quadruped position?
9. Why is side sitting a difficult posture?
10. Why is standing such an important activity?

CASE STUDIES REVIEWING POSITIONING AND HANDLING CARE: JOSH, ANGIE, AND KELLY

For each of the case studies listed here, identify appropriate ways to pick up, carry, feed, or dress the child. Identify any adaptive equipment that could assist in positioning the child for a functional activity. Give an example of how the parent could play with the child.

Case 1
Josh is a 6-month-old with little head control who has been diagnosed as a floppy infant. He does not like the prone position. However, when he is prone, he is able to lift his head and turn it from side to side, but he does not bear weight on his elbows. He eats slowly and well but tires easily.

Case 2
Angie is a 9-month-old who exhibits good head control and fair trunk control. She has low tone in her trunk and increased tone in her lower extremities (hamstrings, adductors, and gastrocnemius-soleus complex). When her mother picks her up under the arms, Angie crosses her legs and points her toes. When Angie is in her walker, she pushes herself backward. Her mother reports that Angie slides out of her high chair, which makes it difficult for her to finger feed.

Case 3
Kelly is a 3-year-old who has difficulty in maintaining any posture against gravity. Head control and trunk control are inconsistent. She can bear weight on her arms if they are placed for her. She can sit on the floor for a short time when she is placed in tailor sitting. When startled, she throws her arms up in the air (Moro reflex) and falls. She wants to help get herself dressed and undressed.

Possible Suggestions

Case 1
Picking up/Carrying: Use maximum head and trunk support, facilitate rolling to the side, and gather him in a flexed position before picking him up. You could carry him prone to increase tolerance for the position and for the movement experience.

Feeding: Use an infant seat.

Positioning for Functional Activity: Position him prone over a half-roll with toys at eye level.

Positioning for Play: Position him on your tummy while you are lying on the floor, make eye contact and noises to encourage head lifting and pushing up on arms. Engage child in vocal play and mouth games (tickling and making bubbles). The caregiver should be face to face on the floor while encouraging and assisting in pushing up in prone as seen in Fig. 5.21.

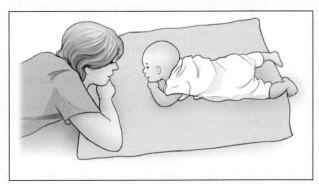

Fig. 5.21 Caregiver encouraging an infant to push up from prone.

Continued

CASE STUDIES REVIEWING POSITIONING AND HANDLING CARE: JOSH, ANGIE, AND KELLY—cont'd

Case 2

Picking up/Carrying: From sitting, pick her up, ensuring lower extremity flexion and separation if possible. Carry her astride your hip, with her trunk and arms rotated away from you.

Feeding: Attach a seatbelt to the high chair. Support her feet so the knees are higher than the hips. Towel rolls can be used to keep the knees abducted. A small towel roll can be used at the low back to encourage a neutral pelvis.

Mobility: Consult with the supervising therapist about the use of a walker for this child.

Positioning for Functional Activity: Sit her astride a bolster to play at a table. A bolster chair with a tray can also be used. A bolster or the caregiver's leg can be used to work on undressing and dressing. Reaching down for clothing and returning to upright sitting can work the trunk muscles.

Positioning for Play: Sit her on a bench and put objects, such as blocks, on a low table in front of her. Practice coming to stand with her feet sufficiently under her to keep her heels on the ground. Help her come to stand and play with the toys or objects on the low table. She could also sit astride a bolster and come to stand to play. Getting on and off the bolster would be fun, as well as picking the objects to reach for. Consider partially hiding objects under a cloth to have the child retrieve a hidden object.

Introduce toys that can be pushed or pulled while in a standing position. Pretend to have tea parties with the use of plastic plates and cups.

Case 3

Picking up/Carrying: Assist her to move into sitting using upper extremity weight bearing for stability. Pick her up in a flexed posture and place her in a corner seat on casters to transport or in a stroller.

Dressing: Position her in ring sitting on the floor, with the caregiver ring sitting around her for stability. Stabilize one of her upper extremities and guide her free arm to assist with dressing. Another option could include sitting on a low dressing bench with her back against the wall and being manually guided to assist with dressing.

Positioning for Functional Activity: Use a corner floor sitter to give a maximum base of support. She could sit in a chair with arms, her feet supported, the table at chest height, and one arm holding on to the edge of the table while the other arm manipulates toys or objects.

Positioning for Play: Seated in a chair with arms and feet on the floor, she can push a large, weighted ball to the parent. Play in tall kneeling with one arm extended for support on a bench while placing puzzle pieces. Engage her in a story related to the theme of the puzzle. Ask her to dramatize an event in her life. Incorporate songs and books into activities requiring static holding and controlling movement transitions.

REFERENCES

Ayres AJ: *Sensory integration and learning disorders*, Los Angeles, 1972, Western Psychological Services.

Barton EE: Teaching generalized pretend play and related behaviors to young children with disabilities, *Except Child* 81:489–506, 2015.

Charman T, Baron-Cohen S: Brief report: prompted pretend play in autism, *J Autism Dev Disord* 27:325–332, 1997.

Chung J, Evans J, Lee C, et al.: Effectiveness of adaptive seating on sitting posture and postural control in children with cerebral palsy, *Pediatr Phys Ther* 20:303–317, 2008.

Costigan FA, Light J: Functional seating for school-age children with cerebral palsy: an evidence-based tutorial, *Lang Speech Hear Serv Sch* 42:223–236, 2011.

de Sousa AM, de Franca Barros J, de Sousa Neto BM: Postural control in children with typical development and children with profound hearing loss, *Int J Gen Med* 5:433–439, 2012.

Dilger NJ, Ling W: The influence of inclined wedge sitting on infantile postural kyphosis, *Dev Med Child Neuro Suppl* 28:23, 1986.

Dusing SC, Harbourne RT: Variability in postural control during infancy: implications for development, assessment, and intervention, *Phys Ther* 90:1838–1849, 2010.

Howes C, Matheson CC: Sequences in the development of competent play with peers: social and social pretend play, *Dev Psychol* 28:961–974, 1992.

Jarrold C: A review of research into pretend play in autism, *Autism* 7:379–390, 2003.

Jennings KD, Connors RE, Stegman CE: Does a physical handicap alter the development of mastery motivation during the preschool years? *J Am Acad Child Adolesc Psychiatry* 27:312–317, 1988.

Koomar JA, Bundy CA: Creating direct intervention from theory. In Bundy AC, Lane SJ, Murray EA, editors: *Sensory integration: theory and practice*, ed 2, Philadelphia, 2002, F. A. Davis, pp 261–308.

Lane SJ: Sensory modulation. In Bundy AC, Lane SJ, Murray EA, editors: *Sensory integration: theory and practice*, ed 2, Philadelphia, 2002, F. A. Davis, pp 101–122.

Levangie P, Chimera M, Johnston M, et al.: Effects of posture control walker versus standard rolling walker on gait characteristics of children with spastic cerebral palsy, *Phys Occup Ther Pediatr* 9:1–18, 1989.

Linder T: *Transdisciplinary play-based intervention*, ed 2, Baltimore, 2008, Brooks.

Livingstone N, McPhillips M: Motor skill deficits in children with partial hearing, *Dev Med Child Neurol* 53(9):836–842, 2011.

Lobo MA, Galloway JC: Enhanced handling and positioning in early infancy advances development throughout the first year, *Child Dev* 83:1290–1302, 2012.

Lobo MA, Harbourne RT, Dusing SC, McCoy SW: Grounding early intervention: physical therapy cannot just be about motor skills anymore, *Phys Ther* 93:94–103, 2013.

Martin SC: *Pretend play in children with motor disabilities* (unpublished doctoral dissertation), Lexington, Kentucky, 2014, University of Kentucky.

Melos RS: Gait performance of children and adolescents with sensorineural hearing losses, *Gait Posture* 57:109–114, 2017.

Miedaner JA: The effects of sitting positions on trunk extension for children with motor impairment, *Pediatr Phys Ther* 2:11–14, 1990.

O'Grady MG, Dusing SC: Assessment position affects problem-solving behaviors in a child with motor impairments, *Pediatr Phys Ther* 28:253–258, 2016.

O'Shea RK, Bonfiglio BS: Assistive technology. In Palisano RJ, Orlin MN, Schreiber J, editors: *Campbell's physical therapy for children*, ed 5, St. Louis, 2017, Elsevier Inc.

Paleg G, Smith B, Glickman L: Systematic review and evidence-based clinical recommendations for dosing of pediatric-supported standing programs, *Pediatr Phys Ther* 25:232–247, 2013.

Paleg G, Smith B, Glickman L: Evidence-based clinical recommendations for dosing of pediatric supported standing programs. Presented at the APTA Combined Sections Meeting, Feb 4, 2014, Las Vegas, NV.

Pfeifer LI, Pacciulio AM, dos Santos CA, dos Santos JL, Stagnitti KE: Pretend play of children with cerebral palsy, *Am J Occup Ther* 31:390–402, 2011.

Rigby PJ, Ryan SE, Campbell KA: Effect of adaptive seating devices on the activity performance of children with cerebral palsy, *Arch Phys Med Rehabil* 90:1389–1395, 2009.

Rosenbaum P, Gorter JW: The 'F-words' in childhood disability: I swear this is how we should think! *Child Care Health Dev* 38(4):457–463, 2011.

Rutherford MD, Young GS, Hepburn S, Rogers SJ: A longitudinal study of pretend play in autism, *J Autism Dev Disord* 37:1024–1039, 2007.

Ryan SE, Campbell KA, Rigby PJ, et al.: The impact of adaptive seating devices on the lives of young children with cerebral palsy and their families, *Arch Phys Med Rehabil* 90:27–33, 2009.

Sochaniwskyz A, Koheil R, Bablich K, et al.: Dynamic monitoring of sitting posture for children with spastic cerebral palsy, *Clin Biomech (Bristol, Avon)* 6:161–167, 1991.

Tassone JC, Duey-Holtz A: Spine concerns in the Special Olympian with Down syndrome, *Sports Med Arthrosc Rev* 16(1):55–60, 2008.

Walls G, Rosen A: Wheelchair seating and mobility evaluation, *PT Magazine Phys Ther* 11:28–31, 2008.

World Health Organization: Motor development study: windows of achievement for six gross motor milestones, *Acta Paediatr Suppl* 450:86–95, 2006.

Cerebral Palsy

OBJECTIVES

After reading this chapter, the student will be able to:

1. Describe the incidence, etiology, and classification of cerebral palsy (CP).
2. Describe the clinical manifestations and associated deficits seen in children with CP throughout the lifespan.
3. Discuss the physical therapy management of children with CP throughout the lifespan.
4. Discuss the medical and surgical management of children with CP.
5. Describe the role of the physical therapist assistant in the treatment of children with CP.
6. Discuss the importance of activity and participation throughout the lifespan of a child with CP.

INTRODUCTION

Cerebral palsy (CP) is a group of permanent disorders of posture and movement that occur secondary to damage to the developing fetal or infant brain. The damage is static but the effects of the damage affect development because the brain is connected to many different areas of the nervous system. Despite the nonprogressive nature of the brain damage in CP, the clinical manifestations of the disorder may appear to change as the child grows older. The motor disorders of CP are highly associated with disturbances of communication, cognition, sensation, perception, and behavior. Accompanying secondary musculoskeletal impairments may include hip displacement, bony torsion, spinal deformities, and contractures, which can produce activity limitations and participation restrictions (Rosenbaum et al., 2007). Although movement demands increase with age, the child's motor abilities may not be able to change quickly enough to meet these demands.

CP is characterized by decreased motor function, activity limitations, and participation restrictions because of delayed and abnormal motor development, impaired muscle tone, and movement patterns. Balance responses are the reverse of what is seen in typically developing children. How the damage to the central nervous system manifests depends on the developmental age of the child at the time of the brain injury, the severity and extent of the lesion, and its location. Poor selective motor control results in excessive motor activity. Too many muscles are activated during a task rather than only those appropriate for the task. Recent research has shown that the lesions occur during the second half of gestation (Hadders-Algra, 2014). Up to 80% of the cases of CP are due to prenatal factors (Longo and Hankins, 2009).

INCIDENCE

CP is the most common motor disability of childhood with a reported incidence of about 2.1 cases per 1000 live births in high-income countries (Oskoui et al., 2013). The prevalence of CP in the United States, or the number of individuals within a population who have the disorder, has recently been reported to range from 2.6 to 2.9 per 1000 children based on two US National Surveys (Maenner et al., 2016). Although prevalence has declined in Australia and Europe (Reid et al., 2016; Sellier et al., 2016), rates tend to be higher in lower to middle-income countries (Blair and Watson, 2006), with more physical disability being related to differences in pre- and perinatal care (Khandaker et al., 2015). Smaller preterm infants are more likely to demonstrate moderately severe CP because the risk of CP is greater with increasing prematurity and lower birth weights (Hintz et al., 2011).

ETIOLOGY

CP can have multiple causes with multiple risk factors interacting across time. Typical causes of CP and the relationship of these causes with prenatal, perinatal, and postnatal occurrences are listed in Table 6.1. The primary risk factor for CP is preterm birth. Intrauterine growth retardation and postnatal inflammation can increase the risk of developing CP in premature infants (Leviton et al., 2013). Premature infants' risk increases when evidence of white matter damage is found on brain imaging or cranial ultrasound (Graham et al., 2016). Vulnerability to CP changes relative to gestational age and type of CP (Nelson, 2008). Prematurity and intrauterine growth restriction are consistently identified as risk factors for CP.

TABLE 6.1 Risk Factors Associated With Cerebral Palsy

Prenatal Factors	Perinatal Factors	Postnatal Factors
Maternal infections	Prematurity	Neonatal infection
• Rubella	Obstetric complications • Twins or multiple births	Stroke
• Herpes simplex	Low birth weight for gestational age	Kernicterus
• Toxoplasmosis		
• Cytomegalovirus		
• Zika		
Placental abnormalities • Inflammation		
Maternal thyroid		
Toxemia		
Brain maldevelopment		

Modified from Glanzman A: Cerebral palsy. In Goodman C, Fuller KS, editors: *Pathology: implications for the physical therapist*, ed 3, Philadelphia, 2015, WB Saunders, p. 1579.

Prenatal Causes

When the cause of CP is known, it is most often related to problems experienced during intrauterine development. A fetus exposed to maternal infections, such as rubella, herpes simplex, cytomegalovirus, or toxoplasmosis, early in gestation can incur damage to the motor centers of the fetus' brain. Children born with congenital Zika syndrome also have a higher risk for CP (Marques et al., 2019). If the placenta, which provides nutrition and oxygen from the mother, does not remain attached to the uterine wall throughout the pregnancy, the fetus can be deprived of oxygen and other vital nutrients. The placenta can become inflamed or develop thrombi, either of which can impair fetal growth. The reader is referred to Nelson (2008) for a review of causative factors in CP, and to Graham et al. (2016) for a review of the epidemiology of CP.

Rh factor is found in the red blood cells of 85% of the population. Rh incompatibility occurs when a mother who is Rh-negative is carrying a baby who is Rh-positive. The mother becomes sensitive to the baby's blood and begins to make antibodies if she is not given RhIg (Rh immunoglobulin). RhIg prevents sensitization. The development of maternal antibodies predisposes subsequent Rh-positive babies to *kernicterus*, a syndrome characterized by CP, high-frequency hearing loss, visual problems, and discoloration of the teeth. Each successive pregnancy requires that RhIg be given. Additional maternal problems that can place an infant at risk for neurologic injury include diabetes and toxemia during pregnancy. In diabetes, the mother's metabolic deficits can cause stunted growth of the fetus and delayed tissue maturation. Toxemia of pregnancy causes the mother's blood pressure to become so high that the baby is in danger of not receiving sufficient blood flow, and therefore oxygen.

Only 10% to 15% of children with CP have brain malformations other than a brain lesion (Korzeniewski et al., 2008), whereas maldevelopment of other organ systems is commonly seen in CP (Himmelmann and Uvebrant, 2011). Fetal inflammation contributes to preterm birth and development of CP (Graham et al., 2016). Genetic mutations and exposure to teratogens can produce brain malformations and increase the risk for CP (MacLennan et al., 2015). A *teratogen* is any agent or condition that causes a defect in the fetus; these include radiation, drugs, bacterial and viral infections, and chronic illness. Exome sequencing has shown that 14% of cases of CP were likely caused by single-gene mutations (McMichael et al., 2015).

Perinatal Causes

Perinatal factors associated with CP in preterm infants include low maternal thyroid hormone levels, intraamniotic infection, and perinatal inflammation that continues postnatally (Kuban et al., 2015; Reuss et al., 1996). An infant may experience birth asphyxia resulting from *anoxia* (a lack of oxygen) during labor and delivery but it only accounts for a very small percentage of CP cases (10% or less) (Ellenberg and Nelson, 2013). Prolonged or difficult labor because of a *breech presentation* (bottom first) or the presence of a prolapsed umbilical cord may contribute to *asphyxia*. The brain may be compressed, or blood vessels in the brain may rupture during the birth process. Perinatal hypoxic-ischemic stroke is now recognized as a cause of CP with the advent of imaging. Hemiplegic CP is the most common type in term-born infants. Inflammation and infection can trigger thrombosis, which can lead to a stroke. Stroke can occur before birth as well as around the time of birth. Risk factors can be related to disorders of the mother, infant, or placenta.

Preterm infants are at risk of developing periventricular leukomalacia (PVL), a necrosis of the white matter in the arterial watershed areas around the ventricles. The fibers of the corticospinal tract to the lower extremities are particularly vulnerable. Decreased blood flow to this area (Fig. 6.1) may result in spastic diplegic CP. The incidence of PVL is inversely related to gestational age. Preterm infants between 23 and 32 weeks of gestation are at particular risk for this problem due to autoregulation of blood flow of the central nervous system (Glanzman, 2015).

Although CP is more likely to be associated with premature birth, the majority of cases of CP occur in full-term infants. Many cases have no clear-cut explanation of the cause (Novak et al., 2017). Although neuroimaging, specifically magnetic resonance imaging (MRI), is predictive for CP in preterm infants (Ashwal et al., 2004; Novak et al., 2017), up to 17% of children clinically diagnosed with CP have normal MRI scans (Reid et al., 2014).

Postnatal Causes

An infant or toddler may acquire brain damage secondary to stroke, trauma, infection, or anoxia. These conditions can be related to motor vehicle accidents, child abuse in the form of shaken baby syndrome, near-drowning, or lead exposure. Meningitis and encephalitis (inflammatory disorders of the brain) account for 60% of cases of postnatal CP (Horstmann and Bleck, 2007).

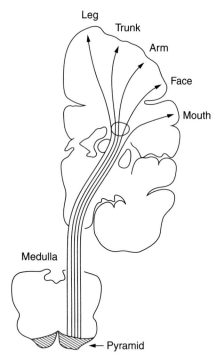

Leg
Trunk
Arm
Face
Mouth
Medulla
← Pyramid

Fig. 6.1 Schematic diagram of corticospinal tract fibers from the motor cortex through the periventricular region into the pyramid of the medulla. The fibers from the lower extremities are most vulnerable to periventricular leukomalacia, which may result in spastic diplegic cerebral palsy. (Modified from Volpe JJ: Hypoxic ischemic encephalopathy: neuropathology and pathogenesis. In Volpe JJ, editor: *Neurology of the neonate*, Philadelphia, 1995, WB Saunders.)

Prevention

There have been advances in prevention of CP in premature infants. Mothers who received magnesium sulfate during labor showed a decrease in percentage of preterm infants diagnosed with CP (Conde-Agudelo and Romero, 2009; Costantine and Weiner, 2009; Jacquemyn et al., 2015). A recent invited review concluded that administration of magnesium sulfate to women before 32 weeks' gestation was a cost-effective intervention that reduced the rate of CP (Chollat et al., 2019). A second prevention, using brain or body cooling for 72 hours in full-term infants with birth asphyxia (hypoxic-ischemic encephalopathy), decreased mortality and risk for CP (Jacobs et al., 2013). Therapeutic hypothermia also reduces the risk of postnatal seizures in newborns with moderate to severe hypoxic-ischemic encephalopathy (Lugli et al., 2018).

CLASSIFICATION

The designation "cerebral palsy" does not convey much specific information about the type or severity of movement dysfunction a child exhibits. CP can be classified at least three different ways: (1) by distribution of involvement or topology; (2) by type of abnormal tone and movement; and (3) by severity, which is best described according to the Gross Motor Function Classification System (GMFCS) (Palisano et al., 1997, 2008) rather than using the terms *mild, moderate,* or *severe.*

Distribution of Involvement (Topology)

The motor defects seen as a result of CP depend on the location of the brain lesion. The term *plegia* is used along with a prefix to designate how much of the body is affected by paralysis or weakness. Children with *quadriplegic* CP have involvement of the entire body, with the upper extremities usually more severely affected than the lower extremities (Fig. 6.2, *A*). These children have difficulty in developing head and trunk control, and they may or may not be able to ambulate. If they do learn to walk, it may not be until middle childhood. In *triplegia,* there is asymmetrical bilateral lower extremity involvement and unilateral upper extremity involvement. Children with *quadriplegia, triplegia,* and *diplegia* have bilateral brain damage. Children with *diplegia* have primarily lower extremity involvement, although the trunk is almost always affected to some degree (Fig. 6.2, *B*). Surveillance of Cerebral Palsy Europe (SCPE) defines *diplegia* as having all four limbs involved, with the lower extremities more severely involved than the upper ones (SCPE, 2000). *Diplegia* is often related to premature birth, especially if the child is born at around 32 weeks of gestation or 2 months premature. For this reason, *spastic diplegia* has been labeled the CP of prematurity. *Monoplegia* designates only one limb is involved and that is usually a lower extremity (SCPE, 2000). Children with *hemiplegia* have one side of the body involved, as is seen in adults after a stroke (Fig. 6.2, *C*). Children with hemiplegia have incurred unilateral brain damage. Although these designations seem to focus on the number of limbs or the side of the body involved, the limbs are connected to the trunk. The trunk is always affected to some degree when a child has CP. The trunk is primarily affected by abnormal tone in hemiplegia and quadriplegia, or it is secondarily affected, as in diplegia or triplegia, when the trunk compensates for lack of controlled movement in the involved lower limbs.

Abnormal Tone and Movement

There are four motor types of CP according to SCPE (2000): (1) spastic, (2) dyskinetic including dystonia and athetosis, (3) ataxic, and (4) hypotonic. The topography and motor type may change during the first 2 years of life. Children with *hypotonia* present as floppy infants (Fig. 6.3); their resting postural tone is below normal. Uncertainty exists regarding the ultimate impairment of tone when an infant presents with *hypotonia* because tone can change over time as the infant attempts to move against gravity. The tone may remain low, may increase to normal, may increase beyond normal to hypertonia, or may fluctuate from high to low to normal. Continual low tone in an infant impedes the development of head and trunk control, and interferes with the development of mature breathing patterns. Tone fluctuations are characteristically seen in the child with an *athetoid* type of CP. Children with hypotonia, dyskinesias, and ataxia have all four limbs and trunk involved. *Dystonia* is characterized by overflow of muscle activation and cocontraction of muscles making it difficult to switch between movements involved in a complicated task. The *spastic* type is most common and is classified by topography, as previously described.

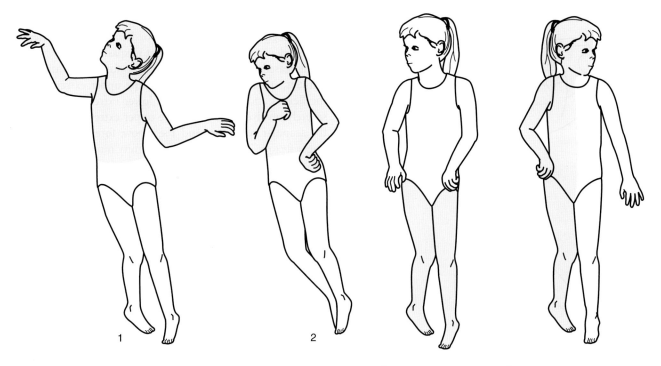

A SPASTIC QUADRIPLEGIA
1 Dominant extension
2 Dominant flexion

B SPASTIC DIPLEGIA   **C RIGHT SPASTIC HEMIPLEGIA**

Fig. 6.2 **(A-C)** Distribution of involvement in cerebral palsy.

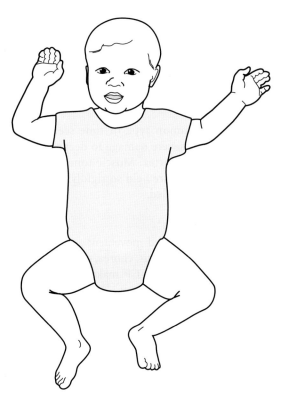

Fig. 6.3 Hypotonic infant.

The abnormal tone manifested in children with CP may be the nervous system's response to the initial brain damage, rather than a direct result of the damage. The nervous system may be trying to compensate for a lack of feedback from the involved parts of the body. The distribution of abnormal muscle tone may change when the child's body position changes relative to gravity. A child whose posture is characterized by an extended trunk and limbs when supine may be totally flexed (head and trunk) when sitting because the child's relationship with gravity has changed (Fig. 6.4). Tonal differences may be apparent even within different parts of the body. A child with spastic diplegia may exhibit hypertonic muscles in the lower extremities and hypotonia in the trunk muscles. The pattern of tone may be consistent in all body positions, or it may change with each new relationship to gravity. The degree or amount of abnormal muscle tone is judged relative to the degree of resistance encountered with passive movement. Rudimentary assessments can be made based on the ability of the child to initiate movement against gravity. In general, the greater the resistance to passive movement, the greater the difficulty is seen in the child's attempts to move.

Spasticity

Spasticity is a velocity-dependent increase in muscle tone. *Hypertonus* is increased resistance to passive motion that may

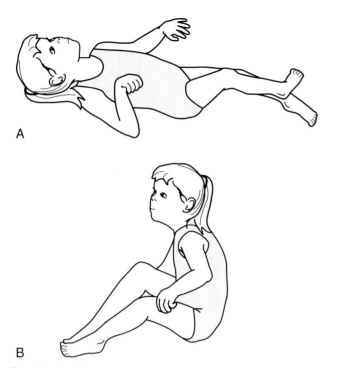

Fig. 6.4 **(A)** Child in extension in the supine position. **(B)** The same child demonstrating a flexed sitting posture.

not be affected by the speed of movement. Hypertonus is the result of several factors, one of which is the reflex stiffness (hyperactive deep tendon reflex), passive stiffness from changes in the muscle itself, and active stiffness because of the increased force needed to change the length of the muscle. Clinically hypertonus and spasticity are often used interchangeably. However, Nahm et al. (2018) consider spasticity a subtype of hypertonia. Spasticity is a classic symptom of an upper motor neuron lesion. Classification and differentiation of the amount of muscle tone above normal are subjective and are represented by a continuum from mild to moderate to severe. The mild and moderate designations usually describe a person who has the ability to move actively through at least part of the available range of motion. Severe hypertonus and spasticity indicate extreme difficulty in moving, with an inability to complete the full range of motion. In the latter instance, the child may have difficulty even initiating movement without use of some type of inhibitory technique. Prolonged increased tone predisposes the individual to contractures and deformities because, in most situations, an antagonist muscle cannot adequately oppose the pull of a spastic muscle. The modified Ashworth scale and the Tardieu scale have been used to measure tone in children with CP. The Tardieu scale was found to be more reliable than the modified Ashworth (Wright and Palisano, 2017). Neither assessment method is universally accepted.

Spasticity may not be present initially at birth, but it can gradually replace low muscle tone as the child attempts to move against gravity. *Spastic paralysis* results from a classic upper motor neuron lesion. A Swedish study showed that spasticity increased until 4 years of age, and then declined until 12 years of age (Hagglund and Wagner, 2008). The

muscles affected depend on the distribution of involvement—quadriplegia, diplegia (bilateral), or hemiplegia (unilateral). Fig. 6.2 depicts typical involvement in spastic CP.

Increased muscle tone tends to be found in antigravity muscles, specifically the flexors in the upper extremity and the flexors and extensors in the lower extremity. The most severely involved muscles in the upper extremity tend to be the scapular retractors and the elbow, forearm, wrist, and finger flexors. The same lower extremity muscles that are involved in children with diplegia are seen in quadriplegia and hemiplegia: hip flexors and adductors; knee flexors, especially medial hamstrings; and ankle plantar flexors. The degree of involvement among these muscles may vary, and additional muscles may also be affected. Trunk musculature may exhibit increased tone as well. Increased trunk tone may impair breath control for speech by hampering the normal excursion of the diaphragm and chest wall during inspiration and expiration.

Transient Dystonia

This temporary condition is seen in as many as 60% of all preterm infants who have a low birth weight and even in some term infants. Although the characteristics seen during the first year life may be transient, they have been linked to behavior deficits later in life in some studies. The characteristics are troubling to a physical therapist because it is often difficult to distinguish these from clinical signs of early CP. The characteristics include increased tone in neck extensor muscles, hypotonia, irritability, and lethargy during the neonatal period; increased tone in extremity muscles, low tone in the trunk muscles, shoulder retraction, and scapular adduction with a persistent asymmetrical tonic neck reflex (ATNR) and persistent + support reflex at age 4 months; and immature postural reactions with minimal trunk rotation, continued trunk hypotonia, and extremity hypertonicity at 6 to 8 months. Children with transient dystonia present with signs similar to CP but they resolve (Calado et al., 2011).

Rigidity

Rigidity is an uncommon type of tone seen in children with CP. It indicates severe damage to deeper areas of the brain rather than the cortex. Muscle tone is increased to the point that postures are held so rigidly that movement in any direction is impeded.

Dyskinesia

Dyskinesia means disordered movement and can be further classified as dystonia, athetosis, chorea, or a mixture of chorea and athetosis. Dyskinetic CP makes up roughly 4% to 17% of all CP (Himmelman et al., 2010; Reid et al., 2011). *Dystonia* coexists with the spastic subtype of CP (Fehlings et al., 2018; Nahm et al., 2018). Seventy percent of children with dyskinetic CP have spasticity (Sun et al., 2018). Involuntary movement due to fluctuating hypertonia results in repetitive abnormal posturing of the extremities, trunk, or neck. The twisting movements impair motor function and can be painful (Lin and Nardocci, 2016). *Athetosis* is characterized by disordered movement of the extremities described classically as slow and writhing, whereas *chorea* is jerky and dance-like. In athetosis, movements in the midrange are especially difficult because of the lack of proximal postural stability on which to superimpose movement. As the limb moves farther away from the body, selective motor control diminishes. Involuntary movements can be observed in the child's entire extremity, distally in the hands and feet, or proximally in the mouth and face. The child with athetosis must depend on external support to improve movement accuracy and efficiency. Difficulty in feeding and in speech can be expected if the oral muscles are involved. Speech usually develops, but the child may not be easily understood. *Athetoid* CP is characterized by decreased static and dynamic postural stability. Children with athetosis lack the postural stability necessary to allow purposeful movements to be controlled for the completion of functional tasks (Fig. 6.5). Muscle tone often fluctuates from low to high to normal to high such that the child has difficulty in maintaining postural alignment in all but the most firmly supported positions and exhibits slow, repetitive involuntary movements. Dystonia and choreoathetosis make up the two subtypes of dyskinetic CP.

Ataxia

Ataxia is classically defined as a loss of coordination resulting from damage to the cerebellum. Children with ataxic CP exhibit loss of coordination and low postural tone. They usually demonstrate a diplegic distribution, with the trunk and lower extremities most severely affected. This pattern of low tone makes it difficult for the child to maintain midline stability of the head and trunk in any posture. Ataxic movements are jerky and irregular. Children with ataxic CP ultimately achieve upright standing, but to maintain this position, they must stand with a wide base of support as a compensation for a lack of static postural control (Fig. 6.6). Postural reactions are slow to develop in all postures, with the most significant balance impairment demonstrated during gait.

Children with *ataxia* walk with large lateral displacements of the trunk in an effort to maintain balance. Their gait is often described as "staggering" because of these wide displacements, which are a natural consequence of the lack of stability and poor timing of postural corrections. Together, these impairments may seem to spell imminent disaster for balance, but these children are able, with practice, to adjust to the wide displacements in their center of gravity and to walk without falling. Wide displacements and slow balance reactions are counteracted by the wide base of support. Arm movements are typically used as a compensatory strategy to counteract excessive truncal weight shifts. The biggest challenge for the clinician is to allow the child to ambulate independently using what looks like a precarious gait. Proper safety precautions

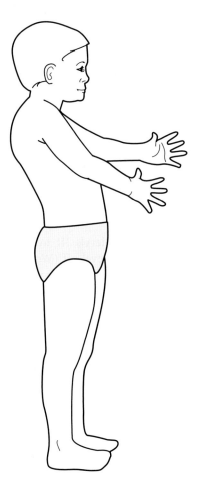

Fig. 6.5 Standing posture in a child with athetoid cerebral palsy.

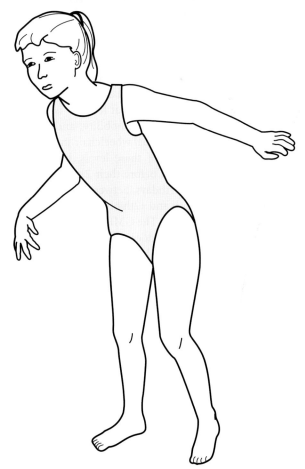

Fig. 6.6 Ataxic cerebral palsy.

should always be taken, and some children may need to wear a helmet for personal safety. Assistive devices do not appear to be helpful during ambulation unless they can be adequately weighted, and even then, these devices may be more of a deterrent than a help.

FUNCTIONAL CLASSIFICATION

In keeping with the World Health Organization's International Classification of Functioning, Disability, and Health, the best way to classify a disorder like CP is to look at the impact on function. The GMFCS (Palisano et al., 1997, 2008) is the preferred way to classify mobility in children with CP. The Manual Ability Classification System (Eliasson et al., 2006) is the preferred way to classify how children with CP use their hands when engaged in activities of daily living (ADLs). There is also the Communication Function Classification System (Hidecker et al., 2011) for children with CP. Interprofessional communication will be enhanced by utilizing these tools, which provide standardized terminology and stratification of levels of function. Use of the classification systems should also enhance communication among parents and professionals when discussing a child's level of function and long-term outcomes. Use of all three classification systems can provide a functional profile of the child (Effgen et al., 2014). Table 6.2 shows a general description of the five levels of each of the classification systems. Only the GMFCS will be discussed in more detail here.

The GMFCS (Palisano et al., 2008) is a five-level scale that determines a motor level for a child with a motor disability. A child at level I walks without limitations; a child at level II walks with limitations; a child at level III walks using a handheld mobility device; a child at level IV is limited in self-mobility and may use power mobility; and a child at level V is transported in a manual wheelchair in all settings. More detailed descriptions of these levels, based on age bands, are used for children before their 2nd birthday, between the 2nd and 4th birthdays, between the 4th and 6th birthdays, between the 6th and 12th birthdays, and between the 12th and 18th birthdays. The GMFCS is based on usual *performance*, what the child does rather than what she is known to be able to do at her best, which is *capability*. The older age bands reflect the potential impact of the environment on function and the personal preference of the child/youth in regard to mobility. A summary of the expectations for the older age bands can be found in Fig. 6.7. A description of all levels and age bands can be found on the CanChild website (www.canchild.ca).

Gross motor function curves were produced by researchers at CanChild Centre for Developmental Disability Research using the GMFCS levels and data from the Gross Motor Function Measure–66. These curves provide the average pattern of development for each of the five levels of the GMFCS and can be used to guide motor expectations for the first 5 years of life. Children at levels I and II progress faster to a maximum motor score then level off,

TABLE 6.2	**Classification Systems for Cerebral Palsy**
Mobility	Gross Motor Classification System
	Level I: Walks without limitations
	Level II: Walks with limitations
	Level III: Walks using a handheld mobility device
	Level IV: Self-mobility with limitations, may use power mobility
	Level V: Transported in a manual wheelchair
Hand use	Manual Ability Classification System
	Level I: Handles objects easily and successfully
	Level II: Handles most objects but with somewhat reduced quality or speed of achievement
	Level III: Handles objects with difficulty, needs help to prepare or modify activities
	Level IV: Handles a limited selection of easily managed objects in adapted situations
	Level V: Does not handle objects and has severely limited ability to perform simple actions
Communication	Communication Function Classification System
	Level I: Effective sender and receiver with unfamiliar and familiar partners
	Level II: Effective but slower-paced sender or receiver with unfamiliar and familiar partners
	Level III: Effective sender and receiver with familiar partners
	Level IV: Sometimes effective sender or receiver with familiar partners
	Level V: Seldom effective sender and receiver even with familiar partners

Data from Eliasson et al., 2006; Hidecker et al., 2011; Palisano et al., 2008.

whereas those children at levels III to V progress more slowly and then decline or level off (Wright and Palisano, 2017). Motor severity in children age 2 years and older can reliably be classified using the five-level GMFCS Extended and Revised (Palisano et al., 1997). Before age 2 years, motor severity is difficult to predict (Novak et al., 2017). The motor function of young children is more likely to be reclassified (Palisano et al., 2018).

The probability of ambulation depends on the child's age and environmental setting. Children at GMFCS level I usually walk by age 3 years based on longitudinal data (Palisano et al., 2010). The probability of walking in children at level II was found to depend on the environment (home, school, and outdoors) with 90% walking outdoors at age 18. The highest percentage of children at level III walked in school at age 9, with 50% walking in all three settings at age 18. As children at level IV got older, they were likely to use wheeled mobility, and children at level V almost all used assisted mobility. Clinical decision-making about mobility involves discussion of options, safety, efficiency, and environmental concerns with the family and the child. The means of mobility that works best for the child in one setting may not be optimal in another. The goal is always for the child to actively participate in life activities.

Diagnosis

Signs and symptoms of CP emerge over the first two years of life with a diagnosis typically made between 12 and 24 months. Many years of research have been devoted to developing sensitive assessment tools that allow pediatricians and pediatric physical therapists to identify infants with CP as early as 4 to 6 months of age. In a recent review, Novak et al. (2017) provide evidence that it is now possible to diagnosis CP before 6 months' corrected age using a combination of assessments. The most sensitive tools to detect CP include neuroimaging (brain MRI), and either the General Movement Assessment or the Hammersmith Infant Neurological Examination (Novak et al., 2017). Despite advances in diagnosis, many children are not formally diagnosed until after 6 months of age. For the first time a US clinical setting demonstrated the feasibility of implementing the international early diagnosis and treatment guidelines for CP (Byrne et al., 2017). There was a significant decrease in the mean age at diagnosis as a result of the implementation of the guidelines.

GMFCS E & R descriptors and illustrations for children between their 6th and 12th birthdays

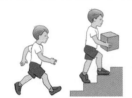

GMFCS Level I

Children walk at home, school, outdoors and in the community. They can climb stairs without the use of a railing. Children perform gross motor skills such as running and jumping, but speed, balance and coordination are limited.

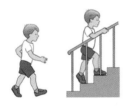

GMFCS Level II

Children walk in most settings and climb stairs holding on to a railing. They may experience difficulty walking long distances and balancing on uneven terrain, inclines, in crowded areas or confined spaces. Children may walk with physical assistance, a hand-held mobility device, or use wheeled mobility over long distances. Children have only minimal ability to perform gross motor skills such as running and jumping.

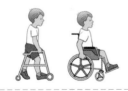

GMFCS Level III

Children walk using a hand-held mobility device in most settings. They may climb stairs holding on to a railing with supervision or assistance. Children use wheeled mobility when traveling long distances and may self-propel for shorter distances.

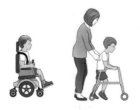

GMFCS Level IV

Children use methods of mobility that require physical assistance or powered mobility in most settings. They may walk for short distances at home with physical assistance or use powered mobility or a body support walker when positioned. At school, outdoors and in the community children are transported in a manual wheelchair or use powered mobility.

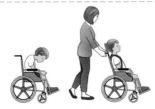

GMFCS Level V

Children are transported in a manual wheelchair in all settings. Children are limited in their ability to maintain antigravity head and trunk postures and control leg and arm movements.

Fig. 6.7 Gross Motor Function Classification System.

**GMFCS E & R descriptors and illustrations for children
between their 12th and 18th birthdays**

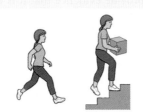

GMFCS Level I

Youth walk at home, school, outdoors and in community. Youth are able to climb stairs without physical assistance or a railing. They perform gross motor skills such as running and jumping but speed, balance and coordination are limited.

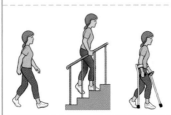

GMFCS Level II

Youth walk in most settings but environmental factors and personal choice influence mobility choices. At school or work they may require a hand-held mobility device for safety and climb stairs holding on to a railing. Outdoors and in the community youth may use wheeled mobility when traveling long distances.

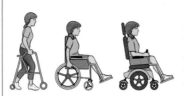

GMFCS Level III

Youth are capable of walking using a hand-held mobility device. Youth may climb stairs holding on to a railing with supervision or assistance. At school they may self-propel a manual wheelchair or use powered mobility. Outdoors and in the community youth are transported in a wheelchair or use powered mobility.

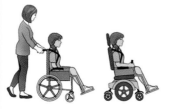

GMFCS Level IV

Youth use wheeled mobility in most settings. Physical assistance of one to two people is required for transfers. Indoors, youth may walk short distances with physical assistance, use wheeled mobility or a body support walker when positioned. They may operate a powered chair, otherwise are transported in a manual wheelchair.

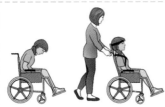

GMFCS Level V

Youth are transported in a manual wheelchair in all settings. Youth are limited in their ability to maintain antigravity head and trunk postures and control leg and arm movements. Self-mobility is severely limited, even with the use of assistive technology.

Fig. 6.7, **cont'd**

PATHOPHYSIOLOGY

Lesions involving the cerebral cortex can involve one or both hemispheres. Depending on which fibers of the corticospinal tract are involved and whether the damage is bilateral or unilateral, the resultant neurologic deficit manifests as quadriplegia, diplegia, or hemiplegia. The stage of brain maturation in which the pathology occurs often determines the site and type of lesion. Preterm infants with low birth weights are at substantially higher risk for PVL damage to white matter around the ventricles due to hypoxia and ischemia. PVL is the most common cause of *spastic diplegia. Spastic hemiplegia*, the most common type of CP, can result from unilateral brain damage secondary to perinatal stroke or to cysts that develop in the preterm infant following white matter damage. The term infants dyskinesia occurring with spastic quadriplegia has been associated with severe asphyxia (Graham et al., 2016). Dystonia is linked to white matter damage, damage to the basal ganglia or thalamus late in

gestation or around the time of birth (Himmelmann et al., 2017). *Athetosis* is most often seen when too high bilirubin levels (kernicterus) cause basal ganglia damage. *Ataxia*, the rarest form of CP, is related to damage to the cerebellum.

ASSOCIATED DEFICITS

The deficits associated with CP are presented in the order in which they may become apparent in the infant with CP (Box 6.1). Early signs of motor dysfunction in an infant often present as problems with feeding and breathing.

Feeding and Speech Impairments

Poor suck-swallow reflexes and uncoordinated sucking and breathing may be evidence of central nervous system dysfunction in a newborn. Persistence of infantile oral reflexes, such as rooting or suck-swallow, or exaggerations of normally occurring reflexes, such as a tonic bite or tongue thrust, can

---

BOX 6.1 Deficits Associated With Cerebral Palsy

Feeding and speech impairments
Breathing inefficiency
Visual impairments
Hearing impairments
Intellectual disability
Seizures

---

indicate abnormal oral motor development. A hyperactive or hypoactive response to touch around and in the mouth is also possible. Hypersensitivity may be seen in the child with spastic hemiplegia or quadriplegia, whereas hyposensitivity may be evident in the child with low-tone CP.

Feeding is considered a precursor to speech, so the child who has feeding problems may well have difficulty in producing intelligible sounds. Lip closure around the nipple is needed to prevent loss of liquids during sucking. Lip closure is also needed in speech to produce "p," "b," and "m" sounds. If the infant cannot bring the lips together because of tonal problems, feeding and sound production will be hindered. The tongue moves in various ways within the mouth during sucking and swallowing and later in chewing; these patterns change with oral motor development. These changes in tongue movements are crucial not only for taking in food and swallowing, but also for the production of various sounds requiring specific tongue placement within the oral cavity.

Breathing Inefficiency

Breathing inefficiency may compound feeding and speech problems. Typically developing infants are belly breathers, and only over time do they develop the ability to use the rib cage effectively to increase the volume of inspired air. Gravity promotes developmental changes in the configuration of the rib cage that place the diaphragm in a more advantageous position for efficient inspiration. This developmental change is hampered in children who are delayed in experiencing being in an upright posture because of lack of attainment of age-appropriate motor abilities, such as head and trunk control. Lack of development in the upright posture can result in structural deformities of the ribs, such as rib flaring, and functional limitations, such as poor breath control and shorter breath length that is inadequate for sound production. Abnormally increased tone in the trunk musculature may allow only short bursts of air to be expelled and produce staccato speech. Low muscle tone can predispose children to rib flaring because of lack of abdominal muscle development. Intellectual disability, hearing impairment, or central language processing impairment may further impede the ability of the child with CP to develop effective oral communication skills.

Intellectual Disability

Children with CP have many other problems associated with damage to the nervous system that also relate to and affect normal development. The most common of these are vision and hearing impairments, feeding and speech difficulties, seizures, and intellectual disability. The classification of intellectual disability is given in Chapter 8, and thus not found in this chapter. Although no direct correlation exists between the severity of motor involvement and the degree of intellectual disability, the percentage of children with CP with intellectual disability has been estimated at between 25% and 45% (Yin Foo et al., 2013). A recent systematic review of population data from high-income countries concluded that 1 in 2 children with CP would have normal intelligence (Novak et al., 2012). Intelligence tests require a verbal or motor response, either of which may be impaired in these children. Mean cognitive scores in children with CP are related to gestational age and birth weight (Accardo, 2008). The risk for intellectual disability increases 1.4-fold when an infant is born between 32 and 36 weeks, and 7-fold if born before 32 weeks of gestation. It is further suggested that children of normal intelligence who have CP may be at risk of having learning disabilities or other cognitive or neurobehavioral impairments. In general, children with spastic hemiplegia or diplegia, athetosis, or ataxia are more likely to have normal or higher than normal intelligence, whereas children with more severe types of CP, such as spastic quadriplegia, or a mixed type, are more likely to exhibit intellectual disability (Hoon and Tolley, 2013). However, as with any generalizations, exceptions always exist. Yin Foo et al. (2013) proposed using a clinical reasoning tool to select appropriate IQ assessments for children with CP. It is extremely important to not make judgments about a child's intellectual status based solely on the severity of the motor involvement.

Seizures

Seizures are more common in children with CP than in typically developing children. The site of brain damage in CP may become the focal point of abnormal electrical activity, which can cause seizures. Epilepsy is a disease characterized by recurrent seizures. Approximately 40% of children with CP experience seizures that must be managed by medication (Nordmark et al., 2001). A smaller percentage may have a single seizure episode related to high fever or increased intracranial pressure. Intellectual impairment and seizures are comorbidities in CP (Gabis et al., 2015). Thirty-two percent of children with severe CP based on the GMFCS level had epilepsy. Intellectual disability was correlated with motor ability and epilepsy (Gabis et al., 2015). Fifty percent of children with hemiplegic CP due to perinatal stroke develop epilepsy but with favorable outcomes (Wanigasinghe et al., 2010). The main seizure types in this group were epileptic spasms and focal seizures. Children with CP due to white matter injury are also at risk for seizures but again they appear to be age-limited epileptic syndromes of childhood, most of which have a favorable outcome (Cooper et al., 2017).

Seizures are classified as generalized, focal, or unclassified and are listed in Table 6.3. *Generalized seizures* are named for the type of motor activity the person exhibits. *Focal seizures* used to be called partial seizures, which were simple or complex, depending on whether the child experiences a loss of consciousness. Focal seizures can have either sensory or motor manifestations or both. *Unclassified seizures* do not fit in any

TABLE 6.3 Classification of Seizures

International Classification of Seizures	Manifestation of Seizures
Generalized seizures	Seizures that are generalized to the entire body; always involve a loss of consciousness
Tonic-clonic seizure	Begin with a tonic contraction (stiffening) of the body, then change to clonic movements (jerking) of the body
Tonic seizure	Stiffening of the entire body
Clonic seizure	Myoclonic jerks start and stop abruptly
Atonic seizure	Sudden lack of muscle tone
Absence seizure	Nonconvulsive seizure with a loss of consciousness; blinking, staring, or minor movements lasting a few seconds
Myoclonic seizure	Irregular, involuntary contraction of a muscle or group of muscles
Focal seizures	Seizures not generalized to the entire body; a variety of sensory or motor symptoms may accompany this type of seizure; the distinction between partial seizures has been eliminated (Berg et al., 2010)
Syndromes	See Berg et al., 2010
Unclassified seizure	Seizures that do not fit into the above categories

Modified from Berg AT, Berkovic SF, Brodie MJ, et al.: Revised terminology and concepts for organization of seizures and epilepsies: report of the ILAE Commission on Classification and Terminology, 2005–2009, *Epilepsia* 51(4):676–685, 2010.

other category. Epilepsy syndromes have common signs and symptoms, electroencephalogram features, characteristics, and the same genetic origin or pathogenesis. The physical therapist assistant should always document any seizure activity observed in a child, including time of occurrence, duration, loss of consciousness, motor and sensory manifestations, and status of the child after the seizure.

Visual Impairments

Vision is extremely important for the development of balance during the first 3 years of life (Shumway-Cook and Woollacott, 2017). Any visual difficulty may exacerbate the inherent neuromotor problems that typically accompany a diagnosis of CP. Eye muscle control can be negatively affected by abnormal tone and can lead to either turning in *(esotropia)* or turning out *(exotropia)* of one or both eyes. *Strabismus* is the general term for an abnormal ocular condition in which the eyes are crossed. Strabismus is present in many children with CP (Salt and Sargent, 2014) along with poor visual acuity and refractive errors. A higher incidence of visual impairment is associated with more severe motor involvement. Children with PVL may also be at risk for visual perception problems not explained by intellectual disability or visual acuity (Fazzi et al., 2009; Fedrizzi et al., 1998).

Nystagmus is most often seen in children with ataxia. In nystagmus, the eyes move back and forth rapidly in a horizontal, vertical, or rotary direction. Normally, nystagmus is produced in response to vestibular stimulation and indicates the close relationship between head movement and vision. The presence of nystagmus may complicate the task of balancing the head or trunk. Some children compensate for nystagmus by tilting their heads into extension, a move that can be mistaken for neck retraction and abnormal extensor tone. The posteriorly tilted head position gives the child the most stable visual input. Although neck hyperextension is generally to be avoided, if it is a compensation for nystagmus, the extended neck posture may not be avoidable. Visual deficits are common in children with hemiplegic CP (Ashwal et al., 2004). These deficits may include *homonymous hemianopia*, or loss of vision in half the visual field. Every child with hemiplegia should have a detailed assessment of vision.

Visual impairments in children with disabilities can interfere with development of head and trunk control and exploration of the immediate surroundings. Visual function should be assessed in any infant or child who is exhibiting difficulty in developing head control or in reaching for objects. Clinically, the child may not follow a familiar face or turn to examine a new face. If you suspect that a child has a visual problem, report your suspicions to the supervising physical therapist.

Hearing, Speech, and Language Impairments

Almost one-third of children with CP have hearing, speech, and language problems. As already mentioned, some speech problems can be secondary to poor motor control of oral muscles or respiratory impairment. Language difficulties in the form of expressive or receptive aphasia can result when the initial damage that caused the CP also affects the brain areas responsible for understanding speech or producing language. For most of the right-handed population, speech centers are located in the dominant left hemisphere. Clinically, the child may not turn toward sound or be able to localize a familiar voice. Hearing loss may be present in any type of CP, but it occurs in a higher percentage of children with quadriplegia. These children should be evaluated by an audiologist to ascertain whether amplification is warranted.

PHYSICAL THERAPY EXAMINATION

The physical therapist conducts a thorough examination and evaluation of the child with CP that includes a history, observation, and administration of specific standardized tests of development. Test selection is based on the reason for the evaluation: screening, information gathering, treatment planning, eligibility determination, or outcomes measurement. A discussion of developmental assessment is beyond the scope of this text; refer to Effgen (2013) for information on specific developmental assessment tools. However, the most commonly used measure of gross motor function in children with CP is the Gross Motor Function Measure (Hanna et al., 2007). The physical therapist assistant needs to have an understanding of the purpose of the examination and awareness of the tools commonly administered and of the process used within a particular treatment setting. For example, an arena assessment may be used when examining a young child or a play-based assessment, whereas a one-on-one examination may be used in the school system.

The physical therapist assistant should be familiar with the information reported by the physical therapist in the child's examination: social and medical history; range of motion; muscle tone, strength, and bulk; reflexes and postural reactions; balance and mobility skills; transfers; ADLs, recreation, type of play, leisure preferences; and adaptive equipment. The assistant needs to be aware of the basis on which the physical therapist makes decisions about the child's plan of care. The physical therapist's responsibility is to make sure that the goals of therapy and the strategies used to implement the treatment plan are thoroughly understood by the physical therapist assistant.

Neuromuscular Impairments, Activity Limitations, and Participation Restrictions

The physical therapy examination should identify the neuromuscular impairments and the present or anticipated functional limitations of the child with CP. Physical impairments, such as too much or too little range of motion or muscle extensibility, are related to delayed and abnormal motor development. CP causes impaired muscle activation and use of immature motor strategies such as cocontraction, which leads to poor selective motor control. Muscle imbalance can occur because the muscles and tendons do not keep up with long bone growth. Muscle imbalance also occurs with hypertonia. Weakness and altered gait biomechanics negatively affect performance of motor tasks. Activity limitations are seen in sitting, standing, or use of the extremities. Activity limitations lead to restrictions in participation. In the spastic type of CP, weakness can cause more disability than spasticity (Kim et al., 2003;

Damiano, 2006). Poor motor function is only partly explained by spasticity. Reducing spasticity does not necessarily lead to positive changes in function (Graham et al., 2016). Gross motor function and functional outcomes are associated with strength. Children with athetoid or ataxic CP may have some of the same functional limitations, but their impairments are related to too much mobility and too little stability. The impairments and activity limitations of the child with hypotonic CP are similar to those of children with Down syndrome; therefore the reader is referred to Chapter 8 for a discussion of intervention strategies.

The Child With Spastic Cerebral Palsy

The child with spasticity often moves slowly and with difficulty. When movement is produced, it occurs in predictable, *stereotypical* patterns that occur the same way every time with little variability. A child with spastic CP at GMFCS levels (IV and V) will have difficulty developing head and trunk control. Children at GMFCS levels (I to III) may have some difficulty with trunk control but will ambulate independently. Most children with CP attain their gross motor ceiling capacity by age 5 years (Hanna et al., 2009; Rosenbaum et al., 2007). Activity limitations in addition to mobility include eating, drinking, dressing, playing, and learning (Table 6.4). Participation may be restricted in social interactions, peer play, school, dating, and finding a job.

Head Control

The child with spasticity can have difficulty in developing head control because of increased tone, persistent primitive reflexes, exaggerated tonic reflexes, or absent or impaired sensory input. Because the child often has difficulty in generating enough muscle force to maintain a posture or to move, substitutions and compensatory movements are common.

TABLE 6.4 Impairments, Activity Limitations, Participation Restrictions, and Focus of Treatment in Children With Spastic or Dystonic Cerebral Palsy

Impairments in Body Structure/Function	Activity Limitations	Participation Restrictions	Focus of Treatment
Movement • Muscle tone • Muscle strength • Skeletal system	Sitting, standing, walking Communication Motor cognition	Social engagement	Educate family about cerebral palsy Teach/coach handling and positioning for function Strength training
Poor selective motor control	Eating, drinking	Self-care	Teach/coach adaptations of task or environment
• Motor recruitment	Dressing	Self-care	Embed in daily routines
• Cocontraction	Mobility	Playing with peers Attending school	Playing with peers Gait training
Postural control • Balance	Any activity	Playing a sport Going to a movie	Self-initiated movement/practice movement transitions
Sensory processing	Dressing/playing Learning and communication Applying knowledge	Playing with peers Attending school Dating Finding a job	Optimize sensorimotor experiences Functional independence
Pain	All activities	Finding a job	Transition planning

For example, an infant who cannot control the head when held upright or supported in sitting may elevate the shoulders to provide some neck stability.

Trunk Control

Lack of trunk rotation and a predominance of extensor or flexor tone can impair the child's ability to roll. Inadequate trunk control prevents independent sitting. In a child with predominantly lower extremity problems, the lack of extensibility at the hips may prevent the attainment of an aligned sitting position. The child compensates by rounding the upper back to allow for sitting (Fig. 6.4, *B*). Trunk rotation can be absent or impaired secondary to a lack of balanced development of the trunk extensors and flexors. Without this balance, controlled lateral flexion is not possible, nor is rotation. Absent trunk rotation makes transitional movements (moving from one posture to another) extremely difficult. The child with spasticity may discover that it is possible to achieve a sitting position by pushing the body backward over passively flexed and adducted legs, to end up in a W-sitting position (Fig. 6.8). This posture should be avoided because its use can impede further development of trunk control and lower extremity dissociation.

Influence of Tonic Reflexes

Tonic reflexes are often obligatory in children with spastic CP. When a reflex is obligatory, it dominates the child's posture. Obligatory tonic reflexes produce increased tone and postures that can interfere with adaptive movement. When they occur during the course of typical development, they do not interfere with the infant's ability to move. The retention of these reflexes and their exaggerated expression appear to impair the acquisition of postural responses (balance) such as head and neck righting reactions and use of the extremities for protective extension. The retention of these tonic reflexes occurs because of the lack of typical development of selective motor control associated with CP. These reflexes are depicted in Fig. 6.8.

The Tonic Labyrinthine Reflex (TLR) affects tone relative to the head's relationship with gravity. When the child is supine, the TLR causes an increase in extensor tone, whereas when the child is prone, it causes an increase in flexor tone (Fig. 6.9, *A,B*). Typically, the reflex is present at birth and then is integrated by 6 months. It is thought to afford some unfolding of the flexed infant to counter the predominance of physiologic flexor tone at birth. If this reflex persists, it can impair the infant's ability to develop antigravity motion (to flex against gravity in supine and to extend against gravity in prone). An exaggerated TLR affects the entire body and can prevent the child from reaching with the arms in the supine position or from pushing with the arms in the prone position to assist in coming to sit. The TLR can affect the child's posture in sitting because the reflex is stimulated by the head's relationship with gravity. If the child loses head control posteriorly during sitting, the labyrinths sense the body as being supine, and the extensor tone produced may cause the child to fall backward and to slide out of the chair. Children who slump into flexion when the head is flexed may be demonstrating the influence of a prone TLR.

The ATNR causes associated upper extremity extension on the face side and flexion of the upper extremity on the skull side (Fig. 6.8, *C*). For example, turning the head to the right causes the right arm to extend and the left arm to bend. This reflex is usually apparent only in the upper extremities in a typically developing child; however, in the child with CP, the lower extremities may also be affected by the reflex. The ATNR is typically present from birth to 4 to 6 months. If this reflex persists and is obligatory, the child will be prevented from rolling or bringing the extended arm to her mouth. The asymmetry can affect the trunk and can predispose the child to scoliosis. In extreme cases, the dominant ATNR can produce hip dislocation on the flexed side.

The symmetrical tonic neck reflex causes the arms and legs to flex or extend, depending on the head position (Fig. 6.9, *D*). If the child's head is flexed, the arms flex and the legs extend; if the head is extended, vice versa. This reflex has the potential to assist the typically developing infant in attaining a four-point or hands-and-knees position. However, its persistence prevents reciprocal creeping and allows the child only to "bunny hop" as a means of mobility in the four-point position. When the symmetrical tonic neck reflex is obligatory, the arms and legs imitate or contradict the head movement. The child either sits back on the heels or thrusts forward. Maintaining a four-point position is difficult, as are any dissociated movements of the extremities needed for creeping. The exaggeration of tonic reflexes and the way in which they may interfere with functional movement are found in Table 6.5. The dysfunctional postures generated by the tonic reflexes should be avoided.

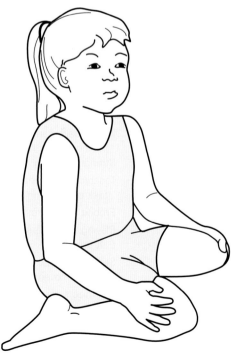

Fig. 6.8 W sitting.

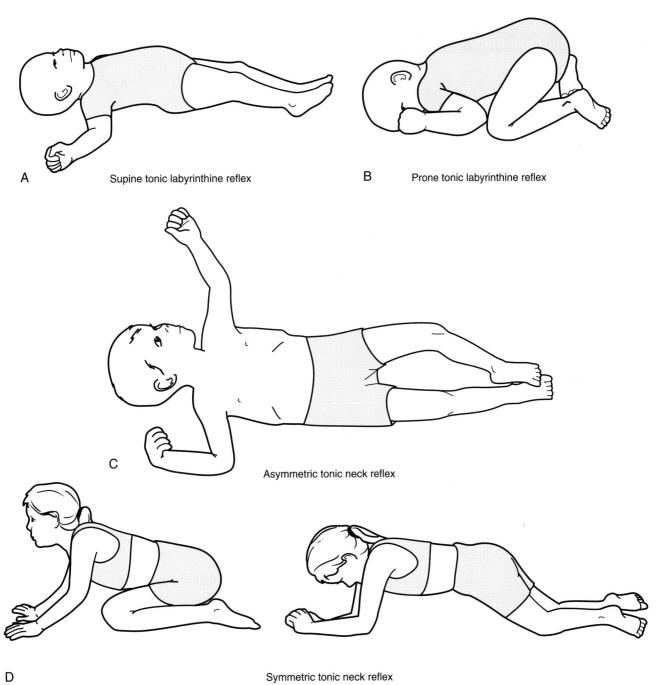

A   Supine tonic labyrinthine reflex

B   Prone tonic labyrinthine reflex

C   Asymmetric tonic neck reflex

D   Symmetric tonic neck reflex

Fig. 6.9 **(A-D)** Tonic reflexes.

Movement Transitions

The child with spastic CP often lacks the ability to control or to respond appropriately to shifts in the center of gravity that should typically result in righting, equilibrium, or protective reactions. These children are fearful and often do not feel safe because they have such precarious static and dynamic balance. In addition, the child's awareness of poor postural stability may lead to an expectation of falling based on prior experience. The inability to generate sufficient muscle activity in postural muscles for static balance is further compounded by the difficulty in anticipating postural changes in response to body movement. These features make performance of movement transitions, such as moving from prone to sitting or the reverse, sitting to prone, more difficult.

Mobility and Ambulation

Impaired lower extremity separation hinders reciprocal leg movements for creeping and walking; therefore, some children learn to move forward across the floor on their hands and knees by using a "bunny hopping" pattern that pulls both legs together. Other ways that the child with spasticity may attempt to move is by "commando crawling," forcefully pulling the arms under the chest and simultaneously dragging stiff legs along the floor. The additional effort by the arms increases

TABLE 6.5 Influence of Tonic Reflexes on Functional Movement

Tonic Reflex	Impairment	Functional Movement Limitation
TLR in supine	Contractures Abnormal vestibular input Limited visual field	Rolling from supine to prone Reaching in supine Coming to sit Sitting
TLR in prone	Contractures Abnormal vestibular input Limited visual field	Rolling from prone to supine Coming to sit Sitting
ATNR	Contractures Hip dislocation Trunk asymmetry Scoliosis	Segmental rolling Reaching Bringing hand to mouth Sitting
STNR	Contractures Lack of upper and lower extremity dissociation Lack of trunk rotation	Creeping Kneeling Walking

ATNR, Asymmetrical tonic neck reflex; *STNR,* symmetrical tonic neck reflex; *TLR,* tonic labyrinthine reflex.

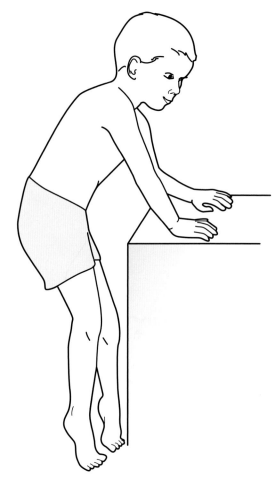

Fig. 6.10 Tiptoe standing.

lower extremity muscle tone in extensor muscle groups and may also interfere when the child tries to pull to stand and to cruise around furniture. The child may attain a standing position only on tiptoes and with legs crossed (Fig. 6.10). Cruising may be hindered by a lack of lower extremity separation in a lateral direction. Walking is also limited by an absence of separation of the legs in the sagittal plane. Adequate trunk control may be lacking to provide a stable base for the stance leg, and inadequate force production may prevent controlled movement of the swing leg. Because of absent trunk rotation, arm movements are often used to initiate weight shifts in the lower extremities or to substitute for a lack of lower extremity movement. The arms may remain in a high-guard position to reinforce weak trunk muscles by sustaining an extended posture, and thus delay the onset of arm swing.

Extremity Usage

Reaching in any position may be limited by an inability to bear weight on an extremity or to shift weight onto an extremity and produce the appropriate balance response. Weight-bearing on the upper extremities is necessary for propped sitting and for protective extension when other balance responses fail. Lower extremity weight-bearing is crucial to independent ambulation.

The child with spastic CP is at risk of contractures and deformities secondary to muscle and joint stiffness, and to muscle imbalances from poor selective motor control. Spasticity may be present only in extremity muscles, whereas the trunk may demonstrate low muscle tone. In an effort to overcome gravity, the child may try to use the abdominal muscles to attain sitting from a supine position. Excessive exertion can increase overall tone and can result in lower extremity extension and possible scissoring (hip adduction) of the legs.

The Child With Athetosis or Ataxia

The most severe impairments and activity limitations in children with athetosis or ataxia are related to the lack of postural stability. These are listed in Table 6.6. The inability to maintain a posture is evident in the lack of consistent head and trunk control. The child exhibits large, uncompensated movements around the long axis of the body or extremities. In contrast to children with spasticity who lack movement, children with athetosis or ataxia lack postural stability. Because of this instability, the child with athetosis or ataxia may use abnormal movements, such as an asymmetric tonic neck posture, to provide additional stability for functional movements, such as using a pointer or pushing a joystick. Overuse of this posture can predispose the child with CP to scoliosis or hip subluxation.

PHYSICAL THERAPY INTERVENTION

Children with CP demonstrate impairments, functional limitations, and movement dysfunction throughout their lifetime. Four stages of care are used to describe the continuum of physical therapy management of the child with CP from

TABLE 6.6 Impairments, Activity Limitations, Participation Restrictions, and Focus of Treatment in Children With Athetoid Cerebral Palsy

Impairments in Body Structure/Function	Activity Limitation	Participation Restriction	Focus of Treatment
Movement • Muscle tone • Muscle strength	Sitting, standing, and walking	Playing with peers	Educate parents on cerebral palsy Increase participation in all activities
Poor selective motor control • Lack of stability	Eating, drinking, and dressing	Increased time to carry out activities of daily living	Teach/coach adaptations of task or environment
• Lack of cocontraction	Unstable walking	Attending school Timed activities	Teach/coach limits of stability
• Poor coordination	Handwriting	School assignments	Occupational therapy
Postural control • Lack of graded response	Balance instability Slow to respond if perturbed in all postures	Playing a sport Finding a job/working	Increase midline holding in postures or use weight-bearing to provide stability

From Glanzman A: Cerebral palsy. In Goodman C, Fuller KS, editors: *Pathology: implications for the physical therapist*, St. Louis, 2015, Saunders, p. 1524.

infancy to adulthood. Physical therapy goals and treatment are presented within the framework of these four stages: early intervention, preschool, school-age and adolescence, and adulthood.

Because the brain damage occurs in a developing motor system, the primary emphasis of physical therapy intervention is to foster motor development and to learn functional motor skills. When a child learns to move for the first time, the infant's own movements provide sensory feedback for the learning process to occur. If the feedback is incorrect or is incorrectly perceived, the movement may be learned incorrectly. Children with CP tend to develop stereotypical patterns of movement because they have difficulty in controlling movement against gravity. These stereotypical patterns interfere with developing functional motor skills. Inaccurate motor learning appears to occur in CP. The child (1) moves incorrectly; (2) learns to move incorrectly; and (3) continues to move incorrectly, thereby setting up a cycle for more and more abnormal movement. By assisting the child to experience more functional movement, the clinician promotes functional movement and allows the child more independence within his or her environment.

The acquisition of motor milestones and of subsequent skills has to be viewed as the promotion of the child's highest possible independent level of function. Although the developmental sequence can act as a guide for formulating treatment goals and as a source of treatment activities, it should not be adhered to exclusively. Just because one skill comes before another in the typical developmental sequence does not mean that it is a prerequisite for the next skill. A good example of this concept is demonstrated by looking at the skill of creeping. Creeping is not a necessary prerequisite for walking. In fact, learning to creep may be more difficult for the child because creeping requires weight shifting and coordination of all four extremities. Little is to be gained by blindly following the developmental sequence. In fact, doing so may make it more difficult for the child to progress to upright standing.

The physical therapist is responsible for formulating and directing the plan of care. The physical therapist assistant implements interventions designed to assist the child to achieve the goals as outlined in the plan of care. Therapeutic interventions may include positioning, developmental activities, and practicing postural control within cognitively and socially appropriate functional tasks. The physical therapist assistant can foster motor development through play and use play to expand the child's ability to self-generate perceptual motor experiences. The physical therapist assistant can model and coach positive social interactions for the caregiver and provide family education.

General Treatment Ideas

Child With Spastic Cerebral Palsy

Treatment for the child with spastic CP focuses on mobility in all possible postures and transitions between these postures. The tendency to develop contractures needs to be counteracted by range of motion, positioning, and development of active movement. Areas that are prone to tightness may include shoulder adductors and elbow, wrist, and finger flexors in children with quadriplegic involvement, whereas hip flexors and adductors, knee flexors, and ankle plantar flexors are more likely to be involved in children with diplegic involvement. Children with quadriplegia can show lower extremity tightness as well. These same joints may be involved unilaterally in hemiplegia. Useful techniques to encourage movement and decrease tone include weight-bearing; weight shifting; slow, rhythmic rocking; and rhythmic rotation of the trunk and body segments. Active trunk rotation, dissociation of body segments, and isolated joint movements should be included in the treatment activities and home program. Appropriate positioning for function and use of manual guidance can increase the likelihood that the child will receive more accurate sensory feedback for motor learning. However, the child must actively participate in movement and explore ways to accomplish various motor skills independently.

Advantages and disadvantages of different positions. The influence of tonic reflexes on functional movement is presented in the earlier section of this chapter. The advantages of using different positions in treatment are now discussed. Both advantages and disadvantages can be found in the previous chapter in Table 5.1. The reader is also referred to Chapter 5 for descriptions of facilitating movement transitions between positions.

Supine. Early weight-bearing can be performed when the child is supine, with the knees bent and the feet flat on the support surface. To counteract the total extension influence of the TLR, the child's body can be flexed by placing the upper trunk on a wedge and the legs over a bolster. Flexion of the head and upper trunk can decrease the effect of the supine TLR. Dangling or presenting objects at the child's eye level can facilitate the use of the arms for play or object exploration.

Side lying. This position is best to dampen the effect of most of the tonic reflexes because of the neutral position of the head. Be careful not to allow lateral flexion with too thick a support under the head. It is also relatively easy to achieve protraction of the shoulders and pelvis, as well as trunk rotation, in preparation for rolling and coming to sit. The side the child is lying on is weight-bearing and should be elongated. This maneuver can be done passively before the child is placed into the side-lying position (Intervention 5.8), or it may occur as a result of a lateral weight shift as the child's position is changed.

Prone. The prone position promotes weight-bearing through the upper extremities, as well as providing some stretch to the hip and knee flexors. Head and trunk control can be facilitated by the development of active extension as well as promoting eye-head relationships. Movement while the child is prone, prone on elbows, or prone on extended arms can promote upper extremity loading and weight shift.

Sitting. Almost no better functional position exists than sitting. Weight-bearing can be accomplished through the extremities while active head and trunk control is promoted. An extended trunk is dissociated from flexed lower extremities. Righting and equilibrium reactions can be facilitated from this position. ADLs such as feeding, dressing, bathing, and movement transitions can all be encouraged while the child is sitting.

Quadruped. The main advantage of the four-point or quadruped position is that the extremities are all weight-bearing, and the trunk must work directly against gravity. The position provides a great opportunity for dissociated movements of limbs from the trunk and the upper trunk from the lower trunk. Movement in and out of quadruped to sitting or from quadruped to kneeling encourages exploration of the environment and develops dynamic postural control.

Kneeling. As a dissociated posture, kneeling affords the child the opportunity to practice keeping the trunk and hips extended while flexed at the knees. The hip flexors can be stretched, and balance responses can be practiced without having to control all lower extremity joints. Playing in kneeling is developmentally appropriate, and with support, the child can also practice moving into half-kneeling. Half-kneeling may be difficult if the child has difficulty moving one leg separately.

Standing. The advantages of standing are obvious from a musculoskeletal standpoint. Weight-bearing through the lower extremities is of great importance for long bone growth. Weight-bearing can produce a prolonged stretch on heel cords and knee flexors while promoting active head and trunk control. Upright standing also provides appropriate visual input for social interaction with peers. Standing programs are an integral part of maintaining good hip health in children with CP, especially in children at GMFCS levels IV to V. See the following for positioning guidelines: http://www.childdevelopment.ca/Libraries/Hip_Health/sunnyhill_clinical_tool_Hip_Health_Full_FINAL.sflb.ashx (accessed March 19, 2019). Hip surveillance should be part of every child's medical management regardless of GMFCS level. The latest clinical care pathway from American Academy of Cerebral Palsy and Developmental Medicine is available at https://www.aacpdm.org/publications/care-pathways/hip-surveillance (accessed March 19, 2019).

Child With Athetosis or Ataxia

Treatment for the child with athetosis focuses on stability in weight-bearing and the use of developmental postures that provide trunk or extremity support. Useful techniques include approximation, weight-bearing, and moving within small ranges of motion with resistance as tolerated. The assistant can use sensory cues that provide the child with information about joint and postural alignment, such as mirrors, weight vests, and heavier toys that provide some resistance but do not inhibit movement. Grading movement within the midrange, where instability is typically the greatest, is the most difficult for the child. Activities that may be beneficial include playing "statues," holding ballet positions, and holding any other fixed posture, such as stork standing. Use of hand support in sitting, kneeling, and standing can improve the child's stability. Visually fixing on a target may also be helpful. As the child grows older, the assistant should help the child to develop safe movement strategies during customary ADLs. If possible, the child should be actively involved in discovering ways to overcome his or her own particular obstacles.

Valued Life Outcomes

Giangreco et al. (2011) identified five life outcomes that should be highly valued for all children, even those with severe disabilities:

1. Being safe and healthy both physically and emotionally.
2. Having a safe, stable home in which to live now and in the future.
3. Having meaningful personal relationships.
4. Having control and choice based on age and culture.
5. Engaging in meaningful activities in a variety of places within a community.

These outcomes can be used to guide goal setting for children with disabilities across the lifespan. Giangreco et al. (2011) continue to support linking educational curriculum to individually determined life outcomes. They provide a guide to education planning that is collaborative and family-centered for young children, and life outcome–based for the school-aged child. School-based interventions must be focused on education needs of the child (Effgen, 2013). However, physical fitness interventions can be implemented through sports programs or community exercise programs (Wright and Palisano, 2017). By having a vision of what life should be like for these children, we can be more future-oriented in planning and giving support to these children and their families. This approach is certainly in keeping with the International Classification of Functioning, Disability, and Health focus on activities and participation of children with disabilities.

First Stage of Physical Therapy Intervention: Early Intervention (Birth to 3 Years)

Theoretically, early therapy can have a positive impact on nervous system development and recovery from injury. The ability of the nervous system to be flexible in its response to injury and development is termed *plasticity*. Infants diagnosed with CP or at risk for CP are candidates for early physical therapy intervention to take advantage of the nervous system's plasticity.

The decision to initiate physical therapy intervention and at what level (frequency and duration) is based on the infant's neuromotor performance during the physical therapy examination and the family's concerns. Several assessment tools designed by physical therapists are used in the clinic to identify infants with CP as early as possible. Pediatric physical therapists need to update their knowledge of such tools continually. As previously stated, a discussion of these tools is beyond the scope of this text because physical therapist assistants do not evaluate children's motor status. However, a list of tools used by pediatric physical therapists can be found at the Academy of Pediatric Physical Therapy website (www.pediatricapta.org). Typical problems often identified during a physical therapy examination at this time include lack of head control, inability to track visually, dislike of the prone position, fussiness, asymmetric postures, primitive reflexes, tonal abnormalities, and feeding or breathing difficulty.

Early intervention usually spans the first 3 years of life. During this time, typically developing infants are establishing trust in their caregivers and are learning how to move about safely within their environment. Parents develop a sense of competence by supporting their infant's development and guiding them in safe exploration of the world. Having a child with a disability is stressful for a family. The goal of early intervention is to improve the child's function and participation within the context of the family. Parents and families collaborate to identify activities that the child enjoys but has difficulty doing. By educating the family about the child's strengths and challenges, the therapy team can empower the family's success. By teaching the family ways to position, carry, feed, and dress the child, the therapist and the therapist assistant practice family-centered intervention. The therapy team must recognize the needs of the family in relation to the child (context-focused therapy), rather than focusing on the child's needs alone (child-focused therapy). Early intervention should strive to maximize the child's movement, cognition, and communication skills by adapting the environment, fostering self-initiated movement exploration, and task-specific practice (Morgan et al., 2013; Novak et al., 2017).

Federal funding to states provides for the screening and intervention from birth to 3 years of age of children who have or are at risk for having disabilities and their families. Periodic assessment by a pediatric physical therapist who comes into the home may be sufficient to monitor an infant's development and to provide parent education. Hospitals that provide intensive care for newborns often have follow-up clinics in which children are examined at regular intervals. Instruction in home management, including specific handling and positioning techniques, is done by the therapist assigned to that clinic. Infants are best served by receiving early intervention services in the home. Physical therapy provides activity-based interventions that are embedded into daily routines and designed to meet the goals of the family as outlined in an individualized family service plan. At 3 years of age, the child may likely transition into an early childhood program in a public school to continue to receive services.

Role of the Family

The family is an important component in the early management of the infant with CP. Family-centered care is best practice in pediatric physical therapy (Chiarello, 2013). Bamm and Rosenbaum (2008) reviewed the genesis, development, and implementation of family-centered care, which was introduced more than 40 years ago. The most frequently delineated concepts of family-centered care in child health literature are:

1. Recognizing the family as a constant in the child's life and the primary source of strength and support for the child.
2. Acknowledging the diversity and uniqueness of children and families.
3. Acknowledging that parents bring expertise.
4. Recognizing that family-centered care fosters competency.
5. Encouraging collaboration and partnership between families and health care providers.
6. Facilitating family-to-family support and networking (McKean et al., 2005).

Families and professionals prioritize important issues differently (Terwiel et al., 2017). The most diverse important ratings involved provision of general information. Families identify communication, availability, and accessibility as the most important issues in contrast to professionals who identify education, information, and counseling as most important. Bamm and Rosenbaum (2008) identified the four barriers and supports to implementing family-centered care. They are attitudinal, conceptual, financial, and political factors that can be viewed negatively or positively in affecting the implementation of family-centered care. Regardless of these factors, family-centered care is the preferred service delivery philosophy for physical therapy in any setting and can be utilized across the lifespan (Chiarello, 2013). In a recent meta-analysis, parents rated that family-centered care was provided to a "fairly great extent" (Almasri et al., 2018).

Role of the physical therapist assistant. The physical therapist assistant's role in providing ongoing therapy to infants is determined by the supervising physical therapist. The neonatal intensive care unit is not an appropriate practice setting for a physical therapist assistant or an inexperienced physical therapist because of the acuity and instability of very ill infants. Specific competencies must be met to practice safely within this specialized environment, and meeting these competencies usually requires additional coursework and supervised work experience. These competencies have been identified and are available from the Academy of Pediatrics of the American Physical Therapy Association.

The role of the physical therapist assistant in working with the child with CP is as a member of the health care team. The makeup of the team varies depending on the age of the child. During infancy, the team may be small and may consist only of the infant, parents, physician, and therapist. By the time the child is 3 years old, the rehabilitation team may have enlarged to include additional physicians involved in the child's medical management and other professionals such as an audiologist, an occupational therapist, a speech pathologist, a teacher, and a teacher's aide. The physical therapist assistant is expected to bring certain skills to the team and to the child, including knowledge of positioning and handling techniques, use of adaptive equipment, management of impaired tone, and developmental activities that foster motor abilities and movement transitions within a functional context. Because the physical therapist assistant may be providing services to the child in the home or at school, the assistant may be the first to observe additional problems or be told of a parental concern. These concerns should be communicated to the supervising therapist in a timely manner.

General goals of physical therapy in early intervention are to:
1. Promote infant-parent interaction.
2. Promote sensorimotor development.
3. Foster child-initiated movements and mobility.
4. Attain and maintain upright orientation.
5. Encourage development of functional skills and play.

Handling and Positioning

Handling and positioning can influence development (Lobo et al., 2013). Parents can be coached in positioning techniques that maximize function and promote symmetry. Handling and positioning in the supine or "en face" (face-to-face) posture should promote orientation of the head in the midline and symmetry of the extremities. A flexed position is preferred so the shoulders are forward, and the hands can easily come to the midline. Reaching is encouraged by making sure that objects are within the infant's grasp. The infant can be encouraged to initiate reaching when in the supine position by being presented with visually interesting toys. Positioning with the infant prone is also important because this is the position from which the infant first moves into extension. Active head lifting when in prone can be encouraged by using toys that are brightly colored or make noise. Some infants do not like being in prone, and the caregiver has to be encouraged to continue to put the infant in this position for longer periods. Carrying the infant in prone can increase the child's tolerance for the position.

The infant should not sleep in prone, however, because of the increased incidence of sudden infant death syndrome in infants who sleep in this position (American Academy of Pediatrics, 1992). Carrying positions should accentuate the strengths of the infant and should avoid as much abnormal posturing as possible. The infant should be allowed to control as much of her body as possible for as long as possible before external support is given. Fig. 6.11 shows a way to hold the child to increase tolerance to prone and to provide gentle movement; refer to Chapter 5 for other carrying positions.

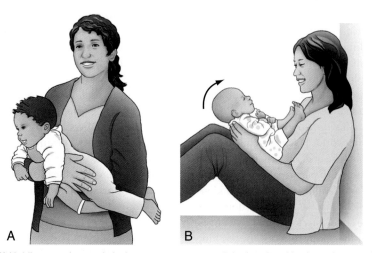

A   B

Fig. 6.11 (A,B) Holding, moving, and playing as a way to control the head and body against gravity. (Redrawn from Shepherd RB: *Cerebral palsy in infancy*, 2014, Elsevier, p. 247.)

Additionally, Fig. 6.11 depicts a way to engage a child in moving and playing.

Most handling and positioning techniques represent the use or modification of the developmental sequence to maximize function of the child with CP. Activity-based approaches should be used to enhance functional motor activity. Skill training should be task specific. Constraint-induced movement therapy (CIMT) for children with hemiplegia has been shown to be efficacious. Neuromotor development occurs at the same time at which the child's musculoskeletal and cognitive systems are maturing. Motor learning must take place if any permanent change in motor behavior is to occur. Affording the infant opportunities to self-generate sensorimotor experiences is an excellent way to promote motor exploration and social play. Practice in the natural environment provides the best carryover. Remember that movement variability is the hallmark of an adaptable neuromuscular system, so trial and error learning is to be encouraged. However, there may be times when the infant's movements need to be guided to maximize sensory input or feedback, but that does not mean practicing only one "correct" movement pattern (Dusing and Harbourne, 2010).

Feeding and Respiration

A flexed posture facilitates feeding and social interaction between the child and the caregiver. The more upright the child is, the easier it is to promote a flexed posture of the head and neck. Although it is not appropriate for a physical therapist assistant to provide oral motor therapy for an infant with severe feeding difficulties, the physical therapist assistant could assist in positioning the infant during a therapist-directed feeding session. One example of a position for feeding is shown in Intervention 6.1A. The face-to-face position can be used for a child who needs trunk support. Be careful that the roll does not slip behind the child's neck and encourage extension. Other examples of proper body positioning for improved oral motor and respiratory functioning during mealtime are depicted in Intervention 6.1B. Deeper respirations can also be

---

INTERVENTION 6.1 Positioning for Feeding

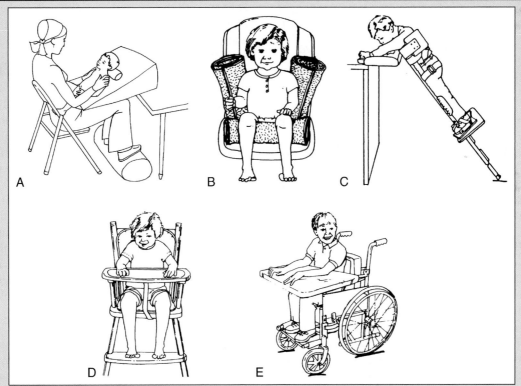

A. The face-to-face position can be used for a child who needs trunk support. Be careful that the roll does not slip behind the child's neck and encourage extension.

B. A young child is positioned for feeding in a car seat with adaptations using towel rolls.

C. A young child positioned on a prone stander is standing for mealtime.

D. A child is positioned in a high chair with adaptations for greater hip stability and symmetry during feeding.

E. A child is positioned in his wheelchair with an adapted seat insert, a tray, and hip stabilizing straps for mealtime.

(A, Reprinted by permission of the publisher from Connor FP, Williamson GG, Siepp JM, editors: *Program guide for infants and toddlers with neuromotor and other developmental disabilities*, New York, 1978, Teachers College Press, p. 201. ©1978 Teachers College, Columbia University. All rights reserved; B to E, From Connolly BH, Montgomery PC: *Therapeutic exercise in developmental disabilities*, ed 2, Thorofare, NJ, 2001, Slack.)

INTERVENTION 6.2 Facilitating Deeper Inspiration

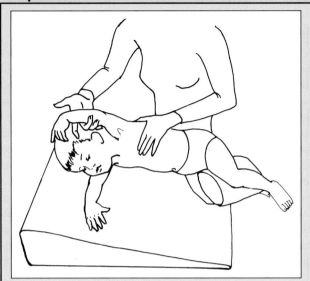

In side lying, slight pressure is applied to the lateral thorax to facilitate deeper inspiration.

(Reprinted by permission of the publisher from Connor FP, Williamson GG, Siepp JM, editors: *Program guide for infants and toddlers with neuromotor and other developmental disabilities,* New York, 1978, Teachers College Press, p. 199. Teachers College, Columbia University. All rights reserved.)

encouraged prior to feeding or at other times by applying slight pressure to the child's thorax and abdominal area prior to inspiration. This maneuver can be done when the child is in the side-lying position, as shown in Intervention 6.2, or with bilateral hand placements when the child is supine. The tilt of the wedge makes it easier for the child to use the diaphragm for deeper inspiration, as well as expanding the chest wall.

Movement Practice

Gentle range-of-motion exercises may be indicated if the infant has difficulty reaching to the midline, has difficulty separating the lower extremities for diapering, or has tight heel cords. Infants do not have complete range of motion in the lower extremities normally, so the hips should never be forced into what would be considered full range of adduction or extension for an adult. Parents can be taught to incorporate range of motion into the daily routines of diapering, bathing, and dressing. The infant needs to see and touch hands and feet and play in the midline. Environmental adaptation may be needed for more motorically involved children in the form of positioning to foster movement. Toys may need to be adapted for easier object play.

Motor Skill Acquisition

The skills needed for age-appropriate play vary. Babies look around and reach first from the supine position and then from the prone position before they start moving through the environment. Adequate time playing on the floor is needed to encourage movement of the body against gravity. Gravity must be conquered to attain upright sitting and standing postures. Body movement during play is crucial to body awareness. Movement within and through the environment is necessary for spatial orientation to the external world. Although floor time is important and is critical for learning to move against gravity, time spent in supine and prone positions must be balanced with the benefits of being in an upright orientation. All children need to be held upright, on the parent's lap, and over the shoulder to experience as many different postures as are feasible. Refer to Chapter 5 for specific techniques that may be used to encourage head and trunk control, upper extremity usage, and transitional movements.

Constraint-Induced Movement Therapy

Young children with CP from 18 months to 3 years who have unilateral upper extremity involvement are good candidates for CIMT. A short arm cast is applied to the noninvolved arm to prevent the child with hemiplegia from using the unaffected extremity, which forces use of the affected arm. Children from ages 3 to 6 may also be treated in the clinic or at home with this intervention, although as the child transitions to school, it may be harder to ensure the child's cooperation. CIMT is one of the most researched interventions used for children with hemiplegic CP (Case-Smith, 2014; Charles et al., 2006; DeLuca et al., 2012). A full description of the intervention is beyond the scope of this text. Physical therapy and occupational therapy are typically part of the protocols with the focus on intensive repetition for motor learning. Results have been very positive, with improvements in arm function (DeLuca et al., 2003; Eliasson et al., 2005) and gait (Coker et al., 2010). A recent systematic review found no difference in effect size of either CIMT or intense bimanual training in the short or long term (Tervahauta et al., 2017). The authors suggested that the family and child's motivation and expertise of the clinician be considered when deciding on either intervention protocol. Both CIMT and bimanual intensive training are effective interventions to improve hand function and decrease disregard of the involved hand and arm in children with hemiplegic CP.

Postural Control and Balance

The two most functional positions for a person are sitting and standing because upright orientation can be achieved with either position. Some children with CP cannot become functional in standing because of the severity of their motor involvement, but almost every child has the potential to be upright in sitting. Function in sitting can be augmented by appropriate seating devices, inserts, and supports. For example, the child with spastic diplegia, as in Fig. 6.12, has difficulty sitting on the floor and playing because of hamstring stiffness, which prevents her from flexing her hips. By having the child sit on a stool with feet on the floor, as in Fig. 6.12, *B,* the child exhibits better arm use in play and a more upright sitting posture. In Fig. 6.12, *C,* having the child sit on a low stool allows her to practice moving her body away from the

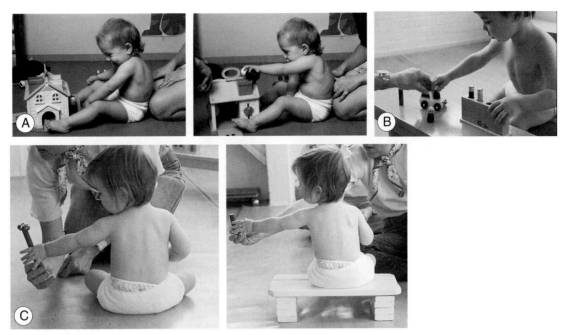

Fig. 6.12. Function in sitting. **(A)** An infant with diplegia has difficulty playing because tight hamstrings prevent adequate hip flexion for sitting squarely on the floor. **(B)** A child is able to play while sitting on a stool with feet on the floor. **(C)** A wide abducted floor sitting posture prevents lateral movement away from the midline, limiting her reach. Sitting on a stool with her feet on the floor enables her to balance as she shifts her body laterally. (From Shepherd RB: *Cerebral palsy in infancy*, 2014, Elsevier, p. 249.)

midline to reach for a toy. This movement was blocked while sitting on the floor by her wide abducted sitting posture.

When motor control is insufficient to allow independent standing, a standing program can be implemented. Upright standing can be achieved by using a supine or prone stander, along with orthoses for distal control. Standers provide lower extremity weight-bearing while they support the child's trunk. The child is free to work on head control in a prone stander and to bear weight on the upper extremities or engage in play. In a supine stander, the child's head is supported while the hands are free for reaching and manipulation. The trunk and legs should be in correct anatomic alignment. Standing programs were typically begun when the child is around 12 to 16 months of age. Standing for at least 60 minutes, four or five times per week is a general guideline with supported standing begun as early at 9 to 10 months (Paleg et al., 2013). The goals are to improve bone density and hip development and to manage contractures. Paleg et al. (2013) recommend 60 to 90 minutes per day for 5 days to positively affect bone mineral density. For hip health, 60 minutes a day with the lower extremities in 30 to 60 degrees of bilateral hip abduction while in a supported stander is recommended. Forty-five to sixty minutes is recommended to affect range of motion of the lower extremity and to affect spasticity.

Independent Mobility

Mobility can be achieved in many ways. Rolling is a form of independent mobility but may not be practical, except in certain surroundings. Sitting and hitching (bottom scooting with or without extremity assistance) are other means of mobility and may be appropriate for a younger child. Creeping on hands and knees can be functional, but upright ambulation is still seen as the most acceptable way for a child to get around because it provides the customary and expected orientation to the world. The use of body-weight support devices has increased as part of gait training of children with CP.

Some early interventions that may be useful for the infant with CP have been suggested by Shepherd (2014). She stresses ways that a typical infant uses her legs during infancy such as when kicking, moving the body up and down on fixed feet as in a squat or crouch, moving from sit to stand to sit, and stepping up and down and walking. Intervention 6.3 is crouching to standing or squatting and crouching. Intervention 6.4 is moving from sit to stand and stand to sit. Weight-bearing through the feet from an early age can assist in keeping the gastrocnemius and soleus muscles lengthened as they tend to stiffen over time and develop a contracture that might require surgery. Intervention 6.5 is stepping up and down. These interventions can be continued throughout this stage of physical therapy management.

Ambulation Predictors

Independent ambulation in children classified at GMFCS levels II and III was predicted by the child's ability to transfer to and from sitting and standing (Begnoche et al., 2016). This task requires dynamic postural control and functional strength. Children with CP at GMFCS level II are expected to walk by 4 to 6 years of age without any assistive device, and those at GMFCS level III are expected to walk by 4 to 6 years with an assistive device. Previous indicators of ambulation potential before the GMFCS or the motor development curves were developed (Hanna et al., 2009) included sitting independently

INTERVENTION 6.3 Squatting and Crouching

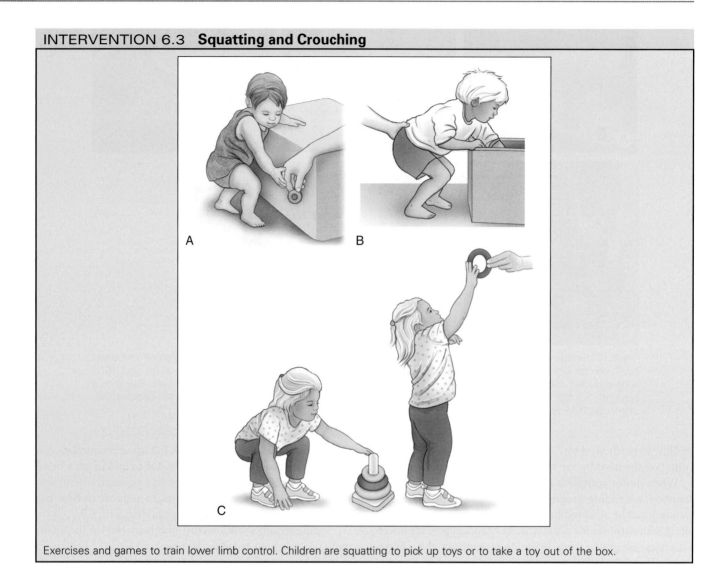

Exercises and games to train lower limb control. Children are squatting to pick up toys or to take a toy out of the box.

before the age of 2 years (Campos de Paz et al., 1994) and pulling to stand at 2 years (Wu et al., 2004). Children with spastic quadriplegia show the largest variability in their potential to walk. Children who display independent sitting or the ability to scoot along the floor on the buttocks by the age of 2 years have a good chance of ambulating (Watt et al., 1989).

A child with CP may achieve independent ambulation with or without an assistive device. Children with spastic hemiplegia or unilateral CP are more likely to ambulate at the high end of the age range for typically developing children to walk, which is 18 months. Other investigators have reported that if ambulation is possible for a child with any level of involvement, it usually takes place by the time the child is age 8 years (Glanzman, 2015).

Most children do not require extra encouragement to attempt ambulation, but they do need assistance and practice in bearing weight equally on their lower extremities, in initiating reciprocal limb movement, and in balancing. Postural reactions involving the trunk are usually delayed, as are extremity protective responses. Impairments in transitional

movements from sitting to standing can impede independence. In children with hemiplegic CP, movements initiated with the involved side of the body may be avoided, with all the work of standing and walking actually accomplished by the uninvolved side. Practicing postural control in standing with reduced hand support could be beneficial in producing more mature balance reactions. "Reduced hand support is a potential indicator of readiness to take steps independently" (Begnoche et al., 2016). The way a child with CP moves is dependent on age, GMFCS level, and environment in which ambulation takes place (home, school, or outdoors).

Body Weight–Supported Treadmill Training

Use of body weight–supported treadmill training has become an acceptable rehabilitation strategy for improving the walking performance of children with CP. A harness can be used to support an infant as she learns to walk, to keep the child safe for walking practice, as seen in Fig. 6.13, or while engaged in another activity. Data on using a harness apparatus to partially support a child's body weight while training ambulation on a treadmill has shown that children at GMFCS

INTERVENTION 6.4   Sitting to Stand and Stand to Sit

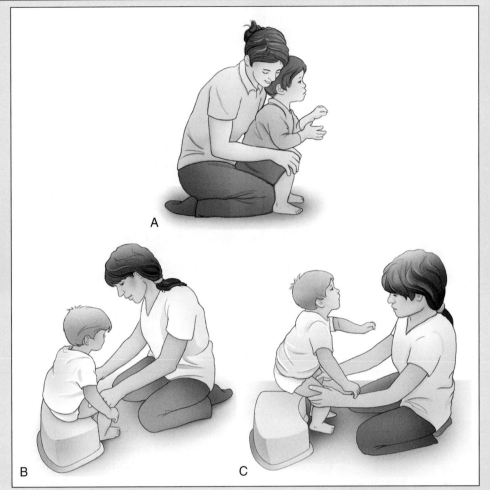

Sit-stand-sit exercise. **(A)** The therapist steadies the infant as he does not yet have the ability to balance throughout the action. **(B)** The therapist moves the infant's knee (and body mass) forward to show him what he must do. **(C)** This little boy needs assistance to initiate knee flexion for sitting.

levels III and IV significantly increased gross motor performance and walking speed (Willoughby et al., 2009). Early task-specific practice is beneficial for acquiring the ability to ambulate. Richards et al. (1997) studied the use of such a system in four children with CP and concluded that it would be possible to train children as young as 19 months of age. In a study of older children, there were positive changes in motor test scores and in the ability to transfer some children (Schindl et al., 2000). A 12-week program performed 2 days a week resulted in improved walking performance in children with CP (Kurz et al., 2011). The changes in stepping kinematics were strongly correlated with changes in step length, walking speed, and Gross Motor Function Measure score. Additional studies have shown that body weight–supported treadmill training improves gait in children with CP functioning at GMFCS levels III, IV, and V (Cherng et al., 2007; Dodd and Foley, 2007; Mattern-Baxter et al., 2009). The latest systematic review of treadmill interventions found that it

may accelerate attainment of motor skills in children with CP (Valentín-Guidol et al., 2017).

The research is equivocal when comparing the effect of treadmill training and overground walking. Willoughby et al. (2010) found no difference between the two groups in walking speed or in walking in the school environment. However, Grecco et al. (2013) found that their treadmill training group demonstrated greater improvement than the overground walking group. The difference was significant after treatment and on follow-up. It should be noted that in the study by Willoughby et al. (2010) partial weight support was used while on the treadmill and the participants were GMFCS levels III or IV, whereas in the study by Grecco et al. (2013) the treadmill was used without partial weight support and the participants were GMFCS levels I to III. Use of a treadmill with or without partial body weight support needs to continue to be researched to develop appropriate protocols for children at different GMFCS levels.

INTERVENTION 6.5   Stepping Up and Down

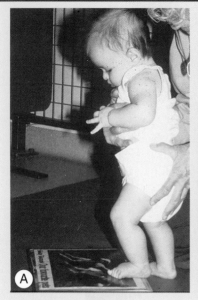 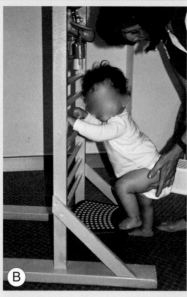 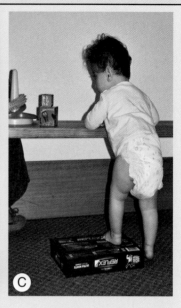

(A) and **(B)** With manual contacts at the pelvis, encourage the infant to place a foot on a small flat object and bring weight forward; repeat with the other leg. Child may support herself on rails or a table while stepping. Gradually increase the height of the object to increase activation of the leg muscles. Assist the infant in stepping forward and up but do not take all of the infant's weight. **(C)** Practice stepping sideways as in cruising. Place an object to either side and encourage stepping up laterally.

(From Shepherd RB: *Physiotherapy in Paediatrics*, ed 3, Oxford, 1995, Butterworth-Heinemann.)

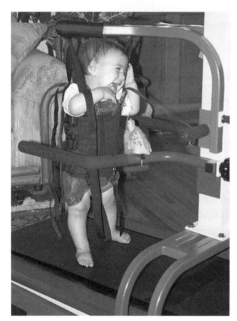

Fig. 6.13. Body-weight support treadmill use. (Treadmill with harness, used with permission from LiteGait, Mobility Research, Tempe, AZ; From Shepherd RB: *Cerebral palsy in infancy*, 2014, Elsevier, p. 7.)

Power Mobility

Mobility within the environment is too important for the development of spatial concepts to be delayed until the child can move independently. Power mobility should be considered a viable option even for a young child. As young as 17 to 20 months, some children with disabilities have learned to maneuver a motorized wheelchair (Butler, 1986, 1991). Just because a child is taught to use power mobility does not preclude working concurrently on independent ambulation. This point needs to be stressed to the family. Early use of power mobility has been shown to have positive effects on young children who are unable to move independently (Guerette et al., 2013). Refer to the first international consensus on power mobility recently published by Livingstone and Paleg (2014). Clinical practice suggestions are made for using power mobility in children with different abilities, needs, and ages. Children with CP who are not mobile but have the cognitive skills of a 12-month-old should be evaluated for power mobility. The mismatch of motor and cognition has the potential to produce negative developmental outcomes (Shepherd, 2014). Other mobility alternatives include devices such as prone scooters, adapted tricycles, battery-powered riding toys, and manual wheelchairs. The independence of moving on one's own teaches young children that they can control the environment around them, rather than being controlled.

Second Stage of Physical Therapy Intervention: Preschool Period

The major emphasis during the preschool period is to promote mobility and functional independence in the child with CP. Depending on the distribution and degree of involvement, the child with CP may or may not have achieved an upright orientation to gravity in sitting or standing during the first 3 years of life. By the preschool period, most children's social sphere has broadened to include daycare attendants, babysitters, preschool personnel, and playmates, so mobility is not merely important for self-control and object interaction; it is a social necessity. All aspects of the child's being—mental, motor, and social-emotional—are developing concurrently during the preschool period in an effort to achieve functional independence.

Physical therapy goals during the preschool period are:
1. Establish or maintain a means of independent mobility.
2. Increase physical activity, functional movement, and ADLs.
3. Promote social interaction and play with peers.
4. Promote communication and learning.

The physical therapist assistant is more likely to work with a preschool-age child than with a child in an early intervention program. Within a preschool setting, the physical therapist assistant implements certain aspects of the treatment plan formulated by the physical therapist. Activities may include promoting postural reactions to improve head and trunk control, teaching transitions such as moving from sitting to standing, positioning to maintain adequate muscle length for function, strengthening and endurance exercises for promoting function and health, and practice of self-care skills as part of the child's daily home or classroom schedule.

Independent Mobility

If the child with CP did not achieve upright orientation and mobility in some form during the early intervention period, now is the time to make a concerted effort to assist the child to do so. For children who are ambulatory with or without assistive devices and orthoses, it may be a period of monitoring and reexamining the continued need for either the assistive or orthotic device. Some children who may not have previously required any type of assistance may benefit from one now because of their changing musculoskeletal status, body weight, seizure status, or safety concerns. Their previous degree of selective motor control may have been sufficient for a small body, but with growth, control may be diminished. Any time the physical therapist assistant observes that a child is having difficulty with a task previously performed without problems, the supervising therapist should be alerted. Although the physical therapist performs periodic reexaminations, the physical therapist assistant working with the child should request a reexamination any time negative changes in the child's motor performance occur. Positive changes should, of course, be thoroughly documented and reported because these too may necessitate updating the plan of care.

Postural Control

Five interventions have been shown to be moderately effective in improving postural control in children with CP (Dewar et al., 2015). Hippotherapy provides sensory and motor information to the child's postural system. Two 1 hour sessions a week for 8 weeks totaling 16 hours was found to improve sitting balance (Kang et al., 2012). Children with less severe involvement are more likely to show improvement than those with more severe involvement (Zadnikar and Kastrin, 2011; Tseng et al., 2013). Trunk targeted strength training on a vibrating platform, treadmill training, gross motor task training, and reactive balance training all were moderately effective. The speed of the treadmill had to be gradually increased to be effective. The gross motor tasks that were trained needed to be task specific and practiced for at least 10 hours to be effective, and the reactive balance training required at least 2 hours to be effective. All of the studies in the Dewar et al. (2015) systematic review involved children with CP (GMFCS I-III) who were ambulatory.

Gait. Walking ability in children with CP is related to muscle strength. Eek and Beckung (2008) found a significant correlation between muscle strength and walking ability as determined by the GMFCS. Children 5 to 15 years of age at GMFCS levels I to III were able to isolate muscle actions for muscle testing with a handheld device. Children at GMFCS level IV were not. Studies of interventions to improve gait speeds in children with CP have found gait training to be the most effective (Moreau et al., 2016). They did not find strength training to be effective. The age of the children in the resistance studies were on average 10 years old. Hoffman et al. (2018) found a positive correlation between percent change in lower extremity strength and improved walking speed in children with CP (GMFCS II and III) ages 6 to 17 years. There was also a significant increase in endurance. The intervention consisted of 30 minutes of treadmill locomotion 3 times a week for 6 weeks. There was a negative correlation between strength and age, which might imply that younger children may benefit more from exercise than older children due to muscle plasticity. The authors suggest that strength changes may be a factor that drives improvements in walking speed.

Children at GMFCS level IV can walk if provided with support of the trunk and pelvis. Wheeled walking devices or gait trainers provide a way to enhance activity and participation. Paleg and Livingstone (2015) conducted a systematic review of the potential impact of using gait trainers at home and in school. Results were mainly descriptive with only one random clinical trial suggesting use of the gait trainer increased distance covered overground. Despite lack of evidence, these trainers provide the potential for greater interaction with others and the surrounding environment.

Specific gait difficulties seen in children with spastic diplegia include lack of lower extremity dissociation, decreased single-limb and increased double-limb support time, and limited postural reactions during weight shifting. Children with spastic diplegia have problems dissociating one leg from the other and dissociating leg movements from the trunk. They often fix (stabilize) with the hip adductors to substitute for the lack of trunk stability in upright necessary for initiation of lower limb motion. Practicing coming to stand over a bolster can provide a deterrent to lower extremity adduction while the child works on muscular strengthening and weight-bearing (Intervention 6.6A). If the child cannot support all the body's weight in standing or during a sit-to-stand transition, have part of the child's body weight on extended arms while the child practices coming to stand, standing, or shifting weight in standing (Intervention 6.6B).

INTERVENTION 6.6   Coming to Stand Over a Bolster

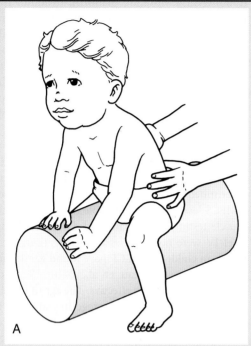
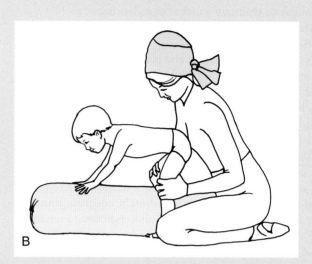

A

B

A. Practicing coming to stand over a bolster can provide a deterrent to lower extremity adduction and can work on lower extremity strengthening and weight-bearing.
B. If the child cannot support all the body's weight in standing or during a sit-to-stand transition, part of the child's body weight can be borne on extended arms while the child practices coming to stand, standing, or weight shifting in standing.

Practicing lateral trunk postural reactions may automatically result in lower extremity separation as the lower extremity opposite the weight shift is automatically abducted (Intervention 6.7). The addition of trunk rotation to the lateral righting may even produce external rotation of the opposite leg. Pushing a toy and shifting weight in step-stance are also useful activities to practice lower extremity separation. As the child decreases the time in double-limb support by taking a step of appropriate length, she can progress to stepping over an object or to stepping up and down off a step. Single-limb balance can be challenged by using a floor ladder or taller steps. Having the child hold on to vertical poles decreases the amount of support and facilitates upper trunk extension (Fig. 6.14). The walkable LiteGait (Mobility Research, Tempe, AZ) could be used to transition someone from treadmill walking to overground walking (Fig. 6.15). Many children can benefit from using an assistive device, such as a rolling reverse walker, during gait training (Fig. 6.16). Orthoses may also be needed to enhance ambulation.

Orthoses. The most frequently used orthosis in children with CP who are ambulatory is some type of ankle-foot orthosis (AFO). A solid AFO is a single piece of molded polypropylene. The orthosis extends 10 to 15 mm distal to the head of the fibula. The orthosis should not pinch the child behind the knee at any time. All AFOs and foot orthoses should support the foot and should try and maintain the subtalar joint in a neutral position. A study by Westberry et al. (2007) reported that static foot alignment was not able to be maintained while wearing prescribed AFO. In general, AFOs have been shown to improve stride length and speed (Aboutorabi et al., 2017). A review by Morris (2002) found that a solid AFO or a hinged AFO with a plantarflexion stop improved gait efficiency. Ground reaction AFOs, also called floor reaction AFOs (FRAFOs) (Fig. 6.17), can be used to improve knee extension, stride length, and walking speed (Rogozinski et al., 2009). Their use is indicated for children with a crouched gait pattern provided they do not have hip and knee flexion contractures greater than 15 degrees (Rogozinski et al., 2009; Aboutorabi et al., 2017). A recent article by Böhm et al. (2018) showed that contractures did not reduce the positive effects of an FRAFO on gait. However, the FRAFOs used in the Böhm study were constructed differently than those used in the Rogozinski study. Dynamic AFOs have a custom-contoured soleplate that provides forefoot and hindfoot alignment. The use of AFOs in children with spastic CP at GMFCS levels I to III controls the ankle and foot during both phases of gait and improves gait efficiency (Morris et al., 2011). The concept of tuning an AFO to provide more

INTERVENTION 6.7 Balance Reaction on a Bolster

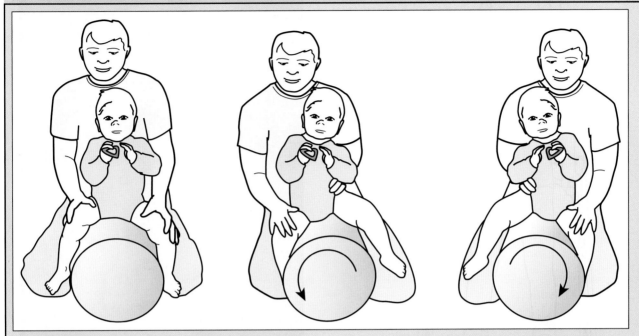

Practicing lateral trunk postural reactions may automatically result in lower extremity separation as the lower extremity opposite the weight shift is automatically abducted.

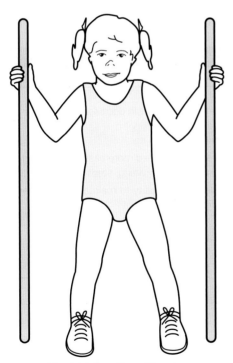

Fig. 6.14 Standing with poles.

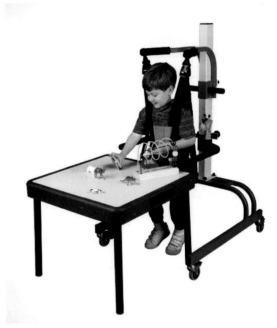

Fig. 6.15 Walkable LiteGait. (Used with permission from LiteGait, Mobility Research, Tempe, AZ; From Shepherd RB: *Cerebral palsy in infancy*, 2014, Elsevier, p. 7.)

individualized solutions to impaired movement is being explored (Owen, 2010).

An AFO may be indicated following surgery or casting to maintain musculotendinous length gains. The orthosis may be worn during both the day and at night. Proper precautions should always be taken to inspect the skin regularly for any

signs of skin breakdown or excessive pressure. The physical therapist should establish a wearing schedule for the child. Areas of redness lasting more than 20 minutes after brace removal should be reported to the supervising physical therapist.

A child with unstable ankles who needs medial lateral stability may benefit from a supramalleolar orthosis (SMO).

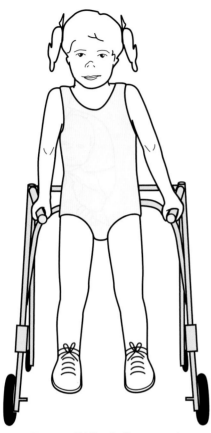

Fig. 6.16 Walker (rolling reverse).

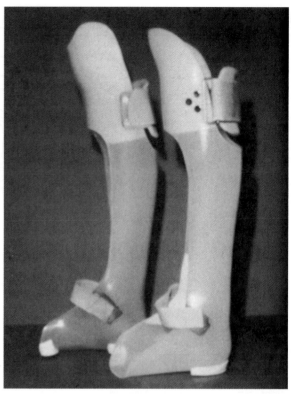

Fig. 6.17 Ground reaction ankle-foot orthoses. (From Campbell SK, editor: *Physical therapy for children*, ed 4, St. Louis, 2012, WB Saunders.)

TABLE 6.7   General Foot and Ankle Splinting Guidelines

Splints	Status	Application
Solid AFO neutral to + 3° DF	Nonambulators, beginning standers	1. Less than 3° of DF 2. Genu recurvatum associated with decreased ankle DF or weakness 3. Need for medial-lateral stability 4. Nighttime/positional stretching
AFO with 90° posterior stop and free DF (hinged AFO)	Clients with some, but limited, functional mobility	Application of 1-4 above, but need more passive DF during movement, such as ambulation, squatting, steps, and sit to stand
Floor reaction AFO (set DF depending on weight line in standing)	Crouch gait Full passive knee extension in standing	For clients with decreased ability to maintain knee extension during ambulation
SMO	Standers/ambulators with pronation at the ankles	1. Need medial-lateral ankle stability 2. Would like opportunity to use active plantar flexion 3. Decreased DF not a problem during gait

AFO, Ankle-foot orthosis; *DF*, dorsiflexion; *SMO*, supramalleolar orthosis.
From Glanzman A: Cerebral palsy. In Goodman CC, Fuller K, editors: *Pathology: implications for the physical therapist*, ed 3, St. Louis, 2015, Saunders, p. 1529.

This orthotic device allows the child to move freely into dorsiflexion and plantar flexion while restricting mediolateral movement. An SMO or a foot orthosis may be indicated for a child with mild hypertonia or foot pronation if the child does not need ankle stabilization. There is some evidence that children with better motor control, that is those with less severe involvement, may do better with less restrictive orthotic designs (Morris, 2002; Morris et al., 2011). In the child with hypotonia or athetoid CP, the SMO or foot orthosis may provide sufficient stability within a tennis shoe to allow ambulation. General guidelines for orthotic use can be found in Table 6.7. A good supportive shoe may also provide sufficient support while allowing variability of movement including use of an ankle strategy.

Assistive devices. Some assistive devices should be avoided in this population. For example, ring walkers that do not require the child to control the head and trunk as much as possible are passive and may be of little long-term benefit. When the use of a walker results in increased lower extremity extension and toe walking, a more appropriate means of encouraging ambulation should be sought such as a gait trainer. Exercise saucers can be as dangerous as walkers. Jumpers should be avoided in children with increased lower extremity muscle tone.

Power mobility. Power options are being explored earlier and earlier for children. Use of power mobility does not necessarily mean that the child does not have the potential to be an overground walker.

Children with more severe involvement, as in quadriplegia, do not have sufficient head or trunk control, let alone adequate upper extremity function, to ambulate independently even with an assistive device. For them, some form of power mobility, such as a wheelchair or other motorized device, may be a solution. For others, a more controlling apparatus such as a gait trainer may provide enough trunk support to allow training of the reciprocal lower extremity movements to propel the device (Fig. 6.18). M.O.V.E. (Mobility Opportunity Via Education, Bakersfield, CA) is a program developed by a special education teacher to foster independent mobility in children who experience difficulty with standing and walking, especially severely physically disabled children. Early work with equipment has been expanded to include a curriculum and an international organization that promotes mobility for all children. Much of the equipment is available at Rifton Equipment (Rifton, NY).

For children already using power mobility, studies have shown that the most consistent use of the wheelchair is at school. When parents and caregivers of children who use power mobility were interviewed, two overriding issues were of greatest concern: accessibility and independence. Although the wheelchair was viewed as a way to foster independence in an otherwise dependent child, most caregivers stated that they had some difficulty with accessibility, either in the home or in other local environments. To increase the benefit derived from a power wheelchair, the environment it is to be used in must be accessible, the needs of the caregiver must be considered, and the child must be adequately trained to develop skill in driving the wheelchair. Livingstone and Paleg (2014) note that power mobility is appropriate even for children who never become competent drivers.

Medical Management

This section presents the medical and surgical management of children with CP because it is during the preschool period that spasticity management is introduced to prevent secondary impairments, such as contractures and pain, to reduce the need for orthopedic surgery. Decreasing spasticity alone will not necessarily improve function (Wright et al., 2008). The presence of coexisting impairments in selective motor control, weakness, as well as environmental and child factors determine function.

Medications. The most common oral medications used to manage spasticity include the benzodiazepines, diazepam (Valium), clonazepam (Klonopin), alpha$_2$ agonists, tizanidine (Zanaflex), baclofen (Lioresal), and dantrolene (Dantrium) (Theroux and DiCindio, 2014). Oral medications trihexyphenidyl and levodopa have been used to treat dystonia (Nahm et al., 2018) but are not licensed for use in children. According to a systematic review, there is insufficient evidence to support use of oral antispasticity medications or botulinum toxin to decrease dystonia (Fehlings et al., 2018). The mechanism of action and potential adverse effects are found in Table 6.8. Sedation, fatigue, and generalized weakness can negatively impact the child's function. Increased drooling has been reported to interfere with feeding and speech (Batshaw et al., 2013). Usefulness of oral medications for spasticity can be limited owing to their various side effects. The use of a pump to deliver baclofen directly to the spinal cord has been promoted because it takes less medication to achieve a greater effect. The youngest age at which a

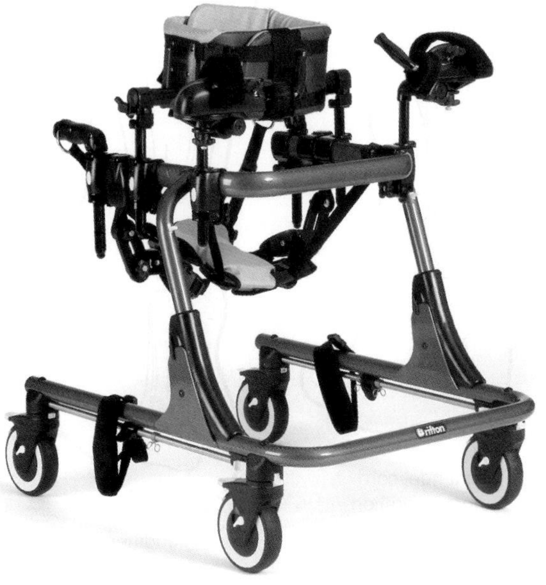

Fig. 6.18 Rifton gait trainer. (Courtesy Rifton Equipment, Rifton, NY.)

TABLE 6.8 Oral Medications for Spasticity

Medication	Mechanism of Action	Side Effects
Benzodiazepine (Valium), (Klonopin)	Inhibits release of excitatory neurotransmitters	Sedation, ataxia, physical dependence, impaired memory
Alpha-2 adrenergic agonist (Zanaflex)	Decreased release of excitatory neurotransmitters	Sedation, hypotension, nausea, vomiting, hepatitis
Dantrolene (Dantrium)	Inhibits release of calcium at sarcoplasmic reticulum	Weakness, nausea, vomiting, hepatitis
Baclofen	Inhibits release of excitatory neurotransmitters in the spinal cord	Sedation, ataxia, weakness, hypotension

Modified from Theroux MC, DiCindio S: Major surgical procedures in children with cerebral palsy, *Anesthesiology Clin* 32:63–81, 2014.

child would be considered for this approach is 3 years. It takes up to 6 months to see functional gains. The procedure is expensive, and the benefits are being studied. Because implantation of the pump is a neurosurgical procedure, further discussion is found under that heading.

Botulinum toxin. Traditionally, spasticity has also been treated in the adult population with injections of chemical agents, such as alcohol or phenol, to block nerve transmission to a spastic muscle. Botulinum bacteria produces a powerful toxin (BoNT-A) that can inhibit a spastic muscle. If a small amount is injected into a spastic muscle group, weakness and decline of spasticity can be achieved for up to 3 to 6 months. These effects can make it easier to position a child, to fit an orthosis, and to improve function. More than one muscle group can be injected. The lack of discomfort and ease of administration are definite advantages over motor point blocks using alcohol or phenol (Gormley, 2001). Use of botox is predicated on the theory that spasticity is the reason for lack of function in a muscle group. Research has found that BoNT-A causes atrophy and weakness of skeletal muscle as well as reducing muscle torque (Fortuna et al., 2011; Minamoto et al., 2015). If weakness is the culprit rather than spasticity, use of botox needs to be studied over the long-term to elucidate the risks and fully assess its benefits.

Surgical Management

Orthopedic surgery is an often inevitable occurrence in the life of a child with CP. Indications for surgery may be to (1) decrease pain, (2) correct or prevent deformity, and (3) improve function. The decision to undergo an operation should be a mutual one among the physician, the family, the child, and the medical, therapy, and educational teams. The therapist should modify the child's treatment plan according to the type of surgical procedure, postoperative casting, and the expected length of time of immobilization. A plan should be developed to address the child's seating and mobility needs, and to instruct everyone how to move and position the child safely at home and school.

Muscles in CP are weak, and do not keep up with skeletal growth. Muscles that cross two joints are especially prone to contracture development. Strategies that are used to prevent fixed deformities include night splints and casting. As children with CP grow range of motion decreases, and despite conscientious intervention contractures developed (Nordmark et al., 2009). Muscle shortening occurs even though the sarcomeres (functional unit of contraction) are lengthened.

Single-event multilevel surgery (SEML) has become the norm for children with CP. SEML is defined as "two or more soft-tissue or bony surgical procedures at two or more anatomical levels during one operative procedure, requiring only one hospital admission and one period of rehabilitation" (McGinley et al., 2012). Outcome of surgery for contractures is more predictable and rarely required before age 6 years (Graham et al., 2016). Surgical procedures to lengthen soft tissues may include Achilles tendon, hamstrings, or adductors. Children who undergo heel cord lengthening at 6 years of age or older do not have a recurrence of tightness (Rattey et al., 1993).

A child with tight heel cords who has not responded to traditional stretching or to plaster casting may require surgical treatment to achieve a flat (plantigrade) foot. Surgical lengthening of the heel cord is done to improve walking (Fig. 6.19). Davids et al. (2011) further stated that surgical lengthening should only be considered for the correction of fixed muscle contractures that did not respond to nonoperative treatments, such as manual stretching, serial casting, and strength training (Damiano et al., 1999). Torsional deformities of long bones are ideally performed between 6 and 12 years of age. The type of surgery should be tailored to the type of CP and be based on data from an instrumented gait analysis to assure evidence-based decision-making.

More complex orthopedic surgical procedures may be indicated in the presence of hip subluxation or dislocation. The risk of hip displacement is linearly related to GMFCS level (Hagglund et al., 2005; Soo et al., 2006). Of the one-third of children who are affected by hip displacement, 90% are at GMFCS level V. The hip may sublux secondary to muscle imbalances from hypertonia or hypotonia. Hip surveillance is necessary. Conservative treatment typically includes appropriate positioning to decrease the influence of the ATNR, passive stretching of tight muscle groups, and an abduction splint at night. If the hip becomes dislocated and produces pain and asymmetry, surgical treatment is indicated. The problem can be dealt with surgically in many ways, depending on its severity and acuity. The most minimal level of intervention involves soft tissue releases of the adductors, iliopsoas muscles, or proximal hamstrings. The next level requires an osteotomy of the femur in which the angle of the femur is changed by severing the bone, derotation of the femur, and internal fixation. By changing the angle, the head of

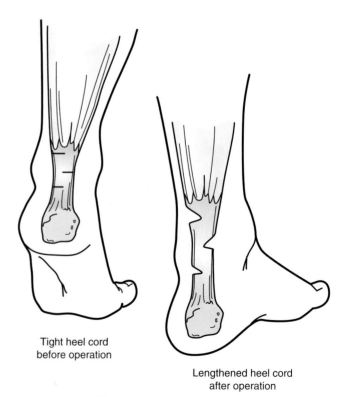

Tight heel cord
before operation

Lengthened heel cord
after operation

Fig. 6.19 Heel cord lengthening.

the femur is put back into the acetabulum. Sometimes, the acetabulum has to be reshaped in addition to the osteotomy. A hip replacement or arthrodesis can be an option. Bony surgical procedures are much more complex and require more lengthy immobilization and rehabilitation.

Gait analysis in a gait laboratory can provide a clearer picture on which to base surgical decisions than visual assessment of gait. Quantifiable information about gait deviations in a child with CP is gained by observing the child walk from all angles and collecting data on muscle output and limb range of motion during the gait cycle. Video analysis and surface electromyography provide additional invaluable information for the orthopedic surgeon.

A study by Marconi et al. (2014) assessed the effect of SEMLs on gait parameters in children with CP. Participants were between the ages of 9 and 16 years with GMFCS levels between I to III. The energy cost of walking was significantly reduced and thought to be because of a reduction in energy cost of muscular work used to maintain the posture rather than to an improvement in mechanical efficiency. According to the systematic review by McGinley et al. (2012), there is a trend toward positive outcomes in gait as a result of SEMLs.

Neurosurgery. Selective posterior or dorsal rhizotomy (SDR) has become an accepted treatment for spasticity in certain children with CP. Peacock et al. (1987) began advocating the use of this procedure in which dorsal roots in the spinal cord are identified by electromyographic response (Fig. 6.20). Dorsal roots are selectively cut to decrease synaptic,

afferent activity within the spinal cord that decreases spasticity. Through careful selection, touch and proprioception remain intact. Ideal candidates for this procedure are children with spastic diplegia or hemiplegia with moderate motor control and an IQ of 70 or above (Cole et al., 2007; Gormley, 2001). Following rhizotomy, a child requires intense physical therapy for several months postoperatively to maximize strength, range of motion, and functional skills (Gormley, 2001). Physical therapy can be decreased to 1 to 2 times a week within 1 year. Once the spasticity is gone, weakness and incoordination are prevalent. Any orthopedic surgical procedures that are still needed should not be performed until after this period of rehabilitation. Cole et al. (2007) excluded any child who had any multilevel surgery. Hurvitz et al. (2010) surveyed adults who had an SDR as children. The majority reported an improved quality of life (QOL) with only 10% reporting a decrease.

Implantation of a baclofen pump is a neurosurgical procedure. The pump, which is the size of a hockey puck, is placed beneath the skin of the abdomen, and a catheter is threaded below the skin around to the back, where it is inserted through the lumbar spine into the intrathecal space. This placement allows the direct delivery of the medication into the spinal fluid. The medication is stored inside the disk and can be refilled by injection through the skin. It is continuously given, with the dosage adjustable and controlled by a computer (Fig. 6.21). According to Brochard et al. (2009), the greatest advantage is the adjustable dosages, with a resulting real decrease in spasticity and the reversibility of the procedure unlike the permanence of SDR. Lower amounts of medication can be given because the drug is delivered to the site of action, with fewer systemic complications. Intrathecal baclofen (ITB) therapy is used mostly with children with

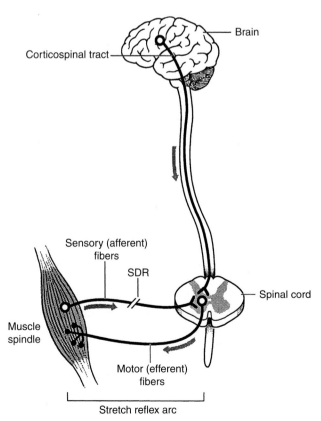

Fig. 6.20 Selective dorsal rhizotomy (SDR). (From Batshaw ML: *Children with developmental disabilities,* ed 4, Baltimore, 1997, Paul H. Brookes.)

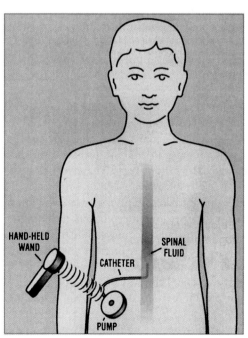

Fig. 6.21 Baclofen pump. (Courtesy Medtronic, Inc.)

spastic quadriplegia. Brochard et al. (2009) studied the effects of ITB therapy on gait of children with CP and found that spasticity was decreased, and gait capacity measured by the Gillette Functional Assessment Questionnaire significantly increased. In a recent systematic review, deep brain stimulation and ITB were found to be somewhat effective in reducing dystonia, but there was inadequate evidence regarding improvement in motor function (Fehlings et al., 2018).

Outcomes following treatment to improve gait are highly variable in children with CP. Some patients benefit whereas others do not. Schwartz et al. (2016) studied 473 children with CP who received various treatments to improve gait. The treatments ranged from single to multiple orthopedic surgeries, dorsal rhizotomy, and conservative (routine physical therapy). Outcome measures studied included gait speed, gait pattern, energy cost of walking, and the Pediatric Outcomes Data Collection Instrument. All children were ambulatory and at GMFCS levels I to III. The researchers found that better dynamic motor control was associated with better treatment outcomes. Having less involvement pretreatment was associated with smaller posttreatment gains. The study is limited because it is retrospective, but it does show that ambulant children with CP who have good motor control tend to have good treatment outcomes, and those with poor motor control do not.

Functional Movement

Strength and endurance are incorporated into functional movements against gravity and can be practiced continuously over the course of a typical day. Kicking balls, carrying objects of varying weights, reaching overhead for dressing or undressing, pulling pants down and up for toileting, and climbing or walking up and down stairs and ramps can be used to promote strength, endurance, and coordination. Endurance can be promoted by having a child who can ambulate use a treadmill (Fig. 6.22) or dance or play tag during recess. Preschool is a great time to increase physical activity so that a high activity level becomes a lifetime habit.

Use of positioning can provide a prolonged static stretch. Manual stretching of the muscles, most likely to develop contractures, should be incorporated into the child's functional tasks. Positions used while dressing, eating, and sleeping should be reviewed periodically by a member of the therapy team with the child's parents. Stretching may need to be part of a therapy program in addition to part of the home program conducted by the parents. The evidence suggests that 6 hours of elongation is needed to produce a change in muscle length (Tardieu et al., 1988). Stretching interventions were found to be yellow interventions meaning that clinicians can use them, but outcomes should be closely measured (Craig et al., 2016). Casting to improve ankle range of motion is a green intervention meaning there is evidence of short-term improvement. The most important positions of function for a preschooler are standing, lying, and sitting on a chair or on the floor to play. Teachers should be made aware of the importance of varying the child's position during the day. If a preschooler cannot stand independently, a standing

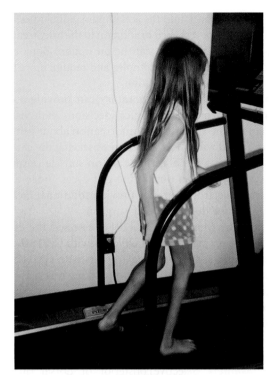

Fig. 6.22 Treadmill.

program should be incorporated into the child's daily routine in the classroom and at home. Standing programs have been found to increase bone mineral density (Craig et al., 2016). Such a standing program may well be carried over from a program started when the child was younger. Standing devices are pictured in Chapter 5.

Activities of Daily Living and Peer Interaction

While the child is in preschool, the ability to perform ADLs may not seem to be an important issue; however, if it takes a child with CP twice as long to toilet than her classmates, what she misses is the social interaction during snack time and when on the playground. Social-emotional development depends on interactions among peers, such as sharing secrets, pretend play, and learning game playing. Making these opportunities available to the child with CP may be one of the most important things we can do in physical therapy because these interactions help form the child's self-image and social competence. Immobility and slow motor performance can create social isolation. Always take the child's level of cognitive ability into consideration when selecting a game or activity to incorporate into therapy. If therapy takes place in an outpatient setting, the clinician should plan an activity that will keep the child's interest and will also accomplish predetermined movement goals. When therapy is incorporated into the classroom, the activity to be carried out by the child may have already been selected by the teacher and will need to address an educational need. The assistant may need to be creative by using an alternative position to assist the child to improve performance within the context of a classroom activity. Some classroom periods such as free play or story time may be more easily adapted for therapeutic intervention.

Physical therapy services provided in the school setting must be educationally relevant and address goals on the student's individual education plan.

Young children with CP and limited mobility have a lower frequency of participation in home, school, and community activities (Chiarello et al., 2012). The lower frequency of participation was explained by the child's physical ability and adaptive behavior, the latter being the biggest determinant. This finding is in keeping with other researches supporting the importance of person-environment interaction as being crucial for children's participation (Majnemer et al., 2008; Palisano et al., 2011). A list of activities that young children with CP participate in can be found in Table 6.9. Chiarello et al. (2014) confirmed that age and gross motor ability contributed to the frequency and enjoyment of participation by children with CP from age 18 to 60 months.

Function in sitting can be augmented by the use of assistive technology such as communication devices and environmental controls. The child can use eye, head, or hand pointing to communicate or to activate other electronic devices. Children with neuromotor dysfunction should also achieve upright orientation to facilitate social interaction. McEwen (1992) studied interactions between students with disabilities and teachers and found that when students with disabilities were in a more upright position, such as sitting on a chair rather than on the floor, the level of interaction increased.

Third Stage of Physical Therapy Intervention: School Age and Adolescence

During the next two major periods of development, the focus of physical therapy intervention is to safeguard all previous gains. This may be easier said than done because the school-age child may be understandably and appropriately more interested in the school environment and in friends than in physical therapy. Rosenbaum and Gorter (2011) address the need for professionals working with children with CP to recognize the five F's: function, family, fun, fitness, and friends. School-age children need to experience play, have fun, get fit, have friends, engage in family routines, and plan for the future. By focusing on activities that the school-age child wants to engage in and modifying the task or the environment to allow the student to actively participate, function and fitness can be promoted, and future possibilities explored.

Activity and Participation

QOL of individuals with CP is similar to peers (Dickinson et al., 2007). However, participation in life activities is decreased relative to the severity of involvement (Orlin et al., 2010). The school-age child should be empowered to take responsibility for the therapy program. An activity record in the form of a calendar may be a way to motivate a younger child to perform physical activities/exercises on a routine basis. A walking program may be used to work on increasing endurance and cardiovascular fitness. Finding an activity that motivates the student to improve performance may be as simple as timing an obstacle course, increasing the time spent on a treadmill, or improving the number of repetitions. Everyone loves a contest. Find out what important motor task the student wants to accomplish or a sport in which she wants to participate. Can the student carry a tray in the cafeteria (Fig. 6.23)? Does she want to be able to dribble a basketball, ride a bicycle, or run a race? Be sure it is something the student wants to do. Pain limits participation and should always be eliminated or alleviated.

TABLE 6.9 Activities Participated in by the Highest and Lowest Percentage of Young Children With Cerebral Palsy		
Activity	**Sample of Activities**	**Percentage**
Play activities	Playing with toys	95
	Watching television or a video	94
Skill development	Listening to stories	99
	Drawing and coloring	91
	Reading or looking at books	91
	Taking swimming lessons	11
	Participating in community organizations	11
	Learning to dance	9
	Doing gymnastics	7
	Taking music lessons	0
Active physical recreation	Doing team sports	1
Social activities	Listening to music	91

Modified from Chiarello LA, et al.: Understanding participation of preschool-age children with cerebral palsy, *J Early Intervention* 34(1):3–19, 2012.

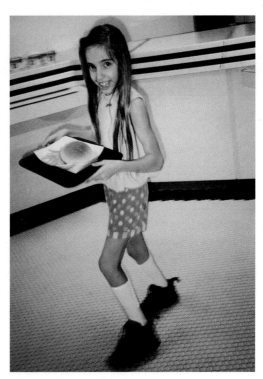

Fig. 6.23 Carrying a tray.

Participation in family and recreational activities in children from 1.5 to 12 years old were studied by Alghamdi et al. (2017). Differences in enjoyment and frequency of participation were found to be based on GMFCS, Manual Ability Classification System, and Communication Function Classification System levels, but not sex or age. A child's communication level had more of an impact on frequency of participation than their motor level. Enjoyment was not related to gross motor level as previously found by Chiarello et al. (2016) but is related to frequency of participation. Earlier provision of mobility aids (Ragonesi and Galloway, 2012) and augmentative communication options (Myrden et al., 2014) fosters psychosocial development in the child (Guerette et al., 2013) and positive social outcomes of families (Tefft et al., 2011). The assistant may notice differences in participation as the child transitions to adolescence.

Adolescents are notorious for ignoring adults' directions, so lack of interest in therapy can be especially trying during this period. However, adolescence can work in favor of compliance with physical therapy goals if the student becomes so concerned about appearances that he or she is willing to work to improve gait efficiency or to minimize a potential contracture. Some teenagers may find it more difficult to ambulate the longer distances required in middle school, or they may find that they do not have the physical stamina to carry books and make multiple trips to and from their lockers and still have energy to focus attention in the classroom. Poor endurance in performing routine self-care and personal hygiene functions can cause difficulty as the teen demands more privacy and seeks personal independence while still requiring physical assistance. By being creative, the therapist can help the teen locate recreational opportunities within the community and tailor goals to meet the individual's needs.

Physical therapy goals during the school years and through adolescence are to:
1. Continue independent mobility.
2. Develop independent ADL and instrumental ADL skills.
3. Participate in a community fitness program.
4. Foster social interaction with peers and a positive self-image.
5. Develop a transition plan for adulthood.

Independence

Strength

Strength is a component of independence, gait, activity performance, and participation in life. Strength training and progressive resistive exercise have been an integral part of the physical therapy program. Strengthening and resistance does not increase spasticity or pain (Gillett et al., 2015). School-aged children and adolescents with CP should be guided by the following when strength training: engage in a minimum of 12 to 16 week program that involves 40 to 50 minute sessions 3 times a week; use rest intervals of greater than 1 minute up to 3 minutes; train single-joint muscles when they are weak or compensations are present in multijoint muscles; and take into consideration National Strength and Conditioning Guidelines for Children (Gillett et al., 2015; Park and Kim, 2014; Verschuren et al., 2011). Verschuren et al. published the first CP-specific guidelines for exercise and physical activity in 2016. Their recommendations based on the available evidence and expert opinion can be found in Table 6.10.

Circuit training (Blundell et al., 2003) used with young children with CP found improvements in gait velocity and strength that were maintained after the training ceased. A

TABLE 6.10	Recommendations for Exercise and Physical Activity in People With Cerebral Palsy			
Exercise	Frequency	Intensity	Time	Type
Resistive	2-4 times a week	1-3 sets of 6-15 reps at 50%-85% repetition maximum	Not indicated 12-16 week training period	Single-joint, machine-based progressing to machine plus free weights, multijoint and closed kinetic change resistance exercise Single-joint exercise indicated for weak muscles or for children, adolescents, or adults who compensate
Aerobic	1-2 times to start progress to 3 times a week	>60% of peak heart rate or 40% of heart rate reserve	Minimum 20 minutes per session/8 or 16 consecutive weeks	Regular exercise involving major muscle groups that is continuous and rhythmic
Physical activity	≥5 days per week	Moderate to vigorous	60 minutes	Variety
Physical activity	7 days per week	Sedentary	Limit to <2 h/day Move for 2 minutes for every 30-60 spent sitting	Leisure-time sedentary, television watching, playing video or computer games

From Verschuren O, Peterson MD, Balemans ACJ, Hurvitz EA: Exercise and physical activity recommendations for people with cerebral palsy, *Dev Med Child Neurol* 58:798-808, 2016.

circuit-training program in the Netherlands (Gorter et al., 2009) demonstrated improved aerobic endurance in children (GMFCS level I or II) 8 to 13 years of age after 9 weeks of twice-a-week training, with every session lasting 30 minutes. More recently, Schranz et al. (2018) found that a home-based high-intensity circuit training program increased strength and participation in teens (majority GMFCS level I) compared with a progressive resistance program. Both groups trained 3 times a week for 8 weeks. Aviram et al. (2017) used functional focused strength training in a group circuit training program for adolescents with CP that was compared to a treadmill intervention. Both groups improved in walking speed and endurance; and the gains were maintained during follow-up.

Rehabilitation has embraced technology such as virtual reality and video games that provide motivation and whole body movement. An interactive video home-based intervention (Bilde et al., 2011) resulted in positive changes in children in sit to stand and step ups in the frontal and sagittal planes as well as endurance. No change in balance, tested using the Romberg, was seen, but visual perceptual abilities significantly increased. The children (GMFCS level I or II) were 6 to 13 years of age and trained about 30 minutes a day with a novel system delivered via the Internet. In the first published study using the Wii gaming system (Nintendo, Kyoto, Japan), Deutsch et al. (2008) reported that using this system was feasible with an 11-year-old with spastic diplegia at GMFCS level III. Positive changes were documented in postural control, functional mobility, and visual-perceptual processing. The program was carried out in a summer school setting. Virtual reality has been combined with robot-assisted devices to improve participation in robot-assisted gait training (Labruyere et al., 2013).

Functional Gait Training

Functional gait training is defined as active practice of walking to improve walking ability. It can be done overground or on a treadmill. Booth et al. (2018) found functional gait training for children and young adults with CP had a more positive effect on walking speed and endurance than standard physical therapy based on their systematic review and meta-analysis. Participant engagement was increased, and the effects magnified when biofeedback and virtual reality was added to the functional gait training. There is no optimal training intensity at this time. Motor learning principles such as duration, intensity, and variability of the intervention contribute to the retention of the effect of the treatment.

Physiologic Changes

Other great potential hazards to continued independent motor performance are the physical and physiologic changes brought on by adolescence. Greater growth of the lower extremities in relation to the trunk and upper body can produce a less stable gait. Growth spurts in which muscle length does not keep up with changes in bone length can cause problems with static balance and dynamic balance.

During periods of rapid growth, bone length may outstrip the ability to elongate the attached muscles, with resulting potential contracture formation. The development of such contractures may contribute to a loss of independent mobility or to a loss in movement efficiency. In other words, the student may have to work harder to move. Some teens may fall with increasing frequency. Others may limit distances walked in an effort to preserve function or to save energy for school-related tasks and learning. Any change in functional ambulation ability should be reported to the supervising physical therapist so the therapist can evaluate the need for a change in the student's treatment plan. The student may benefit from a change in either assistive device or orthosis. In some instances, the loss of functional upright ambulation is a real possibility, and a wheelchair evaluation may be warranted.

Another difficulty that can arise during this period is related to body mass changes secondary to the adolescent's growth. Increasing body weight compared with a disproportionately smaller muscle mass in the adolescent with CP can represent a serious threat to continued functional independence. The adolescent with CP who is sedentary is at greater risk for obesity and premature sarcopenia (loss of muscle mass) (Peterson et al., 2013). Together these conditions can lead to cardiovascular disease. It is imperative that the adolescent/young adult with CP value and engage in lifelong participation in physical activity. Health-related quality of life (HRQOL) in people with CP was studied over many years. The researchers found that people with CP had a lower HRQOL in the areas of motor and social functioning (Tan et al., 2014). The variability in HRQOL between individuals with CP was explained by type of CP, GMFCS level, and intellectual disability.

Fitness. Students with physical disabilities, such as CP, are often unable to fully participate in physical education. If the physical education teacher is knowledgeable about adapting routines for students with disabilities, the student may experience some cardiovascular benefits. The neuromuscular deficits affect the ability of a student with CP to perform exercises. Students with CP have higher energy costs for routine activities. Eken et al. (2016) reported on the relationship of muscle endurance and fatigue, walking capacity, and participation in adolescents with CP. The adolescents were mildly involved (GMFSC I or II). They found that knee extensor muscle endurance was significantly related to subjective reports of fatigue and walking capacity. The reduced muscle endurance had no effect on participation. Slaman et al. (2014) focused on a lifestyle intervention to improve physical fitness in adolescents and young adults. The 6-month intervention included a physical fitness training combined with counseling. The counseling sessions focused on sports participation and physical behavior. The program improved body composition and cardiopulmonary fitness. A sports-specific intervention was successfully used in an adolescent with CP (Kenyon et al., 2010). A cycling-based exercise video-game has been used successfully to promote cardiovascular fitness and participation in youth with CP (Knights et al., 2016; MacIntosh et al., 2017). Australian researchers studied the efficacy of using a participation-focused therapy on habitual physical activity and leisure-time physical activity in children with CP (Reedman et al., 2019). The children were classified as GMFSC I to III. Using the Canadian Occupational Performance Measure and accelerometers, they found that after the 8-week intervention, the intervention group improved in performance of leisure-time physical activity goals compared with controls. There was no change in habitual physical activity. Fitness in all students with disabilities needs to be fostered as part of physical therapy to improve overall health and QOL.

Community integration. Availability of recreation and leisure activities that are appropriate and accessible are easier to come by than in the past. It is no less important for the individual with a disability to remain physically active and to achieve some degree of health-related fitness than it is for a person without disabilities. In fact, it may be more important for the person with CP to work on aerobic fitness as a way to prevent a decline in ambulation in adulthood. Recreational and leisure activities, sports-related or not, should be part of every adolescent's free time. Swim programs at the YMCA, local fitness club, or elsewhere provide wonderful opportunities to socialize, develop and improve cardiovascular fitness, control weight, and maintain joint and muscle integrity. Recent attention has been given to encouraging children and adolescents with CP to participate in aquatic and martial arts programs to improve movement, balance, and self-esteem. Wheelchair athletics are a good option for school-age children or adolescents who live in places with a junior wheelchair sports program.

Accessibility is an important issue in transportation and in providing students with disabilities easy entrance to and exit from community buildings. Accessibility is often a challenge to a teenager who may not be able to drive because of CP. Every effort should be made to support the teenager's ability to drive a motor vehicle because the freedom this type of mobility provides is important for social interaction and vocational pursuits. Van Gorp et al. (2019) found that participation in community life and recreation improves in individuals at GMFCS levels III and IV before age 23.

Fourth Stage of Physical Therapy Intervention: Adulthood

Physical therapy goals during adulthood are to:
1. Be independent in mobility and ADLs.
2. Engage in a healthy lifestyle.
3. Participate in the community.
4. Live independently.
5. Have a job and family.

Even though five separate goals are identified for this stage of rehabilitation, they are all part of the life of an adult. Society expects adults to live on their own and to participate within the community where they live and work. This can be the ultimate challenge for a person with CP or any lifelong disability. Living facilities that offer varied levels of assisted living are available in some communities. Adults with CP may live on their own, in group homes, in institutions, or in nursing homes. Some continue to live at home with aging parents or with older siblings. Transition planning should begin by the student's 16th birthday. Priorities identified

include but are not limited to participation in meaningful activities, protection of health, and having supportive relationships (Rehm et al., 2012).

Employment figures from the National Longitudinal Transition Study-2 (Wagner et al., 2006) found that only 40% of young adults with childhood onset disabilities were employed 2 years out of high school, 20% less than same-age peers without disabilities. Dreamscape Foundation (2019) states that 35% of working-age persons with a disability are employed, whereas the Bureau of Labor statistics (2018) states that the employment/population ratio for people with disabilities is 19.1%. Despite the focus on transition services for the adolescent with CP, employment has not been a major goal for the adult with CP. Factors that determine the ability of an adult with CP to live and work independently are cognitive status, degree of functional limitations, and adequacy of social and financial support. Family and educators play a significant role in providing the child and adolescent with CP with an expectation to participate in work. Clinicians must help the adolescent with CP to transition to adulthood by being aware of and working with vocational rehabilitation services (Huang et al., 2013). Specific services provided by vocational rehabilitation institutes predicted employment outcomes as (1) use of rehabilitation assistive technology, (2) on-the-job support, (3) job placement assistance, (4) on-the-job training, and (5) support services for basic living. Early prior planning between therapist and vocational counselor can provide a foundation for later employment (Vogtle, 2013). Language and communication are keys to developing relationships and employment for adults with CP (Graham et al., 2016).

Liljenqist et al. (2018) looked at utilization of physical therapy services by youth with CP transitioning to adulthood. Their secondary analysis of the National Longitudinal Transition Study-2 data revealed that 59.4% of youth used physical therapy services while in secondary school, but only 33.7% used physical therapy services after leaving secondary school. For youth with CP who had some or many problems accessing disability support services, factors that influenced access were demographic ones: sex, race, poverty status, parental education level, and disability characteristics. For youth with no problems accessing support services, the factors influencing access were disability characteristics. Service providers may lack knowledge that adults with CP need continued monitoring, consultation, or direct services to achieve and maintain mobility skills to support function and participation. Increased awareness and advocacy in this area is a role for everyone involved.

Physical Activity and Participation in Adults

Fatigue

Compared with typically developing peers, individuals with CP are at risk for losing ambulation and mobility skills earlier in the aging process (Benner et al., 2017; Jahnsen et al., 2003; Palisano et al., 2011). In a longitudinal study, Benner et al. (2017) identified pain and severe fatigue as the most common health issues in adults with CP aged 35 to 45 years. High fatigue has been associated with crouch gait and low QOL in adults with CP (Lundh et al., 2018). The researchers recommended identifying risk factors as a way to prevent development of fatigue and gait deterioration. More research is needed to determine the mechanisms involved in aging in persons with CP.

Mobility is crucial for youth with CP as they enter adulthood. Achieving and maintaining mobility skills supports maximum participation in daily life. Youth with CP spend twice as much time as in sedentary behavior than typically developing peers (Carlon et al., 2013). Strength training may prevent the decline in walking ability as a young person with CP transitions to adulthood. One study found an increase in strength but no change in mobility using a progressive resistive exercise program (Taylor et al., 2013). However, a combination of functional anaerobic and strength training over 12 weeks resulted in increased strength, muscle size, and functional capacity in young adults with CP (Gillett et al., 2018). The authors thought the addition of anaerobic training to progressive resistance training assisted in producing an improved functional outcome.

Quality of Life

Two goals of Healthy People 2020 particularly relevant to improving the QOL of people with disabilities are (1) reduce the percentage who report delays in accessing primary and preventive care, and (2) increase the number reporting being engaged in transition planning from pediatric to adult health care (US Department of Health and Human Services). Finding a medical home is crucial to a successful transition to adulthood and adult health care. A medical home is an approach to providing accessible, comprehensive, collaborative, compassionate, and culturally effective care. See the website for the American Academy of Pediatrics for more information (https://medicalhomeinfo.aap.org/Pages/default.aspx). Several medical organizations including the American Academy of Pediatrics have recommended that transition planning begin at age 14 rather than the legally mandated age 16 (American Academy of Pediatrics, 2011). QOL of adults with CP is related to QOL in adolescence (Colver et al., 2015). Variability in both QOL, the holistic sense of well-being and the specific components of HRQOL such as mobility, self-care, and mental health have been associated with the type of CP, GMFCS level, and intellectual disability (Tan et al., 2014; Livingston et al., 2007). QOL was found to predict overall health in nonambulatory children, adolescents, and young adults with CP at GMFCS levels IV and V (Kolman et al., 2018). Communication and social interaction predicted overall QOL more than self-care and transfer mobility. Results also showed that comfort in sitting was associated with a 15-fold higher QOL in this group. These findings reinforce that psychosocial well-being is related to social integration and coping but not physical function (Majnemer et al., 2007; Wake et al., 2003).

CHAPTER SUMMARY

The child with CP and her family present the physical therapist and the physical therapist assistant with a lifetime of opportunities to assist them to accomplish meaningful functional goals. These goals revolve around the child's achievement of some type of mobility and mastery of the environment, including the ability to manipulate objects, to communicate, and to demonstrate as much independence as possible in physical, cognitive, and social functions. The needs of the child with CP and her family change in relation to the child's maturation and reflect the family's priorities at any given time. Physical therapy may be one of many therapies the child receives. Physical therapists and physical therapist assistants are part of the team working to provide family-centered care in the home, school, and community. Regardless of the stage of physical therapy management, families need to be empowered to make informed decisions. Goals need to be meaningful and based on what the family wants the child to learn to do to participate meaningfully in her life and the life of the family. Activities that promote fitness, fun, and planning for the future must be part of physical therapy interventions for children, adolescents, and adults with CP. The long-term goal must always be to promote relationships and new roles across the lifespan to enhance participation in life. Physical therapists collaborate with families at all times but especially during times of transition such as when moving from early intervention to school and beyond. Physical therapist and physical therapist assistants must advocate for good public policy and adequate resources that will help families plan for the future. People with CP need access to medical services that support health and full participation across their lifespan. It is hoped that the end result is an adult who can fully engage in and enjoy all aspects of life.

REVIEW QUESTIONS

1. Why may the clinical manifestations of CP appear to worsen with age even though the pathologic features are static?
2. Name the two greatest risk factors for CP.
3. What is the most common type of muscle tone seen in children with CP?
4. How does muscle development in CP contribute to muscle stiffness?
5. Compare and contrast the focus of physical therapy intervention in a child with spastic CP and in a child with athetoid CP.
6. What is the role of the physical therapist assistant when working with a preschool-age child with CP?
7. What type of orthosis is most commonly used by children with CP who ambulate?
8. When should a fitness program be developed for a child with CP?
9. What medications are used to manage spasticity in children with CP?
10. What are the expected life outcomes that should be used as a guide for goal setting with children with disabilities?

CASE STUDIES REHABILITATION UNIT INITIAL EXAMINATION AND EVALUATION: JC

History
Chart Review
JC is a 6-year-old girl with spastic diplegic cerebral palsy (CP) (Gross Motor Function Classification System [GMFCS] level III). She was born at 28 weeks of gestation, required mechanical ventilation, and sustained a left intraventricular hemorrhage. She received physical therapy as part of an infant intervention program. She sat at 18 months of age. At 3 years of age, she made the transition into a school-based preschool program. She had two surgical procedures for heel cord tendon transfers and adductor releases of the hips. She is now making the transition into a regular first grade. JC has a younger sister. Both parents work. Her father brings her to weekly outpatient therapy. JC goes to daycare or to her grandparents' home after school.

Subjective
JC's parents are concerned about her independence in the school setting.

Objective
Systems Review
Communication/Cognition: JC communicates easily and appropriately. Her intelligence is within the normal range.
Cardiovascular/Pulmonary: Normal values for age.
Integumentary: Intact.
Musculoskeletal: Active range of movement and strength intact in the upper extremities but impaired in the trunk and lower extremities.
Neuromuscular: Coordination within functional limits in the upper extremity, but impaired in the lower extremities.

Tests and Measures
Anthropometrics: Height 46 inches, weight 45 lbs, body mass index 15 (20 to 24 is normal).

Motor Function: JC can roll to either direction and can achieve sitting by pushing up from side lying. She can get into a quadruped position from prone and can pull herself into kneeling. She attains standing by moving into half-kneeling with upper extremity support. She can come to stand from sitting in a straight chair without hand support but adducts her knees for stability.

Neurodevelopmental Status: Peabody Developmental Motor Scales Developmental Motor Quotient = 69, with an age equivalent of 12 months. Fine-motor development is average for her age (Peabody Developmental Motor Scales, Developmental Motor Quotient = 90).

Range of Motion	ACTIVE		PASSIVE	
	R	L	R	L
Hips				
Flexion	0°–100°	0°–90°	0°–105°	0°–120°
Adduction	0°–15°	0°–12°	0°–5°	0°–12°
Abduction	0°–30°	0°–40°	0°–30°	0°–40°
Internal rotation	0°–25°	0°–78°	0°–83°	0°–84°
External rotation	0°–26°	0°–30°	0°–26°	0°–40°
Knees				
Flexion	0°–80°	0°–80°	0°–120°	0°–120°
Extension	−15°	−15°	Neutral	Neutral

Range of Motion	ACTIVE		PASSIVE	
	R	L	R	L
Ankle				
Dorsiflexion	Neutral	Neutral	0°–20°	0°–20°
Plantar flexion	0°–8°	0°–40°	0°–30°	0°–40°
Inversion	0°–5°	0°–12°	0°–5°	0°–20°
Eversion	0°–30°	0°–30°	0°–50°	0°–40°

Reflex Integrity: Patellar 3 +, Achilles 3 +, Babinski present bilaterally. Moderately increased tone is present in the hamstrings, adductors, and plantar flexors bilaterally.

Posture: JC demonstrates a functional scoliosis with the convexity to the right. The right shoulder and pelvis are elevated. JC lacks complete thoracic extension in standing. The pelvis is rotated to the left in standing. Leg length is 23.5 inches bilaterally, measured from anterior superior iliac spine to medial malleolus.

Muscle Performance: Upper extremity strength appears to be within functional limits because JC can move her arms against gravity and take moderate resistance. Lower extremity strength is difficult to determine in the presence of increased tone but is generally less than fair with the left side appearing to be stronger than the right.

Gait, Locomotion, and Balance: JC ambulates independently 15 feet using a reverse-facing walker while wearing solid polypropylene ankle-foot orthoses (AFOs). She can take five steps independently without a device before requiring external support for balance. She goes up and down stairs, alternating feet using a handrail. She can maneuver her walker up and down a ramp and a curb with stand by assist. JC requires standby assistance to move about with her walker in the classroom and when getting up and down from her desk. Incomplete trunk righting is present with any displacement in sitting. No trunk rotation present with lateral displacements in sitting. Upper extremity protective reactions are present in all directions in sitting. JC stands alone for 3 to 4 minutes every trial. She exhibits no protective stepping when she loses her balance in standing.

Sensory Integrity: Intact.

Self-Care: JC is independent in eating and in toileting with grab bars. She requires moderate assistance with dressing secondary to balance.

Play: JC enjoys reading Junie B. Jones books and playing with dolls.

Assessment/Evaluation
JC is a 6-year-old girl with spastic diplegic CP. She is independently ambulatory with a reverse-facing walker and AFOs for short distances on level ground. She is functioning at GMFCS level III and attends a regular first grade class. She is seen for outpatient physical therapy once a week for 45 minutes.

Problem List
1. Dependent in ambulation without an assistive device.
2. Impaired strength and endurance to perform age-appropriate motor activities.
3. Impaired dynamic sitting and standing balance.
4. Dependent in dressing.

Diagnosis: JC exhibits impaired force production and balance, poor selective motor control, and lack of lower extremity dissociation consistent with spastic diplegic CP.

CASE STUDIES REHABILITATION UNIT INITIAL EXAMINATION AND EVALUATION: JC—cont'd

Prognosis: JC will improve her functional independence and motor skills in the school setting. Her rehabilitation potential for the following goals is good.

Short-term Goals (Actions to Be Achieved By Midyear Review)

1. JC will ambulate independently within her classroom.
2. JC will throw and catch a ball with minimal loss of balance.
3. JC will walk on a treadmill with arm support for 10 consecutive minutes.
4. JC will ambulate 25 feet without an assistive device three times a day.
5. JC will don and doff AFOs, shoes, and socks, independently.

Long-term Goals (End of First Grade)

1. JC will ambulate independently without an assistive device on level surfaces.
2. JC will go up and down a set of three stairs, step over step, without holding on to a railing.
3. JC will walk continuously for 20 minutes without resting.
4. JC will dress herself for school in 15 minutes.

Plan

Coordination, Communication, and Documentation

The physical therapist and physical therapist assistant will be in frequent communication with JC's family and teacher regarding her physical therapy program. Outcomes of interventions will be documented on a weekly basis.

Patient/Family Education

JC and her parents will be given suggestions to assist her in becoming more independent at home, such as getting clothes out the night before and getting up early enough to complete the dressing tasks before leaving for school. JC and her family will be instructed in a home exercise program consisting of stretching and strengthening. A reminder calendar will assist her in remembering to perform her exercises four times a week.

Interventions

Increase dynamic trunk postural reactions by using a movable surface to shift her weight and to facilitate balance responses in all directions.

1. Practice coming to stand while sitting astride a bolster. One end of the bolster can be placed on a stool of varying height to decrease the distance needed for her to move from sitting to standing. Begin with allowing her to use hand support and then gradually withdraw it.
2. Practice stepping over low objects, first with upper extremity support followed by gradual withdrawal of support; next practice stepping up and down one step without the railing while giving manual support at the hips.
3. Walk at a slow speed on a treadmill using hand support for 5 minutes. Gradually increase the time. Once she can tolerate 15 minutes, begin to increase speed.
4. Time her ability to maneuver an obstacle course involving walking, stepping over objects, moving around objects, going up and down stairs, and throwing a ball and beanbags. Monitor and track her personal best time. Vary the complexity of the tasks involved, according to how efficient she is at completing them.

Follow-Up

JC is now 12 years old. Secondary to rapid growth, especially in her lower extremities and extensive hip and knee flexion contractures, she is once again ambulating with a reverse-facing wheeled walker. She is able to stand independently for 5 seconds, and to take 13 steps before falling or requiring external support. She has been evaluated for surgical releases, but the gait studies indicate significant lower extremity weakness and increased cocontraction of these muscles during gait. The orthopedist believes that she would not have sufficient strength to ambulate following surgery. Physical therapy goals are to increase hip and knee range of motion, gluteus maximus, quadriceps, and ankle musculature strength, and to regain the ability to ambulate independently without an assistive device. What treatment interventions could be used to attain these functional goals?

Questions to Think About

- What interventions could be part of JC's home exercise program?
- How can fitness be incorporated into her physical therapy program?

REFERENCES

Aboutorabi A, et al.: Efficacy of ankle foot orthoses types on walking in children with cerebral palsy: a systematic review, *Ann Phys Rehab Med* 60(6):393–402, 2017.

Accardo PJ, editor: *Capute & Accardo's neurodevelopmental disabilities in infancy and childhood*, vol 1, ed 3, Baltimore, 2008, Paul H. Brookes.

Alghamdi MS, et al.: Understanding participation of children with cerebral palsy in family and recreational activities, *Res Dev Disabil* 69:96–104, 2017.

Almasri NA, An M, Palisano RJ: Parents' perception of receiving family-centered care for their children with physical disabilities: a meta-analysis, *Phys Occup Ther Pediatr* 38:427–443, 2018.

American Academy of Pediatrics, American Academy of Family Physicians, and America College of Physicians, Transitions Clinical Report Authoring Group: Supporting the health care transition from adolescence to adulthood in the medical home, *Pediatrics* 128(1):182–200, 2011.

American Academy of Pediatrics AAP Task Force on Infant Positioning and SIDS. Positioning and SIDS, *Pediatrics* 90:264, 1992.

Ashwal S, Russman BS, Blasco PA, et al.: Practice parameter. Diagnostic assessment of the child with cerebral palsy: report of the Quality Standards Subcommittee of the American Academy of Neurology and the Practice Committee of the Child Neurology Society, *Neurology* 62(6):851–863, 2004.

Aviram R, et al.: Effects of a group circuit progressive resistance training program compared with a treadmill training program for adolescents with cerebral palsy, *Dev Neurorehabil* 20(6):347–354, 2017.

Bamm EL, Rosenbaum P: Family-centered theory: origins, development, barriers, and supports to implementation in rehabilitation medicine, *Arch Phys Med Rehabil* 89:1618–1624, 2008.

Bar-Or O: Disease-specific benefits of training in the child with a chronic disease: what is the evidence? *Pediatr Exerc Sci* 2:384–394, 1990.

Batshaw ML, Roizen NJ, Lotrecchiano GR: *Children with disabilities*, ed 7, Baltimore, 2013, Paul H Brooks.

Begnoche DM, et al.: Predictors of independent walking in young children with cerebral palsy, *Phys Ther* 96:183–192, 2016.

Benner JL, et al.: Long-term deterioration of perceived health and functioning in adults with cerebral palsy, *Arch Phys Med Rehabil* 98:2196–2205.e1, 2017.

Berg AT, Berkovic SF, Brodie MJ, et al.: Revised terminology and concepts for organization of seizures and epilepsies: report of the ILAE Commission on Classification and Terminology, 2005–2009, *Epilepsia* 51(4):676–685, 2010.

Bilde PE, Kliim-Due M, Rasmussen B, et al.: Individualized, home-based interactive training of cerebral palsy children delivered through the internet, *BMC Neurol* 11:32, 2011.

Blair E, Watson L: Epidemiology of cerebral palsy, *Semin Fetal Neonatal Med* 11(2):117–125, 2006.

Blundell SW, Shepherd RB, Dean CM, et al.: Functional strength training in cerebral palsy: a pilot study of group circuit training class for children aged 4–8 years, *Clin Rehabil* 17(1):48–57, 2003.

Böhm H, et al.: Effect of floor reaction ankle-foot orthosis on crouch gait inpatients with cerebral palsy: What can be expected? *Prosthet Orthot Int* 42:(3):245–253, 2018.

Booth ATC, et al.: The efficacy of functional gait training in children and young adults with cerebral palsy: a systematic review and meta-analysis, *Dev Med Child Neurol* 60:866–883, 2018.

Brochard S, Remy-Neris O, Filipetti P, Bussel B: Intrathecal baclofen infusion for ambulant children with cerebral palsy, *Pediatr Neurol* 40:265–270, 2009.

Buccieri KM: Use of orthoses and early intervention physical therapy to minimize hyperpronation and promote functional skills in a child with gross motor delays: a case report, *Phys Occup Ther Pediatr* 23(1):5–20, 2003.

Bureau of Labor Statistics: *Persons with disability: labor force characteristics-2018*, 2018. Available at: www.bls.gov/news.release/pdf/disabl.pdf. Accessed March, 2019.

Butler C: Effects of powered mobility on self-initiated behaviors of very young children with locomotor disability, *Dev Med Child Neurol* 28:325–332, 1986.

Butler C: Augmentative mobility: Why do st? *Phys Med Rehabil Clin North Am* 2:801–815, 1991.

Byrne R, Noritz G, Maitre NL, NCH Early Developmental Group: Implementation of early diagnosis and intervention guidelines for cerebral palsy in a high-risk follow-up clinic, *Pediatr Neurol* 76:66–71, 2017.

Calado R, Monteiro JP, Fonseca MJ: Transient idiopathic dystonia in infancy, *Acta Paediatr* 100(4):624–627, 2011.

Campos de Paz A, Burnett SM, Braga IW: Walking prognosis in cerebral palsy: a 22-year retrospective analysis, *Dev Med Child Neurol* 36:130–134, 1994.

Carlon SL, et al.: Differences in habitual physical activity levels of young people with cerebral palsy and their typically developing peers: a systematic review, *Disabil Rehabil* 35:647–655, 2013.

Case-Smith J: Using evidence-based clinical guidelines to improve your practice. In *PREPaRE Conference*, Lexington, KY, March 22, 2014, University of Kentucky.

Charles JR, Wolf SL, Schneider JA, Gordon AM: Efficacy of a child-friendly form of constraint-induced movement therapy in hemiplegic cerebral palsy: a randomized control trial, *Dev Med Child Neurol* 48:635–642, 2006.

Cherng RF, Liu CF, Lau TW, Hong RB: Effect of treadmill training with body weight support on gait and gross motor function in children with spastic cerebral palsy, *Am J Phys Med Rehab* 86:548–555, 2007.

Chiarello LA: Family-centered care. In Effgen SK, editor: *Meeting the physical therapy needs of children*, ed 2, Philadelphia, 2013, FA Davis.

Chiarello LA, et al.: Determinants of participation in family and recreational activities of young children with cerebral palsy, *Disabil Rehabil* 38:2455–2468, 2016.

Chiarello LA, Palisano RJ, Orlin MN, et al.: Understanding participation of preschool-age children with cerebral palsy, *J Early Inter* 34(1):3–19, 2012.

Chiarello LA, Palisano RJ, McCoy SW, et al.: Child engagement in daily life: a measure of participation for young children with cerebral palsy, *Disabil Rehabil* 36:1804–1816, 2014.

Chollat C, Sentilhes L, Marret S: Protection of brain development by antenatal magnesium sulphate for infants born preterm, *Dev Med Child Neurol* 61:25–30, 2019.

Colver A, et al.: Self-reported quality of life of adolescents with cerebral palsy: a cross-sectional and longitudinal analysis, *Lancet* 385(9969):705–716, 2015.

Conde-Agudelo A, Romero R: Antenatal magnesium sulfate for the prevention of cerebral palsy in preterm infants less than 34 weeks' gestation: a systematic review and metaanalysis, *Am J Obstet Gynecol* 200:595–609, 2009.

Coker P, Karakostas T, Dodds C, Hsiang S: Gait characteristics of children with hemiplegic cerebral palsy before and after modified constraint-induced movement therapy, *Disabil Rehabil* 32(5):402–408, 2010.

Cole GF, Farmer SE, Roberts A, Stewart C, Patrick JH: Selective dorsal rhizotomy for children with cerebral palsy: the Oswestry experience, *Arch Dis Child* 92:781–785, 2007.

Cooper MS, Mackay MT, Hahey M, et al.: Seizures in children with cerebral palsy and white matter injury, *Pediatrics* 139(3):e20162975, 2017.

Costantine MM, Weiner SJ: Effects of antenatal exposure to magnesium sulfate on neuroprotection and mortality in preterm infants: a meta-analysis, *Obstet Gynecol* 114:354–364, 2009.

Craig J, et al.: Effectiveness of stretch interventions for children with neuromuscular disabilities: evidence-based recommendations, *Pediatr Phys Ther* 28:262–275, 2016.

Damiano DL: Activity, activity, activity: rethinking our physical therapy approach to cerebral palsy, *Phys Ther* 86:1534–1540, 2006.

Damiano DL, Abel MF, Pannunzio M, Romano JP: Interrelationships of strength and gait before and after hamstrings lengthening, *J Pediatr Orthop* 19:352–358, 1999.

Davids JR, Rogozinski BM, Hardin JW, Davis RB: Ankle dorsiflexor function after plantar flexor surgery in children with cerebral palsy, *J Bone Joint Surg Am* 93(23):e1381–e1387, 2011.

DeLuca SC, Echols K, Ramey SL, Taub E: Pediatric constraint-induced movement therapy for a young child with cerebral palsy: two episodes of care, *Phys Ther* 83:1003–1013, 2003.

DeLuca SC, Case-Smith J, Stevenson R, Ramey SL: Constraint-induced movement therapy (CIMT) for young children with cerebral palsy: effects of therapeutic dosage, *J Pediatr Rehabil Med* 5(2):133–142, 2012.

Deutsch JE, Borbely M, Filler J, Huhn K, Guarrera-Bowlby P: Use of a low-cost commercially available gaming console (Wii) for rehabilitation of an adolescent with cerebral palsy, *Phys Ther* 88:1196–1207, 2008.

Dewar R, Love S, Johnston LM: Exercise interventions improve postural control in children with cerebral palsy: a systematic review, *Dev Med Child Neurol* 57:504–529, 2015.

Dickinson HO, et al.: Self-reported quality of life of 8-12-year-old children with cerebral palsy: a cross-sectional European study, *Lancet* 369:2171–2178, 2007.

Dodd KJ, Foley S: Partial body-weight–supported treadmill training can improve walking in children with cerebral palsy: a clinical controlled trial, *Dev Med Child Neurol* 49:101–105, 2007.

Dreamscape Foundation. 2019. Available at: https://dreamscape-foundation.org. Accessed March, 2019.

Dusing S, Harbourne R: Variability in postural control in infancy: implications for development, assessment, and intervention, *Phys Ther* 90:1838–1849, 2010.

Eek MN, Beckung E: Walking ability is related to muscle strength in children with cerebral palsy, *Gait Posture* 28:366–371, 2008.

Effgen SK: *Meeting the physical therapy needs of children*, ed 2, Philadelphia, 2013, FA Davis.

Effgen SK, Myers C, Kleinert J: Use of classification systems to facilitate interprofessional communication. In *5th Annual PREPaRE Conference*, Lexington, KY, March 22, 2014, University of Kentucky.

Eken MM, et al.: Relations between muscle endurance and subjectively reported fatigue, walking capacity and participation in mildly affected adolescents with cerebral palsy, *Dev Med Child Neurol* 58:814–821, 2016.

Eliasson AC, Krumlinde-Sundholm L, Shaw K, Wang C: Effects of constraint-induced movement therapy in young children with hemiplegic cerebral palsy: an adapted model, *Dev Med Child Neurol* 47:266–275, 2005.

Eliasson AC, Krumlinde-Sundholm L, Rosblad B, et al.: The Manual Ability Classification System (MACS) for children with cerebral palsy: scale development and evidence of validity and reliability, *Dev Med Child Neurol* 48:549–554, 2006.

Ellenberg JH, Nelson KB: The association of cerebral palsy with birth asphyxia: a definitional quagmire, *Dev Med Child Neurol* 55:499–508, 2013.

Fazzi E, Bova S, Giovenzana A, et al.: Cognitive visual dysfunctions in preterm children with periventricular leukomalacia, *Dev Med Child Neurol* 51:974–981, 2009.

Fedrizzi E, Anderloni A, Bono R, et al.: Eye-movement disorders and visual-perceptual impairment in diplegic children born preterm: a clinical evaluation, *Dev Med Child Neurol* 40:682–688, 1998.

Fehlings D, Brown L, Harvey A, et al.: Pharmacological and neurosurgical interventions for managing dystonia in cerebral palsy: a systematic review, *Dev Med Child Neurol* 60:356–366, 2018.

Fortuna R, et al.: Changes in contractile properties of muscles receiving repeat injections of botulinum toxin (Botox), *J Biomech* 44:39–44, 2011.

Gabis LV, Tsubary NM, Leon O, Ashkenasi A, Shefer S: Assessment of abilities and comorbidities in children with cerebral palsy, *J Child Neuro* 30(12):1640–1645, 2015. doi:10.1177/0883073815576792.

Giangreco MF, Cloninger CJ, Iverson VS: *Choosing options and accommodations for children (COACH): a guide to educational planning for students with disabilities*, ed 3, Baltimore, 2011, Paul H. Brookes.

Gillett JG, et al.: FAST CP: protocol of a randomised controlled trial of the efficacy of a 12-week combined Functional Anaerobic and Strength Training programme on muscle properties and mechanical gait deficiencies in adolescents and young adults with spastic-type cerebral palsy, *BMJ Open* 5:e008059, 2015.

Gillett JG, Lichtwark GA, Boyd RN, Barber LA: Functional anaerobic and strength training in young adults with cerebral palsy, *Med Sci Sports Exerc* 50:1549–1557, 2018.

Glanzman A: Cerebral palsy. In Goodman C, Fuller KS, editors: *Pathology: implications for the physical therapist*, Philadelphia, 2015, Elsevier, pp 1576–1590.

Gormley ME: Treatment of neuromuscular and musculoskeletal problems in cerebral palsy, *Pediatr Rehabil* 4(1):5–16, 2001.

Gorter H, Holty L, Rameckers E, Elvers H, Oostendorp R: Changes in endurance and walking ability through functional physical training in children with cerebral palsy, *Pediatr Phys Ther* 21:31–37, 2009.

Graham HK, Rosenbaum P, Paneth N, et al.: Cerebral palsy, *Nat Rev Dis Primers* 7(2):15082, 2016. doi:10.1038/nrdp.2015.82.

Grecco L, de Freita T, Satie J, et al.: Treadmill training following orthopedic surgery in lower limbs of children with cerebral palsy, *Pediatr Phys Ther* 25:187–192, 2013.

Guerette P, Furumasu J, Tefft D: The positive effects of early powered mobility on children's psychosocial and play skills, *Assist Technol* 25:39–48, 2013.

Hadders-Algra M: Early diagnosis and early intervention in cerebral palsy, *Front Neurol* 5:1–13, 2014.

Hagglund G, et al.: Prevention of dislocation of the hip in children with cerebral palsy. The first ten years of a population-based prevention programme, *J Bone Joint Sug Br* 87:95–101, 2005.

Hagglund G, Wagner P: Development of spasticity with age in a total population of children with cerebral palsy, *BMC Musculoskelet Disord* 9:150, 2008.

Hanna SE, et al.: Measurement practices in pediatric rehabilitation: a survey of physical therapists, occupational therapists, and speech-language pathologists in Ontario, *Phys Occup Ther Pediatr* 27:25–42, 2007.

Hanna SE, et al.: Stability and decline in gross motor function among children and youth with cerebral palsy aged 2 to 21 years, *Dev Med Child Neurol* 51:295–302, 2009.

Healthy People 2020 [Internet]. Washington, DC, U.S. Department of Health and Human Services, Office of Disease Prevention and Health Promotion .

Hidecker M, Paneth N, Rosenbaum P, et al.: Developing and validating the Communication Function Classification System (CFCS) for individuals with cerebral palsy, *Dev Med Child Neurol* 53(8):704–710, 2011.

Himmelmann K, Hagberg G, Uvebrant P: The changing panorama of cerebral palsy in Sweden. X. Prevalence and origin in the birth-year period 1999-2002, *Acta Pediatr* 99:1337–1343, 2010.

Himmelmann K, Horber V, De La Cruz J, et al.: MRI classification system (MRICS) for children with cerebral palsy: development, reliability, and recommendations, *Dev Med Child Neurol* 59:57–64, 2017.

Himmelmann K, Uvebrant P: Function and neuroimaging in cerebral palsy: a population-based study, *Dev Med Child Neurol* 53(6):516–521, 2011.

Hintz SR, Kendrick DE, Wilson-Costello DE, et al.: Early-childhood neurodevelopmental outcomes are not improving for infants born at <25 weeks' gestational age, *Pediatrics* 127(1):62–70, 2011.

Hoffman RM, et al.: Changes in lower extremity strength may be related to the walking speed improvements in children with cerebral palsy after gait training, *Res Rev Disabil* 73:14–20, 2018.

Hoon AH, Tolley F: Cerebral palsy. In Batshaw ML, Roizen NJ, Lotrecchiano GR, editors: *Children with disabilities*, ed 7, Baltimore, 2013, Paul H. Brookes, pp 423–450.

Horstmann HM, Bleck EE: *Orthopaedic management in cerebral palsy*, ed 2, London, 2007, Mac Keith Press.

Huang IC, et al.: Vocational rehabilitation services and employment outcomes for adults with cerebral palsy in the United States, *Dev Med Child Neurol* 55:1000–1008, 2013.

Hurvitz EA, Fox MA, Haapala HJ, et al.: Adults with cerebral palsy who had a rhizotomy as a child: long-term follow-up, *PM & R* 2(9S):S3, 2010.

Jacobs SE, Berg M, Hunt R, et al.: Cooling for newborns with hypoxic ischaemic encephalopathy, *Cochrane Database Syst Rev* (1):CD003311, 2013.

Jacquemyn Y, et al.: The use of intravenous magnesium in non-preeclamptic pregnant women: fetal/neonatal neuroprotection, *Arch Gynecol Ostet* 291(5):969–975, 2015.

Jahnsen R, et al.: Fatigue in adults with cerebral palsy in Norway compared with the general population, *Dev Med Child Neurol* 45:296–303, 2003.

Kang H, Jung J, Yu J: Effects of hippotherapy on the sitting balance of children with cerebral palsy: a randomized control trial, *J Phys Ther Sci* 24:833–836, 2012.

Kenyon LK, Sleeper MD, Tovin MM: Sport-specific fitness testing and intervention for an adolescent with cerebral palsy: a case report, *Pediatr Phys Ther* 22:234–240, 2010.

Khandaker G, Smithers-Sheedy H, Islam J, et al.: Bangladesh Cerebral Palsy Register (BCPR): a pilot study to develop a national cerebral palsy (CP) register with surveillance of children for CP, *BMC Neurol* 15:173, 2015. doi:10.1186/s12883-015-0427-9.

Kim HS, et al.: Effect of muscle activity and botulinum toxin dilution volume on muscle paralysis, *Dev Med Child Neurol* 45:200–206, 2003.

Knights S, et al.: An innovative cycling exergame to promote cardiovascular fitness in youth with cerebral palsy, *Dev Neurorehabil* 19(2):135–140, 2016.

Kolman SE, et al.: Factors that predict overall health and quality of life in non-ambulatory individuals with cerebral palsy, *Iowa Orthop J* 38:147–152, 2018.

Korzeniewski SJ, Birbeck G, DeLano MC, Potchen MJ, Paneth N: A systematic review of neuroimaging for cerebral palsy, *J Child Neurol* 23:216–227, 2008.

Kuban KC, O'Shea TM, Allred EN, et al.: The breadth and type of systematic inflammation and the risk of adverse neurological outcomes in extremely low gestation newborns, *Pediatr Neurol* 52:42–48, 2015.

Kurz MJ, Stuberg W, DeJong SL: Body weight–supported treadmill training improves the regularity of the stepping kinematics in children with cerebral palsy, *Dev Neuro Rehabil* 14(2):87–93, 2011.

Labruyere R, et al.: Requirements for and impact of a serious game for neuro-pediatric robot-assisted gait training, *Res Dev Disabil* 34:3906–3915, 2013.

Leviton A, et al.: Two-hit model of brain damage in the very preterm newborn: small for gestational age and postnatal systemic inflammation, *Pediatr Res* 73:362–370, 2013.

Liljenqist K, O'Neil ME, Bjornson KF: Utilization of physical therapy services during transition for young people with cerebral palsy: a call for improved care into adulthood, *Phys Ther* 98:796–803, 2018.

Lin JP, Nardocci N: Recognizing the common origins of dystonia and the development of human movement: a manifesto of unmet needs in isolated childhood dystonias, *Front Neurol* 7:226, 2016.

Livingston MH, et al.: Quality of life among adolescents with cerebral palsy: what does the literature tell us? *Dev Med Child Neurol* 49:225–231, 2007.

Livingstone R, Paleg G: Practice considerations for the introduction and use of power mobility for children, *Dev Med Child Neurol* 56:210–222, 2014.

Lobo MA, et al.: Grounding early intervention: physical therapy cannot just be about motor skills anymore, *Phys Ther* 93:94–103, 2013.

Longo M, Hankins GDV: Defining cerebral palsy: pathogenesis, pathophysiology, and new intervention, *Minerva Gynecol* 61:421–429, 2009.

Lugli L, Balestri E, Berardi A, et al.: Brain cooling reduces the risk of post-neonatal epilepsy in newborns affected by moderate to severe hypoxic-ischemic encephalopathy, *Minerva Pediatr* July 2, 2018. doi:10.23736/S0026-4946.18.05224-6.

Lundh S, Nasic S, Riad J: Fatigue, quality of life and walking ability in adults with cerebral palsy, *Gait Posture* 61:1–6, 2018.

MacIntosh A, et al.: Ability-based balancing using the gross motor function measure in exergaming for youth with cerebral palsy, *Games Health J* 6:379–385, 2017.

MacLennan AH, Thompson, SC, Gecz J: Cerebral palsy: causes, pathways, and the role of genetic variants, *Am J Obstet Gynecol* 213(6):779–788, 2015. doi:10.1016/j.ajog.2015.05.034.

Maenner MJ, Blumberg SJ, Kogan MD, et al.: Prevalence of cerebral palsy and intellectual disability among children identified in two U.S. National Surveys, 2011-2013, *Ann Epidemiol* 26(3):222–226, 2016.

Majnemer A, et al.: Determinants of life quality in school-age children with cerebral palsy, *J Pediatr* 151(5):470–475, 2007.

Majnemer A, Shevell M, Law M, et al.: Participation and enjoyment of leisure activities in school-aged children with cerebral palsy, *Dev Med Child Neurol* 50:751–758, 2008.

Marconi V, Hachez H, Renders A, Docquier PL, Detrembleur C: Mechanical work and energy consumption in children with cerebral palsy after single-event multilevel surgery, *Gait Posture* 40:633–639, 2014.

Marques FJP, Teixeira MCS, Barra RR, et al.: Children born with congenital Zika syndrome display atypical gross motor development ad a higher risk for cerebral palsy, *J Child Neurol* 34:81–85, 2019. doi:10.1177/0883073818811234.

Mattern-Baxter K, Bellamy S, Mansoor JK: Effects of intensive locomotor treadmill training on young children with cerebral palsy, *Pediatr Phys Ther* 21:308–318, 2009.

McEwen IR: Assistive positioning as a control parameter of social-communicative interactions between students with profound multiple disabilities and classroom staff, *Phys Ther* 72:534–647, 1992.

McGinley JL, Dobson F, Ganeshalingham R, et al.: Single-event multilevel surgery for children with cerebral palsy: a systematic review, *Dev Med Child Neurol* 54(2):117–128, 2012.

McKean GL, Thurston WE, Scott CM: Bridging the divide between families and health professionals' perspectives on family-centered care, *Health Expect* 8:74–85, 2005.

McMichael G, Bainbridge MN, Haan E, et al.: Whole-exome sequencing points to considerable genetic heterogeneity of cerebral palsy, *Mol Psychiatr* 20:176–182, 2015.

Minamoto VB, et al.: Dramatic changes in muscle contractile and structural properties after two botulinum toxin injections, *Muscle Nerve* 52:649–657, 2015.

Moreau NG, et al.: Effectiveness of rehabilitation interventions to improve gait speed in children with cerebral palsy: systematic review and meta-analysis, *Phys Ther* 96:1938–1954, 2016.

Morgan C, Novak I, Badawi N: Enriched environments and motor outcomes in cerebral palsy: systematic review and meta-analysis, *Pediatrics* 132:e735–e746, 2013.

Morris C: A review of the efficacy of lower limb orthoses used for cerebral palsy, *Dev Med Child Neurol* 44:205–211, 2002.

Morris C, Bowers R, Ross K, Steven P, Phillips D: Orthotic management of cerebral palsy: recommendations from a consensus conference, *Neuro Rehabil* 28:37–46, 2011.

Myrden A, et al.: Trends in communicative access solutions for children with cerebral palsy, *J Child Neurol* 29:1108–1118, 2014.

Nahm NJ, Graham HK, Gormley ME, Georgiadis AG: Management of hypertonia in cerebral palsy, *Curr Opin Pediatr* 30:57–64, 2018.

Nelson KB: Causative factors in cerebral palsy, *Clin Obstet Gynecol* 51:749–762, 2008.

Nordmark E, Hagglund G, Lagergren J: Cerebral palsy in southern Sweden II. Gross motor function and disabilities, *Acta Paediatr* 90(11):1277–1282, 2001.

Nordmark E, et al.: Development of lower limb range of motion from early childhood to adolescence in cerebral palsy: a population study, *BMC Med* 7:65, 2009.

Novak I, Hines M, Goldsmith S, Barclay R: Clinical prognostic messages from a systematic review on cerebral palsy, *Pediatrics* 130(5):e1285–e1312, 2012.

Novak I, Morgan C, Adde L, et al.: Early, accurate diagnosis and early intervention in cerebral palsy: advances in diagnosis and treatment, *JAMA Pediatr* 171(9):897–907, 2017.

Orlin MN, et al.: Participation in home, extracurricular, and community activities among children and young people with cerebral palsy, *Dev Med Child Neurol* 52:160–166, 2010.

Oskoui M, et al.: An update on the prevalence of cerebral palsy: a systematic review and meta-analysis, *Dev Med Child Neurol* 55(6):509–519, 2013.

Owen E: The importance of being earnest about shank and thigh kinematics especially when using ankle-foot orthoses, *Prosthet Orthot Int* 34:254–269, 2010.

Paleg G, Smith B, Blickman L: Systematic review and evidence-based clinical recommendations for dosing of pediatric-supported standing programs, *Pediatr Phys Ther* 25(3):232–247, 2013.

Paleg G, Livingstone R: Outcomes of gait trainer use in home and school settings for children with motor impairments: a systematic review, *Clin Rehabil* 29:1077–1091, 2015.

Palisano RJ, et al.: Content validity of the expanded and revised Gross Motor Function Classification System, *Dev Med Child Neurol* 50:744–750, 2008.

Palisano RJ, et al.: Determinants of intensity of participation in leisure and recreational activities by children with cerebral palsy, *Dev Med Child Neurol* 53:142–149, 2011.

Palisano RJ, et al.: Development and reliability of a system to classify gross motor function in children with cerebral palsy, *Dev Med Child Neurol* 39:214–223, 1997.

Palisano RJ, et al.: Probability of walking, wheeled, and assisted mobility in children and adolescents with cerebral palsy, *Dev Med Child Neurol* 52:66–71, 2010.

Palisano RJ, et al.: Stability of the gross motor function classification system, manual ability classification system, and communication function classification system, *Dev Med Child Neurol* 60:1026–1032, 2018.

Park EY, Kim WH: Meta-analysis of the effect of strengthening interventions in individuals with cerebral palsy, *Res Dev Disabil* 35(2):239–249, 2014.

Peacock WJ, Arens LF, Berman B: Cerebral palsy spasticity: selective dorsal rhizotomy, *Pediatr Neurosci* 13:61–66, 1987.

Peterson MD, Gordon PM, Hurvitz EA: Chronic disease risk among adults with cerebral palsy: the role of premature sarcopoenia, obesity and sedentary behaviour, *Obes Rev* 14(2):171–182, 2013.

Phillips JP, Sullivan KF, Burtner PA, et al.: Ankle dorsiflexion fMRI in children with cerebral palsy undergoing intensive body-weight-supported treadmill training: a pilot study, *Dev Med Child Neurol* 49:39–44, 2007.

Ragonesi CB, Galloway JC: Short-term, early intensive power mobility training: case report of an infant at risk for cerebral palsy, *Pediatr Phys Ther* 24:141–148, 2012.

Rattey TE, Leahey L, Hyndman J, et al.: Recurrence after Achilles tendon lengthening in cerebral palsy, *J Pediatr Orthop* 134:184–147, 1993.

Reedman SE, et al.: Efficacy of participation-focused therapy on performance of physical activity participation goals and habitual physical activity in children with cerebral palsy: a randomized controlled trial, *Arch Phys Med Rehabil* 100(4):676–686, 2019.

Rehm RS, et al.: Parent and youth priorities during the transition to adulthood for youth with special health care needs and developmental disability, *ANS Adv Nurs Sci* 35:e57–e72, 2012.

Reid SM, Carlin JB, Reddihough DS: Distribution of motor types in cerebral palsy: how do registry data compare? *Dev Med Child Neurol* 53:233–238, 2011.

Reid SM, Dagia CD, Ditchfield MR, Carlin JB, Reddihough DS: Population based studies of brain imaging patterns in cerebral palsy, *Dev Med Child Neurol* 56:222–232, 2014.

Reid SM, Meehan E, McIntrye S, et al.: Temporal trends in cerebral palsy by impairment severity and birth gestation, *Dev Med Child Neurol* 58(Suppl 2):25–35, 2016. doi:10.1111/dmcn.13001.

Reuss ML, Paneth N, Pinto-Martin JA, Lorenz JM, Susser M: The relationship of transient hypothryroxinemia in preterm infants to neurologic development at two years of age, *N Engl J Med* 334:821–827, 1996.

Richards CL, Malouin F, Dumas F, et al.: Early and intensive treadmill locomotor training for young children with cerebral palsy: a feasibility study, *Pediatr Phys Ther* 9:158–165, 1997.

Rogozinski BM, et al.: The efficacy of the floor-reaction ankle-foot orthosis in children with cerebral palsy, *J Bone Jt Surg* 91:2440–2447, 2009.

Rosenbaum P, Gorter JW: The 'F-word' in childhood disability: I swear this is how we should think! *Child Care Health Dev* 38(4):457–463, 2011.

Rosenbaum P, Paneth N, Leviton A, et al.: A report: the definition and classification of cerebral palsy April 2006, *Dev Med Child Neurol Suppl* 109:8–14, 2007.

Salt A, Sargent J: Common visual problems in children with disability, *Arch Dis Child* 99:1163–1168, 2014.

Schindl MR, Forstner C, Kern H, Hesse S: Treadmill training with partial body weight support in nonambulatory patients with cerebral palsy, *Arch Phys Med Rehabil* 81:301–306, 2000.

Schranz D, et al.: Does home-based progressive resistance or high-intensity circuit training improve strength, function, activity or participation in children with cerebral palsy? *Arch Phys Med Rehabil* 99(12):2457–2464.e4, 2018.

Schwartz MH, Rozumalski A, Steele KM: Dynamic motor control is associated with treatment outcomes for children with cerebral palsy, *Dev Med Child Neurol* 58:1139–1146, 2016.

Sellier E, Platt MJ, Anderson GL, et al.: Decreasing prevalence in cerebral palsy: a multi-site European population–based study, 1980 to 2003, *Dev Med Child Neurol* 58(1):85–92, 2016.

Shepherd RB, editor: *Cerebral palsy in infancy*, London, 2014, Churchill Livingstone.

Shumway-Cook A, Woollacott MH: Development of postural control. In Shumway-Cook A, Woollacott MH, editors: *Motor control: translating research into clinical practice*, ed 5, Philadelphia, 2017, Wolters Kluwer, pp 183–205.

Slaman J, et al.: Can a lifestyle intervention improve physical fitness in adolescents and young adults with spastic cerebral palsy? A randomized control trial, *Arch Phys Med Rehabil* 95:1646–1655, 2014.

Soo B, et al.: Hip displacement in cerebral palsy, *J Bone Joint Surg Am* 88:121–129, 2006.

Sun D, et al.: Clinical characteristics and functional status of children with different subtypes of dyskinetic cerebral palsy, *Medicine* 97(21):e10817, 2018.

Surveillance of Cerebral Palsy Europe: A collaboration of cerebral palsy surveys and registers. *Dev Med Child Neurol* 42:816–824, 2000.

Tan SS, et al.: Long-term trajectories of health-related quality of life in individuals with cerebral palsy: a multicenter longitudinal study, *Arch Phys Med Rehabil* 95:2029–2039, 2014.

Tardieu C, Lespargot A, Tabary C, Bret MD: For how long must the soleus muscle be stretched each day to prevent contracture? *Dev Med Child Neurol* 30:3–10, 1988.

Taylor NF, et al.: Progressive resistive training and mobility-related function in young people with cerebral palsy: a randomized controlled trial, *Dev Med Child Neurol* 55:806–812, 2013.

Tervahauta MH, Girolami GL, Oberg GK: Efficacy of constraint-induced movement therapy compared with bimanual intensive training in children with unilateral cerebral palsy: a systematic review, *Clin Rehabil* 31:1445–1456, 2017.

Tefft D, Guerette P, Furumasu J: The impact of early powered mobility on parental stress, negative emotions, and family social interactions, *Phys Occup Ther Pediatr* 31:4–15, 2011.

Terwiel M, et al.: Family-centered service: differences in what parents of children with cerebral palsy rate important, *Child Health Care Dev* 43:663–669, 2017.

Theroux MC, DiCindio S: Major surgical procedures in children with cerebral palsy, *Anesthesiology Clin* 32:63–81, 2014.

Tseng SH, Chen HC, Tam KW: Systematic review and meta-analysis of the effect of equine assisted activities and therapies on gross motor outcome in children with cerebral palsy, *Disabil Rehabil* 35:89–99, 2013.

US Department of Health and Human Services: *Healthy People 2020*. Available at: http://www.healthypeople.gov/.

Valentín-Gudiol M, et al.: Treadmill interventions in children under six years of age at risk of neuromotor delay, *Cochrane Database Syst Rev* 7:CD009242, July 29, 2017. doi:10.1002/14651858.CD009242.pub3.

Van Gorp M, et al.: Long-term course of difficulty in participation of individuals with cerebral palsy age 16 to 34 years: a prospective cohort study, *Dev Med Child Neurol* 61:194–203, 2019.

Verschuren O, et al.: Muscle strengthening in children with adolescents with spastic cerebral palsy: consideration for future resistance protocols, *Phys Ther* 91:1130–1139, 2011.

Verschuren O, Peterson MD, Balemans ACJ, Hurvitz EA: Exercise and physical activity recommendations for people with cerebral palsy, *Dev Med Child Neurol* 58:798–808, 2016.

Vogtle LK: Employment outcomes for adults with cerebral palsy: an issue that needs to be addressed, *Dev Med Child Neurol* 55:973, 2013.

Wagner M, Newman L, Cameto R, et al.: *An overview of finding from Wave 2 of the National Longitudinal Transition Study-2 (NLTS2). National Center for Special Education Research*, Menlo Park, CA, 2006, SRI International.

Wake M, Salmon L, Reddihough D: Health status of Australian children with mild to severe cerebral palsy: cross-sectional survey using the Child Health Questionnaire, *Dev Med Child Neurol* 45:194–199, 2003.

Wanigasinghe J, Reid SM, Mackay MT, et al.: Epilepsy in hemiplegic cerebral palsy due to perinatal arterial ischaemic stroke, *Dev Med Child Neurol* 52(11):1022–1027, 2010.

Watt JM, Robertson CM, Grace MG: Early prognosis for ambulation of neonatal intensive care survivors with cerebral palsy, *Dev Med Child Neurol* 31:766–773, 1989.

Westberry DE, et al.: Impact of ankle-foot orthoses on static foot alignment in children with cerebral palsy, *J Bone Jt Surg* 89:806–813, 2007.

Willoughby KL, Dodd KJ, Shields N: A systematic review of the effectiveness of treadmill training for children with cerebral palsy, *Disabil Rehabil* 31(24):1971–1979, 2009.

Willoughby KL, Dodd KJ, Shields N, Foley S: Efficacy of partial body weight–supported treadmill training compared with overground walking practice for children with cerebral palsy: a randomized clinical trial, *Arch Phys Med Rehabil* 91:333–339, 2010.

Wright FV, et al.: How do changes in body functions and structures, activity, and participation relate in children with cerebral palsy? *Dev Med Child Neurol* 50:283–289, 2008.

Wright M, Palisano RJ: Cerebral palsy. In Palisano RJ, Orlin MN, Schreiber J, editors: *Campbell's physical therapy for children*, ed 5, St. Louis, 2017, Elsevier Inc, pp 447–487.

Wu YW, et al.: Prognosis for ambulation in cerebral palsy: a population-based study, *Pediatrics* 114:1264–1271, 2004.

Yin Foo R, Guppy M, Johnston LM: Intelligence assessments for children with cerebral palsy: a systematic review, *Dev Med Child Neurol* 55:911–918, 2013.

Zadnikar M, Kastrin A: Effects of hippotherapy and therapeutic horseback riding on postural control or balance in children with cerebral palsy: a meta-analysis, *Dev Med Child Neurol* 53:684–691, 2011.

Myelomeningocele

After reading this chapter, the student will be able to:

1. Describe the incidence, prevalence, etiology, and clinical manifestations of myelomeningocele (MMC).
2. Describe common complications seen in children with MMC.
3. Discuss the medical and surgical management of children with MMC.
4. Articulate the role of the physical therapist assistant in the treatment of children with MMC.
5. Describe appropriate interventions for children with MMC.
6. Recognize the importance of functional training throughout the lifespan of a child with MMC.

INTRODUCTION

Myelomeningocele (MMC) is a complex congenital anomaly. Although it primarily affects the nervous system, it secondarily involves the musculoskeletal and urologic systems. MMC is a specific form of myelodysplasia that is the result of faulty embryologic development of the spinal cord, especially the lower segments. The caudal end of the neural tube or primitive spinal cord fails to close before the 28th day of gestation (Fig. 7.1, *A*). Definitions of basic myelodysplastic defects can be found in Table 7.1. Accompanying the spinal cord dysplasia (abnormal tissue growth) is a bony defect known as spina bifida, which occurs when the posterior vertebral arches fail to close in the midline to form a spinous process (Fig. 7.1, *C–E*). The normal spine at birth is seen in Fig. 7.1, *B*. The term *spina bifida* is often used to mean both the bony defect and the various forms of myelodysplasia. When the bifid spine occurs in isolation, with no involvement of the spinal cord or meninges, it is called *spina bifida occulta* (Fig. 7.1, *C*). Usually, no neurologic impairment occurs in persons with spina bifida occulta. The area of skin over the defect may be marked by a dimple or tuft of hair and can go unnoticed. In *spina bifida cystica*, patients have a visible cyst protruding from the opening caused by the bony defect. The cyst may be covered with skin or meninges. This condition is also called *spina bifida aperta*, meaning open or visible. If the cyst contains only cerebrospinal fluid (CSF) and meninges, it is referred to as a *meningocele* because the "cele" (cyst) is covered by the meninges (Fig. 7.1, *D*). When the malformed spinal cord is present within the cyst, the lesion is referred to as a *myelomeningocele* (Fig. 7.1, *E*). In MMC, the cyst may be covered with only meninges or with skin. Motor paralysis and sensory loss are present below the level of the MMC. The most common location for MMC is in the lumbar region.

INCIDENCE

The incidence of MMC has declined over the last decade due to better nutrition and increased screening. However, MMC is still the most common neural tube defect (NTD). About 1645 babies are born annually in the United States with MMC according to the Centers for Disease Control and Prevention (2018). Incidence in the United States has decreased to 1.9 per 10,000 live births due to folic acid fortification (Swaroop and Dias, 2011). If a sibling has already been born with MMC, the risk of recurrence in the family is 2% to 3%. Worldwide incidence of all NTDs occurs at a rate of 0.17 to 6.39 per 1000 live births (Bowman et al., 2009a). These figures include defects of closure of the neural tube at the cephalic end, as well as in the thoracic, lumbar, and sacral regions. China continues to have the highest prevalence of NTDs (Zaganjor et al., 2016). Prevalence is the number of people with a disorder in a population.

The lack of closure cephalically results in *anencephaly*, or failure of the brain to develop beyond the brain stem. These infants rarely survive for any length of time after birth. An *encephalocele* results when the brain tissue protrudes from the skull. It usually occurs in the occipital and results in visual impairment. Prevalence of NTDs is highest in Hispanic people (3.80 per 10,000), followed by non-Hispanic whites (3.09 per 10,000), and finally non-Hispanic blacks and African Americans (2.73 per 10,000) (Centers for Disease Control and Prevention, 2018).

ETIOLOGY

NTDs including spina bifida and MMC are multifactorial, that is they are caused by a combination of environmental and genetic factors (Greene and Copp, 2014). Despite the fact that 60% to 70% of NTDs have a genetic component, there is

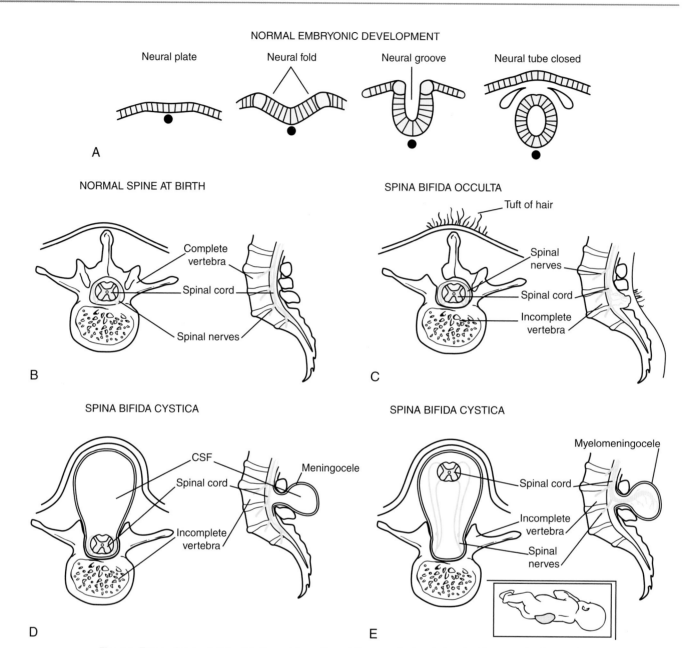

Fig. 7.1 Types of spina bifida. **(A)** Normal formation of the neural tube during the first month of gestation. **(B)** Complete closure with normal development in cross-section on the left and in longitudinal section on the right. **(C)** Incomplete vertebral closure with no cyst, marked by a tuft of hair. **(D)** Incomplete vertebral closure with a cyst of meninges and cerebrospinal fluid (CSF)—meningocele. **(E)** Incomplete vertebral closure with a cyst containing a malformed spinal cord—myelomeningocele.

TABLE 7.1	**Basic Definitions of Myelodysplastic Defects**
Defect	**Definition**
Spina bifida occulta	Vertebral defect in which posterior elements of the vertebral arch fail to close; no sac; vertebral defect usually not associated with an abnormality of the spinal cord
Spina bifida cystica	Vertebral defect with a protruding cyst of meninges or spinal cord and meninges
Meningocele	Cyst containing cerebrospinal fluid and meninges and usually covered with epithelium; clinical symptoms variable
Myelomeningocele	Cyst containing cerebrospinal fluid, meninges, spinal cord, and possibly nerve roots; cord incompletely formed or malformed; most common in the lumbar area; the higher the lesion, the more deficits present

Modified from Ryan KD, Ploski C, Emans JB: Myelodysplasia: the musculoskeletal problem: habilitation from infancy to adulthood, *Phys Ther* 71:935–946, 1991. With permission of the American Physical Therapy Association.

a lag in genetic research in this area. New genetic techniques such as next-generation sequencing and genome association have not yet been used to explore causes of spina bifida and MMC (Lupo et al., 2017). Following mandatory fortification of food with folic acid, prevalence of MMC decreased 31% in the United States (Boulet et al., 2008). This decline has held steady since the initial reduction in 1999–2000 (Williams et al., 2015). It is recommended that a woman with a history of having had a child with an NTD takes 4 mg of folic acid a day at least 3 months before conception, and throughout the first trimester. Those with no positive history should take 0.4 mg of folic acid 3 months before conception. Obesity and diabetes have been identified as risk factors for NTDs (Greene and Copp, 2014). Single-gene disorders and trisomy 13, 18, and 21 have been associated with MMC (Luthy et al., 1991), and a few genes have been identified that may play a role in MMC (Copp and Greene, 2010).

PRENATAL DIAGNOSIS

An NTD can be diagnosed at 18 weeks gestation (Sutton, 2008) prenatally by testing for levels of alpha-fetoprotein. If levels of the protein are too high, it may mean that the fetus has an open NTD. This suspicion can be confirmed by high-resolution ultrasonography to visualize the vertebral defect. When an open NTD is detected, the infant should be delivered by cesarean section before labor begins to decrease the risk of infection and further damage to the spinal cord during the delivery process. This practice has been shown to lessen the paralysis (Hinderer et al., 2017). Chromosome analysis of cells in the amniotic fluid can confirm if there is an associated chromosome error and provide more information to parents who are considering terminating the pregnancy. Because of improved medical care, survival has increased and so has prevalence of MMC in the population, even though the likelihood of having an infant with MMC has declined.

Fetal surgery to repair the defect in MMC has been performed in selected centers since 2003 (Walsh and Adzick, 2003; Tulipan, 2003). The goal of the intrauterine surgery is to decrease the need for placing a shunt for hydrocephalus, which typically develops after closure of the MMC, and to improve lower extremity function. In the recent randomized control trial of prenatal versus postnatal repair, fetal surgery was performed before 26 weeks of gestation (Adzick et al., 2011). The Management of Myelomeningocele Study (MoMS) compared the efficacy and safety between standard postnatal repair and prenatal repair. Results were promising and an effort was made to duplicate results in other centers. The original MoMS results (Adzick et al., 2011) found that the need for shunt surgery was reduced, and improved motor outcomes were demonstrated at 30 months in the group who had prenatal surgical repair. However, the results in the ideal setting were not generalizable to other centers. Fetal repair was associated with increased maternal and fetal risks. The MoMS 2 study is presently looking at long-term outcomes and investigating modifications to closure techniques (Heurer et al., 2017).

CLINICAL FEATURES

Neurologic Defects and Impairments

The infant with MMC presents with motor and sensory impairments as a result of the spinal cord malformation. The extent of the impairment is directly related to the level of the cyst and the level of the spinal cord defect. Unlike in complete spinal cord injuries, which have a relatively straightforward relationship between the level of bony vertebra involvement and the underlying cord involvement, no clear relationship is present in infants with MMC. Some bony defects may involve more than one vertebral level. The spinal cord may be partially formed or malformed, or part of the spinal cord may be intact at one of the involved levels and may have innervated muscles below the MMC. If the nerve roots are damaged or the cord is dysplastic, the infant will have a flaccid type of motor paralysis with lack of sensation, the classic lower motor neuron presentation. However, if part of the spinal cord below the MMC is intact and has innervated muscles, the potential exists for a spastic type of motor paralysis. In some cases, the child may actually demonstrate an area of flaccidity at the level of the MMC, with spasticity present below the flaccid muscles. Either type of motor paralysis presents inherent difficulty in managing range of motion and in using orthoses for ambulation.

Functional Movement Related to Level

In general, the higher the level of the lesion, the greater the degree of muscular impairment and the less likely the child will ambulate functionally. A child with thoracic involvement at T12 has some control of the pelvis because of the innervation of the quadratus and complete innervation of the abdominal muscles. The gluteus maximus would not be active because it is innervated by L5 to S1. A high lumbar level lesion (L1 to L2) affects the lower extremities, but hip flexors and hip adductors are innervated. A midlumbar level lesion at L3 means that the child can flex at the hips and can extend the knees but has no ankle or toe movement. In a low lumbar level of paralysis at L4 or L5, the child adds the ability to flex the knees and dorsiflex the ankles, but only weakly extend the hips. Children with sacral level paralysis at S1 have weak plantar flexion for push-off and good hip abduction. To be classified as having an S2 or S3 level lesion, the child's plantar flexors must have a muscle grade of at least 3/5 and the gluteal muscles a grade of 4/5 on a manual muscle test scale (Hinderer et al., 2017). The lesion is considered "no loss" when the child has normal function of bowel and bladder and normal strength in the lower extremity muscles.

Musculoskeletal Impairments

Muscle paralysis results in an impairment of voluntary movement of the trunk and lower extremities. Children with the classic lower motor neuron presentation of flaccid paralysis have no lower extremity motion, and the legs are drawn into a frog-leg position by gravity. Because of the lack of voluntary movement, the lower extremities assume a position of comfort: hip abduction, external rotation, knee flexion, and ankle

TABLE 7.2 Function Related to Level of Lesion

Level of Lesion	Muscle Function	Potential Deformity
Thoracic	Trunk weakness T7–T9 upper abdominals T9–T12 lower abdominals T12 has weak quadratus lumborum	Positional deformities of hips, knees, and ankles secondary to frog-leg posture
High lumbar (L1–L2)	Unopposed hip flexors and some adductors	Hip flexion, adduction Hip dislocation Lumbar lordosis Knee flexion and plantar flexion
Midlumbar (L3)	Strong hip flexors, adductors Weak hip rotators Antigravity knee extension	Hip dislocation, subluxation Genu recurvatum
Low lumbar (L4)	Strong quadriceps, medial knee flexors against gravity, ankle dorsiflexion and inversion	Equinovarus, calcaneovarus, or calcaneocavus foot
Low lumbar (L5)	Weak hip extension, abduction Good knee flexion against gravity Weak plantar flexion with eversion	Equinovarus, calcaneovalgus, or calcaneocavus foot
Sacral (S1)	Good hip abductors, weak plantar flexors	–
Sacral (S2–S3)	Good hip extensors and ankle plantar flexors	–

plantar flexion. Table 7.2 provides a list of typical deformities caused by muscle imbalances seen with a given level of lesion. Rather than memorizing the table, one would be better served to review the appropriate anatomy and kinesiology and determine in what direction the limbs would be pulled if only certain muscles were innervated. For example, if there was innervation of only the anterior tibialis (L4 motor level) with no opposing pull from the gastrocnemius or posterior tibialis, in what position would the foot be held? It would be pulled into dorsiflexion and inversion, resulting in a calcaneovarus foot posture. In this situation, what muscle is most likely to become shortened? This may be one of the few instances in which the anterior tibialis needs to be stretched to maintain its resting length to allow for a plantigrade foot.

The child with MMC may also have congenital lower limb deformities, in addition to being at risk of acquiring additional deformities because of muscle imbalances. These deformities may include hip dislocation, hip dysplasia and subluxation, genu varus, and genu valgus. Congenital foot deformities associated with MMC are talipes equinovarus or congenital clubfoot, pes equinus or flatfoot, and convex pes valgus or rocker-bottom foot, with a vertical talus. These are depicted in Fig. 7.2. Clubfoot is the most common foot deformity seen in children with MMC (Swaroop and Dias, 2011). The physical therapist may perform taping and gentle manipulation during the early management of this foot problem. The physical therapist assistant may or may not be involved with providing gentle corrective range of motion. Because of pressure problems over the bony prominences, splinting is recommended instead of serial casting. Surgical correction of the foot deformity is probably indicated in all but the mildest cases (Swaroop and Dias, 2011).

Most children with MMC begin to ambulate between 1 and 2 years of age. A plantigrade foot, that is one that is flat and in contact with the ground, is essential to ensure ambulation. In addition, the foot needs to be able to exhibit 10 degrees of dorsiflexion for toe clearance. This does not, however, have to be active range. A plantigrade foot is also important for the nonambulatory child so that the foot can be positioned correctly while seated or in a lying position to prevent undue pressures on an insensate foot.

If the child has a spastic type of motor paralysis, limb movements may result from muscle spasms, but such movements are not under the child's voluntary control. Various limb positions may result, depending on which muscles are spastic. The deforming forces will be stronger if spasticity is present. For example, in a child with an L1 or L2 motor level, the hip flexors and adductors may pull so strongly because of increased tone that the hip is dislocated. Muscle imbalances owing to the level of innervation may be intensified by increased tone. Contractures can interfere with function such as maneuvering a wheelchair, as well as put the person at risk for skin breakdown or interfere with lying down comfortably.

Osteoporosis

As in adults with spinal cord injury, the loss of the ability to produce a muscle contraction is devastating for voluntary movement, but it also has ramifications for the ongoing development and function of the skeletal system. The skeletal system, including the long bones and axial skeleton, depends on muscle pull and weight-bearing to maintain structural integrity and to help balance normal bone loss with new bone production. Children with MMC, like adults with spinal cord injury, are at risk of developing *osteoporosis*. Osteoporosis predisposes a bone to fracture; therefore children with MMC are at greater risk of developing fractures secondary to loss of muscle strength and inactivity (Dosa et al., 2007). Walking ability is a significant determinant of bone

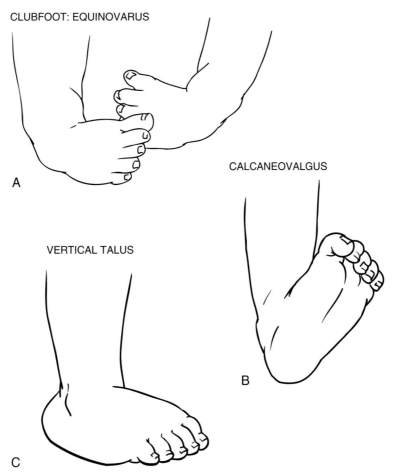

Fig. 7.2 **(A-C)** Common lower extremity deformities.

density in children with MMC (Ausili et al., 2008). A recent review found that the risk of low bone mineral density and fractures was related to higher neurologic levels, inactivity, previous spontaneous fracture, not walking, and contractures (Marrieos et al., 2012). Researchers have found that children who are household or community ambulators have higher bone mineral density than children who walk only therapeutically (Rosenstein et al., 1987).

Three levels of ambulation have been identified by Hoffer et al. (1973): therapeutic, household, and community. These levels describe the type and location in which the ambulation takes place. Therapeutic means that the person requires orthoses, assistive devices, and assistance to ambulate. This level has also been described as "exercise" walking and is usually done within a therapy setting. Household ambulators can walk independently within the home but still require orthoses and assistive devices. They can manage some barriers within the home. The community level indicates that the person is independent in the community and can handle barriers with or without assistive devices or orthoses. Some community ambulators choose to use a wheelchair for long distance.

Neuropathic Fractures

Twenty percent of children with MMC are likely to experience a neuropathic fracture (Lock and Aronson, 1989). *Neuropathic*

fractures relate to the underlying neurologic disorder. Paralyzed muscles cannot generate forces through long bones, so that essentially no weight-bearing takes place, with resulting osteoporosis. Osteoporosis makes it easier for the bone to fracture. Low bone density for age is strongly related to risk for fractures (Yasar et al., 2018). The most common fracture in childhood occurs in the distal femur (Trinh et al., 2017). Fracture risk is greater in nonambulatory children. Proper nutrition is always important but even more so if the child is taking seizure medications that disrupt the metabolism of vitamin D and calcium. Adults with MMC have a lower risk for fracture than children (Trinh et al., 2017).

The following clinical example illustrates another possible situation involving a neuropathic fracture. Once, when placing the lower extremities of a child with MMC into his braces, a clinician felt warmth along the child's tibial crest. The child was biracial, so no redness was apparent, but a definite separation was noted along the tibia. The child was in no pain or distress. His mother later recounted that it had been particularly difficult to put his braces on the day before. A radiograph confirmed the therapist's clinical suspicion that the child had a fracture. The limb was put in a cast until the fracture healed. While the child was in his cast, therapy continued, with an emphasis on upper extremity strengthening and trunk balance. Presence of a cast protecting a fracture is usually not an indication to curtail activity in children with MMC. In fact, it may spark creativity on the part of the rehabilitation team to come up with ways to combat postural insecurity and loss of antigravity muscle strength while the child's limb is immobilized.

Spinal Deformities

Children with MMC can have congenital or acquired *scoliosis*. *Congenital scoliosis* is usually related to vertebral anomalies, such as a hemivertebra, that are present in addition to the bifid spine. This type of scoliosis is inflexible. *Acquired scoliosis* results from muscle imbalances in the trunk, producing a flexible scoliosis. A rapid onset of scoliosis can also occur secondary to a tethered spinal cord or to a condition called hydromyelia. These conditions are explained later in the text. The physical therapist assistant must be observant of any postural changes in treating a child with MMC. Acquired scoliosis should be managed by some type of orthosis until spinal fixation with instrumentation is appropriate. Children with MMC go through puberty at a younger age than typically developing children, and this allows for earlier spinal surgery with little loss of the child's mature trunk height.

Other spinal deformities, such as *kyphosis* and *lordosis*, may also be seen in these children. The kyphosis may be in the thoracic area or may encompass the entire spine, as seen in a baby. The lordosis in the lumbar area may be exaggerated or reversed. Spinal deformities of all kinds are more likely to be present in children with higher-level lesions.

Spinal alignment and potential for deformity must always be considered when one uses developmentally appropriate positions, such as sitting and standing. If the child cannot maintain trunk alignment muscularly, then some type of orthosis may be indicated (Fig. 7.3). The child's sitting posture should be documented during therapy and sitting positions to be used at home should be identified. Spinal

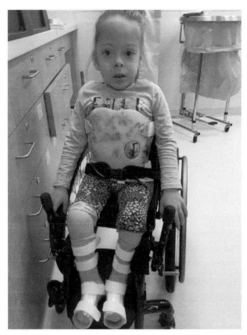

Fig. 7.3 Use of a thoracolumbar orthosis by a child with thoracolumbar myelomeningocele. (From Webster JB, Murphy DP, editors: *Atlas of orthoses and assistive devices*, ed 5, Philadelphia, 2019, Elsevier Inc, p. 356.)

deformities may not always be preventable, but attention must be paid to the effect of gravity on a malleable spine when it is in vulnerable developmental postures.

Arnold-Chiari Malformation

In addition to the spinal cord defect in MMC, most children with this neuromuscular problem have an *Arnold-Chiari type II malformation*. The Arnold-Chiari malformation involves the cerebellum, the medulla, and the cervical part of the spinal cord (Fig. 7.4). Because the cerebellum is not fully

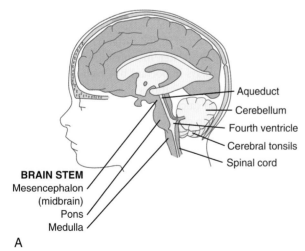

Fig. 7.4 **(A)** Normal brain with patent cerebrospinal fluid circulation. **(B)** Arnold-Chiari type II malformation with enlarged ventricles, a condition that predisposes a child with myelomeningocele to hydrocephalus. The brain stem, the fourth ventricle, part of the cerebellum, and the cerebral tonsils are displaced downward through the foramen magnum, and this leads to blockage of cerebrospinal fluid flow. Additionally, pressure on the brain stem housing the cranial nerves may result in nerve palsies. (From Goodman CC, Boissonnault WG, Fuller KS: *Pathology: implications for the physical therapist,* St. Louis, 2015, WB Saunders.)

developed, the hindbrain is downwardly displaced through the foramen magnum. The flow of CSF is obstructed, thus causing fluid to build up within the ventricles of the brain. The abnormal accumulation of CSF results in hydrocephalus, as shown in Fig. 7.4. A child with spina bifida, MMC, and an Arnold-Chiari type II malformation has a greater than 90% chance of developing hydrocephalus. The Arnold-Chiari type II malformation may also affect cranial nerve and brain stem function because of the pressure exerted on these areas by the accumulation of CSF within the ventricular system. Clinically, this involvement may be manifested by swallowing difficulties.

Hydrocephalus

Hydrocephalus can occur in children with MMC with or without the Arnold-Chiari malformation. Hydrocephalus is treated neurosurgically with the placement of a ventriculo-peritoneal shunt, which drains excess CSF into the peritoneal cavity (Fig. 7.5). You will be able to palpate the shunt tubing along the child's neck as it goes under the clavicle and down the chest wall. All shunt systems have a one-way valve that allows fluid to flow out of the ventricles but prevents backflow. The child's movements are generally not restricted

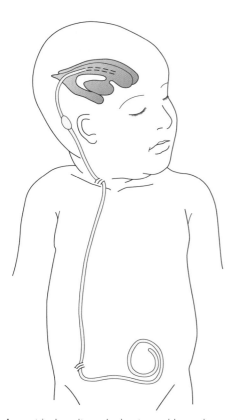

Fig. 7.5 A ventriculoperitoneal shunt provides primary drainage of cerebrospinal fluid from the ventricles to an extracranial compartment, usually either the heart or the abdominal or peritoneal cavity, as shown here. Extra tubing is left in the extracranial site to uncoil as the child grows. A unidirectional valve designed to open at a predetermined intraventricular pressure and to close when the pressure falls below that level prevents backflow of fluid. (From Goodman CC, Boissonnault WG, Fuller KS: *Pathology: implications for the physical therapist,* St. Louis, 2015, WB Saunders.)

unless such restriction is specified by the physician. However, the child should avoid spending prolonged periods of time in a head-down position, such as hanging upside down, because this may disrupt the valve function or may interfere with the flow of the fluid (Williamson, 1987). Knowledge of signs of shunt malfunction is important when working with children with MMC. "Approximately 40% of new shunts fail within a year, and 80% fail within 10 years" (Sandler, 2010).

Shunts can become blocked or infected, so the clinician must be aware of signs that could indicate shunt malfunction. These signs are listed in Table 7.3. Ninety-five percent of children with shunts will have at least one shunt revision (Bowman et al., 2001). Many of the signs and symptoms, such as irritability, seizures, vomiting, and lethargy, are seen regardless of the age of the child. Other signs are unique to the age of the child. Infants may display bulging of the fontanels secondary to increased intracranial pressure. The sunset sign of the eyes refers to the finding that the iris is only partially visible because of the infant's downward gaze. Older children may exhibit personality or memory changes. Shunt malfunction can occur years after implantation even without symptoms (Tomlinson and Sugarman, 1995).

Central Nervous System Deterioration

In addition to being vigilant about watching for signs of shunt malfunction as the child grows, the clinician must investigate any change in motor and sensory status or functional abilities because it may indicate neurologic deterioration. Common causes of such deterioration are hydromyelia and a tethered spinal cord. All areas of the child's function, such as mobility, activities of daily living (ADLs), and school performance, can be affected by either of these two conditions.

TABLE 7.3 **Signs and Symptoms of Shunt Malfunction**			
Sign or Symptom	**Infants**	**Toddlers**	**School-Age Children**
Bulging fontanel	X		
Sunset sign of eyes	X		
Excessive rate of growth of head circumference	X		
Thinning of skin over scalp	X		
Irritability	X	X	X
Seizures	X	X	X
Vomiting	X	X	X
Lethargy	X	X	X
Headaches	X	X	
Edema, redness along shunt tract	X	X	X
Personality changes			X
Memory changes			X

Hydromyelia

Hydromyelia is characterized by an accumulation of CSF in the central canal of the spinal cord. The condition can cause rapidly progressing scoliosis, upper extremity weakness, and increased tone. Other investigators have reported sensory changes and ascending motor loss in the lower extremities (Krosschell and Pesavento, 2013). The incidence of hydromyelia in children with MMC ranges from 20% to 80% (Byrd et al., 1991). Any time a child presents with rapidly progressing scoliosis, alert your supervising therapist, who will inform the child's physician so that the cause of the symptoms can be investigated and treated quickly. Scoliosis in this disorder is often an indication of a progressing neurologic problem.

Tethered Spinal Cord

The relationship of the spinal cord to the vertebral column normally changes with age. At birth, the end of the spinal cord is at the level of L3, rising to L1 in adulthood as a result of skeletal growth. Because of scarring from the surgical repair of the back lesion, adhesions can form and can anchor the spinal cord at the lesion site. The spinal cord is then tethered and is not free to move upward within the vertebral canal as the child grows. Progressive neurologic dysfunction, such as a decline in motor and sensory function, pain, or loss of previous bowel and bladder control, may occur. Other signs may include rapidly progressive scoliosis, increased tone in the lower extremities, and changes in gait pattern. The mean age of onset of tethered cord syndrome is the early 30s to early 40s (Hertzler et al., 2010). Prompt surgical correction can usually prevent any permanent neurologic damage and relieve pain (Schoenmakers et al., 2003; Bowman et al., 2009b). Any deterioration in neuromuscular or urologic performance from the child's baseline or the rapid onset of scoliosis should immediately be reported to the supervising physical therapist.

Sensory Impairment

Sensory impairment from MMC is not as straightforward in children as it is in adults with a spinal cord injury. The sensory losses exhibited by children are less likely to correspond to the motor level of paralysis. Do not presume that because one part of a dermatome is intact, the entire dermatome is intact to sensation. "Skip" areas that have no sensation may be present within an innervated dermatome (Hinderer et al., 2017). Often, the therapist has tested for only light touch or pinprick because the child with MMC is usually unable to differentiate between the two sensations. If the therapist has tested for vibration, intact areas of sensation may be present below those perceived as insensate for either light touch or pinprick (Hinderer and Hinderer, 1990).

The functional implications of loss of sensation are enormous. An increased potential exists for damaging the skin and underlying tissue secondary to extremes of temperature and normal pressure. A child with MMC loses the ability to feel that he has too much pressure on the buttocks from sitting too long. This loss of sensation can lead to the development of pressure ulcers. The consequences of loss of time from school and play and of independent function because of a pressure ulcer can be immeasurable. The plan of care must include teaching skin safety and inspection, as well as pressure-relief techniques. These techniques are essential to good primary prevention of complications. The use of seat cushions and other joint protective devices is advised. Insensitive skin needs to be protected as the child learns to move around and explore the environment. The family needs to be made aware of the importance of making regular skin inspection part of the daily routine. As the child grows and shoes and braces are introduced, skin integrity must be a high priority when one initiates a wearing schedule for any orthotic devices.

Bowel and Bladder Dysfunction

Most children with MMC have some degree of bowel and bladder dysfunction. The sacral levels of the spinal cord, S2 to S4, innervate the bladder and are responsible for voiding and defecation reflexes. With loss of motor and sensory functions, the child has no sensation of bladder fullness or of wetness. The reflex emptying and the inhibition of voiding can be problematic. If tone in the bladder wall is increased, the bladder cannot store the typical amount of urine and empties reflexively. Special attention must be paid to the treatment of urinary dysfunction because mismanagement can result in kidney damage. By the age of 3 or 4 years, most children begin to work on gaining urinary continence by using clean intermittent catheterization. By 6 years, the child should be independent in self-intermittent catheterization. Functional prerequisites for this skill include sitting balance with no hand support and the ability to do a toilet transfer. These functional activities should be incorporated into early and middle stages of physical therapy management.

Latex Allergy

It has been estimated that up to 50% of children with MMC are allergic to latex (Cremer et al., 2002; Sandler, 2010). This may be because the infant with MMC is exposed repeatedly to latex products. Exposure to latex can produce an anaphylactic reaction that can be life-threatening with the risk increasing as the child gets older (Mazon et al., 2000). All contact with latex products should be avoided from the beginning, including catheters, surgical gloves, and Theraband (Akron, OH). Any surgery should be performed in a latex-free environment. Toys that contain latex, such as rubber balls and balloons, should be avoided. With the concentrated effort to avoid all latex, children born more recently have lower rates of latex sensitivity (Blumchen et al., 2010). However, therapists in the community should be aware that children with MMC need to avoid exposure to latex products.

Physical Therapy Intervention

Three stages of care are used to describe the continuum of physical therapy management of the child with myelodysplasia. Although similarities exist between adults with spinal cord injuries and children with congenital neurologic spinal deficits, inherent differences are also present. The biggest difference is that the anomaly occurs during development of the body and its systems. Therefore, one of the major foci of a physical therapy plan of care should be to minimize the impact and ongoing development of bony deformation, postural changes, and abnormal tone. Optimizing development encompasses not only motor development but cognitive and social-emotional development as well. Other therapeutic considerations are the same as for an adult who has sustained a spinal cord injury, such as strengthening the upper extremities, developing sitting and standing balance, fostering locomotion, promoting self-care, encouraging safety and personal hygiene, and teaching functional mobility, pressure relief, and fostering independence.

First Stage of Physical Therapy Intervention

This stage includes the acute care the infant receives after birth and up to the time of ambulation. Initially, after the birth of a child with MMC, parents deal with multiple medical practitioners, each with his or her own contribution to the health of the infant. The neurosurgeon performs the surgery to remove and close the MMC within 24 hours of the infant's birth to minimize the risk of infection. The placement of a shunt to relieve the hydrocephalus may be performed at the same time or may occur within the first week of life. The orthopedist assesses the status of the infant's joints and muscles. The urologist assesses the child's renal status and monitors bowel and bladder function. Depending on the amount of skin coverage available to close the defect, a plastic surgeon may also be involved. Once the back lesion is repaired and a shunt is placed, the infant is medically stabilized in preparation for discharge home. Communication among all members of the team working with the parents and infant is crucial. Information about the infant's present level of function must be shared among all personnel who evaluate and treat the infant.

The physical therapist establishes motor and sensory levels of function; evaluates muscle tone, degree of head and trunk control, and range-of-motion limitations; and checks for the presence of any musculoskeletal deformities. General physical therapy goals during this first stage of care include the following:

1. Prevent secondary complications (contractures, deformities, skin breakdown).
2. Promote age-appropriate sensorimotor development.
3. Prepare the child for ambulation.
4. Educate the family about appropriate strategies to manage the child's condition.

If the physical therapist assistant is involved at this stage of the infant's care, a caring and positive attitude is of utmost importance to foster healthy, appropriate interactions between the parents and the infant. The most important thing to teach the parents is how to interact with their infant. Parents have many things to learn before the infant is discharged from the acute care facility: positioning, sensory precautions, range of motion, and therapeutic handling. Parents need to be comfortable in using handling techniques to promote normal sensorimotor development, especially head and trunk control. Giving parents a sense of competence in their ability to care for their infant is everyone's job and ensures carryover of instructions to the home setting.

Prevention of Deformities: Postoperative Positioning

Positioning after the surgical repair of the back lesion should avoid pressure on the repaired area until it is healed. Therefore the infant initially is limited to prone and side-lying positions. You can show the child's parents how to place the infant prone on their laps and gently rock to soothe and stimulate head lifting. Holding the infant high on the shoulder, with support under the arms, fosters head control and may be the easiest position for the infant with MMC to maintain a stable head. Handling and carrying strategies may be recommended by the physical therapist and practiced by the assistant before being demonstrated to the parents. Parents are naturally anxious when handling an infant with a disability. Use gentle encouragement, and do not hesitate to correct any errors in hand placement. The infant's head should be supported when the infant is picked up and put down. As the child's head control improves, support can gradually be withdrawn. As the back heals, the infant can experience brief periods of supine and supported upright sitting without any interference with wound healing. When the shunt has been inserted, you should always follow any positioning precautions according to the physician's orders.

Prone Positioning

Prone positioning is important to prevent development of potentially deforming hip and knee flexion contractures. Prone is also a position from which the infant can begin to develop head control. Depending on the child's level of motor paralysis and the presence of hypotonia in the neck and trunk, the infant may have more difficulty in learning to lift the head off the support surface in prone than in a supported upright position. Movement in the prone position, as when the infant is placed over the caregiver's lap or when the infant is carried while prone, will also stimulate head control by encouraging lifting the head into extension. Intervention 7.1 demonstrates a way to position an infant in lying prone with lateral supports to maintain proper alignment. Encouraging the infant to use the upper extremities for propping on elbows and for pushing up to extended arms provides a good beginning for upper extremity strengthening.

Effects of Gravity

When the infant is in the supine position, the paralyzed lower extremities will tend to assume positions of comfort, such as hip abduction and external rotation, because of the effect of gravity. In children with partial innervation of the lower extremities, hip flexion and adduction can produce hip flexion contractures and can lead to hip dislocation because of the lack of muscle pull from hip extensors or abductors. Certain postures should be avoided, as listed in Box 7.1. *Genu recurvatum* is seen when the quadriceps muscles are not opposed by equally strong hamstring pull to balance the knee-extension posture. When only anterior tibialis function is present, a

INTERVENTION 7.1   Prone Lying With Support

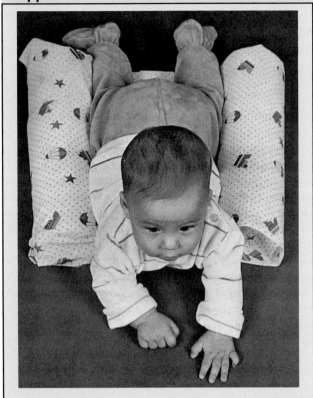

Infant in prone lying position with lateral supports to maintain proper trunk and lower extremity alignment.

(Adapted by permission from Williamson GG: *Children with spina bifida: early intervention and preschool programming*, Baltimore, 1987, Paul H. Brookes.)

BOX 7.1   Positions to be Avoided in Children With Myelomeningocele

Frog-leg position in prone or supine
W sitting
Ring sitting
Heel sitting
Cross-legged sitting

(Modified from Hinderer KA, Hinderer SR, Shurtleff DB: Myelodysplasia. In Campbell SK, Palisano RJ, Orlin MN, editors: *Physical therapy for children*, ed 4, Philadelphia, 2012, WB Saunders, pp. 703–755.)

calcaneovarus foot results. Some of these foot deformities are depicted in Fig. 7.2.

Orthoses for Lower Extremity Positioning

Orthoses may be needed early to prevent deformities, or the caregiver may simply need to position the child with towel rolls or small pillows to help maintain a neutral hip, knee, and ankle position. An example of a simple lower extremity splint is seen in Fig. 7.6. Early on, it is detrimental to adduct the hips completely because the hip joints are incompletely

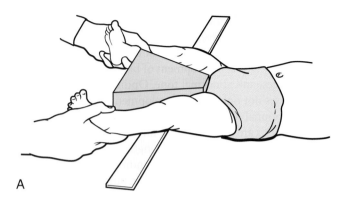

A

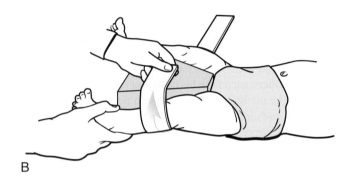

B

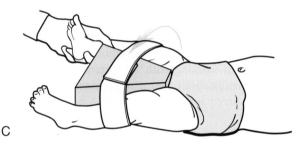

C

Fig. 7.6 Simple abduction splint. **(A)** A pad is placed between the child's legs with a strap underneath. **(B)** The straps are wrapped around the legs and attached with Velcro, **(C)** bringing the legs into neutral hip rotation.

formed and may sublux or dislocate if they are adducted beyond neutral. Maintaining a neutral alignment of the foot is critical for later plantigrade weight-bearing. Children with higher-level lesions may benefit initially from a total body splint to be worn while they are sleeping (Fig. 7.7). Many clinicians recommend night splints for this reason. Any orthosis should be introduced gradually because of lack of skin sensation, and the skin should be monitored closely for breakdown.

Prevention of Skin Breakdown

Lack of awareness of pressure may cause the infant to remain in one position too long, especially once sitting is attained. However, the supine position may pose more danger of skin breakdown over the ischial tuberosities, the sacrum, and the

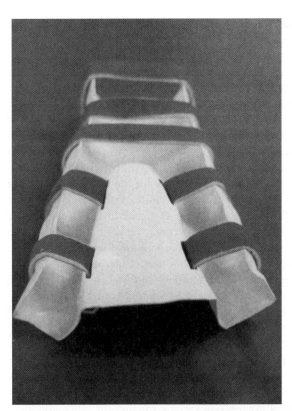

Fig. 7.7 Total body splint. (From Schneider JW, Pesavento MJ: Spina bifida: a congenital spinal cord injury. In Umphred DA, Lazaro RT, Roller ML, Burton GU, editors: *Umphred's neurological rehabilitation,* ed 6, St. Louis, 2013, CV Mosby.)

calcaneus. Side-lying can be a dangerous position because of the excess pressure on the trochanters. Because of the lack of sensation and decreased awareness of excessive pressure from being in one position for too long, the skin of children with MMC must be closely monitored for redness. Infants need to have their position changed often. Check for red areas, especially over bony prominences and after the infant wears any orthosis. If redness persists longer than 20 minutes, the orthosis should be adjusted.

Sensory Precautions

Parents often find it difficult to realize that the infant lacks the ability to feel below the level of the injury. Encouraging parents to play with the infant and to tickle different areas of the child's body will help them understand where the baby has feeling. It is not appropriate to demonstrate the infant's lack of sensitivity by stroking the skin with a pin, even though the therapist may use this technique during formal sensory testing. Socks or booties are a good idea for protecting the feet from being nibbled as the infant finds his toes at around 6 months. Teach the parents to keep the infant's lower extremities covered to protect the skin when the infant is crawling or creeping. Close inspection of the floor or carpet for small objects that could cause an accidental injury is a necessity. Protecting the skin with clothing also helps with temperature regulation, which is impaired. Skin that is anesthetic does not sweat and cannot conserve heat or give off heat, and

therefore must be protected. Parents must always be instructed to test bath water before placing the infant into the tub because a burn could easily result. Proper shoe fit is imperative to prevent pressure areas and abrasions. Children with MMC may continue to have a chubby baby foot, so extra room may be needed in shoes.

Prevention of Contractures: Range of Motion

Passive range of motion should be done two to three times a day in an infant with MMC. To decrease the number of exercises in the home program, exercises for certain joints, such as the hip and knee, can be combined. For example, hip and knee flexion on one side can be combined with hip and knee extension on the other side while the infant is supine. Hip abduction can be done bilaterally, as can internal and external rotation. Performing these movements when the infant is prone provides a nice stretch to the hip flexors.

Range of motion of the foot and ankle should be done individually. Always be sure that the subtalar joint is in a neutral position when doing ankle dorsiflexion range, so that the movement occurs at the correct joint. If the foot is allowed to go into varus or valgus positioning when stretching a tight heel cord, the motion caused by your stretching will take place in the midfoot, rather than the hindfoot. You may be causing a rocker-bottom foot by allowing the motion to occur at the wrong place. Be sure that your supervising physical therapist demonstrates the correct technique to stretch a heel cord while maintaining subtalar neutral.

Range-of-motion exercises should be done gently, with your hands placed close to the child's joints, to provide a short lever arm. Hold the motion briefly at the end of the available range. Even in the presence of contractures, aggressive stretching is not indicated. Serial casting may be needed as an adjunct to therapy if persistent passive range-of-motion exercise does not improve the range of motion. Always keep your supervising therapist apprised of any problems in this area. Range-of-motion exercises are easy to forget when the infant becomes more active, but these simple exercises are an important part of the infant's program. Once able, the child should be responsible for doing her own daily range of motion.

Promotion of Age-Appropriate Sensorimotor Development

Therapeutic handling: development of head control. Any of the techniques outlined in Chapter 5 to encourage head control can be used in a child with MMC. Some early cautions include being sure that the skin over the back defect is well healed and that care is taken to prevent shearing forces on the lower extremities or the trunk when the infant is positioned for head lifting. Additionally, the caregiver should provide extra support if the child's head is larger than normal, secondary to hydrocephalus. The infant can be carried at the caregiver's shoulder to encourage head lifting as the body sways, just as you would with any newborn. The caregiver can also support the infant in the prone position during carrying or gentle rocking on the lap to promote head control using vestibular input. Extra support can be given to the infant's head at the jaw or forehead when the child is in the prone position (Intervention 7.2).

Although head control in infants usually develops first in the prone position, it may be more difficult for an infant with myelodysplasia to lift the head from this position because of hydrocephalus and hypotonic neck and trunk muscles. Extra support from a bolster or a small half-roll under the chest aids in distributing some of the weight farther down the trunk, as well as help in bringing the upper extremities under the body to assume a prone-on-elbows position (Fig. 7.8). Additional support can be provided under the child's forehead, if needed, to give the infant a chance to experience this position. Rolling from supine to side-lying with the head supported on a half-roll also gives the child practice in keeping the head in line with the body during rotation around the long axis of the body. Head control in the supine position is needed to balance the development of axial extension with axial flexion. Positioning the child in a supported supine position on a wedge can encourage a chin tuck or forward head lift into flexion. Every time the infant is picked up, the caregiver should encourage active head and trunk movements on the part of the child. Carrying should also be seen as a therapeutic activity to promote postural control, rather than as a passive action performed by the caregiver. The clinician or caregiver should watch for signs that could indicate medical complications while interacting with and handling a child with MMC and a shunt. Signs of shunt obstruction may include the setting-sun sign and increased muscle tone in the upper or lower extremities.

Therapeutic handling: developing righting and equilibrium reactions. If the infant uses too much shoulder elevation as a substitute for head control, developing righting reactions of the head and trunk becomes more difficult. Try to modify the position to make it easier for the infant to use neck muscles for stability, rather than the elevated shoulder position. In addition, give more support proximally at the child's trunk to provide a stable base on which the head can work. The infant may use an elevated position of the shoulders when in propped sitting, with the arms internally rotated and the scapula protracted. Although this posture may be positionally stable, it does not allow the infant to move within or from the posture with any degree of control, thus making it difficult to reach or to shift weight in sitting.

As the infant with MMC develops head control in prone, supine, and side-lying positions, righting reactions should be seen in the trunk. Head and trunk righting can be encouraged in prone by slightly shifting the infant's weight onto one side of the body and seeing whether the other side shortens. Righting of the trunk occurs only as far down the body as the muscles are innervated. The clinician should note any asymmetry in the trunk because this will need to be considered for planning upright activities that could predispose the child to scoliosis. As the infant is able to lift the head off the supporting surface, trunk extension develops down the back. The extension of the infant's back and the arms should be encouraged by enticing the child to reach forward from a prone position with one or both arms. As the infant becomes stronger and depending on how much of the trunk is innervated, less and less anterior trunk support can be given while still encouraging lifting and reaching with the arms and upper trunk. (The goal is to have the child "fly," as in the Landau reflex.) By placing the infant on a small ball or over a small bolster and shifting weight forward, you may elicit head and trunk lifting (Intervention 7.3, *A*), reaching with arms (Intervention 7.3, *B*), or propping on one extended arm and reaching with the other (Intervention 7.3, *C*). If the infant is moved quickly, protective extension of the upper extremities may be elicited. For the infant with a lower level lesion and hip innervation, hip extension should be encouraged when the child is in the prone position.

Trunk rotation must be encouraged to support the child's transition from one posture to another, such as in rolling from supine to prone and back, and in coming to sit from side-lying. Trunk rotation in sitting encourages the development of equilibrium reactions that bring the center of gravity back within the base of support. Equilibrium reactions are trunk reactions that occur in developmental postures. In prone and supine, trunk incurvation and limb abduction result from a lateral weight shift. Again, the trunk responds only to the degree to which it is innervated, so one should

---

INTERVENTION 7.2 **Prone Carrying**

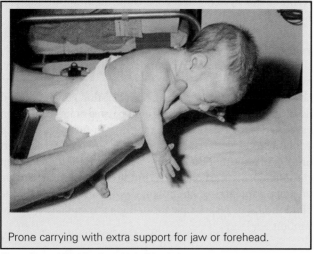

Prone carrying with extra support for jaw or forehead.

(From Burns YR, MacDonald J: *Physiotherapy and the growing child*, London, 1996, WB Saunders.)

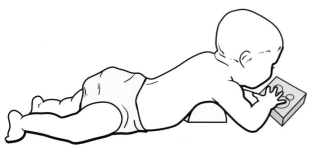

Fig. 7.8 Prone position over a half-roll.

INTERVENTION 7.3 **Ball Exercises**

A. Prone positioning on a ball with the child's weight shifted forward for head lifting.
B. Reaching with both arms over a ball.
C. Reaching with one arm while propping on the other over a ball.

encourage rotation in all directions. Trunk rotation is also used in protective reactions of the upper extremities when balance is lost.

Handling: developing trunk control in sitting. Acclimation to upright sitting is begun as close as possible to the developmentally appropriate time (6 months). Ideally, the infant should have sufficient head control and sufficient ability to bear weight on extended arms. Propped sitting is a typical way to begin developing independence in sitting. Good postural alignment of the back should be maintained when the child is placed in a sitting position. A floor sitter, a type of adaptive equipment, can be used to support the child's back if kyphosis is present. Some floor sitters have extensions that provide head support if head control is inconsistent. Floor sitters with head support allow even the child with poor head control to be placed in a sitting position on the floor to play.

In children with good head control, sitting balance can be trained by varying the child's base of support and the amount of hand support. Often, a bench or tray placed in front of the child can provide extra support and security as confidence is gained while the child plays in a new position. Certain sitting positions should be avoided because of their potentially deforming forces. These positions are listed in Box 7.1.

Once propped sitting is achieved, hand support is gradually but methodically decreased. Reaching for objects while supporting with one hand can begin in the midline, and then the range can be widened as balance improves. Weight shifting at the pelvis in sitting can be used to elicit head and trunk righting reactions and upper-extremity protective reactions. Trunk rotation with extension is needed to foster the ability to protect in a backward direction. Later, the child can work on transferring objects at the midline with no hand support, an ultimate test of balance. Always remember to protect the child's back and skin during weight-bearing in sitting. Skin inspection should be done after sitting for short periods of time. If the child cannot maintain an upright trunk muscularly, an orthosis may be indicated for alignment in sitting and for prevention of scoliosis.

Preparation for ambulation: acclimation to upright and weight-bearing. Acclimation to upright and weight-bearing begins with fostering development of head and trunk control and includes sensory input to the lower extremities despite the lack of sensation. Brief periods of weight-bearing on properly aligned lower extremities should be encouraged throughout the day. These periods occur in supported standing and should be done often. Providing a symmetric position for the infant is important for increasing awareness of body position and sensory input. Handling should promote symmetry, equal weight-bearing, and equal sensory input. Weight-bearing in the upright position provides a perfect opportunity to engage the child in cognitively appropriate play. The physical therapist assistant can serve as a vocal model for speech by making sounds, talking, and describing objects and actions in the child's environment. By interacting with the child, you are also modeling appropriate behavior for the caregiver.

Upper extremity strengthening. During early development, pulling and pushing with the upper extremities are excellent ways to foster increasing upper extremity strength. The progression of pushing from prone on elbows to prone on extended arms and onto hands and knees can provide many opportunities for the child to use the arms in a weight-bearing form of work. Providing the infant with your hands and requesting her to pull to sit can be done before she turns and pushes up to sit. Pulling on various resistances of latex-free Theraband can be a fun way to incorporate upper extremity strengthening into the child's treatment plan. Other objects can be used for pulling, such as a dowel rod or cane. Pushing on the floor on a scooter board can provide excellent resistance training.

Mat mobility. Moving around in supine and prone positions is important for exploring the environment and self-care activities, but mat mobility includes movement in upright sitting. Mat mobility needs to be encouraged once trunk balance begins in supported sitting. The child can be encouraged to pull herself up to sitting by using another person, a rope tied to the end of the bed, or an overhead trapeze. Children can and should use pushup blocks or other devices to increase the strength in their upper extremities (Intervention 7.4). They need to have strong triceps, latissimus dorsi, and shoulder depressors to transfer independently. Moving around on the mat or floor is good preparation for moving around in upright standing or doing push-ups in a wheelchair. Connecting arm motion with mobility early gives the child a foundation for coordinating other, more advanced transfer and self-care movements. Insensate skin requires protection to prevent friction burns on knees and feet. Good bowel and bladder management can decrease potential skin breakdown from ammonia burns secondary to skin soiling in young children.

INTERVENTION 7.4 Strengthening Upper Extremities With Push-Up Blocks

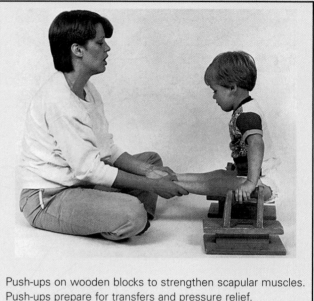

Push-ups on wooden blocks to strengthen scapular muscles. Push-ups prepare for transfers and pressure relief.

(Adapted by permission from Williamson GG: *Children with spina bifida: early intervention and preschool programming,* Baltimore, 1987, Paul H. Brookes.)

Standing frames. Use of a standing frame for weight-bearing can begin when the child has sufficient head control and exhibits interest in attaining an upright standing position. Normally, infants begin to pull to stand at around 9 months of age. By 1 year, all children with a motor level of L3 or above should be fitted with a standing frame (Fig. 7.9) or parapodium (Fig. 7.10) to encourage early weight-bearing. A standing frame is usually less expensive than a parapodium and is easier to apply (Ryan et al., 1991). The tubular frame supports the trunk, hips, and knees and leaves the hands free. Some children with L4 or lower lesions may be fitted with some type of hip-knee-ankle-foot orthosis (HKAFO) to begin standing in preparation for walking. The orthosis pictured in Fig. 7.11 has a thoracic support. Having the child stand four or five times a day for 20 to 30 minutes seems to be manageable for most parents. A more detailed explanation of standing frames is presented later in this chapter.

Family Education

The family must be taught sensory precautions, signs of shunt malfunction, range of motion, handling, and positioning. Most of these activities are not particularly difficult. However, the difficulty comes in trying not to overwhelm the parents with all the things that need to be done. Parents of children with a physical disability need to be empowered to be parents and advocates for their child. Parents are not surrogate therapists and should not be made to think they should be. Literature that may be helpful is available from the Spina Bifida Association of America. As much as possible, many of the precautions, range-of-motion exercises, and developmental activities should become part of the family's everyday routine.

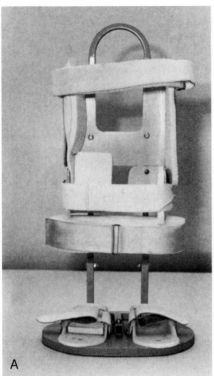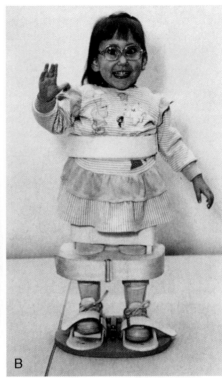

Fig. 7.9 Standing frame. **(A)** Anterior view. **(B)** The frame is adapted to accommodate the child's leg-length discrepancy and tendency to lean to the right. (From Ryan KD, Ploski C, Emans JB: Myelodysplasia: the musculoskeletal problem: habilitation from infancy to adulthood, *Phys Ther* 71:935–946, 1991. With permission of the American Physical Therapy Association.)

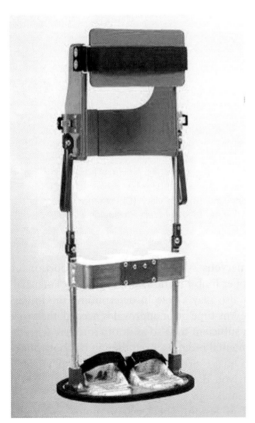

Fig. 7.10 Parapodium. (Parapodium image provided courtesy of Fillauer, LLC © 2010-2017.)

Range-of-motion exercises and developmental activities can be shared between the spouses, and a schedule of standing time can be outlined. Siblings are often the best partners in encouraging developmentally appropriate play.

Second Stage of Physical Therapy Intervention

The ambulatory phase begins when the infant becomes a toddler and continues into the school years. The general physical therapy goals for this second stage include the following:

1. Ambulation and independent mobility.
2. Continued improvements in flexibility, strength, and endurance.
3. Independence in pressure relief, self-care, and ADLs.
4. Promotion of ongoing cognitive and social-emotional development.
5. Identification of perceptual problems that may interfere with learning.
6. Collaboration with family, school, and health care providers for total management.

Box 7.2 lists vital components of a physical therapy program.

Orthotic Management

The health care provider's philosophy of orthosis use may determine who receives what type of orthosis and when. Some clinicians do not think that children with high levels of paralysis, such as those with thoracic or high lumbar (L1 or L2) lesions, should be prescribed orthoses because studies show

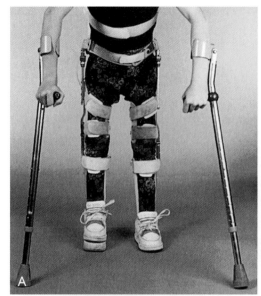

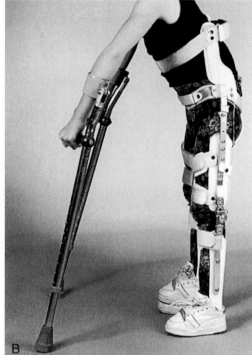

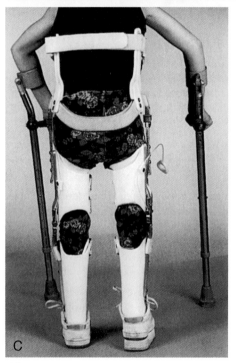

Fig. 7.11 Hip-knee-ankle-foot orthosis with a thoracic strap. **(A)** Front view. **(B)** Side view. **(C)** Posterior view. (From Nawoczenski DA, Epler ME: *Orthotics in functional rehabilitation of the lower limb,* Philadelphia, 1997, WB Saunders.)

that by adolescence these individuals are mobile in a wheelchair and have discarded walking as a primary means of mobility. Others think that all children, regardless of the level of lesion, have the right to experience upright ambulation even though they may discard this type of mobility later.

Orthotic selection. The physical therapist, in conjunction with the orthopedist and the orthotist, is involved with the family in making orthotic decisions for the child with MMC. The main goal of an orthosis is to correct deformities that would interfere with ambulation. Many factors have to be considered when choosing an orthosis for a child who is beginning to stand and ambulate, including level of lesion, age,

central nervous system status, body proportions, contractures, upper limb function, and cognition. Financial considerations also play a role in determining the initial type of orthosis. Any time prior approval is needed, the process must begin in sufficient time so as not to interfere with the child's developmental progress. Even though it is not your responsibility to make orthotic decisions as a physical therapist assistant, you do need to be aware of what goes into this decision-making.

Level of lesion. The level of motor function demonstrated by the toddler does not always correspond to the level of the lesion because of individual differences in nerve root

BOX 7.2 Vital Components of a Physical Therapy Program

Proper positioning in sitting and sleeping
Stretching
Strengthening
Pressure relief and joint protection
Mobility for short and long distances
Transfers and activities of daily living
Skin inspection
Self-care
Play
Recreation and physical fitness
Prevention of secondary complications
Attain independent management of own health care needs

(Modified from Hinderer KA, Hinderer SR, Shurtleff DB: Myelodysplasia. In Campbell SK, Palisano RJ, Orlin MN, editors: *Physical therapy for children*, ed 4, Philadelphia, 2012, WB Saunders, pp. 703–755.)

innervation. A thorough examination needs to be completed by the physical therapist prior to making orthotic recommendations. A chart of possible orthoses to be considered according to the child's motor level is found in Table 7.4. Age recommendations for each device vary considerably among different sources and are often linked to the philosophy of orthotic management espoused by a particular facility or

TABLE 7.4 Predicted Ambulation of Children With Spina Bifida

Motor Level	Orthosis/ Assistive Device	Long-Term Prognosis/ Community Mobility
Thoracic to L2	May use THKAFO or parapodium for limited distance "exercise" walking or for supported standing when young	W/C
L1 to L3	May use HKAFO or RGO with walker or crutches for short distances in house when young	W/C
L3 to L4	May use KAFO with walker or crutches for short distances in house and community	W/C
L4 to L5	May or may not use standard AFOs or ground reaction AFOs and crutches in community	Community, W/C for long distances
S1 to "no loss"	May use FO or SMO in community	Community

AFO, Ankle-foot orthosis; *FO,* foot orthosis; *HKAFO,* hip-knee-ankle-foot orthosis; *KAFO,* knee-ankle-foot orthosis; *RGO,* reciprocating gait orthosis; *SMO,* supramalleolar orthosis; *THKAFO,* trunk-hip-knee-ankle-foot orthosis; *W/C,* wheelchair.
Data from Hinderer et al., 2017.

clinic. Contractures can prevent a child from being fitted with orthoses. The child cannot have any significant amount of hip or knee flexion contractures and must have a planti-grade foot—that is, the ankle must be able to achieve a neutral position or 90 degrees—to be able to wear an orthotic device for standing and ambulation. Standers may be used to counteract hip flexor tightness seen in children with MMC. Addition of a 15-degree wedge to increase passive stretch of the gastrocnemius muscles can be used in conjunction with a stander (Paleg et al., 2014). Children with undergo hip or knee contracture release are less likely to remain ambulatory (Dicianno et al., 2015).

Age. The type of orthosis used by a child with MMC may vary according to age. A child younger than 1 year of age can be fitted with a night splint to maintain the lower extremities in proper alignment. By 1 year, all children should be weight-bearing using either a stander or a parapodium. Most children exhibit a desire to pull to stand at around 9 months of age, and the therapist and the assistant should anticipate this desire and should be ready to take advantage of the child's readiness to stand. When a child with MMC exhibits a developmental delay, the child should be placed in a standing device when her developmental age reaches 9 months. If, however, the child does not attain a developmental age of 9 months by 20 to 24 months of chronologic age, standing should be begun for physiologic benefits. A parapodium is the orthosis of choice in this situation (Fig. 7.10).

The level of MMC is correlated with the child's age to determine the appropriate type of orthotic device. A child with a thoracic or high lumbar (L1, 2) motor level requires an HKAFO with thoracic support (Fig. 7.11). Household ambulation may be possible but at a very high energy cost. "Exercise" walking is more likely to occur in children with thoracic motor involvement. Children with a high motor level should be engaged in activities to prepare them for wheelchair propulsion, such as transfers and increasing upper body strength. A child with high lumbar motor level can begin gait training in a parapodium and progress to a reciprocating gait orthosis (RGO) (Fig. 7.12, *A–B*). A child with a midlumbar (L3 or L4) motor level may begin with a standard bilateral knee-ankle-foot orthoses (KAFOs) (Fig. 7.13), ankle-foot orthosis (AFO) (Fig. 7.14, *A*), or ground reaction AFO (Fig. 7.14, *B*), depending on quadriceps strength. The child in Fig. 7.15 has been fitted with AFOs with twister cables to correct rotational deformities. These can be introduced as early as 2 years and worn until the child is old enough for surgical correction (Swaroop and Dias, 2009). A child with a low motor level, such as L4 to L5 or S2, may begin standing without any device. When learning to ambulate, children with low lumbar motor levels benefit from bilateral AFOs or supramalleolar molded orthoses to support the foot and ankle (Fig. 7.14, *A–C*). A child with an L5 motor level has hip extension and ankle eversion, and may need only lightweight AFOs to ambulate. Although the child with an S2 motor level may begin to walk without any orthosis, she may later be fitted with a foot orthosis.

Types of orthoses. Parapodiums and RGOs are all specially designed HKAFOs. They encompass and control the

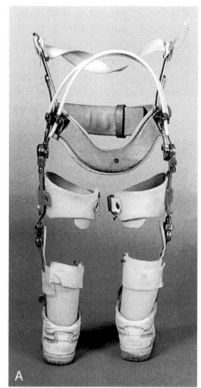

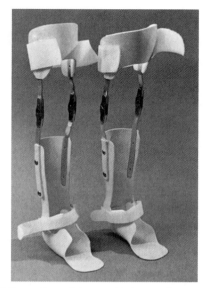

Fig. 7.13 Oblique view of knee-ankle-foot orthoses with anterior thigh cuffs. (From Knutson LM, Clark DE: Orthotic devices for ambulation in children with cerebral palsy and myelomeningocele, *Phys Ther* 71:947–960, 1991. With permission of the American Physical Therapy Association.)

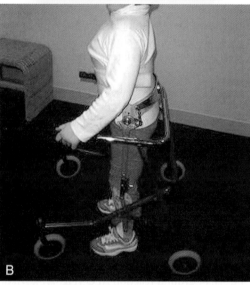

Fig. 7.12 **(A)** Reciprocating gait orthosis with a thoracic strap, posterior view. (From Nawoczenski DA, Epler ME: *Orthotics in functional rehabilitation of the lower limb*, Philadelphia, 1997, WB Saunders.) **(B)** Side view of a reciprocating gait orthosis being used with a rolling reverser walker. (From Swaroop VT, Dias L: Orthopedic management of spina bifida. Part I: hip, knee, and rotational deformities, *J Child Orthop* 3:441–449, 2009).

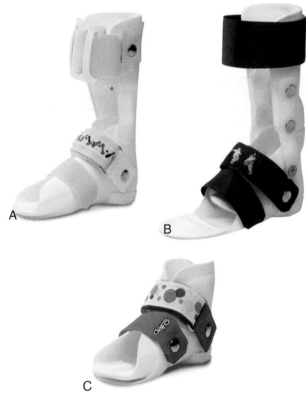

Fig. 7.14 **(A)** Solid ankle-foot orthosis with an ankle strap to restrain the heel (DAFO Cascade); **(B)** Floor reaction DAFO Cascade; **(C)** Supramalleolar orthosis DAFO Cascade. (Courtesy Cascade Dafo, Inc.)

child's hips, knees, ankles, and feet. A traditional HKAFO consists of a pelvic band, external hip joints, and bilateral long-leg braces (i.e., KAFOs). Additional trunk components may be attached to an HKAFO if the child has minimal trunk control or needs to control a spinal deformity. The more extensive the orthosis, the less likely the child will be to continue to ambulate as she grows older. The amount of energy expended to ambulate with a cumbersome orthosis is high.

Although the child is young, she may be highly motivated to move around in the upright position. As time progresses, it may become more important to keep up with a peer group, and she may prefer an alternative, faster, and less cumbersome means of mobility.

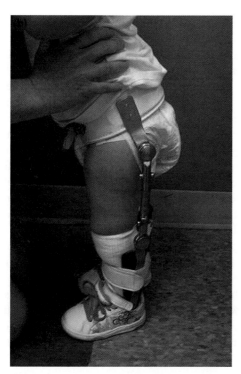

Fig. 7.15 Side view of a child with myelomeningocele wearing ankle-foot orthoses with twister cables. (From Swaroop VT, Dias L: Orthopedic management of spina bifida. Part I: hip, knee, and rotational deformities, *J Child Orthop* 3:441–449, 2009).

Parapodium. The parapodium (Fig. 7.10) can be used as the first orthotic device for standing and ambulating. Its wide base provides support for standing and allows the child to acclimate to upright while leaving the arms free for play. The child's knees and hips can be unlocked for sitting at a table or on a bench, a feature that allows the child to participate in typical preschool activities such as snack and circle time. The Toronto parapodium has one lock for the hip and knee, whereas the Rochester parapodium has separate locks for each joint.

Reciprocating gait orthosis. An RGO can be the orthosis of choice for a child with motor function at L1 to L3. Some centers advocate its use for children with thoracic level function. The RGO is more *energy efficient* than a traditional HKAFO because it employs a cable system to cause hip extension reciprocally on the stance side when hip flexion is initiated on the swing side. An RGO is usually introduced at about 2 years of age (Swaroop and Dias, 2009). The RGO requires use of an assistive device, rolling reverse walker (Fig. 7.12, *B*), Lofstrand crutches, or canes. The energy cost must be considered individually, and recognition that in the long-term community ambulation for children with thoracic to L3 levels is typically accomplished using a wheelchair.

Donning and doffing of orthoses. Ambulating with orthoses and assistive devices requires assistance to don the braces. Teaching donning and doffing of orthoses can be accomplished when the child is supine or sitting. The child may be able to roll into the orthosis by going from prone to supine. Sitting is preferable for independent donning of the orthosis

if the child can boost into the brace. Next, the child places each foot into the shoe with the knees of the orthosis unlocked, laces or closes the foot piece, locks the knees, and fastens the thigh cuffs or waist belt, if the device has one. Cotton knee-high socks or tights should be worn under the orthosis to absorb perspiration and to decrease any skin irritation. It takes a great deal of practice on the part of the child to become independent in donning the orthosis.

Wearing time of orthoses. Caregivers should monitor the wearing time of orthoses, including the gradual increase in time, with periodic checks for any areas of potential skin breakdown. The child can begin wearing the orthosis for 1 or 2 hours for the first few days and can increase wearing time from there. A chart is helpful so that everyone (teacher, aide, family member) knows the length of time the child is wearing the orthosis and who is responsible for checking skin integrity. Check for red marks after the child wears the orthosis and note how long it takes for these marks to disappear. If they do not resolve after 20 to 30 minutes, contact the orthotist about making an adjustment. The orthosis should not be worn again until it is checked by the orthotist.

Factors associated with mobility outcomes in children with MMC have been identified via the National Spina Bifida Patient Registry (Thibadeau et al., 2013). The following factors were found to be inversely related to ambulation status: history of having a shunt for hydrocephalus; having a higher motor level, that is thoracic versus lumbar or sacral; and having had surgical release of hip or knee contractures (Dicianno et al., 2015). It was the authors' hope that these findings would assist in identifying interventions to improve mobility outcomes and explain the reasons for the associations described. The relationship between obesity and ambulation status was not investigated but increasing body weight can often contribute to a decline in ambulation.

Upper Limb Function

Two-thirds of children with MMC exhibit impaired upper limb function that can be linked to structural abnormalities of the cerebellum (Dennis et al., 2009). The difficulties in coordination appear to be related to the timing and smooth control of the movements of the upper extremities. These children do not perform well on tests that are timed and exhibit delayed or mixed hand dominance (Dennis et al., 2009). Children with MMC have hand weakness (Effgen and Brown, 1992), poor hand function (Grimm, 1976), and impaired kinesthetic awareness (Hwang et al., 2002). Difficulties with fine-motor tasks and those related to eye–hand coordination are documented in the literature. Some authors relate the perceptual difficulties to the upper limb incoordination rather than to a true perceptual deficit (Hinderer et al., 2012). Motor planning and timing deficits are documented (Peny-Dahlstrand et al., 2009; Jewell et al., 2010). The low muscle tone often exhibited in the neck and trunk of these children could also add to their coordination problems. The child with MMC must have sufficient upper extremity control to be able to use an assistive device, such as a walker, and the ability to learn the sequence of using a walker for independent gait.

Practicing fine-motor activities has been found to help with the problem and carries over to functional tasks (Fay et al., 1986). Occupational therapists are also involved in the treatment of these children.

Cognition

The child must also be able to understand the task to be performed to master upright ambulation with an orthosis and assistive device. Cognitive function in a child with MMC can vary with the degree of nervous system involvement and hydrocephalus. Results from intelligence testing place them in the low normal range but below the population mean, which is an IQ of greater than 70 (Barf et al., 2004). The remaining 25% are in the mild intellectual disability category, with an IQ of between 55 and 70. Children with MMC are at risk for a myriad of developmental disabilities including what is often called nonverbal learning disability. They can demonstrate better reading than math and often demonstrate impairments in executive function, which includes problem solving, staying on task, and sequencing actions. Some of the poor performance by children with MMC may be related to their attention difficulties, slow speed of motor response, and memory deficits secondary to cerebellar dysgenesis.

Vision and visual perception. Twenty percent of children with MMC have strabismus, which may require surgical correction (Verhoef et al., 2004). Infants with MMC delay in orienting to faces (Landry et al., 2003), and when they are older have difficulty orienting to external stimuli and once engaged cannot easily break their focus (Dennis et al., 2005). In visual perceptual tasks, the child with MMC finds it more difficult if the task is action-based rather than object-based. They may have a more developed "what" neural pathway than a "where" neural pathway. Spatial perception usually depends on moving through an environment, something that may be delayed in the child with MMC. Jansen-Osmann et al. (2008) found that children with MMC had difficulty constructing a situation model of space, which may relate to deficits in figure-ground perception.

Cocktail party speech. You may encounter a child who seems verbally much more intelligent than she really is when formally tested. "Cocktail party speech" can be indicative of "cocktail party personality," a behavioral manifestation associated with cognitive dysfunction. The therapist assistant must be cautious not to mistake verbose speech for more advanced cognitive ability in a child with MMC. These children are often more severely impaired than one would first think based on their verbal conversation. When they are closely questioned about a topic such as performing daily tasks within their environment, they are unable to furnish details, solve problems, or generalize the task to new situations.

Principles of Gait Training

Regardless of the timing and type of orthosis that is used, general principles of treatment can be discussed for this second or middle stage of care. Gait training begins with learning to perform and control weight shifts in standing. If the toddler has had only limited experience in upright standing, a standing program may be initiated simultaneously with practicing weight shifting. If the toddler is already acclimated to standing and has a standing frame, one can challenge the child's balance while the child is in the frame. The therapist assistant moves the child in the frame and causes the child to respond with head and trunk reactions (Intervention 7.5). This maneuver can be a good beginning for any standing session. Parents should be taught how to challenge the child's balance similarly at home. The child should not be left unattended in the frame because she may topple over from too much self-initiated body movement. By being placed at a surface of appropriate height, the child can engage in fine-motor activities such as building block towers, sorting objects, lacing cards, or practicing puzzles.

The physical therapist assistant can play an important role during this second stage of physical therapy management by teaching the child with MMC to ambulate with the new orthosis, usually a parapodium. The child is first taught to shift weight laterally onto one side of the base of the parapodium, and to allow the unweighted portion of the base to pivot forward. This maneuver is called a *swivel gait pattern*.

INTERVENTION 7.5 Weight Shifting in Standing

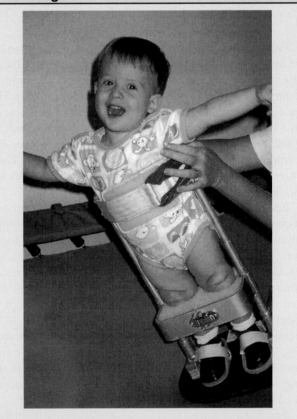

Weight shifting the child while in a standing frame can promote head and trunk righting reactions. These movements prepare the child for later weight shifting during ambulation.

(From Burns YR, MacDonald J: *Physiotherapy and the growing child,* London, 1996, WB Saunders.)

Children can be taught this maneuver in appropriately high parallel bars or with a walker. However, use of the parallel bars may encourage the child to pull rather than push and may make it more difficult to progress to using a walker. The therapist assistant may also be seated on a rolling stool in front of the child and may hold the child's hands to encourage the weight-shifting sequence.

Once the child has mastered ambulation with the new orthosis, consideration can be given to changing the type of assistive device. The child's gait pattern in a parapodium is progressed from a swivel pattern to a swing-to pattern, which requires a walker. A rollator walker may be used as an initial assistive device for gait training a child with MMC because it provides a wide base of stability and two wheels; therefore the child can advance the walker without picking it up. A child should be independent with one type of orthosis and assistive device before moving on to a different orthosis or different device. After success with a swing-to gait pattern using a walker, the child can be progressed to using the same pattern with Lofstrand crutches. Once the child has mastered the gait progression with a parapodium and a walker, plans can be made for progression to a more energy-efficient orthosis or a less restrictive assistive device, but not at the same time. A swing-through gait pattern is the most efficient, but it requires using forearm or Lofstrand crutches. The earliest a child may be able to understand and succeed in using Lofstrand crutches is 3 years of age. The therapist should take the child's cognitive level of function as well as the functional neurologic level of the paralysis to determine when to introduce Lofstrand crutches. Lofstrand crutches provide much greater maneuverability than a walker, so whenever possible, the child should be progressed from a walker to forearm crutches.

If the child has some innervated knee musculature, such as a child with an L3 motor level, ambulation with KAFOs protects the knees. A long-term goal may be walking with the knees unlocked, and if quadriceps strength increases sufficiently, the KAFOs could be cut down to AFOs. If the child is able to move each lower extremity separately, a four-point or two-point gait pattern can be taught. Gait instruction starts on level ground and progresses to uneven ground to elevated surfaces, such as curbs, ramps, and stairs.

Level of Ambulation

The functional ambulatory level for a child with MMC is linked to the motor level. Table 7.4 relates the level of lesion to the child's long-term ambulation potential. Early on, a child with thoracic-level involvement can be a therapeutic ambulator. However, children with high thoracic involvement (above T10) rarely ambulate by the time they are teenagers; they prefer to be independently mobile in a wheelchair to be able to keep up with their peers. Children with high lumbar innervation (L1 or L2) can usually ambulate within the home or classroom but long-term prognosis is ambulation in a wheelchair. At L3 level, the strength of the quadriceps determines the level of functional ambulation in this group. Early on ambulation is household and short distances

in the community, but again wheelchair independence is the long-term prognosis. Children with L4 or below levels of innervation are community ambulators and should be able to maintain this level of independence throughout adulthood. Those at L4, L5, and sacral levels may also use a wheelchair for long distances or for sports participation.

Ambulation is a major goal during early childhood, and most children with MMC are successful. Over 90% of infants with sacral level lesions and 80% of those with low lumbar lesions achieve independent ambulation as compared with 20% with high lumbar lesions (Williams et al., 1999). Nevertheless, many children need a wheelchair to explore and have total access to their environments. Studies have shown that early introduction of wheeled mobility does not interfere with the acquisition of upright ambulation. In fact, wheelchair use may boost the child's self-confidence. It enables the child to exert control over her environment by independently moving to acquire an object or to seek out attention rather than passively waiting for an object to be brought by another person. Movement through the spatial environment is crucial for the development of perceptual cognitive development. Mobility is crucial to the child with MMC who may have difficulty with visual spatial cues, and several options should be made available depending on the child's developmental status. Box 7.3 shows a list of mobility options.

Wheelchair training for the toddler or preschooler should consist of preparatory and actual training activities, as listed in Box 7.4 and Box 7.5. The child should have sufficient sitting balance to use her arms to propel the chair or to operate

---

BOX 7.3 Mobility Options for Children With Myelomeningocele

Caster cart	Manual wheelchair
Prone scooter	Electric wheelchair
Walker	Adapted tricycle
Mobile vertical stander	Cyclone

BOX 7.4 Preparatory Activities for Wheelchair Mobility

Sitting balance
Arm strength
Ability to transfer
Wheelchair propulsion or operating an electric switch or joystick

---

BOX 7.5 Wheelchair Training for Toddlers and Preschoolers

Ability to transfer
Mobility on level surfaces
Exploration of home and classroom
Safety

(From Hinderer KA, Hinderer SR, Shurtleff DB: Myelodysplasia. In Campbell SK, Palisano RJ, Orlin MN, editors: *Physical therapy for children*, ed 4, Philadelphia, 2012, WB Saunders, pp. 703–755.)

an electric switch. Arm strength is necessary to propel a manual chair and to execute lateral transfers with or without a sliding board. Training begins on level surfaces within the home and classroom. Safety is always a number one priority; therefore the child should wear a seat belt while in the wheelchair. A study by Meiser and McEwen (2007) supports use of ultralight, rigid-frame wheelchairs for young children.

Strength, Flexibility, and Endurance

All functional activities in which a child participates require strong upper extremities. Traditional strengthening activities can be modified for the shorter stature of the child, and the amount of weight used can be adjusted to decrease the strain on growing bones. Weights, pulleys, latex-free tubing, and push-up blocks can be incorporated into games of "tug of war" and mat races. Trunk control and strength can be improved by use of righting and equilibrium reactions in developmentally appropriate positions. Refer to the descriptions earlier in this chapter.

Monitoring joint range of motion for possible contractures is exceedingly important at all stages of care. Be careful with repetitive movements because this population is prone to injury from excessive joint stress and overuse. Begin early on to think of joint conservation when the child is performing routine motions for transfers and ADLs. Learning to move the lower extremities by attaching strips of latex-free bands to them can be an early functional activity that fosters learning of self-performed range of motion. Group fitness (Fragala-Pinkham et al., 2006) programs resulted in improvement of all measures, especially functional mobility.

Use of a treadmill to increase endurance and foster earlier ambulation has been reported in the literature (Pantall et al., 2011; Moerchen et al., 2011). Principles of neural plasticity used with infants with Down syndrome to entrain locomotion have been applied to infants with spina bifida. Because infants with MMC do not produce as much spontaneous movement of the lower extremities as typically developing infants, they may benefit from using the treadmill to promote a stepping response. Pantall et al. (2011) used modifications to target sensory input to drive a motor response. Using Dycem (Warwick, Rhode Island) to increase friction and enhanced visual flow seemed to be more effective in producing stepping. Moerchen et al. (2011) reported on the decision-making that was used to develop and progress a home program for a child with low lumbar MMC that resulted in ambulation with a walker after 18 weeks of intervention. Lee and Sansom (2019) recently reported on a pilot study that involved daily parent-administered treadmill stepping in 10 infants with MMC. Feasibility of using the program within 6 months after birth was demonstrated. Participants acquired gross motor milestones 1.5 to 2 months earlier than similar children with MMC and within ranges of typically developing children.

Independence in Pressure Relief

Pressure relief and mobility must also be monitored whether the child is wearing an orthosis or not. When the child has the orthosis on, can she still do a push-up for pressure relief? Does the seating device or wheelchair currently used allow enough room for the child to sit without undue pressure from the additional width of the orthosis, or does it take up too much room in the wheelchair? How many different ways does the child know to relieve pressure? The more ways that are available to the child, the more likely the task is to be accomplished. The obvious way is to do push-ups, but if the child is in a regular chair at school, the chair may not have arms. If the child sits in a wheelchair at the desk, the chair must be locked before the child attempts a push-up. Forward leans can also be performed from a seated position. Alternative positioning in kneeling, standing, or lying prone can be used during rest and play periods. Be creative!

Independence in Self-Care and Activities of Daily Living

Skin care must be a high priority for the child with MMC, especially as the amount of sitting increases during the school day. Skin inspection should be done twice a day with a hand-held mirror. Clothing should be nonrestrictive and sufficiently thick to protect the skin from sharp objects and wheelchair parts and orthoses. An appropriate seat cushion must be used to distribute pressure while the child sits in the wheelchair. Pressure-reducing seat cushions do not, however, decrease the need for performing pressure-relief activities.

Children with MMC do not accomplish self-care activities at the same age as typically developing children (Okamoto et al., 1984; Sousa et al., 1983; Tsai et al., 2002) and are not independent in their daily performance (Peny-Dahlstrand et al., 2009). Children with MMC were found to be "unable to perform self-chosen and well-known everyday activities in an effortless, efficient, safe, and independent manner" (Peny-Dahlstrand et al., 2009). Daily self-care includes dressing and undressing, feeding, bathing, and bowel and bladder care. Interpretation of the data further suggests that the delays may be the result of lower performance expectations. Parents often do not perceive their children as competent compared with typically developing children, and may therefore expect less from them. Parents must be encouraged to expect independence from the child with MMC. Peny-Dahlstrand et al. (2009) suggested that children with MMC need help to learn how to do tasks and encouragement to persevere to complete the task.

By the time the child goes to preschool, she will be aware that her toileting abilities are different from those of her peers of the same age (Williamson, 1987). Bowel and bladder care are usually overseen by the school nurse where available, but everyone working with a child with MMC needs to be aware of the importance of these skills. Consistency of routine, privacy, and safety must always be part of any bowel and bladder program for a young child. Helping a child to maintain a positive self-image while teaching responsible toileting behavior can be especially tricky. The child should be given responsibility for as much of her own care as possible. Even if the child is still in diapers, she should also wash her hands at the sink after a diaper change. Williamson (1987) suggests these ways to assist the child to begin to participate:

1. Indicate the need for a diaper change.
2. Assist in pulling the pants down and in removing any orthotic devices, if necessary.

3. Unfasten the soiled diaper.
4. Refasten the clean diaper.
5. Assist in donning the orthosis if necessary and in pulling up the pants.
6. Wash hands.

Williamson (1987) provides many excellent suggestions for fostering self-care skills in the preschooler with MMC. The reader is referred to the text by this author for more information. ADL skills include the ability to transfer. We tend to think of transferring from mat to wheelchair and back as the ultimate transfer goal, but for the child to be as independent as possible, he should also be able to perform all transfers related to ADLs, such as to and from a bed, a dressing bench or a regular chair, a chair and a toilet, a chair and the floor, and the tub or shower.

Promotion of Cognitive and Social-Emotional Growth

Preschoolers are inquisitive individuals who need mobility to explore their environment. They should be encouraged to explore the space around them by physically moving through it, not just visually observing what goes on around them. Scooter boards can be used to help the child move her body weight with the arms while receiving vestibular input. The use of adapted tricycles that are propelled by arm cranking allows movement through space and they could be used on the playground rather than a wheelchair. Difficulty with mobility may interfere with self-initiated exploration and may foster dependence instead of independence. Other barriers to peer interaction or factors that may limit peer interaction are listed in Box 7.6.

Having a child with MMC can be stressful for the family (Holmbeck and Devine, 2010; Vermaes et al., 2008). Caregivers describe children with MMC as being less adaptable, more negative when initially responding to new or novel stimuli, more distractible, and less able to persist when completing a task compared with same-age peers without MMC (Vachha and Adams, 2005). Parents report that their children with MMC are less competent physically and cognitively than typically developing children (Landry et al., 1993). Clinicians can provide guidance to parents to interpret the child's signals and provide appropriate responses.

Many children with MMC experience healthy emotional development and exhibit high levels of resilience (Holmbeck and Devine, 2010). The task of infancy, according to Erikson, is to develop trust that basic needs will be met. Parents,

primary caregivers, and health care providers need to ensure that these emotional needs are met. If the infant perceives the world as hostile, she may develop coping mechanisms such as withdrawal or perseveration. If the child is encouraged to explore the environment and is guided to overcome the physical barriers encountered, she will perceive the world realistically as full of a series of challenges to be mastered, rather than as full of unsurmountable obstacles. In the case of children with MMC, the motor skills that they have the most difficulty with are those that involve motor planning and adaptation. Parents need to foster autonomy in daily life in their children with MMC.

Identification of Perceptual Problems

School-age children with MMC are motivated to learn and to perform academically to the same extent as any other children. During this time, perceptual problems may become apparent. Children with MMC have impaired visual analysis and synthesis (Vinck et al., 2006, 2010). Visual perception in a child with MMC should be evaluated separately from her visuomotor abilities, to determine whether she truly has a perceptual deficit. For example, a child's difficulty with copying shapes, a motor skill, may be more closely related to her lack of motor control of the upper extremity than to an inaccurate visual perception of the shape to be copied. Perception and cognition are connected to movement. Development of visual spatial perception and spatial cognition can occur because children with MMC have impaired movement. For example, children with MMC have been found to have problems with figure-ground (find the hidden shapes) and route finding as in a maze (Dennis et al., 2002; Jansen-Osmann et al., 2008).

Collaboration for Total Management

The management of the child with MMC in preschool and subsequently in the primary grades involves everyone who comes in contact with that child. From the bus driver to the teacher to the classroom aide, everyone has to know what the child is capable of doing, in which areas she needs assistance, and what must be done for her. Medical and educational goals should overlap to support the development of the most functionally independent child possible, a child whose psychosocial development is on the same level as that of her able-bodied peers and who is ready to fully participate in all aspects of adolescence and adulthood.

Third Stage of Physical Therapy Intervention

The third stage of management involves the transition to adolescence and into adulthood. General physical therapy goals during this last stage are as follows:
1. Reevaluation of ambulation potential including mobility in all settings.
2. Continued improvements in flexibility, strength, and endurance.
3. Independence in ADLs and self-management.
4. Physical fitness and participation in recreational and community activities.

BOX 7.6 Limitations to Peer Interaction

Mobility
Activities of daily living, especially transfers
Additional equipment
Independence in bowel and bladder care
Hygiene
Accessibility

5. Prevention of secondary complications and activity limitations.
6. Preparation for life as an adult with a chronic condition.

As more and more people with MMC are living later into adulthood, there is a need to focus more on prevention of secondary complications such as shunt malfunction, renal health, hypertension, diabetes, obesity, and skin breakdown.

Reevaluation of Ambulation Potential

The potential for continued ambulation needs to be reevaluated by the physical therapist during the student's school years and, in particular, as she approaches adolescence. Children with MMC go through puberty earlier than their peers who are able-bodied. Surgical procedures that depend on skeletal maturity may be scheduled at this time. The long-term functional level of mobility of these students can be determined as their physical maturity is peaking. The assistant working with the student can provide valuable data regarding the length of time that upright ambulation is used as the primary means of mobility. Any student in whom ambulation becomes unsafe or whose ambulation skills become limited functionally should discontinue ambulation except with supervision. Physical therapy goals during this time are to maintain the adolescent's present level of function if possible, to prevent secondary complications, to promote independence, to remediate any perceptual-motor problems, to provide any needed adaptive devices, and to promote self-esteem and social-sexual adjustment.

Developmental changes that may contribute to the loss of mobility in adolescents with MMC are as follows:

1. Changes in length of long bones, such that skeletal growth outstrips muscular growth.
2. Changes in body composition that alter the biomechanics of movement.
3. Progression of neurologic deficit.
4. Immobilization resulting from treatment of secondary problems, such as skin breakdown, neurosurgical intervention, or orthopedic surgery.
5. Progression of spinal deformity.
6. Joint pain or ligamentous laxity.

Physical therapy during this stage focuses on making a smooth transition to primary wheeled mobility if that transition is needed to save energy for more academic, athletic, or social activities. Individuals with thoracic, high lumbar (L1 or L2), and midlumbar (L3 or L4) lesions require a wheelchair for long-term functional mobility. They may have already been using a wheelchair during transport to and from school or for school field trips. School-age children can lose function because of spinal-cord tethering, so they should be monitored closely during rapid periods of growth for any signs of change in neurologic status. An adolescent with a midlumbar lesion can ambulate independently within a house or a classroom but may need aids to be functional within the community. Long-distance mobility is much more energy-efficient if the individual uses a wheelchair. Individuals with lower-level lesions (L5 and below) should be able to remain ambulatory for life, unless too great an increase in body weight occurs, thereby making wheelchair use a necessity. Hinderer et al. (1988) found a potential decline in mobility resulting from progressive neurologic loss in adolescents even with lower-level lesions, so any adolescent with MMC should be monitored for potential progression of neurologic deficit (Mukherjee and Pasulka, 2017). Weight gain can severely impair the teen's ability to ambulate.

Youths with MMC engage in unhealthy behaviors such as less healthy diets, sedentary activities, and less exercise compared with national estimates. Peer interactions may predict community participation and quality of life in adults with MMC. Eighteen- and 19-year-olds are considered emerging adults. One study reported that lower levels of executive dysfunction predicted that the individual with MMC would have a greater number of friends (Zukerman et al., 2011). Social and emotional problems were seen in children and adolescents who had less severe impairments (Stromfors et al., 2017). This paradox may be due to marginality that makes it hard for the person to identify with either healthy or more impaired peers. Marginality is characterized by ambiguous self-perceptions (Friedman, 1988). Studies have found that includes identifying as both a healthy person and as a disabled person.

Wheelchair mobility. When an adolescent with MMC makes the transition to continuous use of a wheelchair, you should not dwell on the loss of upright ambulation as something devastating but focus on the positive gains provided by wheeled mobility. Most of the time, if the transition is presented as a natural and normal occurrence, it is more easily accepted by the individual. The wheelchair should be presented as just another type of "assistive" device, thereby decreasing any negative connotation for the adolescent. The mitigating factor is always the energy cost. The student with MMC may be able to ambulate within the classroom but may need a wheelchair to move efficiently between classes and keep up with her friends. "Mobility limitations are magnified once a child begins school because of the increased community mobility distances and skills required" (Hinderer et al., 2000). This requirement becomes a significant problem once a child is in school because the travel distances increase, and the skills needed to maneuver within new environments become more complicated. A wheelchair may be a necessity by middle school or whenever the student begins to change classes, has to retrieve books from a locker, and needs to go to the next class in a short time. For the student with all but the lowest motor levels, wheeled mobility is a must to maintain efficient function. Johnson et al. (2007) found that 57% to 65% of young adults with MMC use lightweight wheelchairs, both manual and power-assisted.

Environmental Accessibility

All environments in which a person with MMC functions should be accessible: home, school, and community. The Americans with Disabilities Act was an effort to make all public buildings, programs, and services accessible to the general public. Under this Act, reasonable accommodations have to be made to allow an individual with a disability to access public education and facilities. Public transportation, libraries, and grocery stores, for example, should be accessible to everyone. Assistive technology can play a significant role in improving access and independence for the youth with MMC. Timers, cell phones, and computer access can be used to support personal-care routines as well as organization skills (Johnson et al., 2007).

Driver Education

Driver education is as important to a person with MMC as it is to any 16-year-old teenager, and may be even more so. Some states have programs that evaluate the ability of an individual with a disability to drive, after which recommendations to use appropriate devices, such as hand controls and type of vehicle, will be given. A review of car transfers should be part of therapy for adolescents along with other activities that prepare them for independent living and a job. The ability to move the wheelchair in and out of the car is also vital to independent function.

Flexibility, Strength, and Endurance

Prevention of contractures must be aggressively pursued during the rapid growth of adolescence because skeletal growth can cause significant shortening of muscles. Stretching should be done at home on a regular basis and at school if the student has problem areas. Areas that should be targeted are the low back extensors, the hip flexors, the hamstrings, and the shoulder girdle. Proper positioning for sitting and sleeping should be reviewed, with the routine use of the prone position crucial to keep hip and knee flexors loose and to relieve pressure on the buttocks. More decubitus ulcers are seen in adolescents with MMC because of increased body weight, less strict adherence to pressure-relief procedures, and development of adult patterns of sweating around the buttocks.

Strengthening exercises and activities can be incorporated into physical education free time. A workout can be planned for the student that can be carried out both at home and at a local gym. Endurance activities such as wind sprints in the wheelchair, swimming, wheelchair track, basketball, and tennis are all appropriate ways to work on muscular and cardiovascular endurance while the student is socializing. If wheelchair sports are available, this is an excellent way to combine strengthening and endurance activities for fun and fitness. Check with your local parks and recreation department for information on wheelchair sports available in your area.

Hygiene/Health Practices

Adult patterns of sweating, incontinence of bowel and bladder, and the onset of menses can all contribute to a potential hygiene problem for an adolescent with MMC. A good bowel and bladder program is essential to avoid incontinence, odor, and skin irritation, which can contribute to low self-esteem. Adolescents are extremely body conscious, and the additional stress of dealing with bowel and bladder dysfunction, along with menstruation for girls, may be particularly burdensome. Scheduled toileting and bathing and meticulous self-care, including being able to wipe properly and to handle pads and

tampons, can provide adequate maintenance of personal hygiene. In a qualitative study by Stromfors et al. (2017), some adolescents with MMC expressed worrying about urine leakage and missing classroom time at school due to visits. Half of adults with MMC report having a urinary tract infection annually (Dicianno et al., 2015).

Socialization/Sexuality

Adolescents are particularly conscious about their body image, so they may be motivated to maintain a normal weight and to provide extra attention to their bowel and bladder programs. Sexuality is also a big concern for adolescents. Functional limitations based on levels of innervation are discussed in Chapter 13. However, the level of neurologic lesion may not correlate with sexual function in this group. Abstinence, safe sex, use of birth control to prevent pregnancy, and knowledge of the dangers of sexually transmitted diseases must all be topics of discussion with the teenager with MMC. At least one-quarter of patients with MMC report having had sexual intercourse (Lassman et al., 2007; Sawin et al., 2014; Visconti et al., 2012). Information on sexuality comes primarily from health care providers, and it is incumbent on them to encourage adherence to healthy practices by providing accurate information.

Social isolation can have a negative effect on emotional and social development in this population (Holmbeck et al., 2003). Socialization requires access to all social situations at school and in the community. Peer relationships can be predictive of quality of life. Peer interaction during adolescence can be limited by the same things identified as potential limitations early in life, as listed in Box 7.6. Additional challenges to the adolescent with MMC can occur if issues of adolescence such as personal identity, sexuality, and peer relations, and concern for loss of biped ambulation are not resolved. Again, the therapist needs to be aware of a potential condition-severity paradox in that the person with less severe impairment might be at increased risk for developing social and emotional problems (Stromfors et al., 2017). Achieving adult development can be hindered by the development of secondary complications, which can result in more hospitalizations than occurs in the general population. Shunt revisions are associated with lack of independent living, learning to drive a car, employment status.

Independent Living/Autonomy

Basic ADLs (BADLs) are those activities required for personal care such as ambulating, feeding, bathing, dressing, grooming, maintaining continence, and toileting. Instrumental ADLs (IADLs) are those skills that require the use of equipment such as the stove, washing machine, or vacuum cleaner, and they relate to managing within the home and community. Being able to shop for food or clothes and being able to prepare a meal are examples of IADLs. Mastery of both BADL and IADL skills is needed to be able to live on one's own. Functional limitations that may affect both BADLs and IADLs may become apparent when the person with MMC has difficulty in lifting and carrying objects. Vocational counseling and planning should begin during high school or even possibly in middle school. The student should be encouraged to live on her own if possible after high school as part of a college experience or during vocational training.

Persons with MMC often exhibit problems attaining autonomy and living independently. Stromfors et al. (2017) found that participants in their study, persons with MMC between 10 and 17 years of age, did not accurately assess their level of independence nor did they express being strongly motivated to become independent. Even as children, mastery of motivation, that internal drive to increase independence, has been found to be low (Landry et al., 1993; Warschausky et al., 2017). Planning for the future and "launching" of a young adult with MMC has been reported in the literature. Launching is the last transition in the family life cycle in which "the late adolescent is launched into the outside world to begin to develop an autonomous life" (Friedrich and Shaffer, 1986). Challenges during this time include discussion regarding guardianship if ongoing care is needed, placement plans, and a redefinition of the roles of the parents and the young adult with MMC. Employment of only 25% of adults with MMC was reported by Hunt (1990), and few persons described in this report were married or had children. Buran et al. (2004) describe adolescents with MMC as having hopeful and positive attitudes toward their disability. However, they found the adolescents were not engaging in sufficient decision-making and self-management to prepare themselves for adult roles. This lack of preparation might be the reason many individuals with MMC are underemployed and not living independently as young adults (Buran et al., 2004). Each period of the lifespan brings different challenges for the family with a child with MMC. In light of the recent research, more emphasis may need to be placed on decision-making during adolescence.

QUALITY OF LIFE

Locomotion and therefore ambulation potential impact the quality of life of an individual with MMC. Rendeli et al. (2002) found that children with MMC had significantly different cognitive outcomes based on their ambulatory status. Those that walked with or without assistive devices had higher performance IQ than those who did not ambulate. There was no difference between the two groups on total IQ. It has been suggested that self-produced locomotion facilitates development of spatial cognition. Others have found

that independent ambulatory status was the most important factor in determining health-related quality of life (HRQOL) (Schoenmakers et al., 2005; Danielsson et al., 2008). HRQOL is a broad multidimensional concept that usually includes self-reported measures of physical and mental health. Children with MMC were found to have a lower HRQOL than other children with a chronic illness (Oddson et al., 2006). Seventy-two percent of youths and young adults with MMC had decreased participation in structured activities and required assistive technology to assist their mobility (Johnson et al., 2007). The presence of spasticity in the muscles around the hip and knee, quadriceps muscle weakness, level of lesion, and severity of neurologic symptoms affected ambulatory ability and functional ability, which in turn decreased HRQOL (Danielsson et al., 2008). Flanagan et al. (2011) found that the parentally perceived HRQOL of children with MMC differed based on the motor level of the child. Children with motor levels at L2 and above had decreased HRQOL scores compared with children with motor levels at L3 to L5. They used the Pediatric Quality of Life Inventory and the Pediatric Outcomes Data Collection Instrument Version 2.0 as measures of HRQOL. Categories in which there were score differences included sports and physical function, transfers and basic mobility, health, and global function.

In contrast, Kelley et al. (2011) found that participation in children with MMC did not differ based on motor level, ambulation status, or bowel and bladder problems. They divided their subjects into age groups, 2 to 5 years, 6 to 12 years, and 13 to 18 years. There were differences between groups in participation scores for skill-based activities (physical and recreational activities), with younger children participating more in skill-based and physical activities and the middle age group participating more in recreational activities than the older group. Bowel and bladder problems were found to limit the participation of the children of 6 to 12 years old in social and physical activities. Kelley et al. (2011) used different measures for participation than Flanagan et al. (2011). It also appears that a higher percentage of children in the study of Kelley et al. (2011) were at a L3 motor level, which according to the study by Flanagan et al. (2011) have a higher HRQOL. Regardless, physical function does affect the quality of life of individuals with MMC. Clinicians need to be more focused on breaking down community barriers to participation and promoting optimal mobility and health so that children with MMC transition into independent adults.

CHAPTER SUMMARY

The management of the person with MMC is complex and requires multiple levels of intervention and constant monitoring. Early on, intensive periods of intervention are needed to establish the best outcome and to provide the infant and child with MMC the best developmental start possible. Physical therapy intervention focuses primarily on the attainment of head and trunk control within the boundaries of the neurologic involvement. Although the achievement of

independent ambulation may be expected of most people with MMC during their childhood years, this expectation needs to be tempered based on the child's motor level and long-term potential for functional ambulation. Fostering cognitive and social–emotional maturity should occur simultaneously. Mobility in the community is crucial for reaching functional outcomes and ensuring activity and participation. Children with MMC can develop social abilities despite a reduced level of self-care or impaired motor function. However, independence in self-care, transfers, and mobility will ease the transition from adolescence to adulthood. The physical therapist monitors the student's motor progress throughout the school years and intervenes during transitions to a new setting. Each new setting may demand increased or different functional skills. Monitoring the student in school also includes looking for any evidence of deterioration of neurologic or musculoskeletal status that may prevent optimum function in school or access to the community. Examples of appropriate intervention times are occasions when the student needs assistance in making the transition to another level of function, such as using a wheelchair for primary mobility and evaluating a work site

for wheelchair access. The physical therapist assistant may provide therapy to the individual with MMC that is aimed at fostering functional motor abilities or teaching functional skills related to use of orthoses or assistive devices, transfers, and ADLs. The physical therapist assistant can provide valuable data to the therapist during annual examinations, as well as ongoing information regarding function to manage the needs of the person with MMC from birth through adulthood most efficiently. Greater attention needs to be given to prevention of secondary impairments owing to changes in body structure and function with age. Transition to adulthood may be more difficult for persons with MMC if they do not realistically assess their own level of independence or lack sufficient motivation to become independent.

REVIEW QUESTIONS

1. What type of paralysis can be expected in a child with MMC?
2. What complications are seen in a child with MMC that may be related to skeletal growth?
3. What are the signs of shunt malfunction in a child with MMC?
4. What position is important to use in preventing the development of hip and knee flexion contractures in a child with MMC?
5. What precautions should be taken by parents to protect skin integrity in a child with MMC?

6. What determines the type of orthosis used by a child with MMC?
7. What is the relationship of motor level to level of ambulation in a child with MMC?
8. When is the functional level of mobility determined for an individual with MMC?
9. What developmental changes may contribute to a loss of mobility in the adolescent with MMC?
10. What issues should be addressed in a transition program for an individual with MMC?

CASE STUDIES REHABILITATION UNIT INITIAL EXAMINATION AND EVALUATION: PL

History

Chart Review

PL is a talkative, good-natured, 3-year-old boy. He is in the care of his grandmother during the day because both of his parents work. He is the younger of two children. PL presents with a low lumbar (L2) myelomeningocele (MMC) with flaccid paralysis. Medical history includes premature birth at 32 weeks of gestation, bilateral hip dislocation, bilateral clubfeet (surgically repaired at 1 year of age), scoliosis, multiple hemivertebrae, and shunted (ventriculoperitoneal) hydrocephalus (at birth).

Subjective

Mother reports that PL's previous physical therapy consisted of passive and active range of motion for the lower extremities and learning to walk with a walker and braces. She expresses concern about his continued mobility now that he is going to preschool. She lacks confidence in his ability to perform self-care, master toileting, and participate in preschool.

Objective

Systems Review

Communication/Cognition: PL communicates in 5- to 6-word sentences. PL has an IQ of 90.

Cardiovascular/Pulmonary: Normal values for age.

Integumentary: Healed 7-cm scar on the lower back, no areas of redness below L2.

Musculoskeletal: Active range of motion and strength within functional limits in the upper extremities. Active range of motion limitations present in the lower extremities, secondary to neuromuscular weakness.

Neuromuscular: Upper extremities grossly coordinated, lower extremity paralysis.

Tests and Measures

Anthropometric: Height 36 inches, weight 35 lbs, body mass index 19 (20 to 24 is normal).

Circulation: Skin warm to touch below L2, pedal pulses present bilaterally, strong radial pulse.

Integumentary: No ulcers or edema present. Shunt palpable behind right ear.

Motor Function: PL's motor upper extremity skills are coordinated. He can build an 8-cube tower. He sits independently and moves in and out of sitting and standing independently. He is unable to transfer into and out of the tub independently.

Neurodevelopmental Status: Peabody Developmental Motor Scales Developmental Motor Quotient = 69. Age equivalent = 12 months. Fine motor development is average for his age

Continued

CASE STUDIES REHABILITATION UNIT INITIAL EXAMINATION AND EVALUATION: PL—cont'd

(Peabody Developmental Motor Scales Developmental Motor Quotient = 90).

Reflex integrity: Patellar 1 +, Achilles 0 bilaterally. No abnormal tone is noted in the upper extremities; tone is decreased in the trunk, flaccid in the lower extremities.

Range of Motion: Active motion is within functional limits for the upper extremities and for hip flexion and adduction. Active knee extension is complete in side-lying. Passive motion is within functional limits for remaining joints of the lower extremities.

Muscle Performance: As tested using functional muscle testing. If the child could move the limb against gravity and take any resistance the muscle was graded 3 +. If the limb could only move through full range in the gravity-eliminated position, the muscle was graded a 2.

Abdominals	Right	Left
	Partial Symmetrical Curl Up	
Hips		
Iliopsoas	3 +	3 +
Gluteus maximus	0	0
Adductors	3	3
Abductors	0	0
Knees		
Quadriceps	2	2
Hamstrings	0	0
Ankles and feet	0	0

Sensory Integrity: Pinprick intact to L2, absent below.

Posture: PL exhibits a mild right thoracic–left lumbar scoliosis.

Gait, Locomotion, and Balance: PL sits independently and stands with a forward facing walker and bilateral hip-knee-ankle-foot orthoses (HKAFOs). PL can demonstrate a reciprocal gait pattern for approximately 10 feet when he ambulates with a walker and HKAFOs but prefers a swing-to pattern. Using a swing-to pattern, he can ambulate 25 feet before wanting to rest. He creeps reciprocally but prefers to drag-crawl. PL can creep up stairs with assistance and comes down headfirst on his stomach. Head and trunk righting are present in sitting, with upper extremity protective extension present in all directions to either side. PL exhibits minimal trunk rotation when balance is disturbed laterally in sitting.

Self-Care: PL assists with dressing and undressing and is independent in his sitting balance while performing bathing and dressing activities. He feeds himself but is dependent in bowel and bladder care (wears a diaper).

Play/Preschool: PL exhibits cooperative play and functional play but is delayed in pretend play. He presently attends morning preschool 3 days a week and will be attending every day within 1 month.

Assessment/Evaluation

PL is a 3-year-old boy with a repaired L2 MMC, a ventriculoperitoneal shunt. He is currently ambulating with a forward-facing walker and HKAFOs. He is making the transition to a preschool program. He is seen one time a week for 30 minutes of physical therapy.

Problem List

1. Unable to ambulate with Lofstrand crutches.
2. Decreased strength and endurance.
3. Dependent in self-care and transfers.
4. Lacking knowledge of pressure relief.
5. Lacks pretend play.

Diagnosis: PL exhibits impaired force production and sensory deficits associated with MMC. He is at risk for visual perceptual problems and is delayed in development of pretend play.

Prognosis: PL will improve his level of functional independence and functional skills in the preschool setting. He has excellent potential to achieve the following goals within the school year.

Short-Term Objectives (Actions to be Accomplished by Midyear Review)

1. PL will propel a prone scooter up and down the hall of the preschool for 15 consecutive minutes.
2. PL will perform 20 consecutive chin-ups during free play on the playground daily.
3. PL will kick a soccer ball 5 to 10 feet, 4 or 5 attempts during free play daily.
4. PL will wash and dry hands after toileting without cueing.
5. PL will be independent in pressure relief.

Long-Term Functional Goals (End of the First Year in Preschool)

1. PL will ambulate to and from the gym and the lunchroom using a reciprocal gait pattern and Lofstrand crutches daily.
2. PL will exhibit pretend play by verbally engaging in story time 3 times a week.
3. PL will assist in managing clothing during toileting and clean intermittent catheterization.

Plan

Coordination, Communication, and Documentation

The therapist and physical therapist assistant will communicate with PL's mother and teacher on a regular basis. Suggestions regarding increasing PL's play complexity will be shared with the teacher and his mother. Outcomes of interventions will be documented on a weekly basis. He may be a candidate for a reciprocating gait orthosis to improve gait efficiency.

Patient/Client Instruction

PL and his family will be instructed in a home exercise program, including upper extremity and trunk strengthening exercises, practicing trunk righting and equilibrium reactions in sitting and standing, dressing, toileting, transfers, improving standing time, and ambulation using the preferred pattern.

Interventions

1. Mat activities that incorporate prone push-ups, wheelbarrow walking, movement transitions from prone to long sitting, and back to prone, sitting push-ups with push-up blocks, and pressure relief techniques.
2. Using a movable surface such as a ball, promote lateral equilibrium reactions to encourage active trunk rotation.

CASE STUDIES REHABILITATION UNIT INITIAL EXAMINATION AND EVALUATION: PL—cont'd

3. Resistive exercises for upper and lower extremities using latex-free Theraband or cuff weights.
4. Resisted creeping to improve lower extremity reciprocation and trunk control.
5. Increased distances walked using a reciprocal gait pattern by 5 feet every 2 weeks, first with a walker, progressing to Lofstrand crutches.
6. Increased standing time and ability to shift weight while using Lofstrand crutches.
7. Transfer training.
8. Play with peers and engage in play songs using props.
9. Use multiple step motor actions on the playground.

Questions to Think About
- What additional interventions could be used to accomplish these goals?
- Are these goals educationally relevant?
- Which activities should be part of the home exercise program?
- How can fitness be incorporated into PL's physical therapy program?
- Identify interventions that may be needed as PL makes the transition to school.

REFERENCES

Adzick NS, Thom EA, Spong CY, et al.: A randomized trial of prenatal versus postnatal repair of myelomeningocele, *N Engl J Med* 364:993–1004, 2011.

Ausili E, Focarelli B, Tabacco F, et al.: Bone mineral density and body composition in a myelomeningocele children population: effects of walking ability and sport activity, *Eur Rev Med Pharmacol Sci* 12(6):349–354, 2008.

Barf HA, Verhoef M, Post MW, et al.: Educational career and predictors of type of education in young adults with spina bifida, *Int J Rehabil Res* 27(1):45–52, 2004.

Blumchen K, Bayer P, Buck D, et al.: Effects of latex avoidance on latex sensitization, atopy, and allergic diseases in patients with spina bifida, *Allergy* 65(12):1585–1593, 2010.

Boulet SL, Yang Q, Mai C, et al.: National Birth Defects Prevention Network: Trends in the postfortification prevalence of spina bifida and anencephaly in the United States, *Birth Defects Res A Clin Mol Teratol* 82(7):527–532, 2008.

Bowman RM, McLone DG, Grant JA, Tomita T, Ito JA: Spina bifida outcome: a 25-year prospective, *Pediatr Neurosurg* 34(3):114–120, 2001.

Bowman RM, Boshnjaku V, McLone DG: The changing incidence of myelomeningocele and its impact on pediatric neurosurgery: a review from the Children's Memorial Hospital, *Childs Nerv Syst* 25:801–806, 2009a.

Bowman RM, Mohan A, Ito J, et al.: Tethered cord release: a long-term study in 114 patients, *J Neurosurg Pediatr* 3:181–187, 2009b.

Buran CF, Sawin KJ, Brei TJ, Fastenau PS: Adolescents with myelomeningocele: activities, beliefs, expectations, and perceptions, *Dev Med Child Neurol* 46:244–252, 2004.

Byrd SE, Darling CF, McLone DG, et al.: Developmental disorders of the pediatric spine, *Radiol Clin North Am* 29:711–752, 1991.

Centers for Disease Control and Prevention: *Spina bifida.* Available at: www.cdc.gov/ncbddd/spinabifida/data.html/. Accessed November 11, 2018.

Copp AJ, Greene ND: Genetics and development of neural tube defects, *J Pathol* 220:217–230, 2010.

Cremer R, Kleine-Diepenbruck U, Hering F, Holschneider AM: Reduction of latex sensitization in spina bifida patients by a primary prophylaxis programme (five-year experience), *Eur J Pediatr Surg* 12(Suppl 1):S19–S21, 2002.

Danielsson AJ, Bartonek A, Levey E, et al.: Associations between orthopaedic findings, ambulation, and health-related quality of life in children with myelomeningocele, *J Child Orthop* 2:45–54, 2008.

Dennis M, Fletcher JM, Rogers T, et al.: Object-based and action-based visual perception in children with spina bifida and hydrocephalus, *J Int Neuropsychol Soc* 8:95–106, 2002.

Dennis M, Edelstein K, Copeland K, et al.: Covert orienting to exogenous and endogenous cues children with spina bifida, *Neuropsychologia* 43:976–987, 2005.

Dennis M, Salman S, Jewell D, et al.: Upper limb motor function in young adults with spina bifida and hydrocephalus, *Childs Nerv Syst* 25:1447–1453, 2009.

Dicianno BE, Karmarkar A, Houtrow A, et al.: Factors associated with mobility outcomes in a national spina bifida patient registry, *Am J Phys Med Rehabil* 94(2):1015–1025, 2015.

Dosa NP, Eckrich M, Katz DA, et al.: Incidence, prevalence, and characteristics of fractures in children, adolescents, and adults with spina bifida, *J Spinal Cord Med* 30(Suppl 1):S5–S9, 2007.

Effgen SK, Brown DA: Long-term stability of hand-held dynamometric measurements in children who have myelomeningocele, *Phys Ther* 72:458–465, 1992.

Fay G, Shurtleff DB, Shurtleff H, Wolf L: Approaches to facilitate independent self-care and academic success. In Shurtleff DB, editor: *Myelodysplasias and exstrophies: significance, prevention, and treatment*, Orlando, FL, 1986, Grune & Stratton, pp 373–398.

Flanagan A, Gorzkowski M, Altiok H, Hassani S, Ahn KW: Activity level, functional health, and quality of life of children with myelomeningocele as perceived by parents, *Clin Orthop Relat Res* 469:1230–1235, 2011.

Fragala-Pinkham MA, Haley SM, Goodgold S: Evaluation of a community based group fitness program for children with disabilities, *Pediatr Phys Ther* 18:159–167, 2006.

Friedman SB: The concept of "marginality" applied to psychosomatic medicine, *Psychosom Med* 50:447–453, 1988.

Friedrich W, Shaffer J: Family adjustments and contributions. In Shurtleff DB, editor: *Myelodysplasias and exstrophies: significance, prevention, and treatment*, Orlando, FL, 1986, Grune & Stratton, pp 399–410.

Greene ND, Copp AJ: Neural tube defects, *Annu Rev Neurosci* 37:221–242, 2014.

Grief L, Stalmasek V: Tethered cord syndrome: a pediatric case study, *J Neurosci Nurs* 21:86–91, 1989.

Grimm RA: Hand function and tactile perception in a sample of children with myelomeningocele, *Am J Occup Ther* 30:234–240, 1976.

Hertzler DA, DePowell JJ, Stevenson CB, Mangano FT: Tethered cord syndrome: a review of the literature from embryology to adult presentation, *Neurosurg Focus* 29(1):E1, 2010.

Heurer GG, Moldenhauer JS, Adzick S: Prenatal surgery for myelomeningocele: review of the literature and future directions, *Childs Nerv Syst* 33(7):1149–1155, 2017.

Hinderer SR, Hinderer KA: Sensory examination of individuals with myelodysplasia (abstract), *Arch Phys Med Rehabil* 71: 769–770, 1990.

Hinderer SR, Hinderer KA, Dunne K, et al.: Medical and functional status of adults with spina bifida (abstract), *Dev Med Child Neurol* 30(Suppl 57):28, 1988.

Hinderer KA, Hinderer SR, Shurtleff DB: Myelodysplasia. In Campbell SK, Palisano RJ, Vander Linden DW, editors: *Physical therapy for children*, ed 2, Philadelphia, 2000, Saunders, pp 621–670.

Hinderer KA, Hinderer SR, Shurtleff DB: Myelodysplasia. In Palisano RJ, Orlin MN, Schreiber J, editors: *Campbell's physical therapy for children*, ed 5, St. Louis, 2017, Elsevier, pp 542–582.

Hinderer KA, Hinderer SR, Shurtleff DB: Myelodysplasia. In Campbell SK, Palisano RJ, Orlin MN, editors: *Physical therapy for children*, ed 3, Philadelphia, 2012, Saunders, pp 703–755.

Hoffer MM, Feiwell E, Perry R, et al.: Functional ambulation in patients with myelomeningocele, *J Bone Joint Surg Am* 55: 137–148, 1973.

Holmbeck GM, Devine KA: Psychosocial and family functioning in spina bifida, *Dev Disabil Res Rev* 16:40–46, 2010.

Holmbeck GN, Westhoven VC, Philips WS, et al.: A multimethod, multi-informant, and multidimensional perspective on psychosocial adjustment in preadolescents with spina bifida, *J Consult Clin Psychol* 71:782–795, 2003.

Hunt GM: Open spina bifida: outcome for a complete cohort treated unselectively and followed into adulthood, *Dev Med Child Neurol* 32:108–118, 1990.

Hwang R, Kentish M, Burns Y: Hand positioning sense in children with spina bifida myelomeningocele, *Aust J Physiother* 48:17–22, 2002.

Jansen-Osmann P, Wiedenbauer G, Heil M: Spatial cognition and motor development: a study of children with spina bifida, *Percept Mot Skills* 106(2):436–446, 2008.

Jewell D, Fletcher JM, Mahy CEV, et al.: Upper limb cerebellar motor function in children with spina bifida, *Childs Nerv Syst* 26:67–73, 2010.

Johnson KL, Dudgeon B, Kuehn C, Walker W: Assistive technology use among adolescents and young adults with spina bifida, *Am J Public Health* 97:330–336, 2007.

Kelley EH, Altiok H, Gorzkowski JA, Abrams JR, Vogel LC: How does participation of youth with spina bifida vary by age? *Clin Orthop Relat Res* 469:1236–1245, 2011.

Krosschell KJ, Pesavento MJ: Spina bifida: a congenital spinal cord injury. In Umphred DA, Lazaro RT, Roller ML, Burton GU, editors: *Umphred's neurological rehabilitation*, ed 6, St. Louis, 2013, Elsevier, pp 419–458.

Landry SH, Robinson SS, Copeland D, Garner PW: Goal-directed behavior and perception of self-competence in children with spina bifida, *J Pediatr Psychol* 18:389–396, 1993.

Landry SH, Lomax-Bream L, Barnes M: The importance of early motor and visual functioning for later cognitive skills in preschoolers with and without spina bifida, *J Int Neuropsychol Soc* 9:175, 2003.

Lassman J, Garibay Gonzalez F, Melchionni JB, et al.: Sexual function in adult patients with spina bifida and its impact on quality of life, *J Urol* 178(4):1611–1614, 2007.

Lee DK, Sansom JK: Early treadmill practice in infants born with myelomeningocele: a pilot study, *Pediatr Phys Ther* 31:68–75, 2019.

Lock TR, Aronson DD: Fractures in patients who have myelomeningocele, *J Bone Joint Surg Am* 71:1153–1157, 1989.

Lupo PJ, Agopian AJ, Castillo H, et al.: Genetic epidemiology of neural tube defects, *J Pediatr Rehabil Med* 10(3-4):189–194, 2017.

Luthy DA, Wardinsky T, Shurtleff DB, et al.: Cesarean section before the onset of labor and subsequent motor function in infants with myelomeningocele diagnosed antenatally, *N Engl J Med* 324:662–666, 1991.

Marrieos H, Loff C, Calado E: Osteoporosis in paediatric patients with spina bifida, *J Spinal Cord Med* 35(1):9–21, 2012.

Mazon A, Nieto A, Linana JJ, et al.: Latex sensitization in children with spina bifida: follow-up comparative study after two years, *Ann Allergy Asthma Immunol* 84:207–210, 2000.

Meiser MJ, McEwen I: Lightweight and ultralightweight wheelchairs: propulsion and preferences of two young children with spina bifida, *Pediatr Phys Ther* 19:245–253, 2007.

Moerchen VA, Habibi M, Lynett KA, et al.: Treadmill training and overground gait: decision making for a toddler with spina bifida, *Pediatr Phys Ther* 23:53–61, 2011.

Mukherjee S, Pasulka J: Care for adults with spina bifida: current state and future directions, *Top Spinal Cord Inj Rehabil* 23(2):155–167, 2017.

Oddson BE, Clancey CA, McGrath PJ: The role of pain in reduced quality of life and depressive symptomatology in children with spina bifida, *Clin J Pain* 22:784–789, 2006.

Okamoto GA, Sousa J, Telzrow RW, et al.: Toileting skills in children with myelomeningocele: rates of learning, *Arch Phys Med Rehabil* 65:182–185, 1984.

Paleg G, Glickman LB, Smith BA: Evidence-based clinical recommendations for dosing of pediatric supported standing programs. Presented at combined sections meeting of the American Physical Therapy Association, Las Vegas, Feb. 4, 2014, Nevada.

Pantall A, Teulier C, Smith BA, et al.: Impact of enhanced sensory input on treadmill step frequency: infants born with myelomeningocele, *Pediatr Phys Ther* 23:42–52, 2011.

Peny-Dahlstrand M, Ahlander AC, Krumlinde-Sunholm L, Gosman-Hedstrom G: Quality of performance of everyday activities in children with spina bifida: a population-based study, *Acta Paediatr* 98:1674–1679, 2009.

Rendeli C, Salvaggio E, Cannizzaro GS, et al.: Does locomotion improve the cognitive profile of children with myelomeningocele? *Childs Nerv Syst* 18:231–234, 2002.

Rosenstein BD, Greene WB, Herrington RT, et al.: Bone density in myelomeningocele: the effects of ambulatory status and other factors, *Dev Med Child Neurol* 29:486–494, 1987.

Ryan KD, Ploski C, Emans JB: Myelodysplasia—the musculoskeletal problem: habilitation from infancy to adulthood, *Phys Ther* 71:935–946, 1991.

Sandler AD: Children with spina bifida: key clinical issues, *Pediatr Clin North Am* 57:879–892, 2010.

Sawin KJ, Bellin MH, Roux G, et al.: The experience of self-management in adolescent women with spina bifida, *Rehabil Nurs* 34:26–38, 2014.

Schoenmakers MA, Gooskens RH, Gulmans VA, et al.: Long-term outcome of neurosurgical untethering on neurosegmental motor and ambulation levels, *Dev Med Child Neurol* 45:551–555, 2003.

Schoenmakers MA, Uiterwaal CS, Gulmans VA, Gooskens RH, Helders PJ: Determinants of functional independence and quality of life in children with spina bifida, *Clin Rehabil* 19:677–685, 2005.

Sousa JC, Telzrow RW, Holm RA, et al.: Developmental guidelines for children with myelodysplasia, *Phys Ther* 63:21–29, 1983.

Stromfors L, Wilhelmsson S, Falk L, Host GE: Experiences among children and adolescents of living with spina bifida and their visions of the future, *Disabil Rehabil* 39(3):261–271, 2017.

Sutton LN: Fetal surgery for neural tube defects, *Best Pract Res Clin Obstet Gynaecol* 22:175--188, 2008.

Swaroop VT, Dias L: Orthopaedic management of spina bifida – part I: hip, knee, and rotational deformities, *J Child Orthop* 3:441–449, 2009.

Swaroop VT, Dias L: Orthopaedic management of spina bifida – part II: foot and ankle deformities, *J Child Orthop* 5:403–414, 2011.

Thibadeau JK, Ward EA, Soe MM, et al.: Testing the feasibility of a National Spina Bifida Patient Registry, *Birth Defects Res A Clin Mol Teratol* 97(1):36–41, 2013.

Tomlinson P, Sugarman ID: Complications with shunts in adults with spina bifida, *BMJ* 311(7000):286–287, 1995.

Trinh A, Wong P, Brown J, et al.: Fractures in spina bifida from childhood to adulthood, *Osteoporos Int* 28(1):399–406, 2017.

Tsai PY, Yang TF, Chan RC, Huang PH, Wong TT: Functional investigation in children with spina bifida, measured by the Pediatric Evaluation of Disability Inventory (PEDI), *Childs Nerv Syst* 18:48–53, 2002.

Tulipan N: Intrauterine myelomeningocele repair, *Clin Perinatol* 30(3):521–530, 2003.

Vachha B, Adams R: Myelomeningocele, temperament patterns, and parental perceptions, *Pediatrics* 115:e58–e63, 2005.

Verhoef M, Barf HA, Post MW, et al.: Secondary impairment in young adults with spina bifida, *Dev Med Child Neurol* 46(6):420–427, 2004.

Vermaes IPR, Janssens JMAM, Mullaart RA, Vinck A, Gerris JRM: Parent's personality and parenting stress in families of children with spina bifida, *Child Care Health Dev* 34(5): 665–674, 2008.

Vinck A, Maassen B, Mullaart RA, Rottevell J: Arnold-Chiari-II malformation and cognitive functioning in spina bifida, *J Neurol Neurosurg Psychiatry* 77(9):1083–1086, 2006.

Vinck A, Nijhuis-van der Sanden M, Roeleveld N, et al.: Motor profile and cognitive function in children with spina bifida, *Eur J Paediatr Neurol* 14:86–92, 2010.

Visconti D, Noia G, Triarico S, et al.: Sexuality, preconception counseling and urological management of pregnancy for young women with spina bifida, *Eur J Obstet Gynecol Reprod Biol* 162(2):129–133, 2012.

Walsh DS, Adzick NS: Foetal surgery for spina bifida, *Semin Neonatal* 8(3):197–205, 2003.

Warschausky S, Kaufman JN, Evitts M, et al.: Mastery motivation and executive functions as predictors of adaptive behavior in adolescent and young children with cerebral palsy or myelomeningocele, *Rehabil Psychol* 62(3):258–267, 2017.

Williams EN, Broughton NS, Menelaus MB: Age-related walking in children with spina bifida, *Dev Med Child Neurol* 41(7): 446–449, 1999.

Williams J, Mai CT, Mulinare J, et al.: Updated estimates of neural tube defects prevented by mandatory folic acid fortification-United States 1995-2011, *MMWR Morb Mortal Wkly Rep* 64(1):1–5, 2015.

Williamson GG: *Children with spina bifida: early intervention and preschool programming*, Baltimore, 1987, Paul H. Brookes.

Yasar E, Adiguzel E, Arslan M, Mathews DJ: Basics of bone metabolism and osteoporosis in common neuromuscular pediatric disabilities, *Eur J Paediatr Neurol* 22:17–26, 2018.

Zaganjor I, Sekkarie A, Tsang BL, et al.: Describing the prevalence of neural tube defects worldwide: a systematic literature review, *PLoS One* 11(4):e0151586. doi:10.1371/journal.pone.0151586. eCollection 2016.

Zukerman JM, Devine KA, Holmbeck GN: Adolescent predictors of emerging adulthood milestones in youth with spina bifida, *J Pediatr Psychol* 36(3):265–276, 2011.

8

Genetic Disorders

After reading this chapter, the student will be able to:
1. Describe different modes of genetic transmission.
2. Compare and contrast the incidence, etiology, and clinical manifestations of specific genetic disorders.
3. Explain the medical and surgical management of children with genetic disorders.
4. Articulate the role of the physical therapist assistant in the management of children with genetic disorders.
5. Describe appropriate physical therapy interventions used with children with genetic disorders.
6. Discuss the importance of functional activity training through the life span of a child with a genetic disorder.

INTRODUCTION

More than 6000 genetic disorders have been identified to date. Some are evident at birth, whereas others present later in life. Most genetic disorders have their onset in childhood. The physical therapist assistant working in a children's hospital, outpatient rehabilitation center, or school system may be involved in providing physical therapy for these children. Some of the genetic disorders discussed in this chapter include Down syndrome (DS), fragile X syndrome (FXS), Rett syndrome, cystic fibrosis (CF), Duchenne muscular dystrophy (DMD), and osteogenesis imperfecta (OI). After a general discussion of the types of genetic transmission, the pathophysiology and clinical features of these conditions are outlined, followed by a brief discussion of the physical therapy management. A case study of a child with DS is presented at the end of the chapter to illustrate the physical therapy management of children with low muscle tone. A second case study of a child with DMD is presented to illustrate the physical therapy management of a child with a progressive genetic disorder.

Genetic disorders in children are often thought to involve primarily only one body system (muscular, skeletal, respiratory, or nervous) and to affect other systems secondarily. However, genetic disorders typically affect more than one body system, especially when those systems are embryonically linked, such as the nervous and integumentary systems, both of which are derived from the same primitive tissue. For example, individuals with neurofibromatosis have skin defects in the form of café-au-lait spots in addition to nervous system tumors. Genetic disorders that primarily affect one system, such as the muscular dystrophies, eventually have an impact on or stress other body systems, such as the cardiac and pulmonary systems. Because the nervous system is most frequently involved in genetic disorders, similar clinical features are displayed by a large number of affected children.

In addition to the cluster of clinical symptoms that constitute many genetic syndromes, children with genetic disorders often present with what is termed a *behavioral phenotype*. This term has been around quite a while in medical genetics but may not be familiar to the physical therapist assistant; ". . . a behavioral phenotype is a profile of behavior, cognition, or personality that represents a component of the overall pattern seen in many or most individuals with a particular condition or syndrome" (Baty et al., 2011). Just as facial features may be different in children with DS or FXS, there may be behavioral and cognitive differences related to the different genetic syndromes.

GENETIC TRANSMISSION

Genes carry the blueprint for how body systems are put together, how the body changes during growth and development, and how the body operates on a daily basis. The color of your eyes and hair is genetically determined. One hair color, such as brown, is more dominant than another color, such as blond. A trait that is passed on as *dominant* is expressed, whereas a *recessive* trait may be expressed only under certain circumstances. All cells of the body carry genetic material in chromosomes. The chromosomes in the body cells are called *autosomes*. Because each of us has 22 pairs of autosomes, every cell in the body has 44 chromosomes, and two *sex chromosomes*. Reproductive cells contain 23 chromosomes (22 autosomes and either an X or a Y chromosome). After fertilization of the egg by the sperm, the genetic material is combined during *meiosis*, determining the sex of the child by the pairing of the sex chromosomes. Two X chromosomes make a female, whereas one X and one Y make a male. Each gene inherited by a child has a paternal and a maternal contribution. Alleles are alternative forms of a gene, such as H or h. If someone carries identical alleles of a gene, HH or hh, the person is homozygous. If the person carries different alleles of a gene, Hh or hH, the person is heterozygous.

CATEGORIES

The two major categories of genetic disorders are *chromosomal abnormalities* and *specific gene defects*. Chromosomal abnormalities occur by one of three mechanisms: nondisjunction, deletion, and translocation. When cells divide unequally, the result is called a *nondisjunction*. Nondisjunction can cause DS. When part or all of a chromosome is lost, it is called a *deletion*. When part of one chromosome becomes detached and reattaches to a completely different chromosome, it is called a *translocation*. Chromosome abnormalities include the following: *trisomies*, in which three of a particular chromosome are present instead of the usual two; *sex chromosome abnormalities*, in which there is an absence or addition of one sex chromosome; and *partial deletions*. The most widely recognized trisomy is DS, or trisomy 21. Turner syndrome and Klinefelter syndrome are examples of sex chromosome errors, but they are not discussed in this chapter. Partial deletion syndromes that are discussed include cri-du-chat syndrome and Prader-Willi syndrome (PWS).

A specific gene defect is inherited in three different ways: (1) as an autosomal dominant trait, (2) as an autosomal recessive trait, or (3) as a sex-linked trait. *Autosomal dominant inheritance* requires that one parent be affected by the gene or that a spontaneous mutation of the gene occurs. In the latter case, neither parent has the disorder, but the gene spontaneously mutates or changes in the child. When one parent has an autosomal dominant disorder, each child born has a 1 in 2 chance of having the same disorder. Examples of autosomal dominant disorders include OI, which affects the skeletal system and produces brittle bones, and neurofibromatosis, which affects the skin and nervous system.

Autosomal recessive inheritance occurs when either parent is a carrier for the disorder. A *carrier* is a person who has the gene but in whom it is not expressed. The condition is not apparent in the person. The carrier may pass the gene on without having the disorder or knowing that he or she is a carrier. In this situation, the carrier parent is said to be *heterozygous* for the abnormal gene, and each child has a 1 in 4 chance of being a carrier. The heterozygous parent is carrying a gene with alleles that are dissimilar for a particular trait. If both parents are carriers, each is heterozygous for the abnormal gene, and each child will have a 1 in 4 chance of having the disorder and an increased chance that the child will be homozygous for the disorder. *Homozygous* means that the person is carrying a gene with identical alleles for a given trait. Examples of autosomal recessive disorders that are discussed in this chapter are CF, phenylketonuria (PKU), and three types of spinal muscular atrophy (SMA).

Sex-linked inheritance means that the abnormal gene is carried on the X chromosome. Just as autosomes can have dominant and recessive expressions, so can sex chromosomes. In X-linked recessive inheritance, females with only one abnormal allele are carriers for the disorder, but they usually do not exhibit any symptoms because they have one normal X chromosome. Each child born to a carrier mother has a 1 in 2 chance of becoming a carrier, and each son has a 1 in 2 chance of having the disorder. The most common examples of X-linked recessive disorders are DMD and hemophilia, which is a disorder of blood coagulation. FXS is the most common X-linked disorder that causes intellectual disability (ID) in males. Rett syndrome is also X-linked and seen predominately in females.

Genetic Testing

Significant changes have occurred in genetic testing in the last decade. Chromosomal microarray analysis (CMA) is used to discover genetic causes of ID, autism spectrum disorder, developmental delay, and multiple congenital anomalies. CMA is able to diagnose common genetic problems as well as detect severe genetic conditions not detected in a traditional chromosome analysis. Copy number variations can be detected in this manner. CMA is recommended as a first tier test by the American Academy (AA) of Neurology, AA of Pediatrics, and the Child Neurology Society. A discussion of genetically transmitted disorders follows including first chromosome abnormalities and then specific gene defects.

DOWN SYNDROME

DS is the leading chromosomal cause of ID and the most frequently reported birth defect (Centers for Disease Control and Prevention, 2018). Increasing maternal and paternal age is a risk factor. DS occurs in 1 in every 700 live births and is caused by a genetic imbalance resulting in the presence of an extra 21st chromosome or trisomy 21 in all or most of the body's cells. Ninety-five percent of DS cases result from a failure of chromosome 21 to split completely during formation of the egg or sperm (nondisjunction). A *gamete* is a mature male or female germ cell (sperm or egg). When the abnormal gamete joins a normal one, the result is three copies of chromosome 21. Fewer than 5% of children have a third chromosome 21 attached to another chromosome. This type of DS is caused by a translocation. The least common type of DS is a mosaic type in which some of the body's cells have three copies of chromosome 21 and others have a normal complement of chromosomes. The severity of the syndrome is related to the proportion of normal to abnormal cells.

Clinical Features

Characteristic features of the child with DS include hypotonicity, joint hypermobility, upwardly slanting epicanthal folds, and a flat nasal bridge and facial profile (Fig. 8.1). The child has a small oral cavity that sometimes causes the tongue to seem to protrude. Developmental findings include delayed development and impaired motor control. Feeding problems may be evident at birth and may require intervention. Fifty

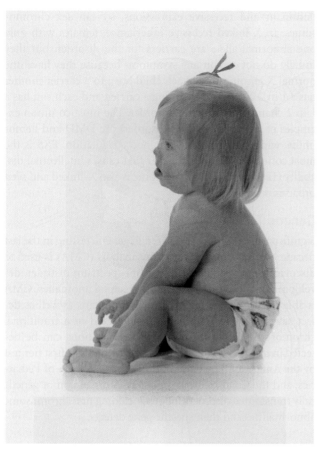

Fig. 8.1 Profile of a child with Down syndrome.

BOX 8.1   Symptoms of Atlantoaxial Instability

- Hyperreflexia
- Clonus
- Babinski sign
- Torticollis
- Increased loss of strength
- Sensory changes
- Loss of bowel or bladder control
- Decrease in motor skills

From Glanzman A: Genetic and developmental disorders. In Goodman CC, Fuller KS, editors: *Pathology: implications for the physical therapist*, ed 2, Philadelphia, 2003, WB Saunders, pp 1161–1210.

---

percent of children with DS also have congenital heart defects of the wall between the atria or the ventricles (Vis et al., 2009), which can be corrected by cardiac surgery. Musculoskeletal manifestations may include pes planus (flatfoot), thoracolumbar scoliosis, and patellar dislocation as well as possible atlantoaxial instability (AAI). The incidence of AAI ranges from 10% to 15% (Mik et al., 2008). Beginning at the age of 2 years, a child's cervical spine can and should be radiographed to determine whether AAI is present. If instability is present, the family should be educated for possible symptoms, which are listed in Box 8.1. The child's activity should be modified to avoid stress or strain on the neck such as that which may occur when diving, doing gymnastics, and playing any contact sport. Most cases are asymptomatic (Glanzman, 2015).

After over a decade of support for screening for AAI in children with DS, the AA of Pediatrics' Committee on Sports Medicine and Fitness withdrew support of this practice in 1995 (AA Pediatrics Committee on Sports Medicine and Fitness, 1995). Others still recommend the practice and support family and community awareness of the potential problems with AAI in children with DS (Bull, 2011; Glanzman, 2015; Pueschel, 1998). As physical therapists and physical therapist assistants working with families of children with DS, we have a responsibility to provide such education and advocate for screening.

Major sensory systems, such as hearing and vision, may be impaired in children with DS. Visual impairments may include nearsightedness (myopia), cataracts, crossing of the eyes (esotropia), nystagmus, and astigmatism. Mild to moderate hearing loss is not uncommon. Either a sensorineural loss, in which the eighth cranial nerve is damaged, or a conductive loss, resulting from too much fluid in the middle ear, may cause delayed language development. These problems must be identified early in life and treated aggressively so as to not hinder the child's ability to interact with caregivers and the environment and to develop appropriate language skills.

Intelligence

As stated earlier, DS is the major cause of ID in children. Intelligence quotients (IQs) within this population range from 25 to 50, with the majority falling in the mild to moderate range of ID (Ratliffe, 1998). To be diagnosed with an ID, a child's IQ has to be 70 to 75 or below. The American Association on Intellectual Developmental Disabilities (AAIDD) has moved away from defining ID based only on IQ scores. The definition of ID means the person is significantly limited in intelligence and in adaptive skills before the age of 18 (Schalock et al., 2010). Adaptive skills can include participation, communication, self-care, and ability to engage in social roles consistent with the International Classification of Functioning, Disability, and Health (ICF) (World Health Organization, 2001).

If effective early intervention programs can be designed and used in the preschool years, the subsequent educational progress of a child with DS may be altered significantly. A person with mild ID is capable of learning such basic skills as reading and arithmetic and is quite capable of self-care and independent living. Those persons with moderate ID may be limited in educational attainments, but they can benefit from training for self-care and vocational tasks.

Development

Motor development is slow, and without intervention the rate of acquisition of skills declines. Difficulty in learning motor skills has always been linked to the lack of postural tone and, to some extent, to hypermobile joints. Ligamentous laxity with resulting joint hypermobility is thought to be caused by a collagen defect. The hypotonia is related not only to

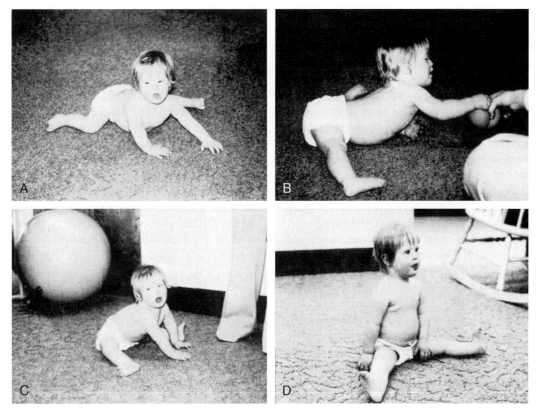

Fig. 8.2 (A–D) Common abnormal prone-to-sitting maneuver pattern noted in children with Down syndrome. (Reprinted from Lydic JS, Steele C: Assessment of the quality of sitting and gait patterns in children with Down syndrome, *Phys Ther* 59:1489–1494, 1979. With permission of the APTA.)

structural changes in the cerebellum but also to changes in other central nervous system structures and processes. These changes are indicative of missing or delayed neuromaturation in DS. As a result of the low tone and joint laxity, it is difficult for the child with DS to attain head and trunk control. Weight-bearing on the limbs is typically accomplished by locking extremity joints such as the elbows and knees. These children often substitute positional stability for muscular stability, as in W sitting, to provide trunk stability in sitting, rather than dynamically firing trunk muscles in response to weight shifting in a position. Children with DS often avoid activating trunk muscles for rotation and prefer to advance from prone to sitting over widely abducted legs (Fig. 8.2). Table 8.1 compares the age at which motor tasks may be accomplished by children with DS and typically developing children. Infant intervention has been shown to have a positive impact on developing motor skills and overall function in these children (Connolly et al., 1993; Hines and Bennett, 1996; Ulrich et al., 2001, 2008).

Individuals with DS can live in group communities that foster independence and self-reliance. Some individuals with DS have been employed in small- and medium-sized offices as clerical workers or in hotels and restaurants. Batshaw et al. (2013) credited the introduction of supported employment in the 1980s with providing the potential for adults with DS to obtain and to hold a job. In supported employment, the individual has a job coach. Crucial to the individual's job success is the early development and maintenance of a positive self-image and a healthy self-esteem, along with the ability to work apart from the family and to participate in personal recreational activities.

Fitness is decreased in individuals with DS. Dichter et al. (1993) found that a group of children with DS had reduced pulmonary function and fitness compared with age-matched controls without disabilities. Other researchers have found children with DS to be less active (Sharav and Bowman,

TABLE 8.1 Predicted Probability (%) of Children With Down Syndrome Achieving Milestones Based on Logistic Regression

Skill	6	12	18	24	30	36	48	60	72
				AGE (MONTHS)					
Roll	51	64	74	83	89	93	97	99	100
Sit	8	78	99	100	100	100	100	100	100
Crawl	10	19	34	53	71	84	96	99	100
Stand	4	14	40	73	91	98	100	100	100
Walk	1	4	14	40	74	92	99	100	100
Run	1	2	3	5	8	12	25	45	67
Steps	0	0	1	1	3	5	18	46	77

From Palisano RJ, Walter SD, Russell DJ, et al: Gross motor function of children with Down syndrome: creation of motor growth curves, *Arch Phys Med Rehabil* 82:494–500, 2001.

1992). Sixty percent of children with DS have been found to be obese and exhibit low levels of fitness (Roizen and Patterson, 2003). Lack of cardiorespiratory endurance and weak abdominal muscles have been linked to the reductions in fitness (Shields et al., 2009). Strength protocols for children with DS have been outlined by Rowland et al. (2015). Because of increased longevity, fitness in every person with a disability needs to be explored as another potential area of physical therapy intervention. Barriers to exercise for people with DS have been identified as lack of a support person and appropriate levels of interaction (Heller et al., 2002; Menear, 2007). When physical therapy students mentored adolescents with DS to exercise, the student's attitudes toward working with a person with disabilities improved considerably. A 4-week community fitness program improved movement security in children with disabilities and provided service learning for students (Schwartzkopf-Phifer and Liang, 2017).

Life expectancy for individuals with DS has increased to 60 years (Bittles et al., 2006). The increase has occurred despite the higher incidence of other serious diseases in this population. Children with DS have a 15% to 20% higher chance of acquiring leukemia during their first 3 years of life. Again, the cure rate is high. The last major health risk faced by these individuals is Alzheimer disease. Every person with DS who lives past 40 years develops pathologic signs of Alzheimer disease, such as amyloid plaques and neurofibrillary tangles. Individuals with DS produce more of the β-amyloid that makes up the plaques because the gene that produces the protein is located on the 21st chromosome (Head and Lott, 2004). Adults with DS over 50 years old are more likely to regress in adaptive behavior than are adults with ID without DS (Zigman et al., 1996). This could be explained by the inability of the adult with DS to counteract oxidative stress from abundance of free radicals in the brain (Pagano and Castello, 2012). Three-fourths of adults who live past 65 years of age have signs of dementia (Lott and Dierssen, 2010).

Child's Impairments, Activity Limitations, Participation Restrictions, and Interventions

The physical therapist's examination and evaluation of a child with DS typically identifies the following issues to be addressed by physical therapy intervention:

1. Delayed psychomotor development
2. Joint laxity, hypotonia, poor postural control
3. Impaired respiratory or cardiac function
4. Impaired exercise tolerance
5. Dependent in self-care, feeding, dressing and activities of daily living (ADLs)
6. Dependent in play

Early physical therapy is important for the child with DS. A case study of a child with DS is presented at the end of the chapter to illustrate general intervention strategies with a child with low muscle tone because the problems demonstrated by these children are similar. These interventions could be used with any child who displays low muscle tone or muscle weakness secondary to genetic disorders such as cri-du-chat syndrome, PWS, and SMA.

Body-Weight Support Treadmill Training

Children with DS walk independently between 18 months and 3 years (Palisano et al., 2001). Research has shown that infants with DS who participant in body-weight support treadmill training walk earlier than typically developing children with DS. Early ambulation in this population is beneficial because it supports development in other areas such as language and cognition. Ulrich et al. (2001) were the first to show that using treadmill training accelerated the developmental outcome of independent ambulation in children with DS. As little as 8 minutes five times a week produced change. When a higher intensity was compared with a lower intensity, the children in the higher intensity group walked 3 months earlier than the children in the lower intensity group (Ulrich et al., 2008). Treadmill training should be considered an appropriate intervention for a child with DS around 10 months of age.

Orthoses

Children with DS have low tone and joint hypermobility. Instability in the lower extremity may not allow the child to experience a stable base while in standing or when attempting to walk. Martin (2004) studied use of supramalleolar orthoses (SMOs) in children with DS to determine the effect of their use on independent ambulation. Children showed significant improvement in standing and walking, running, and jumping on the Gross Motor Function Measure, both at the initial fitting and after wearing the orthoses for 7 weeks. Balance improved at the end of the 7-week period.

Looper and Ulrich (2010) found that too early use of SMOs while the child engaged in treadmill training actually deterred onset of walking. However, to use an orthosis with the children, the treadmill training did not begin until the child pulled to standing, which is a milestone that is delayed in children with DS. Looper et al. (2012) compared the effect of two types of orthoses on the gait of children with DS. They compared a foot orthosis (FO) and an SMO. The results were not clearly in favor of one orthosis over another. There were strong correlations found between the use of each orthosis and specific gait parameters.

Body-weight support treadmill training appears to have a positive effect on achievement of early ambulation; however, use of an orthosis during treadmill training may not be indicated. After achievement of independent ambulation, an orthosis may be needed to address gait deviations, such as foot angle, walking speed, and amount of pronation during stance phase (Selby-Silverstein et al., 2001). As pointed out by Nervik and Roberts (2012), the best practice continues to be individualized recommendations for use of orthoses and trials of different orthoses to make the best decision.

CRI-DU-CHAT SYNDROME

When part of the short arm of chromosome 5 is deleted, the result is the cat-cry syndrome, or cri-du-chat syndrome. The chromosome abnormality primarily affects the nervous system and results in ID. The incidence is 1 in 20,000 to 1 in

50,000 live births (Mainardi, 2006). Characteristic clinical features include a catlike cry, microcephaly, widely spaced eyes, and profound ID. The cry is usually present only in infancy and is the result of laryngeal malformation, which lessens as the child grows. Although usually born at term, these children exhibit the result of intrauterine growth retardation by being small for their gestational age. Microcephaly is diagnosed when the head circumference is less than the third percentile. Together, these features constitute cri-du-chat syndrome, but any or all of the signs can be noted in many other congenital genetic disorders.

Child's Impairments, Activity Limitations, Participation, and Interventions

The physical therapist's examination and evaluation of the child with cri-du-chat syndrome typically identifies the following issues or potential problems to be addressed by physical therapy intervention:
1. Delayed psychomotor development
2. Hyperextensible joints, hypotonia
3. Poor postural control
4. Contractures and skeletal deformities
5. Impaired respiratory or cardiac function
6. Dependent in self-care, ADLs, and play

Musculoskeletal problems that may be associated with cri-du-chat syndrome include clubfeet, hip dislocation, joint hypermobility, and scoliosis. Muscle tone is low, which is a feature that may predispose the child to problems related to musculoskeletal alignment. In addition, motor delays also result from a lack of the cognitive ability needed to learn motor skills. Postural control is difficult to develop because of the low tone and nervous system immaturity. Physically, the child's movements are laborious and inconsistent. Gravity is a true enemy to the child with low tone. Congenital heart disease is also common, and severe respiratory problems can be present (Bellamy and Shen, 2013). Life expectancy has improved to almost normal with better medical care (Chen, 2013).

PRADER-WILLI SYNDROME AND ANGELMAN SYNDROME

PWS is another example of a syndrome caused by a partial deletion of a chromosome, which in this case is a microdeletion of a part of the long arm of chromosome 15. The incidence of this syndrome originally described by Prader et al. (1956) is thought to be about 1 in 10,000 to 1 in 30,000 (Batshaw et al., 2013). The disorder is more common than cri-du-chat syndrome. In fact, it is one of the most common microdeletions seen in genetic clinics (Dykens et al., 2011). Diagnosis is usually made based on the child's behavior and physical features and confirmed by genetic testing. Features include obesity, underdeveloped gonads, short stature, hypotonia, and mild to moderate ID. These children become obsessed with food at around the age of 2 years and exhibit *hyperphagia* (excessive eating). Before this age they have difficulty in feeding secondary to low muscle tone, gain weight slowly, and may be

diagnosed as failure to thrive. Children with PWS are very delayed in attainment of motor milestones during the first 2 years of life and often do not sit until 12 months and do not walk until 24 months (Dykens et al., 2011). Obesity can lead to respiratory compromise with impaired breathing and cyanosis. PWS is the most common genetic form of obesity. Maladaptive behavior is part of the behavioral phenotype of this genetic condition and includes temper tantrums, obsessive compulsive disorder, self-harm, and lability.

If a child inherits the deletion from the father, the child will have PWS, but if the child inherits the deletion from the mother, the child will have Angelman syndrome (AS). This variability of expression depending on the sex of the parent is called *genomic imprinting*. This phenomenon is a result of differential activation of genes on the same chromosome. AS is characterized by significantly delayed development, ID, ataxia, severe speech problems, and progressive microcephaly. Delays are not apparent until around 6 to 12 months of age. There may be problems with sucking and swallowing, drooling, or tongue thrusting in 20% to 80% of children (Bellamy and Shen, 2013). They have a happy affect and display hand-flapping movements. A little over a quarter of children are diagnosed based on clinical findings and have no genetic cause (Van Buggenhout and Fryns, 2009).

Child's Impairments, Activity limitations, Participation Restrictions, and Interventions

The physical therapist's examination and evaluation of the child with PWS typically identifies the following potential problems to be addressed by physical therapy intervention:
1. Impaired feeding (before age 2); obesity (after age 2)
2. Delayed psychomotor development
3. Decreased aerobic capacity
4. Dependent in self-care, ADLs, and play

Intervention must match the needs of the child based on age. The infant may need oral motor therapy to improve the ability to feed. Positioning for support and alignment is necessary for feeding and carrying. Techniques for fostering head and trunk control should be taught to the caregivers. As the child's appetite increases, weight control becomes crucial. The aim of a preschool program is to provide interventions to establish and improve gross-motor abilities. Food control must be understood by everyone working with the child with PWS. Attention in the school years is focused on training good eating habits while improving tolerance for aerobic activity. This is continued throughout adolescence, when behavioral control appears to be the most successful means for controlling weight gain.

"Interventions should be directed toward increasing muscle strength, aerobic endurance, postural control, movement efficiency, function, and respiration to manage obesity and minimize cardiovascular risk factors and osteoporosis" (Lewis, 2000). Suggested activities for strength training at various ages can be found in Table 8.2. These activities would be appropriate for most children with weakness. Aquatic exercise is also an ideal beginning aerobic activity for the child with severe

TABLE 8.2   Activities for Strength Training

Monitor	Ages	ACTIVITIES TO STRENGTHEN			
		Upper Limbs	Lower Limbs	Trunk	Muscles of Respiration
Blood pressure Breath holding Stabilization	Younger children	Wheelbarrow walks Push/pull a wagon Vertical drawing Lifting objects Scooter board	Squats Vertical jumping Stair climbing Walking on toes Ball kicking Walking sideways	Sit-ups Bridges Trunk rotations Stand up from supine Swing a weighted bat	Blowing bubbles Straw sucking Blowing balloons Cotton ball hockey Singing Chair pushups
Blood pressure Breath holding Stabilization	Older children/ younger adolescents	Elastic bands, hand weights, games, music, dance	Elastic bands, ankle weights, games, music, dance Broad jumping	Swiss ball Incline sit-ups Foam rollers	Swimming laps Running sprints
Blood pressure Breath holding Stabilization	Older adolescents/ young adults	Strength training: bicep curls, triceps, latissimus pulls	Strength training: hamstring curls, quadriceps, extensions, squats, toe raises	Strength training: abdominal crunches, obliques	Swimming laps Running laps Running for endurance

Modified from Lewis CL: Prader-Willi syndrome: a review for pediatric physical therapists, *Pediatr Phys Ther* 12:87–95, 2000; Young HJ: The effects of home fitness programs in preschoolers with disabilities. Chapel Hill, NC, Program in Human Movement Science with Division of Physical Therapy. University of North Carolina, Chapel Hill, Thesis, 1996:50.

TABLE 8.3   Activities for Aerobic Conditioning

Ages	Activities
Younger children	Bunny hopping Running long jump Running up and down steps or incline Running up and down hills Riding a tricycle Sitting on a scooter board and propelling with the feet
Older children/ younger adolescents	Bike riding Stationary bike riding Brisk walking Water aerobics Roller skating Roller-blading Ice skating Cross-country skiing Downhill skiing
Older adolescents/ younger adults	Same as above, plus: Dancing Low-impact step aerobics Jazzercise Aerobic circuit training

From Lewis CL: Prader-Willi syndrome: a review for pediatric physical therapists, *Pediatr Phys Ther* 12:87–95, 2000.

obesity (Lewis, 2000). Additional aerobic activities for different age groups are found in Table 8.3. They, too, have general applicability to most children with developmental deficits. Box 8.2 details outcome measures that could be used to document changes in strength and aerobic conditioning in the PWS population. Some of these measures may be applicable with children with other developmental diagnoses, whereas others may be difficult because of lack of motor control.

ARTHROGRYPOSIS MULTIPLEX CONGENITA

Arthrogryposis multiplex congenita (AMC) is defined by the presence of contractures in two or more body areas. Not all cases of AMC have a genetic origin, but hundreds of contracture syndromes have been traced to specific genes. The gene that causes the neuropathic form of AMC is found on chromosome 5 (Tanamy et al., 2001). Another form, distal AMC, which affects primarily hands and feet, is inherited as an autosomal dominant trait with the defective gene mapped to chromosome 9 (Bamshad et al., 1994). AMC is a nonprogressive neuromuscular syndrome that the physical therapist assistant may encounter in practice. AMC results in multiple joint contractures and usually requires surgical intervention to correct misaligned joints. AMC is also known as multiple congenital contractures. The incidence of the disorder is 1 in 3000 to 5000 live births according to Hall (2014), and a 1 in 4300 prevalence has been reported in Canada (Lowry et al., 2010). Pathogenesis has been related to the muscular, nervous, or joint abnormalities associated with intrauterine movement restriction, but despite identification of multiple causes, the exact cause is still unknown.

Pathophysiology and Natural History

As early as 1990, Tachdjian postulated that the basic mechanism for the multiple joint contractures seen in AMC was a lack of fetal movement. That hypothesis has been accepted in that AMC can result from any condition that limits fetal movement (Glanzman, 2015). Fetal akinesia can have myopathic and neuropathic causes. If muscles around a fetal joint

---

BOX 8.2 Clinical Outcome Measures

Measures of Strength Training

- Grip dynamometer: before and after training (average of five trials)
- Myometer of target muscles: before and after training (average of five trials)
- One-repetition or six-repetition maximum (1 RM, 6 RM)[a]: before and after training (average over 3 different days)[a,b]
- Standing long jump distance: before and after training (average of five trials)[†]

Measures of Aerobic Conditioning

- Heart rate: measure the radial pulse or use a heart rate monitor; establish baseline over a 5-day period

- Improved cardiovascular function documented by decreased resting heart rate; decreased heart rate during steady state (2 min into the activity); time it takes for heart rate to return to preactivity level
- Timed performance of activities such as 50-foot sprint, seven sit-ups, stair climbing
- 2-min or 6-min walk/run/lap swim time: maximum distance covered divided by time
- Determine EEI[b,c] of gait: working HR minus resting HR divided by speed

---

[a]One RM is the maximum amount of weight that can be lifted one time; six RM is the maximum amount of weight that can be lifted six times.
[b]From 1985 School Population Fitness Survey. Washington, DC, 1985, President's Council on Physical Fitness and Sports.
[c]Rose J, Gamble J, Lee J, et al: The energy expenditure index: a method to quantitate and compare walking energy expenditure for children and adolescents, *J Pediatr Orthop* 11:571–578, 1991.
EEI, Energy expenditure index; *HR*, heart rate; *RM*, repetition maximum.
From Lewis CL: Prader-Willi syndrome: a review for pediatric physical therapists, *Pediatr Phys Ther* 12:87–95, 2000.

---

do not provide enough stimulation (muscle pull), the result is joint stiffness. If the anterior horn cell does not function properly, muscle movement is lessened, and contractures and soft-tissue fibrosis occur. Muscle imbalances in utero can lead to abnormal joint positions. The first trimester of pregnancy has been identified as the most likely time for the primary insult to occur to produce AMC. Newborns with congenital contractures can be categorized as having amyoplasia (lack of muscle development), which is the most commonly recognized type, a lethal type related to the central nervous system, or a heterogenous group. The latter group consists of various neuromuscular syndromes, contracture syndromes, and skeletal dysplasia. Regardless, the end result is multiple nonprogressive joint contractures. Although the contractures themselves are not progressive, the extent of functional disability they produce is significant, as seen in Fig. 8.3. These two presentations are often noted in the literature. Limitation in mobility and in ADLs can make the child dependent on family members.

Child's Impairments, Activity Limitations, Participation Restrictions, and Interventions

The physical therapist's examination and evaluation of the child with AMC typically identifies the following problems to be addressed by physical therapy intervention:

1. Impaired range of motion
2. Impaired functional mobility and balance
3. Limitations in play and ADLs, including donning and doffing orthoses
4. Participation at home, school, and community

Early physical therapy intervention focuses on assisting the infant to attain head and trunk control. Depending on the extent of limb involvement, the child may have difficulty using the arms for object exploration, support when initially learning to sit, or to catch herself when losing balance. Most of these children become ambulatory, but they may

need some assistance in finding ways to go up and down the stairs. An adapted tricycle can provide an alternative means of mobility before walking is mastered (Fig. 8.4). Functional movement and maintenance of range of motion are the two major physical therapy goals for a child with this physical disability. No cognitive deficit is present; therefore the child with AMC should be able to attend regular preschool and school. Table 8.4 gives an overview of the management of the child with AMC across the life span.

Range of Motion

Range-of-motion exercises and stretching exercises are the cornerstone of physical therapy intervention in children with AMC. Initially stretching needs to be performed three to five times a day. Each affected joint should be moved three to five times and held for 20 to 30 seconds at the end of the available range. Because these children have multijoint involvement, range of motion requires a serious commitment on the part of the family. Incorporating stretching into the daily routine of feeding, bathing, dressing, and diaper changing is warranted. Use of molded thermoplastic splints is seen in Fig. 8.5. Splints for knee flexion contracture management can be removed to allow floor mobility when the skills emerge (Donahoe, 2017a). As the child grows older, the frequency of stretching can be decreased. The school-age child should begin to take over responsibility for his or her own stretching program. Although stretching is less important once skeletal growth has ceased, flexibility remains a goal to prevent further deformities from developing. Joint preservation and energy conservation techniques are legitimate strategies for the adult with AMC.

Positioning

Positioning options depend on the type of contractures present. If the joints are more extended in the upper extremity, this will hamper the child's acceptance of the prone position

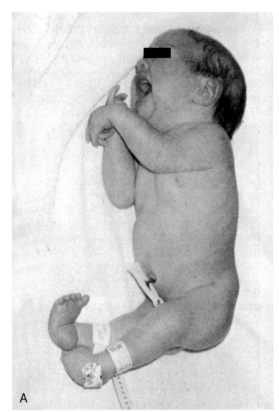
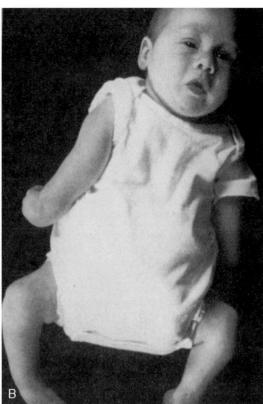

Fig. 8.3 **(A)** Infant with arthrogryposis multiplex congenita (AMC) with flexed and dislocated hips, extended knees, clubfeet (equinovarus), internally rotated shoulders, flexed elbows, and flexed and ulnarly deviated wrists. **(B)** An infant with AMC with abducted and externally rotated hips, flexed knees, clubfeet, internally rotated shoulders, extended elbows, and flexed and ulnarly deviated wrists. (From Donohoe M: Arthrogryposis multiplex congenita. In Campbell SK, Palisano RJ, Orlin MN, editors: *Physical therapy for children*, ed 4, Philadelphia, 2012, Saunders.)

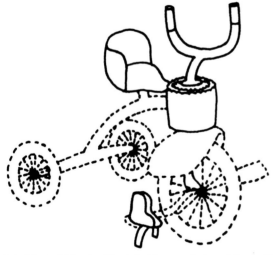

Fig. 8.4 Adapted tricycle. (Reprinted by permission of the publisher from Connor FP, Williamson GG, Siepp JM, editors: *Program guide for infants and toddlers with neuromotor and other developmental disabilities,* New York, 1978, Teachers College Press, p. 361. © 1978 Teachers College, Columbia University. All rights reserved.)

and will require that the chest be supported by a roll or a wedge. Too much flexion and abduction in the lower extremities may need to be controlled by lateral towel rolls or a Velcro strap (Fig. 8.6). Quadruped is not a good posture to use because it reinforces flexion in the upper and lower extremities.

Prone positioning is an excellent way to stretch hip flexion contractures while encouraging the development of the motor abilities of the prone progression. A prone positioning program should be continued throughout the life span.

Functional Activities and Gait

Rolling and scooting on the bottom are used as primary means of floor mobility. Development of independent sitting is often delayed because of the child's inability to attain the position, but most children do by 15 months of age. Placement in sitting and encouragement of static sitting balance with or without hand support should begin early. Object exploration in sitting fosters cognitive development through play and exploration of the environment. For children with impaired upper extremity movement the use of wearable technology such as Playskin Lift is being explored (Hall and Lobo, 2018). Playskin Lift is a wearable exoskeleton that assists a child to lift the arms and encourages reaching behavior.

Focus on dynamic balance and transitions into and out of sitting while using trunk flexion and rotation should follow, although some children may never learn to independently transition from sitting to standing using rotation. Six months is an appropriate age for the child to begin experiencing weight-bearing in standing. They can stand well before they can pull to stand. For children with plantar flexion contractures, shoes can be wedged to allow total contact of the foot

TABLE 8.4 Management of Arthrogryposis Multiplex Congenita or Multiple Congenital Contractures

Time Period	Goals	Strategies	Medical/Surgical	Home Program
Infancy	Maximize strength Increase ROM Enhance sensory and motor development	Teach rolling Floor scooting Strengthening Stretching Positioning	Clubfoot surgery by age 2 years Splints adjusted every 4–6 weeks	Stretching three to five times a day Standing 2 hours a day Positioning Object play
Preschool	Decrease disability Enhance ambulation Maximize ADLs Establish peer relationships	Solve ADL challenges Gait training Stretching, positioning Promote self-esteem	Stroller for community Articulating AFOs Splints	Stretching twice a day Positioning Play groups, sleepovers, sports
School-age and adolescent	Strengthen peer relationships Independent mobility Preserve ROM	Adaptive physical education Environmental adaptations, stretching Compensatory for ADLs	Manual wheelchair for community Power mobility Surgery	Sports, social activities Self-directed stretching and prone positioning Personal hygiene
Adulthood	Independent in ADLs with/without assistive devices Ambulation/mobility Driving	Joint protection and conservation Assess accessibility Assistive technology	Wheelchair	Flexibility Positioning Endurance

ADLs, Activities of daily living; *AFOs,* ankle-foot orthoses; *ROM,* range of motion.
Data from Donohoe M: Arthrogryposis multiplex congenita. In Campbell SK, Palisano RJ, Orlin MN, editors: *Physical therapy for children,* ed 4, Philadelphia, 2012, WB Saunders, pp 313–332.

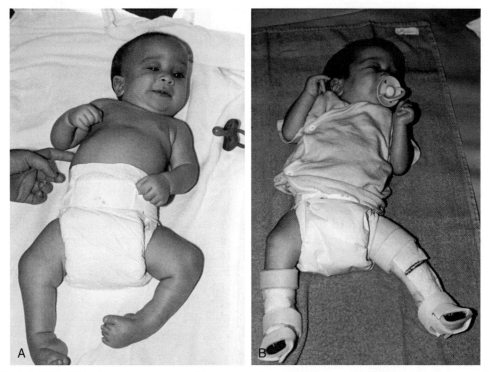

Fig. 8.5 **(A)** A child with arthrogryposis multiplex congenita without leg splint. **(B)** Child with arthrogryposis multiplex congenita wearing a molded knee splint on one leg and ankle foot orthoses to counteract deforming positions. (From Donahoe M: Arthrogryposis multiplex congenital. In Palisano RJ, Orlin MN, Schreiber J, editors: *Campbell's physical therapy for children,* ed 4, St. Louis, 2017, Elsevier.)

with the support surface. In some cases, a standing frame or parapodium, as is used with children with myelomeningocele, can be beneficial (Fig. 8.7). Other children benefit from use of supine or prone standers. The standing goal for a 1-year-old child is 2 hours a day (Donohoe 2017a). Strengthening of muscles needed for key functional motor skills, such as rolling,

sitting, hitching (bottom scooting), standing, and walking, is done in play. Reaching to roll, rotation in sitting and standing, and movement transitions into and out of postures can facilitate carryover into functional tasks. Toys should be adapted with switches to facilitate the child's ability to play, and adaptive equipment should be used to lessen dependence during ADLs.

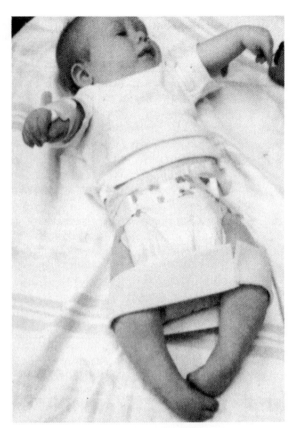

Fig. 8.6 Child with arthrogryposis multiplex congenita is wearing a wide Velcro band strapped around the thighs to keep the legs in more neutral alignment. (From Donohoe M, Bleakney DA: Arthrogryposis multiplex congenita. In Campbell SK, Vander Linden DW, Palisano RJ, editors: *Physical therapy for children*, ed 2, Philadelphia, 2000, WB Saunders.)

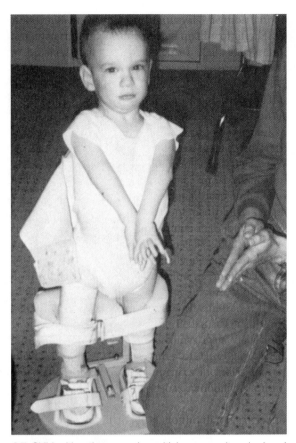

Fig. 8.7 Child with arthrogryposis multiplex congenita who is using a standing frame. (From Donohoe M: Arthrogryposis multiplex congenita. In Campbell SK, Palisano RJ, Orline MN, editors: *Physical therapy for children*, ed 4, Philadelphia, 2012, Saunders.)

Ambulation is achieved by most children with AMC by 18 months of age (Donohoe, 2017a). Because clubfoot is often a part of the presentation in AMC, its presence must be dealt with in the development of standing and walking. Early surgical correction of the deformity often requires later surgical revisions, so investigators have suggested that surgery occur after the child is stronger and wants to walk, at around the end of the first year of life. The operation should be performed by the time the child is 2 years old to avoid the possibility of having to do more bony surgery, as opposed to soft-tissue corrections.

Most children achieve ambulation with orthoses. In children with AMC, the ability to walk depends on the extent of joint range in the hips and knees and achieving a plantigrade foot (Bartonek, 2015). Use of orthoses for ambulation depends on the strength of the lower extremity extensors and the degree of contractures found at the hip, knee, and ankle. Less than fair muscle strength at a joint usually indicates the need for an orthosis at that joint. For example, if the quadriceps muscles are scored less than 3 out of 5 on manual muscle testing, then a knee-ankle-foot orthosis (KAFO) is indicated. Children with knee extension contractures tend to require less orthotic control than those with knee flexion contractures (Donohoe, 2017a). Children with weak quadriceps or knee flexion contractures may need to walk with the knees of the KAFO locked. The reader is referred to Bartonek (2015)

for a review of orthoses and gait analysis of children with AMC.

Functional ambulation also depends on the child's ability to use an assistive device. Because of upper extremity contractures, this may not be possible, and adaptations to walkers and crutches may be needed. Polyvinyl chloride pipe can often be used to fabricate lightweight walkers or crutches to give the child maximal independence (Fig. 8.8). Power mobility may provide easy and efficient environmental access for a child with weak lower extremities and poor upper extremity function. Some school-age children or adolescents routinely use a manual wheelchair to keep up with peers in a community setting.

Participation

Fostering peer interaction throughout the life span is critical for participation of the child, adolescent, and adult with AMC. Limited mobility can hinder participation and impede social interactions in preschool, on the playground, and in the community. Goals that focus on safe, speedy ways to keep up with peers should be part of the plan of care across the lifespan. Adaptive physical education can be an adjunct to physical therapy for reinforcing strength, endurance, and mobility. While most children with AMC achieve household mobility, a scooter or wheelchair (manual or motorized) may be needed for efficient community mobility.

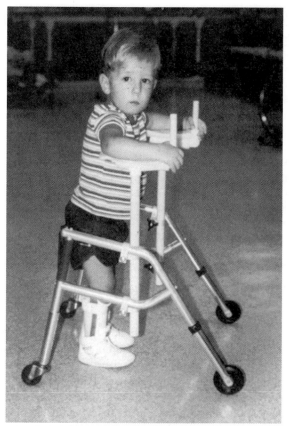

Fig. 8.8 Thermoplastic forearm supports can be customized to the walker for the child with arthrogryposis multiplex congenita. (From Donohoe M: Arthrogryposis multiplex congenita. In Campbell SK, Palisano RJ, Orlin MN, editors: *Physical therapy for children,* ed 4, Philadelphia, 2012, Saunders.)

OSTEOGENESIS IMPERFECTA

OI is an inherited connective tissue disorder secondary to a defect in collagen synthesis. It occurs in around 1 in 15,000 to 25,000 of the population (Semler et al., 2008). The original classification scheme of four types was devised by Sillence et al. (1979) based on clinical examination, x-ray findings, and type of inheritance. Recent research in molecular genetics has resulted in the identification of seven more types, expanding the number of types from 4 to 11 (Glorieux et al., 2000; Valadares et al., 2014). The first four types are listed in Table 8.5. All four types are inherited as an autosomal dominant trait, which occurs in 1 per 10,000 to 20,000 live births. Each type has a different degree of severity. Type V represents only a small percentage of cases and the remaining six types (VI through XI) are autosomal recessive and will not be discussed in detail. Many of the additional types are similar to the original four but are molecularly very different. Type I accounts for 50% of all OI cases and, together with type IV, accounts for 95% of all cases (Martin and Shapiro, 2007). Depending on the type of OI, the infant may be born with multiple fractures or may not experience any broken bones until reaching preschool age. The more fragile the skeletal system, the less likely it is that a physical therapist assistant will be involved in the child's therapy. It would be more likely for an assistant to treat children with types I and IV because these are the most common. Individuals

TABLE 8.5 Classification of Osteogenesis Imperfecta

Type	Characteristics	Severity	Ambulation
I	AD, mild to moderate fragility	Mildest	Community
II	AD, in utero fractures	Most severe (perinatal lethal)	Nonambulatory
III	AD, progressive deformities	Moderately severe	Exercise walking
IV	AD, mild to moderate deformity, short stature	More severe than type I	Household/community

AD, Autosomal dominant.
Data from Donohoe M: Osteogenesis imperfecta. In Campbell SK, Palisano RJ, Orlin MN, editors: *Physical therapy for children,* ed 4, Philadelphia, 2012, WB Saunders, pp 332–352; Engelbert R et al: Osteogenesis imperfecta in childhood: prognosis for walking, *J Pediatr* 37:397–402, 2000; Glanzman, AM: Genetic and developmental disorders. In Goodman CC, Fuller, KS, editors: *Pathology: implications for the physical therapist,* ed 4, Philadelphia, 2015, Saunders, pp 1161–1210.

with OI have "brittle bones." Many also exhibit short stature, bowing of long bones, ligamentous joint laxity, kyphosis, and scoliosis. Average or above-average intelligence is typical.

Pathophysiology

OI is a varied group of disorders distinguished by genetic testing, histologic findings, and clinical presentation. The first four types identified by Sillence have defects in type I collagen caused by mutations in genes located on chromosomes 7 and 17. The remainder of types do not have a defect in type I collagen but present with similar degrees of bone fragility as the types with the collagen defect. The failure is in the way the body translates the type I collagen into bone. Diffuse osteoporosis results in multiple recurring fractures, weak muscles, joint laxity, and spinal and long bone deformities. It is hoped that the medical management can be more individualized by knowing the specific type of OI. The first incidence of OI in a family is typically caused by a spontaneous mutation; thereafter the same type of OI is possible with varying presentation. Genetic counseling can assist in giving parents accurate information about recurrence and how OI presentation can vary within a family.

Child's Impairments, Activity Limitations, Participation Restrictions, and Interventions

The physical therapist's examination and evaluation of the child with OI typically identifies the following problems to be addressed by physical therapy intervention:

1. Impaired strength and range of motion
2. Pathologic fractures, scoliosis, bowing of long bones
3. Limited functional mobility, transfers and ambulation/wheelchair mobility
4. Limitations in self-care skills and play
5. Restricted participation in activities requiring physical endurance
6. Restricted participation in educational and work environments

TABLE 8.6	**Therapeutic Management of Osteogenesis Imperfecta**	
Time Period	**Goals**	**Therapeutic Interventions**
Infancy	Safe handling and positioning Development of age-appropriate skills	Even distribution of body weight Padded carrier Prone, side-lying, supine, sitting positions Pull-to-sit transfer contraindicated
Preschool	Protected weight-bearing Safe independent self-mobility	Use of contour-molded orthoses for compression and support in standing Adaptive devices Light weights, aquatic therapy
School age and adolescence	Maximizing independence Maximizing endurance Maximizing strength Peer relationships	Mobility cart, HKAFOs, clamshell braces, air splints Ambulation without orthoses as fracture rate declines Wheelchair for community ambulation Adaptive physical education Boy Scouts, Girl Scouts, 4-H
Adulthood	Appropriate career placement	Career counseling Job site evaluation

HKAFOs, Hip-knee-ankle-foot orthoses.
Data from Donohoe M: Osteogenesis imperfecta. In Campbell SK, Palisano RJ, Orlin MN, editors: *Physical therapy for children,* ed 4, Philadelphia, 2012, Saunders, pp 333–352.

Children with milder forms of OI are seen for strengthening and endurance training in a preschool or school setting. Every situation must be viewed as being potentially hazardous because of the potential for bony fracture. Safety always comes first when dealing with a potential hazard; therefore orthoses can be used to protect joints, and playground equipment can be padded. No extra force should be used in donning and doffing orthoses. Signs of redness, swelling, or warmth may indicate more than excessive pressure and could indicate a fracture.

> **CAUTION** Fracture risk is greatest during bathing, dressing, and carrying. Baby walkers and jumper seats should be avoided. All trunk or extremity rotations should be active, not passive.

Social interaction may need to be structured if the child with OI is unable to participate in many, if any, sports-related activities. Being the manager of the softball or soccer team may be as close as the child with OI can be to participating in sports. Table 8.6 provides an overview of the management of a child with OI across the life span.

Handling and Positioning

Parents of an infant with OI must be taught to protect the child while carrying him or her on a pillow or in a custom-molded carrier. Handling and positioning are illustrated in Intervention 8.1. All hard surfaces must be padded. Protective positioning must be balanced with permitting the infant's active movement. Sandbags, towel rolls, and other objects may be used. Greatest care is needed when dressing, diapering, and feeding the child. When handling the child, caregivers should avoid grasping the child around the ankles, around the ribs, or under the arms because this may increase the risk of fractures. Clothing should be roomy enough so that it fits easily over the child's head. Temperature regulation is often impaired, so light, absorbent clothing is a good idea. A plastic or spongy basin is best for bathing. Despite all precautions, infants may

still experience fractures. The physical therapist assistant will most likely not be involved in the initial stages of physical therapy care for the infant with OI because of the patient's fragility. The physical therapist should provide a range of carrying positions to allow the infant to develop strength while adapting to postural changes. However, if the physical therapist assistant is involved later, he or she does need to be knowledgeable about what has been taught to the family.

Positioning should be used to minimize joint deformities. Using symmetry with the infant in supine and side-lying positions is good. A wedge can be placed under the chest when the infant is in prone to encourage head and trunk movement while providing support (Fig. 8.9). The child's feet should not be allowed to dangle while sitting but should always be supported. Water beds are not recommended for this population because the pressure may cause joint deformities. Rear-facing car seats should be used as long as possible to ensure utmost safety in the car (Donohoe, 2017b).

Range of Motion and Strengthening

By the time the child is of preschool age, not only are the bones still fragile, the joints lax, and the muscles weak, but the child also has probably developed disuse atrophy and osteoporosis from immobilization secondary to fractures in infancy or childhood. OI has a variable time of onset depending on the type. Range of motion and strengthening are essential. Active movement promotes bone mineralization, and early protected weight-bearing seems to have a positive effect on the condition. Range of motion in a straight plane is preferable to diagonal exercises, with emphasis placed on the shoulder and pelvic girdles initially. Light weights can be used to increase strength, but they need to be placed close to the joint to limit excessive torque.

Pool exercise is good because the water can support the child's limbs, and flotation devices can be used to increase buoyancy. Water is an excellent medium for active movement progressing to some resistance as tolerated. The child's

INTERVENTION 8.1   Handling a Child With Osteogenesis Imperfecta

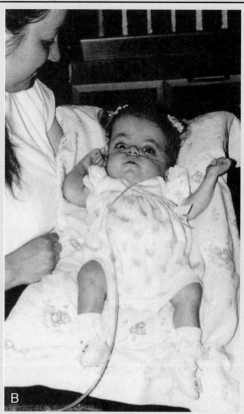
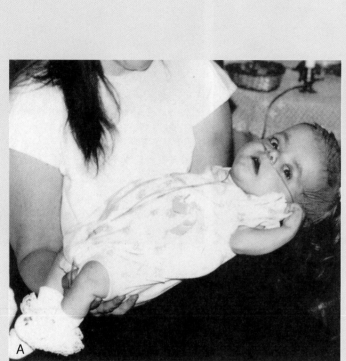

A. In handling a young child with osteogenesis imperfecta, support the neck and shoulders and the pelvis with your hands; do not lift the child from under the arms.

B. Placing the child on a pillow may make lifting and holding easier.

From Myers RS: *Saunders manual of physical therapy practice,* Philadelphia, 1995, WB Saunders.

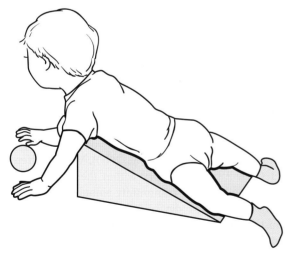

Fig. 8.9 Prone positioning of a child on a wedge encourages head and trunk movement and upper extremity weight-bearing.

respiratory function can be strengthened in the water by having the child blow bubbles and hold his or her breath. Deep breathing is good for chest expansion, which may be limited secondary to chest wall deformities. The water temperature needs to be kept low because of these children's increased metabolism (Donohoe, 2017b). Increased endurance, protected weight-bearing, chest expansion, muscle strengthening, and improved coordination are all potential benefits of aquatic intervention. Initial sessions in the pool are short, lasting for only 20 to 30 minutes (Cintas, 2005).

Functional Activities and Gait

Developmental activities should be encouraged within safe limits (Intervention 8.2). Use proximal points from which to handle the child and incorporate safe, lightweight toys for motivation. Reaching in supine, side-lying, and supported sitting can be used for upper extremity strengthening, as well as for encouraging weight shifting. Rolling is important as a primary means of floor mobility. Prepositioning one upper extremity beside the child's head as the child is encouraged to roll can be beneficial. All rotations should be active, not passive (Brenneman et al., 1995). Performing a traditional pull-to-sit maneuver is contraindicated. The assistant or caregiver should provide manual assistance at the child's shoulders to encourage head lifting and trunk activation when the assistant is helping the child into an upright position. Holding and carrying positions that safely challenge head control should be encouraged.

Sitting needs to be in erect alignment compared with the typical progression of children from prop sitting to no hands

INTERVENTION 8.2   Developmental Activities for a Child With Osteogenesis Imperfecta

A. The emphasis is on sitting with an erect trunk.
B. All rotations should be active.
C. Weight-bearing on the arms and legs is indicated as tolerated.

From Myers RS: *Saunders manual of physical therapy practice,* Philadelphia, 1995, WB Saunders.

because propping may lead to a more kyphotic trunk posture. External support may be necessary to promote tolerance to the upright position, such as with a corner seat or a seat insert. Sling seats in strollers and other seating devices should be avoided because they do not promote proper alignment. Once head control is present, short sitting or sitting straddling the caregiver's leg or a bolster can be used to encourage active trunk righting, equilibrium, and protective reactions. These sitting positions can also be used to begin protected weight-bearing for the lower extremities, such as that seen in Fig. 8.10. Scooting on a bolster or a bench can be the start of learning sitting transfers. Sitting and hitching are primary means of floor mobility for the child with OI after rolling and are used until the child masters creeping. A scooter propelled by a child's arms or legs can be used for mobility (Fig. 8.11).

Transition to Standing

The child with OI should have sufficient upright control to begin standing during the preschool period. Prior to that time, standing and walking with insufficient support will put too much weight on the lower extremities and will produce further bending and bowing of the long bones. Susceptibility to fractures of these long bones is greatest between 2 years and 10 to 15 years (Jones, 2006). Air splints can be used to manage fractures temporarily or may be able to provide sufficient support in a standing device. A child with OI should begin a standing program with appropriate support. Those with moderate to severe OI will need braces to prevent bowing. Hip-knee-ankle-foot orthoses (HKAFOs) may be used in conjunction with some type of standing frame. Lower extremity bracing is not as prevalent since bisphosphonates have been shown to increase bone strength. Ambulation is often begun in the pool because of the protection afforded by the water. The child is then progressed to shallow water. Water also can be used to teach ambulation for the first time or to retrain walking after a fracture, but lightweight plastic splints also should be used. Duffield (1983) suggested the following progression in water: (1) in parallel bars or a standing frame, with a weight shift from side to side, forward, and backward, and (2) forward walking.

Motor skill development is delayed because of fractures and also because muscles are poorly developed and joints are hypermobile. The disease type and ability to sit by 9 or 10 months of age are the best predictors of ambulatory status (Daley et al., 1996; Engelbert et al., 2000). Most children with type I OI will be ambulatory within their household and about half will become community ambulators without the need for any assistive device (Glanzman, 2015). This is in contrast to children with type III, in which almost 50% will depend on power mobility.

Medical Management

Typically developing children without disabilities form 7% more bone than is resorbed when their bones grow and remodel. Children with mild forms of OI only form 3% more bone than they resorb (Batshaw et al., 2013). Pamidronate, a bisphosphonate, is a powerful antiresorptive agent. It has become the standard of care for children with moderate to severe OI (Glorieux, 2007). Studies have found that it

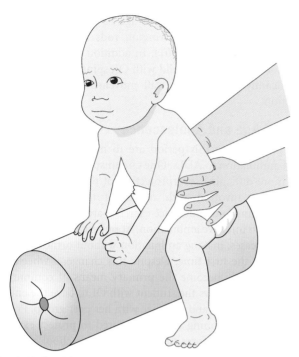

Fig. 8.10 Straddle roll activity of supported sit-to-stand for lower extremity strengthening and weight-bearing. (From Campbell SK, Vander Linden DW, Palisano RJ, editors: *Physical therapy for children,* ed 4, Philadelphia, 2012, WB Saunders, p 343.)

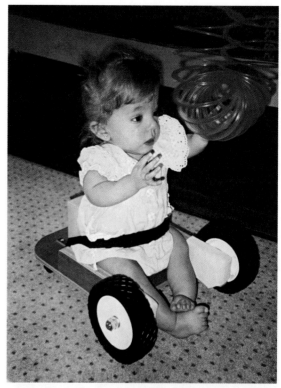

Fig. 8.11 Scooter used for mobility that can be propelled by a child's legs or arms. (From Campbell SK, Vander Linden DW, Palisano RJ, editors: *Physical therapy for children,* ed 4, Philadelphia, 2012, WB Saunders, p 344.)

increases bone density, decreases bone pain, and increases the ability of the patients to ambulate (DiMeglio and Peacock, 2006; Land et al., 2006). There is still limited evidence for a reduction in fracture rate (Dwan et al., 2016). However, long-term use of bisphosphonates in conjunction with orthopedic surgery and physical therapy has resulted in an improved quality of life for those with OI (Biggin and Munns, 2017).

Whole-body vibration (WBV) has been studied as an intervention for immobilized children and adolescents with OI by Semler et al. (2007, 2008). Vibration was delivered by a platform on a tilt table. An increase in the tilt angle of the tilt table was used as a measure of improved mobility. Function as measured by the Brief Assessment of Motor function was improved and mobility as defined by the tilt table angle increased. This intervention is not appropriate for children with a history of joint subluxation or who have telescoping rods.

Two more recent studies found different results with WBV. Hoyer-Kuhn et al. (2014) evaluated the effect of a side alternating WBV on motor function in 53 children with OI. The entire study spanned 12 months and included 6 months of WBV delivered at home in 3-month blocks in addition to physical therapy, resistance training, treadmill training with body weight support, and pool therapy delivered during two inpatient stays lasting a total of 19, 13, and 6 days, respectively. All children with OI were walking and were classified as having types 1, 3, 4, and 5 based on the expanded levels. The children were reassessed 6 months after the completion of the program. Walking distance and Gross Motor Function-66 significantly improved as did bone mineral density. The researchers concluded that this approach should be considered

as a model for children with severe OI. Hogler et al. (2017) compared 5 months of WBV training to usual care in 24 children matched by sex and pubertal stage in a random controlled trial. The children had Sillence type 1 or type 4 OI, were short in stature, and had limited mobility based on the Child Assessment Health Questionnaire and 6 Minute Walk Test. The WBV group received twice daily training, whereas the control group had regular care including physical therapy. The results of this pilot study showed no difference in bone changes in the two groups. The authors concluded that WBV is not practical and questioned the ability of vibration to make changes in the bone–muscle unit. They did suggest that the training period might have not been long enough to see a change.

Orthotic and Surgical Management

Orthoses are made of lightweight polypropylene and are created to conform to the contours of the child's lower extremity. Initially, the orthosis may have a pelvic band and no knee joints for maximum stability. As strength and control increase, the pelvic band may be removed, and knee joints may be used. Some orthoses have a clamshell design that includes an ischial weight-bearing component, which is a feature borrowed from lower extremity prostheses. The ambulation potential of a child with OI is highly variable, as are orthotic choices. From using a standing frame and orthosis, the child progresses to some type of KAFO with the knees locked in full extension (Fig. 8.12). The child first ambulates in the

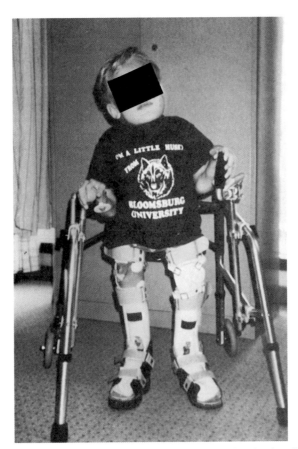

Fig. 8.12 Child with osteogenesis imperfecta who is using long-leg braces and a rollator posture walker. (From Bleakney DA, Donohoe M: Osteogenesis imperfecta. In Campbell SK, Vander Linden DW, Palisano RJ, editors: *Physical therapy for children*, ed 3, Philadelphia, 2006, WB Saunders.)

safety of the parallel bars, then moves to a walker, and finally progresses to crutches as limb strength and coordination improve. "Most children ambulate without braces when the fracture rate decreases" (Donohoe, 2017b, p. 237).

Healing time for fractures in children with OI is normally 4 to 6 weeks, which is the same as in children without the condition. What is not normal is the number of fractures these children can experience. Intramedullary rod fixation is the best way to stabilize fractures that occur in the long, weight-bearing bones. Special telescoping rods developed by Bailey and Dubow (1965) allowed the child's bones to grow with the rod in place. This type of surgical procedure is usually performed after the child is 4 or 5 years of age to allow for sufficient growth of the femur. However, one study suggested that the operation be performed when the child is between the ages of 2 and 3.5 years, potentially to improve the child's neuromotor development (Engelbert et al., 1995). Fortunately, the frequency of fractures tends to decrease after puberty (Glorieux, 2007).

Scoliosis or kyphosis occurs in 50% of children with OI (Tachdjian, 2002). Often, the child cannot use an orthosis to manage a spinal curve because the forces from the orthosis produce rib deformities rather than controlling the spine. Curvatures can progress rapidly after the age of 5 years, with maximum deformity present by age 12 (Gitelis et al., 1983). Surgical fixation with Harrington rods is often necessary (Marini and Chernoff, 2001). In addition to compounding the short stature in the child with OI, spinal deformities can significantly impair chest wall movement and respiratory function.

School Age and Adolescence

The goals during this period are to maximize all abilities from ambulation to ADLs. One circumstance that may make this more difficult is overprotection of the school-age child by anyone involved with managing the student's care. Strengthening and endurance exercises are continued during this time to improve ambulation. At puberty, the rate of fractures decreases, making ambulation without orthoses a possibility for the first time. Despite this change, a wheelchair will most likely become the primary means of community mobility. This allows the student with OI to have the energy needed to keep up and socialize with her peer group. Proper wheelchair positioning must be assured to protect exposed extremities from deformities or trauma. The school-age child with OI has to avoid contact sports, for obvious reasons, but still needs to have some means of exercising to maintain cardiovascular fitness. Swimming and wheelchair court sports, such as tennis, are excellent choices.

Strengthening and fitness programs have been undertaken in children with type I and IV OI that have resulted in functional gains. Van Brussel et al. (2008) conducted a study of a 12-week graded exercise program in children with the mildest forms of OI. In this random control trial, children who participated in 30 sessions of 45 minutes of graded exercise showed significant improvements in aerobic capacity and muscle force and a decrease in subjective fatigue. The improvements were not sustained after the intervention ended, which supports the need for ongoing exercise in this group. Caudill et al. (2010) found that weak plantar flexion in children with type I OI was correlated with function as measured by the Pediatric Outcome Data Collection Instrument, the Gillette Functional Assessment Questionnaire, and the revised Faces Pain Scale. Ambulatory children with OI need to participate in progressive strengthening and functional fitness programs. Children with OI who are not ambulatory need to increase core strength and their ability to sit and hitch or sit-scoot because these are essential for transfers and self-care into adulthood.

Adulthood

The major challenge to individuals with OI as they move into adulthood is dealing with the secondary problems of the disorder. Spinal deformity may be severe and may continue to progress. Scoliosis is present in close to 80% to 90% of teens and adults with OI (Albright, 1981). Spinal fusion is often used to manage scoliosis and kyphosis. Career planning must take into account the physical limitations imposed by the musculoskeletal problems. Travel away from home was found to be the most important factor in an adolescent's ability to participate outside the school environment (Bachman,

1972). Assisting youth with developmental disabilities to transition into the adult care system, work, and community is a relatively new role for the physical therapist (Cicirello et al., 2012) but one that is a vital part of advocacy. By assisting a young adult to learn how to problem solve, she can create strategies to maximize participation. Optimizing academic, social, and physical development can assist persons with OI to become productive members of society (Bleck, 1981).

CYSTIC FIBROSIS

CF is an autosomal recessive disorder of the exocrine glands that is caused by a defect on chromosome 7. The pancreas does not secrete enzymes to break down fat and protein in 85% of these individuals. CF produces respiratory compromise, because abnormally thick mucus builds up in the lungs. This buildup creates a chronic obstructive lung disorder. A parent can be a carrier of this gene and may not express any symptoms. When one parent is a carrier or has the gene, the child has a 1 in 4 chance of having the disorder. The incidence is 1 in 3000 live births in whites. Five percent of the population carries a single copy of the CF gene, which equates to 12 million people in the United States. Newborn screening is mandated in every state.

Diagnosis

CF is the most lethal genetic disease in white patients. Diagnosis can be made on the basis of a positive sweat chloride test. Children with CF excrete too much salt in their sweat, and this salt can be measured and compared with normal values. Values greater than 60 mEq/L indicate CF. Some mothers have even stated that the child tastes salty when kissed. Because of the difficulty with digesting fat, the child may have foul-smelling stools and may not be able to gain weight. Before being diagnosed with CF, the child may have been labeled as failing to thrive because of a lack of weight gain. Prenatal diagnosis is available, and couples can be screened to detect whether either parent is a carrier of the gene.

Pathophysiology and Natural History

Even though the genetic defect has been localized, the exact mechanism that causes the disease is still unidentified. The ability of salt and water to cross the cell membrane is altered, and this change explains the high salt content present when these children perspire. Thick secretions obstruct the mucus-secreting exocrine glands. The disease involves multiple systems including gastrointestinal, reproductive, sweat glands, and respiratory. The two most severely impaired organs are the lungs and the pancreas. Diet and pancreatic enzymes are used to manage the pancreatic involvement. With life expectancy increasing, there has been an increased incidence of CF-related diabetes (CFRD) caused by damage of the beta cells in the pancreas (Moran et al., 2009). The percentage of individuals with CFRD rises with increasing age such that 40% to 50% of adults with CF have this condition.

The structure and function of the lungs are normal at birth. Only after thick secretions begin to obstruct or block

airways, which are smaller in infants than in adults, is pulmonary function adversely affected. The secretions also provide a place for bacteria to grow. Inflammation of the airways brings in infiltrates that eventually destroy the airway walls. The combination of increased thick secretions and chronic bacterial infections produces chronic airway obstruction. Initially, this condition may be reversed with aggressive bronchial hygiene and medications. Eventually, repeated infections and bronchitis progress to bronchiectasis, which is irreversible. Bronchiectasis stretches the breathing tubes and leads to abnormal breathing patterns. Pulmonary function becomes more and more severely compromised over the life span, and the person dies of respiratory failure.

Life expectancy for an individual with CF has increased over the last several decades. The median predicted survival is into the late 40s (Pettit and Fellner, 2014; Volsko, 2009). Increase in longevity can be related to improved medical care, pharmacologic intervention, and heart and lung transplantation. The pulmonary manifestations of the disease are those that result in the greatest mortality. Fifty-four percent of pediatric lung recipients have CF with a median survival of 4.9 years (Benden et al., 2013). Early referral and a preoperative conditioning program are linked to better postoperative outcomes. Walking greater than 229-305 m during a 6 meter walk test predicted a better outcome (Yimlamai et al., 2013). A higher exercise capacity has been linked to improved survival (Schneiderman et al., 2014). Advances in genetic testing for the specific mutation involved has led to the ability to predict how severe the lungs will be affected and therefore the prognosis for survival (Corvol et al., 2015; McKone et al., 2015).

Child's Impairments, Activity Limitations, Participation Restrictions, and Interventions

The physical therapist's examination and evaluation of the child with CF typically identifies the following problems to be addressed by physical therapy intervention:

1. Retained secretions
2. Impaired pulmonary function
3. Limited exercise tolerance
4. Chest wall deformities
5. Nutritional deficits
6. Delayed puberty

Chest Physical Therapy

Central to the care of the child with CF is chest physical therapy (CPT). It consists of bronchial drainage in specific positions with percussion, rib shaking, vibration, and breathing exercises and retraining. Treatment is focused on reducing symptoms. Respiratory infections are to be avoided or treated aggressively. Signs of pulmonary infection include increased cough and sputum production, fever, and increased respiration rate. Additional findings could include increased white blood cell count, new findings on auscultation or radiographs, and decreased pulmonary function test values. Unfortunately, bacteria can become resistant to certain medications over time. Parents are taught to perform postural drainage three to five times a day. Adequate fluid intake is important to keep the mucus hydrated and therefore make it easier to move and be expectorated. The child with CF receives medications to provide hydration, to break up the mucus, to keep the bronchial tubes open, and to prevent bronchial spasms. These drugs are usually administered before postural drainage is performed. Antibiotics are a key to the increased survival rate in patients with CF and must be matched to the organism causing the infection.

Postural Drainage

Postural drainage is the physical act of using gravity or body position to aid in draining mucus from the lungs. The breathing tubes that branch off from the two main stem bronchi are like branches of an upside down tree, each branch becoming smaller and smaller the farther away it is from the main trunk. The position of the body for postural drainage depends on the direction the branch points. Each segment of the lobes of the lungs has an optimal position for gravity to drain the secretions and allow them to travel back up the bronchial tree to be expelled by coughing. Postural drainage or positioning for drainage is almost always accompanied by percussion and vibration. Manual vibration is shown in Intervention 8.3. *Percussion* is manually applied with a cupped hand while the person is in the drainage positions for 3 to 5 minutes. Proper configuration of the hand for percussion is shown in Fig. 8.13. Percussion dislodges secretions within that segment of the lung, and gravity usually does the rest. The classic 12 positions are shown in Fig. 8.14. Percussion and vibration should be applied only to those areas that have retained secretions. Treatment usually lasts no more than 30 minutes total, with the time divided among the lung segments that need to be drained.

Coughing as a form of forced expiration is necessary to clear secretions. Laughing or crying can stimulate coughing.

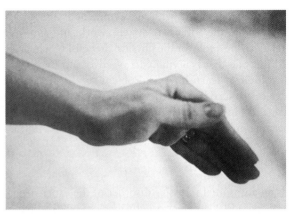

Fig. 8.13 Proper configuration of the hand for percussion. (From Hillegass EA, Sadowsky HS: *Essentials of cardiopulmonary physical therapy*, Philadelphia, 1994, WB Saunders.)

Although most children with CF cough on their own, some may need to be encouraged to do so through laughter. If this technique is unsuccessful, the tracheal "tickle" can be used by placing a finger on the trachea above the sternal notch and gently applying pressure. If you attempt this maneuver on yourself, you will feel the urge to clear your throat. To make coughing more functional and productive, the physical therapist assistant can teach the child a *forced expiration technique* (FET). When in a gravity-aided position, the child is asked to "huff" several times after taking a medium-sized breath. This is followed by several relaxed breaths using the diaphragm. The sequence of huffing and diaphragmatic breathing is repeated as long as secretions are being expectorated. The force of the expirations (huffs) can be magnified by manual resistance over the epigastric area or by having the child actively adduct the arms and compress the chest wall laterally. This technique can be taught to children who are 4 to 5 years of age.

Alternative forms of airway clearance include autogenic drainage (AD), active cycle breathing technique (ACBT), positive expiratory pressure (PEP) delivered by a mask (Fig. 8.15) and oscillating PEP via a Flutter device or Acapella. Use of a Flutter device is seen in Fig. 8.16. Modification of the amount of PEP and oscillations is possible with the Acapella and it is not angle dependent like the Flutter device. AD is a sequence of breathing exercises performed at different lung volumes. It can be used alone or combined with oscillating PEP. However, learning how to perform this type of self-controlled breathing is difficult to teach and learn and is usually not achievable before the age of 12 (Agnew and Owen, 2017). ACBT combines FET with thoracic expansion. FET is the most important component. The reader is referred to Lee et al. (2017) for more detailed descriptions of these breathing techniques. Pryor et al. (2010) found that all forms of airway clearance techniques worked equally well in children with CF, whereas adolescents with CF preferred AD over postural drainage with percussion (McIlwaine et al., 2010).

PEP with a mask has also been studied compared with typical CPT. PEP is easy to use, takes less time than typical CPT, and is accepted by patients (McIlwaine et al., 1997). Most importantly, it is effective in removing secretions

---

INTERVENTION 8.3   Manual Vibration

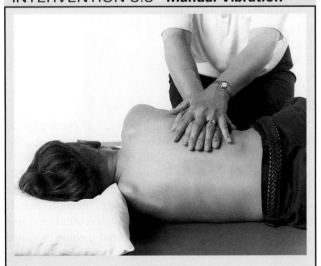

Vibration is used in conjunction with positioning to drain secretions out of the lungs. The chest wall should be vibrated as the child exhales to encourage coughing.

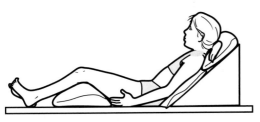

Position 1: Upper lobes, apical segments

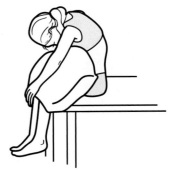

Position 2: Upper lobes, posterior segments

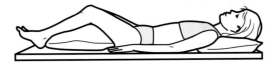

Position 3: Upper lobes, anterior segments

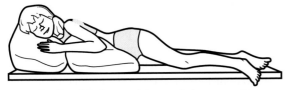

Position 4: Left upper lobe, posterior segments

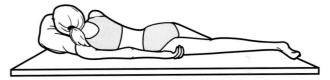

Position 5: Right upper lobe, posterior segments

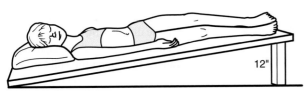

Position 6: Left upper lobe, lingula segment

12"

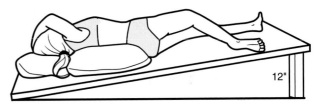

Position 7: Right middle lobe

12"

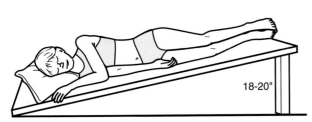

Position 8: Lower lobes, anterior basal segment

18-20"

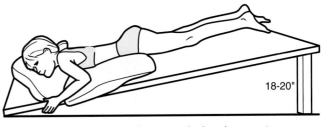

Position 9: Lower lobes, posterior basal segments

18-20"

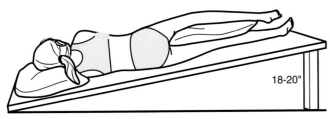

Positions 10 and 11: Lower lobes, lateral basal segments

18-20"

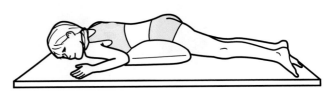

Position 12: Lower lobes, superior segments

Fig. 8.14 Postural drainage positions.

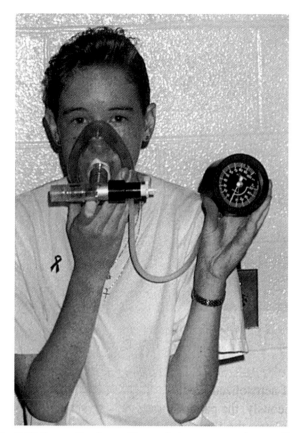

Fig. 8.15 Preparation for positive expiratory pressure therapy. (From Frownfelter D, Dean E: *Principles and practice of cardiopulmonary physical therapy*, ed 3, Philadelphia, 1996, WB Saunders, p 356.)

(Gaskin et al., 1998). "The PEP device maintains pressure in the lungs, keeping the airways open and allowing air to get behind the mucous" (Packel and von Berg, 2014). PEP is combined with the FET, which was described earlier in the section "Postural Drainage." A Cochrane review by McIlwaine et al. (2015) concluded that exacerbation rates

were lower when individuals with CF used a PEP mask rather than ACBT or AD.

The last way that high frequency vibration can be used for airway clearance is through use of an inflatable vest that fits snugly around the chest wall. A pump generates high-frequency oscillations. This technique is called high-frequency chest wall oscillation, or HFCWO, and has been successful in short-term studies (Grece, 2000; Tecklin et al., 2000). However, the results of a multicenter study by McIlwaine et al. (2013) did not support the use of HFCWO as a primary way to clear secretions because of the number of pulmonary exacerbations that occurred during the 12-month randomized controlled trial. Morrison and Innes (2017) concluded that there was no clear evidence that oscillation delivered orally or via chest wall is any better or more effective than other forms of CPT. No one device appeared to be better than another. Patient preference must be taken into consideration to ensure commitment to using the device for secretion management.

Strengthening specific muscles can assist respiration. Target the upper body, with emphasis on the shoulder girdle and chest wall muscles, such as the pectoralis major and minor, intercostals, serratus, erector spinae, rhomboids, latissimus dorsi, and abdominals. Stretches to maintain optimal length-tension relationships of chest wall musculature are helpful. Respiratory efficiency can be lost when too much of the work of breathing is done by the accessory neck muscles.

Part of pulmonary rehabilitation is to teach breathlessness positions, use of the diaphragm, and lateral basal expansion. *Breathlessness positions* allow the upper body to rest to allow the major muscle of inspiration, the diaphragm, to work most easily. Typical postures are seen in Intervention 8.4. *Diaphragmatic breathing* can initially be taught by having the child in a supported back-lying position and by using manual cues on the epigastric area (Intervention 8.5A). The child should be progressed from this position to upright sitting, to standing, and then to walking (see Intervention 8.5, B,C). The diaphragm

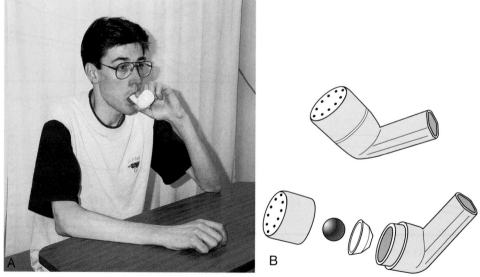

Fig. 8.16 **(A)** Use of Flutter valve. **(B)** Close-up construction of valve. (A, From Frownfelter D, Dean E: *Principles and practice of cardiopulmonary physical therapy*, ed 3, Philadelphia, 1996, WB Saunders, p 356.)

INTERVENTION 8.4 Breathlessness Postures

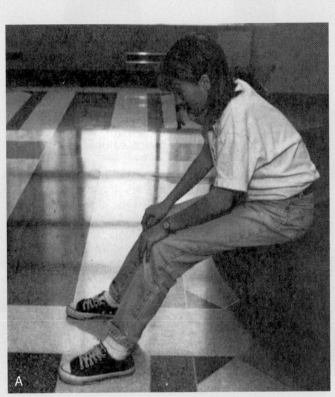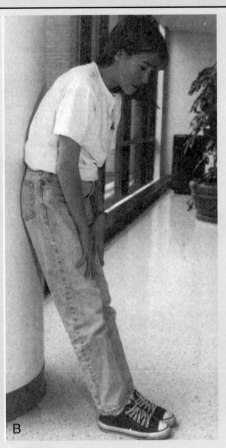

A, B. Breathlessness postures for conserving energy, promoting relaxation, and ease of breathing.

From Campbell SK, Palisano RJ, Orlin MN, editors: *Physical therapy for children*, ed 4, Philadelphia, 2012, Saunders.

works maximally when the child breathes deeply. Manual contacts on the lateral borders of the ribs can be used to encourage full expansion of the bases of the lungs (Intervention 8.6).

Exercise

Most individuals with CF can participate in an exercise program. Exercise tolerance does vary with the severity of the disease. Exercise for cardiovascular and muscular endurance plays a major role in keeping these individuals fit and in slowing the deterioration of lung function. Using exercise early on provides the child with a positive attitude toward exercise and to make a habit of daily physical activity. Bike riding, swimming, tumbling, and walking are all excellent means of providing low-impact endurance training. Making habitual physical activity a family activity is the goal for young children. Age-related recommendations for physical activity are found in Table 8.7. Activities that provide impact forces, such as basketball, volleyball, running, and jumping, help build bone. Collaco et al. (2014) found that self-reported exercise participation rates peaked at age 10. Teens with CF are just as at risk for becoming sedentary as their peers. Exercise programs for those with CF should be based on the results of an exercise test performed by a physical therapist. Long-term

relationships between clinicians and individuals with CF are important to provide support because it takes 6 months or more to elicit behavioral changes in habitual physical activity (Hommerding et al., 2015).

Children with CF may cough while exercising, causing brief oxygen desaturation. Coughing during exercise is not an indication to stop the exercise (Philpott et al., 2010). Some children with CF also have asthma. The results of the exercise test may indicate the need to monitor oxygen saturation using an ear or finger pulse oximeter while the child exercises. Oxygen saturation should remain at 90% during exercise. Exercise improves not only lung function but also the habitual activity of children with CF (Paranjape et al., 2012). Evidence-based guidelines for advising patients with CF on exercise and physical activity are found in Table 8.7 (Swisher et al., 2015).

When monitoring exercise tolerance with an individual with CF, use the perceived exertion rating scale and level of dyspnea scale to assess how hard the child is working. These ratings are found in Tables 8.8 and 8.9. If the child is known to desaturate with exercise, monitoring with an oximeter is indicated. If the oxygen saturation level drops below 90%, exercise should be terminated, and the supervising therapist should be notified before additional forms of exercise are

INTERVENTION 8.5 Diaphragmatic Breathing

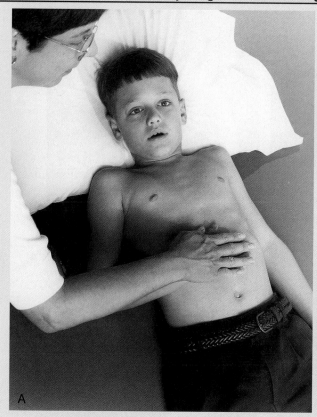

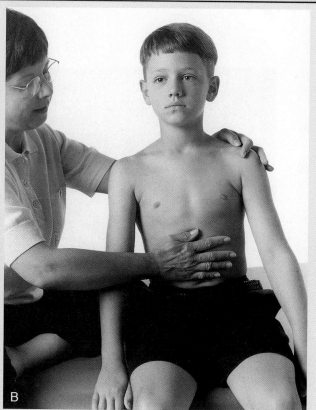

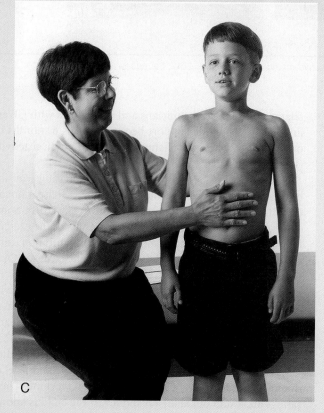

A. Initially, the child can be taught diaphragmatic breathing in a supported back-lying position, with manual cues on the epigastric area.

B, C. Then the child should be progressed to upright sitting, standing, and eventually walking while continuing to use the diaphragm for breathing.

INTERVENTION 8.6 Lateral Basal Chest Expansion

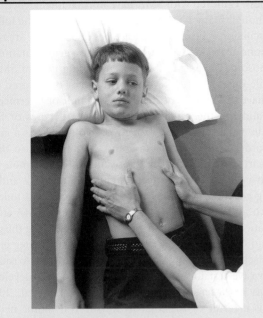

Manual contacts on the lateral borders of the ribs can be used to encourage full expansion of the bases of the lungs.

attempted. Use of a bronchodilator medication 20 minutes prior to exercise may also be beneficial, but again, guidelines for use of any medication should be sought from the supervising therapist in consultation with the child's physician.

As life expectancy has increased, sports and exercise have become an even bigger part of the management of children, adolescents, and adults with CF (Hebestreit et al., 2006; Orenstein et al., 2004; Philpott et al., 2010). Most students with CF can participate in school sports and are able to continue to pursue cycling, swimming, and even running marathons as adults (Webb and Dodd, 1999). However, some may have to change sports because of progressive lung disease. Good nutrition and pulmonary function must always be considered. Caloric intake may need to be increased to avoid weight loss because individuals with CF expend more energy to perform exercises than individuals without CF. Fluid replacement during exercise is crucial and needs to include electrolytes and not just water. Exercise improves airway clearance, delays decline in pulmonary function, delays onset of dyspnea, and prevents decreases in bone density. However, the best reason to exercise is to improve aerobic fitness because it correlates and predicts longevity in CF (Nixon et al., 1992, 2001). It is recommended that all children over the age of 10 undergo maximal exercise tests to determine aerobic capacity (Hebestreit et al., 2015) for that very reason.

TABLE 8.7 Summary of Recommendations for Physical Activity by Age Group

Type of Activity	Young Child (1–6 years)	Child (7–12 years)	Adolescent (13–19 years)	Adult (≥19 years)
Habitual physical activity	60 min daily in developmentally appropriate activities	60 min daily in a variety of activities enjoyed, preferably as a family activity	60 min daily in a variety of activities enjoyed, especially with family and friends	150 min per week or more (preferably 300 min) in a variety of activities of choice
Aerobic exercise	No formal program recommended but should perform full body activities that increase ventilation and heart rate	30–60 min daily of moderate-to-vigorous exercise (at least 70% of maximal heart rate) especially if using for airway clearance (must also perform coughing/huffing to clear secretions)	30–60 min daily of moderate-to-vigorous exercise (at least 70% of maximal heart rate) especially if using for airway clearance (must also perform coughing/huffing to clear secretions)	30–60 min daily of moderate-to-vigorous exercise (at least 70% of maximal heart rate) especially if using for airway clearance (must also perform coughing/huffing to clear secretions)
Resistance/ strengthening exercise	No formal program recommended but should perform activities using body weight to develop strength (e.g., calisthenics)	All activities that use body weight to strengthen muscles and bones (e.g., calisthenics) most days and if interested, begin formal weight training program under good supervision, learning technique first (twice weekly)	Formal resistance training two to three times per week per muscle group, incorporate limb and trunk muscles, one to three sets of 8–12 repetitions at 70%–85% of maximal load (one-repetition maximum)	Formal resistance training two to three times per week per muscle group, incorporate limb and trunk muscles, one to three sets of 8–12 repetitions at 70%–85% of maximal load (one-repetition maximum)
Other comments	Encourage normal motor development, including agility and balance/coordination	Encourage normal motor development, including agility and balance/coordination	Encourage muscle activities to help prevent or minimize adverse postural changes	Adapt for disease-related complications such as CF-related diabetes or low bone density as indicated

CF, Cystic fibrosis.

From Swisher AK, Hebestreit H, Mejia-Downs A, et al: Exercise and habitual physical activity for people with cystic fibrosis: expert consensus, evidence-based guide for advising patients, *Cardiopul Phys Ther J* 26(4):85–98, 2015.

TABLE 8.8 Rating of Perceived Exertion Scale

6	No exertion at all
7	Extremely light
8	—
9	Very light
10	—
11	Light
12	—
13	Somewhat hard
14	—
15	Hard (heavy)
16	—
17	Very hard
18	—
19	Extremely hard
20	Maximal exertion

From Borg RPE scale, © Gunnar Borg, 1970, 1985, 1998, 2006.

TABLE 8.9 Dyspnea Scale

+1	Mild, noticeable to patient but not observer
+2	Mild, some difficulty, noticeable to observer
+3	Moderate difficulty, but can continue
+4	Severe difficulty, patient cannot continue

From American College of Sports Medicine: *Guidelines for exercise testing and prescription*, ed 4, Philadelphia, 1991, Lea & Febiger. Reprinted with permission.

Some sports to be avoided are those such as skiing, bungee jumping, parachute jumping, and scuba diving. These have inherent risks because of altitude, increasing vascular pressure, or air trapping. Sports activities should be curtailed during an infective exacerbation (Packel and von Berg, 2014). Exercising in hot weather is not contraindicated but, again, fluid and electrolytes must be sufficiently replaced. Heavy breathing is a typical response to intense exercise. Deconditioned individuals with CF may demonstrate heavy breathing at lower workloads; this is not pathologic (Orenstein, 2002). In general, individuals with CF should be encouraged to exercise and set their own limits. Quality of life is associated with fitness and physical activity in this population (Hebestreit et al., 2014).

SPINAL MUSCULAR ATROPHY

SMA is a progressive disease of the nervous system inherited as an autosomal recessive trait. Although most of the genetic disorders discussed so far have involved the central nervous system, in SMA the anterior horn cell undergoes progressive degeneration. Children with SMA exhibit hypotonia of peripheral, rather than of central, origin. Damage to lower motor neurons produces low muscle tone or flaccidity, depending on whether some or all anterior horn cells degenerate.

Muscle fibers have little or no innervation from the spinal nerve if the anterior horn cell is damaged, and the result is weakness. Children with SMA have normal intelligence.

Although many types of SMA are recognized, the following discussion is limited to three types of SMA that are really variations of the same disorder involving a gene mutation on chromosome 5q13.2. The earliest occurring type of SMA is infantile-onset or acute SMA. The majority of children with SMA have this type. Type 2 SMA is a chronic or intermediate form and has the mildest presentation. All types of SMA differ in age at onset and severity of symptoms. As a group of disorders, SMA occurs in about 1 in 11,000 live births (Verhaart et al., 2017). It is the second most common fatal recessive genetic disorder seen in children, after CF, and the leading genetic cause of early death in infants and toddlers (Gidaro and Servais, 2018). The prevalence of SMA in the population is 1 in 6000 with 1 in 40 people carrying the gene (Beroud et al., 2003). Carrier detection rate is better in the non-black population (MacDonald et al., 2014). A routine noninvasive test for prenatal diagnosis has been developed that has 100% sensitivity and sensitivity (Parks et al., 2017). SMA is a result of the loss of the survival motor neuron 1 gene (SMN1), which produces a protein that supports basic cellular functions. Lack of the protein leads to apoptosis (programmed cell death). Recent advances in gene therapy are having a significant effect on changing the natural history of SMA (Alfano et al., 2019).

Type 1 SMA

The earliest occurring and therefore the most physically devastating form is type 1, acute infantile SMA. The incidence is about 1 in 10,000 births (MacDonald et al., 2014) with an onset between birth and 2 months. The child's limp, "frog-legged" lower extremity posture is evident at birth, along with a weak cry. Most children have a prenatal history of decreased fetal movements. Deep tendon reflexes are absent, and the tongue may fasciculate (quiver) because of weakness. Most infants are sociable and interact appropriately because they have normal intelligence. Motor weakness progresses rapidly, and death results from respiratory compromise within the first 2 years of life (Finkel et al., 2014). Life may be extended into the first decade of life if the family chooses mechanical ventilation and gastrostomy feedings (Oskoui et al., 2007), but despite aggressive care these children have significant functional impairment.

In the infant with type 1 SMA, positioning and family support have been the most important interventions. Physical therapy is focused on fostering typical developmental activities and providing the infant with access to the environment. Positioning for feeding, playing with toys, and interacting with caregivers are paramount. Poor head control makes positioning in prone too difficult. The prone position may also be difficult for the child to tolerate because it may inhibit diaphragm movement and cause respiratory distress. These infants rely on the diaphragm to breathe because their intercostal and neck accessory muscles are weak. Creative solutions to adaptive equipment needs can often be the result of brainstorming sessions with the entire health care team and

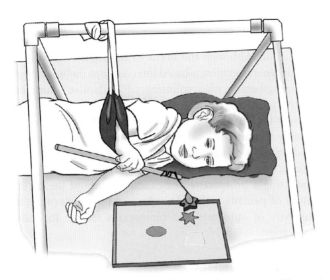

Fig. 8.17 Overhead sling supports the forearm of a youngster with type 1 spinal muscle atrophy and allows her to fish with a magnet puzzle. (Modified from Bach JR: *Management of patients with neuromuscular disease*, Philadelphia, 2004, Hanley & Belfus.)

the family. Positioning in side-lying to play may be very appropriate, as seen in Fig. 8.17, because it allows midline alignment of head and trunk. Toys need to be lightweight with Velcro straps. Slings may help to support limbs for reaching. Development of flexion contractures can be counteracted by a program of range of motion. Because of the poorer prognosis of children with this type of SMA, listening to the family's concerns is an integral part of the role of physical therapy clinicians. The natural history of SMA has recently been changed with the use of gene therapy. The first ever drug for SMA, Nusinersen, was introduced in 2016 and has been approved for use in the United States and Europe after successful trials. Finkel et al. (2016) reported the safety and clinical efficacy of using Nusinersen in infants with SMA type 1. Nusinersen is designed to increase the amount of functional survival motor neuron protein. Infants taking Nusinersen have been documented to make unexpected motor gains (Alfano et al., 2019). Recently in a study comparing Nusinersen to a sham treatment, the trial was stopped because the likelihood of survival was higher in the experimental group than in the sham group (Finkel et al., 2017). The infants in the experimental group also had a higher percentage of motor milestone responses. Nusinersen may have the potential to increase survival in children with type 1 from 10% to 60% (Finkel et al., 2016, 2017).

Type 2 SMA

Chronic type 2 SMA has a later onset, which is reported to occur between 6 and 12 months. This type is characterized by the onset of proximal weakness, similar to the infantile type, and has the same incidence in the population. Most children with this type develop the ability to sit independently, stand, and in some cases walk with KAFOs. Because of trunk muscle weakness, scoliosis is a pervasive problem and may require surgical intervention. Furthermore, with a reported 12% to

15% fracture rate, weight-bearing is also recommended as part of any therapeutic intervention to prevent fractures (Ballestrazzi et al., 1989). Standers and KAFOs have been used to start standing by the age of 12 to 18 months in children with type 2 SMA (Glanzman et al., 2017). A standing program needs to start before the onset of contractures. A supine stander is recommended for children who lack adequate head control (Stuberg, 2012). Weight-bearing is critical for bone health. If adequate trunk alignment is not able to be maintained with adaptive equipment, a corset or thoracic lumbar sacral orthosis (TLSO) with abdominal cutout should be considered. The deforming effect of gravity on the spine needs to be constantly monitored because of the risk of scoliosis. Family members need to be instructed in the proper use of all adaptive equipment used for sitting or standing.

The course of the disease is rapid at first and then stabilizes; therefore the range of disability can be varied. In one study, 58% of toddlers with SMA type 2 were able to demonstrate assisted ambulation with lightweight KAFOs (Granata et al., 1989). Those that ambulated had less severe spinal curvatures than a control group with SMA. Additionally, a lower incidence of contractures and hip dislocation was reported in a supported walking program (Granata et al., 1989). Children participating in a supportive walking program need to be closely monitored because their weakness increases fall risk. Training begins with the parallel bars and progresses to a walker.

Physical therapy goals should be directed toward attaining some independent type of functional mobility. Many children master use of a power wheelchair between 1 and 2 years of age. Some can even propel a lightweight manual chair, but this may not be functional in the long run (Glanzman et al., 2017). Power mobility is indicated for a child who is not strong enough to propel a manual chair. The physical therapist assistant can play a vital role in promoting the child's independence by teaching the child to control a power wheelchair both in and out of the classroom. Appropriate trunk support when seated must be ensured to decrease the progression of spinal deformities. Because of the tendency of the child to lean in the wheelchair even with lateral supports, one should consider alternating placement of the joystick from one side to the other (Stuberg, 2000). Although scoliosis cannot always be prevented, every effort should be made to minimize any progression of deformities and therefore to maintain adequate respiratory function. Any changes or decreases in strength should be reported by the physical therapist assistant to the supervising therapist. As genetic therapy continues to change the natural history of this disease, interventions will need to be modified to support new possibilities for these children.

Intellectually and socially, children with type 2 SMA need to be stimulated just as much as their typically developing peer group. The child's ability to participate in preschool and school is often hampered by inadequate positioning and lack of ability to access play and academic materials. Assistive technology can be very helpful in providing easier access. Goals can be related to improved access using switches, overhead slings, and adaptive equipment.

Life expectancy has improved in type 2 with survival into adulthood being typical. This is likely to improve even more with future advancements in genetic therapy. Survival may still depend on the aggressive management of respiratory compromise, secondary deformities, and monitoring muscle function. Prognosis in this type of SMA has depended on the degree and frequency of pulmonary complications. Postural drainage positioning can be incorporated into the preschool, school, and home routines. Deep breathing should be an integral part of the exercise program. Scoliosis can compound pulmonary problems, with surgical correction indicated only if the child has a good prognosis for survival. Respiratory compromise remains the major cause of death, although cardiac muscle involvement may contribute to mortality.

Type 3 SMA

The third type of SMA has an onset between 1 and 10 years (Glanzman et al., 2017). This is the least involved form with an incidence of 6 in 100,000 live births. Characteristics include proximal weakness, which is greatest in the hips, knees, and trunk. Developmental progress is slow, with independent sitting achieved by 1 year and independent walking by 3 years. The gait is slow and waddling, often with bilateral Trendelenburg signs. These children have good upper extremity strength, which can differentiate this type of SMA from DMD.

The progression of the disease is slow in type 3. Physical therapy goals in the toddler and preschool period are directed toward mobility, including walking. Maintenance of walking throughout the person's life span is a real possibility. Appropriate orthoses for ambulation could include KAFOs, parapodiums, and reciprocating gait orthoses. The reader is referred to Chapter 7 for a discussion of these devices. The physical therapist assistant may be involved in training the child to use and to apply orthotic devices. Orthotic devices assist ambulation, as does the use of a walker. Safety can be a significant issue as the child becomes weaker, so appropriate precautions such as close monitoring must be taken.

Goals for the school-aged child and adolescent with SMA include support of mobility, access to and completion of academic tasks such as using a computer, positioning to prevent scoliosis and promote pulmonary hygiene, and vocational planning. A power scooter or manual wheelchair for long distances may be indicated in some cases when weakness is present before 2 years of age. The physical therapist assistant may not be treating a child with SMA that is in a regular classroom on a weekly basis because therapy may be provided in a consultative service delivery model. However, the assistant may be asked to adjust orthoses, adapt equipment, or teach transfers when guided by the supervising physical therapist. Driver training may be indicated as part of the adolescent's prevocational plan. Children with type 3 SMA usually ambulate and half will maintain the ability past age 12, whereas half will still be walking at age 44 (Russman et al., 1996). The rest become wheelchair dependent (Glanzman, 2015). Life expectancy is normal for individuals with type 3, so vocational planning is realistic.

The physical therapy needs are determined by the specific type of SMA, the functional limitations present, and the age of the child. Although the needs of the child vary with the type, in general, evidence-based interventions include stretching, strengthening, night splinting, CPT, adaptive equipment, assistive technology, and environmental modification. Management includes positioning, functional strengthening and mobility training including power mobility if indicated, standing and walking if possible, adapted sports, pulmonary hygiene, and ventilatory support. Chabanon et al. (2018) are conducting a prospective, longitudinal study of the natural history of patients with SMA type 2 and 3 to determine the sensitivity of outcomes and biomarkers relative to disease progression.

PHENYLKETONURIA

One genetic cause of ID that is preventable is the inborn error of metabolism called PKU. PKU is caused by an autosomal recessive trait that can be detected at birth by a simple blood test. The infant's metabolism is missing an enzyme that converts phenylalanine to tyrosine. Too much phenylalanine causes ID and growth retardation along with seizures and behavioral problems. Once the error is identified, infants are placed on a phenylalanine-restricted diet. If dietary management is begun, the child will not develop ID or any of the other neurologic signs of the disorder. If the error is undetected, the infant's mental and physical development will be delayed, and physical therapy intervention is warranted.

DUCHENNE MUSCULAR DYSTROPHY

DMD is transmitted as an X-linked recessive trait, which means that it is manifested only in boys. Females can be carriers of the gene, but they do not express it, although some sources state that a small percentage of female carriers do exhibit muscle weakness. DMD affects 20 to 30 in 100,000 male births (Glanzman, 2015). Two-thirds of cases of DMD are inherited, whereas one-third of cases result from a spontaneous mutation. Boys with DMD develop motor skills normally. However, between the ages of 3 and 5 years, they may begin to fall more often or experience difficulty in going up and down stairs, or they may use a characteristic Gower maneuver to move into a standing position from the floor (Fig. 8.18). The *Gower maneuver* is characterized by the child using his arms to push on the thighs to achieve a standing position. This maneuver indicates presenting muscle weakness. The diagnosis is usually made during this time. Elevated levels of creatine kinase are often found in the blood as a result of the breakdown of muscle. This enzyme is a measure of the amount of muscle fiber loss. The definitive diagnosis is usually made by muscle biopsy.

Pathophysiology and Natural History

Children with DMD lack the gene that produces the muscle protein *dystrophin*. Absence of this protein weakens the cell membrane and eventually leads to the destruction of muscle

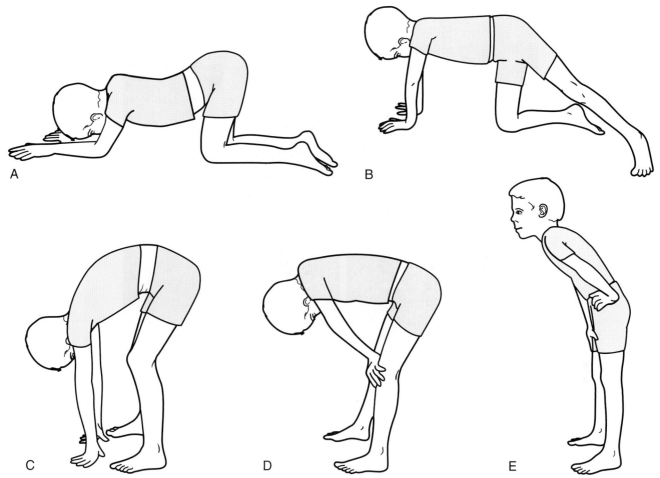

Fig. 8.18 **(A–E)** Gower maneuver. The child needs to push on his legs to achieve an upright position because of pelvic girdle and lower extremity weakness.

fibers. The lack of another protein, *nebulin*, prevents proper alignment of the contractile filaments during muscle contraction. As muscle fibers break down, they are replaced by fat and connective tissue. Fiber necrosis, degeneration, and regeneration are characteristically seen on muscle biopsy. The replacement of muscle fiber with fat and connective tissue results in a *pseudohypertrophy*, or false hypertrophy of muscles that is most readily apparent in the calves (Fig. 8.19). With progressive loss of muscle, weakness ensues, followed by loss of active and passive range of motion. Limitations in range and ADLs begin at around 5 years of age (Hallum and Allen, 2013), an inability to climb stairs is seen between 7 and 10 years of age, and the ability to ambulate independently is usually lost by 10 to 12 years (Glanzman et al., 2017). Intellectual function is less than normal in about one-third of these children.

Smooth muscle also is affected by the lack of dystrophin; 84% of boys with DMD exhibit cardiomyopathy, or weakness of the heart muscle. Cardiac failure results either from this weakness or from respiratory insufficiency. As the muscles of respiration become involved, pulmonary function is compromised, with death from respiratory or cardiac failure usually occurring before age 25. Life can be prolonged by use of mechanical ventilation, but this decision is based on the individual's and the family's wishes. Bach et al. (1991) reported that satisfaction with life was positive in a majority of individuals with DMD who used long-term ventilatory support. Survival is being prolonged by use of noninvasive ventilator support (Bach and Martinez, 2011).

Child's Impairments, Activity Limitations, Participation Restrictions, and Interventions

The physical therapist's examination and evaluation of the child with DMD typically identifies the following impairments, activity limitations, or participation restrictions to be addressed by physical therapy intervention:

1. Impaired strength and range of motion
2. Decreased functional mobility, transfers and gait
3. Limitations in functional abilities
4. Impaired respiratory function
5. Spinal deformities, apparent or potential
6. Potential need for adaptive equipment, orthoses, and wheelchair
7. Emotional trauma of the individual and family

The family's understanding of the disease and its progressive nature must be taken into consideration when the physical

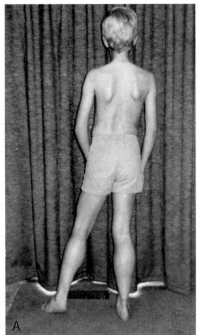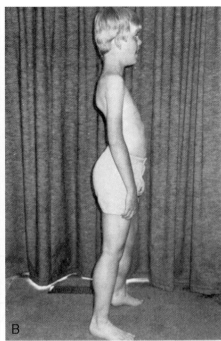

Fig. 8.19 **(A, B)** Pseudohypertrophy of the calves. (From Stuberg W: Muscular dystrophy and spinal muscular atrophy. In Campbell SK, Palisano RJ, Orlin MN, editors: *Physical therapy for children*, ed 4, Philadelphia, 2012, WB Saunders.)

therapist plans an intervention program. The ultimate goal of the program is to provide education and support for the family while managing the child's impairments. Each problem or impairment is discussed, along with possible interventions.

The physical therapy goals are to prevent deformity, to prolong function by maintaining capacity for ADLs and play, to facilitate movement, to assist in supporting the family, and to control discomfort. Management is a total approach requiring blending of medical, educational, and family goals. Treatment has both preventive and supportive aspects.

Weakness

Proximal muscle weakness is one of the major clinical features of DMD and is most clearly apparent in the shoulder and pelvic girdles (see Fig. 8.19). The loss of strength eventually progresses distally to encompass all the musculature. Whether exercise can be used to counteract the pathologic weakness seen in muscular dystrophies is unclear. Strengthening exercises have been found to be beneficial by some researchers and not by others. More important, however, although exercise has not been found to hasten the progression of the disease, the role of exercise remains controversial (Ansved, 2003; Grange and Call, 2007). Some therapists do not encourage active resistive exercises (Florence, 1999) and choose instead to focus on preserving functional levels of strength by having the child do all ADLs. Other therapists recommend that submaximal forms of exercise are beneficial but advocate these activities only if they are not burdensome to the family. Movement in some form must be an integral part of a physical therapy plan of care for the child with DMD.

Theoretically, exercise should be able to assist intact muscle fibers to increase in strength to make up for lost fibers. Key muscles to target, if exercise is going to be used to treat weakness, include the abdominals, hip extensors and abductors, and knee extensors. In addition, the triceps and scapular stabilizers should be targeted in the upper extremities. Recreational activities, such as bike riding and swimming, are excellent choices and provide aerobic conditioning. Even though the exact role of exercise in these children is unclear, clinicians generally agree that overexertion, exercising at maximal levels, and immobility are detrimental to the child with DMD. High resistance and eccentric training also should be avoided (Ansved, 2003; Hu and Blemker, 2015). Exercise capacity is probably best determined by the stage and rate of disease progression (Ansved, 2003; McDonald, 2002). Exercise may be more beneficial early as opposed to later in the disease process.

Mobility status is related to knee extension strength and gait velocity in children with DMD. Boys with less than antigravity (3/5) quadriceps strength lost the ability to ambulate (McDonald, 2002). Walking should be done for a minimum of 2 to 3 hours a day, according to many sources (Siegel, 1978; Ziter and Allsop, 1976). The speed of walking has been used to predict the length of time that will pass before a child with DMD will require the use of a wheelchair. A high percentage of boys who walked 10 m in less than 6 seconds were more than 2 years away from using a wheelchair, whereas all of the boys who took 12 seconds or more to walk 10 m required a wheelchair within a year (McDonald et al., 1995). The longer a child can remain ambulatory, the better.

INTERVENTION 8.7 Stretching of the Iliopsoas, Iliotibial Band, and Tensor Fasciae Latae

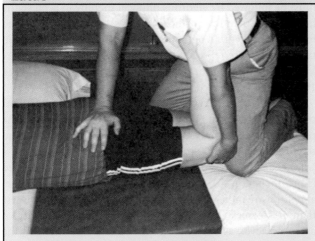

Prone stretching of the hip flexors, iliotibial band, and tensor fasciae latae. The hip first is positioned in abduction and then is moved into maximal hip extension and then hip adduction. The knee can be extended to provide greater stretch for the iliotibial and tensor muscles.

From Campbell SK, Vander Linden DW, Palisano RJ, editors: *Physical therapy for children*, ed 3, Philadelphia, 2006, WB Saunders.

Range of Motion

The potential for muscle contractures is high, and every effort should be made to maintain range of motion at all joints. Specifically, attention should be paid to the gastrocnemius-soleus complex and the tensor fasciae latae. Tightness in these muscle groups results in gait deviations and a widened base of support. Stretching of the iliopsoas, iliotibial band, and tensor fasciae latae is demonstrated in Intervention 8.7. Although contractures cannot be prevented, their progression can be slowed (Stuberg, 2012). A prone positioning program is crucial for managing the detrimental effect of gravity. Time in prone counteracts the potential formation of hip and knee flexion contractures, which develop from too much sitting. The physical therapist assistant may teach a home program to the child's parents and may monitor position changes within the classroom. Prolonged sitting can all too quickly lead to lower extremity flexion deformities that can hinder ambulation.

Alternatives to a sitting position should be scheduled several times a day. When the child is in preschool, the prone position can be easily incorporated into nap or rest time. A prone stander can be used during class time when the child is standing and working on the blackboard can be incorporated into the child's daily classroom routine. Prone positioning over a wedge can also be used. At home, sleeping in the prone position should be encouraged as long as it does not compromise the child's respiratory function.

Skin Care

Skin integrity must always be monitored. Pressure relief and use of a cushion must be part of the daily routine once the child is using a wheelchair for any length of time. If the child is using a splint or orthosis, wearing times must be controlled and the skin must be inspected on a routine basis.

Gait

Children with DMD ambulate with a characteristic waddle because the pelvic girdle muscles weaken. Hip extensor weakness can lead to compensatory lordosis, which keeps the center of mass posterior to the hip joint, as seen in Fig. 8.19. Excessive lateral trunk lean during gait may be seen in response to bilateral Trendelenburg signs indicative of hip abductor weakness. Knee hyperextension may be substituted for quadriceps muscle strength, and it can further increase the lumbar lordosis. Failure to keep the body weight in front of the knee joint or behind the hip joint results in a loss of the ability to stand. Plantar flexion contractures can compromise toe clearance, can lead to toe walking, and may make balance even more precarious.

Functional rating scales can be helpful in documenting the progression of disability, and several are available. Box 8.3 depicts simple scales for the upper and lower extremities. The Pediatric Evaluation of Disability Inventory (Haley et al., 1992) or the School Function Assessment (Coster et al., 1998)

BOX 8.3 Vignos Classification Scales for Children With Duchenne Muscular Dystrophy

Upper Extremity Functional Grades
1. Can abduct arms in a full circle until they touch above the head
2. Raises arms above the head only by shortening the lever arm or using accessory muscles
3. Cannot raise hands above the head but can raise a 180-mL cup of water to mouth using both hands, if necessary
4. Can raise hands to mouth but cannot raise a 180-mL cup of water to mouth
5. Cannot raise hands to mouth but can use hands to hold a pen or pick up a coin
6. Cannot raise hands to mouth and has no functional use of hands

Lower Extremity Functional Grades
1. Walks and climbs stairs without assistance
2. Walks and climbs stairs with aid of railing
3. Walks and climbs stairs slowly with aid of railing (more than 12 s for four steps)
4. Walks unassisted and rises from a chair but cannot climb stairs
5. Walks unassisted but cannot rise from a chair or climb stairs
6. Walks only with assistance or walks independently in long-leg braces
7. Walks in long-leg braces but requires assistance for balance
8. Stands in long-leg braces but is unable to walk even with assistance
9. Must use a wheelchair
10. Bedridden

Data from Vignos PJ, Spencer GE, Archibald KC: Management of progressive muscular dystrophy in childhood, *JAMA* 184:89–96, 1963. ©1963 American Medical Association.

can be used to obtain more specific information about mobility and self-care. The supervising physical therapist may use this information for treatment planning, and the physical therapist assistant may be responsible for collecting data as part of the ongoing assessment. The physical therapist assistant also provides feedback to the primary therapist for appropriate modifications to the child's plan of care.

Medical Management

No known treatment can stop the progression of DMD. However, recently updated standards of care are available (Birnkrant et al., 2018a–c); see Korinthenberg (2019) for a review of the highlights. Steroid therapy has been used to slow the progression of both the Duchenne and Becker forms of muscular dystrophy. Becker is a milder form of muscular dystrophy with a later onset, slower progression, and longer life expectancy. Use of corticosteroids is recommended as appropriate care of persons with DMD (Gloss et al., 2016; Korinthenberg, 2019). Use of steroids such as prednisone and deflazacort has been shown to improve the strength of muscles, prolong walking, and improve pulmonary and cardiac function (Biggar et al., 2006; Korinthenberg, 2019). One study even showed improvements in psychomotor function with corticosteroid therapy (Sato et al., 2014). Recently, corticosteroids were found to have a measurable impact on muscle strength 6 to 24 months after starting treatment (Schreiber et al., 2018). Furthermore the motor function measure (MFM) was found to be a valid outcome measure in those with DMD receiving corticosteroid treatment. A pharmacologic approach using tadalafil has been shown to counteract muscle hypoxia (lack of oxygen) (Nelson et al., 2014) and to slow the development of cardiomyopathy in animals (Hammers et al., 2016). However, in a phase 3 trial, tadalafil did not slow the decline in ambulation in children with DMD (Victor et al., 2017). The program has been terminated for lack of effect. It is recommended that the use of corticosteroids be continued as long as side effects do not negate the benefits. Side effects include weight gain with increased appetite, cataracts, stunted growth, osteoporosis, and adrenal insufficiency or suppression. Gene therapy research continues in this area with ongoing clinical trials. Increased knowledge of the genetic and pathophysiology of DMD has led to potentially promising compounds that change gene translation. Simply put, one drug has been found to change a DMD to a milder Becker phenotype; however, individual variability in DMD continues to be a challenge for researchers.

Surgical and Orthotic Management

As the quality of the child's functional gait declines, medical management of the child with DMD is broadened. Surgical and orthotic solutions to the loss of range or ambulation abilities are by no means universal. Many variables must be factored into a final decision whether to perform surgery or to use an orthosis. Some clinicians think that it is worse to try to postpone the inevitable, whereas others support the child's and family's right to choose to fight for independence as long as resources are available. Surgical procedures that have been used to combat the progressive effects of DMD are Achilles tendon lengthening procedures, tensor fasciae latae fasciotomy, tendon transfers, and tenotomies. These procedures must be followed by vigorous physical therapy to achieve the best gains. Ankle-foot orthoses (AFOs) are often prescribed following heel cord lengthening. Use of KAFOs has also been tried; one source reported that early surgery followed by rehabilitation negated the need for KAFOs (Bach and McKeon, 1991).

Daytime use of AFOs should be used to maintain heel cord length while the patient is ambulating. To prevent the progression of equinovarus contractures, osteoporosis and scoliosis, a standing program with standing devices or a wheelchair with upright positioning should be used (Korinthenberg, 2019). Custom molded AFO night splints set at neutral are indicated when passive ankle dorsiflexion is less than 10 degrees (Korinthenberg, 2019). In the majority of cases, however, as the quadriceps muscles lose strength, the child develops severe lordosis as compensation. This change keeps the body weight in front of the knee joints and allows gravity to control knee extension. The child's gait becomes lurching, and if the ankles do not have sufficient range to keep the feet plantigrade, dynamic balance becomes impaired. Surgical release of the Achilles tendon followed by use of polypropylene AFOs may prolong the length of time a child can remain ambulatory. However, once ambulation skills are lost, the child will require a wheelchair. A motorized scooter may be indicated prior to a wheelchair because it is more likely to be accepted as an alternative means of mobility before ambulation is lost.

Development of scoliosis is a major concern in muscular dystrophy because up to 80% of teens have a significant scoliosis. Visual examination of the back annually is sufficient while the child is ambulatory. If a curve is detected on visual exam, then an x-ray is indicated to determine the degree of the curve. Once a child is no longer ambulatory, the spine should be visually inspected every 6 months and an x-ray taken. If there is a scoliosis, referral to a surgeon is warranted if the curve is greater than 20 degrees. Because bracing does not stop progression and may interfere with respiratory function, it is not recommended. Surgery is recommended if the curve is progressive and cardiac and respiratory functions are stable (Archer et al., 2016; Birnkrant et al., 2018b).

Adaptive Equipment

The physical therapist assistant may participate in the team's decision regarding the type of wheelchair to be prescribed for the child with DMD. The child may not be able to propel a manual wheelchair because of upper extremity weakness, so consideration of a lighter sports wheelchair or a power wheelchair may be appropriate. Energy cost and insurance or reimbursement constraints must be considered. The child may be able to propel a lighter wheelchair during certain times of the day or use it to work on endurance, but in the long term, he may be more mobile in a power wheelchair, as seen in Fig. 8.20. If reimbursement limitations are severe and only one wheelchair is possible, power mobility may be a

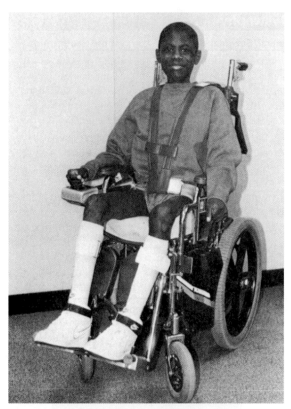

Fig. 8.20 Boy with Duchenne muscular dystrophy using a power chair. (From Stuberg W: Muscular dystrophy and spinal muscular atrophy. In Campbell SK, editor: *Physical therapy for children,* Philadelphia, 1994, WB Saunders.)

INTERVENTION 8.8   Chest Wall Stretching

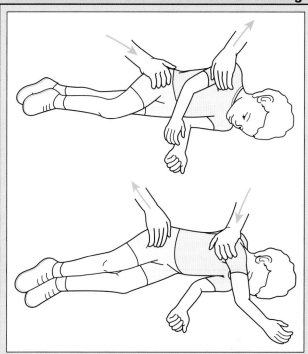

Chest wall mobility can be promoted by active trunk rotation, passive counterrotation, and manual stretching. Stretching counteracts the tendency to tightness that occurs as the child becomes more sedentary.

more functional choice. Other adaptive equipment such as mobile arm supports for feeding or voice-activated computer and environmental controls may also be considered to augment the child's level of function.

Respiratory Function

Respiratory function must be targeted for aggressive management. Breathing exercises and range of motion should be part of a home exercise program and incorporated into any therapy session. Flexion of the arms or legs can be paired with inspiration, whereas extension can be linked to expiration. Diaphragmatic breathing is more efficient than use of accessory muscles and therefore should be emphasized along with lateral basal chest expansion. Chest wall tightness can be discouraged by active trunk rotation, passive counterrotation, and manual stretching (Intervention 8.8). On occasion, postural drainage with percussion may be needed to clear the lungs of retained secretions. Children often miss school because of respiratory involvement. Parents should be taught appropriate airway clearance techniques, as described in the section on CF.

Activities that promote cardiovascular endurance are as important as stretching and functional activities. Always incorporate deep breathing and chest mobility into the child's upper extremity or lower extremity exercises. Wind sprints can be done when the child is in a wheelchair. These are fast, energetic pushes of the wheelchair for set distances.

The child can be timed and work to improve or maintain his best time. An exercise program for a child with DMD needs to include an aerobic component because the respiratory system ultimately causes the child to die from the effects of the disease. Swimming is an excellent aerobic exercise for children with DMD.

At least biannual reexaminations are used to document the inevitable progression of the disease. Documenting progression of the disease is critical for timing of interventions as the child declines from one functional level to another. Whether to have surgical treatment or to use orthotic devices remains controversial. Accurate data must be kept to allow one to intervene aggressively to provide adequate mobility and respiratory support for the individual and his family. Table 8.10 outlines some of the goals, strategies, and interventions that could be implemented over the life span of a person with DMD.

BECKER MUSCULAR DYSTROPHY

Children with Becker muscular dystrophy (BMD) have an onset of symptoms between 5 and 10 years of age. This X-linked dystrophy occurs in 5 per 100,000 males, so it is rarer than DMD. Dystrophin continues to be present but in lesser amounts than normal. Laboratory findings are not as striking as in DMD; one sees less elevation of creatine kinase levels and less destruction of muscle fibers on biopsy.

TABLE 8.10 Management of Duchenne Muscular Dystrophy

Time Period	Goals	Strategies	Medical/Surgical	Home Program
School age	Prevent deformity Preserve independent mobility Preserve vital capacity	Stretching Strengthening Breathing exercises	Splints/AFOs Monitor spinal alignment Manual wheelchair as walking becomes difficult Motorized scooter	ROM program Night splints Cycling or swimming Prone positioning Blow bottles
Adolescence	Manage contractures Maintain ambulation Assist with transfers and ADLs	Stretching Guard during stair climbing or general walking Positioning ADLs, ADL modifications Strengthening shoulder depressors and triceps	AFOs/KAFOs before ambulation ceases Surgery to prolong ambulatory ability Proper wheelchair fit and support Surgery for scoliosis management	ROM program Night splints Prone positioning Blow bottles Assistance with transfers and ADLs
Adulthood	Monitor respiratory function Manage mobility and transfers	Breathing exercises, postural drainage, assisted coughing Assistive technology	Mechanical ventilation Monitoring oxygen saturation Power mobility	Hospital bed Ball-bearing feeder Hoyer lift

ADLs, Activities of daily living; *AFOs,* ankle-foot orthoses; *KAFOs,* knee-ankle-foot orthoses; *ROM,* range of motion.
From Stuberg WA: Muscular dystrophy and spinal muscular atrophy. In Campbell SK, Vander Linden DW, Palisano RJ, editors: *Physical therapy for children,* ed 2, Philadelphia, 2000, WB Saunders, pp 339–369.

Another significant difference from DMD is the lower incidence of ID with the Becker type of muscular dystrophy. Physical therapy management follows the same general outline as for the child with DMD; however, the progression of the disorder is much slower. Greater potential and expectation exist for the individual to continue to ambulate until his late teens and even twenties. Emery and Skinner (1976) stressed that by definition a person with a diagnosis of BMD should continue to ambulate without braces beyond the age of 16. Prevention of excessive weight gain must be vigorously pursued to avoid use of a wheelchair too early because life expectancy reaches into the 40s. Providing sufficient exercise for weight control may be an even greater challenge in this population because the use of power mobility is more prevalent. Sveen et al. (2008) have shown that a cycling program increased endurance and lower extremity strength after 12 weeks without evidence of muscle damage. A follow-up study (Sveen et al., 2013) focused on resistance training with positive results, but the most appropriate training intensity has not yet been determined.

The transition from adolescence to adulthood is more of an issue in BMD because of the longer life expectancy. Individuals with BMD live into their 40s with death secondary to pulmonary or cardiac failure (Glanzman, 2015). Vocational rehabilitation can be invaluable in assisting with vocational training or college attendance, depending on the patient's degree of disability and disease progression. Regardless of vocational or avocational plans, the adult with BMD needs assistance with living arrangements. Evaluation of needs should begin before the completion of high school.

FRAGILE X SYNDROME

FXS is the leading inherited cause of ID. It occurs in 1 per 4000 males and 1 per 8000 females (Jorde et al., 2010). Detection of

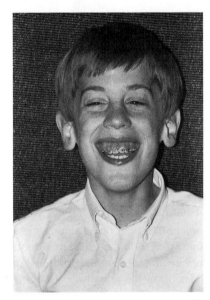

Fig. 8.21 A 6-year-old boy with fragile X syndrome. (From Hagerman R: Fragile X syndrome. In Allen PJ, Vessey JA, and Schapiro NA, editors: Primary care of the child with a chronic condition, ed 5, St. Louis, 2010, Mosby, pp 514–526.)

a fragile site on the X chromosome at a cellular level makes it possible to confirm this entity as the cause of a child's ID. The fragile X gene (FMR) codes for a fragile X mental retardation protein (FMRP). FXS is characterized by ID, unusual facies, poor coordination, a generalized decrease in muscle tone, and enlarged testes in male patients after puberty. These children may have a long, narrow face with a prominent forehead, jaw, and ears (Fig. 8.21). The clinical manifestations of the disorder vary depending on the completeness of the mutation. The FMR gene determines the number of repeats of a series of three amino acids. When the FMR gene is inherited the number of repeats can go from normal (6 to 40 repeats) to a permutation (50 to 200 repeats) to a full-blown mutation of greater than 200 repeats. In the full-blown mutation almost no FMRP is produced. The less FMRP produced, the more severe is the ID. Over successive generations there is an increased risk of the number of repeats expanding so that the disease appears to worsen in successive generations. Genetic counseling for the family of a child with fragile X is extremely important for them to understand the reproductive risks.

Connective tissue involvement can include joint hypermobility, flatfeet (pes planus), inguinal hernia, pectus excavatum, and mitral valve prolapse (Goldstein and Reynolds, 2011). Symptoms in girls are not as severe as in boys. Girls do not usually present with dysmorphic features (structural differences often seen in the face) or connective tissue abnormalities. Females with fragile X are more likely to have normal intelligence but may have a learning disability. Children of female carriers, however, have a greater risk of the disorder than those of male carriers, which again reinforces the importance of genetic counseling for this condition. Behavioral characteristics of both males and females with FXS include a short attention span, impulsivity, tactile defensiveness, hyperactivity, and perseveration in speech and motor actions (Goldstein and Reynolds, 2011).

FXS is the most common single gene defect associated with autism spectrum disorder. Thirty percent of children with FXS will be diagnosed with autism (Harris et al., 2008). Most children with FXS demonstrate autistic-like behavior. There appears to be a shared molecular overlap between autism, FXS, and fragile X permutation (Gurkan and Hagerman, 2012). There is greater impairment of cognition, language, and adaptive behavior in those with FXS and autism compared with those with FXS without autism (Hagerman et al., 2008). Autism is discussed in Chapter 9 of this text.

Intelligence

ID in children with FXS can range from severe to borderline normal. The average IQ falls between 20 and 60, with a mean of 30 to 45. Additional cognitive deficits may include attention deficit-hyperactivity disorder, learning disability, and autistic-like mannerisms. In fact, girls may be incorrectly diagnosed as having infantile autism or may exhibit only a mild cognitive deficit, such as a learning disability (Batshaw et al., 2013).

Motor Development

Gross and fine motor development is delayed in the child with FXS. The average age of walking is 2 years (Levitas et al., 1983), with 75% of boys exhibiting a flatfooted and waddling gait (Davids et al., 1990). The child's motor skills are at the same developmental age level as the child's mental ability. Even before the diagnosis of FXS is made, the physical therapist may be the first to recognize that the child has more problems than just delayed development. Maintaining balance in any developmental posture is a challenge for these

children because of their low tone, joint hypermobility, and gravitational insecurity. Individuals who are mildly affected may present with language delays and behavioral problems, especially hyperactivity (Schopmeyer and Lowe, 1992).

Tactile Defensiveness

Regardless of the severity of the disorder, 90% of these children avoid eye contact and 80% display tactile defensiveness. The characteristics of tactile defensiveness are listed in Table 8.11. Touch can be perceived as aversive, and light touch may elicit a withdrawal response rather than an orienting response. Treatment involves the use of different-textured surfaces on equipment that the child can touch during play. Vestibular stimulation, firm pressure, and increasing proprioceptive input through weight-bearing and movement are helpful (Schopmeyer and Lowe, 1992).

Sensory Integration

In addition to tactile defensiveness, other sensory integration problems are evident in the decreased ability of these children to tolerate being exposed to multiple sensory inputs at one time. These children become easily overwhelmed because they cannot filter out environmental stimuli. When gaze aversion occurs, it is thought to be related to the child's high degree of anxiety, rather than to autism or social dysfunction. Because low tolerance for frustration often leads to tantrums in these children, always be alert to the child's losing control and institute appropriate behavior modification responses that have been decided on by the team.

TABLE 8.11	Tactile Defensiveness
Major Symptom	**Child's Behavior**
Avoidance of touch	Avoids scratchy or rough clothing, prefers soft material, long sleeves or pants
	Prefers to stand alone to avoid contact with other children
	Avoids play activities that involve body contact
Aversive responses to nonnoxious touch	Turns away or struggles when picked up, hugged, or cuddled
	Resists certain ADLs, such as baths, cutting fingernails, haircuts, and face washing
	Has an aversion to dental care
	Has an aversion to art materials such as finger paints, paste, or sand
Atypical affective responses to nonnoxious tactile stimuli	Responds aggressively to light touch to arms, face, or legs
	Increased stress in response to being physically close to people
	Objects to or withdraws from touch contact

ADLs, Activities of daily living.

From Royeen CB: Domain specifications of the construct of tactile defensiveness, *Am J Occup Ther* 39:596–599, 1985. ©1985 American Occupational Therapy Association. Reprinted with permission.

Learning

Visual learning is a strength of children with FXS, so using a visual cue with a verbal request is a good intervention strategy. Teaching any motor skill or task should be done within the context in which it is expected to be performed, such as teaching handwashing at a sink in the bathroom. Examples of inappropriate contexts are teaching tooth brushing in the cafeteria or teaching ball kicking in the classroom. The physical, social, and emotional surroundings in which learning takes place are significant for the activity to make sense to the child. Teaching a task in its entirety, rather than breaking it down into its component parts, may help to lessen the child's difficulty with sequential learning and tendency to *perseverate,* or repeating an action over and over.

RETT SYNDROME

Rett syndrome is a neurodevelopmental disorder that almost exclusively affects females. It occurs in approximately 1 in 12,000 females. The presentation in females suggests an X-linked dominant means of inheritance, but this has been disproven (Goldstein and Reynolds, 2011). Males with Rett syndrome have been described in the literature (Clayton-Smith et al., 2000; Moog et al., 2003).

Rett syndrome is characterized by ID, ataxia, and growth retardation. It is a major cause of ID in females (Shahbazian and Zoghbi, 2001). Despite the ID, Rett syndrome is not a neurodegenerative disorder (Zoghbi, 2003). It represents a failure of postnatal development caused by a mutation in the MECP2 gene, which is responsible for development of synaptic connections in the brain. ID is in the severe, profound range. There is a prestage in which the child's development appears normal. This prestage lasts 6 months and is followed by four stages of decline. Stage 1 has been characterized as early-onset stagnation in which there is loss of language and motor skills between 6 and 18 months. Stage 2 is rapid destruction of previously acquired hand function. It is during this stage that children develop stereotypical hand movements, such as flapping, wringing, and slapping, as well as mouthing. Decline in function during childhood includes a decreased ability to communicate; seizure activity; and later, scoliosis. There is a plateau during stage 3, which lasts until around the age of 10 years, followed by late motor deterioration in stage 4. Expression of the syndrome varies in severity. Girls with Rett syndrome live into adulthood (Goldstein and Reynolds, 2011).

COHEN SYNDROME

Cohen syndrome is a rare autosomal recessive cause of hypotonia in children (Wang et al., 2006). Diagnosis is based on clinical findings; however, no consensus has been reached as to diagnostic criteria. A diagnosis of Cohen syndrome can be made on the basis of molecular genetic testing and the presence of six of the following eight cardinal features: retinal dystrophy and high myopia, microcephaly; developmental delay, joint hypermobility, typical Cohen syndrome facial features, truncal obesity with slender extremities, overly sociable behavior, and neutropenia (Kolehmainen et al., 2004). Characteristic facial features include hypotonic appearance, thick hair and eyebrows, long eyelashes, smooth or short philtrum, broad nasal tip, and wave-shaped palpebral fissures. Attainment of motor milestones such as sitting and standing are significantly delayed; however, once they are achieved there is no regression of psychomotor skills (Chandler et al., 2003; Kivitie-Kallio and Norio, 2001; Nye et al., 2005). Language is also delayed with 20% in the National Cohen Syndrome Database (NCSD) unable to verbally communicate (Nye et al., 2005). Similar to children with PWS, infants with Cohen syndrome exhibit failure to thrive early and continue to be underweight in early childhood. In late childhood rapid weight gain occurs in the trunk. Unlike children with PWS, however, there is no appreciable decline in activity and appetite and food intake do not increase.

Medically, children with Cohen syndrome need to be assessed by a pediatric ophthalmologist because of potential of abnormal retinal findings (Wang et al., 2006) and progressive visual impairments. Neutropenia or decreased number of neutrophils can increase risk of infections. Because of delayed motor and speech development, children with Cohen syndrome are excellent candidates for early intervention. Additionally, physical therapy can focus on acquiring age-appropriate skills, postural control and motor coordination. The microcephaly results in variable cognitive abilities that fall usually into the moderate to profound range. Independence is low but sociability is a positive characteristic. However, some children with Cohen syndrome display autistic behavior.

GENETIC DISORDERS AND INTELLECTUAL DISABILITY

One to three percent of the total population of the United States has psychomotor or ID. *Intellectual disability* is defined by the American Association on Intellectual and Developmental Disabilities as "a significant limitation in both intellectual functioning and adaptive behavior as expressed in conceptual, social, and practical adaptive skills originating before the age of 18" (Schalock et al., 2010). A person must have an IQ of 70 to 75 or less to be diagnosed as having ID. The foregoing definition emphasizes the effect that a decreased ability to learn has on all aspects of a person's life. Educational definitions of ID may vary from state to state because of differences in eligibility criteria for developmental services. An IQ score tells little about the strengths of the individual and may artificially lower the expectations of the child's capabilities. Despite the inclusion of the deficits in adaptive abilities seen in individuals with ID, four classic levels of ID are reported in the literature. These levels are best understood by looking at the learning rate associated with each level compared with a typically developing person. Individuals with mild ID learn at about a 50% to 66% rate, individuals with moderate ID learn at about a 33% to 50% rate, individuals with severe ID learn at a 24% to 33% rate, and those with profound ID learn at about a 25% rate.

The two most common genetic disorders that produce ID are DS and FXS. DS results from a trisomy of one of the chromosomes, chromosome 21, whereas FXS is caused by a defect on the X chromosome. This major X-linked disorder explains why the rate of ID is higher in males than females. The defect on the X chromosome is expressed in males when no normal X chromosome is present. Most genetic disorders involving the nervous system produce ID, and children present with low muscle tone as a primary clinical feature.

Child's Impairments, Activity Limitations, Participation Restrictions, and Interventions

The physical therapist's examination and evaluation of the child with low muscle tone secondary to a genetic problem, regardless of whether the child has associated ID, typically identifies similar problems or potential problems to be addressed by physical therapy intervention:

1. Delayed psychomotor development (only motor delay in SMA)
2. Hypotonia/muscle weakness, joint laxity
3. Poor postural control
4. Contractures and skeletal deformities
5. Impaired respiratory or cardiac function
6. Dependent in self-care activities and play
7. Restricted participation in home, school, and community

Interventions to address these impairments, activity limitations, and participation restrictions are discussed here both generally and within the context of a case study. *Intellectual disability* is the preferred term rather than *mental retardation*.

Psychomotor Development

Promotion of psychomotor development in children with genetic disorders resulting in delayed motor and cognitive development is a primary focus of physical therapy intervention. Children with ID are capable of learning motor skills and life skills. However, children with ID learn fewer things, and those things take longer to learn. Principles of motor learning can and should be used with this population. Practice and repetition are even more critical in the child with ID than in a child with a motor delay without ID. The clinician must always ensure that the skill or task taught is part of the child's everyday function, which is in the appropriate context. Usually, breaking the task into its component parts improves the potential for learning the original task and for that task to carry over into other skills. However, the ability to generalize a skill to another task is decreased in children with ID. Each task is new, no matter how similar we may think it is, and the process of teaching must start again. Skills that are not practiced on a regular basis will not be maintained, which is another reason for tasks to be made relevant and applicable to everyday life.

Hypotonia and Delayed Postural Reactions

Early in therapy, functional goals are focused on the development of postural control. The child must learn to move through the environment safely and to perform tasks such as manipulating objects within the environment. The ID, hypotonia, joint hypermobility, and delayed development characteristically seen in children with genetic disorders such as DS interact to produce poor postural control. The child with low postural tone cannot easily support a posture against gravity, move or shift weight within a posture, or maintain a posture to use limbs efficiently. Making the transition from one posture to another is accomplished only with a great deal of effort and unusual movement patterns. By improving postural tone in therapy, the therapist provides the child with a foundation for movement. Children with DS benefit from being taught or trained to achieve motor milestones and to improve postural responses. Table 8.2 lists the ages at attainment of developmental milestones in children with DS compared with the typical age at attainment of the same skills.

AG, as shown in Fig. 8.22, is a 17-month-old child with DS. She provides a model for treatment of children with genetic disorders in which hypotonia and delayed motor development are the overriding impairments. AG is seen weekly for physical therapy. She creeps and pulls to stand but is not yet walking independently. Although AG undresses, the therapist encourages AG's ability to balance while her weight is shifted to one side (see Fig. 8.22). In addition, typical help with sock removal is greatly appreciated (Fig. 8.23).

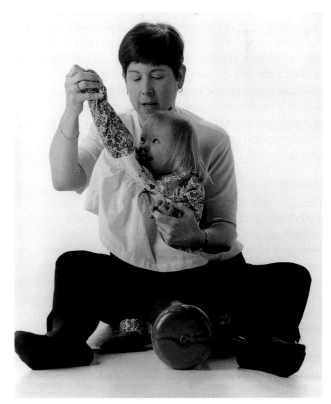

Fig. 8.22 Trunk weight shift while undressing.

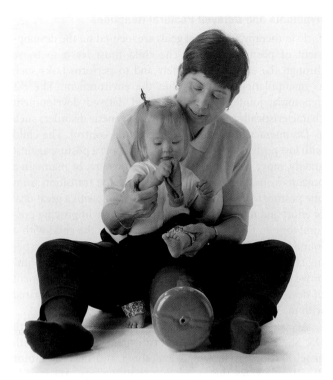

Fig. 8.23 Child with Down syndrome removing her sock.

Stability

Preparation for movement in children consists of weight-bearing in appropriate joint alignment. Splints of various materials may be used to maintain the required alignment without any mechanical joint locking if the child is unable to on her own. Gentle intermittent approximation by manual means helps prepare a body part to accept weight. Approximation is shown in Intervention 8.9. Approximation through the extremities during weight-bearing can reinforce the maintenance of a posture and can provide a stable base on which to superimpose movement, in the form of a weight shift or a movement transition. Intervention 8.10 shows the therapist guiding AG's movement from sitting to upper extremity weight-bearing and AG reaching with a return to sitting.

Mobility

The child with ID needs to be mobile to explore the environment. Manual manipulation of objects and the ability to explore the surrounding environment are assumed to contribute positively to the development of cognition, communication, and emotion. Even if motor and cognition develop separately, they facilitate one another, so by fostering movement, understanding of an action is made possible. AG is encouraged to come to stand at a bench to play both by pulling up and by coming to stand from sitting on the therapist's knee (Intervention 8.11). The use of postural supports such as a toy shopping cart can entice the child into walking (Intervention 8.12). Mobility options facilitate the child's mastery of the environment.

Alternative means of mobility, such as a power wheelchair, a cart, an adapted tricycle, or a prone scooter, can be used to give the child with moderate to severe ID and impaired motor abilities a way to move independently. McEwen (2000) stated that children with ID who have vision and cognition at the level of an 18-month-old are able to learn how to use a powered means of mobility. The rate of learning can vary and may depend on the child's spatial abilities and problem solving (Jones et al., 2012; Nilsson, 2010; Tefft et al., 1999). Orientation in an upright position is important for social interaction with peers and adults. McEwen (1992) also found that teachers interacted more with children who were positioned nearer the normal interaction level of adults (in a wheelchair) than with children who were positioned on the floor.

Postural Control

The child with low tone should be handled firmly, with vestibular input used when appropriate to encourage development of head and trunk control. Joint stability must always be taken into consideration when the clinician uses vestibular sensation or movement to improve a child's balance. The therapist and family should use carrying positions that incorporate trunk support and allow the child's head either to lift against gravity or to be maintained in a midline position. An infant can be carried over the adult's arm, at the adult's shoulder, or with the child's back to the adult's chest (Intervention 8.13). Gathered-together positions in which the limbs are held close to the body and most joints are flexed promote security and reinforce midline orientation and symmetry. Prone on elbows, prone on extended arms, propping on arms in sitting, and four-point are all good weight-bearing positions. When the child cannot fully support the body's weight, the use of an appropriate device, such as a wedge, a bolster, or a half-roll, can still allow the physical therapist assistant to position the child for weight-bearing. Upright positioning can enhance the child's arousal and therefore can provide a more optimal condition for learning than being recumbent (Guess et al., 1988). A recent case study demonstrated a positive effect of upright supported positioning on problem-solving behaviors (O'Grady and Dusing, 2016).

To develop postural control of the trunk, the clinician must balance trunk extensor strength with trunk flexor strength. Trunk extension can be facilitated when the child is in the prone position over a ball by asking the child to reach for an object (Intervention 8.14A). Protective extension of the upper extremities can also be encouraged at the same time, as seen in Intervention 8.14, B. The ball can also be used to support body weight partially for standing after the hips have been prepared with some gentle approximation (Intervention 8.15). A balanced trunk allows for the possibility of eliciting balance reactions. These reactions can be attempted on a movable surface (Intervention 8.16). The reader is referred to Chapter 5 for descriptions of additional ways to encourage development of motor milestones and ways to facilitate protective, righting, and equilibrium reactions within developmental postures.

INTERVENTION 8.9 **Approximation**

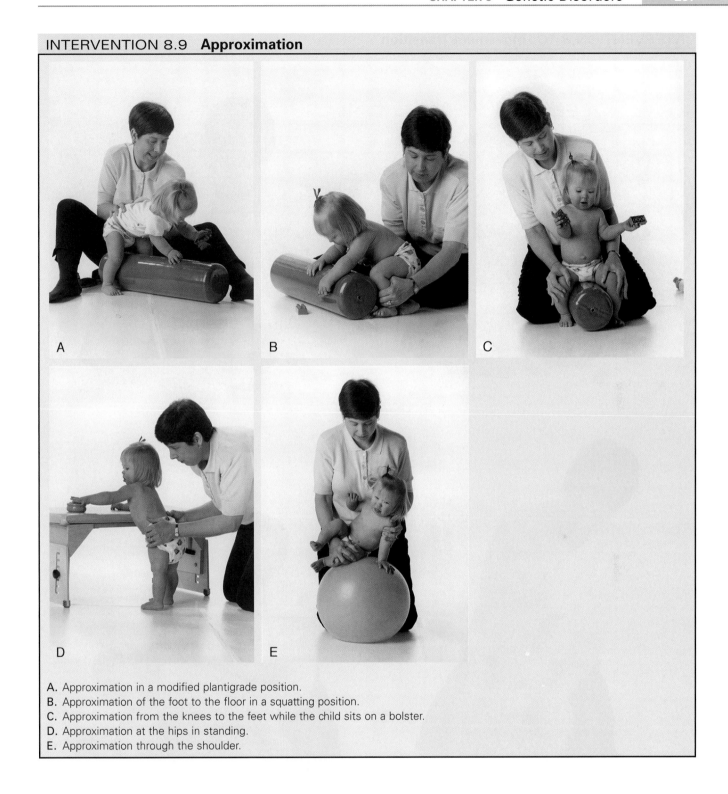

A. Approximation in a modified plantigrade position.
B. Approximation of the foot to the floor in a squatting position.
C. Approximation from the knees to the feet while the child sits on a bolster.
D. Approximation at the hips in standing.
E. Approximation through the shoulder.

When trunk extension is not balanced by abdominal strength, trunk stability may have to be derived from hip adduction and hip extension by using the hamstrings (Moerchen, 1994). If a child has such low tone that the legs are widely abducted in the supine position, the hip flexors will quickly tighten. This tightness impairs the ability of the abdominal oblique muscles to elongate the rib cage. The result is inadequate trunk control, a high-riding rib cage, and trunk rotation.

Inadequate trunk control in children with low tone not only impairs respiratory function but also impedes the development of dynamic postural control of the trunk, usually manifested in righting and equilibrium reactions.

Contractures and Deformities

Avoiding contractures and deformities may seem to be a relatively easy task because these children exhibit increased

INTERVENTION 8.10 Movement Transition

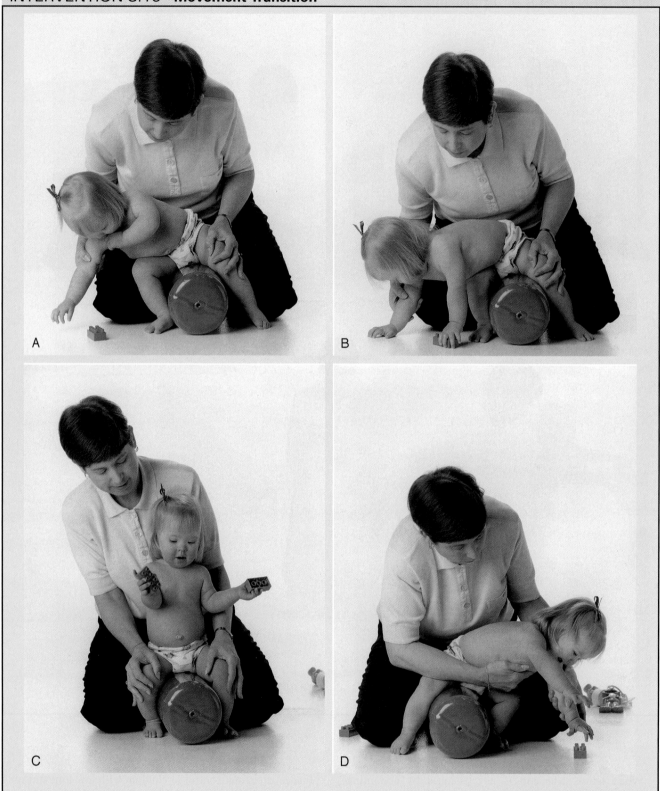

A–D. The child practices active trunk rotation within a play task. Guided movement from sitting to upper extremity weight-bearing and reaching with a return to sitting.

INTERVENTION 8.11 Coming to Stand

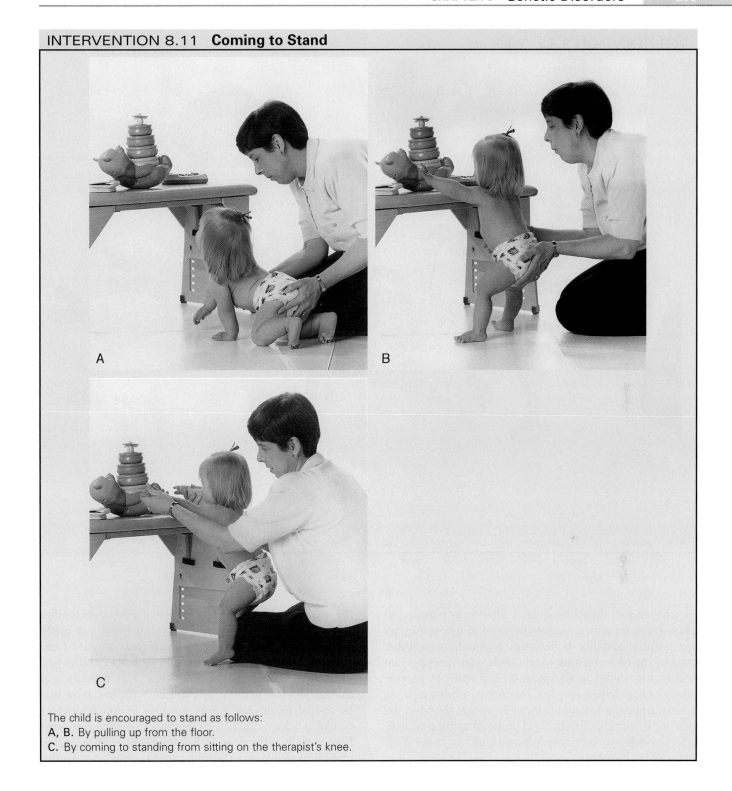

The child is encouraged to stand as follows:
A, B. By pulling up from the floor.
C. By coming to standing from sitting on the therapist's knee.

mobility. However, muscles can shorten in overly lengthened positions. Because of low tone and excessive joint motion, the child's limbs are at the mercy of gravity. When the child is supine, gravity fosters external rotation of the limbs and the tendency for the head to fall to one side, making it difficult for the child with low tone to maintain the head in midline. Simple positioning devices such as a

U-shaped towel roll can be used to promote a midline head position.

Intervention should be aimed at normal alignment and maintenance of appropriate range of motion for typical flexibility and comfort. Positions that provide stability by utilizing excessive range, such as wide abducted sitting, propping on hyperextended arms in sitting, or standing with knee

INTERVENTION 8.12   **Walking**

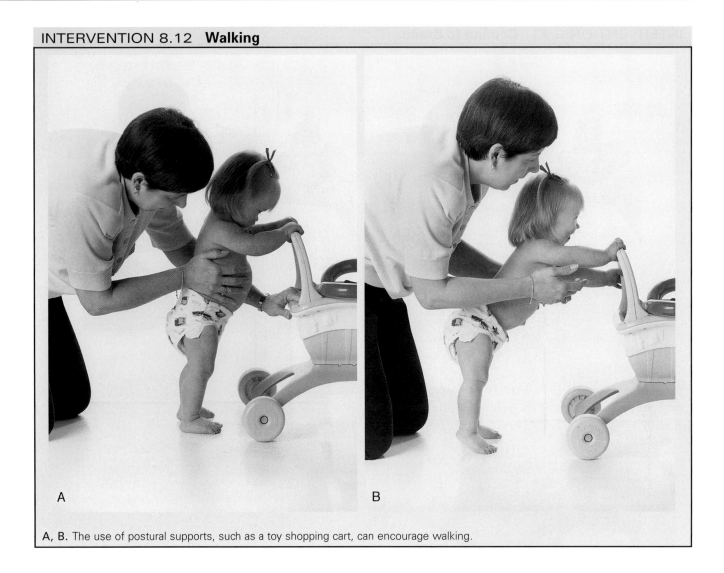

A   B

A, B. The use of postural supports, such as a toy shopping cart, can encourage walking.

hyperextension, should be avoided. Modify the positions to allow for more typical weight-bearing and use of muscles for postural stability rather than maintaining position. Narrow the base of sitting when the child sits with legs too widely abducted. Use air splints or soft splits to prevent elbow or knee hyperextension. Another possibility is to use a vertical stander to support the child so that the knees are in a more neutral position. Good positioning can positively affect muscle use for maintaining posture, for easier feeding, and for breathing.

Respiratory Function

Chest wall tightness may develop in a child who is not able to sit supported at the appropriate time developmentally (6 months). Gravity normally assists in changing the configuration of the chest wall in infants from a triangle to more of a rectangle. If this change does not occur, the diaphragm will remain flat and will not work as efficiently. The child may develop rib flaring as a consequence of the underuse of all the abdominal muscles or

the overuse of the centrally located rectus abdominis muscle. If the structural modifications are not made, the diaphragm cannot become an efficient muscle of respiration. The child may continue to belly breathe and may never learn to expand the chest wall fully. Fatigue during physical activity in children with low tone may be related to the inefficient function of the respiratory system (Dichter et al., 1993). Because these children work harder to breathe than other children, they have less oxygen available for the muscular work of performing functional tasks.

Any child with low muscle tone may have difficulty in generating sufficient expiratory force to clear secretions. Children who are immobile because of the severity of their neuromuscular deficits, such as those with SMA or late-stage muscular dystrophy, can benefit greatly from CPT including postural drainage with percussion and vibration. The positions for postural drainage are found in Fig. 8.11. Additional expiratory techniques are described in the section of this chapter dealing with CF.

INTERVENTION 8.13 Carrying Positions

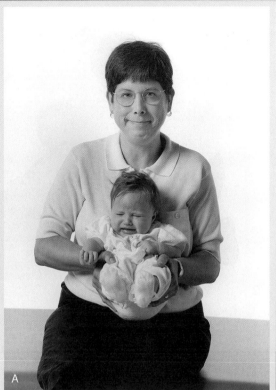
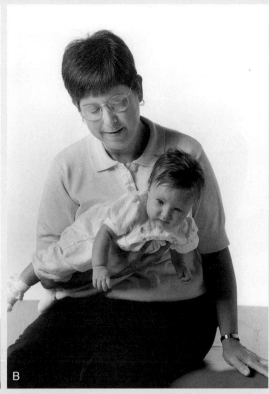

A. Carrying the child with her back to the adult's chest promotes stability.

B. Carrying the child over the arm promotes head lifting and improves tolerance for the prone position.

INTERVENTION 8.14 Trunk Extension and Protective Extension

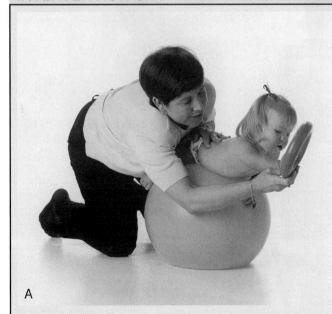
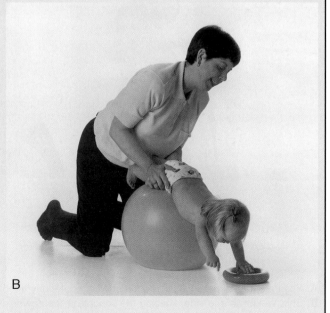

A. Trunk extension can be facilitated with the child in the prone position over a ball by asking the child to reach for an object. The difficulty of the task can be increased by having more of the child's trunk unsupported.

B. Protective extension of the upper extremities can also be encouraged from the same position over a ball if the child is moved quickly forward.

INTERVENTION 8.15   Standing With Support From the Ball

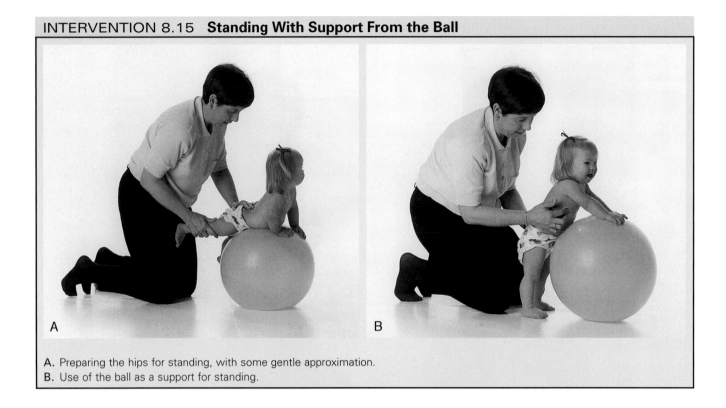

A. Preparing the hips for standing, with some gentle approximation.
B. Use of the ball as a support for standing.

INTERVENTION 8.16   Eliciting Balance Reactions

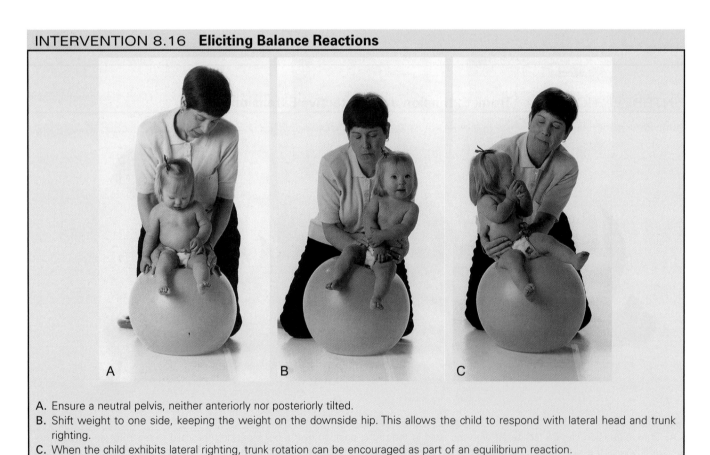

A. Ensure a neutral pelvis, neither anteriorly nor posteriorly tilted.
B. Shift weight to one side, keeping the weight on the downside hip. This allows the child to respond with lateral head and trunk righting.
C. When the child exhibits lateral righting, trunk rotation can be encouraged as part of an equilibrium reaction.

CHAPTER SUMMARY

Working with children with genetic disorders can be challenging and rewarding because of the many variations exhibited within the different disorders. The commonality of clinical features exhibited by children with these disorders, such as low muscle tone, delayed development, and some degree of ID, except for the children with SMA, allows for discussion of some almost universally applicable interventions. Because motor development in children with genetic disorders is generally characterized by immature patterns of movement rather than by abnormal patterns, as seen in children with cerebral palsy, physical therapy management is geared to fostering the typical sequence of sensorimotor development including postural reactions while safeguarding joint alignment. Because of the progressive nature of some of the genetic disorders, physical therapy management must also be focused on preserving motor function or on optimizing function in any body system that is compromised. The physical therapist assistant can play a valuable role in implementing physical therapy interventions for children with any of the genetic disorders discussed in this chapter.

REVIEW QUESTIONS

1. What is the leading cause of inherited ID?
2. When one parent is a carrier for CF, what chance does each child have of being affected?
3. What genetic disorder produces muscle weakness without cognitive impairment?
4. What are the three mechanisms by which chromosome abnormalities occur?
5. What are the two most common clinical features in children with most genetic disorders involving the central nervous system?
6. What principles of motor learning are important to use when working with children with cognitive impairment?
7. What types of interventions are appropriate for a child with low tone?
8. What interventions can be used to prevent secondary complications in children with low tone?
9. What interventions are most often used with a child with OI?
10. What are the age-related physical activity recommendations for people with cystic fibrosis?
11. When is power mobility indicated for a child with a disability?

CASE STUDIES REHABILITATION UNIT INITIAL EXAMINATION AND EVALUATION: AG

History

Chart Review

AG is a 17-month-old girl with DS. AG and her parents have been participants in an infant program since she was 3 months old. AG was born at term with a pneumothorax. During her stay in the neonatal intensive care unit, the DS diagnosis was confirmed by genetic testing. She has had no rehospitalizations. Her health continues to be good. Immunizations are up to date.

Subjective

The child's mother reports that AG laughs and sings. She smiles easily and is a good eater. She previously had difficulty with choking on food. Her mother's biggest concern is knowing when to expect AG to walk.

Objective

Systems Review

Communication/Cognition: AG has 10 words in her vocabulary. She understands "no." AG's mental development index on the Bayley scale is <50, based on a raw score of 75, which is mildly delayed performance.

Cardiovascular/Pulmonary: Values normal for age.

Integumentary: Skin intact, no scars or areas of redness.

Musculoskeletal: AROM greater than normal, strength decreased throughout.

Neuromuscular: Coordination and balance impaired.

Test and Measures

Anthropometric: Height 32", weight 30 lb, BMI 21 (20 to 24 is normal).

Motor Function: AG rolls from supine to prone and pushes herself into sitting over her abducted legs. She pulls to stand by furniture but is unable to come to stand from sitting without pulling with her arms. AG sits independently with a wide base of support. She is unable to stand from a squat.

Neurodevelopmental Status: PDMS DMQ is below average (DMQ = 65), age equivalent is 9 months. Fine Motor DMQ = 69, with an age equivalent of 9 months.

Range of Motion: PROM is WFL in all joints, with joint hypermobility present in the hips, knees, and ankles of the lower extremities and in the shoulders and elbows of the upper extremities. No asymmetry is noted.

Reflex Integrity: Biceps, patellar, and Achilles 1+ bilaterally. Low muscle tone is present throughout her extremities and trunk. No asymmetry is noted.

Cranial Nerve Integrity: AG turns her head toward sound. Visually, she tracks in all directions, although she tends to move

Continued

CASE STUDIES REHABILITATION UNIT INITIAL EXAMINATION AND EVALUATION: AG—cont'd

her head with her eyes. Quick changes in position such as when she is being picked up or in an inverted position are tolerated without crying. She has no difficulty swallowing liquids or solids by parent report.

Sensory Integrity: Sensation appears to be intact to light touch.

Posture: When she is ring sitting on the floor, her trunk is kyphotic. Her posture is slightly lordotic in quadruped position.

Gait, Locomotion, and Balance: AG creeps on her hands and knees for up to 30 feet. She pivots in sitting. AG occasionally exhibits trunk rotation when making the transition from hands-and-knees to side sitting. AG exhibits head-righting reactions in all directions. Trunk-righting reactions are present, but equilibrium reactions are delayed and are incomplete in sitting position and quadruped position. Upper extremity protective reactions are present in all directions in sitting but are delayed. Balance in standing requires support of a person or object. She leans forward, flexing her hips and keeping her knees hyperextended.

Self-care: AG finger-feeds. She assists with dressing by removing some clothes.

Play: AG plays with toys appropriate for a 9 to 12 month old. She looks at pictures in a book and squeezes a doll to make it squeak.

Assessment/Evaluation

AG is a 17-month-old girl with DS who is functioning below her age level in gross and fine motor development and cognitive development. She is creeping reciprocally and pulling to stand but not walking independently. She is classified at a GMFCS level 1. She has a supportive family and is involved in an infant intervention program. Frequency of treatment is one time a week for an hour.

Problem List
1. Delayed gross and fine motor development, secondary to hypotonia
2. Hypermobile joints
3. Dependent in ambulation
4. Delayed postural reactions

Diagnosis

AG demonstrates impaired neuromotor development and problems with force production and postural control. Down syndrome is a genetic syndrome that is characterized by delays in all aspects of development including cognition.

Prognosis

AG will improve her level of functional independence and functional skills in her home. Her potential is good for the following goals.

Short-Term Goals (1 Month)
1. AG will walk while pushing an object 20 feet 80% of the time.

2. AG will demonstrate trunk rotation when moving in and out of side sitting 80% of the time.
3. AG will rise to standing from sitting on a stool without pulling with her arms 80% of the time.

Long-Term Goals (6 Months)
1. AG will ambulate independently without an assistive device for unlimited distances.
2. AG will independently ascend stairs using alternating feet while holding on to a rail.
3. AG will assist in dressing and undressing as requested.
4. AG will exhibit beginning pretend play by substituting one object for another while playing with a doll.

Plan

Coordination, Communication, and Documentation
The physical therapist and physical therapist assistant will be in frequent and constant communication with the family and the early childhood educator regarding AG's program. Outcomes of interventions will be documented on a weekly basis.

Patient/Client Instruction
Discuss family instruction regarding positions to avoid and a home exercise program. The program is to include movement/games that encourage exploration and play in postural positions that challenge AG's balance.

Interventions
1. Using a small treadmill, the parents will support AG as she is encouraged to take steps 15 minutes twice a day.
2. Using appropriate verbal and manual cues, AG will assist with removing her clothes before therapy and putting them back on after therapy.
3. Work on movement transitions from four-point to kneeling, kneeling to half-kneeling, half-kneeling to standing, standing from sitting on a stool, standing to a squat, and returning to standing.
4. Use weight-bearing through the upper and lower extremities in developmentally appropriate postures such as four-point, kneeling, and standing to increase support responses. Maintain joint alignment to prevent mechanical locking of joints and encourage muscular holding of positions.
5. Use alternating isometrics and rhythmic stability in sitting, quadruped, and standing positions to increase stability.
6. AG will be encouraged to push a weighted toy shopping cart during play.
7. AG will be engaged in play with a doll and functional objects, such as a cup and spoon.

Questions to Think About
- What activities could be part of AG's home exercise program?
- How can fitness be incorporated into AG's physical therapy program?

AROM, Active range of motion; *BMI,* body mass index; *DMQ,* Gross Motor Developmental Motor Quotient; *GMFCS,* Gross Motor Functional Classification System; *PDMS,* Peabody Developmental Motor Scales; *PROM,* passive range of motion; *WFL,* within functional limitations.

CASE STUDIES REHABILITATION UNIT INITIAL EXAMINATION AND EVALUATION: DJ

History
Chart Review
DJ is an 8-year-old boy diagnosed with DMD at the age of 3. He attends a regular school and is in the second grade. He has had one recent hospitalization for pneumonia which lasted 3 days. He continues on an antibiotic for the recent lung infection and has just begun taking prednisone.*

Subjective
DJ's mother reports that he lives with his parents and one younger sister. He ambulates independently and wants to play basketball with his classmates during recess. He is being seen in school for physical therapy one time a week. His mother and father are active participants in his home exercise program, which consists of active and PROM and aerobic exercise. DJ's orthopedist is considering surgery to release his tight heel cords.

Objective
Systems Review
Communication/Cognition: DJ is talkative and friendly. His IQ is 80.

Cardiovascular/Pulmonary: RR is 20 beats/min with adventitious breath sounds. HR and BP are normal for age.

Integumentary: Intact.

Musculoskeletal: AROM and PROM impaired. Strength impaired proximally.

Neuromuscular: Coordination diminished.

Tests and Measures
Appearance and Anthropometric: Height 50", weight 49 lb, BMI 14 (20 to 24 is normal). Pseudohypertrophy noted in calf muscles bilaterally.

Cardiovascular/Pulmonary: Rales and crackles evident at bases bilaterally. Diaphragm strength is fair with a functional cough. Vital capacity is 75% of predicted for age.

Motor Function: DJ ambulates independently but fatigues easily. Starting with arms at the sides, he can abduct his arms in a full circle until they touch above his head. He can lift a 10-lb weight to a shelf above eye level. He stands up from lying supine in 60 seconds demonstrating a Gower sign. He climbs stairs with the aid of a railing foot over foot.

Muscle Performance: Muscle testing is performed in sitting unless otherwise specified as per standard manual muscle testing procedures (Berryman, 2005).

	R	L
Shoulders		
• Flexors	4	4
• Abductors	4	4
Elbow		
• Flexors	5	5
• Extensors	4+	4+
Wrist		
• Flexors	5	5
• Extensors	5	5
Hip		
• Flexors	4	4
• Extensors	3–	3– (tested in prone)
• Abductors	4–	4– (tested in side-lying)

	R	L
Knee		
• Extensors	4–	4–
• Flexors	4	4 (tested in prone)
Ankle		
• Plantar flexors	4+	4+ (tested in standing)
• Dorsiflexors	3–	3–

Range of Motion: Active and PROM is WFL except for 15-degree hip flexion contracture bilaterally. He exhibits iliotibial band tightness and 5-degree plantar flexion contractures with 15 degrees of active dorsiflexion bilaterally.

Reflex Integrity: Patellar 2+, Achilles 1+, Babinski is absent bilaterally.

Sensory Integrity: Intact.

Posture: In standing, DJ exhibits a forward head and lordosis; weight is shifted forward onto the toes and his heels are off the ground.

Gait, Locomotion, and Balance: He walks with no arm swing, does not run easily or well. He walks a total of 60 feet in 3 minutes with one rest of 1-minute duration. He can walk 30 feet as fast as he can without falling in 2 minutes. On average, he walks 2.5 hours a day. He takes a protective step in any direction when standing balance is disturbed.

Self-care: DJ dresses, feeds, and toilets himself independently.

Play: He plays with videogames, likes action figures, and is involved in cub scouts. He reads at grade level. He enjoys swimming, going to the zoo, and riding his bicycle around the neighborhood. He participates in physical education at school.

Assessment/Evaluation
DJ is an 8-year-old boy with DMD who attends school regularly and receives physical therapy in the school setting as needed to prevent pulmonary complications and maintain present level of function. He recently had an upper respiratory infection that required hospitalization. He is ambulatory but has lower extremity contractures that are beginning to interfere with upright function. His physician is considering surgical intervention to release his heel cords. He is being seen once a week for 30 minutes and is participating in a home exercise program.

Problem List
1. Lower extremity contractures
2. Decreased strength and endurance
3. Decreased pulmonary function
4. At risk for decreased locomotion

Diagnosis
DJ exhibits impaired force production secondary to the genetic myopathy—Duchenne's muscular dystrophy. He is at risk for loss of movement and cardiovascular/pulmonary impairment that will significantly limit his activities and participation.

Prognosis
DJ will improve or maintain his present level of function and prevent a recurrence of respiratory infection, which might lead

Continued

CASE STUDIES REHABILITATION UNIT INITIAL EXAMINATION AND EVALUATION: DJ—cont'd

to permanent respiratory compromise. His potential is fair for the following goals.

Short-Term Goals (Actions to be Accomplished by Midyear Review)

1. DJ will increase active and passive dorsiflexion to 20 degrees bilaterally so that he can stand to write math problems on the board.
2. DJ will play on the playground equipment safely.
3. DJ will be independent in breathing exercises.
4. DJ's family will demonstrate correct postural drainage and assisted coughing techniques.
5. DJ will ambulate 50 feet times 3 with custom molded AFOs during the school day with only one rest.

Long-Term Goals (End of 2nd Grade)

1. DJ will maintain lower extremity muscle strength.
2. DJ will swim across the pool, breathing every other stroke.
3. DJ will exhibit no decline in vital capacity.
4. DJ will ambulate 50 feet times 4 with AFOs during the school day.
5. DJ will increase total standing time by 30 minutes a day.

Plan

Coordination, Communication, and Documentation

The physical therapist and physical therapist assistant will be in frequent and constant communication with DJ's family and his teacher. The therapist will communicate with the physician and orthotist prior to and after surgery to lengthen his heel cords. If another therapist/assistant is involved during the acute care phase, the school therapist would need to establish and maintain communication. Outcomes of interventions will be documented on a weekly basis.

Patient/Client Instruction

Teach how to don and doff AFOs independently following surgery, implement wearing schedule, and check for skin integrity. Teach safety on the playground. Teach and review techniques of chest wall stretching, diaphragmatic breathing, inspiratory and expiratory muscle training, postural drainage, and assistive cough. Have DJ stand a total of 3 hours a day, part of which should occur at home.

Interventions

1. Positioning
   a. Standing on a small wedge for increasing amounts of time to stretch heel cords.
   b. Use a prone stander for one or two class periods to provide stretch to hip and knee flexors and dorsiflexors.
   c. Wear lower extremity night splints before and after surgery.
   d. Monitor for development of scoliosis.
2. Strengthening
   a. Do concentric movements of quadriceps, hamstrings, and dorsiflexors against gravity; add manual resistance or Theraband if suitable.
   b. Use marching, kicking, and heel walking.
   c. Pull on Theraband with upper extremities.
   d. Monitor for change in strength.
3. Aerobic and functional activities
   a. Move through an obstacle course while being timed. Include activities such as walking up an incline ramp to increase dorsiflexion range but avoid going down; vary the speed of movement using music.
   b. Schedule therapy sessions on the playground.
   c. Ride bicycle every day.
   d. Swim twice a week.
   e. Monitor for changes in respiratory or musculoskeletal status.

Questions to Think About

- What activities could DJ engage in that will increase his standing time?
- What sports activities can DJ engage in?
- What signs or symptoms would indicate respiratory or musculoskeletal deterioration?
- DJ's frequency of care is anticipated to change as the disease progresses. When might some episodes of care be considered physical therapy maintenance and others considered prevention?

*Prednisone has been shown to increase strength and delay loss of ambulation. (From Biggar WD et al., Long-term deficits of deflazacort for treatment for boys with Duchenne muscular dystrophy in their second decade, *Neuromuscul Disord* 16:249–255, 2006.)
AFO, Ankle-foot orthosis; *AROM,* active range of motion; *BMI,* body mass index; *BP,* blood pressure; *HR,* heart rate; *IQ,* intelligence quotient; *PROM,* passive range of motion; *RR,* respiratory rate; *WFL,* within functional limitations.

REFERENCES

Agnew JL, Owen B: Cystic fibrosis. In Palisano RJ, Orlin MN, Schrieber J, editors: *Campbell's physical therapy for children*, ed 5, St. Louis, 2017, Elsevier, pp 614-637.

Albright JA: Management overview of osteogenesis imperfecta, *Clin Orthop Relat Res* 159:80-87, 1981.

Alfano LN, Miller NF, Iammarino M, Lowes LP: *Spinal muscular atrophy: a new year of evaluation and treatment*, Combined Sections Meeting, APTA, Washington, DC, January 2019.

American Academy of Pediatrics Committee on Sports Medicine and Fitness: Atlantoaxial instability in Down syndrome: subject review, *Pediatrics* 96:151-154, 1995.

Ansved T: Muscular dystrophies: influence of physical conditioning on the disease evolution, *Curr Opin Clin Nutr Metab Care* 6(4):435-439, 2003.

Archer JE, Gardner AC, Roper HP, Chilermane AA, Tatman AJ: Duchenne muscular dystrophy: the management of scoliosis, *J Spine Surg* 2:185-194, 2016.

Bach JR, Campagnolo DI, Hoeman S: Life satisfaction of individuals with Duchenne muscular dystrophy using long term mechanical ventilatory support, *Am J Phys Med Rehabil* 70:129-135, 1991.

Bach JR, Martinez D: Duchenne muscular dystrophy: continuous noninvasive ventilator support prolongs survival, *Respir Care* 56(6):744-750, 2011.

Bach JR, McKeon J: Orthopedic surgery and rehabilitation for the prolongation of brace-free ambulation of patients with Duchenne muscular dystrophy, *Am J Phys Med Rehabil* 70:323-331, 1991.

Bachman WH: Variables affecting post school economic adaptation of orthopedically handicapped and other health-impaired students, *Rehabil Lit* 3:98, 1972.

Bailey RW, Dubow HI: Experimental and clinical studies of longitudinal bone growth: utilizing a new method of internal fixation crossing the epiphyseal plate, *J Bone Joint Surg Am* 47:1669, 1965.

Ballestrazzi A, Gnudi A, Magni E, et al: Osteopenia in spinal muscular atrophy. In Merlini L, Granata C, Dubowitz V, editors: *Current concepts in childhood spinal muscular atrophy*, New York, 1989, Springer-Verlag, pp 215-219.

Bamshad M, Watkins WS, Zenger RK, et al: A gene for distal arthrogryposis type I maps to the pericentromeric region of chromosome 9, *Am J Hum Genet* 55:1153-1158, 1994.

Bartonek A: The use of orthoses and gait analysis in children with AMC, *J Child Orthop* 9:437-447, 2015.

Batshaw ML, Roizen NJ, Lotrecchiano GR: *Children with disabilities*, ed 7, Baltimore, MD, 2013, Paul H. Brookes.

Baty BJ, Carey JC, McMahon WM: Neurodevelopmental disorders and medical genetics: an overview. In Goldstein S, Reynolds CR, editors: *Handbook of neurodevelopmental and genetic disorders in children*, ed 2, New York, 2011, Guilford Press, pp 33-57.

Bellamy SG, Shen E: Genetic disorders: a pediatric perspective. In Umphred DA, Lazaro RT, Roller ML, Burton GU, editors: *Umphred's neurological rehabilitation*, ed 6, St. Louis, 2013, Elsevier, pp 345-378.

Benden C, Edwards LB, Kucheryavaya AY, et al: The registry of the International Society for Heart and Lung Transplantation: sixteenth official pediatric lung and heart-lung transplantation report-focus theme: age, *J Heart Lung Transplant* 32(10): 989-997, 2013.

Beroud C, Karliova M, Bonnefont JP, et al: Prenatal diagnosis of spinal muscular atrophy by genetic analysis of circulating fetal cells, *Lancet* 361(9362):1013-1014, 2003.

Berryman RN: *Muscle and sensory testing*, ed 2, Philadelphia, 2005, WB Saunders.

Biggar WD, Harris VA, Eliasoph L, Alman B: Long-term benefits of deflazacort for treatment for boys with Duchenne muscular dystrophy in their second decade, *Neuromuscul Disord* 16:249-255, 2006.

Biggin A, Munns CF: Long-term bisphosphonate therapy in osteogenesis imperfecta, *Curr Osteoporos Rep* 15(5):412-418, 2017.

Birnkrant DJ, Bushby K, Bann CM, et al: Diagnosis and management of Duchenne muscular dystrophy, part 1: diagnosis, and neuromuscular, rehabilitation, endocrine, and gastrointestinal and nutritional management, *Lancet Neurol* 17:251-267, 2018a.

Birnkrant DJ, Bushby K, Bann CM, et al: Diagnosis and management of Duchenne muscular dystrophy, part 2: respiratory, cardiac, bone health, and orthopaedic management, *Lancet Neurol* 17:347-361, 2018b.

Birnkrant DJ, Bushby K, Bann CM, et al: Diagnosis and management of Duchenne muscular dystrophy, part 3: primary care, emergency management, psychosocial care, and transitions of care across the lifespan, *Lancet Neurol* 17:445-455, 2018c.

Bittles AH, Bower C, Hussain R: The four ages of Down syndrome, *Eur J Public Health* 17:221-225, 2006.

Bleck EE: Nonoperative treatment of osteogenesis imperfecta: orthotic and mobility management, *Clin Orthop* 159:111-122, 1981.

Brenneman SK, Stanger M, Bertoti DB: Age-related considerations: pediatric. In Myers RS, editor: *Saunders manual of physical therapy*, Philadelphia, 1995, WB Saunders, pp 1229-1283.

Bull M: Clinical report-health supervision for children with Down syndrome, *Pediatrics* 128:393-406, 2011.

Caudill A, Flanagan A, Hassani S, et al: Ankle strength and functional limitations in children and adolescents with type I osteogenesis imperfecta, *Pediatr Phys Ther* 22:288-295, 2010.

Centers for Disease Control and Prevention: *National estimates for 21 selected major birth defects, 2004-2006* (website). Available at: www.cdc.gov/ncbddd/birthdefects/data.html. Accessed September 17, 2018.

Chabanon A, Sefereian AM, Daron A, et al: Prospective and longitudinal natural history study of patients with type 2 and 3: baseline and NatHis-SMA study, *PLoS One* 13(7):e0201004, 2018.

Chandler KE, Kidd A, Al-Gazali L, et al: Diagnostic criteria, clinical characteristics, and natural history of Cohen syndrome, *J Med Genet* 40:233-241, 2003.

Chen H: *Cri-du-chat syndrome, WebMD* (website). Updated June 26, 2013. Available at: http://emedicine.medscape.com/article/942897-overview. Accessed September 27, 2014.

Cicerello NA, Doty AK, Palisano RJ: Transition to adulthood for youth with disabilities. In Campbell SK, Palisano RJ, Orlin MN, editors: *Physical therapy for children*, ed 4, Philadelphia, 2012, pp 1030-1058.

Cintas HL: Aquatics. In Cintas HL, Gerber LH, editors: *Children with osteogenesis imperfecta: strategies to enhance performance*, Gaithersburg, MD, 2005, Osteogenesis Imperfecta Foundation.

Clayton-Smith J, Watson P, Ramsden S, Black GCM: Somatic mutation in MECP2 as a non-fatal neurodevelopmental disorder in males, *Lancet* 356(9232):830-832, 2000.

Collaco JM, Blackman SM, Raraigh KS, et al: Self-reported exercise and longitudinal outcomes in cystic fibrosis: a retrospective cohort study, *BMC Pulm Med* 14:159, 2014.

Connolly BH, Morgan SB, Russell FF, et al: A longitudinal study of children with Down syndrome who experienced early intervention programming, *Phys Ther* 73:170-181, 1993.

Coster W, Deeney T, Haltiwanger J, Haley S: *School function assessment*, San Antonio, 1998, Therapy Skill Builders.

Corvol H, Blackman SM, Boelle PY, et al: Genome-wide association meta-analysis identifies five modifier loci of lung disease severity in cystic fibrosis, *Nat Commun* 6:8382-8382, 2015.

Daley K, Wisbeach A, Sanpera I Jr, et al: The prognosis for walking in osteogenesis imperfecta, *J Bone Joint Surg Br* 78:477-480, 1996.

Davids JR, Hagerman RJ, Eilkert RE: Orthopaedic aspects of fragile X syndrome, *J Bone Joint Surg Am* 72:889-896, 1990.

Dichter CG, Darbee JC, Effgen SK, et al: Assessment of pulmonary function and physical fitness in children with Down syndrome, *Pediatr Phys Ther* 5:3-8, 1993.

DiMeglio LA, Peacock M: Two-year clinical trial of oral alendronate versus intravenous pamidronate in children with osteogenesis imperfecta, *J Bone Miner Res* 21(1):132-140, 2006.

Donohoe M: Arthrogryposis multiplex congenita. In Palisano RJ, Orlin MN, Schrieber J, editors: *Campbell's physical therapy for children*, ed 5, St. Louis, 2017a, Elsevier, pp 207-223.

Donohoe M: Osteogenesis imperfecta. In Palisano RJ, Orlin MN, Schrieber J, editors: *Campbell's physical therapy for children*, ed 5, St. Louis, 2017b, Elsevier, pp 224-241.

Duffield MH: Physiological and therapeutic effects of exercise in warm water. In Skinner AT, Thomson AM, editors: *Duffield's exercise in water*, ed 3, London, 1983, Bailliere Tindall.

Dwan K, Phillipi CA, Steiner RD, Basel D: Bisphosphonate therapy for osteogenesis imperfecta, *Cochrane Database Syst Rev* 10:CD005088, 2016.

Dykens EM, Cassidy SB, DeVries ML: Prader-Willi syndrome. In Goldstein S, Reynolds CR, editors: *Handbook of neurodevelopmental and genetic disorders in children*, ed 2, New York, 2011, Guilford Press, pp 484-511.

Emery AEH, Skinner R: Clinical studies in benign (Becker-type) X-linked muscular dystrophy, *Clinic Genet* 10:189-201, 1976.

Engelbert R, Uiterwaal C, et al: Osteogenesis imperfecta in childhood: prognosis for walking, *J Pediatr* 137:397-402, 2000.

Engelbert RH, Helders PJ, Keessen W, et al: Intramedullary rodding in type III osteogenesis imperfecta: effects on neuromotor development in 10 children, *Acta Orthop Scand* 66:361-364, 1995.

Finkel RS, Chiriboga CA, Vajsar J, et al: Treatment of infantile-onset spinal muscular atrophy with Nusinersen: a phase 2, open-label, dose-escalation study, *Lancet* 388:3017-3026, 2016.

Finkel RS, McDermott MP, Kaufmann P, et al: Observational study of spinal muscular atrophy type I and implications for clinical trials, *Neurology* 83:810-817, 2014.

Finkel RS, Mercuri BT, Carras AM, et al: Nusinersen versus sham control in infantile-onset spinal muscular atrophy, *N Engl J Med* 2:377(18):1724-1734, 2017.

Florence JM: Neuromuscular disorders in childhood and physical therapy intervention. In Tecklin SJ, editor: *Pediatric physical therapy*, ed 3, Philadelphia, 1999, JB Lippincott, pp 223-246.

Gaskin L, Shin J, Reisman J, et al: Long term trial of conventional postural drainage and percussion vs. positive expiratory pressure, *Pediatr Pulmonol* 15(Suppl):345a, 1998.

Gidaro T, Servais L: Nusinersen treatment of spinal muscular atrophy: current knowledge and existing gaps, *Dev Med Child Neurol* 61:19-24, 2018.

Gitelis S, Whiffen J, DeWald RL: Treatment of severe scoliosis in osteogenesis imperfecta, *Clin Orthop* 175:56-59, 1983.

Glanzman AM: Genetic and developmental disorders. In Goodman CC, Fuller KS, editors: *Pathology: implications for the physical therapist*, ed 4, Philadelphia, 2015, Saunders, pp 1161-1210.

Glanzman AM, Kusler A, Stuberg WA: Muscular dystrophies and spinal muscle atrophy. In Palisano RJ, Orlin MN, Schrieber J, editors: *Campbell's physical therapy for children*, ed 5, St. Louis, 2017, Elsevier, pp 242-271.

Gloss D, Moxley RT, Ashwal S, Oskoui M: Practice guideline update summary: corticosteroid treatment of Duchenne muscular dystrophy: report of the Guideline Development Subcommittee of the American Academy of Neurology, *Neurology* 86:465-472, 2016.

Glorieux FH: Experience with bisphosphonates in osteogenesis imperfecta, *Pediatrics* 119:S163-S165, 2007.

Glorieux FH, Rauch F, Plotkin H, et al: Type V osteogenesis imperfecta: a new form of brittle bone disease, *J Bone Miner Res* 15:1650-1658, 2000.

Goldstein S, Reynolds CR: *Handbook of neurodevelopmental and genetic disorders in children*, ed 2, New York, 2011, Guilford Press.

Granata C, Magni E, Sabattini L, et al: Promotion of ambulation in intermediate spinal muscle atrophy. In Merlini L, Granata C, Dubowitz V, editors: *Current concepts in childhood spinal muscular atrophy*, New York, 1989, Springer-Verlag, pp 127-132.

Grange RW, Call JA: Recommendations to define exercise prescription for Duchenne muscular dystrophy, *Exerc Sport Sci Rev* 35:12-17, 2007.

Grece CA: Effectiveness of high frequency chest compression: a 3-year retrospective study, *Pediatr Pulmonol* 20(Suppl):302, 2000.

Guess D, Mulligan-Ault M, Roberts S, et al: Implications of biobehavioral states for the education and treatment of students with the most profoundly handicapping conditions, *J Assoc Pers Sev Handicaps* 13:163-174, 1988.

Gurkan CK, Hagerman RJ: Targeted treatments in autism and fragile X syndrome, *Res Autism Spectr Disord* 6(4):1311-1320, 2012.

Hagerman RJ, Rivera SM, Hagerman PF: The fragile X family of disorders: a model for autism and targeted treatments, *Curr Pediatr Rev* 4(1):40-52, 2008.

Haley SM, Coster WF, Ludlow LH, et al: *The pediatric evaluation of disability inventory: development standardization and administration manual*, Boston, 1992, New England Medical Center Publications.

Hall JG: Arthrogryposis (multiple congenital contractures): diagnostic approach to etiology, classification, genetics, and general principles, *Eur J Med Genet* 57:464-472, 2014.

Hall ML, Lobo MA: Design and development of the first exoskeletal garment to enhance arm mobility for children with movement impairments, *Assist Technol* 30:251-258, 2018. doi:10.1080/10400435.2017.1320690.

Hallum A, Allen DD: Neuromuscular diseases. In Umphred DA, Lazaro RT, Roller ML, Burton GU, editors: *Umphred's neurological rehabilitation*, ed 6, St. Louis, 2013, Elsevier, pp 521-570.

Hammers DW, Sleeper MJ, Forbes SC, et al: Tadalafil treatment delays the onset of cardiomyopathy in dystrophin-deficient hearts, *J Am Heart Assoc* 5(8):pii:e003911, 2016.

Harris SW, Goodlin-Jones B, Nowicki ST, et al: Autism profiles of young males with fragile X syndrome, *Am J Ment Retard* 113:427-438, 2008.

Head E, Lott IT: Down syndrome and beta-amyloid deposition, *Curr Opin Neurol* 17:95-100, 2004.

Hebestreit H, Arets H, Aurora P, et al: Statement on exercise testing in cystic fibrosis, *Respiration* 90(4):332-351, 2015.

Hebestreit H, Kieser S, Rudiger S, et al: Physical activity is independently related to aerobic capacity in cystic fibrosis, *Eur Respir J* 28:734-739, 2006.

Hebestreit H, Schnid K, Kieser S, et al: Quality of life is associated with physical activity and fitness in cystic fibrosis, *BMC Pulm Med* 14:26, 2014.

Heller T, Hsieh K, Rimmer J: Barriers and supports for exercise participation among adults with Down syndrome, *J Gerontol Soc Work* 38:161-178, 2002.

Hines S, Bennett F: Effectiveness of early intervention for children with Down syndrome, *Ment Retard Dev Disabil Res Rev* 2:96-101, 1996.

Hogler W, Scott J, Bishop N, et al: The effect of whole body vibration training on bone and muscle function in children with osteogenesis imperfecta, *J Clin Endocrinol Metab* 102(8):2734-2743, 2017.

Hommerding PX, Baptista RR, Makarewic GT, et al: Effects of an educational intervention of physical activity for children and adolescents with cystic fibrosis: a randomized controlled trial, *Respir Care* 60:81-87, 2015.

Hoyer-Kuhn, H, Semler O, Stark C, et al: A specialized rehabilitation approach improves mobility in children with osteogenesis imperfecta, *J Musculoskelet Neuronal Interact* 14(4):445-453, 2014.

Hu X, Blemker SS: Musculoskeletal stimulation can help explain selective muscle degeneration in Duchenne muscular dystrophy, *Muscle Nerve* 52(2):174-182, 2015.

Jones KL: *Smith's recognizable patterns of human malformation*, ed 6, Philadelphia, 2006, Elsevier.

Jones MA, McEwen IR, Neas BR: Effects of power wheelchairs on the development and function of young children with severe motor impairments, *Pediatr Phys Ther* 24(2):131-140, 2012.

Jorde LB, Carey JC, Bamshad MC: *Medical genetics*, ed 4, Philadelphia, 2010, Mosby.

Kivitie-Kallio S, Norio R: Cohen syndrome: essential features, natural history, and heterogeneity, *Am J Med Genet* 102:125-135, 2001.

Kolehmainen J, Wilkinson R, Lehesjoki AE, et al: Delineation of Cohen syndrome following a large-scale genotype-phenotype screen, *Am J Hum Genet* 75:122-127, 2004.

Korinthenberg R: A new era in the management of Duchenne muscular dystrophy, *Dev Med Child Neurol* 61:292-297, 2019.

Land C, Rauch F, Montpetit K, Ruck-Gibis J, Glorieux FH: Effect of intravenous pamidronate therapy on functional abilities and level of ambulation in children with osteogenesis imperfecta, *J Pediatr* 148:456-460, 2006.

Lee AL, Button BM, Tannenbaum EL: Airway-clearance techniques in children and adolescents with chronic suppurative lung disease and bronchiectasis, *Front Pediatr* 5:2, 2017. doi:10.3389/fped.2017.00002.

Levitas A, Braden M, Van Norman K, et al: Treatment and intervention. In Hagerman RJ, McBogg P, editors: *The fragile X syndrome: diagnosis, biochemistry, and intervention*, Dillon, CO, 1983, Spectra Publishing, pp 201-226.

Lewis CL: Prader-Willi syndrome: a review for pediatric physical therapists, *Pediatr Phys Ther* 12:87-95, 2000.

Looper J, Benjamin D, Nolan M, Schumm L: What to measure when determining orthotic needs in children with Down syndrome: a pilot study, *Pediatr Phys Ther* 24:313-319, 2012.

Looper J, Ulrich DA: Effect of treadmill training and supramalleolar orthosis use on motor skill development in infants with Down syndrome: a randomized clinical trial, *Phys Ther* 90:382-390, 2010.

Lott IT, Dierssen M: Cognitive deficits and associated neurological complications in individuals with Down syndrome, *Lancet Neurol* 9:623-633, 2010.

Lowry RB, Sibbald B, Bedard T, Hall JG: Prevalence of multiple congenital contractures including arthrogryposis multiplex congenital in Alberta, Canada, and a strategy for classification and coding, *Birth Defects Res A Clin Mol Teratol* 88(12):1057-1061, 2010.

MacDonald WK, Hamilton D, Kuhle S: SMA carrier testing: A meta-analysis of differences in test performance by ethnic group, *Prenat Diagn* 34(12):1219-1226, 2014.

Mainardi PC: Cri du chat, *Orphanet J Rare Dis* 1:33, 2006.

Marini JC, Chernoff EJ: Osteogenesis imperfecta. In Cassidy SB, Allanson JE, editors: *Management of genetic syndromes*, New York, 2001, Wiley-Liss, pp 281-300.

Martin E, Shapiro JR: Osteogenesis imperfecta: epidemiology and pathophysiology, *Curr Osteoporos Rep* 5:91-97, 2007.

Martin K: Effects of supramalleolar orthoses on postural stability in children with Down syndrome, *Dev Med Child Neurol* 46:406-411, 2004.

McDonald CM: Physical activity, health impairments, and disability in neuromuscular disease, *Am J Phys Med Rehabil* 81(11 Suppl):S108-S120, 2002.

McDonald CM, Abresche RT, Carter GT, et al: Profiles of neuromuscular diseases. Duchenne muscular dystrophy, *Am J Phys Med Rehabil* 74:S70-S92, 1995.

McEwen I: Assistive positioning as a control parameter of social-communicative interactions between students with profound multiple disabilities and classroom staff, *Phys Ther* 72:534-647, 1992.

McEwen I: Children with cognitive impairments. In Campbell SK, Vander Linden DW, Palisano RJ, editors: *Physical therapy for children*, ed 2, Philadelphia, 2000, WB Saunders, pp 502-532.

McIlwaine M, Alarie N, Davidson GF, et al: Long-term multicenter randomised controlled study of high frequency chest wall oscillation versus positive expiratory pressure mask in cystic fibrosis, *Thorax* 68(8):746-751, 2013.

McIlwaine M, Button B, Dwan K: Positive expiratory pressure physiotherapy for airway clearance in people with cystic fibrosis, *Cochrane Database Sys Rev* 17(6):CD003147, 2015. doi:10.1002/14651858.CD003147.pub4.

McIlwaine PM, Wong LT, Chilvers M, Davidson GF: Long term comparative trial of two different chest physiotherapy techniques: postural drainage with percussion and autogenic drainage, in the treatment of cystic fibrosis, *Pediatr Pulmonol* 45(11):1064-1069, 2010.

McIlwaine PM, Wong LT, Peacock D, Davidson AG: Long-term comparative trial of conventional postural drainage and percussion versus positive expiratory pressure physiotherapy in the treatment of cystic fibrosis, *J Pediatr* 131(4):570-574, 1997.

McKone EF, Velentgas P, Swenson AJ, Goss CH: Association of sweat chloride concentration at time of diagnosis and CFRT genotype with mortality and cystic fibrosis phenotype, *J Cyst Fibros* 14(5):580-586, 2015.

Menear KS: Parents' perceptions of health and physical activity needs of children with Down syndrome, *Down Syndr Res Pract* 12:60-68, 2007.

Mik G, Gholbe PA, Scher DM, Widmann RF, Green DW: Down syndrome: orthopedic issues, *Curr Opin Pediatr* 20(10):30-36, 2008.

Moerchen V: Respiration and motor development: a systems perspective, *Neurol Rep* 18:8-10, 1994.

Moog U, Smeets EE, van Roozendaal KE, et al: Neurodevelopmental disorders in males related to the gene causing Rett syndrome in females (MECP2), *Eur J Paediatr Neurol* 7(1):5-12, 2003.

Moran A, Dunitz J, Nathan B, et al: Cystic fibrosis related diabetes: current trends in prevalence, incidence, and mortality, *Diabetes Care* 32:1626-1631, 2009.

Morrison L, Innes S: Oscillating devices for airway clearance in people with cystic fibrosis, *Cochrane Database Sys Rev* 5:CD006842, 2017. doi:10.1002/14651858.CD006842.pub4.

Nelson MD, Rader F, Tang X, et al: PDES inhibition alleviates functional muscle ischemia in boy with Duchenne muscular dystrophy, *Neurology* 82(23):2085-2091, 2014.

Nervik D, Roberts T: Clinical Bottom Line, Commentary on "What to measure when determining orthotic needs in children with Down syndrome": a pilot study, *Pediatr Phys Ther* 24:320, 2012.

Nilsson L: Training characteristics important for growing consciousness of joystick-use in people with profound cognitive disabilities, *Int J Ther Rehabil* 17:588-594, 2010.

Nixon PA, Orenstein DM, Kelsey SF: Habitual physical activity in children and adolescents with cystic fibrosis, *Med Sci Sports Exerc* 33:30-35, 2001.

Nixon PA, Orenstein DM, Kelsey SF, et al: The prognostic value of exercise testing in patients with cystic fibrosis, *N Engl J Med* 327:1785-1788, 1992.

Nye L, Renner J, Wang H: Initiation and preliminary analysis of National Cohen Syndrome Database. Poster session 622/F. Salt Lake City, UT: American Society of Human Genetics 55th Annual Meeting, 2005.

O'Grady MG, Dusing SC: Assessment position affects problem-solving behaviors in a child with motor impairments, *Pediatr Phys Ther* 28:253-258, 2016.

Orenstein DM: Pulmonary problems and management concerns in youth sports, *Pediatr Clin North Am* 49:709-721, 2002.

Orenstein DM, Hovell MF, Mulvihill M, et al: Strength vs aerobic training in children with cystic fibrosis, *Chest* 126:1204-1214, 2004.

Oskoui M, Levy G, Garland CJ, et al: The changing natural history of spinal muscular atrophy type 1, *J Neurol* 69:1931-1936, 2007.

Packel L, von Berg K: The respiratory system. In Goodman CC, Fuller KS, editors: *Pathology: implications for the physical therapist*, ed 4, St. Louis, 2014, Saunders, pp 772-861.

Pagano G, Castello G: Oxidative stress and mitochondrial dysfunction in Down syndrome, *Adv Exp Med Biol* 724:291-299, 2012.

Palisano RJ, Walter SD, Russell DJ, et al: Gross motor function of children with Down syndrome: creation of motor growth curves, *Arch Phys Med Rehabil* 82:494-500, 2001.

Paranjape SM, Barnes LA, Carson KA, et al: Exercise improves lung function and habitual activity in children with cystic fibrosis, *J Cyst Fibros* 11:18-23, 2012.

Parks M, Court S, Browns B, et al: Non-invasive prenatal diagnosis of spinal muscle atrophy by relative haplotype dosage, *Eur J Hum Genet* 25(4):416-422, 2017.

Pettit RS, Fellner C: CFTR modulators for the treatment of cystic fibrosis, *P T* 39(7):500-511, 2014.

Philpott J, Houghton K, Luke A, Canadian Paediatric Society, Healthy Living and Sports Medicine Committee, Canadian Academy of Sport Medicine, Paediatric Sport and Exercise Medicine Committee: Physical activity recommendations for children with specific chronic health conditions: juvenile idiopathic arthritis, hemophilia, asthma, and cystic fibrosis, *Paediatr Child Health* 15:213-218, 2010.

Prader A, Labhart A, Willi H: Ein syndrome von adipositas, kleinwuchs, kryptochismus und oligophrenie nach myatonieartigem zustand im neurgeborenenalter, *Schweiz Med Wschr* 86:1260-1261, 1956.

Pryor J, Tannenbaum E, Scott S, et al: Beyond postural drainage and percussion: airway clearance in people with cystic fibrosis, *J Cyst Fibros* 9:187-192, 2010.

Pueschel SM: Should children with Down syndrome be screened for atlantoaxial instability? *Arch Pediatr Adolesc Med* 152:123-125, 1998.

Ratliffe KT: *Clinical pediatric physical therapy*, St. Louis, 1998, CV Mosby.

Roizen NJ, Patterson D: Down syndrome, *Lancet* 361:1281-1289, 2003.

Rowland JL, Fragala-Pinkham M, Miles C, O'Neil M: The scope of pediatric physical therapy practice in health promotion and fitness for youth with disabilities, *Pediatr Phys Ther* 27:2-15, 2015.

Russman BS, Buncher CR, White M, Samaha FJ, Iannaccone ST: Function changes in spinal muscular atrophy II and III. The DCN/SMA Group, *Neurology* 47(4):973-976, 1996.

Sato Y, Yamauchi A, Urano M, Kondo E, Saito K: Corticosteroid therapy for Duchenne muscular dystrophy: improvement of psychomotor function, *Pediatr Neurol* 50(1):31-37, 2014.

Schalock RL, Borthwick-Duffy S, Bradley V, et al: *Intellectual disability: definition, classification, and systems of supports*, ed 11, Washington, DC, 2010, American Association on Intellectual Disabilities.

Schneiderman JE, Wilkes DL, Atenafu EG, et al: Longitudinal relationship between physical activity and lung health in patients with cystic fibrosis, *Eur Respir J* 43(3):817-823, 2014.

Schopmeyer BB, Lowe F, editors: *The fragile X child*, San Diego, 1992, Singular Publishing Group.

Schreiber A, Brochard S, Rippert P, et al: Corticosteroids in Duchenne muscular dystrophy: impact on the motor function measure sensitivity to change and implications for clinical trials, *Dev Med Child Neurol* 60:185-191, 2018.

Schwartzkopf-Phifer K, Liang LY: A pilot study to explore the effect of a 4-week exercise program on physical fitness, exercise self-efficacy and exercise behavior in children with disabilities, Academy of Pediatric Physical Therapy Annual Conference, Louisville, KY, November, 2017.

Selby-Silverstein L, Hillstrom HJ, Palisano RJ: The effect of foot orthoses on standing foot posture and gait of young children with Down syndrome, *NeuroRehabilitation* 16:183-193, 2001.

Semler O, Fricke O, Vezyroglou K, et al: Preliminary results on the mobility after whole body vibration in immobilized children and adolescents, *J Musculoskelet Neuronal Interact* 7(1):77-81, 2007.

Semler O, Fricke O, Vezyroglou K, Stark C, Schoenau E: Results of a prospective pilot trial on mobility after whole body vibration in immobilized children and adolescents with osteogenesis imperfecta, *Clin Rehabil* 22:387-394, 2008.

Shahbazian MD, Zoghbi HY: Molecular genetics of Rett syndrome and clinical spectrum of MECP2 mutations, *Curr Opin Neurol* 14(2):171-176, 2001.

Sharav T, Bowman T: Dietary practices, physical activity, and body mass index in a selected population of Down syndrome children and their siblings, *Clin Pediatr* 31:341-344, 1992.

Shields N, Dodd K, Abblitt C: Children with Down syndrome do not perform sufficient physical activity to maintain good health or optimize cardiovascular fitness, *Adapt Phys Activ Q* 26:307-320, 2009.

Siegel IM: The management of muscular dystrophy: a clinical review, *Muscle Nerve* 1:453-460, 1978.

Sillence DO, Senn A, Danks DM: Genetic heterogeneity in osteogenesis imperfecta, *J Med Genet* 16:101-116, 1979.

Stuberg W: Muscular dystrophy and spinal muscular atrophy. In Campbell SK, Vander Linden DW, Palisano RJ, editors: *Physical therapy for children*, ed 2, Philadelphia, 2000, WB Saunders, pp 339-369.

Stuberg W: Muscular dystrophy and spinal muscular atrophy. In Campbell SK, Palisano RJ, Orlin M, editors: *Physical therapy for children*, ed 4, Philadelphia, 2012, WB Saunders, pp 353-384.

Sveen ML, Anderson SP, Ingelsrud LH, et al: Resistance training in patients with limb-girdle and Becker muscular dystrophies, *Muscle Nerve* 47(2):163-169, 2013.

Sveen ML, Jeepesen TD, Hauerslev S, et al: Endurance training improves fitness and strength in patients with Becker muscular dystrophy, *Brain* 131:2824-2831, 2008.

Swisher AK, Hebestreit H, Mejia-Downs A, et al: Exercise and habitual physical activity for people with cystic fibrosis: expert consensus, evidence-based guide for advising patients, *Cardiopulm Phys Ther J* 26(4):85-98, 2015.

Tachdjian M, editor: *Pediatric orthopedics*, vol 2, ed 2, Philadelphia, 1990, WB Saunders.

Tachdjian M, editor: *Pediatric orthopedics*, vol 2, ed 3, Philadelphia, 2002, WB Saunders.

Tanamy MG, Magal N, Halpern GJ, et al: Fine mapping places the gene for arthrogryposis multiplex congenital neuropathic type between D5S394 and D5S2069 on chromosome 5qter, *Am J Med Genet* 104(2):152-156, 2001.

Tecklin JS, Clayton RG, Scanlin TF: High frequency chest wall oscillation vs. traditional chest physical therapy in DF: a large, 1-year, controlled study, *Pediatr Pulmonol* 20(Suppl):304, 2000.

Tefft D, Guerette P, Furumasu J: Intellectual predictors of young children's readiness for powered mobility, *Dev Med Child Neurol* 41:665-670, 1999.

Ulrich DA, Lloyd MC, Tiernan CW, et al: Effects of intensity of treadmill training on developmental outcomes and stepping in infants with Down syndrome: a randomized trial, *Phys Ther* 88:114-122, 2008.

Ulrich DA, Ulrich BD, Angulo-Kinzler RM, Yun J: Treadmill training of infants with Down syndrome: evidence-based developmental outcomes, *Pediatrics* 108:E84, 2001.

Valadares ER, Carneiro TB, Santos PM, et al: What is new in genetics and osteogenesis imperfecta classification? *J Pediatr (Rio J)* 90:536-541, 2014.

Van Brussel M, Takken T, Uiterwaal C, et al: Physical training in children with osteogenesis imperfecta, *J Pediatr* 152:111-116, 2008.

Van Buggenhout GJ, Fryns JP: Angelman syndrome, *Eur J Hum Genet* 17:1367-1373, 2009.

Verhaart IEC, Roberston A, Wilson IJ, et al: Prevalence, incidence and carrier frequency of 5q-linked spinal muscular atrophy-a literature review, *Orphanet J Rare Dis* 12(1):124, 2017. doi:10.1186/s13023-017-0671-8.

Victor RG, Sweeney HL, Finkel R, et al: A phase 3 randomized placebo-controlled trial of tadalafil for Duchenne muscular dystrophy, *Neurology* 89(17):1811-1820, 2017.

Vis JC, Duffels MG, Winter MM, et al: Down syndrome: a cardiovascular perspective, *J Intellect Disabil Res* 53(5):419-425, 2009.

Volsko TA: Cystic fibrosis and the respiratory therapist: a 50-year perspective, *Respir Care* 54:587-593, 2009.

Wang H, Falk MJ, Wensel C, Traboulsi EI: Cohen syndrome. In Adam MP, Ardinger HH, Pagon RA, Wallace SE, Bean LJH, Stephens K, Amemiya A, editors: *GeneReviews® [Internet]*, Seattle (WA): 1993-2018, University of Washington, Seattle, 2006 Aug 29 [updated 2016 Jul 21].

Webb AK, Dodd ME: Exercise and sport in cystic fibrosis: benefits and risks, *Br J Sports Med* 33(2):77-78, 1999.

World Health Organization: *International classification of function, disability, and health*, Geneva, Switzerland, 2001, World Health Organization.

Yimlamai D, Freiberger DA, Gould A, et al: Pretransplant six-minute walk test predicts peri- and post-operative outcomes after pediatric lung transplantation, *Pediatr Transplant* 17(1):34-40, 2013.

Zigman W, Silverman W, Wisniewski HM: Aging and Alzheimer's disease in Down syndrome: clinical and pathological changes, *Ment Retard Dev Disabil Res Rev* 2:73-79, 1996.

Ziter FA, Allsop K: The diagnosis and management of childhood muscular dystrophy, *Clin Pediatr* 15:540-548, 1976.

Zoghbi HY: Postnatal neurodevelopmental disorders: meeting at the synapse? *Science* 302(5646):826-830, 2003.

9

Autism Spectrum Disorder

Suzanne "Tink" Martin, Elizabeth Ennis

OBJECTIVES

After reading the chapter, the student will be able to:

1. Describe the criteria for autism spectrum disorder according to the *Diagnostic and Statistical Manual of Mental Disorders-5.*
2. Describe risk factors for and early signs and symptoms of autism spectrum disorder.
3. Discuss the role of physical therapy in the diagnosis and treatment of persons with autism spectrum disorder.
4. Describe a range of interventions available for individuals with autism spectrum disorder.
5. Discuss appropriate motor interventions for persons with autism spectrum disorder across the lifespan.

INTRODUCTION

Autism spectrum disorder (ASD) is a complex neurodevelopmental disorder characterized by difficulties with social interaction, communication, and repetitive behaviors. ASD is the most common pediatric diagnosis in the United States (Bhat et al., 2011) and the fastest growing developmental disability. According to the Centers for Disease Control and Prevention, the prevalence of ASD has risen to 1 in 59 children (Centers for Disease Control and Prevention, 2019), which is 15% higher than the 1 in 68 prevalence reported in 2016. Males are much more likely to be affected than females (4-5:1 ratio). In the fourth edition of the *Diagnostic and Statistical Manual of Mental Disorders* (DSM-IV), ASD consisted of five diagnostic subcategories: autistic disorder, Asperger disorder, Rett disorder, childhood disintegrative disorder, and pervasive developmental disorder not otherwise specified. In the new DSM-5, the previous subcategories are included under the broad term ASD, with the criteria describing the severity of the difficulties in functioning, that is amount of support needed, and presence of comorbidities.

Children on the spectrum are being diagnosed earlier than ever before. The rapid increase in diagnosis may mean more children have ASD or there is better recognition of signs by physician and health care providers. Wright (2017) concluded that changes in the diagnostic criteria and the growing awareness of autism were the explanation for the rise in prevalence. Although the core features of relate to problems with social interaction and communication, there is mounting evidence that children with demonstrate motor delays early on. ASD remains prevalent in all racial, ethnic, social, economic, and national groups despite strides in genetics to elucidate its etiology. Having a child with ASD significantly stresses the family and produces a burden on society to provide multidisciplinary services. Exercise and physical activities are accepted evidence-based interventions that result in functional improvements and reduction of negative behaviors (Wong et al., 2015). Therefore it is important for physical therapists and physical therapist assistants to be able to recognize signs and symptoms and risk factors of ASD, and to participate in the care of individuals with ASD across the lifespan.

Core Clinical Features

Diagnostic criteria for ASD in the DSM-5 include two major areas: impaired social communication and atypical patterns of behavior (American Psychiatric Association, 2013). Three deficits in social communication and a minimum of two symptoms in restricted range of behaviors/activities are required for diagnosis. Social communication deficits are manifest as poor social-emotional reciprocity such as carrying on a conversation or sharing emotions; poor nonverbal communication including gestures, body language, facial expressions; and difficulty with relationships including adjusting behavior, imaginative play, and making friends. Restricted, repetitive patterns of behavior, interests and activities are manifested by lining up toys, flipping objects, and echolalia. Echolalia is the repetition of words or phrases someone says. For example, if a therapist asks, "What is your name?" the child will repeat the question rather than answer the question. Children with ASD insist on sameness and inflexibly adhere to routines or ritualized patterns of verbal or nonverbal behavior. They seem to be in their own world. Finally, they may be hyper- or hyporeactive to sensory input, or display an unusual interest in sensory aspects of their environment. Children with ASD display significant functional impairments, and approximately 45% have an intellectual disability (Lai et al., 2014).

Sensory Processing

Sensory processing problems are present in more than 80% of children with ASD (Ben-Sasson et al., 2009). In fact, occupational therapy has played a major role in assessment and treatment of children with ASD because of their knowledge of sensory development and processing. Dunn (2014) postulates that there are two continua of responses to environmental stimuli: threshold and self-regulation. Threshold is the speed of reaction to a stimulus (slow versus quick to detect), whereas self-regulation relates to the level of response to a stimulus (under versus over responsiveness). Children with ASD may demonstrate sensory-seeking behavior, as well as increased responsiveness to or avoidance of sensory input (Baranek et al., 2006; Ben-Sasson et al., 2009; Miller et al., 2007). Hyporeactivity in social situations is the most common type of sensory modulation disorder seen in children with ASD (Baranek et al., 2006). Sensory processing patterns in children with ASD and attention-deficit/hyperactivity disorder (ADHD) were shown to overlap in a recent study (Little et al., 2018). The authors suggested that the overlap of sensory behaviors in these two conditions might indicate that similar intervention strategies could be used for both.

ASSOCIATED FEATURES OF AUTISM SPECTRUM DISORDER

Atypical Language Development

Associated features of ASD not reflected in the DSM-5 criteria are atypical language development and motor abnormalities (Lai et al., 2014). Poor language development has historically been linked to autism. Language delays were a defining feature of autism in the DSM-IV. Deficits in nonverbal communication used for social interaction are still part of the DSM-5 criteria. A child with ASD may present with delayed and deviant speech comprehension as an associated problem. Although two-thirds of children with autism have difficulty with expressive language at age 6, development of expressive language by age 5 has been considered a good prognostic sign (Billstedt et al., 2005). The inability to relate to people may lead to anxiety and aggression and further impede developing, maintaining, and understanding relationships.

Motor Abnormalities

Motor abnormalities in children with ASD were described as early as 1943 by Leo Kanner, a child psychiatrist. He noted motor clumsiness in the children he saw. Although stereotypical movements such as body rocking and hand flapping are part of the criteria for ASD, gross and fine motor delays are not. Lai et al. (2014) identified motor delay, coordination deficits, and hypotonia as *associated* features in ASD. Research shows that motor delays are common in children with ASD (Downey and Rapport, 2012; Green et al., 2009; Lloyd et al., 2013). Green et al. (2009) reported that 79% of children with ASD demonstrated motor impairments on the Movement Assessment Battery for Children. Ament et al. (2015) found that children with ASD had difficulty using visual and temporal information together to perform tasks such as standing on one foot or catching a ball. People with ASD use visual information differently than people without ASD.

Postural Control

Multiple sensory processing and sensorimotor deficits can be present in ASD. Impairments in sensory processing seen in children with ASD negatively affect postural control (Lim et al., 2017). Postural instability was produced when visual or somatosensory inputs were manipulated in a study of children with ASD (Minshew et al., 2004). Stins et al. (2015) found no difference in postural sway at baseline in children with mild ASD, but with eyes closed sway increased in the medial-lateral direction. In a study of a group of adults with ASD and a control group, the differences in postural instability increased as the sensory information became more unreliable (Doumas et al., 2016). A review by Lim et al. (2017) proposed that perinatal alteration in sensory development might explain the variations in how different sensory conditions affect standing postural control. There was a tendency for individuals with ASD to be more susceptible to postural instability when using visual information compared with somatosensory information (Lim et al., 2017; Morris et al., 2015).

Cooccurring Conditions

Over 70% of individuals with ASD have associated or cooccurring conditions, which can significantly affect prognosis and make clinical management more difficult (Lai et al., 2014). These conditions can be developmental such as intellectual disability seen in ~45% (Lai et al., 2014), general medical such as epilepsy (Woolfenden et al., 2012), or psychiatric such as personality disorders and behavioral disorders. The reader is referred to Lai et al. (2014) for a complete list of common cooccurring conditions. If the cooccurring medical conditions are severe, diagnosis of ASD may be delayed (Levy et al., 2010) or the cooccurring condition may be overlooked and not treated if the diagnosis of ASD is made at a younger age (Gillberg and Fernell, 2014). The prevalence of the associated conditions ranges from 10% for psychiatric disorders including anxiety, depression, and schizophrenia (Levy et al., 2010) to 41% to 95% for ADHD (Antshel and Hier, 2014). A recent study found that 92% of individuals with ASD had at least two other cooccurring problems. The most common were ADHD symptoms, learning difficulties, and emotional problems (Posserud et al., 2018). Furthermore, having cooccurring problems was related to the level of impairment and need for services.

Etiology

As with the majority of developmental disabilities, there is no single cause of ASD. It appears to be the result of a complex interaction between genetic predisposition and environmental factors (Hyman and Levy, 2013; Lai et al., 2014). ASD is more common in children with certain genetic syndromes. Prevalence estimates of ASD have been reported for Fragile X (males only 30%), Rett syndrome (females only 61%), Angelman syndrome (34%), and Cohen syndrome (54%) (Richards et al., 2015). See Chapter 8 for a description of these genetic syndromes. The likelihood of having autism symptoms with these syndromes is significantly higher than in the general population. High heritability has been confirmed in twin studies (Ronald and Hoekstra, 2011). After having a child diagnosed with ASD there is an increased risk (2% to 18% chance) of having a second child with ASD (Waye and Cheng, 2018). Chawarska et al. (2007) report siblings of children diagnosed with ASD are 14.7 times more likely to be diagnosed with ASD than siblings of children without ASD. The genetics of autism is not simple with over 1000 genes being implicated in its etiology of ASD (Murdoch and State, 2013). Genetic mutations have been linked to defects in synapse formation, transcription regulation, pathway remodeling, and connectivity (Waye and Cheng, 2018; Hu et al., 2014). A summary of the latest research on the genetics and some epigenetic findings in ASD can be found in Waye and Cheng (2018).

Teratogens such as thalidomide and valproic acid have been linked to ASD (Hyman and Levy, 2013). Teratogens are agents that can cause damage to a developing fetus. After much public concern, research has shown that vaccines are safe and do not cause ASD. Consistent risk factors were identified in a scoping review and categorized as physiologic risks such as advanced parental age, preterm birth, low birth weight, and hyperbilirubinemia; environmental risk such as air pollution from traffic; and social risk such as maternal immigrant status (Michelle et al., 2017). However, lack of specificity and consistency of associations between and environmental factors prevents establishing any causal relationships at this time.

Multiple differences in brain architecture and function have been described in ASD. The areas involved include the frontal lobe, temporal lobe, brainstem, and cerebellum. For a review of the functions of these brain areas the reader is referred to Chapter 2. Thirty percent of children with ASD have macrocephaly, which is a head circumference that is 2 standard deviations above the norm for age. Ninety percent of toddlers with ASD have larger than normal brain volume (Enticott et al., 2009). Changes in cortical thickness vary with age in children with ASD. Rapid growth in early childhood is followed by accelerated thinning of the cortex in later childhood and adolescence and a final decelerated thinning in early adulthood (Zielinski et al., 2014). Changes in cortical thickness are region-specific with social and communication scores being correlated with the thickness of the function-related brain region (Doyle-Thomas et al., 2013). Multiple abnormal neurodevelopmental trajectories exist in children with ASD that may help explain the heterogenous presentations seen in this disorder (Sussman et al., 2015).

Disturbed patterns of connectivity have been reported for the mirror neuron system in children with ASD (Theoret et al., 2005). The mirror neuron system is involved in imitation of movement and is crucial for adequate motor planning. Atypical motor cortex activation has been reported during simple finger movements in individuals with ASD. Structural differences in the brain pathways linking sensory and motor regions interferes with information transfer that must occur when learning and performing motor sequences (Moseley and Pulvermüller, 2018). Children with ASD who have poor motor timing were found to have the greatest motor and praxis deficits (Miller et al., 2014). Praxis refers to the ability to motor plan. Dyspraxia is an inability to motor plan and is often seen in children with coordination disorders. Researchers suggest that "dyspraxia in autism involves cerebellar mechanisms of movement control and the integration of these mechanisms with the cortical networks implicated in praxis" (Miller et al., 2014). Balance regulation requires cooperation between higher centers such as the cerebellum, vestibular cortex, brainstem, and motor cortex, all of which are brain structures involved in ASD. Regardless of the lack of a clear etiology, brain changes ultimately result in the manifestation of symptoms that constitute ASD.

Screening

Routine screening is recommended at 18 and 24 months of age by the American Academy of Pediatrics (Johnson and Myers, 2007). Age appropriate screening tools are available that only take a short time to administer. The most commonly used for young children are the infant toddler checklist (6 to 24 months), checklist for autism in toddlers (18 months), and a modified checklist for autism in toddlers (16 to 30 months). These questionnaires are completed by the parent/caregiver except in the case of the checklist for autism in toddlers, which is completed by a primary health care provider.

Diagnosis

Some researchers think that ASD can be reliably diagnosed by 18 months of age (Noyes-Grosser et al., 2018), whereas others report that 24 months is the earliest an accurate diagnosis can be made (Daniels et al., 2014). Early signs of autism in toddlers may include delayed or absent joint attention (shared focus on an object/task), delayed development of pretend or symbolic play, decreased response to own name, extreme variation in temperament, decreased imitation or gesturing, motor delay, unusual visual-motor exploration, and an inability to disengage visual attention.

Early motor delays may provide a diagnostic clue in ASD. Harris (2017) recently reviewed both prospective and retrospective studies that support the possibility that motor delays are apparent before other early social and behavioral signs of ASD are manifest. Using the Alberta Infant Motor Scale, Bhat et al. (2012) showed that a greater number of infant siblings of children with ASD demonstrated delayed motor abilities at 3 and 6 months of age than a group of typically developing (TD) low-risk infants. LeBarton and Iverson (2016) found similar results. Not only were motor skills delayed in toddlers with ASD (Lloyd et al., 2013), the motor delays increased as the child got older. The researchers suggested that the motor development deficits in toddlers with ASD may generate a cycle whereby "poor motor skills constrain social interactions and poor social interactions constrain motor skill development" (Lloyd et al., 2013).

Danish researchers prospectively interviewed 76,441 mothers about their children's development at 6 and 18 months of age (Lemcke et al., 2013). The study design controlled for selection and recall bias. At the 6-month interview, the only question that related to an increased prevalence of

ASD was "cannot sit up straight when put on lap." Language and social development predictors of ASD were found at 18 months of age. Iranian parents retrospectively reported motor delays in their children after being diagnosed with ASD (Arabameri and Sotoodeh, 2015). The children were significantly delayed in sitting and standing without support and independent walking compared with World Health Organization standards (see Chapter 4 on motor development). Unlike the Lemcke et al. (2013) study, there could have been recall bias as the findings were based on parent reports. In a study of infants at risk for ASD because of having an older sibling with ASD, parental concerns about motor abilities at 6 months of age were significant predictors of an ASD diagnosis, whereas social communication concerns and stereotypical motor behaviors were not predictive of ASD until after 12 months of age (Sacrey et al., 2015). These results reinforce the importance of taking parents' concerns about their child's development seriously.

Low cognitive ability may contribute to delays in motor skill development seen in children with ASD. However, the results of the Lloyd et al. (2013) study support the findings of Ozonoff et al. (2008) that the motor deficits are not caused by decreased cognitive ability. MacDonald et al. (2013) studied the relationship between motor skills and social communication skills. Weaker motor skills were associated with greater social communication skills in school-aged children with ASD. A recent study by Kaur et al. (2018) found that children with ASD, regardless of their IQ scores, had lower gross and fine motor scores.

Early Intervention

Early identification is crucial to early intervention (EI). Japanese researchers found that 28 of 47 children under the age of 2 years who were referred for motor delays were ultimately diagnosed with a neurodevelopmental disorder, and 36.7% of those referred were diagnosed with ASD (Hatakenaka et al., 2016). The children diagnosed with ASD were found to be delayed in sitting, crawling, and supported standing. The researchers concluded that early motor delay may be considered a red flag for global developmental disorders or for a specific disorder such as autism.

Screening should be done early and use developmentally appropriate standardized assessment tools. Practice recommendations most relevant to physical therapy practice are presented in Table 9.1. Physical therapists need to become more familiar with and utilize autism-specific screening tools to use them reliably. The American Academy of Pediatrics recommends screening begin at 18 months of age; however, motor abnormalities may be seen as early as 6 months of age. Recognition of motor stereotypies as well as abnormalities of motor control can be improved by consistently practicing observation skills during free play. Particular attention should be paid to the presence of postural reactions such as righting reactions of the head and trunk during movement transitions (rolling, coming to sit and stand) or postural perturbations (Teitelbaum et al., 1998). Upper extremity protective extension reactions may be absent in sitting and indicate lack of postural control. See Chapter 3 for a description of postural reactions. North American experts recommend that delayed motor development and atypical body movements should be considered as possible early markers for ASD (Zwaigenbaum et al., 2015a).

Hedgecock et al. (2018) recently analyzed the associations among problem behaviors, quality of life, and gross motor functioning in 2- to 6-year-old children with ASD. They found that gross motor delay was independently associated with problematic daytime behavior. Problematic daytime behaviors are typically categorized as either internalizing (anxious, withdrawn, inhibited) or externalizing (aggressive, hyperactive, poor inhibition) (Fig. 9.1). Children with ASD who exhibited cooccurring internalized behaviors had greater motor delays than children without internalized problem

TABLE 9.1 Practice Recommendations for Early Identification of Motor Symptoms in Autism Spectrum Disorder

Recommendation	Age	Recommended Tool
Developmental surveillance of all infants and children	Birth to 10 years	Infant-Toddler Checklist Modified Checklist for Autism in Toddlers Communication[3,6]
Screen for fine motor delays	6-15 months[5]	Peabody–2
Screen for gross motor delays	3-10 months	Alberta Infant Motor Scale[1]
Screen for abnormalities in motor control	Persistent head lag at 6 months[7] Delay in bringing hands to midline at 4-6 months[2] Delay in protective extension in sitting[5] and moving freely in sitting at about 6 months[4]	Observation
Screen for motor stereotypies such as hand flapping[6], and atypical arm and foot movements during walking[7]	18-24 months < 24 months	Observation Observational Gait Analysis

[1]Bhat et al., 2012, [2]Heathcock et al., 2015, [3]Lai et al., 2014, [4]Nickel et al., 2013, [5]Teitelbaum et al., 1998, [6]Zachor and Curatolo, 2014, [7]Zwaigenbaum et al., 2015a.
Modified from Harris SR: Early motor delays as diagnostic clues in autism spectrum disorder. *Eur J Pediatr* 176:1261, 2017.

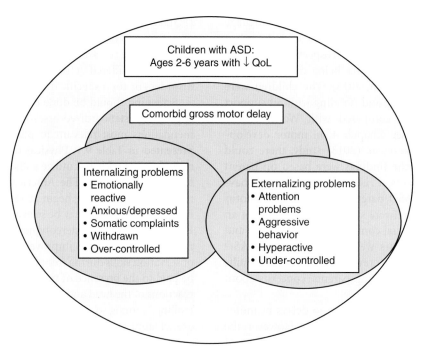

Fig. 9.1 Proposed associations among gross motor delay, internalizing and externalizing problem daytime behaviors, and health-related quality of life in young children with autism spectrum disorder. *QoL,* Quality of life. (From Hedgecock JB, Dannemiller LA, Shui AM, et al: Associations of gross motor delay, behavior, and quality of life in young children with autism spectrum disorder, *Phys Ther* 98:251–259, 2018.)

behaviors. The researchers concluded that identifying the children with ASD and internalizing behavior problems should be a priority for early evaluation and intervention by physical therapists. Gross motor delays as well as problematic daytime behaviors were also found to negatively affect quality of life.

School Age

Motor deficits in infants and toddlers with ASD present as poor postural control and will eventually affect the development of more fundamental motor skills such as running, jumping, hopping, and skipping. See Chapter 4 for a description of these skills. Poor timing and coordination impair balance in children with ASD (Stins and Emck, 2018). School-age children with ASD demonstrate difficulty with running, jumping, and ball throwing (MacDonald et al., 2013). They have lower scores than TD peers on standardized tests of motor skills including balance (Emck et al., 2011; Liu and Breslin, 2013; Paquet et al., 2016). Fournier et al. (2010) found a large effect size for motor coordination deficits in children with in a meta-analysis and concluded that motor problems may be a core feature of ASD.

Kaur et al. (2018) assessed children between 5 and 12 years of age with ASD using the Bruininks-Oseretsky Test of Motor Proficiency Second Edition and the Bilateral Motor Coordination subtests of the Sensory Integration and Praxis Tests. They found two types of praxis errors: *overflow* and *rhythmicity.* Both types of errors were strongly correlated with autism severity. *Overflow* is a spatial error defined as additional movements toward the end of an action sequence beyond what the tester performed. *Rhythmicity* is a temporal (timing) error

and is the inability to imitate rhythm of the action sequence. Motor deficits are more prevalent when the developmental assessment tool includes items that assess postural control and mobility. Adolescents with are more unstable when balancing on one leg (Travers et al., 2013). Asymmetry in two-legged standing predicted the severity and presence of repetitive behaviors in the study. Postural dynamics are altered during social challenges. Children with demonstrated increased postural sway in standing when presented with pictures of faces but not an object (Ghanouni et al., 2017). A similar study showed children with ASD had more sway in standing when shown sad or happy faces (Gouleme et al., 2017).

Motor and Social Skills

Development of movement complements the development of social skills in early childhood (Bar-Haim and Bart, 2006). Motor and sensory differences seen in individuals with ASD can significantly impact the ability to relate and participate in social interactions (Donnellan et al., 2013). Changes in development occur because of the interaction between the perceptual-motor experiences and the environment. Movement allows or affords opportunities for object exploration, social interaction, and communication, thus impacting development of cognition and language. LeBarton and Iverson (2016) found that at-risk siblings of children diagnosed with ASD showed delays in sitting and prone development that were related to gesturing and babbling. Holloway et al. (2018) found moderately high correlations between overall gross motor and social skills in a group of young boys with ASD. Specific motor impairments in object manipulation, stability, and motor accuracy predicted social function. Although motor ability differed by the severity of autism symptoms, participants' motor scores may have underestimated their abilities (Allen et al., 2017; Liu and Breslin, 2013).

Role of Physical Therapy

Physical therapists and physical therapy assistants may engage in different roles across the lifespan of an individual with ASD. Table 9.2 provides a brief outline of possible roles and potential interventions that can be utilized. The remainder of the chapter will focus on interventions that are most appropriate for physical therapy. A multidisciplinary approach is recommended that includes a combination of behavioral and developmental approaches. Physical therapists should be motor advocates, treating the whole child, not just a symptom such as toe walking or impaired gait. A large number of evidence-based interventions have been identified for individuals with ASD (Wong et al., 2015). The majority of interventions over the last 20 years have focused on preschool and school-age children with ASD. The interventions that target social communication fall into two general categories: (1) behavioral/naturalistic, and (2) developmental/relationship based. Applied behavioral analysis (ABA), prompting, and modeling are examples of the first category, whereas imitation and following the child's lead are examples of the latter category. There can be overlap, and many interventions combine the two categories. Multisystem interventions are being examined as a way to take advantage of children's inherent strengths (Srinivasan et al., 2015a), and to capitalize on fun ways to incorporate movement.

As more research has accumulated regarding interventions for children under 3 years of age, Zwaigenbaum et al. (2015b) proposed recommendations for best practice and research. Intervention should start as early as possible for children under 3 years of age with either a suspected or confirmed diagnosis of ASD. Parents should play a central role in providing interventions for infants and toddlers with ASD. Learning activities should be embedded in everyday life, taking advantage of "teachable moments" that will facilitate the generalization of skills outside the home. The working group recommended a combination of behavioral and developmental approaches be used and started as early as possible. Because sensory processing problems, motor delays, and challenging behaviors are common in children with ASD, these areas should be targeted in EI. Sensory and motor concerns should always be addressed because they may be a source of the anxious and disruptive behavior seen in children with ASD. Research has shown that the sensory and motor systems provide a substrate for development of cognition and social communication that is so lacking in individuals with ASD (Leonard and Hill, 2014; Moseley and Pulvermüller, 2018; Thelen, 2005).

Early Intervention Strategies

Warreyn et al. (2014) recommend that EI and preschool programs target three abilities that underpin development of language and social function: joint attention, imitation, and play. Imitation is an important form of communication in preverbal children. A positive association has been found between imitation and play and subsequent language development (Charman et al., 2003; Thurm et al., 2007). Interventions such as parent training and caregiver-mediated joint engagement have been found to improve social engagement (Kasari et al., 2008; Kasari et al., 2010), joint attention (Landa et al., 2011; Kasari et al., 2010), imitation (Ingersoll and Dvortcsak 2010; Landa et al., 2011) and play (Kasari et al., 2010).

Research supports combining interventions at the same time to provide an additive effect (Landa et al., 2011). Kasari et al. (2012) added interventions targeting joint attention and play to an ABA program for toddlers with ASD. Early intensive behavioral intervention usually heads the list of acceptable and well-established treatments for ASD (Reichow et al., 2018). Children exposed to the additional interventions showed an increase in joint attention and play in generalized contexts, which predicted greater language outcomes than the children only engaged in an ABA program.

Noyes-Grosser et al. (2018) conducted a large study of outcomes of a community-based EI program for infants/toddlers with and without ASD and their families. They reported that the children with ASD accounted for 13% of all EI

TABLE 9.2	Role of Physical Therapy and Possible Interventions Across the Lifespan	
Life Stage	**Role**	**Intervention**
Infant/toddler	Screen, evaluate motor skills	Foster early motor skills: head control, sitting posture, postural control Reach and grasp/object exploration/ play Walking for environmental exploration
Childhood/preschool	Screen, evaluate motor skills, fitness level, peer interaction, play skills, monitor activity level	Refine postural control, remediate gait, develop fundamental movement skills: running, jumping, hopping, skipping Foster pretend play, physical play, games with peers, use rhythmic movements, aquatic activities
School/adolescence	Evaluate fitness, activity level, advocate for active community engagement	Modify and adapt motor skill training, foster community participation in meaningful activities, plan for transition to adulthood
Adulthood	Evaluate physical fitness and health-related fitness	Group exercise programs, support healthy lifestyle choices

participants. The children with ASD made some developmental gains and decreased maladaptive behaviors. More of the families of children with ASD achieved recommended standards than families of children with other disabilities. This may be explained by the fact that the level of intensity of services was higher for children with ASD compared with those with other disabilities. The most effective level of intensity of EI has yet to be determined. EI behavioral intervention intensity for ASD can range from 20 to 40 hours per week (Reichow et al., 2018). The Noyes-Grosser et al. (2018) study concluded that results-driven accountability can be used to identify outcome measures for large subpopulations in EI such as children with ASD and their families.

Pretend or symbolic play is facilitated by joint attention, social referencing, and parental scaffolding (Lillard, 2007). Object play is related to language acquisition as well as cause and effect. Parents can encourage grasping by scaffolding reaching experiences using sticky mittens (Libertus and Landa, 2014). Pretend play develops once a child learns cause and effect and is a natural progression from functional play. See Chapter 5 for a discussion of play development. Play is an effective tool to foster participation of children with autism in inclusive settings (Kossyvaki and Papoudi, 2016). Children with ASD can be taught to engage in pretend play (Barton and Pavlanis, 2012) using a system of least prompts. A prompting sequence starts with presenting an object, observing, and imitating the child before prompting play. A second level of prompt might be to provide a choice either between a physical model of pretend play or a choice of two toys. A third level would be to prompt expansion of the play sequence to include more than one action such as feeding a baby a bottle, wrapping the baby in a blanket, and putting the baby to bed. A study by Barton et al. (2019) supports using response-prompting sequences to teach pretend play in children who do not demonstrate such behaviors.

Use of peer modeling of play has been successful in improving social communication in young children with ASD (Barber et al., 2016; National Autism Center, 2015). The Early Start Denver Model (Dawson et al., 2010) fuses developmental and behavioral principles of treatment using a play-based approach. Kasari et al. (2008) compared the effect of joint attention and play interventions on language outcomes of 3- and 4-year-olds with ASD. These interventions were added to an ABA program that did not target these developmental skills. Both interventions resulted in positive change. The researchers hypothesized that joint attention and play represent a common mechanism to foster engagement between parent and child that ultimately affects language acquisition. In a 5-year follow-up study involving these same children, 80% were using spoken language functionally by age 8 to 9 years (Kasari et al., 2012). The primary predictor was baseline play level. Other predictors of spoken language included earlier enrollment in the intervention, initiating more joint attention, and receiving the experimental interventions focused on joint attention or play. Cognitive scores at age 8 years were only predicted by baseline play complexity. This study further supports the relevance of object play skills in the development of language and cognition. Please refer to Table 5.4 for Play Development and Box 5.4 for Principles to Support Play Complexity.

Exercise/Physical Activity

Exercise was identified as an evidence-based practice for all ages of individuals with ASD in a review by Wong et al. (2015). Exercise has been classified as an emerging evidence-based intervention for children under 22 years of age by the National Standards Project, phase 2 (National Autism Center, 2015). Some exercise interventions focus on autism-specific impairments such as stereotypical repetitive behaviors, whereas others focus on perceptual-motor skills or academics. Various forms of exercise have been used including cycling, jogging, horseback riding, walking, and swimming. Exercise can provide short-term decreases in repetitive behaviors based on a systematic review by Petrus et al. (2008). Two of the studies in the review showed that a higher intensity exercise such as jogging was more effective in decreasing self-stimulation. High-intensity exercise such as roller-skating, jogging, and exergames (games involving exercises such as a Wii) was found to lessen the frequency of stereotypical behaviors (Anderson-Hanley et al., 2011). A 37% improvement in behavior and academic performance was reported in a meta-analysis of the effects of physical exercise (Sowa and Meulenbroek, 2012). In fact, the amount of physical activity a child with ASD engages in has been positively correlated with engagement in the classroom (Nicholson et al., 2011).

Physical activity levels of individuals with ASD may be lower than TD peers because of lack of social engagement with peers. In addition, sensory and motor impairments common in ASD can compound difficulties in participation in group games and sports. Obesity is a possible result of low activity levels and has been identified as a potential cooccurring medical problem. Intense interventions such as ABA are sedentary and may leave little time for physical activity within a child's daily routine. Physical therapists have been involved in studying and promoting fitness in children with ASD (Fragala-Pinkham et al., 2011; Oriel et al., 2011). However, at this time there is limited evidence regarding the efficacy of exercise in individuals with ASD to treat obesity and improve physical fitness (Srinivasan et al., 2014), despite promising studies. It is still recommended that motor activities be imbedded into an ABA or speech intervention.

Physical therapists are uniquely qualified to develop motor skill training interventions for children with ASD. Physical therapy should be offered to children with autism as it affords them the opportunity to explore their environment and participate in their world. Physical therapists and physical therapist assistants can promote a healthy lifestyle for children with ASD across the lifespan by ensuring that physical activity and exercise are included in their comprehensive intervention program (Long and Holloway, 2017). The reader is referred to Table 9.3: Specific Exercise Session Recommendations for Children with Autism Spectrum Disorder. Exercise groups can be used in preschool and adapted physical activities in school. Finding leisure activities that are

TABLE 9.3 Specific Exercise Session Recommendations for Children with Autism Spectrum Disorder

Domain	Specific Recommendations
Structure of the environment	1. Follow a familiar exercise schedule. 2. Conduct sessions in the same space.[1] 3. Exercise in a thermoneutral environment.[2] 4. Use visual cues to indicate child's place and space. 5. Minimize sensory distractions such as bright lights or loud noises. 6. Use visual pictures to provide structure to the session.[3] 7. Allow time for child to adapt to any new activity.
Exercise considerations	1. Use adapted equipment to accommodate any motor impairment.[4,5] 2. Use heart rate monitors if possible or pictorial exertion scales such as pediatric OMNI.[2,6] 3. Individual sessions may be indicated for lower functioning children, whereas higher functioning children can benefit from group exercise sessions. 4. Progress gradually based on the child's abilities. 5. Provide breaks to avoid overwhelming the child. 6. Provide sufficient warm-up and cool-down within a session. 7. Establish a way for the child to stop an activity before negative behavior occurs. Ask caregivers about the best way to manage negative behavior.[7,8] 8. Encourage parents to incorporate physical activity into the daily routine by having the child help with daily chores. 9. Provide activities that the child enjoys and that will foster success.
Instructions, feedback, and reinforcement	1. Be brief and clear when using verbal instructions. 2. Combine verbal and visual instructions when possible, such as "do this" along with a pictorial depiction of the action. 3. Provide manual guidance during the requested motor activity as needed. 4. Exercising with a peer/sibling can be motivation for the child. 5. Provide gestural and verbal reinforcement such as high-fives and good jobs.[8] 6. Provide breaks from activity to do favorite sensory activities. Use small toys, stickers, or healthy edibles to ensure adherence to exercise.

[1]Mesibov GB, Shea V, Schopler E: *The TEACCH approach to autism spectrum disorders,* New York, 2004, Springer. [2]American College of Sports Medicine: *ASCM's guidelines for exercise testing and prescription,* ed 8, Baltimore, 2009, Lippincott William & Wilkins. [3]Bondy A, Frost A: Communication strategies for visual learners. In Lovaas OI, editor: *Teaching individuals with developmental delays: basic intervention techniques,* Austin, TX, 2003, Pro-Ed, pp 291–304. [4]Hayakawa K, Kobayashi K: Physical and motor skill training for children with intellectual disabilities, *Percept Mot Skills* 112:573–580, 2011. [5]MacDonald M, Esposito P Hauchk J, et al.: Bicycle training for youth with Down syndrome and autism spectrum disorder (ASD), *Focus Autism Other Dev Disabl* 27:12–21, 2012. [6]Utter AC: Children's OMNI scale of perceived exertion: walking/running evaluation, *Med Sci Sports Exerc* 34:139–144, 2002. [7]Landa R: Early communication development and intervention for children with autism, *Ment Retard Dev Disabil Res Rev* 13:16–25, 2007. [8]Lovaas OI: Behavioral treatment and normal educational and intellectual functioning in young autistic children, *J Consult Clin Psychol* 55:3–9, 1987.
Modified from Srinivasan SM, Pescatello LS, Bhat AN: Current perspectives on physical activity and exercise recommendations for children and adolescents with autism spectrum disorders, *Phys Ther* 94:875–889, 2014.

pleasurable as well as physically active can help with the transition from adolescence to adulthood. Group exercise programs for adults can be developed at community centers or through private clinics or hospitals to promote and advocate for physical activity and social interaction.

Aquatics

Aquatic activities have been used as an intervention for children with ASD since the early 90s (Dulcy, 1992). Research has shown that aquatics can improve social interaction (Mortimer et al., 2014) and sleep (Oriel et al., 2016). Oriel et al. (2017) found that a twice a week aquatic exercise program for 3- to 11-year-olds with ASD resulted in improvements in behavior. Quality of life improved in children with ASD following a 10-week aquatic program (Ennis, 2011). There was a carryover effect 10 weeks postintervention in the studies included in a systematic review by Mortimer et al. (2014). More

improvement was made by the children with ASD who were assisted by trained peers/siblings than untrained peers/siblings in the study by Chu and Pan (2012). The children were observed to have decreased physical interaction with teachers, which initially might be thought to be a negative outcome but may well be positive as the children were less dependent on adults and more eager to interact with peers. Therefore the pool can provide a rich sensory environment to promote play and social interaction. Playfulness was increased in young children with ASD after engaging in an aquatic playgroup for 12 weeks (Fabrizi, 2015). Aquatic therapy shows potential as a treatment intervention to improve social behaviors and interactions in children with ASD.

Aquatic activities can be therapeutic, playful, and instructive such as swimming. The aquatic environment may provide a more supportive environment for attaining movement skills than being in a gym setting (Prupas et al., 2006). The buoyancy of water can support movement and facilitate practice of motor as well as play skills. Engagement in swimming as a leisure activity may increase the bond between parent and child as they participate in a fun activity (Eversole et al., 2016) and improve the quality of life of the child (Ennis, 2011). Children with ASD were found to enjoy swimming more than TD peers. Difficulty with complex movements can be addressed using swimming instruction (Yanardag et al., 2015). The researchers used a system of prompting to teach 6-year-old children with ASD advanced movement skills.

Caputo et al. (2018) reported that swimming skills were learned during a 10-month program of aquatic therapy using a multisystem approach. They saw significant improvements in activity level, adaptation to change, and emotional response. Their three phase program begins with establishing a secure base followed by teaching swimming skills using adaptive techniques and ending with traditional group activities. Water safety is always a concern for children and should be included in any aquatic intervention. As little as 8 hours of intervention was needed to show improved water safety skills in children with ASD (Alainz et al., 2017) using group therapy. The research supports the use of aquatic therapy as an intervention to promote physical and social development and to increase participation and fun.

Sensory Integration/Sensory-Based Interventions

Sensory integration (SI) uses sensory exploration in child-directed activities to provide a just-right challenge to produce an adaptive response to the sensory experience. Despite a few positive effects seen in small randomized controlled trials, there is little evidence to support the efficacy of using SI in this population. Sensory-based interventions, such as the use of therapy balls or weighted vests to modify a child's arousal state, have not been shown to be effective. The problem is that the protocols for the use of both SI and sensory-based interventions are not consistent across therapists (Case-Smith et al., 2015).

Using Dunn's model of sensory processing, therapists can help parents understand the sensory impairments that are interfering with acquisition of functional life skills (Dunn, 2014). Parental competence and child outcomes improved when contextually based interventions were used to manage the negative effects of sensory processing difficulties in children with ASD (Dunn et al., 2012). A recent cross-sectional study suggested that children with ADHD and ASD demonstrate similar sensory processing patterns (Little et al., 2018). The overlap may have implications for interventions. Consider that children with ASD may increase repetitive behaviors during an activity that results in hyperresponsiveness. The lack of focus may be related to lack of registration of the stimuli, which could be supplemented by giving extra verbal or physical cues. Little et al. (2018) agree that use of visual supports with children with ASD is effective. Visual support could include watching a peer perform an activity.

Positive Behavior Support

A complete discussion of all the possible interventions that can be used to support positive behavior in individuals with ASD is beyond the scope of this chapter. Physical therapists and physical therapist assistants need to incorporate positive behavioral supports into their therapy sessions. Examples of positive supports are seen in Fig. 9.2. These supports include but are not limited to a timer, choice board, clearly communicating what the person is working for, and use of appropriate behavioral reinforcement. Refusal may not always be a negative or noncompliant response. As the child with ASD gains independence in an action, the child may refuse help. When a child refuses, try to ascertain the reason: is the action/activity too hard, too challenging or the opposite, does the activity not have meaning for the child, or does the child not need help? Does the environment engender anxiety? Are peers present that are supportive? Can you build on a previous positive response to scaffold a repeat performance or successive approximation of the requested action? See the Case Study at the end of the chapter for further considerations.

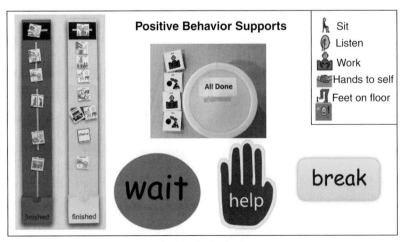

Fig. 9.2 Positive behavior supports.

Social Communication Support: Play

Acquisition of knowledge, cognitive skills, and behavior regulation occurs through interactions we have in the social world, where this knowledge has meaning and function (Donnellan et al., 2013). Engaging in peer-motor play can provide an opportunity for boys with ASD to integrate social and gross motor skills (Holloway et al., 2018). Therapists need to recognize that motor play can be used to promote communication and social skills in children with ASD. Social skills groups and video modeling are evidence-based practice (Reichow and Volkmar, 2010). Pairing a peer without ASD with a child with ASD when playing together can be used to assist the child with ASD to learn new motor skills or to play at a higher level. Children can learn new skills by imitating more advanced peers during play routines. Play provides a social context for embedded instruction. It also affords the child the opportunity to interact socially and communicate with peers, caregivers, and teachers (Barton and Pavilanis, 2012). The system of least prompts is an example of an antecedent-based teaching strategy that can be used with young children with autism. It has been used to increase the frequency and diversity of pretend play. Prompts may include choice, modeling, visual cues, hand over hand, or giving a toy and a verbal prompt. See Barton and Pavilanis (2012) for an example of a prompt sequence.

Kossyvaki and Papoudi (2016) reviewed play interventions for school-age children with autism. The majority of the studies supported play as a valuable intervention but there was concern that maturation of the participants might have influenced the outcome. The studies used a mix of behavioral/naturalistic and developmental/relationship approaches to foster play. Prompting and modeling was used to shape behavior and following the child's lead along with imitation was used to mimic typical development. Some studies targeted specific types of play such as pretend, whereas others focused on specific play scripts like teaching gardening. Still other studies aimed to increase responses during play.

Integrated play groups (IPG) have been used as a model for intensive intervention in school-age children with ASD (Wolfberg et al., 2015). Forty-eight children with ASD completed a 12-week after school program. The play group consisted of two children with ASD and three TD peers who met twice a week for 60 minutes. An IPG guide facilitated a minimum of 40 minutes of participation between an opening and closing script. Play behaviors were coded from the least complex to most complex, that is, from not engaged to engaged in symbolic/pretend play. Social behaviors were coded similarly from isolated to sharing a common goal. Results showed an increase in play complexity and social engagement that generalized to being able to play with unfamiliar peers. IPG appears to be a robust intervention for producing change in play complexity and social behavior. Research needs to continue to determine if changes in pretend play, a social activity, may drive developmental changes in social play. Therapists should consider guiding children with ASD and TD children using pretend play scripts while challenging posture and balance.

Play interventions have also been implemented with preschool children with ASD. These interventions include Picture Me Playing (Murdock and Hobbs, 2011), using the iPad to increase play dialogue (Murdock et al., 2013), and Stay, Play, Talk (Barber et al., 2016). The two former studies used an intervention designed to assist preschoolers with autism to visualize a sequence of imaginative play constructed from photographs of action figures or play sets. Dialogue was provided when engaging with peers. Results showed a significant increase in play dialogue and most importantly there was generalization to an unscripted play opportunity with novel toys (Murdock and Hobbs, 2011). The second study using the iPad and play story had a very small sample size but did show moderate to strong effects across the intervention phase that were mostly maintained after 3 weeks. Barber et al. (2016) used TD peers paired with a child with autism to increase social reciprocations. The TD peers were taught to *stay* with their friend, *play* with their friend, and *talk* to their friend. The pairs played together twice for 20 minute sessions for 6 to 8 weeks. All of the friends increased the frequency of their responses and social reciprocations. However, these gains were not maintained at 2 months postintervention.

Deficits in pretend play have been closely linked to social and cognitive deficits (Hobson et al., 2013; Manning and Wainright, 2010; Rutherford et al., 2007). Lower levels of social engagement have been found to correlate with less developed pretend play skills in a group of younger siblings of children with ASD (Campbell et al., 2018). Changes in pretend play were observed in a high-risk group of toddlers who had older siblings diagnosed with ASD, and a low-risk group of toddlers of TD siblings at 22, 28, and 34 months of age. Those high-risk children diagnosed with ASD at 3 years of age were poorer at pretending at each age despite similar growth trajectories among the three groups: high risk with ASD, high risk no ASD, and low risk. The high-risk ASD group showed delays in play on all measures. Cognitive ability did not account for group differences. Parents of children in all groups were highly engaged with their children, but the children with ASD showed less engagement with both parents and examiner during play.

Motor Interventions: Infants/Toddlers

Physical therapy interventions should focus on development of postural control and balance if motor delays are present. Head control can be assisted by supporting the child in sitting as seen in Fig. 5.11. The caregiver should be at the same eye level as the infant to encourage joint attention. Intervention 5.14 A,B depicts positions to encourage head control. Head control can be further encouraged by using a modified pull-to-sit maneuver as seen in Intervention 5.15. Prone positioning can facilitate the infant's head and neck strength, pushing up, and postural control. Fig. 5.21 encourages pushing up from prone. Furthermore, the prone position allows for upper extremity weight-bearing, development of shoulder stability, and an opportunity to weight shift and reach (Fig. 4.30, Fig. 4.33). Transitioning from prone to sitting is seen in Intervention 5.1.

Once sitting with some upper extremity support is possible, trunk responses called righting reactions can be facilitated by having the child on a moveable surface such as a bolster (Intervention 6.7) or on a ball (Intervention 8.16). The child's trunk responses can also be elicited while sitting on the caregiver's lap. Active trunk rotation can be practiced moving in and out of a side sitting position or within a play task as seen in Intervention 8.10.

Bhat et al. recommend that motor play be part of any intervention with an infant or toddler with ASD or at risk for ASD (Ries, 2018). Furthermore, these children may have low postural tone and may not move or change body position as often as TD peers, and exhibit less movement variability (Ries, 2018). Weight-bearing and approximation can be used to counteract low postural tone. Time spent in four-point or quadruped helps build shoulder and pelvic girdle stability and allows the trunk to work against gravity. Coming to stand can be practiced as seen in Intervention 8.11, and lower limb control can be improved with squatting and crouching (Intervention 6.3). Object play and spatial language such as up/down, in/out can be incorporated with movement. Pushing a weighted object such as a toy grocery cart can encourage walking for a child with low postural tone (Intervention 8.12).

Motor Interventions: Childhood

Interventions in childhood should focus on fundamental movement skills such as running, jumping, hopping, and skipping. See Chapter 4 for a description of the acquisition of these fundamental movement skills. These may need to be modified due to coordination and balance issues or motor planning impairments. Imitation of gestures can be helpful starting with mirror movements and progressing to opposites when right and left are mastered. Pairing movement with verbal spatial directions can help the child develop a sense of internal reference such as moving an arm or leg forward, to the side, and back. The therapist can give the direction and have the child move in the requested direction with the appropriate limb; the child can verbally repeat what the movement was and eventually can learn the sequence of movements in a particular order.

Researchers are beginning to study the effectiveness of motor skills intervention on motor outcomes. Bremer and Lloyd (2016) used a fundamental motor skill intervention consisting of two 6-week blocks to teach object control and locomotor skills to 3- to 7-year-olds with autism-like characteristics. The children improved in both motor and social skills. Bremer et al. (2014) demonstrated significant gains in gross motor skills on the Peabody-2 in a group of 4-year-olds with ASD after a 12 week-intervention. Ketcheson et al. (2017) targeted 4- to 6-year-olds with ASD with an intensive motor skill intervention utilizing Classroom Pivotal Response Teaching (Stahmer et al., 2011). The experimental group received 4 hours of intervention daily, 5 days a week for 8 weeks during the summer. The intervention was not provided to the control group. Results showed statistically significant differences in all motor outcomes between the groups in locomotion, gross motor quotient, and object control. Movement

games such as red light/green light and Twister can be used to increase listening and movement skills. Learning to ride a bike can be very functional for a child with ASD and provides an opportunity for family and community participation.

All of the following motor interventions foster strength, coordination, postural control, and balance. Intervention 9.1. Walking and Standing Challenges: A. Heel walking, B. Crab walking, C. Wheelbarrow walking, D. Tiltboard walking, E. Standing one foot on a ball; Intervention 9.2. Activities on a Prone Scooter Board: A. Lawn mower, B. Back-up; Intervention 9.3. Floor Activities: A. Knees to nose, B. Roll up, C. London bridge, D. Bird dog. Bird dog is much like table in yoga with either one arm or leg extended. As balance and core strength increase, opposite arm and leg extension can be added. Intervention 9.4. Games for Two: A. King on one knee, B. Back to back ball pass. Some of the walking challenges can be performed on different floor surfaces, keeping in mind that processing of proprioceptive and kinesthetic information may be challenging for children with ASD. Visual fixation may be used to assist in maintaining balance when standing on one leg. When walking on a balance beam, lowering the center of gravity as in a mini squat may provide additional postural stability. Rhythmic movements, singing while moving or dancing in various postures can be fun and improve balance while engaging the child to participate with peers. Yoga poses have also been used to increase participation in preschool (O'Neil et al., 2016) and school-age children with ASD (Seiden and Tartick, 2018). See Fig. 9.3 for examples of some yoga poses.

Successful interventions use tenets of motor learning such as positive expectancy, support for autonomy (choices), and externally directed attention rather than focusing on the body's movement (Wulf and Lewthwaite, 2016). Embodied interventions are ones predicated on the theory that cognition emerges from an interaction between the agent and the sensorimotor experiences encountered within the environment (Smith and Gasser, 2005; Thelen, 2000). Srinivasan et al. (2015a, 2015b, 2016a, 2016b) studied the effects of rhythm and robotic interventions on several behavioral and motor issues seen in 5- to 12-year-old children with ASD and a comparison group who received standard care. Rhythmic interventions, although initially challenging for children with ASD, can lead to improved behavioral skills, positive affect, and verbal and nonverbal communication (Srinivasan et al., 2016a). Social attention patterns, measured as joint attention, improved in school-age children using an embodied rhythm intervention (Srinivasan et al., 2016b). The groups that were treated with movement, either rhythm or robotic interventions, showed improvements in gross motor imitation, balance, and bilateral coordination following an 8-week intervention (Srinivasan et al., 2015a). The robot's movements were limited, less precise, and not conducive to performing complex movements such as jumping, galloping, or skipping. Use of the robot was recommended only as an adjunct therapy. In conclusion, the researchers encourage clinicians to add music and movement-based active play activities to the standard treatment of children with ASD.

INTERVENTION 9.1 Walking and Standing Challenges

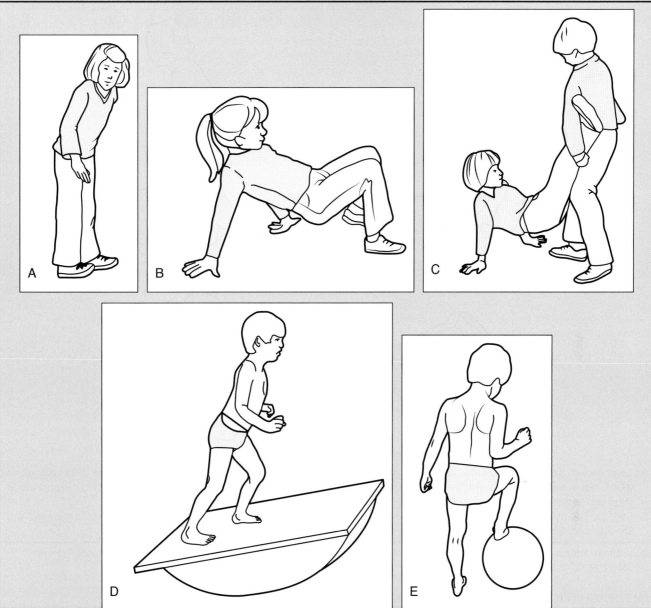

A. **Heel walking.** The child is encouraged to lean back on the heels with a posterior pelvic tilt with contraction of the abdominal muscles.

B. **Crab walking.** The child begins sitting on the floor leaning back on hands. Instruct the child to lift her bottom off the floor maintaining hands and feet contact with the floor. Ask the child to walk backward with the hands leading.

C. **Wheelbarrow walking.** One child begins sitting on the floor while another child faces the first child. The child who is standing lifts the feet of the child who is sitting so that only his hands are touching the floor and his feet are supported by the second child. The children can do a forward or backward wheelbarrow walk.

D. **Tiltboard walking** (the child must demonstrate adequate postural reactions before attempting this intervention). If the child can stand safely on a large tiltboard, instruct the child to walk up and down on the tiltboard slowly while maintaining balance. The therapist or assistant must be prepared to assist if the child loses balance.

E. **Standing one foot on a ball.** The child is instructed to stand with one foot on the ground and the other on a small ball. The therapist or assistant may need to begin by holding the ball if the child has poor righting or equilibrium reactions. If a moveable surface is not feasible, the other leg could be placed on a small stool.

INTERVENTION 9.2   Activities on a Prone Scooter Board

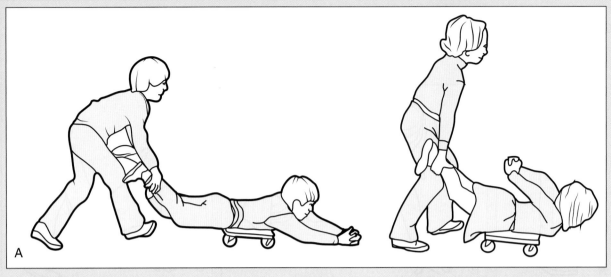

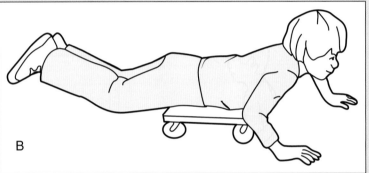

A. **Lawn mower.** One child lies prone on a scooter board while another child standing behind holds his feet. The child holding the feet is instructed to push forward. The child on the scooter board may hold arms forward off the ground or hold clasped hands lifted behind the back.

B. **Back-up.** The child is prone on a scooter board. Instruct the child to push backward with his hands while keeping his head and shoulders up. Legs must be held up as well.

INTERVENTION 9.3   Floor Activities

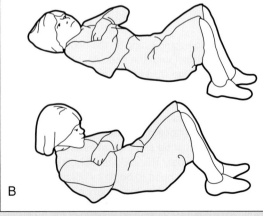

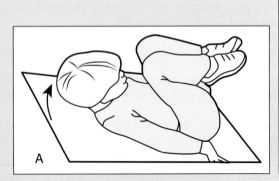

A. **Knees to nose.** The child lies on his back with arms on the floor (easier) or folded across the chest (harder). The child is instructed to lift his head and bring his knees into his chest and hold. Encourage the child to touch his knees to his nose. Once this is possible, have the child alternate bringing one knee toward the nose followed by the other leg. Remind the child to not hold his breath.

B. **Roll up.** The child lies on his back in hook lying (knees bent, feet on the floor). Instruct the child to bring chin to chest; shoulders should come off the floor. Arms are across the chest and the motion should be a slow roll up and down without the back arching.

INTERVENTION 9.3 Floor Activities—cont'd

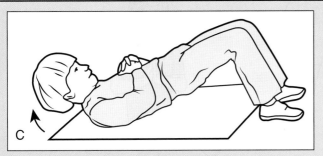

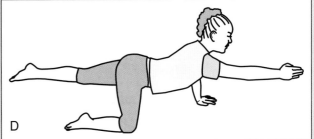

C. London bridge. The child begins on his back in hook lying. Instruct the child to first raise his chin to the chest and then by pushing with his legs make a bridge, that is, lift the hips and hold.

D. Bird dog. The child begins on hands and knees. Hands should be under the shoulders and knees under the hips. Begin lifting one extremity at a time and holding; progress to holding right arm and left leg straight out at the same time. Repeat straightening the opposite diagonals, the left arm and right leg.

INTERVENTION 9.4 Games for Two

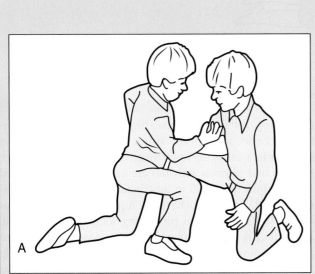

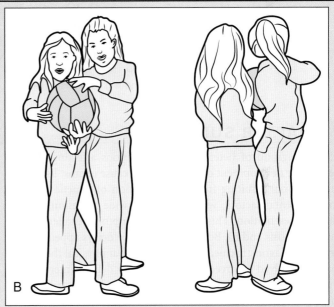

A. King on one knee. Two children kneel in front of each other about 2 feet apart. Instruct each child to raise the right knee so that he is in half-kneeling with the right foot forward. Have the children shake their right hands and attempt to pull each other off balance. Change to the left foot and left hand and repeat.

B. Back to back ball pass. Two children stand back to back. Give the ball to one child and instruct the child to turn and hand it to her partner who must turn the other way to return the ball. The ball will go around in a circle. The feet should remain stationary during the ball pass.

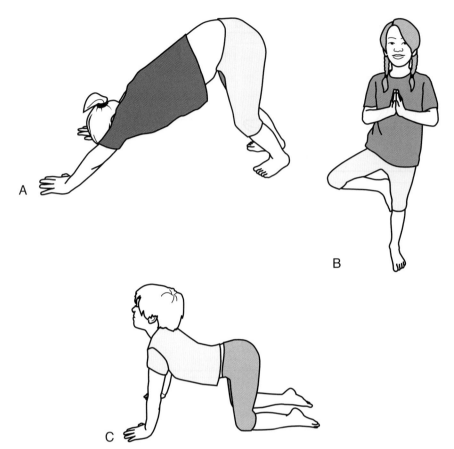

Fig. 9.3 Children performing yoga poses. **(A)** Downward dog pose. **(B)** Tree pose. **(C)** Cow pose.

CHAPTER SUMMARY

ASD is a group of heterogeneous conditions affecting the neurologic development of children. The cause is most likely multifactorial resulting from an interaction of genetic and environmental factors, which produces wide variations in clinical presentation. This diversity of symptoms challenges early diagnosis and EI. Because early motor delays appear to provide a diagnostic clue, it is imperative that physical therapists be involved in screening and EI. Motor deficits interfere with completion of functional tasks and possibly contribute to poor social functioning. Limited social interaction is replaced by repetitive behaviors that prevent participation in critical aspects of childhood such as play and activities of daily living. Interventions have historically focused on managing behavior and sensory issues, but now motor and play interventions are being implemented with promising results. Exercise and physical activities are accepted evidence-based interventions that result in functional improvements and reduction of negative behaviors. Aquatic intervention has shown to be effective in promoting social and motor skill acquisition. A multidisciplinary team approach is required to provide comprehensive interventions for the increasing numbers of children diagnosed with ASD. Physical therapists and physical therapist assistants should be an integral part of the team working with children with ASD and their families.

REVIEW QUESTIONS

1. What is the prevalence of ASD in the US population?
2. Name the major problem areas seen in infants and children with ASD.
3. When should a child be screened for ASD?
4. What sensory processing patterns can be exhibited by children with ASD?
5. Discuss the role of physical therapy in working with children with ASD.
6. What combination of treatment interventions has been shown to improve acquisition of language in children with ASD?
7. How are problem daytime behaviors related to gross motor delays in children with ASD?
8. List the benefits of aquatic therapy for children with ASD.
9. Discuss motor interventions for infants, toddlers, and children with ASD.
10. Which positive behavioral supports are identified in the case study?

CASE STUDIES EXAMINATION AND EVALUATION: BA

History
Review
BA is a 6-year-old boy born full term after an uneventful pregnancy. Early in his development, his parents noted he had difficulty nursing, reduced eye contact, and delays in motor and play skills. He was diagnosed on the autism spectrum at age 2 years. He received early intervention services in the home and community until age 3 years. BA exhibits a delay in expressive language. He has been healthy, with only typical childhood illnesses. He is presently on a gluten-free, dairy-free diet. BA has two older siblings and both parents work. He receives occupational and speech services in the school, as well as ABA and outpatient speech and occupational therapy services.

Subjective
BA's parents are interested in using aquatic therapy to improve his participation in peer activities, tolerance to showering, and motor planning.

Objective
Systems Review
Communication/Cognition: BA communicates his wants and needs using gestures and single words, as well as a picture board for making choices. He makes brief eye contact and follows simple commands when verbal requests are combined with gestures. He is very interested in dinosaurs to the exclusion of other objects. IQ testing results were not available at the time of evaluation, but BA is in an age-appropriate classroom with supports.

Cardiovascular/Pulmonary: Normal values for age. No atypical breathing patterns.

Musculoskeletal: Active range of motion within functional limits for age. He moves against gravity without difficulty.

Neuromuscular: Impaired bilateral coordination and motor planning of complex movements.

Integumentary: Intact.

Tests and Measures
Anthropometrics: Height 48 inches, weight 55 pounds, body mass index 16.8 (20 to 24 is normal).

Motor Function: BA walks without difficulty. He prefers to move quickly using a gallop rather than a run or skip, keeping his eyes down. Occasionally, he will go up on his toes. He can climb a ladder slowly and has difficulty hopping on either foot,

sustaining rhythm, and occasionally initiating movement. BA gets from floor to stand through half kneeling, but tends to place his second foot quickly and pushes up with both legs. Movements are clumsy and uncoordinated with little or no trunk rotation. Hand function is adequate for feeding and simple dressing. He has difficulty tying his shoes and buttoning clothing.

Posture: BA stands leaning forward with shoulder and head in a forward position.

Gait/Locomotion/Balance: BA walks with a reciprocal gait but limited arm swing. He goes up on his toes when he increases his gait speed. He has difficulty climbing structures and walking on unstable surfaces. Single limb stance times are 1 to 2 seconds at most, with eyes open or closed, due to increased trunk movement during the activity.

Play: BA exhibits solitary object play with repetitive actions such as lining up his dinosaurs. He uses single words to describe the actions of the dinosaurs. He tends to use items separately, rather than combining them during play, and although he will play alongside another child for brief periods, he becomes overwhelmed by their activity quickly and moves off to play by himself. BA has difficulty taking turns in group play, and pretend play is significantly limited as evidenced by stereotypical use of objects rather than scenario-based play using objects as intended. For example, BA will line up cars rather than play with them by driving them across the floor or up and down ramps (roads).

Sensory: It is difficult for BA's family to get him into the shower. He dislikes clothes with tags and being messy. BA becomes fearful when asked to walk on an unstable surface like the bridge of a climbing structure. A child Sensory Profile was completed by BA's parents and showed that BA is much more likely to be overwhelmed by sensory experiences than others, and that BA detects more sensory cues than others (Table 9.4).

Bruininks-Oseretsky Test of Motor Proficiency Second Edition
BA was administered a Bruininks-Oseretsky Test of Motor Proficiency Second Edition with modifications to allow BA to fully participate in the items. Results for gross motor subtests are shown in Table 9.5, with upper limb coordination and strength as higher scoring areas, even though the age equivalents in these areas were 6 to 10 months below BA's age. Manual dexterity, bilateral coordination, balance, and running speed/agility were all significantly below age norms.

TABLE 9.4 Sensory Profile Scores

Quadrant	Much Less than Others	Less than Others	Just Like the Majority of Others	More than Others	Much More than Others	
Seeking/seeker	0–6	7–19	20–47	48–60	61–95	BA is just as interested in sensory experiences as the majority of others.
Avoiding/avoider	0–7	8–20	21–46	47–59	60–100	BA is much more likely to be overwhelmed by sensory experiences than others.
Sensitivity/sensor	0–6	7–17	18–42	43–53	54–95	BA detects more sensory cues than others.
Registration/ bystander	0–6	7–18	19–43	44–55	56–110	BA notices sensory cues just like the majority of others.

Continued

CASE STUDY EXAMINATION AND EVALUATION: BA—cont'd

TABLE 9.5 Bruininks-Oseretsky Test of Motor Proficiency Second Edition, Results of Subtests 3-8

Subtest	Raw Score	Scaled Score (mean = 15)	Age Equivalent
Manual dexterity	12	9	4.8
Upper-limb coordination	18	14	5.10
Bilateral coordination	4	8	<4
Balance	9	5	<4
Running speed/agility	12	8	4.2
Strength	12	12	5.4

Assessment/Evaluation

BA is a 6-year-old boy on the autism spectrum who demonstrates repetitive behaviors, communication issues, and anxiety. He has difficulty with balance, bilateral coordination, motor planning, and complex play. His toe walking is not due to limited range of motion. His sensory issues, as well as altered kinesthesia/proprioception, contribute to the problems seen with balance and activities of daily living (ADL). Use of aquatics as an intervention should be considered to increase strength, coordination, body perception, tolerance to water, and participation in swimming and play activities with peers.

Problem List

1. Decreased functional strength, especially in midrange
2. Decreased bilateral coordination and balance
3. Dependent in bathing/showering, face washing, and dressing
4. Decreased play complexity
5. Decreased participation in age-appropriate activities with peers in the pool, playground, and classroom

Diagnosis: BA exhibits impaired motor function, ADL, and social communication skills consistent with autism spectrum disorder.

Prognosis: BA will improve functional skills within all environments. Prognosis is good.

Short-Term Goals (1 to 3 Months)

1. BA will participate fully in a 30-minute aquatic session with minimal redirection.
2. BA will participate in bathing/showering activities without significant distress.
3. BA will consistently reciprocally climb a ladder with minimal verbal cues.
4. BA will demonstrate appropriate play with two objects for 5 minutes.

Long-Term Goals (6 Months)

1. BA will climb on playground equipment (stable and unstable) without assistance.
2. BA will participate in swimming activities with his family at the local pool for 30 minutes without distress.

3. BA will be able to play near peers, either on the playground or in the pool, for 15 minutes without distress.
4. BA will participate in a brief play scenario with toys, like his dinosaurs, with a peer for 5 minutes.

Plan

Coordination, Communication, and Documentation

A weekly aquatic therapy intervention will be implemented to address concerns with movement through space, kinesthetics, and tolerance of water, strength, coordination, and balance. The physical therapist will communicate and coordinate with all other clinicians working with BA to share strategies. Once BA establishes a routine in the pool, the family will be invited to a pool session and encouraged to help progress activities, especially putting his face in the water and getting hair wet, as these relate to bathing and showering. Outcomes of intervention will be documented weekly.

Client Instruction

All interventions will utilize principles from the best practices guidelines on types of feedback, methods of providing information, and amount of repetition (Wong et al., 2015). New activities will be introduced gradually using positive behavioral support such as choices, reinforcement, and rest breaks (Fig. 9.2). Modeling of ADL will be initiated by the therapist who will train the parents to follow through at home. The physical therapist will provide modeling for pool and playground activities and may consider teaching peers to model activities in the pool and on the playground.

Interventions

Pool Program: A sample initial session is provided:

1. Work at edge of pool or on steps to gradually introduce water. The therapist could use dinosaurs and create a story about them swimming to encourage entrance into the water.
2. Walk the dinosaurs down the ramp or steps and back up again, pushing them through the water as they move the water with their movement.
3. Use a float mat as a surface for the dinosaurs to live on and BA could climb up to be with them, moving across the surface and creating a waterfall with a bucket doing dump and fill activities.
4. Move the dinosaurs to the side of the pool and monkey walk along the side to climb through the jungle to reach them.
5. Using a step in a shallow area, walk over and progress to jumping over the trees in the jungle to reach the dinosaurs or help them to get home to family.

Activities in the water that would increase bilateral coordination could include wall crawling, step-ups, and jumping. The pool program may be progressed to having BA go underwater and eventually participate in an obstacle course. Future pool sessions could string steps together and add complexity. Once BA is comfortable with the pool routine, the parents can come to a pool session to learn the routine and encourage BA to use the shower at the pool without getting hair or face wet. These activities may translate to improved tolerance to showering at home and could be incorporated into a visit to the community pool.

Land Program: An initial playground session:

1. Simple walk around the structures, discussing options of activities to complete.

CASE STUDIES EXAMINATION AND EVALUATION: BA—cont'd

2. Present two options on story board and allow BA to choose the first one, stating that both will be done.
3. Complete first activity, maybe a simple climbing activity with a motivator at the top.
4. Use board to move to second activity—walking across bridge with support as needed.
5. Put two more activities on the board during a break, and then discuss these with choice offered.
6. Complete the two activities as previously described.

BA can be prepared for activities in a new environment by using social stories and picture boards. Intervention with BA should begin at a time when there are not a lot of children on the playground. A peer could be used to model climbing, sliding, swinging, and exploring the equipment. However, if a peer is not available, BA could be shown pictures or videos of the activities before engaging in the activity. Gradual introduction to these activities is advised with a slow increase in the sequence. Complexity can be increased by putting two or more related activities together, followed by putting together unrelated activities. Make sure activities can be successful with support but still challenge BA to increase success and learning.

Follow-Up

Once goals have been achieved, BA will be discharged from physical therapy. Periodic follow-up with the family is recommended to assist them with problem-solving any new situations that arise as BA participates more fully in his ADL, and engages with others in typical peer situations.

Questions to Think About

- How can pretend play be incorporated into BA's aquatic therapy?
- How would you use a peer model in BA's activities?
- What signs would indicate that BA is getting overwhelmed? What could your response be?

Resources

Physical Therapist's Guide to Autism Spectrum Disorder: www.moveforwardpt.com/symptomsconditions.aspx
American Academy of Pediatric Physical Therapy: www.pediatricapta.org
Autism Speaks: www.autismspeaks.org
Autism Society: www.autism-society.org/
Centers for Disease Control and Prevention: Act Early: www.cdc.gov/actearly

REFERENCES

Alainz M, Rosenberg S, Beard N, Rosario E: Effectiveness of aquatic group therapy for improving water safety and social interactions in children with ASD: a pilot program, *J Autism Dev Disord* 47(12):4006-4017, 2017.

Allen KA, Bedero B, Van Damme ET, et al.: Test of Gross Motor Development-3 (TGMD-3) with the use of visual supports for children with autism spectrum disorder; validity and reliability, *J Autism Dev Disord* 47(3):813-833, 2017.

American Psychiatric Association: *Diagnostic and statistical manual of mental disorders*, ed 5, Washington DC, 2013, American Psychiatric Association.

Ament K, Mejia A, Buhlman R, et al.: Evidence for specificity of motor impairments in catching and balance in children with autism, *J Autism Dev Disord* 45:742-751, 2015.

Anderson-Hanley C, Tureck K, Schneiderman RL: Autism and exergaming: effects on repetitive behaviors and cognition, *Psychol Res Behav Manag* 4:129-137, 2011.

Antshel K, Hier B: Attention deficit hyperactivity disorder (ADHD) in children with autism spectrum disorders. In Patel VB, Preedy VR, Martin CR, editors: *Comprehensive guide to autism*, New York, 2014, Springer, pp 1013-1029.

Arabameri E, Sotoodeh MS: Early developmental delay in children with autism: a study from a developing country, *Infant Behav Dev* 39:118-123, 2015.

Baranek GT, David FJ, Poe MD, et al.: Sensory experiences questionnaire: discriminating sensory features in young children with autism, developmental delays, and typical development, *J Child Psych* 47:591-601, 2006.

Barber AB, Saffo RW, Gilpin AT, Craft LD, Goldstein H: Peers as clinicians: examining the impact of Stay Play Talk on social communication in young preschoolers with autism, *J Comm Disord* 59:1-15, 2016.

Bar-Haim Y, Bart O: Motor function and social participation in kindergarten children, *Soc Dev* 15(2):296-310, 2006.

Barton EE, Choi G, Mauldin EG: Teaching sequences of pretend play to children with disabilities, *J Early Int* 41(1):13-29, 2019.

Barton EE, Pavilanis MS: Teaching pretend play to young children with autism, *Young Excep Child* 15(1):5-17, 2012.

Ben-Sasson A, Hen L, Fluss R, et al.: A meta-analysis of sensory modulation symptoms in individuals with autism spectrum disorders, *J Autism Dev Disord* 39:1-11, 2009.

Bhat AN, Landa RJ, Galloway JC: Current perspectives on motor functioning in infants, children, and adults with autism spectrum disorders, *Phys Ther* 91:1116-1129, 2011.

Bhat AN, Galloway JC, Landa R: Relation between early motor delay and later communication delay in infants at risk for autism, *Infant Behav Dev* 35:838-846, 2012.

Billstedt E, Gillberg IC, Gillberg C: Autism after adolescence: population-based 13- to 22-year follow-up study of 120 individuals with autism diagnosed in childhood, *J Autism Dev Disord* 35:351-360, 2005.

Bremer E, Balogh R, Lloyd M: Effectiveness of a fundamental motor skill intervention for 4-year-old children with autism spectrum disorder: a pilot study, *Autism* 19(8):9980-9991, 2014.

Bremer E, Lloyd M: School-based fundamental-motor-skill intervention for children with autism-like characteristics: an exploratory study, *Adapt Phys Act Quart* 33:66-88, 2016.

Campbell SB, Mahoney AS, Northrup J, et al.: Developmental changes in pretend play from 22-to 34-months in younger siblings of children with autism spectrum disorder, *J Abnorm Child Psychol* 46:639-654, 2018.

Caputo G, Ippolito G, Mazzotta M, et al.: Effectiveness of a multisystem aquatic therapy for children with autism spectrum disorders, *J Autism Dev Disord* 48:1945-1956, 2018.

Case-Smith J, Weaver LL, Fristad MA: A systematic review of sensory processing interventions for children with autism spectrum disorders, *Autism* 19(2):133-148, 2015. doi:10.1177/1362361313517762.

Centers for Disease Control and Prevention: *Data & statistics on autism spectrum disorder*, 2019. https://www.cdc.gov/ncbddd/autism/data.html. Accessed June 10, 2019.

Charman T, Baron-Cohen S, Swettenham J, et al.: Predicting language outcome in infants with autism and pervasive developmental disorder, *Int J Lang Commun Disord* 38:265-285, 2003.

Chawarska K, Paul R, Klin A, Hannigen S, Dichtel LE, Volkmar F: Parental recognition of developmental problems in toddlers with autism spectrum disorders, *J Autism Dev Disord* 37:62-72, 2007.

Chu CH, Pan CY: The effect of peer- and sibling-assisted aquatic program on interaction behaviors and aquatic skills of children with autism spectrum disorders and their peers/siblings, *Res Autism Spec Disord* 6:1211-1223, 2012.

Daniels AM, Halladay AK, Shih A, Elder LM, Dawson G: Approaches to enhancing the early detection of autism spectrum disorders: a systematic review of the literature, *J Am Acad Child Adolesc Psychiatry* 53:141-152, 2014.

Dawson G, Rogers S, Munson J, et al.: Random clinical trial of an intervention for toddlers with autism: the Early Start Denver Model, *Pediatrics* 125(1):e17-e23, 2010.

Donnellan AM, Hill DA, Leary MR: Rethinking autism: implications of sensory and movement differences for understanding and support, *Front Integr Neurosci* 6:124, 2013.

Doumas M, McKenna R, Murphy B: Postural deficits in autism spectrum disorder: the role of sensory integration, *J Autism Dev Disord* 46:853-861, 2016.

Downey R, Rapport MJ: Motor activity in children with autism: a current review of current literature, *Pediatr Phys Ther* 24:2-20, 2012.

Doyle-Thomas KA, Duerden EG, Taylor MJ, et al.: Effects of age and symptomatology on cortical thickness in autism spectrum disorder, *Res Autism Spectr Disord* 7:141-150, 2013.

Dulcy FH: An integrated developmental aquatic program (IDAP) for children with autism, *Nat Aquatics J* 8(2):7-10, 1992.

Dunn W: *Sensory profile-2*, San Antonio, TX, 2014, Pearson Publishing.

Dunn W, Cox J, Foster L, Mische-Lawson L, Tanquary J: Impact of contextual intervention on child participation and parent competence among children with autism spectrum disorders: a pretest-posttest repeated-measures design, *Am J Occup Ther* 66:520-528, 2012.

Emck C, Bosscher RJ, van Wieringen PC, Doreleijers T, Beek PJ: Gross motor performance and physical fitness in children with psychiatric disorders, *Dev Med Child Neurol* 53:150-155, 2011.

Ennis E: The effects of a physical therapy-directed aquatic program on children with autism spectrum disorders, *J Aquat Phys Ther* 19:4-10, 2011.

Enticott PG, Bradshaw JL Iansek R, Tonge BJ, Rinehart NJ: Electrophysiological signs of supplementary-motor-area deficits in high-functioning autism but not Asperger syndrome: an examination of internally cued movement-related potentials, *Dev Med Child Neurol* 51(10):787-791, 2009.

Eversole M, Collins DM, Karmarkar A, et al.: Leisure activity enjoyment in children with autism spectrum disorders, *J Autism Dev Disord* 46(1):10-20, 2016.

Fabrizi SE: Splashing our way to playfulness! An aquatic playgroup for young children with autism, a repeated measures design, *J Occup Ther Schools Early Int* 8:292-306, 2015.

Fournier KA, Hass CJ, Naik SK, Lodha N, Cauraugh JH: Motor coordination in autism spectrum disorders: a synthesis and meta-analysis, *J Autism Dev Disord* 40:1227-1240, 2010.

Fragala-Pinkham M, Haley SM, O'Neil ME: Group swimming and aquatic exercise programme for children with autism spectrum disorders: a pilot study, *Dev Neurorehabil* 14:230-241. 2011.

Ghanouni P, Memari AH, Gharibzadeh S, Eghlidi J, Moshayedi P: Effect of social stimuli on postural responses in individuals with autism spectrum disorder, *J Autism Dev Disord* 47:1305-1313, 2017.

Gillberg C, Fernell E: Autism plus versus autism pure, *J Autism Dev Disord* 44:3274-3276, 2014.

Gouleme N, Scheid L, Peyre H, et al.: Postural control and emotion in children with autism spectrum disorders, *Transl Neurosci* 8:158-166, 2017.

Green D, Charman T, Pickles A, et al.: Impairment in movement skills of children with autistic spectrum disorders, *Dev Med Child Neurol* 51:311-316, 2009.

Harris SR: Early motor delays as diagnostic clues in autism spectrum disorder, *Eur J Pediatr* 176:1259-1262, 2017.

Hatakenaka Y, Kotani H, Yasumitsu-Lovell K, et al.: Infant motor delay and early symptomatic syndromes eliciting neurodevelopmental clinical examinations in Japan, *Pediatr Neurol* 54:55-63, 2016.

Heathcock JC, Tanner K, Robson D, Young R, Lane AE: Retrospective analysis of motor development in infants at high and low risk for autism spectrum disorder, *Am J Occcup Ther* 69(5):6905185070, 2015.

Hedgecock JB, Dannemiller LA, Shui AM, et al.: Associations of gross motor delay, behavior, and quality of life in young children with autism spectrum disorder, *Phys Ther* 98:251-259, 2018.

Hobson JA, Hobson RP, Malik S, Bargiota K, Calo S: The relationship between social engagement and pretend play in autism, *Brit J Dev Psych* 31:114-127, 2013.

Holloway JM, Long TM, Biasini F: Relationships between gross motor skills and social function in young boys with autism spectrum disorder, *Pediatr Phys Ther* 30:184-190, 2018.

Hu WF, Chahrour MH, Walsh CA: The diverse genetic landscape of neurodevelopmental disorders, *Ann Rev Genom Human Genet* 5:195-213, 2014.

Hyman S, Levy S: Autism spectrum disorders. In Batshaw M, et al., editors: *Children with disabilities*, ed 7, Baltimore, MD, 2013, Paul H. Brookes, pp 345-367.

Ingersoll B, Dvortcsak A: *Teaching social communication: a practitioner's guide to parent training for children with autism*, New York, 2010, Guilford Press.

Johnson CP, Myers SM: Identification and evaluation of children with autism spectrum disorder, *Pediatrics* 120:1183-1215, 2007.

Kanner L: Autistic disturbances of affective contact, *Nervous Child* 2:217-250, 1943.

Kasari C, Gulsrud A, Freeman S, Paparella T, Hellemann G: Longitudinal follow-up of children with autism receiving targeted interventions on joint attention and play, *J Am Acad Child Adolesc Psychiatry* 51(5):487-495, 2012.

Kasari C, Gulsrud A, Wong C, Kwon S, Locke J: Randomized controlled caregiver mediated joint engagement intervention for toddlers with autism, *J Autism Dev Disord* 40:1045-1056, 2010.

Kasari C, Paparella T, Freeman S, Jahroomi LB: Language outcome in autism: randomized comparison of joint attention and play interventions, *J Consult Clin Psychol* 76:125-137, 2008.

Kaur M, Srinivasan S, Bhat AN: Comparing motor performance, praxis, coordination, and interpersonal synchrony between children with and without autism spectrum disorder, *Res Dev Disabil* 72:79-95, 2018.

Ketcheson L, Hauck J, Ulrich D: The effects of an early motor skill intervention on motor skills, levels of physical activity, and socialization in young children with autism spectrum disorder: a pilot study, *Autism* 21(4):481-492, 2017.

Kossyvaki L, Papoudi D: A review of play interventions for children with autism in school, *Int J Disabil Dev Ed* 63:45-63, 2016.

Lai MC, Lombardo MV, Baron-Cohen S: Autism, *Lancet* 383(9920):896-910, 2014.

Landa RJ, Holman KC, O'Neill AH, Stuart EA: Intervention targeting development of socially synchronous engagement in toddlers with autism spectrum disorder: a randomized controlled trial, *J Child Psychol Psychiatry* 52:13-21, 2011.

LeBarton ES, Iverson JM: Associations between gross motor and communication development in at-risk infants, *Infant Behav Dev* 44:59-67, 2016.

Lemcke S, Juul S, Parner ET, Lauritsen MB, Thorsen P: Early signs of autism in toddlers: a followup study in the Danish national birth cohort, *J Autism Dev Disord* 43:2366-2375, 2013.

Leonard HC, Hill EL: Review: the impact of motor development on typical and atypical social cognition and language: a systematic review, *Child Adolesc Ment Health* 19:163-173, 2014.

Levy SE, Giarelli E, Lee LC, et al.: Autism spectrum disorder and co-occurring developmental, psychiatric and medical conditions among children in multiple populations of the United States, *J Dev Behave Pediatr* 31:267-275, 2010.

Libertus K, Landa RJ: Scaffolded reaching experiences encourage grasping activity in infants at high risk for autism, *Front Psychol* 5:1071, 2014.

Lillard A: Pretend play in toddlers. In Brownell CA, Kopp CB, editors: *Socioemotional development in the toddler years: transitions and transformations*, New York, 2007, Guildford Press, pp 149-176.

Lim YH, Partridge K, Girdler S, Morris SL: Standing postural control in individuals with autism spectrum disorder: systematic review and meta-analysis, *J Autism Dev Disord* 47(7):2238-2253, 2017.

Little LM, Dean E, Tomchek S, Dunn W: Sensory processing patterns in autism, attention deficit hyperactivity disorder, and typical development, *Phys Occup Ther Pediatr* 3:243-254, 2018.

Liu T, Breslin CM: The effect of a picture activity schedule on performance of the MABC-2 for children with autism spectrum disorder, *Res Q Exerc Sport* 84(2):206-212, 2013.

Long T, Holloway JM: Children with autism spectrum disorder. In Palisano RJ, Orlin MN, Schreiber J, editor: *Campbell's physical therapy for children*, ed 5, Philadelphia, 2017, Elsevier, pp 583-599.

Lloyd M, MacDonald M, Lord C: Motor skills of toddlers with autism spectrum disorders, *Autism* 17:133-146, 2013.

MacDonald M, Lord C, Ulrich DA: The relationship of motor skills and social communicative skills in school-aged children with autism spectrum disorder, *Adapt Phys Act Quart* 30:271-282, 2013.

Manning MM, Wainright LD: The role of high level play as a predictor of social functioning in autism, *J Autism Dev Disord* 40:523-533, 2010.

Michelle NG, DeMontigny JG, Ofner M, Do MT: Environmental factors associated with autism spectrum disorders: a scoping review for the years 2003-2013, *Health Promot Chronic Dis Prev Can* 37(1):1-23, 2017.

Miller LJ, Anzlone ME, Lane SF, Cermak SA, Osten ET: Concept evolution in sensory integration: a proposed nosology for diagnosis, *Am J Occup Ther* 61:135-140, 2007.

Miller M, Chukoskie L, Zinni M, Townsend J, Trauner D: Dyspraxia, motor function and visual-motor integration in autism, *Behav Brain Res* 269:95-102, 2014.

Minshew NJ, Sung K, Jones BL, Furman JM: Underdevelopment of the postural control system in autism, *Neurology* 63:2056-2061, 2004.

Morris SL, Foster CJ, Parsons R, Falkmer M, Falkmer T, Rosalie SM: Differences in the use of vision and proprioception for postural control in autism spectrum, *Neuroscience* 29:273-280, 2015.

Mortimer R, Privopoulos M, Kumar S: The effectiveness of hydrotherapy in the treatment of social and behavioral aspects of children with autism spectrum disorders: a systematic review, *J Mult Healthcare* 7:93-104, 2014.

Moseley RL, Pulvermüller F: What can autism teach us about the role of sensorimotor systems in higher cognition? New clues from studies on language, action semantics, and abstract emotional concept processing, *Cortex* 100:149-190, 2018.

Murdock LC, Ganz J, Crittendon J: Use of an iPad play story to increase play dialogue of preschoolers with autism spectrum disorder, *J Autism Dev Disord* 43:2174-2189, 2013.

Murdock LC, Hobbs JQ: Picture me playing: increasing pretend play dialogue of children with autism spectrum disorders, *J Autism Dev Disord* 41:870-878, 2011.

Murdoch JD, State MW: Recent developments in the genetics of autism spectrum disorders, *Curr Opin Genet Dev* 23:310-315, 2013.

National Autism Center: Findings and conclusions: National Standards Project: phase 2, 2015.

Nicholson HK, Bray TJ, Heest MA, Van J: The effects of antecedent physical activity on the academic engagement of children with autism spectrum disorder, *Psychol Schools* 48:198-213, 2011.

Nickel AR, Thatcher AR, Keller F, Wozniak RH, Iverson JM: Posture development in infants at heightened vs. low risk for autism spectrum disorder, *Infancy* 18(5):639-661, 2013.

Noyes-Grosser DM, Elbaum B, Wu Y, et al.: Early intervention outcomes for toddlers with autism spectrum disorder and their families, *Infants Young Children* 31:177-199, 2018.

O'Neil ME, Ideishi RI, Benedetto M, Ideishi SK, Fragala-Pinkham M: A yoga program for children in Head Start and early intervention: a feasibility study, *J Yoga Phys Ther* 6:238, 2016. doi:10.4172/2157-7595.1000238.

Oriel KN, George CL, Peckus R, Semon A: The effects of aerobic exercise on academic engagement in young children with autism spectrum disorder, *Pediatr Phys Ther* 23:187-193, 2011.

Oriel KN, Kanupka JW, DeLong KS, Noel K: The impact of aquatic exercise on sleep behaviors in children with autism spectrum disorder: a pilot study, *Focus Autism Other Dev Disabl* 11(4):254-261, 2016.

Oriel KN, Kanupka JW, George CL, et al.: The impact of participation in a structured aquatic exercise program on parents' perceptions of behavior in children with autism spectrum disorder, *J Aquat Phys Ther* 25:12-21, 2017.

Ozonoff S, Young GS, Goldring S, et al.: Gross motor development, movement abnormalities and early identification of autism, *J Autism Dev Disord* 38(4):644-656, 2008.

Paquet A, Olliac B, Bouvard M-P, Golse B, Vaivre-Douret L: Semiology of motor disorders in autism spectrum disorders as highlighted from a standardized neuro-psychomotor assessment, *Front Psychol* 7:1292, 2016.

Petrus C, Adamson SR, Blok L, et al.: Effect of exercise interventions on stereotypic behaviors in children with autism spectrum disorder, *Physiother Can* 60:134-145, 2008.

Posserud M, Hysing M, Helland W, Gillberg C, Lundervold AJ: Autism traits: the importance of "co-morbid" problems for impairment and contact with services. Data from the Bergen Child Study, *Res Dev Disabil* 72:275-283, 2018.

Prupas A, Harvey WJ, Benjamin J: Early intervention aquatics: a program for children with autism and their families, *JOPERD* 77:46-51, 2006.

Reichow B, Hume K, Barton EE, Boyd BA: Early intensive behavioural intervention (EIBI) for young children with autism spectrum disorders (ASD), *Cochrane Database Syst Rev* 5:CD009260, 2018. doi:10.1002/14651858.CD009260.pub3.

Reichow B, Volkmar FR: Social skills interventions for individuals with autism: evaluation for evidence-based practices within a best evidence synthesis framework, *J Autism Dev Disord* 40:149-166, 2010.

Ries E: Physical therapy for people with autism: PTs explain why their role-nonexistent not so long ago-is vitally important today. *PT in Motion* 10(6):26-34, 2018. https://search.ebscohost.com/login.aspx?direct=true&db=rzh&AN=130455649&site=ehost-live. Accessed October 30, 2019.

Richards C, Jones C, Groves L, Moss J, Oliver C: Prevalence of autism spectrum disorder phenomenology in genetic disorders: a systematic review and meta-analysis, *Lancet Psychiatry* 2(10):909-916, 2015.

Ronald A, Hoekstra RA: Autism spectrum disorders and autistic traits: a decade of new twin studies, *Am J Med Genet B Neuropsychiatr Genet* 156B:255-274, 2011.

Rutherford MD, Young GS, Hepburn S, Rogers SJ: A longitudinal study of pretend play in autism, *J Autism Dev Disord* 37:1024-1039, 2007.

Sacrey LA, Zwaigenbaum L, Bryson S, Brian J, Smith IM, Roberts W, et al.: Can parent concerns predict autism spectrum disorder? A prospective study of high-risk siblings from 6 to 36 months of age, *J Am Acad Child Adolesc Psychiatry* 54(6), 470-478, 2015.

Seiden A, Tartick K: Hey! That's my territory! An interdisciplinary approach to evidence-based practice for students with autism spectrum disorder. Presented at Annual Conference of the Academy of Pediatric Physical Therapy, APTA, Chattanooga, TN, Nov. 2018.

Smith LB, Gasser M: The development of embodied cognition: six lessons from babies, *Artificial Life* 11:13-30, 2005.

Sowa M, Meulenbroek R: Effects of physical exercise on autism spectrum disorders: a meta-analysis, *Res Autism Spect Dis* 6:46-57, 2012.

Srinivasan SM, Eigsti IM, Gifford T, Bhat AN: The effects of embodied rhythm and robotic interventions on the spontaneous verbal communication skills of children with autism spectrum disorder (ASD): a further outcome of a pilot randomized control trial, *Res Autism Spectr Disord* 27:73-87, 2016a.

Srinivasan SM, Eigsti IM, Neely LB, Bhat AN: The effects of embodied rhythm and robotic interventions on the spontaneous and responsive social attention patterns of children with autism spectrum disorder (ASD): a pilot randomized controlled trial, *Res Autism Spectr Disord* 27:54-72, 2016b.

Srinivasan SM, Kaur M, Park IK, et al.: The effects of rhythm and robotic interventions on the imitation/praxis, interpersonal synchrony, and motor performance of children with autism

spectrum disorder (ASD): a pilot randomized controlled trial, *Autism Res Treat* 736516, 2015a. doi:10.1155/2015/736516.

Srinivasan SM, Park IK, Neely LB, Bhat AN: A comparison of the effects of rhythm and robotic interventions on repetitive behaviors and affective states of children with autism spectrum disorder (ASD), *Res Autism Spectr Disord* 18:51-63, 2015b.

Srinivasan SM, Pescatello LS, Bhat AN: Current perspectives on physical activity and exercise recommendations for children and adolescents with autism spectrum disorders, *Phys Ther* 94:875-889, 2014.

Stahmer A, Surheinrich J, Reed S, et al.: *Classroom pivotal response teaching*, New York, 2011, Guilford Press.

Stins JF, Emck C: Balance performance in autism: a brief overview, *Front Psychol* 9:901, 2018.

Stins JF, Emck C, de Vries EM, Doop S, Beek PJ: Attentional and sensory contributions to postural sway in children with autism spectrum disorder, *Gait Posture* 42:199-203, 2015.

Sussman D, Leung RC, Vogan VM, Lee W, Trelle S, Lin S, et al.: The autism puzzle: diffuse but not pervasive neuroanatomical abnormalities in children with ASD, *Neuroimag Clin* 15(8):170-179, 2015.

Teitelbaum P, Teitelbaum O, Nye J, Fryman J, Maurere RG: Movement analysis in infancy may be useful for early diagnosis of autism, *Proc Natl Acad Sci USA* 95(23):13982-13987, 1998.

Thelen E: Grounded in the world: developmental origins of the embodied mind, *Infancy* 11:3-28, 2000.

Thelen E: Dynamic systems theory and the complexity of change, *Psychoanal Dialogues* 15:255-283, 2005.

Theoret EH, Kobayashi M, Fregni F, Tager-Flusberg H, Pascual-Leone P: Impaired motor facilitation during action observation in individuals with autism spectrum disorder, *Curr Biol* 15(3):194-282, 2005.

Thurm A, Lord C, Lee LC, Newschaffer C: Predictors of language acquisition in preschool children with autism spectrum disorders, *J Autism Dev Disord* 37:1721-1734, 2007.

Travers BG, Powell PS, Klinger LG, Klinger MR: Motor difficulties in autism spectrum disorder: linking symptom severity and postural stability, *J Autism Dev Disord* 43:1568-1583, 2013.

Warreyn P, Van Der Paelt S, Roeyers H: Social-communicative abilities as treatment goals for preschool children with autism spectrum disorder: the importance of imitation, joint attention, and play, *Dev Med Child Neurol* 56:712-716, 2014.

Waye MM, Cheng HY: Genetics and epigenetics of autism: a review, *Psychiatry Clin Neurosci* 72:228-244, 2018.

Wolfberg P, DeWitt M, Young GS, Nguyen T: Integrated play groups: promoting symbolic play and social engagement in typical peers in children with ASD across settings, *J Autism Dev Disord* 45:830-845, 2015.

Wong C, Odom SL, Hume KA, et al.: Evidence-based practices for children, youth and young adults with autism spectrum disorder: a comprehensive review, *J Autism Dev Disord* 45(7):1951-1966, 2015.

Woolfenden S, Sarkozy V, Ridley G, Coory M, Williams K: A systematic review of two outcomes in autism spectrum disorder - epilepsy and mortality, *Dev Med Child Neurol* 54:302-312, 2012.

Wright B: The real reasons autism rates are up in the US, *Scientific American*. March 3, 2017. https://www.scientificamerican.om/article/the-real-reasons-autism-rates-are-up-in-the-us/. Accessed June 10, 2019.

Wulf G, Lewthwaite R: Optimizing performance through intrinsic motivation and attention for learning: the OPTIMAL theory of motor learning, *Psychon Bull Rev* 23(5):1382-1414, 2016.

Yanardag M, Erkann M, Yilmaz I, Arican E, Duzkantar A: Teaching advance movement exploration skills in water to children with autism spectrum disorders, *Res Autism Spec Disord* 9:121-129, 2015.

Zachor DA, Curatolo P: Participants of Italian-Israeli consensus conference: recommendations for early diagnosis and intervention in autism spectrum disorders: an Italian-Israeli consensus conference, *Eur J Paediatr Neurol* 18(2):107-118, 2014.

Zielinski BA, Prigge MB, Nielsen JA, Foehlich AL, Abildskov TJ, Anderson JS, et al.: Longitudinal changes in cortical thickness in autism and typical development, *Brain* 137(Pt 6):1799-1812, 2014.

Zwaigenbaum L, Bauman ML, Stone WL, Yirmiya N, Estes A, Hansen RL, et al.: Early identification of autism spectrum disorder: recommendations for practice and research, *Pediatrics* 136(Suppl 1):S1-S9, 2015a.

Zwaigenbaum L, Bauman ML, Choueiri R, Kasari C, Carter A, Granpeesheh D, et al.: Early intervention for children with autism spectrum disorder under 3 years of age: recommendations for practice and research, *Pediatrics* 136(Suppl 1):S60-S81, 2015b.

10

Proprioceptive Neuromuscular Facilitation*

Tzurei Chen and Kevin Chui

OBJECTIVES

After reading this chapter, the learner will be able to:

1. State the philosophy of proprioceptive neuromuscular facilitation.
2. List the proprioceptive neuromuscular facilitation patterns for the extremities and trunk.
3. Describe applications of extremity and trunk patterns in neurorehabilitation.
4. Explain the use of proprioceptive neuromuscular facilitation patterns and techniques within postures of the developmental sequence.
5. Identify which proprioceptive neuromuscular facilitation techniques are most appropriate to promote the different stages of motor control.
6. Understand the rationale for using the proprioceptive neuromuscular facilitation approach in neurorehabilitation to address movement impairment.
7. Discuss the motor learning strategies used in proprioceptive neuromuscular facilitation.
8. Discuss evidence to support the use of the proprioceptive neuromuscular facilitation approach in select patient populations.
9. Discuss which outcome measures you will use to examine the effectiveness of proprioceptive neuromuscular facilitation in different patient populations.

INTRODUCTION

The purpose of this chapter is to present one of the most frequently used treatment interventions in neurologic rehabilitation, proprioceptive neuromuscular facilitation (PNF). PNF can be used to (1) improve performance of functional tasks by increasing strength, flexibility, and range of motion, gait, and balance; (2) reduce pain; (3) improve patient satisfaction; and (4) improve health-related quality of life (Westwater-Wood et al., 2010). Integration of these gains assists the patient to (1) establish head and trunk control, (2) initiate and sustain movement, (3) control shifts in the center of gravity (COG), and (4) control the pelvis and trunk in the midline while the extremities move. Using the developmental sequence as a guide, the goal of these techniques is to promote achievement of progressively higher levels of proficiency and functional independence in bed mobility, transitional movements, sitting, standing, and walking.

HISTORY OF PROPRIOCEPTIVE NEUROMUSCULAR FACILITATION

Dr. Herman Kabat, a medical physician, applied his background in neurophysiology to conceptualize this therapeutic approach in the early 1940s. He was joined by two physical therapists,

Margaret Knott in 1947 and Dorothy Voss in 1953. The team collaborated in expanding and refining treatment techniques and procedures to improve motor function. Several years later in 1956, Knott and Voss authored the first book introducing PNF.

The initial focus of these founders was on development and application of integral concepts including resistance, stretch reflexes, approximation, traction, and manual contacts to facilitate movement. Their goal and the goal of their treatment approach was to promote improvement in patient efficiency in motor function and independence in activities of daily living (Kabat, 1961). PNF was based on the understanding of the central nervous system at the time and grew to become a viable treatment method. Kabat, Knott, and Voss continued to treat patients, review the literature, and refine their approach during the ensuing years. Today, clinicians and researchers continue to provide input that allows PNF to grow and evolve. This chapter presents a combination of the traditional interventions used by clinical practitioners and the tenets embraced by the International PNF Association (International Proprioceptive Neuromuscular Facilitation Association, 2015).

---

*The Editors would like to acknowledge Cathy Jeremiason Finch, PT and Terry Chambliss, PT, MHS, OCS for their foundational work on this chapter in previous editions.

TABLE 10.1 Essential Components of Proprioceptive Neuromuscular Facilitation

Manual contacts
Body position and body mechanics
Stretch
Manual resistance
Irradiation
Joint facilitation
Timing of movement
Patterns of movement
Visual cues
Verbal input

BASIC PRINCIPLES OF PROPRIOCEPTIVE NEUROMUSCULAR FACILITATION

Motor learning is enhanced through skilled application of 10 essential components (Knott and Voss, 1968). These concepts are often referred to as the key elements of PNF (Table 10.1).

Manual Contacts

Placing the hands on the skin stimulates pressure receptors and provides information to the patient about the desired direction of movement. Optimally, manual contacts are placed on the skin overlying the target muscle groups and in the direction of the desired movement (Adler et al., 2014). For example, to facilitate shoulder flexion, one or both of the clinician's hands are placed on the anterior and superior surface of the upper extremity (UE); to facilitate trunk flexion, the hands contact the anterior surface of the trunk. A lumbrical grip is preferred to control movement and provide optimal resistance, especially regarding rotation, while avoiding excessive pressure or producing discomfort (Fig. 10.1).

Body Position and Body Mechanics

Dynamic clinician movement that mirrors the patient's direction of movement is essential to effective facilitation. The pelvis, shoulders, arms, and hands of the clinician should be placed in line with the movement. When this is not possible, the arms and hands of the clinician should be in alignment with the movement. Resistance is created through use of the clinician's body weight while the hands and arms remain relatively relaxed (Adler et al., 2014).

Stretch

Kabat proposed that the stretch reflex could be used to facilitate muscle activity. He hypothesized that if the muscle is placed in an elongated position, a stretch reflex could be elicited by producing slight movement farther into the elongated range. A stretch facilitates the muscle that is elongated, synergistic muscles at the same joint and facilitates other associated muscles (Loofbourrow and Gellhorn, 1949). Although quick stretch tends to increase motor response, prolonged stretch can potentially decrease muscle activity; therefore patient response should be closely monitored. More recently, studies have questioned the adequacy of previous neurophysiologic rationales for PNF techniques and proposed alternative hypotheses for consideration (Burke et al., 2000; Chalmers, 2004; Hindle et al., 2012; Mitchell et al., 2009).

The presence of joint hypermobility, fracture, or pain contraindicates the use of facilitatory stretch. Stretch, especially quick stretch, should be applied with caution in the presence of spasticity because individual responses vary, and it may result in undesired motor activity.

Manual Resistance

Resistance is defined by Sullivan and Markos (1995) as "an internal or external force that alters the difficulty of moving." The status of the involved tissue regarding stiffness, length, and neurologic influences dictates the internal resistance that

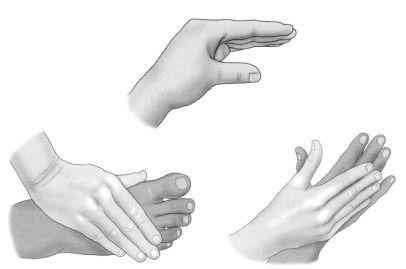

Fig. 10.1 Lumbrical grip. A lumbrical grip is one in which the metacarpophalangeal joints are flexed and adducted while the fingers are in relaxed extension. This position allows flexion forces to be generated through the clinician's hand without squeezing (which provides ambiguous sensory stimulation regarding muscle group and direction) or exerting excessive pressure. This grip provides optimal control of the three-dimensional movements that occur in proprioceptive neuromuscular facilitation patterns.

the patient encounters during movement. Manual, mechanical, or gravitational forces can be used to apply resistance external to the body surface. Some PNF procedures focus on reducing internal resistance by altering neural firing patterns; other activities or techniques provide external resistance to increase motor unit recruitment. Therefore, in the context of PNF, resistance may be considered either a means of neuromuscular facilitation or a tool through which muscle strengthening can be promoted. An 8-week PNF resistance training program demonstrated improvement in strength and alterations in the mean cross-sectional area of the vastus lateralis (Kofotolis et al., 2002, 2005). Through complex interactions among neural and contractile components, resistance may influence movement initiation, postural stability, timing of functional movement patterns, motor learning, endurance, and muscle mass (Sullivan and Markos, 1995).

Appropriate resistance facilitates the maximum motor response that allows proper completion of the defined task (Knott and Voss, 1968). If the goal of intervention is mobility, appropriate resistance is the greatest amount of resistance that allows the patient to move smoothly and without pain through the available range of motion (Kisner and Colby, 2018). The amount and direction of the applied force must adapt to the changes in muscle function and patient ability that may occur throughout the range. If the goal of intervention is stability, appropriate resistance is the greatest amount that allows the patient to isometrically maintain the designated position.

Irradiation

Irradiation is a neurophysiologic phenomenon defined as an increase in activity in related muscles in response to external resistance. By stimulating strong and intact muscles, irradiation facilitates muscle activations in weak and injured muscles (Chiou et al., 2016). This term is often used synonymously with overflow and reinforcement (Adler et al., 2014; Sullivan et al., 1982). The magnitude of the response increases as the stimulus increases in intensity and duration (Sherrington, 1947). Irradiation is a useful technique when the target muscle cannot be strengthened directly (Chiou et al., 2016). Each person's response to resistance varies; therefore different patterns of overflow occur among individuals. By watching patient response, the clinician can identify the manual contacts and amount of resistance that maximize a patient's ability to generate the desired movement. Examples of activities and typical patterns of response include the following:

1. Resistance to trunk flexion produces overflow into the hip flexors and ankle dorsiflexors (Gontijo et al., 2012).
2. Resistance to trunk extension produces overflow into the hip and knee extensors (Gontijo et al., 2012).
3. Resistance to UE extension and adduction produces overflow into the trunk flexors.
4. Resistance to hip flexion, adduction, and external rotation produces overflow into the dorsiflexors.

Traction and Approximation

Traction and approximation stimulate receptors within the joint and periarticular structures. Traction creates elongation of a body segment, which can be used to facilitate motion and decrease pain (Sullivan et al., 1982). Approximation produces compression of body structures, which can be used to promote weight-bearing and muscle cocontraction (Adler et al., 2014). Individual responses to traction and approximation vary. These forces may be applied during performance of extremity patterns or superimposed on body positions.

Timing of Movement

Normal movement requires smooth sequencing and gradation of muscle activation. Timing of most functional movements occurs in a distal to proximal direction, as in picking up a pencil. The pencil is grasped in the hand and then positioned for use by actions of the elbow and shoulder. A related consideration is that development of postural control proceeds from cephalad to caudal and from proximal to distal (Shumway-Cook and Woollacott, 2017). These issues must be considered when assessing, facilitating, and teaching movement strategies in the neurologically impaired individual (Carr and Shepherd, 2014). Adequate muscle strength and joint range of motion may be present to allow execution of a specified functional task; however, sequencing of the components within a movement pattern may be faulty. Also, sufficient control of the trunk and proximal extremity joints must be attained before mastery of tasks that require precise movements of the distal joints.

Patterns of Movement

PNF is characterized by its unique diagonal patterns of movement. Kabat and Knott recognized that groups of muscles work synergistically in functional contexts. They combined these related movements to create PNF patterns. Furthermore, because muscles are spiral and diagonal in both structure and function, most functional movements do not occur in cardinal planes. For example, reaching with an UE and walking are two common activities that occur as triplanar versus uniplanar movements. PNF patterns, therefore, more closely simulate the demands incurred during functional movements.

Visual Cues

Visual cues can help an individual control and correct body position and movement. Eye movement influences head and body position. Feedback from the visual system may be used to promote a stronger muscle contraction (Adler et al., 2014) and to facilitate proper alignment of body parts, such as the head and trunk, through postural reactions.

Verbal Input

A verbal command is used to provide information to the patient. The command should be concise and should provide a directional cue. The verbal command consists of three phases: preparation, action, and correction. The preparatory phase readies the patient for action. The action phase provides information about the desired action and signals the patient to initiate the movement. The correction phase tells the patient how to modify the action if necessary. PNF uses

TABLE 10.2 Proprioceptive Neuromuscular Facilitation Checklist for Clinical Use

Component	Correct	Incorrect
Patient position		
Clinician position		
Clinician's body mechanics		
Manual contacts		
Desired movement		
Stretch		
Verbal command		
Resistance		

the knowledge of the effects of voice volume and intonation to promote the desired response, such as relaxation or greater effort (Adler et al., 2014).

Application of Proprioceptive Neuromuscular Facilitation Principles

When considered as a group, the preceding principles provide a template for the clinical application of PNF techniques. The clinician's hands are placed on the surface of the patient's body in the direction of the desired diagonal movement using a lumbrical grip (see Fig. 10.1). The clinician positions the patient to allow for dynamic movement by aligning the patient's body with the diagonal movement pattern. The body segment is elongated before requesting the patient to move, and a quick stretch is applied if appropriate. A concise verbal command is given and timed to coincide with the initiation of the desired movement. The amount of resistance is graded (increased or decreased to match the patient's ability to generate force) to allow for the desired response. Normal timing is considered and reinforced during the movement pattern. The clinician monitors the patient's response and may add a visual cue to enhance the response. Table 10.2 lists key points to use as a tool for clinical application. This checklist may help the clinician select specific PNF techniques to address individual patient needs.

BIOMECHANICAL CONSIDERATIONS

Other considerations that affect relative ease or difficulty of movement include biomechanical factors such as the base of support (BOS), COG, number of weight-bearing joints, and length of lever arm. The BOS involves both the body surface in contact with the supporting surface and the area enclosed by the contacting body segments. COG refers to the distance of the center of mass of the patient's body to the supporting surface (Shumway-Cook and Woollacott, 2017; Ward et al., 2019). The number of weight-bearing joints involved indicates the complexity and degree of control inherent in the activity. In general, the greater the number of joints through which the line of force passes, the greater is the degree of muscle control required to efficiently perform a related task.

The lever arm is affected by gravity, body weight, and the site of application of the resistive force. The resultant force on the moving segment increases as the distance between the applied force and the target muscles increases. All of these factors must be considered when selecting and progressing activities and techniques within a therapeutic exercise program. A relative increase in difficulty is experienced by the patient when the height of the COG, number of weight-bearing joints, and length of lever arm are increased or the BOS is decreased (Shumway-Cook and Woollacott, 2017). Within the developmental sequence, the natural progression of postures is that of increasing challenge to the stabilizing muscles. Quadruped, therefore, is a more demanding position than prone-on-elbows because of COG location relative to the support surface and differences in surface area within the BOS.

PATTERNS

Early development of PNF techniques included analysis of typical movement strategies (Knott and Voss, 1968). The results of these observations were integrated into specific combinations of joint movements called *patterns*. Although often combined in clinical practice, patterns focus on either the extremities or the trunk. All PNF patterns consist of a combination of motions occurring in three planes. The rotation component is especially important and should be recruited during the beginning range of the pattern. Early rotation reinforces normal distal to proximal timing of extremity movements while recruiting greater participation of the trunk musculature.

Extremity Patterns

The two extremity diagonal patterns are diagrammed in Fig. 10.2. These are named *diagonal 1 (D1)* and *diagonal 2 (D2)*. Extremity patterns are named for the direction of movement occurring in the proximal joint and represent the movement that results from performing the pattern. Each diagonal is further subdivided into *flexion* and *extension* directions. For example, in D_1 flexion in the UE, the shoulder moves into flexion, and in D_1 extension, the shoulder moves into extension. The middle or intermediate joint may be flexed or extended. Straight arm and leg patterns are used to emphasize the proximal component of the pattern and recruit greater trunk activity. When the intermediate joints are flexed, more emphasis can be placed on the intermediate or distal components. The UE patterns will be described in a supine position. Fig. 10.2 illustrates and identifies the components of the UE patterns.

Upper Extremity Patterns

The UE D_1 flexion pattern consists of shoulder flexion/adduction/external rotation. The arm begins in an extended position slightly out to the side, about one fist width from the hip. The shoulder is extended/abducted/internally rotated with the forearm pronated, and the wrist ulnarly deviated. The clinician requests that the patient "squeeze my hand and

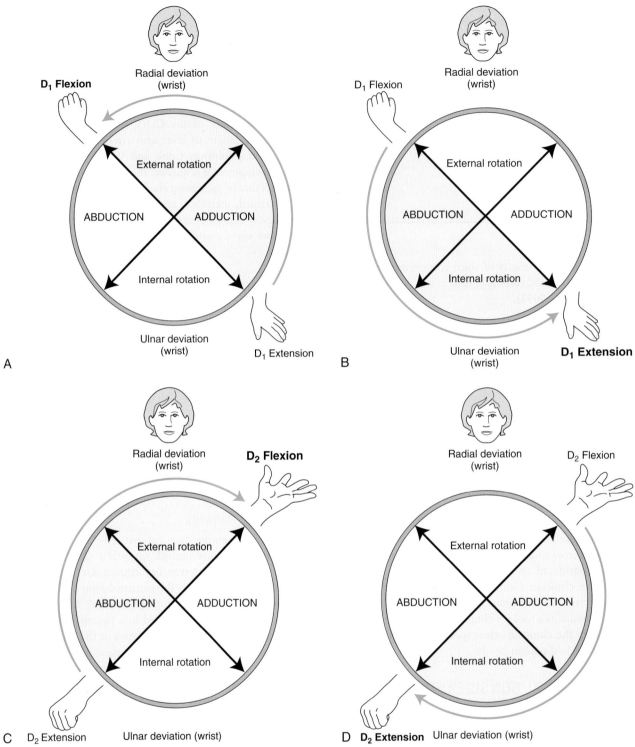

Fig. 10.2 Upper extremity diagonal patterns. The two major diagonal patterns (D_1 and D_2) of the upper extremity are depicted in the four diagrams. The reader should orient herself to the illustration as if the reader is the person (patient role) moving the left arm with the head at the top of the diagram. The posture of the hands is used to help the reader guide the movements in the correct combinations. The shaded areas represent the shoulder components of the pattern in bold type: (A) D_1 flexion, (B) D_1 extension, (C) D_2 flexion, and (D) D_2 extension. For example, to perform D_1 flexion, the reader begins with the hand in the D_1 extension hand position in which the left hand is thrust slightly out from the left side of the body as if in preparation to stop a fall and performs the shaded movements depicted in (A), i.e., shoulder external rotation and adduction, so that the hand ends up in the D_1 hand position (the left hand has performed a movement similar to grasping a scarf and bringing it across the body and over the right shoulder). To perform D_1 extension, the reader looks at (B) and starts in the D_1 flexion hand position, performing the shaded movements in a reverse sequence. To perform D_2 flexion, the reader starts with the left hand curled in a fist next to the right hip with the arm across the body and then moves the arm up and to the left as if in preparation to throw something over the left shoulder. D_2 extension is performed in a reverse sequence.

TABLE 10.3 Upper Extremity D₁ Flexion–Flexion/Adduction/External Rotation–Elbow Extended

Joint	Starting Position	Ending Position
Scapula	Posterior depression	Anterior elevation
Shoulder	Extension/abduction/internal rotation	Flexion/adduction/external rotation
Elbow	Extension	Extension
Forearm	Pronation	Supination
Wrist	Extension/ulnar deviation	Flexion/radial deviation
Fingers	Extension	Flexion

TABLE 10.4 Upper Extremity D₁ Extension–Extension/Abduction/Internal Rotation–Elbow Extended

Joint	Starting Position	Ending Position
Scapula	Anterior elevation	Posterior depression
Shoulder	Flexion/adduction/external rotation	Extension/abduction/internal rotation
Elbow	Extension	Extension
Forearm	Supination	Pronation
Wrist	Flexion/radial deviation	Extension/ulnar deviation
Fingers	Flexion	Extension

pull up." It may be helpful for the clinician to suggest that the patient think about reaching up to bring a scarf over the opposite shoulder.

The UE D₁ extension pattern is the reverse of the flexion pattern and consists of extension/abduction/internal rotation. The patient starts with the arm flexed with the elbow across the midline of the body at about the nose level. The forearm is supinated with the wrist and fingers flexed and the wrist radially deviated. The clinician requests that the patient "open your hand and push down and out." The UE D₁ flexion diagonal pattern is often thought of as functional for feeding and the UE D₁ extension pattern as functional for performing a protective reaction when in a sitting position. Detailed descriptions of the UE D₁ flexion pattern and the UE D₁ extension pattern are found in Tables 10.3 and 10.4, respectively. Performance of the UE D₁ flexion pattern and UE D₁ extension pattern are depicted in Interventions 10.1 and 10.2, respectively.

The D₂ flexion pattern consists of shoulder flexion/abduction/external rotation. The arm begins extended across the body with the elbow crossing the midline, forearm pronated, wrist and fingers flexed, and wrist ulnarly deviated. The clinician asks the patient to "lift your wrist and arm up." The UE D₂ extension pattern is the reverse of the flexion pattern and consists of shoulder extension/adduction/internal rotation. The arm begins in flexion about one fist width lateral to the ipsilateral ear. The shoulder is externally rotated with the

forearm supinated, wrist and fingers extended, and the wrist radially deviated. The clinician requests that the patient "squeeze my hand and pull down and across."

Students can remember these diagonals functionally by thinking of D₂ flexion as throwing a wedding bouquet over the same shoulder and D₂ extension as placing a sword in its sheath. Detailed descriptions of the UE D₂ flexion pattern and UE D₂ extension pattern are found in Tables 10.5 and 10.6, respectively. Performance of the UE D₂ flexion pattern and UE D₂ extension pattern are depicted in Interventions 10.3 and 10.4, respectively.

The following associations may help students remember the movement combinations in the UE. Flexion patterns are always paired with shoulder external rotation, forearm supination, and radial deviation of the wrist. Conversely, UE extension patterns are always paired with shoulder internal rotation, forearm pronation, and ulnar deviation of the wrist.

Scapular Patterns

The scapula moves in diagonal patterns in keeping with scapulohumeral biomechanics. The scapular pattern associated with D₁ flexion is *anterior elevation*. The scapula elevates and protracts as the arm comes across the body. The scapular pattern associated with D₁ extension is the opposite of anterior elevation or *posterior depression*. The scapula is depressed and retracted. To help visualize these movements, consider shrugging your shoulder forward toward your ear as being associated with the UE D₁ flexion pattern and putting the inferior angle of your right scapula in the left hip pocket as related to D₁ extension. These patterns are pictured in Interventions 10.5 and 10.6, respectively.

The scapular pattern associated with D₂ flexion is *posterior elevation*. As the arm is lifted up and externally rotated, the scapula is posteriorly elevated. Shrugging with the shoulder held back is approximately the same motion as the scapula is elevated and retracted. Scapular *anterior depression* is part of the D₂ extension pattern and is the opposite of posterior elevation. The scapula is depressed and protracted as when pushing up to sitting from side-lying. These patterns are shown in Interventions 10.7 and 10.8, respectively.

A clock is a useful way to visualize the scapula moving on the thorax. The patient is positioned in left side-lying. Twelve o'clock is toward the patient's head, and six o'clock is toward the feet. Fig. 10.3 depicts the placement of the scapular diagonals on a clock face. Posterior elevation is at eleven o'clock, and diagonally opposite at five o'clock is anterior depression. Anterior elevation is at one o'clock, and diagonally opposite at seven o'clock is posterior depression.

Lower Extremity Patterns

The lower extremity (LE) patterns are illustrated and explained in supine position but will be related to functional movements in sitting and standing (Fig. 10.4). Analogous to the UE, four LE patterns along two diagonals will be described. The D₁ flexion pattern in the LE includes hip flexion/adduction/external rotation. The pattern begins with the leg resting on the support surface with heel in line with

INTERVENTION 10.1   Upper Extremity D₁ Flexion

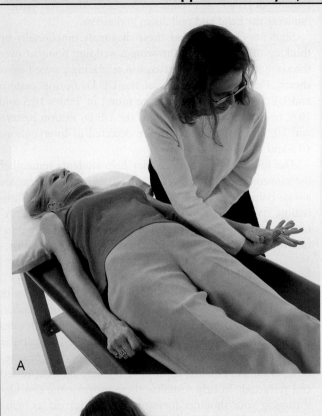

A

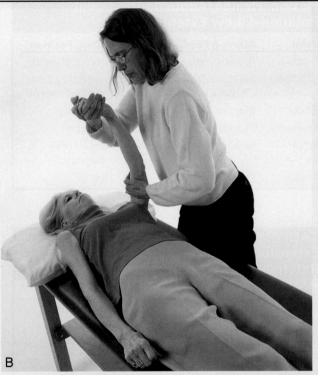

B

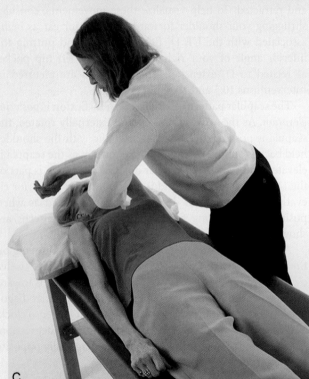

C

The pattern begins in the lengthened position of the primary muscles involved (extension) and ends in the shortened position of the same muscle groups (flexion). The patient's left upper extremity is being treated. The clinician's right hand is placed distally; her left hand proximally.

A. Beginning. The clinician stands in the diagonal position and faces the patient's feet. The clinician's right palm contacts the patient's left palm, similar to holding hands as if going for a walk. The palmar surface of the clinician's left hand is placed on the anterior aspect of the patient's arm just proximal to the elbow. The verbal command is given to "turn your hand up and pull up and across your body."

B. Midrange. As the patient pulls the left upper extremity across the body, the clinician remains in the diagonal position while pivoting to face the patient. Manual contacts may shift slightly to accommodate patient effort.

C. End range. The patient completes the range with hand placements consistent with the previous description of midrange.

ipsilateral shoulder. The hip is abducted and internally rotated. The foot is plantar flexed and everted. The patient is requested to "pull your foot up and in and pull your leg across." Knee flexion frequently accompanies associated functional movements and is, therefore, the most common direction of movement for the intermediate joint during this pattern. This is the motion used to cross one leg over the other in sitting or to bring the foot up to the opposite hand to take off a shoe. If the person is supine, the LE no longer contacts the surface as the knee and foot move toward the contralateral hip.

INTERVENTION 10.2 Upper Extremity D₁ Extension

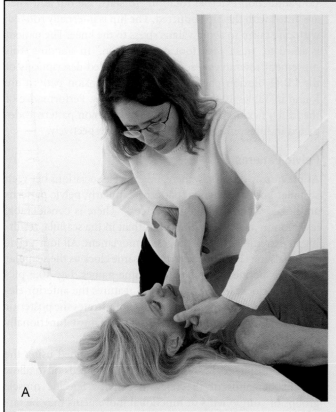

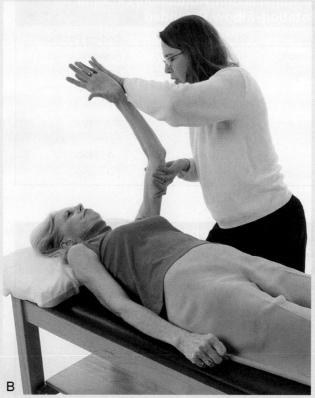

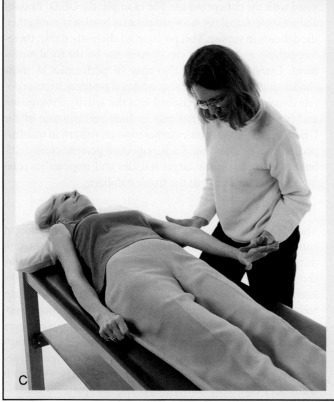

A

B

C

The pattern begins in the lengthened range of the involved muscle groups (flexion) and ends in the shortened range (extension). The patient's left upper extremity is treated. The clinician's left hand contacts the dorsal aspect of the patient's hand, including the fingers. The clinician's right palm contacts the patient's dorsal arm, just proximal to the elbow.

A. Beginning. The clinician stands in the diagonal position and faces the patient. The given verbal command is "turn your hand down and push down and out to the side." The patient extends the wrist and fingers and pronates the forearm, as if pushing the clinician away. Note that some clinicians prefer to face the patient's feet in the starting position of this pattern.

B. Midrange. The clinician shifts body weight and position to accommodate movement through the range. Manual contacts continue on the dorsal hand or fingers and the dorsal and distal aspect of the patient's humerus.

C. End range. The clinician pivots toward the patient's feet while remaining in the diagonal position. Manual contacts remain as previously. It is important that during the latter part of this pattern that as the clinician facilitates or resists wrist extension, the force is parallel to the patient's forearm.

CAUTION: Care must be taken to avoid application of force perpendicular to the forearm, which can result in resistance to the shoulder flexors. This input disrupts the flow of the pattern and often confuses the patient as to the intent of the movement.

TABLE 10.5 Upper Extremity D₂ Flexion–Flexion/Abduction/External Rotation–Elbow Extended

Joint	Starting Position	Ending Position
Scapula	Anterior depression	Posterior elevation
Shoulder	Extension/adduction/ internal rotation	Flexion/abduction/ external rotation
Elbow	Extension	Extension
Forearm	Pronation	Supination
Wrist	Flexion/ulnar deviation	Extension/radial deviation
Fingers	Flexion	Extension

TABLE 10.6 Upper Extremity D₂ Extension–Extension/Adduction/Internal Rotation–Elbow Extended

Joint	Starting Position	Ending Position
Scapula	Posterior elevation	Anterior depression
Shoulder	Flexion/abduction/ external rotation	Extension/adduction/internal rotation
Elbow	Extension	Extension
Forearm	Supination	Pronation
Wrist	Extension/radial deviation	Flexion/ulnar deviation
Fingers	Extension	Flexion

The D_1 extension pattern is a hip extension/abduction/ internal rotation and follows the same diagonal but in the opposite direction as D_1 flexion. The pattern begins with the hip externally rotated and the hip and knee flexed. The foot is dorsiflexed and inverted. The patient is requested to "push your foot down and out." This motion is similar to the stance phase of gait and coming to stand from a seated position. At the end of the pattern, the hip and knee are extended with the ankle in plantar flexion and eversion. Detailed descriptions of LE D_1 flexion pattern and LE D_1 extension pattern are found in Tables 10.7 and 10.8, respectively. Performance of the LE D_1 flexion pattern and LE D_1 extension pattern are depicted in Interventions 10.9 and 10.10, respectively.

Two additional patterns follow the second LE diagonal (D_2); hip components of the D_2 flexion pattern include hip flexion/abduction/internal rotation. The leg begins in hip and knee extension with external rotation of the hip. To position the knee past the midline of the body, the leg not involved in the pattern is abducted. The foot is plantar flexed and inverted. The patient is requested to "pull your foot up and out." This pattern has euphemistically been called the *fire hydrant* as the end position resembles the movement used by an animal to relieve itself. D_2 flexion is not used as frequently as the other LE patterns but does provide a means to elicit eversion with dorsiflexion, which is a movement combination that is often difficult for patients who have had a stroke.

The LE D_2 extension pattern is characterized by hip extension/adduction/external rotation. To start, the hip and knee are flexed with the hip abducted. The hip is internally rotated, with care taken to avoid valgus stress to the knee. The patient is asked to "push your foot down and in." In standing, this movement resembles a soccer kick. Detailed descriptions of the LE D_2 flexion pattern and LE D_2 extension pattern are found in Tables 10.9 and 10.10, respectively. Performance of the LE D_2 flexion pattern and LE D_2 extension pattern is depicted in Interventions 10.11 and 10.12, respectively.

Pelvic Patterns

As previously discussed, there are direct associations between scapular and UE diagonal patterns. Similarly, pelvic patterns are linked with LE diagonal patterns. There is considerably less motion available in the pelvis than in the scapula, resulting in extremely narrow ranges of movement. All four pelvic diagonals may be visualized on the same clock as the scapular diagonals because they have the same names. Fig. 10.3 pictures this clock. Intervention 10.13 features the anterior elevation pattern and Intervention 10.14 illustrates the posterior depression pelvic pattern. These are the most functionally relevant pelvic patterns.

Patterns and basic principles may be modified using the PNF philosophy to address specific patient needs or to allow for the demands of the relevant activity. Specific muscle groups or components of functional movements may be targeted with the patient supine. For example, the UE D_2 flexion/ abduction/external rotation pattern may be used to strengthen the deltoids in supine. This position is inherently stable; therefore patient and clinician can concentrate on the focal movement. Extremity patterns also may be performed in more challenging postures, such as quadruped position, to incorporate dynamic total body control into the activity. Progression and functional integration may include performance of the UE D_2 flexion/abduction/external rotation pattern in quadruped, sitting, or standing. Each respective posture creates different demands on the target muscles and imposes increasingly greater challenge to the trunk stabilizers.

Trunk Patterns

The PNF approach recognizes the trunk as the foundation of controlled movement. To maximize recruitment of the trunk musculature, patterns are used that emphasize either the shoulder or pelvic girdles, or bilateral extremity patterns. *Bilateral extremity patterns* and *trunk patterns* are synonymous terms that will be considered in detail in the following section. The scapula and pelvis are the connecting segments between the trunk and the respective extremities. Thus scapular and pelvic patterns are used to improve the quality, sequence, strength, range of motion, and coordination of both trunk and extremity movements. Scapular patterns directly influence UE function and alignment of the cervical and thoracic spine, whereas pelvic patterns influence LE function and alignment of the lumbar spine. Scapular and pelvic movements may be targeted as components of related extremity patterns or performed in a more isolated manner.

INTERVENTION 10.3 Upper Extremity D₂ Flexion

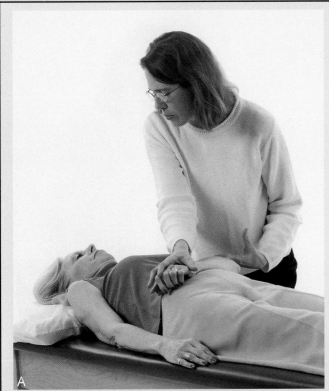

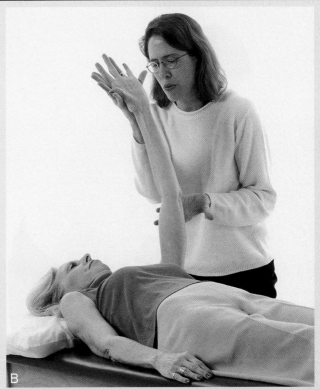

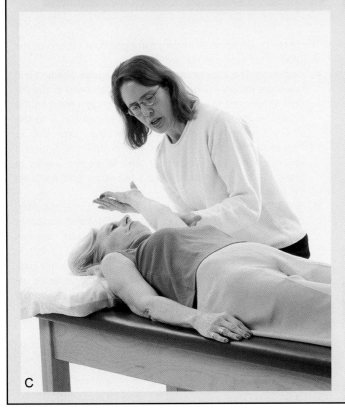

The pattern is pictured as applied to the patient's left upper extremity. The clinician's right hand contacts the dorsal aspect of patient's hand, with the left hand on the dorsal humeral region.

A. Beginning. The clinician stands in the diagonal position and faces the patient's left hip. The clinician's right palm contacts the patient's dorsal hand, and then places the dorsal aspect of her left hand against the patient's dorsal humerus, just proximal to the elbow. The given command is "open your hand and lift your thumb up and out."

B. Midrange. As the patient moves into midrange, the clinician shifts backward. The clinician's left hand naturally supinates with the movement, allowing the palm to now contact the patient's dorsal arm. The clinician's right thumb may be used to facilitate or resist thumb abduction.

C. End range. Movement continues through range with manual contacts remaining similar to those at midrange. The clinician shifts farther posteriorly as needed to accommodate patient movement.

INTERVENTION 10.4 Upper Extremity D₂ Extension

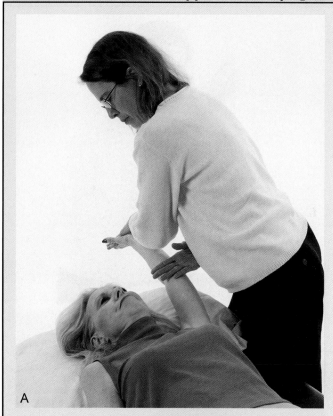

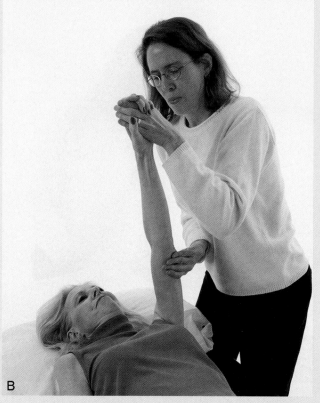

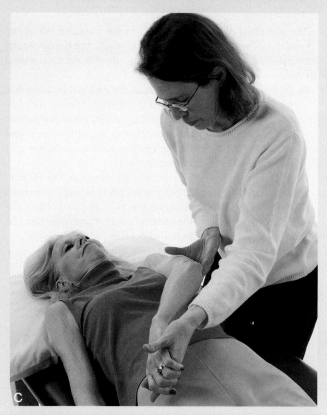

The patient's left upper extremity participates, starting with the shoulder in a flexed position overhead.

A. Beginning. The clinician stands in the diagonal position and faces the patient. She then places the left hand in the patient's palm and the dorsal aspect of the right hand on the anterior surface of the patient's arm, just proximal to the elbow. The pattern commences on the command to "squeeze my hand, turn your thumb down and toward your opposite hip." The patient then flexes her fingers to grasp the clinician's hand, flexes the wrist, and pronates the forearm.

B. Midrange. As the patient extends and adducts her shoulder, the clinician pivots to face the patient's feet and supinates the forearm such that the patient's dorsal arm now lies within the clinician's open hand.

C. End range. The patient completes the motion as the clinician shifts her weight backward to resist the patient's efforts as appropriate. The clinician maintains similar manual contacts as described for midrange.

INTERVENTION 10.5 Scapular Anterior Elevation

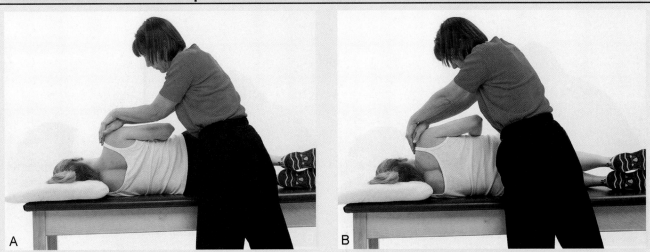

The patient is pictured in left side-lying with the cervical spine in neutral position. The right scapular region is addressed. The clinician stands behind the patient, approximately at level with the patient's pelvis. The clinician stands in the diagonal position and faces the patient's head.

A. Beginning. The clinician's right hand contacts the patient's right acromial region. The clinician's left hand is placed on top of and reinforces her right. The patient is asked to "shrug your shoulder forward toward your ear."

B. End. The patient completes the motion while the clinician shifts her body weight onto the forward foot, mirroring patient movement.

INTERVENTION 10.6 Scapular Posterior Depression

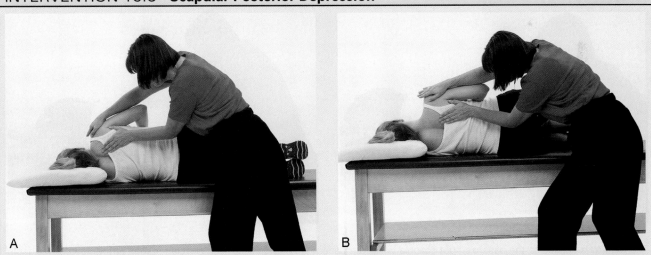

The patient is lying on the left side and the right shoulder region is treated. The clinician stands in the diagonal position, behind the patient and facing her head.

A. Beginning. The clinician's right hand is placed on the patient's right acromion with her left hand contacting the inferior and medial border of the scapula. The pattern begins on the command "pull your shoulder blade down and back."

B. End. As the patient continues through the range, the clinician shifts her body weight onto the back leg to counter patient effort.

INTERVENTION 10.7   Scapular Posterior Elevation

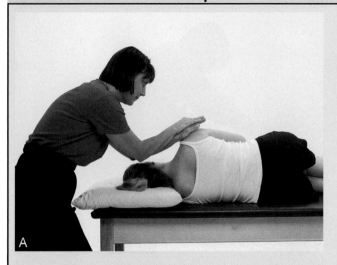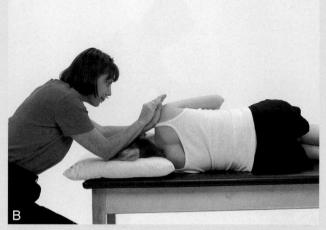

The pattern is performed with the right scapula with the patient lying on the left side. The clinician stands in the diagonal position at the end of the table adjacent and slightly posterior to the patient's head.

A. Beginning. The clinician's left hand is placed slightly posterior to the patient's right acromion; the right hand covers the left hand. The patient is asked to "shrug your shoulder up and back."

B. End. As the patient elevates and adducts the scapula, the clinician shifts her body weight backward.

INTERVENTION 10.8   Scapular Anterior Depression

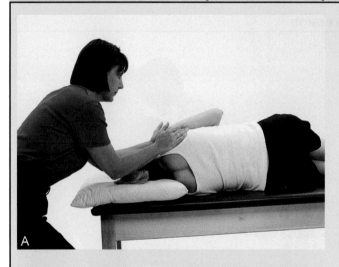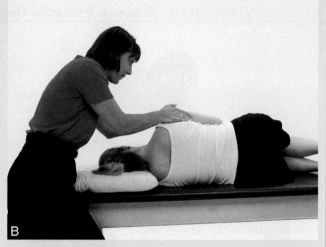

The pattern is applied to the patient's right scapula while the patient is left side-lying. The clinician stands at the head of the table adjacent and slightly posterior to the patient's head.

A. Beginning. Manual contacts are positioned slightly anterior to the patient's right acromion with the left hand under the right. The verbal command "push your shoulder blade down and forward" is given.

B. End. The clinician shifts her weight forward as the patient depresses and adducts the scapula.

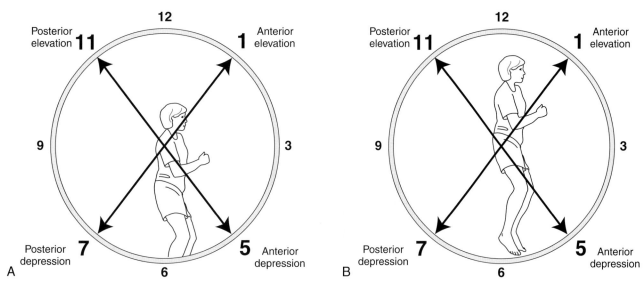

Fig. 10.3 Scapula and pelvic diagonal patterns. Visualizing a clock is a useful way to understand the scapular and pelvic diagonals. (A) The axis for the scapular diagonals occurs at the right shoulder. Posterior elevation is diagonally opposite anterior depression, whereas anterior elevation is diagonally opposite posterior depression. (B) The axis of motion is at the right hip.

Side-lying is an excellent position for performing scapular and pelvic patterns because it provides ease of access for the clinician and unrestricted movement for the patient. The scapular and pelvic PNF patterns are components of functional activities such as rolling, reciprocal arm movements, scooting in supine and sitting, and gait. As previously described, there are two diagonal patterns for both the scapula and the pelvis. These diagonals are narrow, and excessive spinal rotation should be avoided.

Upper Trunk Patterns

Although Knott and Voss described both upper and lower trunk patterns, practical considerations minimize the application of lower trunk patterns. Proper performance of lower trunk patterns entails considerable physical demands on both the patient and the therapist, rendering their clinical use much more infrequent than those patterns targeting the upper trunk. The remaining discussion will address upper trunk patterns only. The term *upper trunk patterns* refers to synchronous performance of PNF patterns with both UEs. This therapeutic tool can promote activation of the trunk musculature, especially the rotators. The two extremities are in contact with each other. One hand holds the other extremity at the wrist. The extremity in which the hand is free may also be referred to as the *lead arm* (Adler et al., 2014; Sullivan et al., 1982). The movement of the lead arm determines the specific name of the trunk pattern. If the lead arm follows the D_2 flexion pattern, the movement is termed a *lifting pattern*. This pattern is depicted in Intervention 10.15.

Facilitatory manual contacts may be used and vary according to the patient abilities and impairments. The combination of two extremities working together increases the irradiation or overflow into the trunk musculature. Resistance may be used to promote isotonic movement throughout the

entire range or to enhance isometric contraction in a desired position. Holding the end range position of a lift can facilitate trunk extension, elongation on one side of the trunk, and a weight shift. The downward motion from the lift position is traditionally referred to as a *reverse lift*. In a reverse lift, the lead arm performs a D_2 extension pattern. This trunk pattern is pictured in Intervention 10.16.

The other upper trunk pattern created by concurrent movement of the upper extremities is called a *chopping pattern*. The extremities are in contact as previously described. The extremity with the free hand, or the lead arm, is again used for naming the pattern. In a chop, the lead arm follows and moves through the D_1 extension pattern, as seen in Intervention 10.17. This combination of UE patterns facilitates trunk flexion, shortening of the trunk on one side, and a weight shift. The upward motion returning from the chop may be referred to as a *reverse chop* (Adler et al., 2014; Sullivan et al., 1982), which is shown in Intervention 10.18. The direction of the weight shift during both chopping and lifting differs from patient to patient. The clinician is encouraged to vary the position of the arms and to use both traction and approximation forces to determine the optimal response for each individual.

PROPRIOCEPTIVE NEUROMUSCULAR FACILITATION TECHNIQUES

The goal of PNF techniques is to promote functional movement through facilitation, inhibition, strengthening, or relaxation of muscle groups (Adler et al., 2014; Sharman et al., 2006). These techniques are designed to promote or enhance specific types of muscle activity associated with a target pattern, posture, or task. Some techniques focus on isometric contractions to increase stability in a chosen position; others

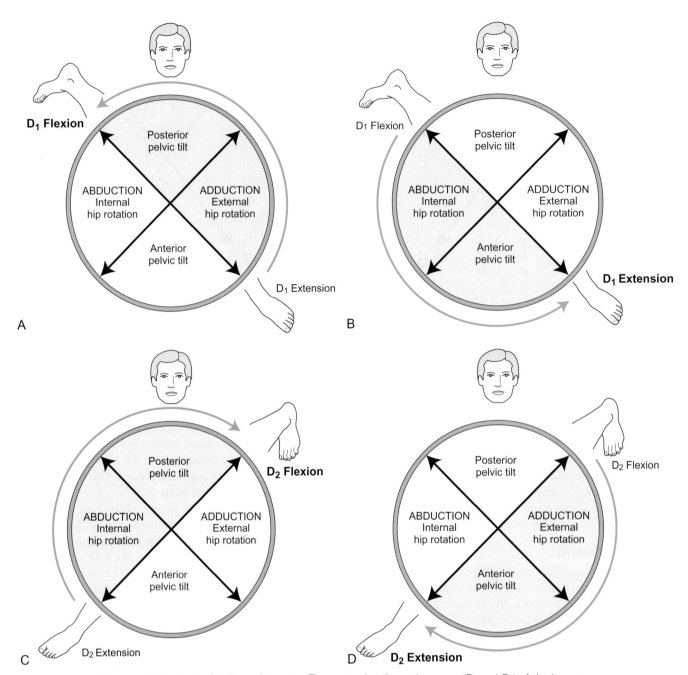

Fig. 10.4 Lower extremity diagonal patterns. The two major diagonal patterns (D₁ and D₂) of the lower extremity are depicted. The reader should orient himself or herself to the illustration as if the reader is the person moving the left leg with the head at the top of the diagram. The posture of the feet is used to help the reader guide his movements in the correct combinations. Unlike the upper extremity, hip internal rotation is *always* paired with abduction, and hip external rotation is *always* paired with adduction. The shaded areas represent the components of the pattern: (A) D₁ flexion, (B) D₁ extension, (C) D₂ flexion, and (D) D₂ extension. For example, to perform D₁ flexion, the reader places the foot in the D₁ extension position (which is out to the side as if taking a protective step) and performs the shaded movement, as depicted in (A) so that the foot ends up in the D₁ flexion position, with the bottom of the foot turned up (as if about to cross the left leg over the right). To perform D₁ extension, the reader looks at (B) and places the foot in the D₁ foot position, then performs the shaded movements in a reverse sequence. To perform D₂ flexion, the reader places the left foot in the D₂ extension position. To get to the D₂ foot position, the reader moves the right leg out to the side, allowing the left foot to cross the midline of the body. The reader performs the shaded movements in (C) so the foot ends up in the D₁ flexion foot position, much like a dog lifting its leg at a fire hydrant. D₂ extension is performed in a reverse sequence, as in a soccer kick.

TABLE 10.7 Lower Extremity D₁ Flexion–Flexion/Adduction/External Rotation–Knee Flexed

Joint	Starting Position	Ending Position
Pelvis	Posterior depression	Anterior elevation
Hip	Extension/abduction/internal rotation	Flexion/adduction/external rotation
Knee	Extension	Flexion
Ankle	Plantar flexion/eversion	Dorsiflexion/inversion

TABLE 10.8 Lower Extremity D₁ Extension–Extension/Abduction/Internal Rotation–Knee Extended

Joint	Starting Position	Ending Position
Pelvis	Anterior elevation	Posterior depression
Hip	Flexion/adduction/external rotation	Extension/abduction/internal rotation
Knee	Flexion	Extension
Ankle	Dorsiflexion/inversion	Plantar flexion/eversion

promote movement through a functional range, using isotonic contractions. Techniques can be used to alleviate impairments in motor-control characteristic of specific stages, such as mobility, stability, controlled mobility, and skill (Table 10.11).

Some techniques address tissue shortness, which limits joint range of motion; others enhance movement initiation. Names assigned to the techniques indicate the focus of that technique. These names have evolved over the last several decades. This process has caused confusion because a specific technique may be referred to by more than one name. The names of techniques presented in this chapter are those most commonly used by clinicians. If the International PNF Association has proposed a different term, it is given in parentheses. The techniques will be presented according to the primary stage of motor control that each promotes, beginning with the *mobility* stage.

Rhythmic Initiation

Rhythmic initiation is a technique that focuses on improving *mobility* that is impaired by deficits in movement initiation, coordination, or relaxation. This technique involves sequential application of first passive, then active assisted, then active or slightly resisted motion. Passive movement is used to encourage relaxation and teach the movement or task. Once relaxation is achieved, the patient is asked to assist. The clinician constantly monitors the patient's movement strategies. If appropriate recruitment patterns are noted, the progression continues such that manual contacts remain in place, but no assistance is provided by the clinician. Slight resistance may then be added to promote further muscle contraction and reinforce the movement pattern. This technique can be used

successfully with any pattern or activity, particularly as a teaching tool. It is frequently used with lower level functional tasks, such as rolling. Patients with hypertonicity who have difficulty initiating functional movements are especially appropriate candidates for this technique.

Rhythmic initiation may be used successfully to promote efficient patterns of rolling. The patient begins supine with the head turned toward the side to which he or she intends to roll. The UE on that side is prepositioned so that it is away from the body. The therapist passively moves the patient into a side-lying position using manual contacts on the trunk and extremities while asking the patient to feel the movement. The clinician then asks the patient to move toward the clinician's manual contacts. The goal is for the patient to continue to increase motor recruitment and desired movement. Facilitatory manual contacts remain in place, but assistance is gradually withdrawn. When appropriate, the clinician may apply slight resistance to the rolling movement through manual contacts on the trunk or extremities.

Rhythmic Rotation

Rhythmic rotation is characterized by application of passive movement in a rotational pattern. The movement is slow and rhythmic in an attempt to promote total body relaxation or tone reduction. The goal is to lessen spasticity to allow further active or passive joint *mobility*. The clinician applies slow rotary movements about the longitudinal axis of the part. The patient is instructed to relax and allow the clinician to perform these movements without assistance. The technique can affect both resting muscle tone and hypertonicity that presents during attempts at active movement (Sullivan et al., 1982).

Lower trunk rotation in hook-lying is an example of rhythmic rotation. The patient is positioned supine with the hips and knees flexed and the feet flat on the surface. The clinician kneels and faces the patient with his or her knees on either side of the patient's feet to help stabilize the LE. Manual contacts are placed on the lateral aspect of the knees or another suitable position on the thighs to allow adequate control. With the clinician's trunk moving as a unit with the patient's lower body, the patient's knees are moved side to side, producing lower trunk rotation.

Hold Relax Active Movement

The hold relax active movement (replication) technique enhances functional *mobility* by facilitating recruitment of muscle contraction in the lengthened range of the agonist. Only one direction of a movement pattern is emphasized. A resisted isometric contraction of the agonist pattern in a shortened range is used to increase muscle spindle sensitivity. Once an optimal contraction is achieved, the patient is asked to relax. The clinician then passively moves the part toward the lengthened position in increments according to patient response. A quick stretch may be applied concurrently with a command for the patient to move into the agonist pattern. Light resistance is often applied as a facilitatory element, although resistance is not mandatory.

INTERVENTION 10.9 **Lower Extremity D₁ Flexion**

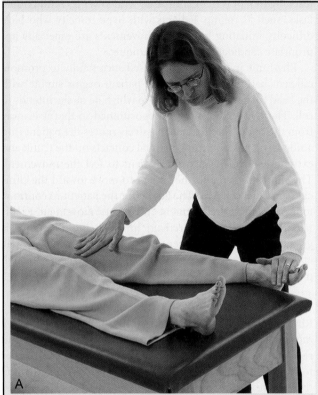

A

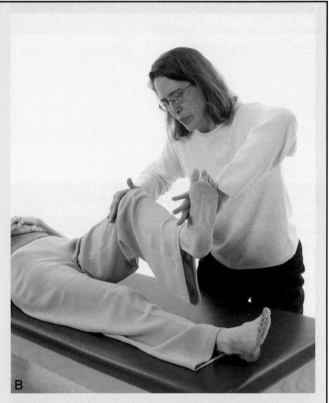

B

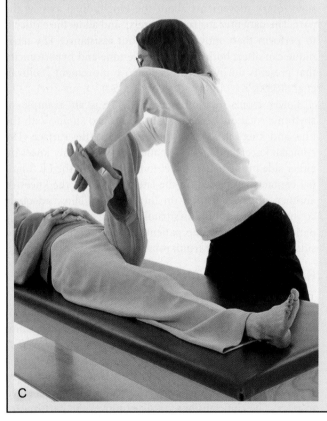

C

The pattern is applied to the patient's left lower extremity, beginning with the primary muscles in a lengthened position (extension). The patient may be requested to maintain isometric knee extension throughout the pattern, or as pictured here, to flex the knee as the hip flexes.

A. Beginning. The clinician stands in the diagonal position and faces the patient's feet. Alternatively, the clinician may begin facing the patient's head. The clinician places her left hand on the patient's dorsomedial foot and her right hand on the anteromedial thigh. The patient is requested to "pull your foot up and in, and lift your leg across the other leg." The clinician facilitates ankle dorsiflexion and inversion, then hip flexion with adduction and medial rotation. The knee is pictured as flexing but may remain extended, depending on the goals for this patient.

B. Midrange. As the patient moves toward midrange of the pattern, the clinician pivots to face the patient's head. The distal hand placement remains consistent. The proximal hand shifts as appropriate to facilitate or resist as needed to address the individual patient's needs.

C. End range. As the patient completes the pattern, the clinician remains in the diagonal position and shifts her body weight onto the back foot. This allows for more efficient application of resistance, if needed. Manual contacts continue as previously described; however, the proximal hand may be shifted to promote the optimal combination of hip flexion, adduction, and medial rotation for this patient.

INTERVENTION 10.10 Lower Extremity D₁ Extension

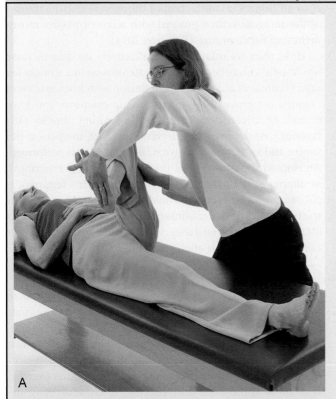

A

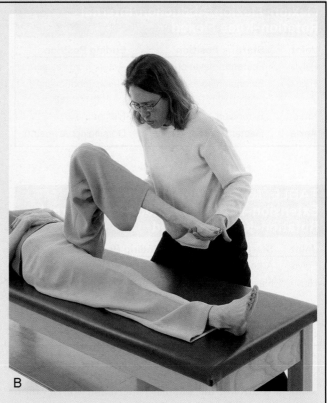

B

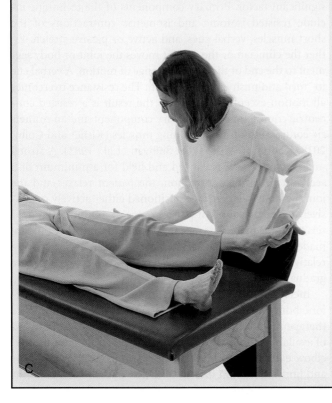

C

The pattern begins with primary muscle groups involved in a lengthened position (flexion). The knee is shown moving from a flexed to an extended position, although the knee may remain extended throughout as appropriate for the individual patient. The left limb is being treated. The clinician stands close to the plinth in the diagonal position and faces the patient.

A. Beginning. The clinician's left hand contacts the plantar surface of the patient's foot, with the right hand on the postero-lateral thigh. When asked to "step down and out into my hand," the patient plantar flexes and everts the foot while extending the hip and knee.

B. Midrange. The clinician's left hand may pivot about the plantar surface of the patient's foot to promote optimal plantar flexion and eversion. The clinician shifts her body weight as needed to accommodate patient movement and effort.

C. End range. The patient completes the pattern to rest on the plinth. Manual contacts are similar to those described at midrange. The clinician continues to shift her weight as needed within the diagonal position. The patient may be positioned closer to the edge of the plinth to allow movement into further hip extension.

TABLE 10.9 Lower Extremity D₂ Flexion–Flexion/Abduction/Internal Rotation–Knee Flexed

Joint	Starting Position	Ending Position
Pelvis	Posterior elevation	Anterior depression
Hip	Extension/adduction/external rotation	Flexion/abduction/internal rotation
Knee	Extension	Flexion
Ankle	Plantar flexion/inversion	Dorsiflexion/eversion

TABLE 10.10 Lower Extremity D₂ Extension–Extension/Adduction/External Rotation–Knee Extended

Joint	Starting Position	Ending Position
Pelvis	Anterior depression	Posterior elevation
Hip	Flexion/abduction/internal rotation	Extension/adduction/external rotation
Knee	Flexion	Extension
Ankle	Dorsiflexion/eversion	Plantar flexion/inversion

Patient control of the scapular pattern anterior elevation may be enhanced through use of hold relax active movement. The patient is side-lying with the clinician kneeling behind. The patient's scapula is passively placed in anterior elevation, and he or she is asked to hold this position. The clinician provides resistance to the isometric contraction. The patient is then told to relax and is moved back slightly toward posterior depression. The patient is told to "pull up" and moves back into anterior elevation. This motion can be performed actively or with resistance. The patient holds the end position of anterior elevation once again, relaxes on verbal command, and then is moved further back toward posterior depression. This cycle is repeated as the patient moves through a greater range each time until he or she completes the entire pattern.

Hold Relax

The purpose of the hold relax technique is to increase passive joint *mobility* and decrease movement-related pain. Main components of the technique include resisted isometric contraction, verbal cues, and active or passive stretch. The patient or clinician moves the joint or body segment to the limit of pain-free motion. The patient maintains this position while the therapist resists an isometric contraction of the antagonist muscle group, with the muscles restricting the desired direction of movement. A verbal cue of "hold" is given as the clinician gradually increases the amount of applied resistance. A command is given for the patient to slowly relax. When possible, the joint or body segment is moved through a greater range of motion. The clinician may perform the movement passively; however, active patient-controlled movement is preferred, especially when pain is a factor. All steps are repeated until there is no further improvement in range of motion. A variation in the traditional method is to elicit an isometric contraction of the agonist muscle, instead of the antagonist, then proceed with active or passive movement into further range (Prentice, 2014).

Hold relax technique can be effectively used to increase hip flexion with concurrent knee extension as in a straight leg raise (Bonnar et al., 2004). If hip flexion with knee extension (agonist movement) is limited, the hip extensors and knee flexors, or hamstrings, would be the limiting muscles (antagonist). As depicted in Intervention 13.19, the person lies supine and an active or passive straight leg raise is performed. An isometric contraction of the hip extensors (hamstrings), or alternatively the hip flexors (iliopsoas/rectus femoris), is elicited through a request to hold the position. After the contraction is held for a minimum of 5 seconds, the patient is asked to relax as resistance is slowly withdrawn. Further range of hip flexion is attempted either actively or passively.

Contract Relax

The contract relax technique provides another method to increase passive joint range and soft tissue length (Kay et al., 2015). A review study conducted by Hindle et al. (2012) concluded that PNF stretching techniques, including contract relax, improve both range of motion and muscle performance, especially when performed consistently after exercise. It is most appropriate and effective when addressing decreased length in two-joint muscles and when pain is not a significant factor. Primary components of the technique include resisted isotonic and isometric contractions of the short muscles, verbal cues, and active or passive stretch. Either the clinician or the patient moves the joint or body segment to the end of the available range of motion. A verbal cue to "turn and push or pull" is given. The resistance overcomes all motion except rotation; thus the result is a resisted concentric contraction of the rotary component and an isometric contraction of the remaining muscles (Kisner and Colby, 2018; Knott and Voss, 1968; Sullivan et al., 1982). A strong muscle contraction is elicited and held for a minimum of 5 seconds. After the contraction, the patient relaxes and the joint or body segment is repositioned either actively or passively to the new limit of passive range of motion. As in hold relax, the sequence is repeated until no further gains are made. Changes in muscle tension with this technique are relatively abrupt, although those used during hold relax are gradual.

Increasing shoulder range of motion into D₂ flexion, flexion/abduction/external rotation is an example of appropriate therapeutic use of contract relax. The arm is placed at the end of available range of the D₂ flexion pattern. The shoulder and elbow extensors are identified as the muscles that are short and limiting motion into flexion. The patient is asked to lift the arm up and out to the side into the D₂ flexion pattern. An isometric contraction of the shoulder extensors and adductors is held for a minimum of 5 seconds while resisted rotation through available range is allowed to occur. A command to "relax" is then given. The arm is moved into further flexion, abduction, and external rotation by either the patient or

INTERVENTION 10.11 Lower Extremity D₂ Flexion

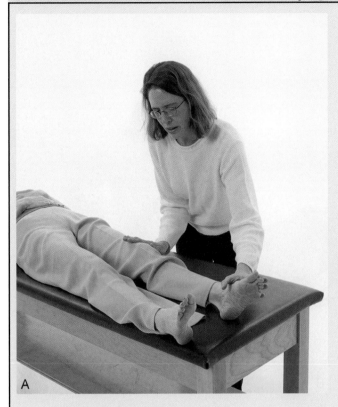

A

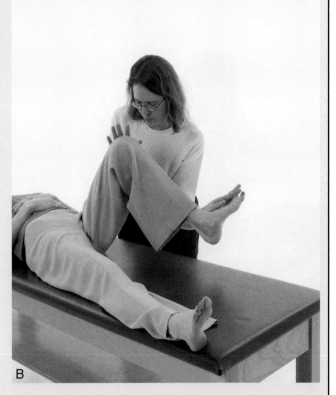

B

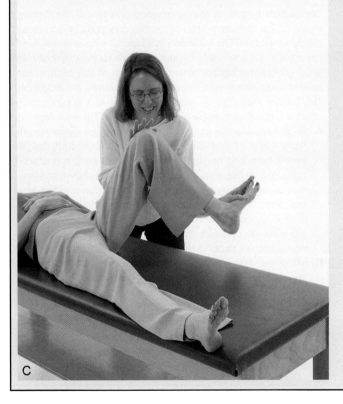

C

The pattern is presented on the left lower extremity. The clinician stands in the diagonal position and faces the patient's feet, with her left hand on the patient's foot and her right hand on the thigh.

A. Beginning. The clinician contacts the patient's dorsolateral foot with her left hand and the patient's anterolateral thigh with her right hand. The patient is requested to "pull your foot up and out and lift your leg out to the side." Near-full-range ankle dorsiflexion and eversion should be achieved early in the range to promote normal timing of the movement pattern. This also provides a "handle" for the clinician that improves her ability to control the patient's limb.

B. Midrange. The clinician remains in the diagonal position and shifts her body weight to optimize patient effort. The proximal contact (right hand) may shift in position to enhance the quality of the movement. For example, if inadequate hip medial rotation is produced, the clinician may move her hand to the medial thigh.

C. End range. As the patient completes the pattern, the clinician may continue to make subtle adjustments in her body and hand positions to enhance the patient's motor response.

INTERVENTION 10.12   Lower Extremity D₂ Extension

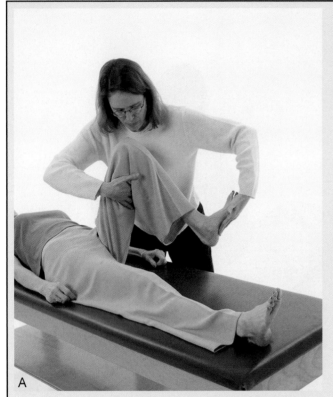

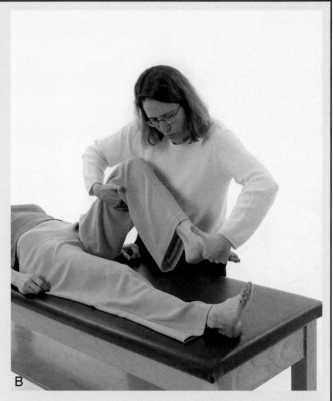

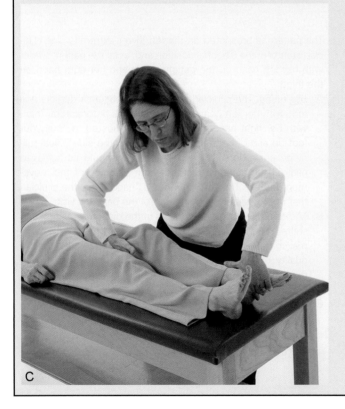

The pattern begins in the lengthened position of the pattern (flexion). The clinician stands in the diagonal position and faces the patient's feet. The clinician's left hand is placed distally and her right hand proximally on the patient's lower extremity. To allow for greater hip adduction at the end of the pattern, the patient's stationary limb may be prepositioned in abduction. The patient may also lie close to the edge of the plinth or in side-lying position to allow a greater range of hip extension.

A. Beginning. Manual contacts are such that the clinician's left hand is placed on the medial and plantar aspect of the patient's foot, and her right hand is placed on the posterior thigh. In this example, the clinician's hand is shown postero-medial, which helps to facilitate hip adduction and the general direction of the pattern. If the patient has difficulty producing hip lateral rotation, a posterolateral contact may enhance the patient's effort. The verbal command to "step down into my hand" initiates the movement pattern.

B. Midrange. Full or nearly full ankle motion and hip rotation should be attained by midrange of the pattern. The clinician may pivot her left hand and shift her body weight to accommodate patient movement and effort.

C. End range. The pattern ends as the moving limb contacts the stationary limb. Alternatively, the patient may be prepositioned to allow for greater range of movement into hip extension and adduction, as previously described.

INTERVENTION 10.13 Pelvic Anterior Elevation

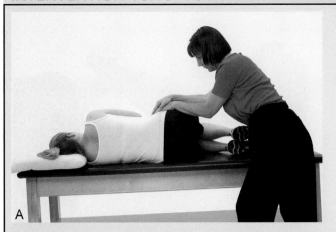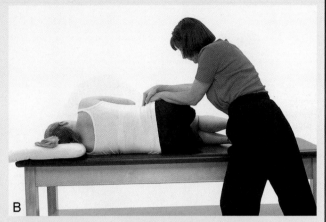

The pelvic pattern of anterior elevation is pictured with the patient in left side-lying position. The clinician stands in the diagonal position, behind and facing the patient. The clinician flexes her hips and knees to adjust her position according to the plinth height.
A. The clinician's left hand contacts the patient's right anterior superior iliac spine with her right hand reinforcing the left. The patient is requested to "pull your pelvis up and forward."
B. The clinician's body follows the line of the pattern as the patient completes the movement.

INTERVENTION 10.14 Pelvic Posterior Depression

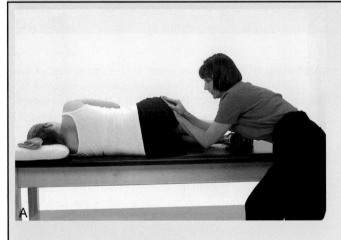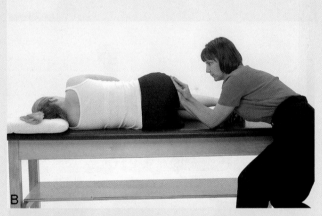

The pelvic pattern of posterior depression is also pictured with the patient in left side-lying position.
A. The clinician's left hand contacts the patient's right ischial tuberosity, and the right hand is placed over the left. The patient is asked to "sit back into my hands."
B. The clinician shifts weight onto her back leg as the patient moves to the end of the range.

the clinician, establishing the new limit to motion. The technique is repeated until there is no further improvement. The arm is then resisted through the UE D_2 patterns of flexion/abduction/external rotation and extension/adduction/internal rotation to help integrate the new range into functional movements.

Alternating Isometrics

The alternating isometrics (isotonic stabilizing reversals, alternating holds) technique promotes *stability*, strength, and endurance in identified muscle groups or in a specific posture. Isometric contractions of both agonist and antagonist muscle groups are facilitated in an alternating manner. Manual contacts and verbal cues are the primary facilitatory elements. Because proximal extremity joint or trunk stability is a common focus, this technique is often applied in developmental postures; however, it may also be used with bilateral or unilateral extremity patterns.

Manual resistance is imparted to encourage isometric contraction of agonist muscles. Once an optimal response is

INTERVENTION 10.15 Lifting Pattern

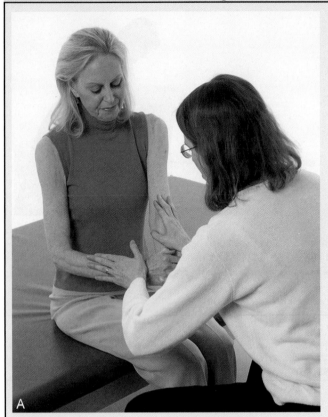

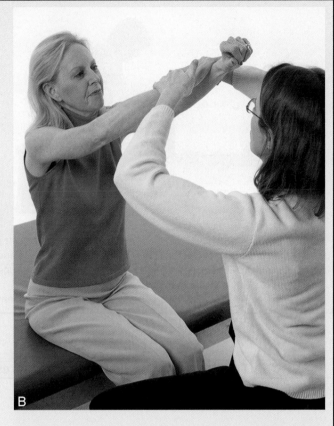

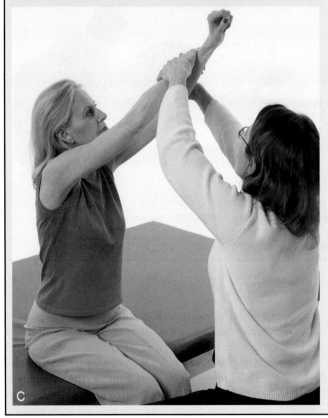

A left lifting pattern is shown, which involves movement of the left lead arm through the D_2 flexion pattern. Many options exist for appropriate manual contacts. Both the clinician and patient sit and face each other; however, the activity may be performed in various positions, including supine, kneeling, and standing. Hand placements on the patient's distal upper extremities are shown. The patient is encouraged to watch her hands as she moves through all trunk patterns.

A. Beginning. The clinician facilitates the D_2 flexion pattern in the left lead arm through manual contact on the dorsal forearm; she also promotes the D_1 flexion pattern in the right upper extremity through contact with the anterior forearm. The command is given to "turn your left hand up and lift your arms over your left shoulder."

B. Midrange. The clinician actively maintains an upright trunk as she observes the patient's trunk position throughout the range of the pattern. Additional verbal cues or changes in manual contacts may be used to enhance trunk extension and rotation.

C. End range. The patient completes the range of the pattern including trunk extension with rotation while the clinician mirrors the movement and applies resistance as indicated to promote optimal patient response.

INTERVENTION 10.16 Reverse Lifting Pattern

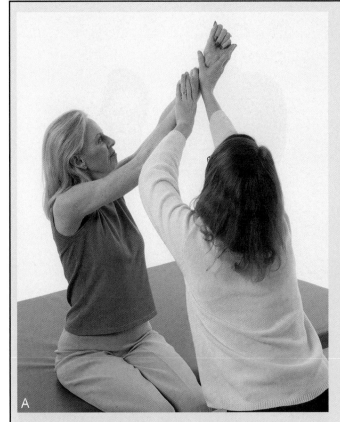

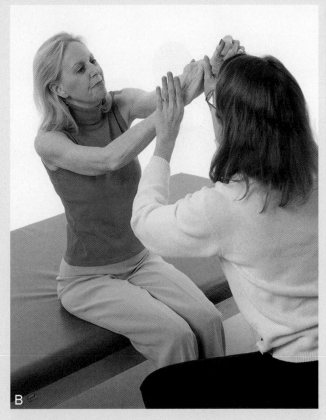

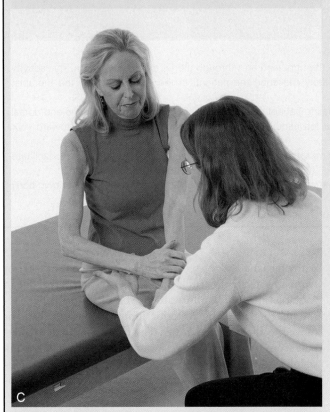

A left reverse lift is pictured involving movement of the left lead arm through the D_2 extension pattern. Both the clinician and patient are shown in sitting. Manual contacts at the distal upper extremities are used in this example.

A. Beginning. The clinician places one hand on the right dorsal forearm and the other on the left anterior forearm or wrist. The request is made for the patient to "make a fist with your left hand, turn your thumb down, and bring your arms down toward your right hip."

B. Midrange. The clinician shifts her body weight to accommodate patient movement. Manual contacts may also shift slightly to adjust to changes in the patient's upper-extremity position. The clinician monitors the patient's trunk and provides verbal or manual cues to promote the desired amounts of flexion and rotation.

C. End range. The patient completes the appropriate range of upper extremity and trunk movement, as the therapist adjusts her body weight and hand positions to evoke optimal patient response.

INTERVENTION 10.17   **Chopping Pattern**

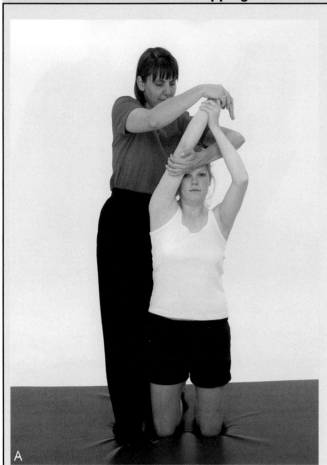 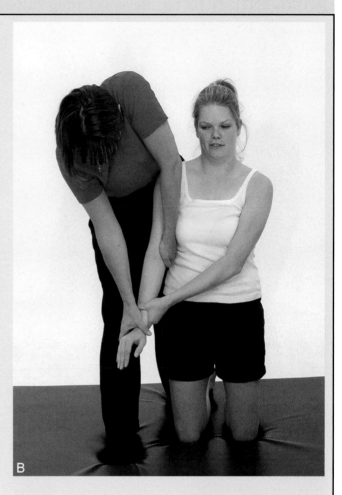

Picture shows right chopping pattern, which involves movement of the right lead arm through the D₁ extension pattern. This activity may be performed in various developmental postures to appropriately challenge the patient. In the given example, the therapist stands in stride stance behind the kneeling patient.

A. Beginning. The therapist stands in stride stance behind the kneeling patient. Manual contacts are on the dorsal hand and dorsal distal humerus. A request is made for the patient to "open your left hand, turn your thumb down, and push down toward your right hip as if chopping wood."

B. Midrange. The patient moves through the pattern as the clinician mirrors patient movement and shifts her body weight to facilitate optimal motor strategies.

C. End range. The patient completes the range of trunk and upper extremity movement. The clinician continues to alter her own body position to accommodate patient effort.

Special note: The patient's left wrist and fingers should extend as the pattern proceeds, which is not depicted in picture B.

achieved, the clinician changes one hand to a new location over the antagonist muscles and gradually increases resistance in the appropriate direction. The second hand may be moved to the new location or removed from the surface until the next change in direction of resistance is initiated. Manual contacts are smoothly adjusted to encourage gradual shifting of contractions between agonist and antagonist muscle groups.

Alternating isometrics may be used to promote trunk stability in unsupported sitting. The clinician resists trunk flexion with manual contacts on the anterior trunk. The initial verbal command of "don't let me push you backward" is given. Once the trunk flexors contract, input is maintained

with one hand and the second hand is moved to the posterior trunk to activate the trunk extensors. A second verbal cue of "don't let me pull you forward" is voiced. As the patient responds to the initial posterior input, the second hand is moved to the posterior trunk. The hands continue to alternate from the anterior to posterior trunk, challenging trunk stability in the sagittal plane. Intervention 10.19 shows this technique being used to increase trunk stability in unsupported sitting.

Rhythmic Stabilization

Rhythmic stabilization (isometric stabilizing reversals) enhances *stability* through cocontraction of muscles surrounding

INTERVENTION 10.18 Reverse Chopping Pattern

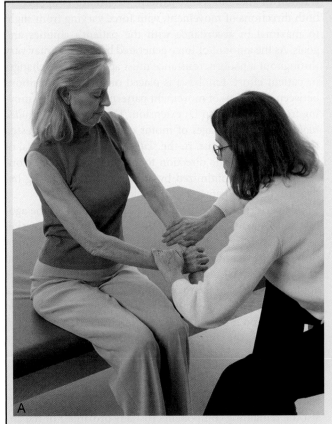

A

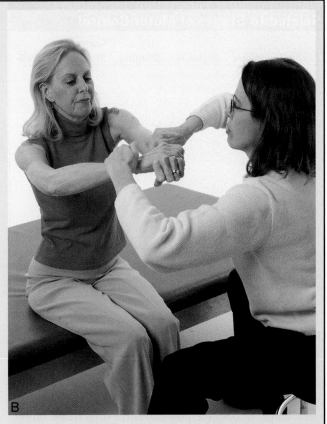

B

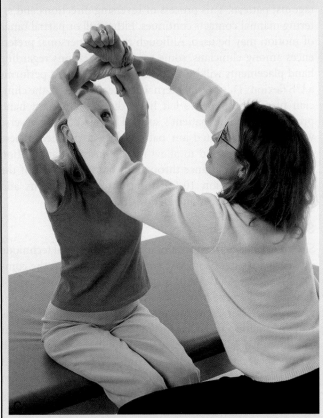

The left or reverse chopping pattern involves movement of the left lead arm through the D₁ flexion pattern. The clinician and patient sit and face each other. Manual contacts at the distal forearms are shown.

A. Beginning. The clinician places one hand on the anterior surface of the patient's left forearm and the other hand on the dorsal surface of the right forearm. The patient is asked to "make a fist with your left hand, turn your thumb up, and pull your arms toward your right shoulder." Special note: The patient's wrist and fingers should be extended when initiating the pattern, which is not shown here.

B. Midrange. The clinician observes the patient's trunk and provides manual or verbal cues as needed. The clinician shifts her body weight to adapt to patient movements.

C. End range. The patient completes the desired range of movement of the trunk and upper extremities. The clinician mirrors patient movement and alters her body and hand positions to optimize patient efforts.

TABLE 10.11   Proprioceptive Neuromuscular Facilitation Techniques Related to Stages of Motor Control

Stage/Technique	Mobility	Stability	Controlled Mobility	Skill
Agonistic reversal	—	—	X	X
Alternating isometrics	—	X	—	—
Contract relax	X	—	—	—
Hold relax	X	—	—	—
Hold relax active movement	—	—	—	—
Rhythmic initiation	X	—	—	—
Rhythmic rotation	X	—	—	—
Rhythmic stabilization	—	X	—	—
Slow reversal hold	—	X	X	X
Slow reversals	—	—	X	X

the target joint(s). Resistance is applied to promote isometric contraction. Often the goal is to enhance the patient's ability to maintain a specific developmental position. A rotary force is emphasized to encourage simultaneous contraction of the primary stabilizers about the involved joints. The patient is asked simply to hold the position. Force is increased slowly, emphasizing the rotary component of the motion and matching patient effort. When the patient has built up muscular force in one direction, the clinician changes the position of one hand and begins to slowly apply force in a different direction, again emphasizing rotation. Depending on the demands of the clinical situation, rhythmic stabilization may be used to promote stability and balance, decrease pain on movement, and increase range of motion and strength.

Rhythmic stabilization may also be applied to promote trunk stability in unsupported sitting. Rotation of the trunk is resisted with the clinician placing one hand on the anterior trunk and the other hand on the posterior trunk. The patient is expected to isometrically hold an erect trunk position. A verbal cue of "hold; don't let me move you" is used. The relative positions of the right and left hands are sequentially adjusted so that opposing rotational forces are created. There is no intention of movement on the part of the patient. The patient matches the resistance provided by the clinician and dynamically maintains the position. Intervention 10.20 depicts the use of rhythmic stabilization to promote trunk stability in sitting.

Slow Reversal

Slow reversal (reversal of antagonists, dynamic reversals) is a versatile technique that may be used to address a variety of patient problems, such as muscle weakness, joint stiffness, or impaired coordination. Concentric contraction of muscles in an agonist pattern is facilitated through manual contacts and verbal cues. At the desired end of range, manual contacts of one or both hands are changed to facilitate concentric contraction of the antagonist pattern. Resistance is applied to both directions of movement, with force varying from slight to maximal in accordance with the patient's abilities and goals. As the amount of force generated by a patient may vary throughout a pattern, resistance must accommodate changes in patient effort. Emphasis is placed on smooth transitions between directions of movement patterns such as when moving from D_2 flexion to D_2 extension. The *mobility, controlled mobility,* and *skill* stages of motor control can be addressed through this technique. In the *skill* stage, smooth reversal of movement from one direction to another is a primary concern. Fatigue is minimized by rhythmically alternating between agonist and antagonist muscle groups.

For performance of the UE D_2 flexion pattern as the agonist and D_2 extension, extension/adduction/internal rotation as the antagonist is an example of therapeutic application of slow reversal technique. Beginning in the lengthened position of the agonist (D_2 flexion) pattern, appropriate resistance is applied through both proximal and distal manual contacts. The flexion pattern is initiated by the command to "open your hand and lift the arm up and out." Near the completion of the pattern, the clinician's proximal hand is moved to resist the distal component of the antagonist (D_2 extension) pattern. The verbal cue to "squeeze my hand and pull down" is timed with the change in direction. As the patient starts to move into extension, the clinician's other hand moves to resist the remaining components (usually proximal) of the antagonist pattern. This process of reversing directions and altering manual contacts continues. Either full or partial range of motion may be used. Although there are personal preferences among clinicians, some specific suggestions regarding hand placements will be offered. When the patient performs a UE flexion (D_1 or D_2) pattern with the right hand, the clinician places the patient's left hand distally and right hand proximally on the patient's arm. The placements reverse when D_1 or D_2 extension patterns are performed. These manual contacts tend to allow more consistent application of appropriate resistance throughout both directions of the pattern. Intervention 10.1 demonstrates the patterns and manual contacts recommended with this technique.

Slow Reversal Hold

Slow reversal hold is a variation of the slow reversal technique in which a resisted isometric contraction is held at the completion of range in each direction of the chosen pattern or activity. Movement may proceed through the available joint range or a lesser excursion may be used, depending on the patient situation or goal. Movement occurs as described for the slow reversal; however, at the desired end point in each direction, a resisted isometric contraction of all involved muscles is elicited. This technique aids in the transition from the *mobility* to *stability* stages of motor control by promoting increased strength, balance, and endurance. Studies examined the treatment effect of slow reversal and slow reversal hold found increased antagonist tension after agonist contraction (Gabriel et al., 2001; Kamimura et al., 2009). The

INTERVENTION 10.19 Alternating Isometrics to Increase Trunk Stability in Sitting

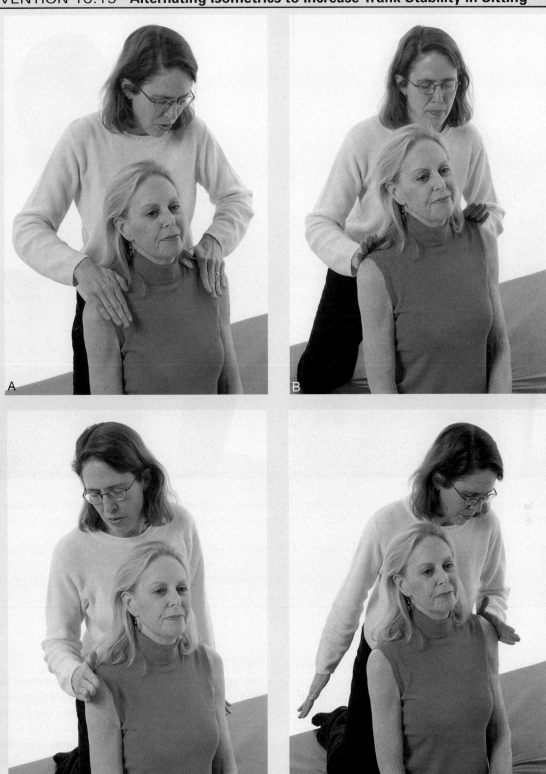

A. Resistance is provided to trunk flexion through symmetrical manual contacts on the anterior shoulder. The verbal cue "don't let me push you backward" is given as the clinician leans posteriorly using her body weight to produce the resistance.

B. The clinician places her hands bilaterally on the superior aspect of the patient's scapulae. The command "don't let me push you forward" is given as the clinician shifts her body weight anteriorly.

C. The clinician provides resistance to right trunk lateral flexion through placement of her right hand on the patient's right shoulder. The verbal command "don't let me push you to the left" is given as the clinician shifts her weight to the right to produce the resistance.

D. Resistance is provided to left trunk lateral flexion through placement of the clinician's left hand on the patient's left shoulder.

INTERVENTION 10.20   Rhythmic Stabilization to Increase Trunk Stability in Sitting

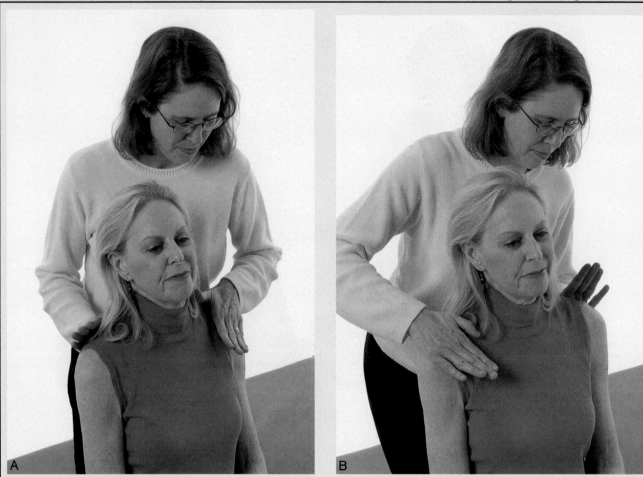

The patient sits on the edge of table. The clinician kneels behind the patient. Suggested manual contacts allow the clinician to resist flexion, extension, and rotation simultaneously or sequentially as placements are rhythmically shifted between the two options pictured.

A. The clinician places her left hand on the anterior aspect of the patient's left shoulder and her right hand on the posterior right shoulder.

B. Manual contacts are shifted to vary the forces applied to the patient. The clinician's left hand is now posterior and her right hand is anterior.

slow reversal hold is appropriate for use with single extremity or trunk patterns as well as functional movements.

Performance of the UE D₂ flexion as agonist pattern in kneeling is an example of clinical application of the slow reversal hold technique. Concentric contraction of the muscles involved in the D_2 flexion (agonist) pattern is resisted throughout the desired range. Without changing manual contacts, the patient is requested to hold the chosen end position using all muscles within the flexion pattern. The distal then proximal hand placements are carefully reestablished to facilitate a smooth transition into the D_2 extension pattern. Graded resistance is applied throughout the D_2 extension pattern. An isometric contraction of the D_2 extension pattern is held at the desired point within the pattern.

Agonistic Reversals

The agonistic reversal technique (combination of isotonics) is used to facilitate functional movement throughout a pattern or task. Both concentric and eccentric contractions of the agonist musculature are used. The focus of the technique is to promote functional stability in a smooth, controlled manner (*controlled mobility*). Other goals include increasing muscle strength and endurance, improving coordination, and training eccentric control. A randomized control study examined the efficacy of agonistic reversal and rhythmic initiation for improving sit-to-stand performance in older women and compared this with two other training protocols (functional training and traditional strengthening) and a control group. The PNF and the functional training group demonstrated significant improvements in the Ten Times Sit-to-Stand test,

Timed Up and Go test, and Functional Reach test when compared with the strengthening group and the control group (Cilento et al., 2013).

To implement the technique, a concentric contraction of the agonist muscle group(s) is resisted through a specific direction and range of the chosen pattern or task. At the desired endpoint of the movement, the patient holds isometrically against resistance. The clinician then resists the patient's slow, controlled return toward the beginning of the movement pattern, promoting an eccentric contraction. The patient holds again at the completion of the eccentric phase to further encourage stability in this range. In summary, the technique begins with resistance to a concentric contraction, followed by a stabilizing hold, resistance to an eccentric contraction, and another stabilizing hold. The agonist muscle groups are targeted throughout this sequence (Saliba et al., 1993).

Bridging is often an appropriate activity with which to superimpose the agonistic reversal technique. The patient lifts the pelvis into a bridge against resistance from the clinician (concentric phase). Manual contacts are on the anterolateral pelvis with force directed posteriorly. The patient is requested to hold the pelvis in this position (stabilizing hold) and then asked to slowly lower the pelvis toward the bed while the clinician's manual contacts and direction of resistance remain consistent (eccentric phase). The clinician instructs the patient to hold the new position (stabilizing hold). Intervention 10.21 depicts this technique as used with bridging.

Resisted Progression

The resisted progression technique focuses on the *skill* level task of locomotion. Resistance is used to increase strength and endurance, develop normal timing, or reinforce motor learning. This technique may be applied during crawling, creeping, or walking. Manual contacts are selected according the desired emphasis, including upper or lower trunk, extremities, pelvis, and scapula (Sullivan et al., 1982).

INTERVENTION 10.21   Agonistic Reversal Technique During Bridging

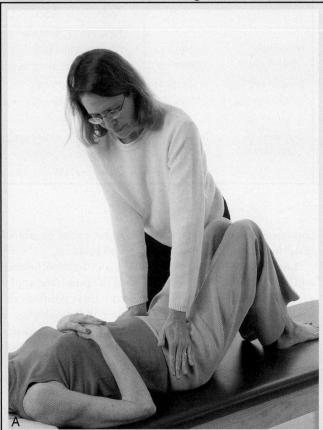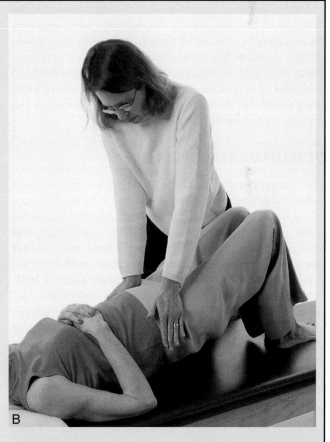

Manual contacts are consistent throughout the activity. The clinician places the heel of each hand on the patient's anterior superior iliac spine with resistance applied in line with the patient's ischial tuberosities.

A. The patient begins in hook-lying position. On the command "lift your buttocks," the patient pushes the pelvis upward, performing a resisted concentric contraction of the hip extensors.

B. When reaching a full bridge position, the patient is requested to "hold" this position briefly. The final command is to "let me push you down slowly" as the patient lowers the buttocks to the surface by eccentrically contracting the hip extensors against resistance.

Resisted progression may be applied effectively to promote proper recruitment hip extensors and pelvic rotators during backward locomotion in quadruped (creeping). Backward progression may occur by moving each extremity separately or by moving contralateral UE and LE simultaneously. This choice is dependent on the motor abilities, coordination, trunk control, strength, and cognitive status of the patient. Typical manual contacts include the posterior thigh, posterior humerus, ischial tuberosity, and inferior angle of the scapula. Any combination of contacts may be used, depending on the intended focus. For example, the clinician's hands may be placed on the ischial tuberosities bilaterally, on the right posterior humerus and left posterior thigh, or on the left scapula and right ischial tuberosity. The clinician kneels beside or behind the patient and faces the patient's head.

Application of Proprioceptive Neuromuscular Facilitation Techniques

The physical therapist examines each patient and determines an individualized plan of care. Specific interventions are selected to meet individual patient's needs; however, there are some typical combinations of PNF basic principles and techniques that are used to address certain impairments. Table 10.12 matches specific impairments with suggested PNF techniques. The use of these techniques in appropriate clinical situations has already been discussed in the sections about techniques. Clinicians should always follow the basic principles of PNF when using any of these techniques while being mindful of those principles that are emphasized in the management of particular impairments.

DEVELOPMENTAL SEQUENCE

PNF patterns and principles of intervention may be used within the different postures that constitute the developmental sequence. The fundamental motor abilities represented within the developmental sequence are interrelated and universal. Most typically developing infants learn to roll (supine ⟷ prone), to move in the prone position, to assume a sitting position, to stand erectly, walk, and run. Individual variations occur in the method of performance, sequence, and rate of mastery. Typical movement patterns emerge from the maturation and interaction of multiple body systems. Developmental postures and patterns of movement can provide a basis for restoration of motor function in persons with neuromuscular impairments and related functional deficits. A review of the developmental process and patterns can be found in Chapter 4.

The developmental sequence provides a means to progress from simple to complex movements and postures (McGraw, 1962). The supine progression and the prone progression compose the developmental sequence. Supine progression consists of the following positions: supine, hook-lying, side-lying, propping up on one elbow, pushing up to one hand, sitting, and standing. Prone progression

TABLE 10.12 Use of Proprioceptive Neuromuscular Facilitation Techniques to Treat Impairments

Impairment	Goal	Technique
Pain	Decrease pain	Alternating isometrics
		Hold relax
		Rhythmic stabilization
Decreased strength	Increase strength	Agonistic reversal
		Rhythmic stabilization
		Slow reversal
Decreased range of motion	Increase range of motion	Alternating isometrics
		Contract relax
		Hold relax
		Hold relax active motion
		Rhythmic initiation
Decreased coordination	Increase coordination	Alternating isometrics
		Agonistic reversal
		Rhythmic initiation
		Slow reversal
Decreased stability	Increase stability	Alternating isometrics
		Agonistic reversal
		Rhythmic stabilization
Movement initiation	Initiate movement	Rhythmic initiation
		Hold relax active motion
Muscle stiffness/ hypertonicity	Promote tone reduction	Rhythmic initiation
		Rhythmic rotation
		Hold relax
Decreased endurance	Increase endurance	Alternating isometrics
		Rhythmic stabilization
		Slow reversal

consists of the following positions: prone, prone on elbows, quadruped, kneeling, half-kneeling, and standing.

Impairments in strength, flexibility, coordination, balance, and endurance can be addressed using the prone and supine progressions. The patient is familiar with these positions and understands the movements; therefore the progression is relevant and functional. Within the developmental sequence, the natural progression of postures is that of increasing challenge to the stabilizing muscles. For example, in prone-on-elbows position, a broad surface area is in contact with the supporting base; the COG is very close to the surface; and only the shoulder and cervical spine segments bear significant weight. Therefore this position is very stable and requires relatively minimal muscular effort to maintain. This biomechanical situation may be ideal to address scapular stabilization in the individual with poor global trunk control. In quadruped, however, the demands placed on the muscles are much greater. The BOS is reduced. The COG is higher. The muscles about the hips, shoulders, and elbows must work in a coordinated fashion to sustain the position, both statically and during superimposed activity.

These biomechanical changes create greater motoric demands which, in the appropriate client, can produce more efficient therapeutic and functional outcomes. Each posture within the developmental sequence fosters achievement of motor skills that serve as a foundation for more advanced functional activities. The stronger components of a total pattern are used to augment the weaker components (Voss et al., 1985). Greater demands may be placed on the patient within each position by considering the stages of motor control and applying these principles in developmental postures. The following section addresses selected postures as to possible treatment progression strategies.

Supine Progression

Working in a *hook-lying* position prepares the patient for bridging and scooting, which are essential for bed mobility. Weight-bearing through the feet facilitates cocontraction of the trunk and LE muscles, which is needed to maintain the position. Unilateral and bilateral LE PNF patterns are used to facilitate acquisition of the hook-lying position. Initial focus within any position is on the *mobility* stage, which is defined as the ability to assume a stated position. Sufficient joint range of motion and muscular strength in the pertinent body regions are prerequisite to mastering this stage.

Use of PNF patterns helps the patient gain the ability to position the legs into a hook-lying position independently. LE D_1 flexion with knee flexion is an appropriate pattern to use. Please refer to Intervention 10.7 for a review of the pattern and manual contacts. Mass flexion of the LE (hip/knee flexion and ankle dorsiflexion without significant rotation) may also be used to aid in assuming hook-lying as pictured in

Intervention 10.22. Resisted movement of the uninvolved extremity can enhance muscular activity through irradiation into the trunk and involved LE.

Once the patient has achieved hook-lying position, stability can be promoted by applying alternating isometrics and rhythmic stabilization. Both of these techniques use facilitation of isometric contractions to sustain a position. Manual contacts may be applied from proximal thigh to ankle as appropriate to vary the lever arm and thus the demand on the patient. The *stability* stage of motor control is reached when the patient can independently maintain the hook-lying position. The third stage of motor control, *controlled mobility*, then becomes the focus of treatment. Controlled mobility involves superimposing proximal mobility on a stable position. Activities in hook-lying that contribute to functional gains in this stage include hip abduction/adduction and lower trunk rotation.

Slow reversal, slow reversal hold, and agonistic reversals may be applied with either activity. Both slow reversal and slow reversal hold include resisted alternating concentric contractions of agonist and antagonist patterns (e.g., hip abduction and adduction, or D_1 flexion and D_1 extension). Slow reversal hold adds a held isometric contraction in the shortened range of each muscle group or pattern. Agonistic reversal focuses on one muscle group only, the designated agonist, and concentric then eccentric contractions are facilitated. The medial and lateral femoral condyles provide effective manual contacts for hip abduction/adduction and lower trunk rotation, with care taken to facilitate the desired direction of movement. The clinician positions himself or herself in front of the patient, or off to one side in the diagonal. The diagonal position may produce a different patient response including increased recruitment of trunk muscles.

INTERVENTION 10.22 Mass Flexion Pattern of the Lower Extremity to Assist in Achieving Hook-Lying Position

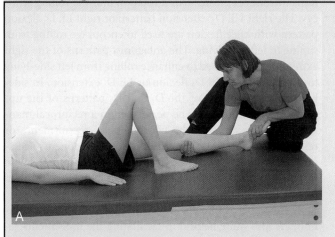
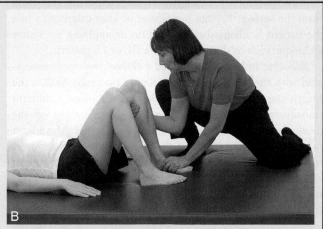

A. The clinician kneels to one side, approximately at level with the patient's knees. Beginning in supine, manual contacts are placed on the dorsal foot and posterior calf and are used to facilitate flexion throughout the lower extremity.

B. The patient completes the flexion movement of first one lower extremity, then the other to assume the hook-lying position.

Bridging is a prerequisite to many functional activities including dressing, toileting, scooting in bed, and weight shifting for pressure relief. The motion of bridging also includes hip extension and pelvic rotation, which are both components of the stance phase of gait. Bridging increases weight-bearing through the plantar surface of the foot and can reduce extensor tone in a patient with hypertonicity. Bridging addresses balance, coordination, and strength while activating multiple muscle groups in a functional context. Bridging is an example of the third stage of motor control.

Bridging is facilitated by use of manual contacts on the patient's anterior pelvis near the anterior superior iliac spine (ASIS). Manual contacts and an appropriate level of assistance are provided to teach proper movement strategies to achieve the *mobility* stage of motor control. It is noted that some individuals may be able to maintain hip extension (*stability* stage) if assisted to the bridge position. The PNF technique hold relax active movement may be used to effectively promote active assumption of a bridge posture in persons for whom this task is particularly challenging. Once this position is achieved either actively or with assistance, techniques such as alternating isometrics or rhythmic stabilization may be applied at the pelvis, then progressively more distally to enhance *stability*. For patients who are weaker on one side, resistance is given to the stronger side while assistance is offered to the weaker side. Once the patient no longer requires assistance to achieve a bridge position, agonistic reversals may be used to promote *controlled mobility*. Eccentric lowering of the pelvis in a smooth coordinated manner is often difficult for patients. *Agonistic reversal* technique is used with bridging to address coordination and strength in both the concentric and eccentric components of the movement. Refer to Intervention 10.18 for illustrations of this technique as used with bridging. The clinician may vary the challenge of bridging by altering the BOS or hold duration. Complexity and functional applicability may be enhanced by combining bridging with various extremity movements. Examples include removing one limb from the surface through hip flexion or knee extension while the patient holds the bridge position or applying a resistive technique such as slow reversal to a UE or LE pattern.

Scooting in bed is considered a *skilled* movement associated with the hook-lying and bridging positions. Skill is the fourth stage of motor control. Scooting is often a difficult transitional movement and requires coordination of the head, upper trunk, lower trunk, and extremities. Movement may be initiated with either the upper trunk, LEs, or lower trunk. Manual contacts facilitate the direction of movement and offer assistance or resistance to the component movements as appropriate. Manual contacts may be used below the clavicles to facilitate upper trunk flexion while verbal cues are given for head and neck flexion. Manual contacts on the pelvis similar to those used to facilitate bridging promote recruitment of the lower trunk.

Rolling

Many components of gait and other higher level activities are found in movements associated with rolling. Additionally, rolling stimulates cutaneous receptors, the vestibular and reticular systems, and proprioceptors within the joints and muscles. Rolling can influence muscle tone, level of arousal/alertness, and body awareness. Rolling is an excellent total body activity that provides opportunities to improve strength, coordination, and sensation in the trunk and extremities.

There are several key points to consider when incorporating rolling into a therapeutic program. As with all complex functional activities, individuals use various strategies to accomplish this task including flexion movements, extension movements, or pushing/pulling with one arm or leg (Richter et al., 1989). The ability to roll in either direction is an important functional and foundational task. Rolling to the involved side may be easier in individuals with hemiplegia because a frequently used strategy involves initiation of trunk rotation to the hemiplegic side through movements of the uninvolved UE or LE. *Prepositioning* in hook-lying or side-lying encourages use of certain components or methods of rolling. In hook-lying, a shorter lever arm is created for initiation of LE and trunk movements with emphasis on the lower trunk and hip musculature. Side-lying provides an ideal position in which to focus on trunk rotation or to minimize the effects of gravity on extremity patterns. The clinician may choose specific extremity or trunk patterns as well as certain PNF techniques to optimally use the patient's abilities and promote maximal function. Rolling is also an effective task through which to enhance head control and eye–hand coordination. Basic prepositioning and one example of manual contacts are shown in Intervention 10.23.

Because of the transitional nature of this activity, the stages of motor control are less useful in providing a clear path of functional treatment progression; therefore treatment applications will focus on tools to enhance rolling in general. Mass flexion and extension trunk patterns provide an initial means to facilitate rolling from supine to side-lying and side-lying to supine, respectively. Use of extremity patterns introduces greater trunk rotation into the rolling strategy. The right UE D_2 extension pattern or right LE D_1 flexion pattern with knee flexion are used to encourage rolling from supine to left side-lying. The antagonist patterns of the right extremities can be used to enhance rolling from left side-lying to supine, that is, UE D_2 flexion or LE D_1 extension. In side-lying, both directions of the D_1 and D_2 patterns of the uppermost extremities may be performed in a reciprocal manner to improve strength, coordination, recruitment, or reinforcement of the trunk and extremity components necessary for rolling. Use of the D_1 pattern with the left LE to promote rolling from supine to right side-lying is pictured in Intervention 10.24.

Trunk patterns, such as chops, lifts, and lower trunk rotation, are also quite helpful in facilitating the movements required to roll. For example, rolling supine to left side-lying may be assisted by using a left chop in which the left UE moves through the D_1 extension pattern. A left lift in which the left UE moves through the D_2 flexion pattern may also be used to roll from supine to left side-lying. Determining which pattern depends on patient abilities. When a person's

INTERVENTION 10.23 Prepositioning and Manual Contacts to Facilitate Rolling Supine to Right Side-Lying

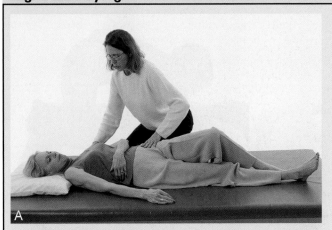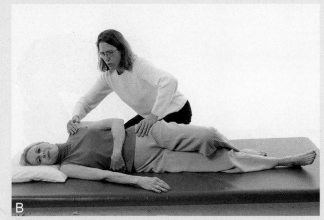

A. Beginning position. In preparation to roll to the right, the patient turns her head to the right. The left hip and knee are flexed. The left upper extremity is placed in flexion with the shoulder adducted. The left upper extremity is positioned away from the body in extension and adduction.

B. End position. Through manual contacts at the left anterior shoulder and pelvis, the patient is assisted, facilitated, or resisted, as appropriate, to aid in assumption of right side-lying position.

preferred strategy is to initiate rolling with the LEs, incorporating lower trunk rotation in hook-lying is advantageous. This activity has been described previously in relation to the hook-lying developmental posture.

Rhythmic initiation is often used when teaching a patient to roll. Movement progresses from passive to assistive to active or slightly resisted. Supine or hook-lying may be used as the starting position. Review the section on rhythmic initiation for a complete description of promoting rolling. The technique hold relax active movement also may be an effective tool to enhance the patient's ability to roll. Initially, the patient is placed in side-lying position and asked to hold while the clinician applies resistance to the patient's trunk, as if trying to roll the patient back toward supine. The command to relax is given and the patient is passively rolled slightly back toward supine. The patient is then requested to actively roll toward side-lying as appropriate resistance is applied. This sequence is repeated with the clinician progressively taking the patient through greater range of motion until the patient is able to roll from supine to side-lying against resistance. Slow reversal, slow reversal hold, and agonistic reversals may then be incorporated into rolling with emphasis on efficient movement strategies, normal timing, trunk control, and effective use of extremity patterns.

Prone Progression

Lying prone and prone on elbows are the foundational postures of the prone progression. Use of an external support, such as a wedge, pillow, or towel roll, may be necessary to promote comfort because of joint or soft tissue restrictions or respiratory dysfunction. The progression begins with the patient moving from lying prone to prone on elbows

(*mobility*). The prone-on-elbows position provides minimal biomechanical stresses because of the low COG, large BOS, and minimal number of weight-bearing joints. This situation provides an ideal opportunity for early weight-bearing on the UEs. Lifting one arm reduces the BOS, providing greater biomechanical challenge to the patient. Patients often fatigue quickly in the prone-on-elbows position; therefore the patient should be monitored carefully for discomfort and proper postural alignment. Frequent verbal and manual cues may be needed to help the patient maintain appropriate cervical and thoracic spine extension, scapular adduction, and shoulder alignment; otherwise, excessive strain may be placed on the periarticular structures of the shoulder, such as the capsule and ligaments. Activities such as weight shifting and reaching form a natural functional progression and promote cocontraction of the upper trunk and shoulder girdle muscles, encourage asymmetrical use of the arms, and establish a foundation for crawling or bed mobility in prone.

Rhythmic initiation uses manual cues and graded assistance to teach the patient to transition from lying prone to prone on elbows (see the section "Proprioceptive Neuromuscular Facilitation Techniques"). Once the patient has learned to assume the position, alternating isometrics and rhythmic stabilization may be applied to the shoulder girdle or head to create *stability*. *Controlled mobility* may be facilitated first through lateral or diagonal weight shifting and then through use of unilateral UE patterns with slow reversal and slow reversal hold techniques.

Commando style crawling is defined as a *skill* level activity in this position. Manual cues at the anterior humerus to guide directional movement or on the scapula to promote stability may assist in developing effective movement

INTERVENTION 10.24   D₁ Pattern With the Left Lower Extremity to Promote Rolling Supine to Right Side-Lying

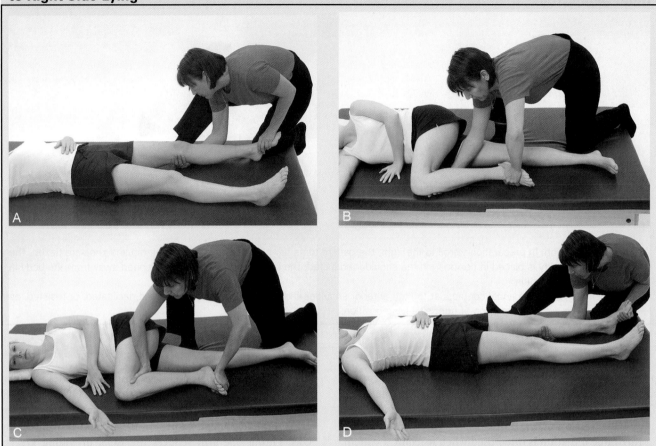

A. The clinician positions into half-kneeling just left of the patient's left lower extremity. The clinician contacts on the patient's dorsal foot with her left hand and the posterior tibia with the right hand.

B. The clinician shifts her body weight forward as the patient completes the left lower extremity D₁ flexion pattern to assist in rolling to right side-lying.

C. To return to supine, the patient performs the D₁ extension pattern with the left lower extremity. The clinician places her right hand on the patient's posterior knee region and the left hand on the plantar surface of the foot.

D. The patient moves through the D₁ extension pattern with the left lower extremity and completes the transition back to supine position. The clinician shifts weight onto her back leg during the transition.

strategies. This task also provides an opportunity to introduce reciprocal pelvic and lower trunk rotation early in the prone progression.

Quadruped

Quadruped represents the first posture in the developmental sequence in which the COG is a significant distance from the supporting surface. The higher COG combined with less body surface contact and a greater number of weight-bearing joints make this posture much more challenging from a biomechanical perspective than the preceding postures within the prone progression. The added biomechanical stresses in addition to weight-bearing on all four extremities create unique opportunities to pursue gains in strength, range of motion, balance, coordination, and endurance throughout the body. Musculoskeletal dysfunction and pain may prohibit

or limit the therapeutic use of this posture, especially regarding the knees, shoulders, and hands. Padding the palms or knees and altering the amount of hip and shoulder flexion through forward or backward weight shifting can improve patient comfort. This position may also place additional stress on the cardiovascular system; therefore patients must be carefully screened for preexisting conditions and monitored for signs of intolerance.

To obtain quadruped position from prone on elbows, patients may begin by moving their upper or lower trunk, or one LE. This transition *(mobility)* can be enhanced through rhythmic initiation by using carefully selected manual contacts at the shoulders or pelvis. Individuals with poor control of the lower trunk will have more difficulty completing this transition. Manual contacts near the ischial tuberosities, as demonstrated in Intervention 10.25, help

INTERVENTION 10.25   Transition From Prone-on-Elbows to Quadruped

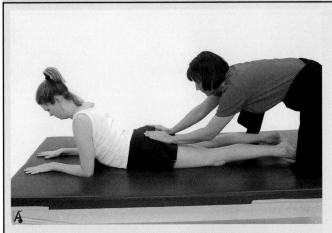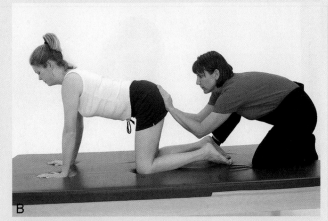

A. Beginning. The patient lies prone, propped on the elbows. The clinician is positioned in half-kneeling, straddling the patient's lower legs. Manual contacts are at the posterior pelvis, near the ischial tuberosities. The patient is requested to "push up on your arms and sit back into my hands."

B. End. The clinician shifts her body weight back to accommodate patient movement into the quadruped position while providing facilitation or resistance as appropriate.

guide the movement of the pelvis, as well as allowing the clinician to provide assistance as needed. Alternating isometrics and rhythmic stabilization are appropriate to establish *stability* within this position. Examples of manual contacts are shown in Intervention 10.26. Only the creativity of the clinician limits the array of activities in this posture, especially during the *controlled mobility* stage of motor control. Some possibilities include forward, backward, and diagonal weight shifts; single extremity patterns; and contralateral arm/leg lifts. Movement-oriented techniques such as slow reversal, slow reversal hold, and agonistic reversals may be applied as indicated by patient abilities and impairments. Intervention 10.27 pictures the use of slow reversal in facilitation of rocking backward. Intervention 10.28 provides examples of activities using the extremities to promote this stage of motor control. Combinations of techniques can be very effective in maximally challenging the patient. One example would be application of rhythmic stabilization to the trunk while the slow reversal technique is applied to an extremity pattern; such hybrid approaches are motorically challenging to the clinician but represent innovative ways to maximally benefit the individual.

Kneeling

Kneeling provides functional progression from quadruped by freeing the UEs for environmental exploration. Therapeutically, biomechanical and neurophysiologic considerations must be addressed. Kneeling is the first developmental position in the prone progression to allow axial loading of the spine and hip joints. Number of weight-bearing joints and potential level arm are greatly increased. The hips are extended and knees flexed, which lessens the influence of an extensor synergy pattern in the LEs. Weight-bearing through

the LEs also can decrease excessive extensor tone. These changes provide functional challenges and therapeutic opportunities. Impairments in hip/knee range of motion, trunk/LE strength, and balance are efficiently addressed either sequentially or concurrently.

The transition from quadruped to kneeling *(mobility)* may be considered a continuation of the process of moving from prone on elbows to quadruped. Because the two transitions share key components, facilitation techniques are similar. Manual contacts are adjusted throughout the movement to facilitate most effectively shifting of the body posteriorly, as portrayed in Intervention 10.29. The transition to upright is cued by traction or approximation to the upper trunk or approximation to the pelvis. The applied force is small because the patient is already lifting his or her body weight against gravity. Once the patient is in a kneeling position with the trunk erect, alternating isometrics or rhythmic stabilization is used to create *stability* with suggested manual contacts, as pictured in Intervention 10.30. Manual contacts may be applied on the pelvis or on the lower or upper trunk, depending on the desired focus and lever arm.

There are many ways to promote *controlled mobility* in the kneeling position. Initial therapeutic activities emphasize active maintenance of a stable upright trunk. Examples include weight shifting in all directions with the trunk upright, chopping and lifting, and moving in and out of heel sitting or side sitting. Intervention 10.31 presents a sample of activities that may be used to enhance achievement of the controlled mobility stage in kneeling. Further progression promotes dynamic stabilization of the trunk during sagittal and then transverse plane movements. Slow reversal, slow reversal hold, and agonistic reversals are frequently used to apply appropriate resistance to selected patterns and movements of

INTERVENTION 10.26   Alternating Isometrics and Rhythmic Stabilization to Promote Stability in Quadruped

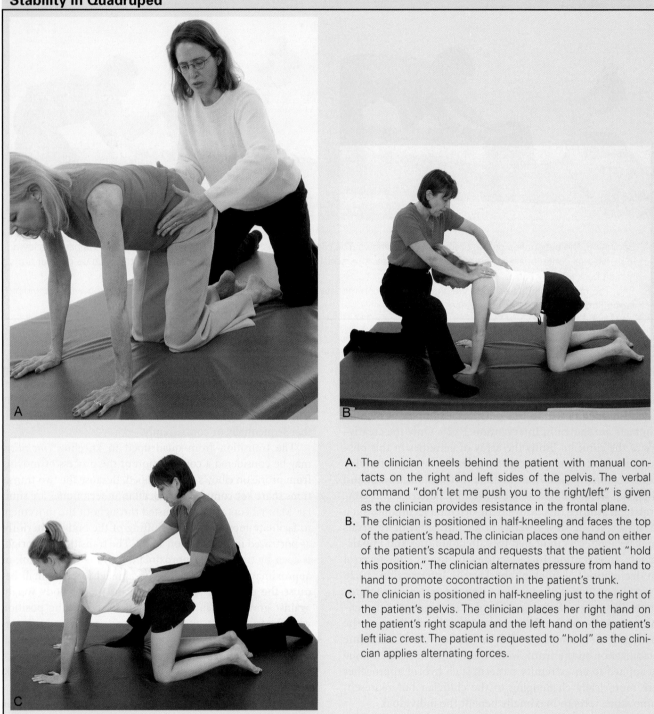

A. The clinician kneels behind the patient with manual contacts on the right and left sides of the pelvis. The verbal command "don't let me push you to the right/left" is given as the clinician provides resistance in the frontal plane.
B. The clinician is positioned in half-kneeling and faces the top of the patient's head. The clinician places one hand on either of the patient's scapula and requests that the patient "hold this position." The clinician alternates pressure from hand to hand to promote cocontraction in the patient's trunk.
C. The clinician is positioned in half-kneeling just to the right of the patient's pelvis. The clinician places her right hand on the patient's right scapula and the left hand on the patient's left iliac crest. The patient is requested to "hold" as the clinician applies alternating forces.

the UEs or trunk. Foundational motor components of higher level functional tasks, particularly sit to/from stand transfers, are recruited and reinforced through activities in kneeling.

The developmental level defined as *skill* in kneeling is represented by independent movements of the UEs while trunk and pelvic stability is actively maintained. Functional movements such as throwing or catching and writing on a chalkboard are categorized as skilled tasks that may be performed

while kneeling. These and other similar functional activities target impairments in strength, core stability, balance, endurance, and UEs and eye–hand coordination.

Half-kneeling is the last posture in the prone progression and enhances efficiency of transition from floor to standing. In cases of unilateral or asymmetrical impairment, either of the LEs may assume the forward position because there are therapeutic benefits associated with either placement.

INTERVENTION 10.27   Slow Reversal Technique to Promote Rocking in Quadruped

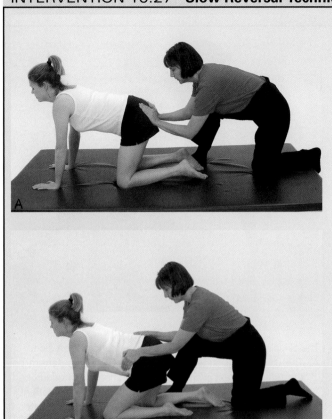

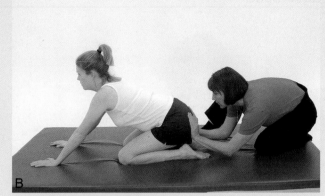

A. The clinician assumes half-kneeling behind the patient and places the heels of her hands over the ischial tuberosities. The patient is requested to "push back into my hands."

B. The patient continues the weight shift until the buttocks approximate the heels or through the desired excursion. The clinician shifts her body weight to accommodate patient's movement.

C. The clinician changes her manual contacts to the anterior superior iliac spine region bilaterally and provides the verbal command "pull your pelvis forward" as the patient returns to quadruped position.

The asymmetrical positioning of the LEs encourages dissociation of hip and knee musculature with the potential for functional carryover to higher level activities such as walking, stair climbing, and certain athletic endeavors associated with kneeling, which may be applied successfully in half-kneeling to enhance the *stability* and *controlled mobility* stages of motor control.

Sitting

Sitting is the primary position for many functional tasks, as well as the midpoint of the transition between recumbency and standing. The sitting position frees both UEs and loads the trunk in an erect position. Learning to weight shift and control the midline position of the trunk and pelvis helps to develop the balance, strength, and neuromuscular control necessary for efficient gait. Multiple combinations of trunk and extremity movements are possible in sitting, allowing patients to develop both mobility and stability in different body regions concurrently. Balance reactions also can be facilitated in this position.

Ideal sitting posture is one in which the pelvis and spine are in neutral positions; the head is aligned with the sternum; and the feet are firmly on the floor. Attention to these details will enhance the effectiveness of sitting activities and their carryover into functional tasks in more challenging postures.

Because many persons, especially those with neurologic dysfunction, tend to sit with the thoracic and lumbar spine flexed and the pelvis posteriorly tilted, facilitation is often required to assist patients in achieving an erect trunk. Postural correction should occur at the pelvis first because it is the foundation for upright sitting. The heels of the clinician's hands are placed between the iliac crest and ASIS, with the fingers pointing down and back toward the ischial tuberosities. The clinician may passively move the patient's pelvis from a posterior to an anterior tilt to help the patient gain awareness of the desired movements. To facilitate assumption of an anterior tilt position, the clinician may passively move the pelvis into a posterior tilt and give resistance down and back as the patient attempts to move the pelvis up and forward. Verbal cues such as "sit up tall" or "push your hips toward me" are used. Approximation or traction through the scapulae or shoulders provides a stimulus to move into an upright posture. Assistance is given if necessary for the patient to successfully achieve an upright posture. The therapist may be able to resist the stronger side and assist the weaker side, using the principle of overflow. Intervention 10.32 demonstrates methods of facilitating erect sitting posture using a variety of manual contacts.

Rhythmic initiation and hold relax active movement are effective techniques to teach patients to assume an upright

INTERVENTION 10.28   Extremity Patterns to Facilitate the Controlled Mobility Stage in Quadruped

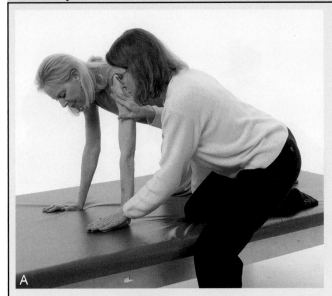

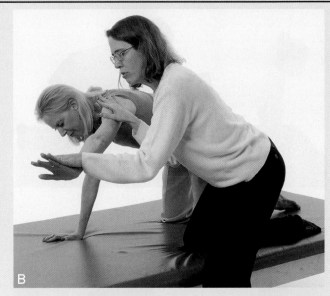

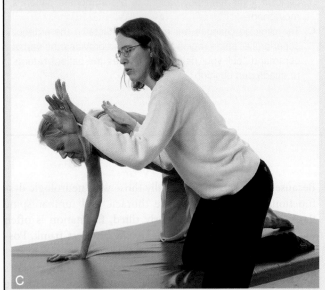

The clinician kneels or half-kneels on the patient's left side.

A. The clinician facilitates or resists the D_2 flexion pattern on the left upper extremity while the patient is in quadruped position. The clinician places her left hand on the patient's dorsal wrist and the right hand on the patient's anterolateral shoulder. The clinician asks the patient to "lift your arm up and out."

B. The patient continues through the pattern and shifts body weight to accommodate the change in base of support. The clinician mirrors patient movement.

C. As the patient nears end range of the pattern, the clinician may shift the right hand to the patient's left scapular region to promote greater scapular and trunk control as shown. The clinician continues to shift body weight to follow the patient's movement.

symmetrical sitting posture *(mobility)*. Intervention 10.33 depicts use of the latter technique. Manual contacts are placed in the direction of the desired movement, unless assistance is needed during early rehabilitation. Once the patient has achieved vertical posture, *stability* is created or reinforced by application of alternating isometrics or rhythmic stabilization. UE weight-bearing activities, with or without facilitatory techniques, may be appropriate in sitting, especially during the stability stage of motor control. Further progression into the *controlled mobility* stage includes lateral weight shifts on the pelvis, unilateral UE patterns, trunk movements in cardinal or diagonal planes, and chops and lifts. Recommended techniques for promoting dynamic trunk control include slow reversal, slow reversal hold, and agonistic reversal.

Emphasis may be placed on trunk rotation by incorporating lifting and chopping patterns. The combination of two extremities working together increases irradiation into the trunk musculature. Lifting pattern facilitates trunk extension, elongation on one side of the trunk, and a weight shift. Chopping pattern promotes trunk flexion, shortening of the trunk on one side, and a weight shift. The direction of the weight shift with either movement pattern varies. Resistive techniques (slow reversal, slow reversal hold, agonistic reversal) are applied as appropriate to increase strength, motor control, endurance, and coordination in the trunk and UEs. See Intervention 10.15 for an example of the use of trunk patterns in promoting erect sitting posture.

INTERVENTION 10.29   Transition From Quadruped to Kneeling

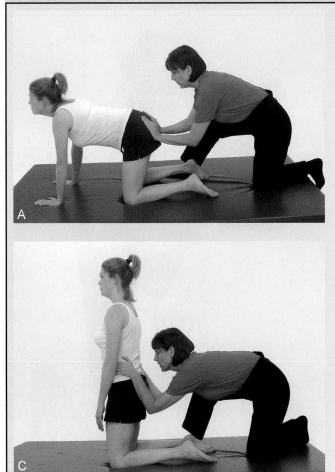

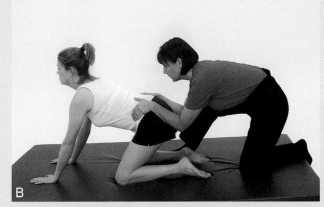

The clinician positions into half-kneeling to one side of the patient. The front foot is at level with the patient's knees.

A. The clinician places the heels of her hands on the patient's ischial tuberosities. The verbal command "sit back into my hands and push off your hands" is given.

B. The patient shifts weight backward to unload the upper extremities. Manual contacts are moved to the iliac crest and posterior pelvis to facilitate continued posterior weight shift.

C. The patient is then requested to "straighten your hips and trunk." Manual contacts shift, as needed, to promote hip and trunk extension. The transition is completed with the patient assuming the kneeling position.

Scooting

The key to successful scooting is the weight shift that occurs before advancing the pelvis forward. For any attempt at reciprocal scooting to be successful, a weight shift to the left must occur to unweight the right side of the pelvis. The right pelvis may then be advanced forward. The weight shift right occurs in a lateral and slightly forward direction with elongation of the left trunk and shortening of the trunk on the right. Left trunk lengthening is facilitated by placing one hand on the patient's left anterior superior shoulder and the other hand on the right anterior superior pelvis. The clinician stands in front of and to the left of the patient. An approximation force is applied concurrent with a verbal cue to "shift to me." The patient responds by lengthening the trunk on the left and shortening the trunk on the right. A manual contact on the right side of the pelvis is used to facilitate the advancement of the right pelvis. The clinician assists the pelvis forward if the patient is unable to perform the movement. The sequence is repeated to obtain elongation to the right side of the trunk and advancement of the left pelvis. The clinician switches position from side to side as the motion of scooting is facilitated. If the patient is unable to perform the motion of

reciprocal scooting, the clinician can isolate component parts, assisting as needed. Rhythmic initiation and hold relax active movement are useful tools that can assist in the process of teaching the patient the motions necessary for scooting. Once each component has been facilitated, the entire motion is then practiced to ensure motor learning of the task as a whole. Because scooting and sit-to-stand transfers (to be considered in the following section) are, by definition, movements, identification of developmental stages is irrelevant.

Sit to Stand

Moving from a seated position into standing requires the patient to move the COG over the BOS and lift the body against gravity. This task is quite challenging for many patients. Forward inclination of an extended trunk with the hips flexed and the knees anterior to the feet brings the COG over the feet and enables the weight of the body to be shifted forward and upward (Carr and Shepherd, 2014). As the person continues to lean forward, the buttocks are lifted off the chair. Ultimately, the hips and knees are extended as the trunk moves into an erect posture, and standing is achieved. Either assistance or resistance can effectively facilitate the

INTERVENTION 10.30   Alternating Isometrics and Rhythmic Stabilization Techniques to Promote Stability in Kneeling

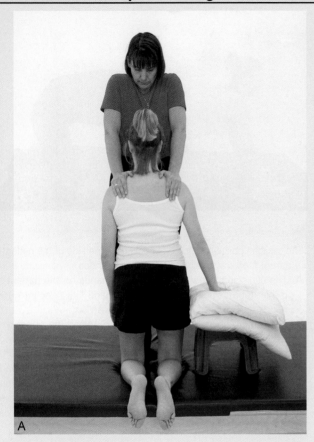

A

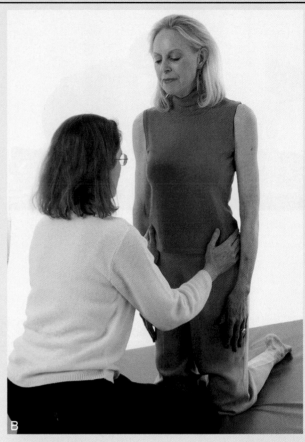

B

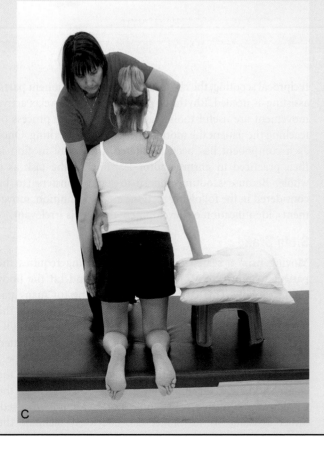

C

A. The patient kneels at the edge of the mat table with the feet extending off the surface. The right hand is supported on a stool. The clinician stands on the mat table and faces the patient. The verbal command "don't let me move you forward" is given. Symmetrical manual contacts are used to facilitate trunk extension. The clinician alternates between anterior and posterior hand placements to apply the alternating isometrics technique to enhance trunk stability.

B. The clinician kneels in front of the patient and places her hands on the patient's anterior pelvis. The verbal command "don't let me push you back" is given. Resistance is applied to match patient effort as alternating isometrics is applied. The clinician alternates between anterior and posterior manual contacts to sequentially facilitate both the trunk flexors and extensors.

C. The clinician stands in front of the patient and applies her hands to scapula and anterolateral pelvis. She requests that the patient "hold" the position as forces are applied to promote cocontraction of the trunk musculature during the rhythmic stabilization technique.

INTERVENTION 10.31   Activities to Promote Controlled Mobility in Kneeling

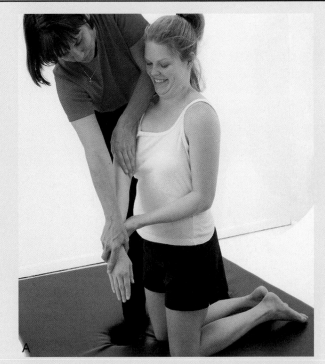

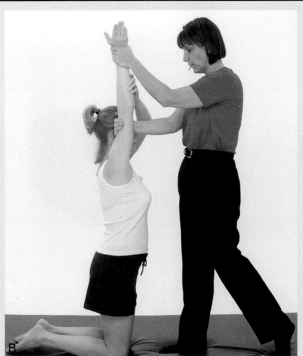

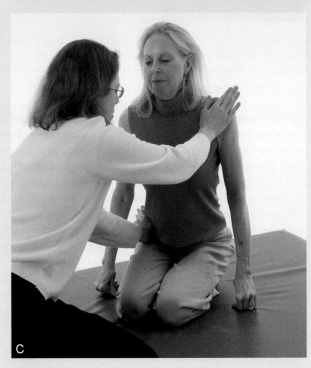

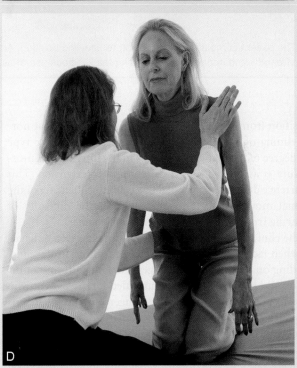

A. Right lifting pattern. The clinician stands behind the patient, adjacent to the right lead arm. The clinician places her right hand on the dorsal surface of the patient's right hand and the left hand on the patient's anterior humerus. The command "turn your right hand up and lift your arms over your right shoulder" initiates the pattern.

B. As the patient moves through the right lifting pattern, the clinician also moves through the diagonal position to accommodate the patient's movements and to maintain effective manual contacts. Optimally, patient gaze follows her lead hand.

C. Rising from heel sitting to kneeling. The clinician kneels (shown) or half-kneels and faces the patient. She contacts the anterior aspect of the patient's left shoulder and right pelvis. The patient's trunk should be erect and the arms at the sides. A request is made for the patient to "straighten your hips."

D. The patient proceeds through midrange of the transition, maintaining manual contacts, and the clinician shifts body position as needed to enhance patient effort.

Continued

INTERVENTION 10.31   **Activities to Promote Controlled Mobility in Kneeling—cont'd**

E. The patient completes the transition to kneeling position. Alternative manual contacts may be used to address individual patient strengths and impairments, including the judicious use of assistance and resistance at the thigh, pelvis, trunk, and head.

transition from sitting to standing. It is important that normal timing of the movement occurs regardless of the type and degree of facilitation. Weakness in the hip extensor musculature is associated with premature knee extension. This occurrence disrupts the normal timing and sequencing of the optimal movement pattern and increases the difficulty of achieving trunk extension in an efficient manner.

The clinician stands in front of the patient or on a diagonal when facilitating the transition from sitting to standing. Standing on a diagonal encourages a weight shift in that direction and is particularly recommended for the patient who tends to push up only with the stronger limb. Manual contacts vary based on the patient's needs and abilities. Hand placements on the upper trunk are effective for patients who have the ability to stand but need cues for the correct sequencing or timing of the movement. Manual contacts on the pelvis are more appropriate for patients who require greater facilitation to successfully complete this transfer (Cilento et al., 2013). The clinician's hands are placed on both sides of the pelvis in the space between the ASIS and the iliac crest. During the transitional movement, the clinician mirrors the forward movement expected from the patient. To maximize patient success, the clinician must deliberately plan and execute his or her own body movements. Posterior weight shift, synchronization of clinician and patient movements, and precise grading of resistance are crucial. The

verbal command consists of "lean toward me and stand up." Once initiated, the sit-to-stand transition must proceed without delay during any phase; otherwise, the patient will experience greater difficulty generating sufficient force to complete the transfer (Carr and Shepherd, 2014). Manual contacts on the pelvis, the clinician's movements, and concise verbal cues inform the patient as to which direction to move. Lifting patterns may be incorporated into the movement to enhance forward weight transfer and maintenance of erect trunk posture, as pictured in Intervention 10.34.

If assistance is needed only on the weaker side, the clinician can maintain manual contact on the pelvis on the strong side and assist the weaker side through a manual contact on the posterolateral iliac crest or at the buttocks. If the patient requires more assistance, both of the clinician's hands are placed on the buttocks to assist the patient into standing, maintaining appropriate timing during the transition. Initial use of an elevated surface, such as a raised hi-lo mat table or lift chair, lessens the demands of the activity to promote early success. Resistive LE patterns, bridging, and controlled mobility activities in sitting or kneeling help the patient to develop the requisite strength, coordination, and motor control to successfully perform sit-to-stand transfers.

Efficient return to sitting from the standing position with efficient eccentric control is also a relevant functional skill. Patients must constantly counteract the downward force of

INTERVENTION 10.32 Erect Sitting Posture

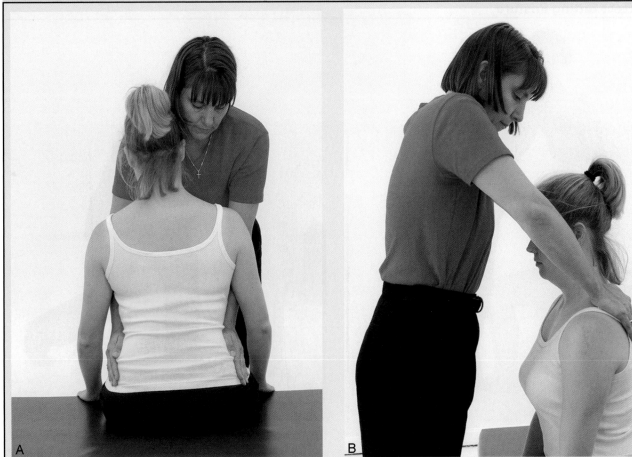

The clinician stands and faces the patient, who is seated on the edge of the mat table with feet on the floor.

A. The clinician may use the lower extremities to stabilize the patient's lower extremities as needed. The clinician uses manual contacts on the pelvis to facilitate an anterior pelvic tilt as a component of upright sitting posture. The clinician requests that the patient "bring your pelvis up and forward into my hands." The patient starts in a slouched sitting position. The end position of the requested movement is shown in the picture.

B. The patient sits on the mat table with feet on the floor. The clinician faces the patient with manual contacts on the scapulae. The patient is requested to "sit up tall" while the clinician applies approximation in a downward and posterior direction.

gravity to complete a controlled slow descent to the sitting position; therefore further resistance is rarely needed therapeutically. Carefully chosen and timed verbal cues and manual contacts, however, effectively improve the quality of this transitional movement. PNF techniques may be adapted and applied to both directions of the sit-to-stand transfer to improve quality, efficiency, and stability including hold relax active movement, slow reversal hold, and agonist reversal.

Standing

Safety and stability in standing are paramount to functional independence. Standing provides the foundation for many higher level functional tasks, such as gait, stand-pivot transfers, activities of daily living, cleaning or cooking tasks, and work-related skills. The transition from sitting position to standing is the *mobility* stage of motor control

and was addressed in the previous section. Once the patient has achieved erect standing, approximation may be used at the pelvis to enhance cocontraction of the muscles in the LEs and create *stability*. The clinician stands and faces the patient on a diagonal with one foot forward while applying approximation. A lumbrical grip (see Fig. 10.1) is used with the thenar eminence on the anterior superior aspect of the patient's iliac crest and fingers pointing toward the ischial tuberosities. Approximation is given through both sides of the pelvis equally and directed downward and backward at a 45-degree angle toward the patient's heels. Suggested hand placements are pictured in Intervention 10.35. The clinician gradually increases the amount of force used as the patient responds. Further *stability* can be developed through the use of alternating isometrics or rhythmic stabilization. The clinician may stand

INTERVENTION 10.33   Hold Relax Active Movement Technique to Promote Assumption of Erect Sitting Posture

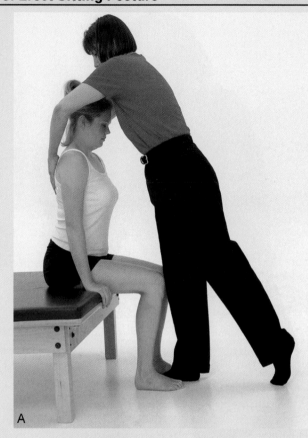

A

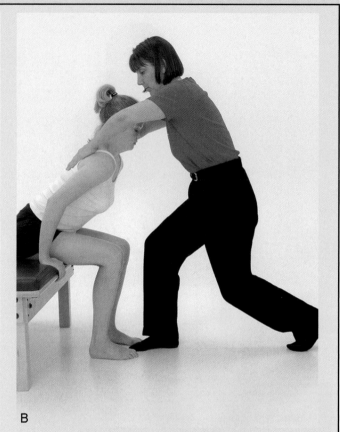

B

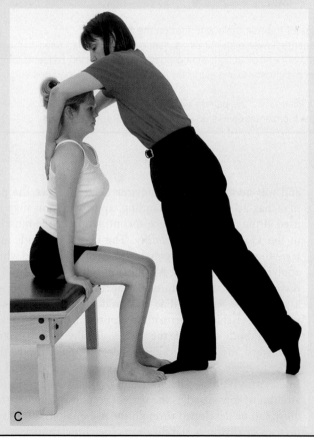

C

The patient sits without external support on the edge of the mat table with feet securely on the floor. The clinician stands in midstance position and faces the patient.

A. Manual contacts are placed on the patient's posterior trunk in the intrascapular area. The clinician resists an isometric hold of the trunk extensors in the shortened range.

B. On the command "relax," the clinician passively moves the patient into the lengthened range of trunk extensors. The clinician shifts body weight posteriorly during the movement.

C. The patient actively returns to the upright sitting position while the clinician facilitates or resists concentric contraction of the trunk extensors. The clinician shifts weight forward as the patient moves into erect sitting.

INTERVENTION 10.34   Activities to Promote Independent Standing in Symmetrical Stance Position

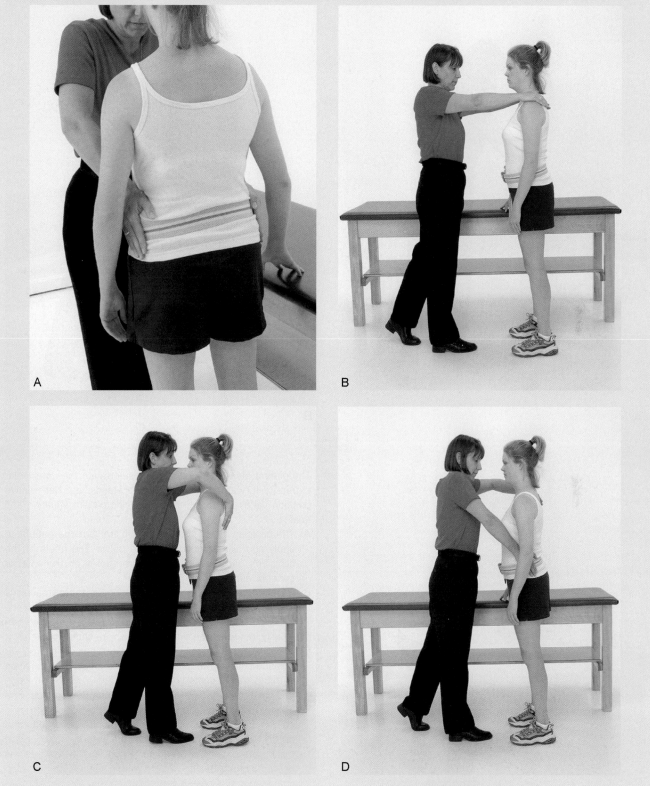

The patient stands with symmetrical foot placement. The clinician stands in midstance position and faces the patient.
A. The clinician applies approximation at the pelvis through manual contacts at the iliac crest. A verbal cue to "stand up straight" may be given.
B. The clinician applies approximation through the superior aspect of the shoulder girdle to promote upright trunk posture.
C. The clinician applies traction through hand placements over the scapula to promote upright standing.
D. Rhythmic stabilization is applied with asymmetrical manual contacts at the shoulder and the pelvis. Emphasis is on application of rotary forces to promote trunk cocontraction to enhance upright standing posture.

INTERVENTION 10.35   Activities to Promote Stability and Pelvic Control While Standing in Midstance Position

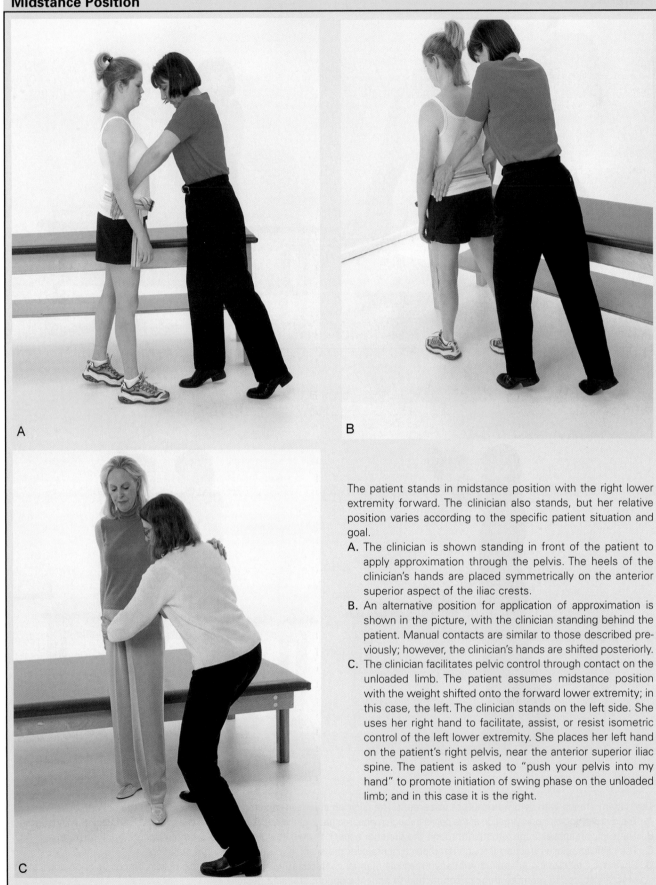

A

B

C

The patient stands in midstance position with the right lower extremity forward. The clinician also stands, but her relative position varies according to the specific patient situation and goal.

A. The clinician is shown standing in front of the patient to apply approximation through the pelvis. The heels of the clinician's hands are placed symmetrically on the anterior superior aspect of the iliac crests.

B. An alternative position for application of approximation is shown in the picture, with the clinician standing behind the patient. Manual contacts are similar to those described previously; however, the clinician's hands are shifted posteriorly.

C. The clinician facilitates pelvic control through contact on the unloaded limb. The patient assumes midstance position with the weight shifted onto the forward lower extremity; in this case, the left. The clinician stands on the left side. She uses her right hand to facilitate, assist, or resist isometric control of the left lower extremity. She places her left hand on the patient's right pelvis, near the anterior superior iliac spine. The patient is asked to "push your pelvis into my hand" to promote initiation of swing phase on the unloaded limb; and in this case it is the right.

directly in front of the patient or on a diagonal while applying these techniques.

Varying manual contacts assists in providing the amount of resistance that appropriately challenges the patient's abilities through changes in lever arm. The least resistance is experienced through use of contacts on the pelvis, and an intermediate amount through contacts on the thigh and lower trunk. The greatest resultant force is produced through hand placements on the lower leg, ankle, shoulder girdle, or UE.

Static positioning in single limb stance provides an excellent intermediate progression between bilateral LE standing and dynamic pregait activities. Techniques that promote stability, such as alternating isometrics and rhythmic stabilization as previously described for the typical standing position, are equally appropriate in single limb stance. Alterations in position or use of additional devices may be advantageous to maximize patient performance or safety, including placement of weight-bearing or non–weight-bearing limb on a stool, provision of a bar or surface for UE support, and positioning of patient perched on the corner of an elevated mat table with only one limb contacting the floor.

The *controlled mobility* stage of development is represented by weight-shifting and squatting activities through partial range, with the LEs assuming various positions. The crucial role of these activities in establishing a foundation for the acquisition of motor components involved in locomotion justifies the need for more detailed analysis and delineation in the following section.

Pregait Activities

In standing, *controlled mobility* activities are targeted at acquiring the skills needed to walk. Weight shifting is a fundamental movement that must be mastered before actual steps are attempted. Symmetrical standing may be used initially, with progression to midstance position (one foot forward) as soon as indicated by patient status. The midstance position in itself facilitates a weight shift from one limb to the other. Assumption of a lunge position with the forward limb flexed at the knee creates additional loading of the forward limb. Procedurally, the clinician uses contacts on the anterior pelvis similar to those used for scooting and the transition from sitting to standing. Intervention 10.36 shows several options for application of approximation and facilitation of pelvic control. Light hand support on a table or bar serves to increase patient stability, safety, and confidence. An additional staff member also may guard the patient to further ensure safety.

Rhythmic initiation assists the patient with the act of weight shifting by using a sequence of passive, active-assisted, active, and slightly resisted motions. Slow reversal hold can be an effective tool that simulates the sequence of isotonic then isometric muscle contractions used during gait. Lever arm may be varied through manual contacts at the pelvis, thigh, lower leg, or trunk. Contacts and resistance may be applied symmetrically or asymmetrically as indicated by patient abilities or responses. For example, appropriately strong resistance may be used through contact on the left midanterior thigh to produce overflow, whereas less resistance is applied on the left anterior pelvis to facilitate movement.

Some patients tolerate only short periods of time in the upright position because of multiple factors including cardiovascular status, balance, trunk control, coordination deficits, and cognitive impairment. Musculoskeletal conditions, such as arthritis in the hips, knees, or spine, also may limit tolerance to standing. It is often appropriate to determine alternative activities in lower level developmental positions to simulate the movements or muscle contractions required during standing and walking. Bridging and weight shifting in quadruped position or half-kneeling represent *controlled mobility* activities with direct functional carryover into components of the gait process. Slow reversal hold and agonistic reversals facilitate and reinforce the types of muscle contractions and movement strategies most crucial to upright locomotion. These techniques also serve to strengthen key muscles important to the process of initiating, sustaining, and refining gait patterns. Depending on the patient's unique abilities and needs, other suggested interventions include resisted extremity patterns in quadruped; rhythmic stabilization or alternating isometrics in quadruped, kneeling, or half-kneeling; and resisted LE patterns in side-lying, especially D_1 extension with emphasis on pelvic control. Some of these activities also may be adapted for inclusion in a home program.

After the patient achieves an adequate weight shift in the midstance position, further stability can be developed, especially in the forward limb through use of rhythmic stabilization. Manual contacts may be altered to focus on control of the pelvis, knee, or ankle. The importance of stability in the stance phase of gait cannot be overemphasized. Efficient progression, or swing through, of the unloaded limb occurs only when the stance limb provides adequate support and security. Once stance limb stability is deemed sufficient, swing phase of the unloaded limb may be facilitated by an applied stretch to ipsilateral pelvis through a lumbrical grip on the ASIS. The direction of the force is posterior and inferior, toward the ischial tuberosity. Application of the stretch is timed with the verbal cue, "step forward." Judiciously applied resistance may also facilitate greater movement. When the patient demonstrates satisfactory control of the pelvis, manual contacts may be moved to the anterior thigh to facilitate further hip flexion. As the foot again contacts the surface, the process of weight shifting and stabilization of the forward limb resumes. Many options exist for continued gait preparation and training. Suggested manual contacts are shown in Intervention 10.36. Dependent on the patient's responses, several typical routes are pursued. Repeated forward and backward stepping may be practiced with or without applied stretch. The procedure for facilitating backward or lateral stepping is similar to that of forward stepping, with the therapist's hands adjusted to facilitate muscle contraction or the desired direction of movement. The therapist may also alternate focus on the swing and stance limb through the procedures previously described. Resisted progression with manual contacts on the trunk, pelvis, or LE is introduced when facilitation through stretch is no longer needed.

INTERVENTION 10.36   Methods of Facilitating and Assisting With Swing Phase of Gait

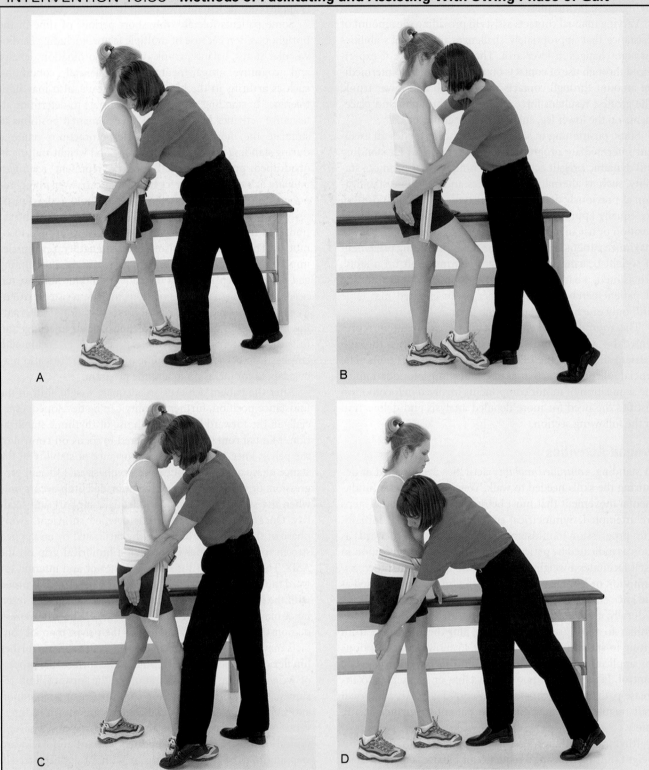

The clinician and patient both stand in midstance position and face each other.

A. The clinician facilitates initiation of the swing phase of gait through manual contacts and appropriate assistance at the ischial tuberosity. The clinician's other hand facilitates trunk extension.

B. The clinician assists the patient's right lower extremity through midswing. She steps backward during the movement to mirror the patient's progression.

C. The clinician facilitates weight transfer onto the right lower extremity through manual contacts at the posterior pelvis. The clinician repositions her body as needed.

D. The clinician demonstrates use of manual contacts at the posterior thigh to assist and facilitate initiation of swing phase.

INTERVENTION 10.36   **Methods of Facilitating and Assisting With Swing Phase of Gait—cont'd**

E

F

E. The patient progresses through midswing. The clinician shifts her manual contacts and body weight to accommodate patient movement.

F. The clinician promotes weight transfer onto the right lower extremity through manual contacts at the posterior thigh.

Retraining of a safe, efficient gait pattern in individuals with neurologic impairments is challenging for both the individual and the clinician. Although no one strategy is optimally effective for every client, the following progression may prove helpful:

- Approximation and stability exercises in standing with feet symmetrically placed
- Approximation and stability exercises in midstance and then with the patient's weight shifted forward onto the front limb
- Application of resistance at the pelvis of the advancing limb as the patient steps forward
- Repetitive stepping forward and backward with one limb
- Reciprocal gait with manual contacts at the pelvis and facilitatory stretch to the hip flexors at the initiation of swing phase
- Resistive reciprocal gait with manual contacts at the pelvis, then the trunk and lower extremities

Stair ambulation with or without an assistive device or handrail may be an appropriate goal for patients who demonstrate the requisite stability and strength. The progression of manual contacts and techniques suggested for level surface ambulation may be successfully adapted to the stair environment.

Deliberate choices regarding LE sequence and method (alternating versus nonalternating) are critical to both patient success and optimal challenge. Step descension provides a functional opportunity for development of eccentric control of the hip and knee extensor musculature. Use of step stools or stacking step platforms within the parallel bars may offer a more protected situation for preparatory training before use of an actual staircase.

PROPRIOCEPTIVE NEUROMUSCULAR FACILITATION AND MOTOR LEARNING

Motor learning is defined as "a set of processes associated with practice or experience leading to relatively permanent changes in the capability for producing skilled action" (Schmidt, 1988). From its conception, the intended outcome of PNF as a therapeutic approach has been to develop and refine functional movement strategies. In the preface to the second edition of their classic text, *Proprioceptive Neuromuscular Facilitation: Patterns and Techniques,* Margaret Knott and Dorothy Voss stated repeatedly that development and application of the PNF approach was targeted at maximizing motor learning. The following excerpt summarizes their perceptions:

All of the procedures suggested for the facilitation of total patterns have a common purpose: to promote motor learning. Oddly this term strikes some physical therapists as new or foreign, yet we have always tried to "teach the patient" to perform a motor act and have been pleased when the patient has learned (Knott and Voss, 1968).

A positive environment that nurtures an interactive relationship between clinician and patient sets the stage for optimal learning and relearning of motor skills. This environment creates a place in which the patient is motivated by realistic demands, clearly articulated expectations, and functionally relevant outcomes. Auditory, tactile, and proprioceptive input are crucial elements in promoting and reinforcing the motor performance that contributes to the acquisition of the pertinent functional skills. The continual process of implementing techniques and patterns matched with the patient's current abilities, observing the patient's responses, and making appropriate modifications is key to optimal achievement of the patient's functional goals.

Evidence for Proprioceptive Neuromuscular Facilitation

A growing body of evidence has examined the effectiveness of PNF techniques on select populations including those with stroke, transtibial amputation, and transfemoral amputation. In addition, evidence exists to support the use of PNF techniques on conditions that are not typically associated with this intervention, such as low back pain. Collectively, these studies consisted of a variety of research methods and designs, including case series, randomized controlled trials, and narrative systematic reviews. In addition, these studies demonstrated improvements in patient outcomes such as function, disability, health-related quality of life, pain, and muscle activity, among other variables, without adverse effects.

Stroke

In a recent case series by Cayco et al. (2019), researchers examined the effects of PNF techniques on four older adults with chronic stroke (Cayco et al., 2019). Summaries of PNF interventions (e.g., stabilizing reversals in sitting and standing) and progressions (e.g., rhythmic initiation to dynamic reversal) were provided for each patient. Outcomes included a battery of self-reported and performance-based measures: Upright Motor Control Test, Five Times Sit-to-Stand test, Activities-Specific Balance Confidence, Mini Balance Evaluation Systems Test, Limits of Stability, and self-selected and fast walking speeds. Findings after 18 intervention sessions (three times per week for 6 weeks) included varied findings that were interpreted in the context of published minimal detectible change and minimal clinically important difference values. Results indicated positive outcomes in all patients, and the researchers concluded that PNF improved multiple fall risk factors in patients with chronic stroke.

Slupska et al. (2019) examined the effects of PNF on accessory respiratory muscles using electromyography in patients after ischemic stroke (chronic poststroke phase). Patients were randomly assigned to a PNF group or a posi-

tion group, which was used as a reference for comparison (Slupska et al., 2019). The PNF group received PNF stretching techniques to stimulate their diaphragm and costal inferolateral regions. Although there were some differences in findings between the affected and unaffected sides, there were significant decreases in accessory muscle activity (i.e., abdominal external oblique, sternocleidomastoid, and pectoralis major muscles) in the PNF group. These findings suggested that PNF interventions can be used to help normalize breathing patterns in patients after ischemic stroke.

In a recent systematic review, researchers examined the effectiveness of PNF techniques on gait parameters in patients with stroke, when compared with routine physical therapy (Gunning and Uszynski, 2019). Their review yielded five studies of varied quality (PEDro scale and the Quality Assessment Tool for Quantitative Studies) with the majority (3/5) examining patients with chronic stroke (>6 months poststroke). PNF interventions varied and included mat activities, gait training, and techniques in standing and sitting positions. One study also examined the effects of early versus delayed PNF intervention. Although all studies examined gait, specific outcome measures used were different in each study making direct comparison difficult. All studies reported significant improvements in gait parameters for groups that received PNF (e.g., velocity, cadence, symmetry, maximum ankle dorsiflexion during swing, Rivermead Mobility Index, 6 Minute Walk Test, among others). The researchers concluded that PNF is an effective intervention for improving gait in patients with stroke.

Amputation

In a randomized controlled trial by Sahay et al (2014), patients with transtibial amputation were randomly assigned to a traditional prosthetic training group (control) or a PNF group (experimental) (Sahay et al., 2014). The control group received weight-bearing, weight-shifting, balance, and gait exercises. The PNF group received the same treatment as the control group with the addition of PNF principles and techniques including joint approximation, slow reversal, rhythmic stabilization, and pelvic patterns. Outcome measures of interest included select spatial and temporal gait parameters and the Locomotor Capabilities Index (LCI). There were significant between-group findings in favor of the PNF group for stride width and the LCI. This study demonstrated that an intervention using PNF is more effective than traditional prosthetic training in improving gait in patients with transtibial amputation.

In an often cited study, Yiğiter et al. (2002) compared the effects of traditional prosthetic training (control) with PNF training (experimental) for patients with transfemoral amputation. The control group received an intervention consisting of dynamic balance exercises, stool stepping, gait exercises, and stair training. The experimental group received similar interventions with the addition of PNF principles and techniques including resistance in the antagonistic direction, joint approximation, and rhythmic initiation, among other examples. The researchers examined numerous spatial and temporal parameters of gait and weight-bearing percentage. Both groups demonstrated numerous significant improvements in select gait parameters and weight-bearing percentage after treatment. However, the PNF group demonstrated significantly better improvements on all variables examined when compared with the control group, including: weight-bearing percentage, stride length, step length on side of amputation, step length on sound side, step width, cadence at self-selected walking speed, cadence at fast walking speed, self-selected walking speed, and stride length/lower limb length. These findings demonstrated that PNF techniques are better at improving weight-bearing and gait parameters in patients with transfemoral amputation than traditional training methods.

Chronic Low Back Pain

A recent review article by Paolucci et al. (2019) on chronic low back pain and postural rehabilitation exercise synthesized evidence on five different treatment techniques, including PNF. Paolucci et al. (2019) concluded that evidence supporting the use of PNF to treat chronic low back pain was promising because of the multiple positive effects and can benefit from further investigation to confirm its efficacy.

Areeudomwong et al. (2017) examined the effects of PNF on patients with chronic low back pain. Participants were randomly assigned to one of two groups. The control group received an educational booklet, which consisted of information on anatomy, causes of low back pain, an active self-management approach, and rehabilitative exercises. The PNF group received a program consisting on the following three phases: (1) alternating isometric contractions of the trunk flexors and extensors against maximum resistance, (2) alternating concentric and eccentric contractions of trunk agonists without relaxation, and (3) bilateral diagonal limb movements with maximum resistance. Patients that received PNF demonstrated significant improvements in pain (11-point numeric rating scale), disability (Roland-Morris Disability Questionnaire), patient satisfaction, health-related quality of lift (physical component summary of the SF-36), and muscle activity (electromyography of the lumbar erector spinae muscles) at the end of the intervention period

(4 weeks) and at follow-up (12 weeks), when compared with the control group.

In a similar study by Young et al. (2015) on patients with chronic low back pain, researchers compared the effects of a proprioceptive neuromuscular facilitation integration pattern (PIP) and Swiss ball training. Outcome measures included laboratory and clinical-based measures of static and dynamic balance and pain. Participants were older adults and randomly assigned to either treatment group. Those in the PIP group performed pattern and return pattern training, whereas those in the Swiss ball group performed balance training on the Swiss ball. After 6 weeks of intervention, both groups demonstrated significant improvements in static balance under different test conditions (Good Balance System), dynamic balance (Functional Reach test and Timed Up and Go test), and pain (visual analog scale). There were no significant differences between groups; therefore either treatment can be considered when trying to improve balance and pain in older adults with chronic low back pain.

Kim and Lee (2017) examined the effects of abdominal muscle strength training (AMST) using PNF on pulmonary function (FEV_1), pain (VAS), and function (Oswestry Disability Index [ODI]) in patients with chronic low back pain. Patients were randomly assigned to a control group (i.e., hot pack, interfacial current therapy, and ultrasound) or an experimental group (i.e., ASMT-PNF) for 6 weeks of treatment. The AMST-PNF intervention included exercises that used various positions (e.g., supine, side lying, sitting), patterns (e.g., bilateral asymmetrical LE, chopping, bilateral symmetrical UE), and techniques (e.g., rhythmic stabilization, combination of isotonics, contract-relax). Results indicated a significant within-group improvement in FEV_1 for the ASMT-PNF group only. Both groups demonstrated significant within-group improvements in VAS and ODI. The ASMT-PNF group, however, demonstrated significantly greater improvements in VAS and ODI when compared with the control group. These findings indicated that ASMT-PNF was effective at improving pulmonary function, pain, and disability in patients with chronic low back pain.

CHAPTER SUMMARY

Kabat and Knott created an approach to patient treatment in the 1940s that continues to grow and evolve today. The PNF treatment is an evidence-based approach that has clinical application to a wide variety of populations including people with stroke, amputation, and low back pain. It consists of a philosophy and basic principles, which can be adapted and applied by clinicians to any functional activity. By incorporating the basic principles of PNF, clinicians broaden their repertoire of intervention

strategies and are better able to customize therapeutic exercise programs to each patient's unique needs. When using PNF principles to create specific activities and patterns of movement for individual clients, a checklist ensures that the basic principles are being followed. Such care allows the clinician to incorporate PNF techniques to address specific problems and enhance patient performance. When the emphasis of treatment is on function, PNF is a viable and safe treatment option.

REVIEW QUESTIONS

1. Define the term *appropriate resistance* according to the PNF approach.
2. What is irradiation? Describe how this phenomenon may be used to promote movement in individuals with hemiplegia.
3. What two PNF techniques are frequently applied to increase stability?
4. What activities, patterns, or techniques are appropriate to use when the outcome is improvement of the functional ability to roll to the left in a patient who has sustained a

right brain stroke? How would clinician strategies change when teaching rolling to the right in the same individual?

5. A patient is having difficulty weight-bearing on the right lower extremity after a left brain stroke. What interventions are appropriate to enhance the patient's ability regarding right stance during gait?

6. A patient has weakness in the right gluteals. Identify activities to strengthen these muscles eccentrically. What PNF technique is most appropriate to address an eccentric deficit?

7. Hamstring shortness is limiting a patient's ability to sit with the knees extended (long sitting position). What PNF technique promotes lengthening of this muscle group?

8. For which other patient populations is there evidence to support the use of PNF techniques? Which specific interventions would you use for each population? Which outcome measures would you use to examine the effectiveness of PNF for each population?

REFERENCES

Adler SS, Beckers D, Buck M: *PNF in practice: an illustrated guide*, ed 4, Heidelberg, 2014, Springer.

Areeudomwong P, Wongrat W, Neammesri N, Thongsakul T: A randomized controlled trial on the long-term effects of proprioceptive neuromuscular facilitation training, on pain-related outcomes and back muscle activity, in patients with chronic low back pain, *Musculoskeletal Care* 15:218–229, 2017.

Bonnar BP, Deivert RG, Gould TE: The relationship between isometric contraction durations during hold-relax stretching and improvement of hamstring flexibility, *J Sports Med Phys Fitness* 44:258–261, 2004.

Burke DG, Culligan CJ, Holt LE: The theoretical basis of proprioceptive neuromuscular facilitation, *J Strength Cond Res* 14:496, 2000.

Carr J, Shepherd R: *Neurological rehabilitation: optimizing motor performance*, ed 2, Edinburgh, 2014, Churchill Livingstone/Elsevier.

Cayco CS, Gorgon EJR, Lazaro RT: Proprioceptive neuromuscular facilitation to improve motor outcomes in older adults with chronic stroke, *Neurosciences (Riyadh)* 24:53–60, 2019.

Chalmers G: Re-examination of the possible role of Golgi tendon organ and muscle spindle reflexes in proprioceptive neuromuscular facilitation muscle stretching, *Sports Biomech* 3:159–183, 2004.

Chiou SY, Wang RY, Liao KK, Yang YR: Facilitation of the lesioned motor cortex during tonic contraction of the unaffected limb corresponds to motor status after stroke, *J Neurol Phys Ther* 40:15–21, 2016.

Cilento M, Nóbrega, ACL, Araújo A: Evaluation of the efficacy of training protocols for the sit-to-stand activity in elderly women. In Ferraresi C, Parizotto NA, editors: *Muscle strength development, assessment and role in disease*, New York, 2013, Nova Science.

Gabriel DA, Basford JR, An KN: The reversal of antagonists facilitates the peak rate of tension development, *Arch Phys Med Rehabil* 82:342–346, 2001.

Gontijo LB, Pereira PD, Neves CD, Santos AP, Machado D, Bastos VH: Evaluation of strength and irradiated movement pattern resulting from trunk motions of the proprioceptive neuromuscular facilitation, *Rehabil Res Pract* 2012:281937, 2012. doi:10.1155/2012/281937.

Gunning E, Uszynski MK: Effectiveness of the proprioceptive neuromuscular facilitation method on gait parameters in patients with stroke: a systematic review, *Arch Phys Med Rehabil* 100(5):980–986, 2019. doi:10.1016/j.apmr.2018.11.020.

Hindle K, Whitcomb T, Briggs W, Hong J: Proprioceptive neuromuscular facilitation (PNF): its mechanisms and effects on range of motion and muscular function, *J Hum Kinet* 31:105–113, 2012.

International Proprioceptive Neuromuscular Facilitation Association: *PNF literature*, 2015, IPNFA. Available at: https://www.ipnfa.org/index.php/pnf-literature.html.

Kabat H: Proprioceptive facilitation in therapeutic exercise. In Licht S, Johnson EW, editors: *Therapeutic exercise*, ed 2, Baltimore, 1961, Waverly Press.

Kamimura T, Yoshioka K, Ito S, Kusakabe T: Increased rate of force development of elbow flexors by antagonist conditioning contraction, *Hum Mov Sci* 28:407–414, 2009.

Kay AD, Husbands-Beasley J, Blazevich AJ: Effects of contract–relax, static stretching, and isometric contractions on muscle–tendon mechanics, *Med Sci Sports Exerc* 47:2181–2190, 2015.

Kim BR, Lee HJ: Effects of proprioceptive neuromuscular facilitation-based abdominal muscle strengthening training on pulmonary function, pain, and functional disability index in chronic low back pain patients, *J Exerc Rehabil* 13:486–490, 2017.

Kisner C, Colby LA: *Therapeutic exercise: foundations and techniques*, ed 7, Philadelphia, 2018, FA Davis.

Knott M, Voss D: *Proprioceptive neuromuscular facilitation: patterns and techniques*, ed 2, New York, 1968, Harper & Row.

Kofotolis N, Vrabas I, Kalogeropoulou E, Sambanis M, Papadopoulos C, Kalogeropoulos I: Proprioceptive neuromuscular facilitation versus isokinetic training for strength, endurance and jumping performance, *J Hum Mov Stud* 42:155–165, 2002.

Kofotolis N, Vrabas I, Vamvakoudis E, Papanikolaou A, Mandroukas K: Proprioceptive neuromuscular facilitation training induced alterations in muscle fibre type and cross sectional area, *Br J Sports Med* 39(3):e11, 2005.

Loofbourrow GN, Gellhorn E: Proprioceptive modification of reflex patterns, *J Neurophys* 12:435–446, 1949.

McGraw MB: *The neuromuscular maturation of the human infant*, New York, 1962, Columbia University Press.

Mitchell UH, Myrer JW, Hopkins JT, Hunter I, Feland JB, Hilton SC: Neurophysiological reflex mechanisms' lack of contribution to the success of PNF stretches, *J Sport Rehabil* 18:343–357, 2009.

Paolucci T, Attanasi C, Cecchini W, Marazzi A, Capobianco SV, Santilli V: Chronic low back pain and postural rehabilitation exercise: a literature review, *J Pain Res* 12:95–107, 2019.

Prentice WE: Proprioceptive neuromuscular facilitation techniques in rehabilitation. In Hoogenboom B, Voight ML, Prentice WE, editors: *Musculoskeletal interventions: techniques for therapeutic exercise*, New York, 2014, McGraw Hill Education, pp 311–338.

Richter RR, VanSant AF, Newton RA: Description of adult rolling movements and hypothesis of developmental sequences. *Phys Ther* 69:63–71, 1989.

Sahay P, Prasad SK, Anwer S, Lenka PK, Kumar R: Efficacy of proprioceptive neuromuscular facilitation techniques versus traditional prosthetic training for improving ambulatory function in transtibial amputees. *Hong Kong Physiother J* 32:28–34, 2014. doi:10.1016/j.hkpj.2013.02.002.

Saliba V, Johnson G, Wardlaw C: Proprioceptive neuromuscular facilitation. In Basmajian J, Nyberg R, editors: *Rational manual therapies*, Baltimore, 1993, Williams & Wilkins, pp 243–284.

Schmidt RA: *Motor control and learning: a behavioral emphasis*, ed 2, Champaign, IL, 1988, Human Kinetics Publishers, pp 346.

Sharman MJ, Cresswell AG, Riek S: Proprioceptive neuromuscular facilitation stretching, *Sports Med* 36:929–939, 2006.

Sherrington C: *The integrative action of the nervous system*, ed 2, New York, 1947, Yale Press.

Shumway-Cook A, Woollacott MH: *Motor control: translating research into clinical practice*, ed 5, Philadelphia, 2017, Wolters Kluwer.

Slupska L, Halski T, Żytkiewicz M, et al.: Proprioceptive neuromuscular facilitation for accessory respiratory muscles training in patients after ischemic stroke. *Adv Exp Med Biol* 1160:81–91, 2019. doi:10.1007/5584_2018_325.

Sullivan PE, Markos PD: *Clinical decision making in therapeutic exercise*, Norwalk, CT, 1995, Appleton & Lange.

Sullivan PE, Markos PD, Minor MA: *An integrated approach to therapeutic exercise: theory and clinical application*, Reston, VA, 1982, Reston Publishing.

Voss D, Ionta M, Meyers B: *Proprioceptive neuromuscular facilitation: patterns and techniques*, ed 3, New York, 1985, Harper & Row.

Ward SR, Shahidi B, Barry D: Biomechanical applications to joint structure and function. In Levangie PK, Norkin CC, Lewek MD, editors: *Joint structure and function: a comprehensive analysis*, Philadelphia, 2019, FA Davis.

Westwater-Wood S, Adams N, Kerry R: The use of proprioceptive neuromuscular facilitation in physiotherapy practice, *Phys Ther Rev* 15:23–28, 2010.

Yiğiter K, Sener G, Erbahçeci F, Bayar K, Ulger OG, Akdoğan S: A comparison of traditional prosthetic training versus proprioceptive neuromuscular facilitation resistive gait training with transfemoral amputees, *Prosthet Orthot Int* 26:213–217, 2002.

Young KJ, Je CW, Hwa ST: Effect of proprioceptive neuromuscular facilitation integration pattern and Swiss ball training on pain and balance in elderly patients with chronic back pain, *J Phys Ther Sci* 27:3237–3240, 2015.

11

Stroke

Mary Kessler, Meghan Bretz

OBJECTIVES

After reading this chapter, the student will be able to:

1. Discuss the etiology and clinical manifestations of stroke.
2. Identify common complications seen in patients who have sustained a stroke.
3. Discuss the Core Set of Outcome Measures.
4. Describe appropriate treatment interventions for patients who have experienced strokes.
5. Recognize the importance of functional training for patients poststroke.
6. Discuss the evidence and application of locomotor training.

INTRODUCTION

Strokes or cerebrovascular accidents are the most common and disabling neurologic condition of adult life, with approximately 15% to 30% of those individuals impacted permanently disabled. The Centers for Disease Control and Prevention estimates that 4 million Americans are living with the effects of stroke, and that 795,000 new strokes occur annually. This equates to someone in the United States sustaining a stroke every 40 seconds (Centers for Disease Control and Prevention, 2017a). Of that number, 610,000 are first attacks and 185,000 are individuals who have sustained a previous stroke. It is estimated that by 2030, 34 million adults in the United States will have had a stroke. Strokes continue to be the fifth leading cause of death in the United States, with a mortality rate of approximately 133,000 individuals annually. It should also be noted that after more than 4 decades of declining stroke rates, the rate of decline has slowed and has been actually increased in certain areas of the country, the South, and in certain ethnic groups (Hispanic men) (Centers for Disease Control and Prevention, 2018a, 2017a, 2017b). With these numbers, one can appreciate the significant financial impact of stroke management. It is estimated that the cost for treating individuals with stroke was $66 billion in 2015 and is projected to be approximately $143 billion by 2035 (American Stroke Association, 2017).

Definition

A *stroke* or *cerebrovascular accident* may be defined as the sudden onset of neurologic signs and symptoms resulting from a disturbance of blood supply to the brain. The onset of the symptoms provides the physician with information regarding the vascular origin of the condition. The individual who sustains a stroke may have a temporary or permanent loss of function as a result of injury to cerebral tissue.

ETIOLOGY

The two major types of strokes are ischemic and hemorrhagic. Approximately 87% of all strokes are caused by ischemia, and 13% are caused by hemorrhage. Hemorrhagic strokes account for 30% of all stroke deaths (National Stroke Association, 2017).

Ischemic Cerebrovascular Accidents

Ischemia is a condition of hypoxia or decreased oxygenation to tissue and results from poor blood supply. Ischemic strokes can be subdivided into two major categories: those that result from thrombosis and those that result from an embolus.

Thrombotic strokes are most frequently a consequence of atherosclerosis. In atherosclerosis, the lumen (opening) of the artery decreases in size as plaque is deposited within the vessel walls. As a result, blood flow through the vessel is reduced, thereby limiting the amount of oxygen that is able to reach cerebral tissues. If an atherosclerotic deposit completely occludes the vessel, the tissue supplied by the artery will undergo death or cerebral infarction. A *cerebral infarct* is defined as the actual death of a portion of the brain.

Strokes of *embolic* origin are frequently associated with cardiovascular disease, specifically atrial fibrillation, myocardial infarction, or valvular disease. In embolic strokes, a blood clot breaks away from the intima, or inner lining of the artery, and is carried to the brain. The embolus can lodge in a cerebral blood vessel, occlude it, and as a result cause death or infarction of cerebral tissue.

The brain relies on constant blood perfusion to maintain neuronal function. If cerebral blood flow is lower than 20 mL/100 mg of tissue per minute, there is disruption in neurologic functioning. If perfusion is less than 8 to 10 mL/100 mg, cell death occurs (Fuller, 2015).

The area surrounding the infarcted cerebral tissue is called the *ischemic penumbra* or transitional zone. Neurons in this area are vulnerable to injury because cerebral blood flow is diminished, and as a result cannot support neuronal function (Fuller, 2015). Changes to neurotransmitters are thought to cause further injury after the ischemic insult. *Glutamate* is a neurotransmitter present throughout the central nervous system (CNS) and stored at synaptic terminals. The amount released at the synapse is regulated so that the level of glutamate is minimal. However, following an ischemic injury, the cells that control glutamate levels are compromised, which leads to overstimulation of postsynaptic receptors. This excessive level of glutamate in the extracellular space facilitates the entry of calcium ions into the cell. Calcium ions enter the cells and further propagate cellular destruction and death. Various destructive (catabolic) enzymes are activated by these calcium ions. As a consequence of tissue hypoxia and changes in tissue perfusion pressure, free radicals (neurotoxic by-products) are released leading to additional damage of vital cellular structures. Thus, damage to cerebral tissue may extend beyond the initial site of infarction (Fuller, 2015).

Hemorrhagic Cerebrovascular Accidents

Hemorrhagic strokes, including those that are caused by intracerebral and subarachnoid hemorrhage and arteriovenous malformation (AVM), result from abnormal bleeding from rupture of a cerebral vessel. The incidence of *intracerebral hemorrhage* (ICH) is low among persons less than 45 years old and increases after age 65. ICH is a major cause of morbidity and death accounting for 30% of all stroke deaths (National Stroke Association, 2017; Fuller, 2015). The incidence of ICH is higher for blacks and individuals of Asian descent (30%) as compared with 10% to 15% in whites. Common causes of spontaneous ICH include vessel malformation and changes in the integrity of cerebral vessels precipitated by the effects of hypertension and aging. Secondary causes of ICH include trauma, exposure to toxins, impaired coagulation, or some type of lesion (Fuller, 2015).

Subarachnoid hemorrhages are a consequence of bleeding into the subarachnoid space. The subarachnoid space is located under the arachnoid membrane and above the pia mater. Aneurysms, which can be defined as a ballooning or outpouching of a vessel wall, and vascular malformations are the primary causes of subarachnoid hemorrhages. These types of conditions tend to weaken the vasculature and can lead to rupture. Approximately 90% of subarachnoid hemorrhages are caused by berry aneurysms. A *berry aneurysm* is a congenital defect of a cerebral artery in which the vessel is abnormally dilated at a bifurcation (Fuller, 2015).

AVMs are congenital anomalies that affect the circulation in the brain. In AVMs, the arteries and veins communicate directly without a conjoining capillary bed (Fuller, 2015). Blood vessels become dilated and form masses within the brain. These defects weaken the blood vessel walls, which in time can rupture and cause a stroke. Hemorrhagic strokes that occur in individuals younger than 40 are often caused by AVMs (Fuller, 2015).

Transient Ischemic Attacks

Transient ischemic attacks (TIAs), which are frequently called mini strokes, resemble a stroke in many ways. When a patient experiences a TIA, the blood supply to the brain is temporarily interrupted. A patient complains of neurologic dysfunction, including loss of motor, sensory, or speech function. These deficits, however, resolve within 24 hours. The patient does not usually experience any residual brain damage or neurologic dysfunction. TIAs are, however, a serious warning sign that the individual is at risk for a future stroke. Approximately 40% of individuals who have a TIA will sustain a stroke and almost half of all strokes occur within a few days after a TIA. Treatment of TIAs includes lifestyle changes (diet changes, increasing physical activity, limiting alcohol intake, and smoking cessation) and pharmacologic interventions for hypertension, hyperlipidemia, and cardiac disease (National Stroke Association, 2019a).

MEDICAL INTERVENTION

Diagnosis

Medical management of a patient who has experienced a stroke includes hospitalization to determine the etiology of the infarct. The physician completes a physical examination to evaluate motor, sensory, speech, and reflex function. Additionally, an evaluation of the patient's cardiac status should be completed. Subjective information received from the patient or a family member regarding the time of onset of symptoms is also important. Neuroimaging by either a computed tomography scan or magnetic resonance imaging (MRI) scan is performed to determine whether the stroke is the result of ischemic or hemorrhagic injury and that information guides medical treatment. However, computed tomography scans that are performed initially do not always show small lesions and may not be able to detect an acute embolic stroke, whereas MRI can diagnose an ischemic event within 2 to 6 hours after the initial onset (Fuller, 2015). Diffusion-weighted imaging, a type of MRI, measures the movement of water in cerebral tissue and is useful in providing information regarding the brain's response to ischemia and to identify strokes in evolution (Fuller, 2015).

Acute Medical Management

Acute care management consists of monitoring the patient's neurologic function and preventing the development of secondary complications. Regulation of the patient's blood pressure, cerebral perfusion, and intracranial pressure is recommended. Pharmacologic interventions to manage hypertension including diuretics, beta-blockers, and angiotensin-converting enzyme inhibitors may be prescribed. Thrombolytic agents such as recombinant tissue plasminogen activator (rt-PA) can be administered to dissolve blood clots, improve blood flow, and minimize tissue damage (Fuller, 2015). This medication must, however, be administered within 4.5 hours of the event to maximize effectiveness. Patients treated with rt-PA within 90 minutes of their first symptom "are 25% less likely to die in the hospital, 28% less likely to" sustain an intracranial hemorrhage, and "33% more likely to be discharged home" (American Stroke Association, 2017). Because of its anticoagulant properties, rt-PA is not recommended for patients with cerebral hemorrhage or those with significant hypertension (Fuller, 2015). Unfortunately, only 25% of patients experiencing a stroke reach a hospital in time for the medication to be administered (American Stroke Association, 2017).

Neuroprotective agents minimize tissue damage when adequate blood supply does not exist. Medications that modify or interfere with glutamate release or enhance recovery from calcium overload have shown promise. Clinical trials continue to determine whether these drugs will be effective for patients with acute stroke (Fuller, 2015).

The medical management of ICH includes prompt diagnosis, decreasing blood pressure, and controlling intracranial pressure. Surgical intervention may be indicated in patients with large lobar insults or cerebellar hemorrhages (Fuller, 2015). "Endovascular thromboaspiration, sonothrombolysis, angioplasty, or stent placement can be performed" (Fuller, 2015). A carotid endarterectomy may be suggested in individuals 80 years and younger with carotid artery occlusion (Fuller, 2015).

RECOVERY FROM STROKE

Many survivors of stroke sustain permanent neurologic damage resulting in disability and are unable to resume previous social roles and functions. The most significant recovery in neurologic function occurs within the first 3 to 6 months after the injury, although movement patterns may be able to be improved with goal-directed activities for up to 5 years after the initial injury (Edwardson, 2019; Cumming et al., 2011; Fuller, 2015). General recovery guidelines estimate that 10% of the individuals who have a stroke recover almost completely, 25% have mild impairments, 40% experience moderate to severe impairments requiring care, 10% require placement in an extended-care facility, and 15% die shortly after the incident (National Stroke Association, 2019b). Specific data regarding functional outcome following strokes do vary. Data obtained from the Framingham Heart Study indicated that 69% of individuals who had a stroke were independent in activities of daily living (ADLs), 80% were independent in functional mobility tasks, and 84% had returned home. Despite independence in self-care and functional mobility skills, 71% of the study subjects had decreased vocational function, 62% had reduced opportunities for socialization in the community, and 16% were institutionalized (Roth and Harvey, 1996). Stroke severity, age, comorbidities, and socioeconomic status have all been associated with lower rates of recovery and functional potential (Edwardson, 2019; Cumming et al., 2011).

Ambulation abilities are a primary factor in the determination of discharge destination and whether patients are able to return to previous levels of social and vocational activities (Hornby et al., 2011). It has been reported that 3 months after

stroke, 20% of individuals remain dependent on their wheelchair for mobility and that approximately 80% of patients experience significant gait deficits (Hornby et al., 2011; Mehrholz et al., 2017). Gait velocity is a "reliable, valid, sensitive measure of recovery of poststroke mobility that discriminates the effects of stroke and is related to the potential for rehabilitation recovery" (Schmid et al., 2007). Gait speed has also been reported to be a strongly related to an individual's perception of balance and self-efficacy (Shumway-Cook and Woollacott, 2017).

PREVENTION OF CEREBROVASCULAR ACCIDENTS

Although progress has been made in the medical management of patients after stroke, more attention has been given to the area of prevention. Individuals can reduce their risk of stroke by recognizing the medical and lifestyle risk factors associated with the condition. Everyone has some risk for the development of stroke, including age (being over the age of 55). It has been reported that your risk of stroke doubles every 10 years after the age of 55 although one in seven strokes occurs in adolescents and adults ages 15 to 49 (Centers for Disease Control and Prevention, 2018c). One's race is also a risk factor as blacks, Hispanics, and American Indians have a greater incidence of stroke. Sex is also a risk factor as 55,000 more women than men sustain strokes annually (Centers for Disease Control and Prevention, 2018c; American Stroke Association, 2017).

Medical risk factors include previous stroke, TIA, cardiac disease, diabetes, atrial fibrillation, and hypertension. Hypertension is defined as a blood pressure of 160/95, although the Centers for Disease Control and Prevention recommend blood pressure readings of less than 140/90. Lowering one's diastolic blood pressure by 5 to 6 mm Hg results in a reduction of stroke risk by 40% (Fuller, 2015). Risk factors associated with lifestyle include smoking, obesity, alcohol and drug use, and inactivity. Approximately 80% of all strokes are preventable through changes in one's lifestyle and following the recommendations of your health care provider (Centers for Disease Control and Prevention, 2018b).

Unfortunately, most individuals do not recognize that strokes are preventable and that medical interventions are available. Only 25% of patients with stroke arrive at the hospital within 3.5 hours after the onset of symptoms (American Stroke Association, 2017). The window of opportunity for administration of medications that enhance patient outcomes is exceeded within this time frame. In an effort to educate the public, support to rename stroke as a *brain attack* has continued. The National Stroke Association has also developed the educational program F.A.S.T. to assist the public in recognizing the warning signs of a stroke: F-Face: Ask the person to smile and note any drooping of the facial muscles; A-Arms: Ask the person to lift both upper extremities and note muscle weakness and symmetry; S-Speech: Ask the person to repeat a simple phrase or sentence and note any speech difficulties; T-Time: If you note any of these signs, individuals are encouraged to activate the emergency medical system (call 911) immediately (American Stroke Association, 2017). Additionally, it is important to record the time of onset of the first symptom. Other signs and symptoms that may be evident include numbness in the face or extremities, confusion, double vision, dizziness, loss of balance, difficulty walking, and/or a severe headache. It is hoped that this education strategy (similar to that used during a myocardial infarction) will lead to earlier entry into the medical system and improved outcomes for individuals with strokes.

STROKE SYNDROMES

To understand the clinical manifestations seen in an individual who has sustained a stroke, it is necessary to know the structure and function of the various parts of the brain, as well as the distribution of the cerebral circulation. A review of this information can be found in Chapter 2. Because specific arteries supply blood to various parts of the cortex and brain stem, a blockage or hemorrhage in one of the vessels results in fairly predictable clinical findings. Individual differences, however, do occur. Table 11.1 provides a review of common stroke syndromes.

Anterior Cerebral Artery Occlusion

A blockage in the anterior cerebral artery is uncommon and is most frequently caused by an embolus (Fuller, 2015). The anterior cerebral artery supplies the superior border of the frontal and parietal lobes of the brain. A patient who has an anterior artery occlusion will have contralateral weakness and sensory loss, primarily in the lower extremity, aphasia, incontinence, and apraxia.

Middle Cerebral Artery Occlusion

Middle cerebral artery infarcts, which are the most common type of stroke, can result in contralateral sensory loss and weakness in the face and upper extremity. Patients with middle cerebral artery infarcts often have less involvement

in their lower extremities. Infarction of the dominant hemisphere can lead to global aphasia. *Homonymous hemianopia*, which is a defect or loss of vision in the temporal half of one visual field and the nasal portion of the other, may be evident. A patient may also experience a loss of *conjugate eye gaze*, which is the movement of the eyes in parallel.

Vertebrobasilar Artery Occlusion

Complete occlusion of the vertebrobasilar artery is often fatal and if the patient survives bilateral brainstem symptoms can be evident. Cranial nerve involvement including *diplopia* (double vision), *dysphagia* (difficulty in swallowing), *dysarthria* (difficulty in forming words secondary to weakness in the tongue and muscles of the face), *deafness*, and *vertigo* (dizziness) may be present. In addition, infarcts to areas supplied by this vascular distribution may lead to *ataxia*, which is characterized by uncoordinated movement, equilibrium deficits, and headaches.

Blockage of the basilar artery can cause the patient to experience *locked-in syndrome*. Patients with this type of stroke have significant motor impairments. The patient is alert and oriented but is unable to move or speak because of weakness in all muscle groups. Eye movements are the only type of active movement possible, and thus become the patient's primary means of communication (Fuller, 2015).

Posterior Artery Occlusion

Occlusion of the proximal component of the posterior artery results in injury to the subthalamus, medial thalamus, and midbrain. Abnormal perception of pain, temperature, touch, and proprioception is noted. The posterior cerebral artery also supplies the occipital and temporal lobes. Occlusion in this artery can lead to contralateral sensory loss; pain; memory deficits; homonymous hemianopia; *visual agnosia*, which is an inability to recognize familiar objects or individuals; and *cortical blindness*, which is the inability to process incoming visual information even though the optic nerve remains intact (Fuller, 2015).

TABLE 11.1	**Cerebral Circulation and Resultant Stroke Syndromes**	
Artery	**Distribution**	**Patient Deficits**
Anterior cerebral	Supplies the superior border of the frontal and parietal lobes.	Contralateral weakness and sensory loss primarily in the lower extremity, incontinence, aphasia, and apraxia.
Middle cerebral	Supplies the surface of the cerebral hemispheres and the deep frontal and parietal lobes.	Contralateral sensory loss and weakness in the face and upper extremity, less involvement in the lower extremity, homonymous hemianopia, and aphasia.
Vertebrobasilar	Supplies the brainstem and cerebellum.	Cranial nerve involvement (diplopia, dysphagia, dysarthria, deafness, vertigo), ataxia, equilibrium disturbances, headaches, and dizziness.
Posterior cerebral	Supplies the occipital and temporal lobes, thalamus, and upper brainstem.	Abnormal perception of pain, temperature, touch and proprioception (proximal component of the artery). Contralateral sensory loss, pain, memory deficits, homonymous hemianopia, visual agnosia, and cortical blindness (posterior component of the artery).

Lacunar Infarcts

Lacunar infarcts are most often encountered in the deep regions of the brain, including the internal capsule, thalamus, basal ganglia, and pons. The term *lacuna* is used because a cystic cavity remains after the infarcted tissue is removed. These infarcts are common in individuals with diabetes and hypertension, and result from small vessel arteriolar disease. Clinical findings can include contralateral weakness and sensory loss, ataxia, and dysarthria.

Other Stroke Syndromes

Other stroke syndromes may occur in patients. The neurologic impairments are closely related to the area of the brain affected. For example, a stroke within the parietal lobe can cause inattention or neglect, which is manifested as a disregard for the involved side of the body; an impaired perception of vertical, visual, spatial, and topographic relationships; and motor perseveration. *Perseveration* is the involuntary persistence of the same verbal or motor response regardless of the stimulus or its duration. Patients who demonstrate perseveration may repeat the same word or movement over and over. It is often difficult to redirect these patients to a new idea or activity.

The resultant patient findings also depend on the hemisphere of the brain affected, although motor and sensory functions are attributed to both hemispheres. Reviewing information covered in Chapter 2, the left hemisphere of the brain is the verbal and analytic side. The left hemisphere allows individuals to process information sequentially and to solve problems. Speech and reading comprehension are also functions of the left hemisphere. The right hemisphere of the brain allows individuals to look at information holistically, to process visual information, to perceive emotions, and to be aware of body image and impairments (Deutsch and O'Sullivan, 2019).

Thalamic Pain Syndrome

Thalamic pain syndrome can occur following an infarction or hemorrhage in the lateral thalamus, the posterior limb of the internal capsule, or the parietal lobe. The patient experiences intolerable burning pain and sensory perseveration. The sensation of the stimulus remains long after the stimulus has been removed or terminated. The patient also perceives the sensation as noxious and exaggerated.

Pusher Syndrome

Patients with strokes in the right or left posterolateral thalamus may demonstrate *pusher syndrome* (Karnath and Broetz, 2003). The prevalence of this condition is approximately 10% to 16% (Abe et al., 2012). Patients with pusher syndrome actively push and lean toward their hemiplegic side and are at increased risk for balance deficits and falls (Abe et al., 2012). Efforts to passively correct the patient's posture are met with resistance (Roller, 2004). Davies (1985) identified the clinical presentation of patients with this condition as: (1) cervical rotation and lateral flexion to the right; (2) absent or significantly impaired tactile and kinesthetic awareness; (3) visual deficits; (4) truncal asymmetries; (5) increased weight-bearing on the left during sitting activities, with resistance encountered when attempts are made to achieve an equal weight-bearing position; and (6) difficulties with transfers as the patient pushes backward and away with the right (uninvolved) extremities. Patients with pusher syndrome frequently report sitting or standing upright when in fact they are actually tilted approximately 18–20 degrees toward their hemiparetic side (Karnath and Broetz, 2003). Patients experience a mismatch between their perception of vertical and the body's orientation to the environment and gravity (Karnath and Broetz, 2003). Specific treatment interventions for patients with this syndrome are discussed later in the chapter.

Summary

In summary, although a description of the different stroke syndromes and a classification system for right hemisphere and left hemisphere disorders have been provided, each patient will have different clinical signs and symptoms. Patients should be viewed and treated as individuals and should not be classified on the basis of which side of the body is impaired. The information presented regarding the functional differences between the right and left hemispheres is meant to serve only as a guide or framework in understanding possible patient impairments and selecting appropriate treatment interventions.

CLINICAL FINDINGS: PATIENT IMPAIRMENTS

A patient who has sustained a stroke may have a number of different impairments. The extent to which these impairments interfere with the patient's functional capabilities and participation in life roles is dependent on the nature of the stroke, the amount of nervous tissue damaged, and the potential for neuroplastic changes. In addition, any preexisting medical conditions, the amount of family support available, and the patient's financial resources may affect the patient's recovery and eventual outcome (Edwardson, 2019).

Motor Impairments

One of the primary and most prevalent of all clinical manifestations seen in patients following stroke is the spectrum of motor problems resulting from damage to the motor cortex. Approximately 70% of all patients with stroke experience persistent motor impairments (Hornby et al., 2011). Initially, a patient may be in a state of low muscle tone or flaccidity. *Flaccid* muscles lack the ability to generate muscle contractions and to initiate movement. This condition of relative low muscle tone is usually transient, and the patient soon develops characteristic patterns of hypertonicity or spasticity. *Spasticity* is a motor disorder characterized by exaggerated deep tendon reflexes (DTRs) and velocity-dependent increased muscle tone. Clinically, the patient with spasticity has increased resistance to passive stretching of the involved muscle, hyperreflexia of DTRs, posturing of the extremities in flexion or extension, cocontraction of muscles, and stereotypical movement patterns called *synergies*.

Spasticity

Theories regarding the development of spasticity have evolved as research in the area of motor behavior has increased. The classic theory of spasticity development centers around the idea that spasticity develops in response to an upper motor neuron injury. This view of spasticity incorporates a hierarchic view of the nervous system and the development of motor control and movement. Investigators had previously postulated that spasticity developed from hyperexcitability of the monosynaptic stretch reflex. This theory is based on muscle spindle physiology. Increased output from the muscle spindle afferents or sensory receptors controls alpha motor neuron activity in the gray matter of the spinal cord. Uninterrupted activity of the gamma efferent or motor system is thought to account for continuous activation of the afferent system by maintaining the muscle spindle's sensitivity to stretch (Craik, 1991).

Research raises questions regarding the validity of this theory. Investigators have postulated that the stretch reflex is not strong enough to control all alpha motor neuron activity. In today's view of spasticity, hypertonicity or increased muscle tone is thought to develop from abnormal processing of the afferent (sensory) input after the stimulus reaches the spinal cord. In addition, investigators have proposed that a defect in inhibitory modulation from higher cortical centers and spinal interneuron pathways leads to the presence of spasticity in many patients (Craik, 1991).

Assessment of Tone

The Modified Ashworth Scale is a clinical tool used to assess the presence of abnormal tone/spasticity in individuals with CNS injuries. A 0 to 4 ordinal scale is used. A score of 0 equates to no increase in muscle tone, whereas a score of 4 indicates that the affected area is fixed in either flexion or extension (Bohannon and Smith, 1987; Rehabilitation Measures Database, 2016a). Table 11.2 describes each of the grades. Clinicians who wish to learn more about this scale may access the tool at www.sralab.org/rehabilitation-measures.

The Rehabilitation Measures Database provides information on over 400 outcome measures and includes guidelines for tool administration, clinical utility, and psychometric properties of the various instruments represented. The reader is advised to become familiar with the database as it is a useful resource for both students and clinicians.

Stages of Motor Recovery

Signe Brunnstrom did much to describe the characteristic stages of motor recovery following stroke. Brunnstrom observed many patients who had sustained strokes and noted a characteristic pattern of muscle tone development and recovery (Sawner and LaVigne, 1992). Table 11.3 gives a description of each of the Brunnstrom stages of recovery.

Brunnstrom reported that, initially, the patient experienced flaccidity in involved muscle groups. As the patient recovered, flaccidity was replaced by the development of spasticity. Spasticity increased and reached its peak in stage 3. At this time, the patient's attempts at voluntary movements were limited to the flexion and extension synergies (Sawner and LaVigne, 1992).

A synergy is defined as a group of muscles that work together to provide patterns of movements. These patterns initially occur in flexion and extension combinations. The movements produced are stereotypical and primitive and can be elicited either as a reflexive or a volitional movement response. Flexion and extension synergies have been described for both the upper and lower extremities (Sawner and LaVigne, 1992). Table 11.4 provides a description of the upper extremity and lower extremity flexion and extension patterns.

In the later stages of Brunnstrom's recovery patterns, spasticity begins to decline, and the patient's movements are dominated to a lesser degree by the synergy patterns. An individual may be able to combine movements in both the flexion and extension patterns and may have increased voluntary control of movement combinations. In the final stages of recovery, spasticity is essentially absent, and isolated movement is possible. The patient is able to control speed and direction of movement with increased ease, and fine motor skills improve. Brunnstrom reported that a patient passes through all of the stages and that a stage would not be skipped. However, variability in a patient's clinical presentation at any stage is possible. The patient may, in fact, move through a stage quickly, and thus observation of its typical characteristics may be difficult. Brunnstrom also postulated

TABLE 11.2 Modified Ashworth Scale for Grading Spasticity

Grade	Description
0	No increase in muscle tone.
1	Slight increase in muscle tone, manifested by a catch and release or by minimal resistance at the end of the range of motion when the affected part is moved in flexion or extension.
1 +	Slight increase in muscle tone, manifested by a catch, followed by minimal resistance throughout the remainder (less than half) of the range of motion.
2	More marked increase in muscle tone through most of the range of motion, but affected part easily moved.
3	Considerable increase in muscle tone, passive movement difficult.
4	Affected part rigid in flexion or extension.

From Bohannon RW, Smith MB: Interrater reliability of a modified Ashworth scale of muscle spasticity, *Phys Ther* 67:207, 1987. With permission from the American Physical Therapy Association.

TABLE 11.3 Brunnstrom Stages of Recovery

Stage	Description
I. Flaccidity	No voluntary or reflex activity is present in the involved extremity.
II. Spasticity begins to develop	Synergy patterns begin to develop. Some of the synergy components may appear as associated reactions.
III. Spasticity increases and reaches its peak	Movement synergies of the involved upper or lower extremity can be performed voluntarily.
IV. Spasticity begins to decrease	Deviation from the movement synergies is possible. Limited combinations of movement may be evident.
V. Spasticity continues to decrease	Movement synergies are less dominant. More complex combinations of movements are possible.
VI. Spasticity is essentially absent	Isolated movements and combinations of movements are evident. Coordination deficits may be present with rapid activities.
VII. Return to normal function	Return of fine motor skills.

TABLE 11.4 Components of the Brunnstrom Synergy Patterns

	Flexion	Extension
Upper extremity	Scapular retraction and/or elevation, shoulder external rotation, shoulder abduction to 90 degrees, elbow flexion, forearm supination, wrist and finger flexion.	Scapular protraction, shoulder internal rotation, shoulder adduction, full elbow extension, forearm pronation, wrist flexion with finger flexion.
Lower extremity	Hip flexion, abduction and external rotation, knee flexion to approximately 90 degrees, ankle dorsiflexion and inversion, toe extension.	Hip extension, adduction, and internal rotation, knee extension, ankle plantar flexion and inversion, toe flexion.

(Modified from Sawner KA, LaVigne JM: *Brunnstrom's movement therapy in hemiplegia, ed 2*, Philadelphia, 1992, JB Lippincott, pp. 41–42.)

that a patient could plateau at any stage, and consequently full recovery would not be possible (Sawner and LaVigne, 1992). As mentioned previously, each patient is unique and progresses through the stages at different rates. Therefore a patient's long-term prognosis and functional outcome are difficult to predict in the early stages of rehabilitation.

Despite the fact that therapists do not use the Brunnstrom stages as much as we once did, they are helpful, especially to students, in the recognition of hemiplegic movement patterns and motor recovery in our patients. Additionally, the stages are utilized as part of the assessment of upper and lower extremity function in the Fugl-Meyer Assessment of Motor Recovery After Stroke, which is a widely used clinical and research tool to quantify recovery in patients with stroke (Rehabilitation Measures Database, 2016b).

Development of Spasticity in Proximal Muscle Groups

Spasticity often initially develops in the muscles of the shoulder and pelvic girdles. At the shoulder, one can see adduction and downward rotation of the scapula. The scapular depressors, as well as the shoulder adductors and internal rotators, can develop muscle stiffness. As upper extremity muscle tone increases, tone in the biceps, forearm pronators, and wrist and finger flexors may also become evident. This pattern of tone produces the characteristic upper extremity posturing seen in patients who have sustained strokes. Fig. 11.1 illustrates this positioning.

Anterior tilting or hiking is common at the pelvis. The pelvic retractors, hip adductors, and hip internal rotators can develop spasticity. In addition, the knee extensors or quadriceps, the ankle plantar flexors and supinators, and the toe flexors can become hypertonic. This pattern of abnormal tone development produces the characteristic lower extremity extensor positioning seen in many patients. As the patient attempts to initiate movement, the presence of abnormal tone and synergies can lead to the characteristic flexion and extension movement patterns.

Other Motor Impairments

Additional motor problems can become evident in this patient population. The impact of muscle weakness or paresis is receiving new emphasis in the literature. Approximately 75% to 80% of patients who have a stroke are often unable to generate normal levels of muscular force, tension, or torque to initiate and control functional movements or to maintain a posture. After a stroke, patients may have difficulty in maintaining a constant level of force production to control movements of the extremities (Ryerson, 2013). Atrophy of remaining muscle fibers on the involved side, abnormal recruitment and timing of muscle activation, and motor units that are more easily fatigued are common findings (Craik, 1991; Light, 1991). One additional point that must be made is that a stroke does not affect only one side of the body. The muscles on the uninvolved side can also exhibit mild weakness (Deutsch and O'Sullivan, 2019; Craik, 1991).

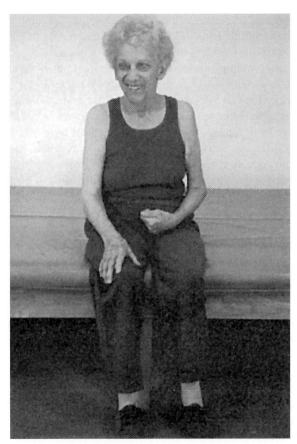

Fig. 11.1 Characteristic upper extremity posturing seen in patients following cerebrovascular accident. The patient has increased tone in the shoulder adductors and internal rotators, biceps, forearm pronators, and wrist and finger flexors. (From Ryerson S, Levit K: *Functional movement reeducation: a contemporary model for stroke rehabilitation*, New York, 1997, Churchill Livingstone.)

Motor Planning Deficits

Motor planning problems may be present in patients who have sustained a stroke. These problems are most frequently noted in patients with involvement of the left hemisphere because of its primary role in the sequencing of movements. Patients can exhibit difficulty in performing purposeful movements, although no sensory or motor impairments are noted. This condition is called *apraxia*. Patients with apraxia may have the motor capabilities to perform a specific movement combination such as a sit-to-stand transfer, but they are unable to determine or remember the steps necessary to achieve this movement goal. Apraxia may also be evident when the patient performs self-care activities. For example, the patient may not remember how to don a piece of clothing or what to do with an item, such as a comb or a brush.

Sensory Impairments

Sensory deficits can also cause the patient many difficulties. Patients who sustain strokes of the parietal lobe may demonstrate sensory dysfunction. Individuals may lose their tactile (touch) or proprioceptive capabilities. *Proprioception* is defined as the patient's ability to perceive position sense. The way in which the physical therapist (PT) evaluates a patient's proprioception is to move a patient's joint quickly in a certain direction. Up-and-down movement is most frequently used. With eyes closed, the patient is asked to identify the position of the joint. Accuracy and speed of response are used to determine whether proprioception is intact, impaired, or absent. Many patients with strokes tend to have partial impairments, as opposed to total loss of sensory integrity. These sensory impairments may also affect the patient's ability to control and coordinate movement. Patients may lose the ability to perceive an upright posture during sitting and standing, which can lead to difficulties in weight shifting, sequencing motor responses, and eye–hand coordination.

Communication Impairments

Infarcts in the frontal and temporal lobes of the brain can lead to specific communication deficits. Approximately 33% of all patients with strokes have some degree of language dysfunction (National Aphasia Association, 2019). *Aphasia* is an acquired communication disorder caused by brain damage and is characterized by impairment of language comprehension, oral expression, and use of symbols to communicate ideas. Several different types of aphasia are recognized. Patients can have an expressive disorder called *Broca aphasia*, a receptive aphasia known as *Wernicke aphasia*, or a combination of both expressive and receptive deficits termed *global aphasia*. Patients with expressive aphasia have difficulty speaking. These patients know what they want to say but are unable to form the words to communicate their thoughts. Individuals with expressive aphasia frequently become frustrated when they are unable to articulate their wants and needs verbally. Patients with receptive aphasia do not understand the spoken word. When attempting to communicate with a patient with receptive aphasia, the patient may not understand what you are trying to say or may misinterpret your words. Working with these patients can be challenging because you will not be able to rely on verbal instructions to direct activity performance. Patients with global aphasia have severe expressive and receptive dysfunction. These individuals do not comprehend spoken words and are unable to communicate their needs, and frequently they also have difficulties understanding gestures that have communicative meaning. Developing a rapport with the patient and trying to establish some method of communicating basic needs can be challenging. Time and patience are needed so the patient will begin to trust the therapist and for a therapeutic relationship to develop. The clinician should also work with the speech-language pathologist in implementing the communication system developed for the patient.

Other Communication Deficits

Other communicative deficits include dysarthria and emotional lability. *Dysarthria* is a condition in which the patient has difficulty articulating words as a result of weakness and inability to control the muscles associated with speech production. *Emotional lability* may be evident in patients who have sustained right hemispheric infarcts. These patients exhibit difficulties in controlling emotions. A patient who is emotionally labile may cry or laugh inappropriately without cause. The patient is often unable to inhibit the emergence of these spontaneous emotions. Active listening, reassurance, and redirection provided by the therapist can be helpful during these moments.

Orofacial Deficits

A patient's orofacial function may also be affected by the stroke. These deficits are often associated with cranial nerve involvement, which can occur with strokes of the brainstem or midbrain region. Frequent findings include facial asymmetries resulting from weakness in the facial muscles, muscles of the eye, and muscles around the mouth. Weakness of the facial muscles can affect the patient's ability to interact with individuals in the environment. The inability to smile, frown, or initiate other facial expressions such as anger or displeasure affects a person's ability to use body language as an adjunct to verbal communication. Inadequate lip closure can lead to problems with control of saliva and fluids during swallowing. Weakness of the muscles that innervate the eye can lead to drooping or ptosis of the eyelid. The patient may also be unable to close the eye to assist with lubrication.

Orofacial dysfunction can be manifested in a patient's difficulty or inability to swallow foods and liquids, also known as *dysphagia*. In the acute phase, approximately 50% of patients experience dysphagia (Edwardson, 2019). Dysphagia can result from muscle weakness, inadequate motor planning capabilities, and poor tongue control. Patients with dysphagia may be unable to move food from the front of the mouth to the sides for chewing and back to the midline for swallowing. Many of these patients may pocket food within their oral cavities.

A final problem seen in patients with orofacial dysfunction is poor coordination between eating and breathing. Such difficulty can lead to poor nutrition and possible aspiration of food into the lungs. Aspiration frequently leads to pneumonia and other respiratory complications, including atelectasis (collapse of a part of the lung tissue). It is important to note that many patients with dysphagia are initially placed on fluid and dietary restrictions to minimize the possibility of aspiration. Fortunately, swallowing impairments often improve over time (Edwardson, 2019).

Respiratory Impairments

Lung expansion may be decreased following a stroke because of decreased control of the muscles of respiration, specifically the diaphragm. A stroke can affect the diaphragm just as it can affect any other muscle in the body. Hemiparesis of the diaphragm or external intercostal muscles may be apparent and can affect the individual's ability to expand the lungs. Poor lung expansion leads to a decrease in an individual's vital capacity. Therefore, to meet the oxygen demands of the body, the patient is forced to increase her respiration rate. Pulmonary complications including pneumonia and atelectasis may develop if shallow breathing continues. Lack of

lateral basilar expansion can also lead to the foregoing pulmonary complications. Cough effectiveness may be impaired secondary to weakness in the abdominal muscles.

Lung volumes are decreased by approximately 30% to 40% in patients who have had a stroke (Watchie, 1994). The capacity for exercise (peak oxygen consumption, VO2 peak) is decreased after acute stroke and is 60% lower than that of the general population (Tang and Eng, 2014; Billinger et al., 2012). Impairments in the neuromuscular, respiratory, and cardiovascular systems lead to a decreased tolerance to exercise and a decrease in peak aerobic performance of 50% as compared with the general public (Macko, 2016; Billinger et al., 2012). Oxygen consumption is increased, leading to muscle and cardiopulmonary fatigue. Fatigue is a major complaint among patients with strokes. Patients frequently ask to rest or stay in bed instead of participating in physical therapy. Although it is necessary to monitor the patient's cardiovascular and pulmonary responses, the patient and family should be advised that participation in exercise and functional activities will improve the patient's tolerance for activity, and that a certain level of intensity is needed to induce neural plasticity and functional recovery (Hornby et al., 2011).

Reflex Activity

Primitive spinal and brainstem reflexes may appear following a stroke. Both types of reflexes are present at birth or during infancy and become integrated by the CNS as the child ages, usually within the first 4 months of life. Once integrated, these reflexes are not present in their pure forms. They do, however, continue to exist as underlying components of volitional movement patterns. In adults, it is possible for these primitive reflexes to reappear when the CNS is damaged or if an individual is experiencing extreme fatigue or stress.

Spinal Reflexes

Spinal level reflexes occur at the level of the spinal cord and result in overt movement of a limb. Frequently, these reflexes are facilitated by a noxious stimulus experienced by the patient. Table 11.5 provides a list of the most common spinal level reflexes seen in patients with CNS dysfunction. Family members must be educated regarding the true meaning of these reflexes. The presence of a spinal level reflex, such as a flexor withdrawal, does not indicate that the patient is demonstrating volitional (voluntary) movement. These reflexive movements often occur when a patient is unresponsive. For example, if a caregiver inadvertently stimulates the patient's foot, the patient may flex the involved lower extremity. This does not, however, mean that the patient is exhibiting conscious control of the limb.

Deep Tendon Reflexes

Patients who have experienced a stroke may also have altered DTRs. DTRs are stretch reflexes that can be elicited by striking the muscle tendon with a reflex hammer or the examiner's fingers. Common DTRs assessed include the biceps, brachioradialis, triceps, quadriceps/patellar, and gastrocnemius soleus/Achilles.

TABLE 11.5 Spinal Reflexes

Reflex	Stimulus	Response
Flexor withdrawal	Noxious stimulus applied to the bottom of the foot.	Toe extension, ankle dorsiflexion, hip and knee flexion.
Cross extension	Noxious stimulus applied to the ball of the foot with the lower extremity prepositioned in extension.	Flexion and then extension of the opposite lower extremity.
Startle	Sudden loud noise.	Extension and abduction of the upper extremities.
Grasp	Pressure applied to the ball of the foot or the palm of the hand.	Flexion of the toes or fingers, respectively.

TABLE 11.6 Brainstem Reflexes

Reflex	Response
Symmetric tonic neck reflex	Flexion of the neck results in flexion of the arms and extension of the legs. Extension of the neck results in extension of the arms and flexion of the legs.
Asymmetric tonic neck reflex	Rotation of the head to the left causes extension of the left arm and leg and flexion of the right arm and leg. Rotation of the head to the right causes extension of the right arm and leg and flexion of the left arm and leg.
Tonic labyrinthine reflex	Prone position facilitates flexion. Supine position facilitates extension.
Tonic thumb reflex	When the involved extremity is elevated above the horizontal, thumb extension is facilitated with forearm supination.

TABLE 11.7 Associated Reactions

Reaction	Response
Souques phenomenon	Flexion of the involved arm above 150 degrees facilitates extension and abduction of the fingers.
Raimiste phenomenon	Resistance applied to hip abduction or adduction of the uninvolved lower extremity causes a similar response in the involved lower extremity.
Homolateral limb synkinesis	Flexion of the involved upper extremity elicits flexion of the involved lower extremity.

The patient's response to the tendon tap is assessed on a 0 to 4 + scale: 0, no response; 1 +, minimal response; 2 +, normal response; 3 +, hyperactive response; and 4 +, clonus. Examination and evaluation of the patient's DTRs by the PT gives valuable information about the presence of abnormal muscle tone. Flaccidity or hypotonia may cause the reflexes to be hypoactive or absent. Spasticity or hypertonia may cause DTRs to be exaggerated or hyperactive. Clonus may also be present when the muscle tendon is tapped or stretched and is described as alternating periods of muscle contractions and relaxation. Clonus is frequently seen in the ankle or wrist and occurs in response to a quick stretch.

Brainstem Reflexes

Brainstem reflexes occur and are integrated at the level of the midbrain. As with all primitive reflexes, these reflexes may initially be present in infants but become integrated during the first year of life. In adult patients with CNS disorders, brainstem level reflexes may become apparent during times of significant stress or fatigue. Brainstem reflexes are primitive reflexes that alter the posture or position of a part of the body. These reflexes frequently serve to alter or affect muscle tone. Table 11.6 lists examples of common brainstem level reflexes.

Associated Reactions

Associated reactions are automatic movements that occur as a result of active or resisted movement in another part of the body. Table 11.7 describes common associated reactions seen in patients with hemiplegia. As stated previously, associated reactions can be misinterpreted as voluntary movement by either the patient or the patient's family member. All individuals interacting with the patient should recognize the meaning of a patient's involuntary movements and be able to communicate their significance to family members.

Bowel and Bladder Dysfunction

Patients who have had a stroke may also exhibit bowel and bladder dysfunction. Incontinence or the inability to control urination may be initially seen secondary to muscle paralysis or inadequate sensory stimulation to the bladder. For adults, incontinence can be extremely problematic and embarrassing. Early weight-bearing through either bridging or standing activities can assist the patient with regaining bladder control. Movement and activity assists in the regulation of bowel function. Attention to the patient's bowel and bladder program by all members of the rehabilitation team can be beneficial in assisting the patient in relearning these important ADLs.

Functional Limitations

Patients often exhibit functional limitations after strokes. Individuals may lose the ability to perform ADLs, such as feeding or bathing, or may be unable to roll over in bed, sit up, or walk. Functional limitations are the result of motor and/or sensory deficits caused by the stroke. Patients may lack the volitional movement needed in the involved upper extremity to wash their faces or comb their hair. The presence of spasticity in the involved lower extremity may limit the patient's ability to ambulate.

Great emphasis during treatment is placed on function and an individual's ability to participate in life roles. The purpose of physical therapy is to help patients achieve their optimal level of physical functioning and to improve their quality of life. Treatment goals and intervention plans must be functionally relevant and meaningful to the patient. For example, if a patient who has had a stroke has decreased active dorsiflexion in the involved ankle, an appropriate goal would be for the patient to demonstrate active dorsiflexion during the heel strike phase of the gait cycle 50% of the time with verbal cueing while ambulating a certain distance on level surfaces. The goal of improving active dorsiflexion has been incorporated into performance of a functional task.

COMPLICATIONS SEEN FOLLOWING STROKE

Abnormal Posturing and Positioning

Patients can develop certain complications following a stroke. As stated previously, spasticity often develops in specific muscle groups and can lead to the development of contractures and deformities. Patients may have flexion contractures of the elbow, wrist, and fingers as a result of spasticity in the flexor muscle groups. This condition can lead to the characteristic upper extremity posturing often seen in patients who have had a stroke. Hygiene and other self-care activities become extremely difficult in the presence of wrist and finger contractures. The patient may not be able to open the fist to wash the palm of the hand or to perform nail care.

Spasticity in the gastrocnemius-soleus complex can lead to plantar flexion contractures of the involved ankle. Ankle contractures make ambulation and transfers difficult by preventing the patient from bearing weight on a flat or plantigrade foot. A plantar flexed foot also impedes foot clearance during the swing phase of the gait cycle.

Several oral medications are available for patients with significant spasticity, including baclofen (Lioresal), tizanidine (Zanaflex), Diazepam, and dantrolene sodium (Dantrium). A major disadvantage associated with several of these medications is that they decrease CNS activity and promote lethargy (Lundy-Ekman, 2018). These are undesirable side effects for patients with neurologic dysfunction. Additionally, the medications do not ameliorate the underlying problem. Instead, they provide a temporary change in the level of muscle tone. Of the medications discussed here, dantrolene sodium is less likely to cause lethargy or cognitive changes. The drug intervenes at the muscular level and decreases the force production of muscle units. Side effects include hepatotoxicity and generalized muscle weakness (Lundy-Ekman, 2018).

Other pharmacologic interventions are available to minimize the effects of spasticity. Botulinum toxin type A can be injected directly into a spastic muscle and produces selective muscle weakness by blocking the release of acetylcholine at the neuromuscular junction (Ryerson, 2013). The effects of an injection can last from 2 to 6 months and side effects are limited. Intrathecal baclofen is administered via a subcutaneous pump. The pump is implanted within the abdominal cavity and a catheter administers the baclofen into the subarachnoid space. The medication inhibits stretch reflex activity within the spinal cord by "decreasing calcium influx into the presynaptic terminals of primary afferent fibers and by stabilizing the postsynaptic membrane" (Lundy-Ekman, 2018).

In some situations, the presence of spasticity is advantageous for the patient. Extensor tone in the lower extremity may allow a patient to weight bear on her involved lower extremity and may provide some lower extremity stability during ambulation. Increased tone around the shoulder joint may limit the patient's predisposition for shoulder subluxation. Clinicians are advised to determine if the patient is using abnormal muscle tone to improve function before requesting pharmacologic or surgical interventions to minimize its effects.

Shoulder pain is extremely common in patients with hemiplegia. Decreased muscle tone and muscle weakness can reduce the support provided by the rotator cuff muscles, specifically the supraspinatus. Consequently, the joint capsule and the ligaments of the shoulder become the sole supporting structures for the head of the humerus within the glenoid fossa. In time, the effects of this weakness combined with the effects of gravity can lead to shoulder subluxation.

Spasticity or increased muscle tone can also lead to shoulder dysfunction and pain. Spasticity within the scapular depressors, retractors, and downward rotators contributes to poor scapular position and joint alignment. Abnormal positioning of the scapula causes secondary tightness in the ligaments, tendons, and joint capsule of the shoulder and can lead to a decrease in the patient's ability to move the involved shoulder. Shoulder pain and loss of upper extremity function can develop as a consequence of changes in the orientation of anatomic structures within the shoulder girdle.

Complex Regional Pain Syndrome

Several terms, including *shoulder/hand syndrome* and *reflex sympathetic dystrophy,* have been used to describe the condition now known as *complex regional pain syndrome* (CRPS). The etiology of the condition is unknown although it is thought to be the result of autonomic nervous system dysfunction. CRPS is characterized by the following signs and symptoms: pain, autonomic nervous system signs and symptoms, edema, movement disorders, weakness, and atrophy. Three distinct stages have been identified. Stage I is characterized by intermittent pain often initially reported in the shoulder; stiffness and loss of range of motion; changes in skin color and temperature; and hypersensitivity to sensation. Stage II is characterized by a decrease in overall pain; thin, brittle nails; and thin, cool skin. Osteoporosis may also be evident on x-ray. Patients in stage III experience irreversible, atrophic skin changes, as well as wrist and finger contractures, and muscle atrophy. Management of the condition is based on prevention through proper positioning and handling, patient and family education, and the encouragement of active functional use of the hand. In addition, elevation, compression, loading the limb through weight-bearing, and pharmacologic interventions including analgesics and steroids may be used to treat this condition (Deutsch and O'Sullivan, 2019).

Additional Complications

Other complications seen after a stroke include the following: (1) increased risk of trauma and falls because of impaired upper extremity and lower extremity protective reactions; (2) increased risk of thrombophlebitis secondary to decreased efficiency of the calf skeletal muscle pump; (3) pain in specific muscles and joints; and (4) depression. Falls are a common complication after stroke as approximately 7% of all individuals experience a fall during their first week after stroke, and 73% of people sustain a fall sometime during the first year (Verheyden et al., 2013). It is also estimated that approximately one-third of stroke survivors experience varying degrees of depression, sadness, anxiety, fear, frustration, and helplessness (Gordon et al., 2004; National Stroke Association, 2019b). A review of the physical therapy interventions used to decrease the risk of these complications is provided later in this chapter.

Outcome Measures

The assessment of patient outcomes has been an important component of physical therapy practice for some time and is a requirement for reimbursement. PTs administer many outcome measures to predict a patient's potential for recovery (prognosis), discriminate (identify individuals at risk for fall vs. those without balance deficits), categorize (household vs. community ambulators), and monitor a patient's response to selected interventions. Use of standardized outcome measures also provides for improved communication among clinicians, a mechanism to examine the effectiveness of interventions, and increases the efficiency of patient care (Moore et al., 2018).

To achieve the goals of outcome measure usage, from 2009–2015, six Academy of Neurologic Physical Therapy Evidence Database to Guide Effectiveness task forces were convened to identify recommended outcome measures for utilization in specific neurologic patient populations including stroke, multiple sclerosis, Parkinson disease, traumatic brain injury, spinal cord injury, and vestibular dysfunction. These groups also provided recommendations regarding when these measures should be utilized in clinical practice, research, and what specific measures should be taught to students in entry-level physical therapy programs.

In 2018, a Core Set of Outcome Measures for Adults with Neurologic Conditions Undergoing Rehabilitation was published. This clinical practice guideline has been endorsed by the Academy of Neurologic Physical Therapy for adults with acute, chronic stable, and chronic progressive neurologic conditions. Given the overwhelming number of outcome measures that are available, many of which are diagnosis specific, this core set was developed to limit variation in neurologic physical therapy practice (Moore et al., 2018). These outcome measures can be used across all practice settings and focus on the construct areas of "balance, gait, transfers, and patient-stated goals" (Moore et al., 2018). These specific construct areas were selected based on feedback from a variety of stakeholders including PTs and patients receiving physical therapy care. The construct areas of balance, gait, transfers, and patient-stated goals were felt to be the most important and were cited as a primary reason for seeking physical therapy services in both stakeholder groups.

Specific goals of the Core Set of Measures are to (1) provide standardization of outcome measures in neurologic physical therapy; (2) provide opportunity for comparison of interventions, therapists, and patients; (3) improve the quality of patient care; (4) facilitate evidence-based practice; (5) ensure standardization of documentation to assist in justifying the need for physical therapy; and (6) enhance the education of physical therapy students by including the core measures in entry-level education (Moore et al., 2018).

The outcome measures identified in the Core Set include the Berg Balance Scale for those "who have goals to improve static and dynamic sitting and standing balance; and have the capacity to change in this area"; the Functional Gait Assessment for those "who have goals to improve balance while walking and have the capacity to change in this area" (Moore et al., 2018); the 10 Meter Walk Test for those who have the capacity and goals to improve walking speed; the 6 Minute Walk Test for those who have the capacity and goals to improve in walking distance; the Five Times Sit to Stand Test for those who have the capacity and goals to improve in transfer ability; and the Activities Specific Balance Confidence Scale for those who have the capacity and goals to improve their balance confidence. It is also recommended that health care organizations administer a patient-stated goals assessment, such as the Goal Attainment Scale or the Patient Specific Functional Scale (Moore et al., 2018). Additionally, results of these assessments should be discussed with the patient using a shared decision-making approach. Integration of the "patient's goals, priorities and values into the plan of care" is important and will hopefully "encourage patient engagement in the rehabilitation process" (Moore et al., 2018).

The Knowledge Translation task force, assigned to the Core Outcome Measure Clinical Practice Guideline (CPG), has developed multiple resources and tools to assist clinicians in the implementation of the outcome measures in the Core Set. This Knowledge Translation task force has created summary references of the CPG, as well as a set of standardized administration protocols for each recommended measure with consideration for the most recent evidence. It is important to note that students and clinicians alike must administer the individual assessments following the exact instructions provided to ensure standardization of delivery. Failure to do so decreases the reliability of the individual assessments, limiting the ability to accurately assess patient function, and the patient's responses to our interventions.

As stated previously, there are many other outcome measures available for use. Although a detailed description of all of the tools available is outside the scope of this text, several of the tools most frequently used in the examination and treatment of patients with neurologic deficits and stroke are discussed here. Readers are encouraged to search the Academy of Neurologic Physical Therapy and the Rehabilitation Measures Database for more specific information.

Furthermore, the Academy of Neurologic Physical Therapy StrokeEDGE task force has recommended that all entry-level physical therapy students learn to administer the following outcome measures: Functional Independence Measure (FIM), Fugl-Meyer Assessment (Motor Performance), the Postural Assessment Scale for Stroke Patients, the Stroke Impact Scale, and the Trunk Impairment Scale. This set of tools is in addition to the core measures recommended for all adults with neurologic disorders that we presented in the preceding paragraphs (Academy of Neurologic Physical Therapy, 2018).

The FIM was developed in the early 1980s in response to the need for a national data system that could be used to differentiate among various clinical services and to establish the efficacy of services provided. The FIM measures physical, psychological, and social functions, as well as the patient's burden of care (how much assistance is needed to care for the individual). Specific items tested in the FIM include self-care, transfers, locomotion, communication, and cognition. A seven-point ordinal scale is used to score the various categories. A score of 1 equates to complete dependence, and a score of 7 indicates that a patient is completely independent during performance of the activity. Scores range from 18 to 126. The FIM is available for purchase through the Uniform Data System for Medical Rehabilitation and requires evaluator training before instrument administration (Rehabilitation Measures Database, 2015; Uniform Data System for Medical Rehabilitation, 2012). The primary PT is responsible for completing the FIM at the time of the patient's initial examination and also at the patient's discharge. The physical therapist assistant (PTA) may score the FIM at other intervals to provide the rehabilitation team with updates regarding the patient's progress.

The Centers for Medicare and Medicaid Services (CMS) have changed the tool clinicians use to assess assist level needed by patients in inpatient rehabilitation facilities as of October 1, 2019. The Quality Indicator Tool assesses a patient's mobility including rolling, supine to sit, sit to stand, transfers including car and commode, walking capabilities, curb and stair climbing, and the ability to pick an object up off the floor. Levels of assistance are recorded on a 6 point scale with 01 representing dependent and a 06 indicating that a patient is independent

and does not require any assistance from a helper. A significant difference for practicing clinicians is that the tool does not use minimal assistance as a patient assist level. Patients who require supervision, verbal cueing, or touching assistance would receive a score of 04 (supervision or touching assistance) (Centers for Medicare and Medicaid Services, 2019 a, 2019b). Following this federal mandate, it is expected that there will be updates to the list of outcome measures recommended for student and clinician mastery.

The Fugl-Meyer Assessment of Motor Recovery After Stroke is one of the most widely used instruments to quantify motor functioning following stroke. In addition, the tool can be used to analyze the efficacy of treatment interventions provided. The Fugl-Meyer Assessment evaluates passive joint range of motion, pain, light touch, proprioception, motor function, and balance. The tool is easy to administer and can be completed in 20 to 30 minutes (Baldrige, 1993; Duncan and Badke, 1987). Limitations of the instrument include increased weighting of upper extremity scores, limited evaluation of finger function, and the availability of better outcomes measures to assess balance (Rehabilitation Measures Database, 2016b). The tool does, however, remain a highly recommended clinical and research assessment instrument that measures motor impairments poststroke.

TREATMENT PLANNING

When the primary PT develops the patient's short- and long-term functional treatment goals and the plan of care, she must do so in consultation with the patient and the patient's family. The patient must be actively engaged in the planning and delivery of care received. Information must be gathered regarding the patient's previous level of function, the patient's goals for resuming those activities, and the patient's goals regarding the rehabilitation process. If a patient did not, for example, perform housework or gardening before her stroke, it would not be realistic to expect that the patient would perform those tasks after such an event. The PT should select interventions that are meaningful to the patient, to assist the patient in returning to previous levels of function. Interventions that address bed mobility, transfers, ambulation, stair negotiation, wheelchair propulsion (if appropriate), and safety issues should be included in the plan of care. Patient and family education is also necessary and must be included. If it appears that the patient may not be able to resume her previous level of function, instruction of the patient's family will become even more important. A more detailed discussion of patient and family education occurs in the section of this chapter on discharge planning.

ACUTE CARE SETTING

Depending on the severity of the individual's stroke, a PTA may or may not be involved in the patient's treatment in the acute care setting. Average lengths of hospitalization following a stroke are approximately 2 to 4 days. In certain geographic areas, patients may not be admitted to an acute care facility unless a strong medical need exists. Patients who have sustained uncomplicated strokes may be evaluated by their physician and instructed to begin outpatient or home-based therapies. Once the patient is medically stable, the physician may determine that it is appropriate for the patient to begin rehabilitation.

DIRECTING INTERVENTIONS TO A PHYSICAL THERAPIST ASSISTANT

Following the patient's initial examination, the supervising PT may determine that a patient who has sustained a stroke is an appropriate candidate to share with a PTA. The supervising PT needs to evaluate the patient carefully for the appropriateness of directing specific interventions to a PTA. Factors to consider when using the PTA to provide specific components or selected interventions are outlined in Chapter 1 and include acuteness of the patient's condition, special patient problems (including medical, cognitive, or emotional), and the patient's current response to physical therapy. Before the PTA's initial visit with the patient, the supervising PT should review the patient's examination and evaluative findings with the PTA. In addition, the PT must also discuss the patient's plan of care including patient goals with the PTA. Any precautions, contraindications, or special instructions should also be provided (American Physical Therapy Association, 2018).

A discussion of the patient's discharge plans should begin at the time of the initial examination. As lengths of stay have decreased, it has become necessary to begin planning for discharge the first time the patient is seen. The supervising PT's responsibility is to begin the discharge planning process. Although state practice acts do not prohibit a PTA from engaging in the planning and preparation for the patient's discharge, the guidelines of the American Physical Therapy Association regarding direction and supervision of PTAs state that it is the responsibility of the supervising PT to conclude the patient's episode of care (American Physical Therapy Association, 2018).

With input from the supervising PT, the PTA may find herself responsible for providing many of the patient's treatment interventions. Requirements for contact with the primary therapist differ from state to state. The PTA is advised to review the state practice act and to adhere to any specific requirements regarding therapist supervision or patient reevaluations that may be required by state jurisdictions.

EARLY PHYSICAL THERAPY INTERVENTION

Cardiopulmonary Retraining

An area of physical therapy practice that often receives limited attention in patients who have sustained strokes is cardiopulmonary retraining. Individuals who have had strokes frequently have significant cardiac and pulmonary medical histories. Previous myocardial infarctions, hypertension, and chronic obstructive pulmonary disease are common findings in this patient population. In addition, diaphragmatic weakness, generalized deconditioning, decreased endurance, and fatigue may affect the patient's ability to participate in rehabilitation by decreasing pulmonary capabilities.

Diaphragmatic Strengthening

The diaphragm is a muscle and may respond to therapeutic techniques designed to improve strength and endurance. Diaphragmatic strengthening is accomplished by having the therapist place one hand on the patient's upper abdomen. Initially, the patient is directed to try, during inspiration, to lift the weight of the clinician's hand. A semireclined position may be the easiest for the patient because the patient will not have to contract the diaphragm directly against gravity. A quick stretch applied to the diaphragm before an active inspiratory movement can facilitate a stronger contraction. As the patient performs these exercises with increased ease, the clinician can make the exercise more challenging by increasing manual resistance, changing the patient's position, or incorporating the performance of a functional task during the exercise. Expansion of the lateral lobes of the lungs should also be practiced. The therapist places her hands on the patient's lateral lower rib cage and encourages the patient to breathe out against the manual pressure. Initially, the weight of the clinician's hands may be sufficient resistance. As the patient progresses, increased resistance can be applied during this activity.

Other Cardiopulmonary Activities

Other activities that can be performed to improve cardiopulmonary functioning include deep-breathing exercises, the use of incentive spirometers, and stretching activities to the lateral trunk, especially in the presence of lateral chest wall tightness. Breathing exercises improve the efficiency of air intake. Breath support is important as the patient tries to perform activities and talk at the same time. The patient's speech-language pathologist can assist the patient in coordinating breathing during speaking and eating activities. As the patient progresses in rehabilitation, the rehabilitation team will need to be cognizant of the patient's cardiopulmonary function and medications. For patients with complicated medical histories, it will be necessary to monitor vital signs including patient reports of perceived exertion during activity performance. All patients should be instructed to avoid breath holding during activity performance because this phenomenon is known to increase blood pressure.

Positioning

One of the most important components of physical therapy interventions is the proper positioning of the patient. Positioning should be started immediately following the patient's stroke and should continue throughout all phases of the patient's recovery. Positioning is the responsibility of the patient and all members of the rehabilitation team. Proper positioning out of the characteristic synergy patterns assists in stimulating motor function, increases sensory awareness, improves respiratory and oromotor functions, and assists in maintaining normal range of motion in the neck, trunk, and extremities. Additionally, common musculoskeletal deformities and the potential for pressure ulcers can be minimized with proper patient positioning.

The patient should be alternately positioned on the back, the involved side, and the uninvolved side. Areas of the patient's body that require special attention and should be addressed first are the shoulder and pelvic girdles. The rhomboids and gluteus maximus muscles frequently become tight and contribute to retraction at the shoulder and pelvic girdles. Therefore both the shoulder and pelvis should be positioned in slight protraction to minimize the effects of muscle spasticity and tightness.

Supine Positioning

When the patient is in the supine position, the clinician will want to place small towel rolls (approximately 1.5 inches thick) underneath the patient's scapula and pelvis on the involved side to promote protraction. The towels should encompass approximately two-thirds of the bony structures (the rolls should not extend all the way to the vertebral column). Care must be taken to avoid placing too much toweling under the scapula and pelvis because this will cause excessive rotation and asymmetry. The involved upper extremity should be externally rotated, abducted approximately 30 degrees, and extended with the forearm supinated. In addition, a neutral or slightly extended wrist position with finger extension and thumb abduction is desirable. Placement of a pillow under the involved upper extremity assists in maintaining this position and can help with venous return.

Pelvic protraction, coupled with hip and knee flexion and ankle dorsiflexion, is the preferred position for the lower extremity. A pillow can be placed under the patient's leg to help maintain this posture. Intervention 11.1 illustrates supine positioning for the patient with hemiplegia. Positioning the patient in the supine position as described previously is beneficial because it counteracts the strong flexion and extension synergies that develop in the upper extremity and lower extremity, respectively.

In addition to the emphasis placed on the shoulder and hip, the clinician must also be aware of the position of the patient's head and neck. Often, in an effort to make the patient more comfortable, family members place extra pillows under the patient's head. This type of positioning promotes cervical flexion and can accentuate forward head posturing. A single pillow under the neck is sufficient unless a patient's medical condition warrants a more elevated neck and upper trunk position. The patient should also be encouraged to look toward the involved side to enhance visual awareness.

Side-Lying Positioning

As stated previously, positioning the patient on both sides should be incorporated. When the patient is lying on the uninvolved side, the patient's trunk should be straight, the involved upper extremity should be protracted on a pillow, the patient's elbow should be extended, and the forearm should be in a neutral position. The patient's wrist should also be in a neutral or slightly extended position, and the fingers should

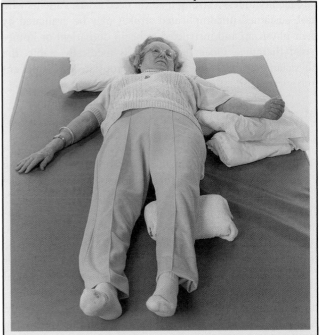

INTERVENTION 11.1 **Supine Positioning**

Protraction of the scapula, external rotation of the shoulder, and elbow extension are emphasized in the upper extremity. Pelvic protraction with slight hip and knee flexion is used to decrease extensor tone in the lower extremity.

be relaxed. The lower extremity should be positioned with the pelvis protracted, the hip and knee flexed, and the ankle in dorsiflexion. Intervention 11.2 illustrates positioning of the patient in a side-lying position on the uninvolved side.

Positioning the patient on the involved side is also beneficial because it increases weight-bearing and proprioceptive input into the involved extremities. When preparing the patient for this activity, one should ensure that the patient's involved shoulder is protracted and well forward, thus preventing the patient from lying directly on the shoulder and causing impingement. It is again optimal to have the elbow extended and the forearm supinated. The pelvis should be protracted, with the involved hip extended and the knee slightly flexed. The uninvolved limbs (both the upper and lower extremities) should be supported with pillows.

Minimizing the Development of Abnormal Tone and Patient Neglect

The positioning examples previously described have other variations. Many of the positioning alternatives are the results of clinicians' attempts to minimize the effects of abnormal tone or spasticity that develop in patients who have had strokes. Positions need to be altered as the patient's mobility improves and tightness develops in various muscle groups. Regardless of the specific positioning techniques employed, special attention must be placed on the achievement of symmetry, midline orientation, and protraction of the scapula and pelvis. Care must also be taken to avoid the potential development of patient neglect of the involved extremities. Neglect of the involved side of

INTERVENTION 11.2 Side-Lying Positioning (Uninvolved Side)

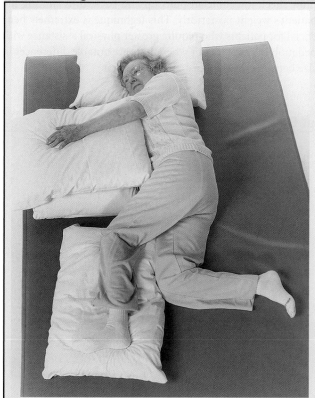

Scapular protraction with elbow extension is desired. Hip and knee flexion with ankle dorsiflexion is the preferred position for the lower extremity.

the body and visual field is often present when the right cerebral hemisphere is damaged. This neglect may be described as an impairment of the patient's awareness of body image or body parts. In addition, if the sensory cortex has been injured, the patient may be unable to perceive sensory stimulation applied to the involved extremities. Both of these situations can lead to the patient's inability to attend to the involved side or may cause the patient to neglect the involved upper or lower extremity. Positioning the patient in a side-lying position on the involved side decreases the effects of this neglect by increasing sensory input into the affected joints and muscles and by enhancing visual awareness of that side of the body.

Leaving Items Within Reach

When leaving the patient in any of the previously described positions, one should place needed items, such as the nurse's call light, the bedside table, and the telephone, within the patient's reach and visual field. Therapists often instruct families to place commonly used objects on the patient's involved side to increase awareness and attention given to that side of the body. This practice should not, however, be employed if it creates a safety concern for the patient or family members. Families and caregivers alike should be encouraged to interact with the patient on her involved side because it reinforces the importance of visually attending to the side of involvement.

Other Considerations

Family members frequently suggest placing a washcloth or soft, squeezable ball in the patient's palm. Many individuals believe that this activity improves hand control. On the contrary, squeezing a soft object often increases tightness (spasticity) in the wrist and finger flexors and facilitates the palmar grasp reflex. A resting hand splint for the involved hand may be beneficial. For patients who have significant extensor tone in the lower extremity and are at risk for the development of a plantar flexion contracture, a resting night splint may be recommended for static positioning at night. Family members should also be encouraged to bring in a pair of low-top tennis shoes for the patient to wear because they provide a better alternative for positioning the foot.

Early Functional Mobility Tasks

Physical therapy treatment interventions that facilitate movement should be initiated while the patient is still in bed. The hip and shoulder are the areas that should be targeted first because proximal control and stability are essential for distal movement.

Bridging and Bridging With Approximation

Examples of early treatment activities that can be performed with the lower extremities include *bridging* and *bridging with approximation*. *Approximation* or *compression* occurs when joint surfaces are brought together. These compressive forces activate joint receptors and facilitate postural holding responses. Approximation applied downward through the knee before the patient's attempt to lift the buttocks prepares the foot for early weight-bearing. Intervention 11.3 illustrates this technique. Approximation

INTERVENTION 11.3 Preparation for Bridging

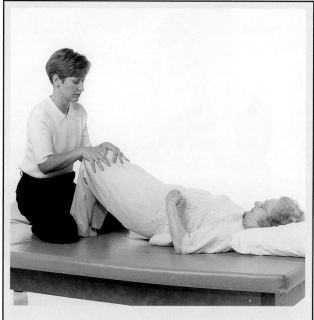

Gentle approximation is applied downward through the patient's knees in preparation for bridging.

can also be administered superiorly through the hip in preparation for bridging. The therapist must observe the quality of the patient's bridge. Weakness in the gluteus maximus muscle and lack of lower extremity control may be evident. This condition can result in asymmetric lifting and lagging of the involved side. Tactile assistance under the buttocks may need to be provided. Intervention 11.4 demonstrates bridging with

assistance. Intervention 11.5 depicts a PT/PTA helping a patient with bridging by using a draw sheet. Holding on to the draw sheet, the clinician pulls up and back, thus shifting the patient's weight posteriorly. This technique is extremely beneficial for patients who require greater physical assistance with bed mobility activities or when there are notable differences in size between the therapist and the patient.

INTERVENTION 11.4 Using Tactile Cues to Assist Bridging

The therapist may need to help the patient with bridging. Tactile cues (tapping) applied to the patient's gluteal muscles will assist the patient with lifting her buttocks.

INTERVENTION 11.5 Using a Draw Sheet to Assist Bridging

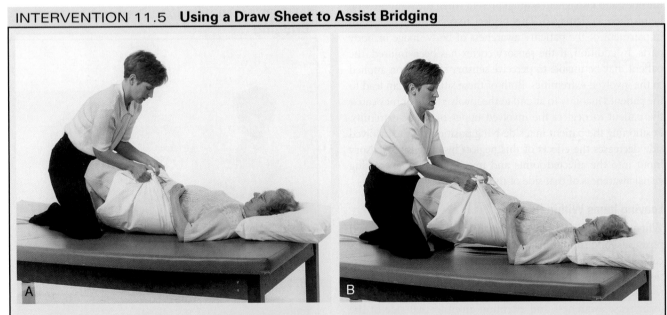

A draw sheet placed under the patient's hips can be used to assist the patient with bridging.
A. The therapist places her forearms along the patient's femurs to maintain positioning of the patient's lower extremities and to provide proprioceptive input.
B. The therapist uses a posterior weight shift of her body to help lift the patient's buttocks.

Other Bedside Activities

Other bedside exercises include hip extension over the edge of the bed or mat and straight leg raising with the uninvolved lower extremity while the involved lower extremity is flexed. Intervention 11.6 and Intervention 11.7 illustrate these exercises. One of the benefits of these exercises is that they facilitate early activation of the gluteus maximus and hamstring muscles. Other early treatment interventions that promote movement and control of the hip musculature include lower trunk rotation, scooting from one side of the bed to the other,

and retraining the hip flexors. Lower trunk rotation provides for separation of the trunk and pelvis, assists in promoting general relaxation, and facilitates pelvic protraction, which is necessary for functional activities, such as rolling, supine-to-sit transfers, and ambulation. Lower trunk rotation is depicted in Intervention 11.8. Facilitation of active hip flexion can be achieved by passively flexing the patient's hip and knee and then working on active hip flexion within various points in the range of motion (Intervention 11.9). As the patient is able to perform this exercise actively and as the quality of the

---

INTERVENTION 11.6   Hip Extension Over the Edge of a Surface

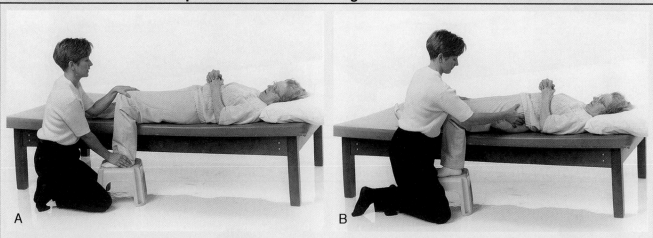

Hip extension can be accomplished over the edge of the bed or mat table. The patient must scoot to the edge of the mat.

A. The therapist may need to help the patient with moving the involved leg off the support surface. The plantar surface of the patient's foot must be supported. A small step stool, a garbage can, or the therapist's leg can be used. The patient pushes down with the involved lower extremity.

B. The clinician palpates the gluteus maximus muscle to assess the strength of the patient's efforts.

INTERVENTION 11.7   Straight Leg Raising (Uninvolved Lower Extremity)

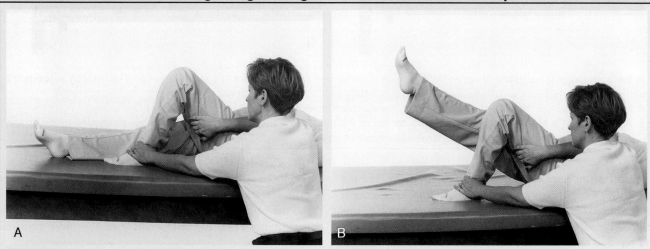

A. The patient is instructed to perform a straight leg raise with the uninvolved lower extremity.

B. As the patient lifts her leg, the therapist palpates the hamstring musculature of the involved side. Contraction of the involved hamstrings should be felt as the patient lifts the uninvolved leg.

INTERVENTION 11.8   Lower Trunk Rotation

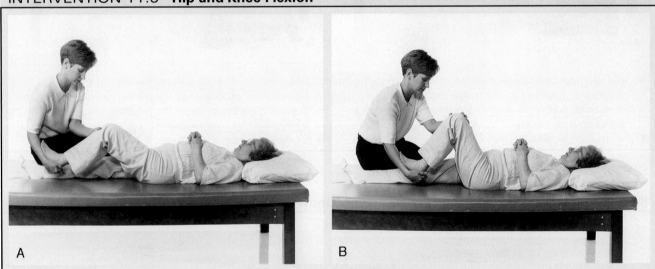

The therapist guides the patient's lower extremities as the patient performs lower trunk rotation in hook lying.

INTERVENTION 11.9   Hip and Knee Flexion

In the acute stages, facilitation of hip and knee flexion is performed with the patient in a supine position. The clinician supports the entire plantar surface of the patient's foot to avoid stimulating a plantar flexion response.
A. Initially, the therapist may need to support the patient's entire lower extremity.
B. As the patient is able to assume more active control of the movement, the therapist can use a more anterior handhold slightly above the patient's patella to guide the lower extremity movement.

movement improves, the exercise can be advanced, and the patient can begin to work on active hip and knee flexion with voluntary ankle dorsiflexion. A final progression of this exercise is to have the patient reverse the movement and work on hip and knee extension with ankle dorsiflexion. The patient's ability to perform this movement combination demonstrates an ability to combine various components of the lower extremity flexion and extension synergy patterns. Intervention 11.10 shows the therapist using a more distal handhold at the toes to prevent excessive toe flexion and to promote ankle dorsiflexion. It should be remembered that the use of distal joints to guide movement implies that the patient possesses adequate control of the more proximal components.

Importance of Movement Assessment

Any time the patient moves, the clinician should observe the quality of the patient's movement. Although no universally

INTERVENTION 11.10   Inhibiting Toe Flexion and Promoting Ankle Dorsiflexion

A. The therapist uses her fingers to abduct (separate) the patient's toes. This positioning combined with slight traction applied to the toes will inhibit toe clawing and facilitate ankle dorsiflexion.

B. A more distal handhold can be used to guide the patient's lower extremity movement.

accepted quality indicators are available in the physical therapy literature to describe movement, the following characteristics should be considered: (1) timing of the movement; (2) sequencing of muscle responses; (3) amount of force generated by the muscle during the movement; and (4) reciprocal release of muscle activity. To address these areas in treatment, the therapist should select motor tasks that demand the proper muscle response. For example, having a patient work on sit-to-stand movement transitions in which the timing of hip and knee extension is coordinated is beneficial. Flexion of the elbow followed by a controlled release of the biceps into elbow extension is another example of an activity that addresses the quality of the patient's motor response.

Scapular Mobilization

Treatment interventions for the upper extremity must be included at all times. Scapular mobilization performed in a side-lying position is extremely beneficial. This type of mobilization should not be confused with the orthopedic mobilization techniques described by Maitland (1977). Scapular mobilization for patients with hemiplegia can be thought of as a range-of-motion or mobility exercise. The goal of the mobilization is to keep the scapula moving on the thorax so that upper extremity function is not lost. Intervention 11.11 demonstrates gentle protraction (abduction) of a patient's scapula. The therapist's hand is placed along the border of the patient's scapula. From that position, the clinician guides the patient's scapular movement. The scapula can also be mobilized in the directions of the proprioceptive neuromuscular facilitation (PNF) diagonals, including elevation, abduction, and upward rotation, which are the scapular components of the D_1 flexion pattern, elevation, adduction, and upward

rotation, demonstrating the scapular movements observed in the D_2 flexion pattern. Care should be taken to stabilize the trunk properly to avoid compensatory motion. Scapular mobility is essential in maintaining the normal scapulohumeral rhythm necessary for upper extremity range of motion and functional reaching. If the scapula is unable to move on the rib cage, the upper extremity will become tightly fixed to the side of the body, thereby limiting the patient's ability to use the arm. In addition, individuals who have had a stroke often develop tightness or increased tone in the scapular elevators and retractors (rhomboids, upper trapezius, and teres minor). This condition can lead to abnormal scapular positioning and upper extremity posturing.

Other Upper Extremity Activities

The patient should be instructed in the performance of self-directed upper extremity elevation with external rotation (double-arm elevation), as illustrated in Intervention 11.12. This movement combination assists in maintaining function of the shoulder and can limit the development of spasticity in the latissimus dorsi muscle, which has been noted to contribute to abnormal posturing (Johnstone, 1995). Passive range-of-motion exercises performed to the patient's involved shoulder, elbow, wrist, and fingers should also be performed during this early stage of rehabilitation. These exercises are absolutely essential, especially in the absence of volitional upper extremity movement because they prevent the development of upper extremity joint contractures.

Facilitation and Inhibition Techniques

Depending on the patient's motor control, the presence or absence of abnormal tone, and the quality of volitional

INTERVENTION 11.11   **Scapular Mobilization**

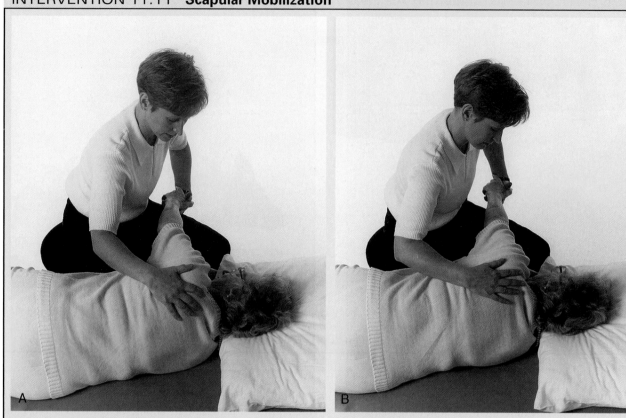

With her hand on the patient's scapula, the therapist gently protracts the involved scapula. A handshake grasp is used to support the patient's involved hand.

INTERVENTION 11.12   **Double-Arm Elevation**

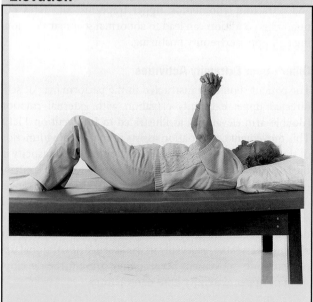

The patient clasps her hands together. The involved thumb should be outermost to maintain the web space and to inhibit abnormal tone.

movement present, performance of facilitation or inhibitory activities in preparation for active attempts of functional activities may be necessary.

Facilitation techniques. The use of primitive (spinal) or tonic (brainstem) reflexes, quick stretching, tapping, vibration, approximation, and weight-bearing have been used to prepare the patient for the performance of functional activities.

Primitive or spinal level reflexes. Primitive or spinal level reflexes have limited usefulness assisting patients in their abilities to perform functional movements. These reflexes may, however, be administered to establish the patient's level of responsiveness. A noxious stimulus applied to the bottom of the patient's foot may elicit extension of the toes, with dorsiflexion of the ankle and flexion of the hip and knee (a flexor withdrawal). Maintained pressure applied to the palm of the hand or ball of the foot can cause the patient to flex the fingers (palmar grasp) or toes (plantar grasp). Eliciting these spinal level reflexes should be avoided in treatment. More important is the education provided to the patient's family members regarding the correct meaning of these reflexes. Individuals often misinterpret this type of reflexive response as volitional movement and may develop unrealistic expectations regarding the patient's current status or eventual functional outcome.

Using brainstem or tonic reflexes. The use of brainstem reflexes, such as the asymmetric tonic neck reflex, to elicit patient responses is also controversial. However, if a patient is not responding to conventional treatment interventions, other avenues must be employed. The use of the asymmetric tonic neck reflex, the symmetric tonic neck reflex, and the tonic labyrinthine reflexes can affect the patient's muscle tone by increasing tone in otherwise flaccid or hypotonic extremities. Having the patient rotate the head to one side causes increased extension in the face arm and increased flexor tone in the skull arm. Flexing the patient's head may also elicit flexion in the upper extremities and increased extensor tone in the lower extremities. Positioning a patient in supine or prone can increase extensor or flexor tone, respectively.

Manual contacts. A quick stretch applied to a muscle will facilitate the muscle spindle to fire and cause a contraction of the muscle fibers. A quick stretch followed by a verbal request to the patient to complete a specific movement may also facilitate a motor response. Once the patient is able to recruit a muscle actively, this technique should be discontinued. Tapping, vibration, approximation, and weight-bearing are other facilitatory treatment techniques. Gentle tapping over a muscle belly often assists in preparing the muscle for activation. Tapping and vibration can be performed to both the agonist and antagonist of a given muscle group. The sensory stimulus should be applied from the muscle's insertion to its origin. Effects of vibratory stimulation last only as long as the stimulus is applied. Vibration can be applied for 1 to 2 minutes, and then the stimulus should be removed. In the presence of significant muscle tone, tapping or vibration administered to the muscle's antagonist often provides insufficient muscle activation to overcome the increased tone. Approximation and weight-bearing are other types of facilitation techniques that provide the patient with proprioceptive input to the joint and muscle receptors. Approximation and early weight-bearing activities applied at the shoulder and hip may stimulate muscle activation around the joint and assist in the development of joint stability.

For patients with increased tone, inhibitory techniques should be employed. Slow, rhythmic rotation can assist in reducing tone in spastic body parts. As stated previously, beginning these activities in proximal body segments is important if the desired outcome is to change the tone more distally. Weight-bearing is another useful inhibitory technique. Prolonged ice applied with an ice pack or iced towels or static stretch applied in conjunction with pressure administered to a tendon of a spastic muscle can assist in decreasing tone in hypertonic muscle groups. Once the tone is at a more manageable level, the patient must then attempt a movement or functional task.

> **CAUTION** Caution must be exercised when using ice to inhibit abnormal tone. The duration of the icing should not exceed 20 minutes, and during its application the patient's skin should be inspected periodically.

Treatment adjunct. Air (pressure) splints can be employed to assist with positioning, tone reduction, and sensory awareness. For some patients, air splints are used as an adjunct during treatment, and for others the therapist may recommend an air splint as a necessary piece of equipment for a patient's home exercise and positioning program.

Johnstone (1995) described the use of air splints. Inflatable air splints are available for a number of different body parts, such as full-length arm and leg splints; splints for the elbow, forearm, and hand; and a splint for the foot and ankle. These splints can be applied to the involved joint or extremity and can assist with positioning and tone management. The dual-channeled air splints are inflated by the therapist. Warm air from the therapist's lungs allows the inner sleeve to contour to the patient, and thus provides constant sensory feedback. The splint must be firmly applied, with the pressure reaching between 38 and 40 mm Hg. Numbness or tingling while wearing the splint may indicate overinflation. Splints should not be worn for longer than 1 hour at a time, although they can be reapplied throughout the day or during the course of a treatment session. A thin cotton sleeve can be applied under the splint to protect the patient's skin (Johnstone, 1995).

Long arm splint. The long arm splint is frequently used for patients poststroke. The splint is applied to the patient's involved upper extremity. Maintaining the patient's hand in a handshake grasp during application of the splint assists in the process. Intervention 11.13 shows a clinician applying a long arm splint to a patient. As the patient's arm is placed through the splint, the patient's fifth finger should be on the side of the splint with the zipper. Positioning of the hand in this manner allows for ulnar weight-bearing, which facilitates forearm pronation and radial opening of the patient's hand. Once the splint is on, the patient's fingers should rest securely within the confines of the splint.

Initially, the therapist may want to use the splint for static positioning. After the splint is applied, the upper extremity is positioned in external rotation, and the patient wears the splint during supine activities, as depicted in Fig. 11.2. The splint allows the arm to be maintained in the antispasm or recovery position. The air splint can also be worn during treatment interventions. With the patient in a side-lying position, the scapula is protracted. Intervention 11.14 illustrates this activity. The splint inhibits the development of abnormal tone, which can develop as the patient attempts active movements of the arm. The patient may also wear the splint as she works on upper extremity elevation exercises. As the patient develops control of the shoulder musculature, placing and holding of the arm at various points within the range of motion can be initiated. Intervention 11.15 shows a patient wearing the long arm splint for upper extremity treatment activities.

Elbow and hand splint. The elbow or hand splint may be used for patients who lack more distal control and movement. The elbow splint can be applied as the patient works on upper extremity weight-bearing activities. The splint holds the elbow passively in extension. The hand splint is especially

INTERVENTION 11.13   Applying a Long Arm Splint

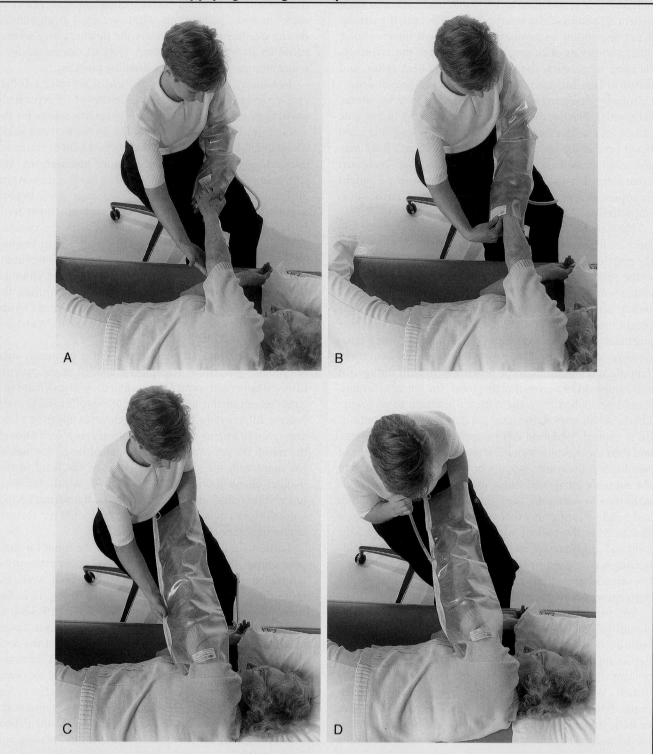

A. With the zipper of the splint closed, the therapist gathers the splint on her own arm. A handshake grasp is used to inhibit tone in the involved hand.

B and C. The splint is applied to the patient's involved upper extremity. The zipper remains on the ulnar or little finger side of the forearm. Inhibition of the wrist and fingers continues.

D. Once in place, the splint is inflated.

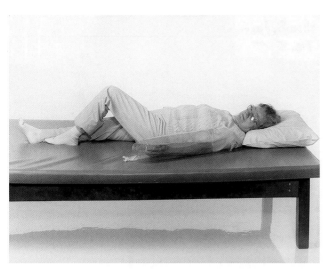

Fig. 11.2 A patient wearing an air splint while lying in bed. The splint can be used as a static positioning device, or it can be applied before treatment to prepare the involved extremity for task-specific activities.

useful for patients who demonstrate increased flexor tone in the involved wrist and fingers during functional activities. As stated previously, these splints can also be used as static positioning devices when necessary. For example, a patient may be working on a high-level developmental sequence activity, such as kneeling. A hand splint can be applied to the involved hand to decrease the effects of increased flexor tone in the wrist and fingers that may be present while the patient practices this task.

Long leg splint. The lower extremity splint can be used during early pregait activities for individuals who lack control or movement in their legs. When the splint is inflated, the patient does not have to be concerned that the involved lower extremity will collapse or buckle when weight is applied. The anterior and posterior chambers of the splint also provide the clinician with the ability to position the patient's knee in slight flexion before beginning standing activities. It is important to note that the lower extremity splint is not to be used for actual gait training activities.

INTERVENTION 11.14 Scapular Protraction With a Splint

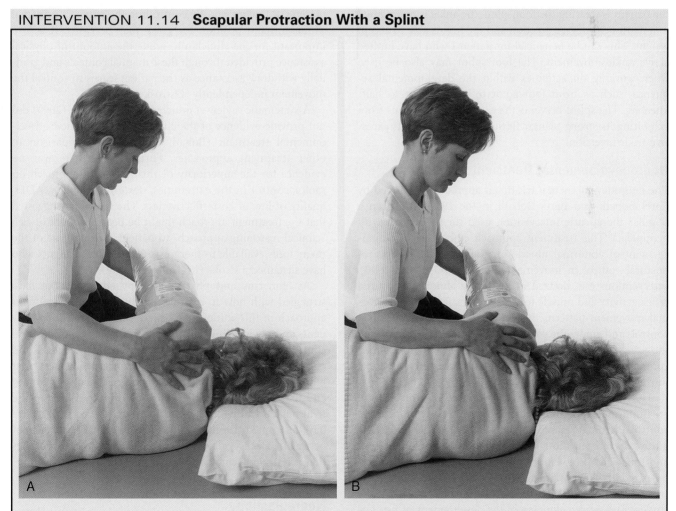

Scapular protraction exercises can be practiced with the patient wearing a long arm splint. The clinician guides the movement of the scapula.

INTERVENTION 11.15 Double Arm Elevation With a Splint

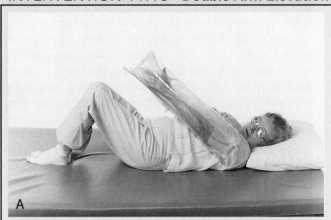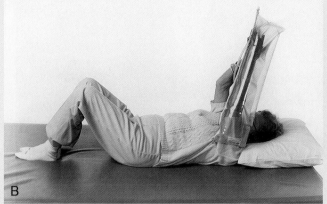

The patient is practicing double-arm elevation exercises while wearing a long arm air splint.

Foot splint. The foot splint can be used for static positioning and the development of lower extremity control. When the patient is wearing the foot splint, the ankle is maintained in a neutral 90-degree position and the heel is able to accept weight. This can be beneficial for patients who have limited active ankle movement. The foot splint may also be used when working on activities within the developmental sequence, such as from four-point to tall-kneeling to half-kneeling. The splint prevents the gastrocnemius soleus from exhibiting its strong plantar flexion action and limits excessive ankle inversion.

Neurodevelopmental Treatment Approach

The neurodevelopmental treatment approach, developed by Karel Bobath and Berta Bobath in the 1940s, has been a popular therapeutic intervention used for individuals with hemiplegia. This treatment approach emphasizes the management of abnormal muscle tone and the importance of postural control in movement initiation (Ostrosky, 1990). Interventions are directed at inhibiting abnormal postural reflex activity and muscle tone and then superimposing normal movement patterns. In a clinical context, the therapist controls and guides the patient's motor performance through the use of manual contacts applied at key points of control (proximal joints) while the patient completes a functional movement transition.

The use of manual contacts or key points of control is still an important component in the development of postural control. Proximal key points, such as the shoulder and pelvic girdles, have been thought to influence postural alignment and tone. The use of more distal key points such as the elbows, hands, knees, and feet can affect movements of the trunk (Bobath, 1990). The use of manual contacts assists the student and novice clinician in the development of psychomotor skills necessary to assist patients in their acquisition of functional movement. Through the use of manual contacts, therapists are able to provide patients with the necessary control and stability to initiate movement in other areas. For example, by providing a manual point of control at the pelvis, the patient may be able to improve trunk posturing or foot placement during gait. By controlling the patient's proximal shoulder, hand position for grasp may be easier. It is also important for the clinician to grade the amount of physical assistance provided through these manual contacts and gradually withdraw assistance as the patient learns to control the movement independently (Ostrosky, 1990).

A systematic review conducted by Kollen et al. (2009) did not provide evidence of the effectiveness of the neurodevelopmental treatment (Bobath concept) in comparison to other treatment approaches. Furthermore, there was no evidence for the superiority of this treatment approach on motor control in the extremities, dexterity, mobility, ADLs, quality of life, or cost-effectiveness. The reviewers suggested that the treatment approach might be better thought of as a "clinical reasoning approach" to patient care and one of the many tools available to therapists as they treat patients who have sustained a stroke (Kollen et al., 2009).

As clinicians and physical therapy educators, we have struggled with how to approach inclusion of the treatment approach in this edition. We believe there is benefit for students and novice clinicians to appreciate the role of postural control and its contributions to movement execution and efficiency. We also embrace the significant advances that have occurred in the body of knowledge related to the brain and its recovery capabilities and how this translates to the treatment of individuals with neurologic impairments. We have attempted throughout this text to provide the current best evidence, as well as treatment adjuncts and approaches that can provide clinicians with a number of different interventions to utilize with their patients.

Neuroplasticity

Newer evidence-based approaches and recovery-based interventions are integral in our treatment of patients with neurologic dysfunction. Current motor control and motor learning theories, as well as principles of neuroplasticity and training, focus less on the actual techniques and more on the process used to maximize patient function. These theories emphasize the need for the patient to be an active participant in learning or relearning movement strategies. Patients must become active problem solvers of their own movement deficits and learn to perform movements in different environments and within multiple contexts if function is to be improved (Whiteside, 1997).

There is a significant body of research regarding the recovery of motor function following stroke. Activity-dependent or task-specific training of appropriate intensity has proven to result in positive patient outcomes and produce cortical adaptations and reorganization (Teasell and Hussein, 2016a, 2016b; Kleim and Jones, 2008). Partial body-weight support treadmill ambulation and constraint-induced movement therapy (CIMT) are examples of such activities. Supported ambulation allows patients, even those that are unable to stand independently, the opportunity to practice stepping in a safe environment (Hornby et al., 2011). For example, if the desired outcome is an improvement in the patient's ambulation potential then clinicians must have the patient practice gait repetitively. Additionally, patients must be engaged in tasks that are meaningful and are at an appropriate intensity if the brain is to engage in repair through cortical reorganization and activation and adaptation of previously unaffected neurons (Kleim and Jones, 2008).

In the sections that follow, we will attempt to identify the tasks critical to patient function and interventions that can assist in achieving those goals. We will emphasize current motor learning and motor development principles, as well as an evidence-based practice perspective in our approach to patient care. We will, however, continue to address the need for the use of manual contacts as patients relearn important motor skills and as students develop their psychomotor skills in the treatment of adults and children with neuromuscular deficits. Reliance on a single approach or technique would be a disservice to our patients, and in the end would not promote best practice.

Functional Activities

In the following sections, the reader will be provided with a step-by-step guide to assist patients in the performance of basic functional activities.

Rolling

During the period of early rehabilitation (including the time spent in acute care), the patient should begin practicing functional movements. Rolling to the right and left should begin immediately. The patient must be instructed in methods to assist in active performance of this activity.

Rolling to the involved side. Rolling to the involved side is often easier because the patient initiates the movement with the uninvolved side of the body. The activity begins with the patient turning the head to the side toward which the patient is going to roll. Head and eye movements provide strong cues to the body to prepare for movement. Head turning also helps to unweight the opposite upper extremity and

facilitates upper trunk rotation. The patient should be encouraged to use the uninvolved upper and lower extremities to assist with the transition from supine to side-lying on the involved side. Patients often want to reach and hold on to the bed rails to assist with rolling. This practice should be discouraged by all members of the patient's rehabilitation team and by the patient's family because few patients return home with hospital beds. To roll over, the patient reaches across the body with the uninvolved upper extremity and flexes and adducts the uninvolved hip and knee. This provides the patient with the momentum needed to complete the roll.

Rolling to the uninvolved side. Rolling to the uninvolved side is usually more challenging for the patient. Again, the activity must be initiated with rotation of the head to the side toward which the patient is rolling. Patients with neglect often have a difficult time initiating cervical rotation for head turning. The patient should be encouraged to look in the direction in which she is moving. It is also important to note the position of the patient's eyes during this activity. If neglect is significant, it may be difficult for the patient to move her eyes past midline to focus on items, tasks, or individuals on the involved side. To initiate rolling to the uninvolved side, the patient is encouraged to assist as much as possible. If the patient is able to initiate any active movement in the involved extremities, the sequence will be similar to that presented for rolling to the involved side. If the patient's extremities are flaccid or essentially hypotonic, the following preparatory activities are often beneficial in assisting the patient. The patient should clasp both hands together with the involved thumb outermost. Thumb abduction is an inhibitory technique used to promote relaxation in the patient's hand. The clasping of the patient's hands also facilitates finger abduction and extension. With the hands clasped, the patient flexes the shoulders to approximately 90 degrees. Slight shoulder adduction should also be present. The patient's lower extremities should then be positioned in hook lying. If the patient is unable to flex the involved lower extremity actively, the therapist can assist with positioning by unweighting the involved leg and encouraging the patient to flex the hip and the knee while the therapist approximates through the femur and into the hip. Intervention 11.16 illustrates a patient rolling in this manner.

A compensatory strategy frequently used by patients involves hooking the uninvolved lower extremity under the involved leg and bringing the two legs up into hook-lying position together.

An alternative technique is to place the uninvolved lower extremity on top of the involved leg and bring both legs up into the hook-lying position as a unit. The patient is encouraged to do this independently or assisted by the therapist. The advantage of this technique over the one mentioned previously is that proprioceptive input is applied into the anterior shin of the involved lower extremity, and the patient is required to use the involved leg as much as possible. The more sensory input that can be applied through the involved lower extremity, the better. Once the patient has her upper and lower extremities in flexion, the patient is asked to turn the

INTERVENTION 11.16   Rolling to the Uninvolved Side

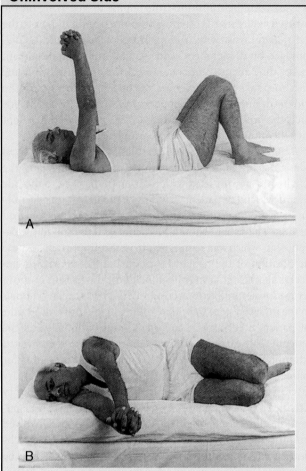

A

B

The patient is rolling to side-lying with the upper extremities clasped and the lower extremities in hook lying. (From Bobath B: *Adult hemiplegia: evaluation and treatment,* ed 3, Boston, 1990, Butterworth-Heinemann.)

head and eyes to the uninvolved side to initiate the roll. The PT/PTA must assess the patient's ability to perform the activity and assist the patient with verbal and tactile cues as needed. PNF techniques can also be incorporated when assisting the patient with rolling. Techniques such as slow reversals and hold-relax active movement can be incorporated into rolling activities.

Scooting

Another bed mobility activity that should be practiced is scooting in the supine position. Patients who are able to move independently in bed possess greater freedom because they do not require assistance from health care personnel to reposition themselves. The patient needs to be able to scoot the hips to both sides but must also be able to move the upper trunk in the same direction as the hips. Having the patient flex the head and neck is the first step when trying to move the shoulders for scooting. Cervical flexion also assists with activation of the patient's core. Placement of one's hands

under the patient's scapulae can assist with moving the upper trunk to the side. Positioning the patient's lower extremities in a hook-lying position assists with moving the patient's lower trunk in the desired direction. As the patient is able to initiate more of the movement independently, the therapist must decrease her manual contacts.

Movement Transitions

Other early functional mobility tasks include movement transitions from supine to sitting and from sitting to supine. Because of shorter hospital and rehabilitation stays, the patient's physical therapy plan of care must address the performance of functional activities during the first treatment session.

Supine-to-sit transfer. Transitions from supine to sitting should be practiced from both the patient's involved and uninvolved sides. Too often, patients are taught to perform activities in a single, structured way and then find it difficult to generalize the task to other environmental conditions. Based on a patient's living arrangements, it may not always be possible for the patient to transfer to the stronger, less involved side. Examples of ways to facilitate movement from supine to sitting include having the patient roll to the uninvolved side, as previously described, followed by moving the lower extremities off the bed. From that point, the patient can use the uninvolved upper extremity to push up into an upright sitting position. The therapist provides appropriate manual assistance at the patient's shoulders and pelvis. As the patient is able to assume a greater degree of independence in the performance of this activity, the clinician decreases the manual assist provided and allows the patient more control over the movement transition. Intervention 11.17 shows a patient performing a supine-to-sit transfer with assistance.

Care must be taken to ensure that distractional forces are not applied to the involved upper extremity during performance of this activity. Frequently, one observes health care workers and family members using both of the patient's upper extremities to assist with coming to sit and other movement transitions. Distraction applied to the shoulder joint can lead to subluxation and can promote the development of painful upper extremity conditions, including CRPS and frozen shoulder. All family members and health care personnel should receive instruction in proper transfer techniques, including protection of the involved upper extremity.

Supine-to-sit transfers can also be facilitated in other ways. Patients can be taught to use diagonals versus straight plane movements to perform this transition. Supine-to-sit transfers performed in a diagonal pattern can be practiced from either the involved or uninvolved side. Most able-bodied individuals perform functional activities in diagonal movement patterns. Diagonal movement patterns tend to be more functional and are also more energy-efficient. To assist the patient with this type of transition, place the patient's lower extremities in a hook-lying position. The legs are then brought off the bed or mat surface. The patient is asked to tuck the chin and, with the uninvolved upper extremity, reaches forward. This technique enables patients to activate

INTERVENTION 11.17 Supine-to-Sit Transfer

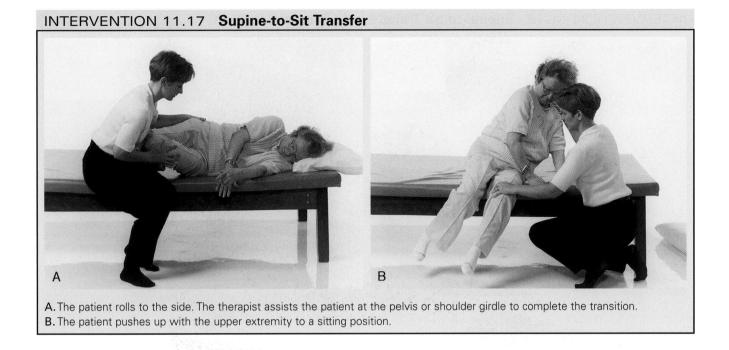

A. The patient rolls to the side. The therapist assists the patient at the pelvis or shoulder girdle to complete the transition.
B. The patient pushes up with the upper extremity to a sitting position.

their abdominal muscles (core) to assist in the achievement of upright sitting. Intervention 11.18 demonstrates a patient performing this transition. The PT/PTA may raise the head of the bed or prop the patient on pillows or a wedge to make the task easier if the abdominal musculature is weak. This technique provides the patient with a mechanical advantage and decreases the work the abdominals need to perform. As the patient is able to complete the transition with increased ease, the degree of inclination can be decreased.

Some patients require increased physical assistance for supine-to-sit transfers. The technique is essentially the same when a second person is used. Often, it is easiest to divide the work and have one person control and assist at the patient's trunk while the other is responsible for the patient's lower extremities. Both individuals must be clear about who is leading the activity and who is responsible for providing the verbal directions. Patients should not be allowed under any circumstance to pull up on the therapist's neck during the performance of supine-to-sit transition. This practice can create a safety concern for both the clinician and the patient.

Wheelchair-to-bed/mat transfers. Once the patient has made the transition from supine to sitting, transfers to the wheelchair are attempted. A stand-pivot transfer is the most common. Initially, therapists may have the patient transfer to the stronger side, as this does not require the patient to step with the involved lower extremity. Over time the patient will need to be able to transfer to both the right and left sides and to various surfaces to maximize independence. To begin the transfer, the patient must scoot forward in the wheelchair or on the mat table to ensure that both feet are flat on the floor. If the patient is sitting in a wheelchair, it is not uncommon for the patient to lean against the back of the chair to scoot the hips forward. Weight shifting from one

side to the next is the preferred technique and should be encouraged. On moving the left hip forward, the patient shifts her weight to the right. This weight shift should be accompanied by elongation of the trunk musculature on the right side. The patient repeats this sequence with movement of the right hip forward and a weight shift to the left. Once the patient's feet are flat on the floor, the gait belt is applied, and the involved upper extremity is prepositioned. The patient performs an anterior weight shift and is instructed to stand. The PT/PTA guards the patient closely and uses her knees to block the patient's hemiplegic knee if necessary. Weakness or spasticity in the involved lower extremity may cause the knee to buckle as weight is transferred to the limb. The patient steps with the uninvolved leg and pivots on the involved lower extremity to the mat table or bed. The position of the involved ankle must be carefully monitored to avoid instability or inadvertent weight-bearing on the lateral malleolus. Intervention 11.19 depicts a patient performing a stand-pivot transfer from the wheelchair to the mat table.

Early mobilization including transferring the patient out of bed and the performance of upright sitting activities has been shown to improve ambulation abilities and may lead to an earlier discharge to a patient's home (Cumming et al., 2011).

Summary

Treatment interventions that can be performed by the patient in the early stages of rehabilitation have been presented. Before more advanced interventions are discussed, a summarized list of techniques that may be part of the initial treatment plan is provided.
- Positioning
- Bridging and bridging with approximation

INTERVENTION 11.18   Supine-to-Sit Transfer on a Diagonal Pattern

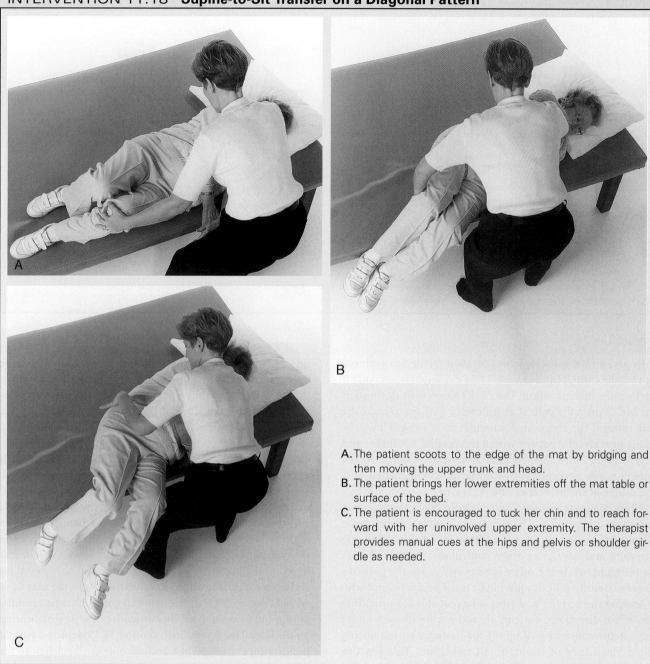

A. The patient scoots to the edge of the mat by bridging and then moving the upper trunk and head.
B. The patient brings her lower extremities off the mat table or surface of the bed.
C. The patient is encouraged to tuck her chin and to reach forward with her uninvolved upper extremity. The therapist provides manual cues at the hips and pelvis or shoulder girdle as needed.

- Hip extension over the edge of the mat or bed
- Hamstring cocontraction (modified straight leg raising)
- Lower trunk rotation and lower trunk rotation with bridging
- Hip flexor retraining
- Hip and knee extension with ankle dorsiflexion
- Scapular mobilization
- Upper extremity elevation

- Functional activities including rolling, scooting, and supine-to-sit and wheelchair-to-bed transfers. Transfers to other surfaces including the commode and bedside chairs should also be practiced.

Adjuncts to treatment at this phase include air splints, the use of spinal and brainstem level reflexes, and various facilitation and inhibition techniques. The treatment of the patient in other functional positions will now be discussed.

INTERVENTION 11.19 Stand-Pivot Transfer

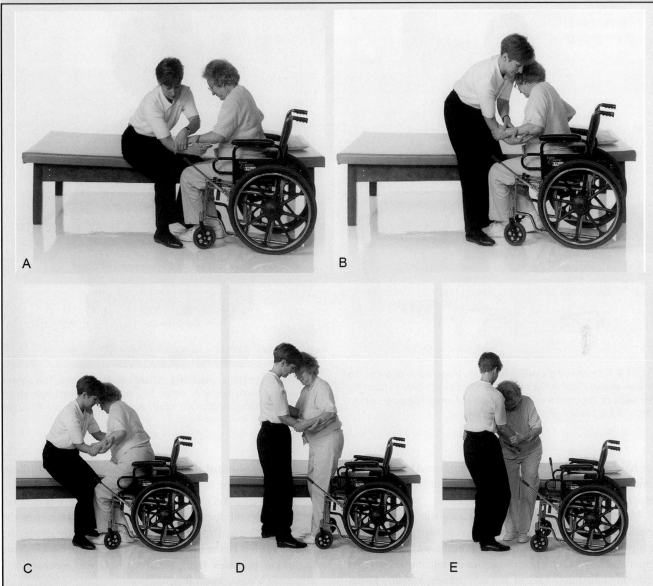

A. The patient weight shifts forward in the chair so her feet are supported and are in a plantigrade position on the floor.

B. The involved arm is prepositioned for safety.

C. The patient is encouraged to perform an anterior weight shift to come to standing. The clinician guards the involved knee to prevent buckling.

D. The patient stands erect.

E. The patient pivots on her feet to sit down. Some patients may require continuous support/guarding of the involved knee to prevent buckling during performance of stand-pivot transfers.

Other Functional Positions

Sitting

Once the patient is able to achieve a short-sitting position, which is defined as sitting on a surface such as a bed or mat table with one's hips and knees flexed and one's feet supported on the floor, the clinician can begin to work on sitting posture and balance activities with the patient. Fig. 11.3 shows a patient who exhibits fair sitting posture and balance. With increased clinical experience, it will become apparent that some patients with hemiplegia have poor or nonfunctional sitting balance. Patients with an altered sense of midline and motor control deficits often lose their balance. In this case, it may be necessary for the PT/PTA to seek help from another clinician or an aide. The second person can be positioned behind the patient and assist with the patient's trunk control. The clinician in front of the patient attempts to establish eye contact and to control the patient's head and trunk position. If not guarded properly, the patient can lose

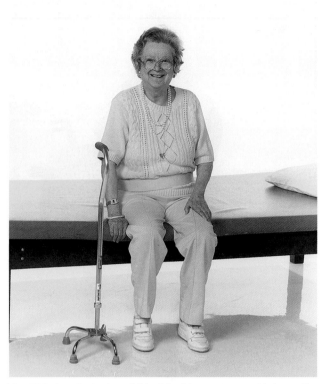

Fig. 11.3 A patient who exhibits fair sitting posture and balance. The clinician should observe the position of the patient's pelvis and trunk, the height of the shoulders, the symmetry of weight-bearing on both hips, and the position of the patient's feet.

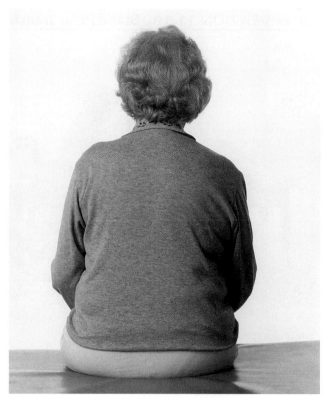

Fig. 11.4 A posterior view of a patient's sitting posture. The patient sits with a slight posterior pelvic tilt, increased weight-bearing on the right without associated trunk elongation, and right shoulder depression.

her balance and fall off the support surface. Therefore, patients functioning at a low level often benefit from treatment sessions with more than one individual.

Motor control. The first problem area that must be addressed is the patient's sitting posture. A patient cannot progress to functional movements of the limbs without a stable upper and lower trunk from which to initiate movement and perform skilled activities of the extremities. *Stability* is defined as the ability to fix or maintain a position or posture in relation to gravity, and it is a prerequisite for the more advanced stages of motor development, including controlled mobility and skilled activities. *Controlled mobility* refers to the ability to maintain postural stability while moving. An example of this would be weight shifting in a quadruped (four-point) position with the hands fixed and the proximal joints moving, in this example, the shoulders. *Skilled activities* are described as coordinated, purposeful movements that are superimposed on a stable posture. These tasks are the ones our patients most often aspire to achieve. Ambulation and fine motor activities of the hand are two common examples of skilled activities.

Sitting posture: positioning the pelvis. The position of the patient's pelvis must be assessed initially. Fig. 11.4 provides a posterior view of the patient's sitting posture. Clinicians often ignore the pelvis and try to initially correct deviations noted in the trunk. A patient will be unable to maintain adequate trunk and/or head control if she is unable to achieve a neutral position of the pelvis. A posteriorly tilted pelvis

creates a bias toward thoracic kyphosis and a forward head position. This type of posturing is common in our everyday world, and as a consequence, many patients have these premorbid postural deviations. By placing one's hands over the lumbar paraspinal musculature, one can gently guide the patient's pelvis in the direction of an anterior pelvic tilt. This technique provides the patient with tactile feedback for achieving a more neutral pelvic position. Intervention 11.20 depicts this activity. Care must be taken to avoid excessively tilting the pelvis and locking the patient in an anterior pelvic tilt. An anterior tilt puts the spine in extension, thus creating a closed-pack position and preventing movement. This closed-pack position limits the patient's abilities to perform functional movement transitions that require lateral weight shifts and rotation.

Achieving pelvic tilts in supine. For individuals who are having difficulty isolating pelvic movements, the patient can work on achieving anterior and posterior pelvic tilts in the supine position. A large therapy ball can be placed under the patient's lower extremities. While stabilizing the patient's legs on the ball, the therapist gently moves the ball forward and backward. This technique allows the patient to feel the movement of the pelvis in a controlled and secure position.

Positioning the trunk. Once the patient is able to move the pelvis actively and maintain a neutral pelvic position in sitting, attention is given to the trunk musculature. Alignment of the shoulders over the hips is desired for an erect sitting posture. Gentle extension of the trunk should be encouraged

INTERVENTION 11.20 **Achieving a Neutral Pelvis**

A. The therapist provides tactile cues to the patient's paraspinals to achieve a neutral pelvis.
B. Tension within the intrinsic finger musculature provides tactile feedback to the patient. Care is taken to avoid poking the patient with the clinician's fingertips. The little fingers are positioned on the patient's abdominals to facilitate movement back into a posterior pelvic tilt.

by having the patient look up and bring the shoulders back. Initially, the patient may require tactile cues to be able to extend the trunk and contract the abdominal muscles. While maintaining a tactile cue on the patient's low back region, the clinician may place her other hand under the patient's clavicles and move the patient's upper trunk into extension. Eventually, the patient must be taught to self-correct her own positioning in sitting. Recognizing when posture should be corrected facilitates motor learning of this task and enables the patient to assume this posture during other functional activities such as standing. If the patient has difficulty maintaining an upright sitting posture, increasing the patient's visual input through the use of a mirror may be beneficial. It may also be necessary to work jointly with another clinician (the occupational therapist) or an aide to provide adequate manual contacts for equal weight-bearing over both hips and to maintain an erect trunk position.

Positioning the head. Poor pelvic positioning often contributes to misalignment of the patient's head. The patient must be able to hold the head erect to orient to the environment. An inability to maintain an upright position of the head causes visual and postural deficits through incorrect input into the vestibular system. Forward flexion of the cervical spine causes the patient's gaze to be directed toward the floor. This condition can affect arousal and the patient's ability to attend to persons or events within the environment. Excessive flexion of the head also biases the patient toward increased thoracic kyphosis and posterior tilting of the pelvis. If the patient is unable to maintain an upright position of the head and neck, facilitation techniques must be employed to correct the deficit. Quick icing or gentle tapping to the posterior cervical muscles produces cervical extension. At times, it is necessary for the PT/PTA to provide manual cues to maintain the patient's head upright. A second person may be needed to achieve this outcome. Once the patient is able to maintain her head positioning independently, the therapist should decrease manual support.

> SPECIAL NOTE Patients who are able to maintain their sitting balance for 30 seconds and are able to initiate muscle contractions in their involved lower extremity within the first 72 hours after their stroke have a 98% probability of achieving independent ambulation within 6 months. For patients who are not able to perform these activities, their likelihood of independent ambulation is only 27% (Edwardson, 2019).

Additional sitting balance activities: weight-bearing on the involved hand. Once the patient is able to maintain an upright sitting posture with minimal to moderate assistance, progression to additional balance activities is warranted. An early sitting activity that promotes sitting balance and upper-extremity function is weight-bearing on the involved hand. The patient's upper extremity should be placed in neutral rotation and abducted approximately 30 degrees, the elbow should be extended, and the wrist and fingers should also be extended, as depicted in Intervention 11.21. Care must be taken to avoid excessive external rotation of the shoulder. Extreme external rotation of the shoulder causes the elbow to become anatomically locked, thus eliminating the need for the patient to use the triceps actively to maintain elbow extension. Extension of the wrist and fingers with thumb abduction assists in decreasing spasticity in the wrist and finger flexors. Some patients, however, find this position uncomfortable or painful secondary to tightness in the wrist and fingers or because of arthritic changes. Thus modifications of this position can be used. Weight-bearing on a flexed elbow with the forearm resting on a bolster or half-roll offers the same benefits. Weight-bearing stimulates joint and muscle proprioceptors to contract and assists in the development of muscle control around a joint. It is especially beneficial to patients who have flaccid or hypotonic upper extremity musculature and who demonstrate glenohumeral subluxation. Use of an upper extremity air splint may also be helpful to assist with stabilizing the arm during weight-bearing activities.

Shoulder subluxation. A subluxation is the separation of the articular surfaces of bones from their normal position in a joint. Shoulder subluxation is relatively common in patients who have sustained strokes. If the upper extremity is flaccid, the scapula can assume a position of downward rotation. This orientation causes the glenoid fossa to become oriented posteriorly. Loss of muscle tone, stretch on the capsule, and abnormal bony alignment results in an inferior shoulder subluxation. Strong hypertonicity in the scapular and shoulder musculature and truncal rotational asymmetries can predispose the patient to an anterior subluxation (Ryerson, 2013). Prevention of shoulder subluxation through proper positioning in sitting, standing, and gait, as well as muscle reeducation activities and patient education, is important.

To determine whether a patient has a subluxation, place the patient's upper extremity in a non–weight-bearing position and palpate the acromion process. Moving distally from the border of the acromion, you should be able to palpate whether a separation exists between the process and the head of the humerus. Fig. 11.5 depicts a shoulder subluxation. Compare the involved shoulder with the uninvolved joint. Measure the separation in terms of finger widths with the fingers oriented horizontally to the acromion. The extent of the separation can vary from one-half finger width up to a separation of four or more. In addition to the resulting bony malalignment, subluxations also lead to ligamentous laxity around the joint. Weight-bearing temporarily moves the head of the humerus back up into the glenoid fossa and assists in the realignment of the joint. Weight-bearing offers only temporary remediation of the condition, however. Active control of the middle deltoid and rotator cuff muscles is necessary to bring the head of the humerus back into proper alignment permanently. Alternative treatments that assist in reducing subluxations include functional electrical stimulation, biofeedback, and slings. The use of functional electrical stimulation and biofeedback for the purposes of muscle reeducation is beyond the scope of this text. Slings can be prescribed for patients who need support of the shoulder joint. However, clinicians disagree regarding the use of slings in patients with hemiparesis. Many slings do not fit the patient properly and consequently do little to support the shoulder.

INTERVENTION 11.21 Weight-Bearing on the Involved Hand

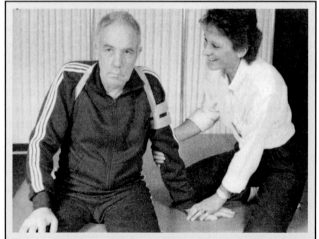

Sitting with the involved upper extremity extended. The patient is wearing a Bobath arm sling with a humeral cuff to prevent subluxation of the shoulder. The clinician assists in stabilizing the patient's elbow and fingers in extension. (From O'Sullivan SB, Schmitz TJ, editors: *Physical rehabilitation: assessment and treatment*, Philadelphia, 2007, FA Davis.)

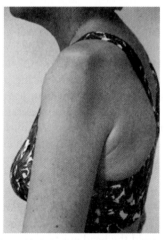

Fig. 11.5 Shoulder subluxation. (From Ryerson S, Levit K: *Functional movement reeducation: a contemporary model for stroke rehabilitation*, New York, 1997, Churchill Livingstone.)

In addition, slings promote neglect and disregard of the involved upper extremity and facilitate asymmetry within the trunk and upper extremities. There has, however, been some advancements in sling design in recent years. The GivMohr sling is used for the flaccid upper extremity and provides joint compression (sensory input) into the hemiparetic limb. The sling maintains the upper extremity in a functional position (shoulder abduction with external rotation and elbow extension). The sling provides protection to the involved arm and facilitates weight shifting during ambulation (Dieruf, 2005). Fig. 11.6 shows a patient wearing a GivMohr sling.

Weight shifting activities. A gradual progression of sitting activities includes weight shifting in both anteroposterior and mediolateral directions. Weight shifting activities are performed with the patient's upper extremities in a weight-bearing position, or with the arms resting in the lap. Initially, patients should relearn to shift their weight within their base of support. Patients with hemiplegia often exhibit difficulties with weight shifting, especially toward the involved side because many patients lack the ability to control their trunk musculature actively. A lateral weight shift to the right requires the ability to elongate the trunk muscles on the right and to shorten the trunk muscles on the left, thus maintaining the weight of the body within the base of support. In addition, the head turns to the right in an attempt to keep the eyes vertical and the mouth horizontal. Patients with spasticity or hypotonia may not be able to activate their neck or trunk muscles in such a way. An attempt to shift weight to the right frequently results in a collapse of the head and trunk

into right lateral flexion. As a consequence, the patient experiences increased weight-bearing on the right side. This, however, is not a controlled weight-bearing condition. Fig. 11.7 shows a patient performing a weight shift to the right side with trunk shortening on the weight-bearing side. A patient's inability to perform weight shifts while sitting may affect her ability to perform ADLs, which include self-care tasks, feeding, and dressing.

In an effort to assist the patient in relearning the appropriate trunk strategies, tactile cues can be provided to the trunk musculature. Intervention 11.22 depicts a therapist who is facilitating trunk elongation on the patient's weight-bearing side. This activity should be practiced to both the right and left sides.

Sitting balance activities to improve trunk control. Once the patient is able to maintain a stable sitting position with proper alignment, additional static sitting balance activities can be practiced. The clinician can apply manual resistance (alternating isometrics) at the shoulders or pelvis in an anteroposterior or mediolateral direction to promote cocontraction around the joints. Manual resistance with a rotational component (rhythmic stabilization) can also be performed to promote trunk stability.

Assessing protective reactions. While the patient is sitting, the therapist may also want to observe the patient's protective reactions. Patients should demonstrate protective reactions laterally, anteriorly, and posteriorly. Protective extension, characterized by extension and abduction, is evident in the upper extremities when a patient's balance is quickly disturbed and the patient realizes that she may fall. Often,

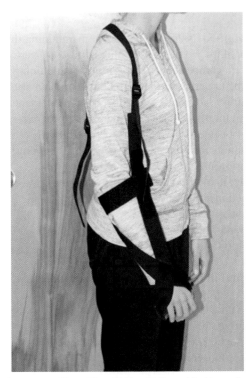

Fig. 11.6 GivMohr Sling. (From Tubbs JT, Pound D: Upper limb orthoses for persons with spinal cord injuries and brachial plexus injuries. In Webster JP, Murphy DP, editors: *Atlas of orthoses and assistive devices*, ed 5, Philadelphia, 2019, Elsevier, p. 168.)

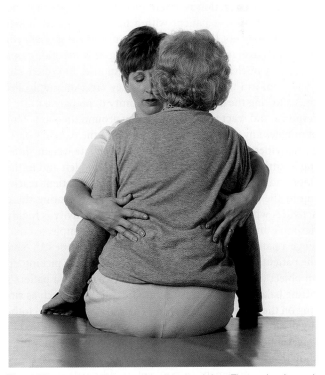

Fig. 11.7 Weight shifting to the right in sitting. The patient's trunk should elongate on the weight-bearing side.

INTERVENTION 11.22 **Facilitating Weight Shifts**

The therapist facilitates weight shifts to the right and left in sitting. Tactile cues are applied to the patient's paraspinals to facilitate the desired trunk response.

this protective reaction is absent or delayed in patients who have had strokes. A patient with a flaccid or spastic upper extremity may not be able to elicit the motor components of the protective response. When testing this reaction, one should try to elicit an unanticipated response. Too often, clinicians inform the patient of what they are planning to do, thus allowing the patient an opportunity to prepare a muscle response and react with cocontraction around the joint. This eliminates any spontaneous movement on the patient's part.

Activities that can be performed to facilitate weight shifting in sitting include reaching to the right and left and to the floor and ceiling. Intervention 11.23 depicts a patient reaching to the left with her hands clasped. Incorporating these activities within the context of a functional activity is highly desirable and therapeutically beneficial. For example, to challenge a patient's ability to shift weight forward, one can have the patient practice putting on shoes and socks or picking up an object off the floor. Other tasks that challenge a patient's sitting balance include the performance of ADLs, such as sitting on the edge of the bed or in a chair to don items of clothing or sitting in a chair to reach for a cup, as demonstrated in Intervention 11.23, *B* and *C*. Reaching activities in sitting should also incorporate trunk rotation. Rotation is a frequently lost movement component in older patients. Passive or active-assisted lower trunk rotation performed in the

supine position assists the patient in maintaining the necessary flexibility in the trunk musculature to perform this movement component. Furthermore, maintaining separation of the upper and lower parts of the trunk assists the patient's ability to rotate and dissociate movements of the shoulder and pelvic girdles. As the patient progresses, performance of bilateral PNF patterns (chops and lifts) can be used to facilitate trunk rotation. These exercises are illustrated in Intervention 11.24.

Sitting activities. A summary of interventions to be performed in sitting includes the following:
- Pelvic positioning
- Trunk positioning
- Head positioning
- Weight-bearing on the involved upper extremity
- Weight shifting in anteroposterior and mediolateral directions
- Alternating isometrics
- Rhythmic stabilization
- Functional reaching to a target or specific item (goal-directed movement)

Standing

As the patient is able to tolerate more treatment activities during sitting, the patient should be progressed to upright

INTERVENTION 11.23 Reaching Activities

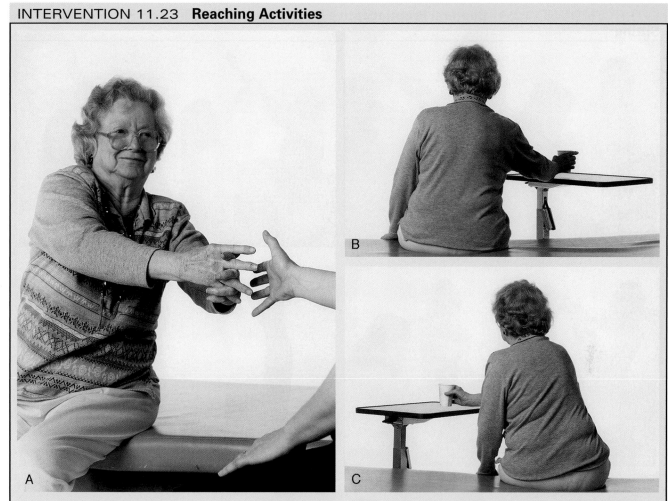

A. Reaching with the hands clasped. Patients should practice reaching to the right, left, and to the floor.

B and C. Reaching with the uninvolved upper extremity to the right and left. The involved arm is in a weight-bearing position during performance of the activity. If the patient has active movement in the involved arm, she can perform reaching tasks with it.

standing. It is not necessary to perfect one posture or activity before advancing the patient to a more challenging one. Patients should work in all possible postures to reach the highest functional level. While working on sitting activities, the patient should also advance to supported standing and gait activities. The primary PT should evaluate the patient's standing and walking abilities before the PTA guides the patient to standing for the first time.

Position of the therapist in relation to the patient. A common question asked by students is where to position oneself when assisting the patient from sitting to standing. Much depends on the patient and the patient's current level of motor control and function. Sitting in front of the patient as she transfers to standing gives the patient more space to move into and also offers the clinician the opportunity to assess the patient's posture in standing. This transition is illustrated in Intervention 11.25. The clinician may also elect to start from a squat position in front of the patient and move to standing with her. If this method is employed, the PT/PTA must allow the patient physical space to perform the forward weight shift

that accompanies trunk flexion before lifting the buttocks off the support surface. Often, clinicians guard the patient so closely that it is nearly impossible for the patient to complete the necessary movement sequences and weight shifts. Standing on the patient's uninvolved side should be avoided because it can promote excessive weight shift to that side. Guarding the patient from the involved side may also be employed as it allows the therapist to encourage weight shifting and weight-bearing on the hemiplegic side, as illustrated in Intervention 11.26. In addition to the therapist's position relative to the patient, a safety belt must always be used. Use of safety belts is standard in most facilities. Even if a patient insists that she does not need a gait belt, it is always in the patient's and the clinician's best interest to apply one.

Sit-to-stand transition. The transition from sitting to standing is the first part of the standing progression. The patient must initially be able to maintain the lower extremities in flexion at the hips, knees, and ankles. In addition, the patient must be able to achieve and maintain a neutral or slightly anterior tilt of the pelvis during a forward weight

INTERVENTION 11.24   Bilateral Proprioceptive Neuromuscular Facilitation Patterns While Sitting

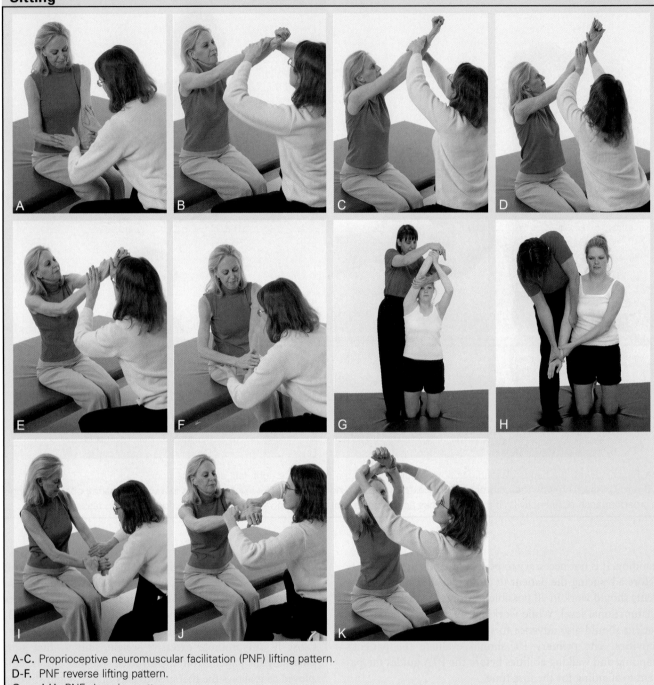

A-C. Proprioceptive neuromuscular facilitation (PNF) lifting pattern.
D-F. PNF reverse lifting pattern.
G and H. PNF chopping pattern.
I-K. PNF reverse chopping pattern.

shift over the fixed feet. It therefore becomes essential that the patient be able to advance the tibias over the feet. Patients with plantar flexion contractures of the ankles or increased tone in the gastrocnemius-soleus complex may not be able to achieve the amount of passive ankle dorsiflexion necessary to complete this activity. In people without neurologic deficits, the ascent to standing is accomplished by combining knee extension with hip extension. Frequently, patients are unable

to perform this part of the movement smoothly and exhibit difficulty maintaining a neutral hip position once they are upright because of lack of strength in their hip extensors. These patients often appear to be in a crouched or flexed position, or they use strong knee hyperextension to lock the knees into extension while coming to stand.

Other deviations noted during sit to stand include excessive reliance on the uninvolved lower extremity. This may be

INTERVENTION 11.25 Sit-to-Stand Transition

A.

B.

A. Prepositioning of the patient is important before a sit-to-stand transition is performed. The patient must be able to weight shift to scoot forward on the mat or wheelchair so that only half of the femurs are supported. The patient's feet should be shoulder-width apart.

B. The clinician sits in front of the patient with her hands on the patient's paraspinals to facilitate an anterior weight shift. The patient should be encouraged to push up with both lower extremities equally to promote symmetrical weight-bearing. Gait belts should be applied during sit-to-stand and standing activities.

caused by lower extremity weakness, insecurity, and a fear of falling. This reliance is evident by increased weight-bearing on the uninvolved leg and truncal asymmetry. The problem can be accentuated if the patient is allowed to push up with the upper extremity. Intervention 11.27 shows a patient coming to stand with the use of the upper extremity. Continued performance of sit-to-stand transitions in this manner results in the patient's inability to bear weight on the involved leg and can intensify the patient's insecurity about stability of the involved lower extremity. Patients with hemiplegia must be encouraged to perform sit-to-stand transitions with equal weight-bearing on both lower extremities. Symmetric foot placement, with feet shoulder-width apart and the patient's feet flat on the floor, can assist in the achievement of equal weight-bearing.

The patient's upper extremity must be carefully monitored during a sit-to-stand transfer. The involved arm should not be allowed to hang down at the patient's side. In this situation, gravity applies a distractional force that can predispose an individual to shoulder subluxation. Intervention 11.28 shows prepositioning the upper extremity on the patient's knee or the clinician's arm. In some instances, a sling may be

necessary to give additional support, or the patient may be advised to place the involved hand in a pocket. By prepositioning the upper extremity in these ways, one is supporting the shoulder and applying a minimal amount of approximation to the shoulder joint and surrounding musculature.

During the sit-to-stand transition, the clinician needs to carefully gauge the amount of physical assistance required by the patient. The PT/PTA can provide manual cues over the patient's gluteus maximus muscle to promote hip extension. As previously stated, if the patient is unable to extend the hips, the patient will often assume a forward flexed posture. It may be necessary to physically move the patient's hips into extension to achieve an upright position. Intervention 11.29 illustrates a therapist who is providing a manual contact at the patient's gluteal muscles.

In addition to monitoring the position of the patient's hips, one must observe the alignment of the patient's involved knee and ankle for proper positioning. If the ankle musculature is flaccid and unstable, the patient may bear weight on the malleolus or the lateral aspect of her foot, with resulting long-term ligamentous injury. To avoid this complication, preposition the patient's foot or block the patient's

INTERVENTION 11.26   Guarding the Patient From the Side During a Sit-to-Stand Transition

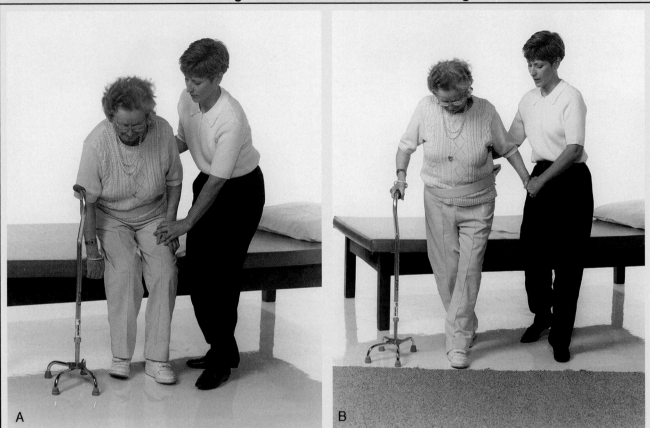

Patients with fair to good static and dynamic standing balance can also be guarded from their involved side.

A. The therapist provides a tactile cue to the patient's upper extremity to inhibit abnormal tone. Note the position of the patient's involved lower extremity during the transition. The left leg is positioned in front of the right leg. This position reinforces reliance on the uninvolved lower extremity to assume the standing position. Ideally, both lower extremities should be positioned symmetrically. Approximation is also provided to the involved lower extremity to encourage weight-bearing.

B. Once the patient is standing, an inhibitory handhold can be used to decrease flexor tone, which is present in the patient's elbow, wrist, and fingers.

ankle to keep it from turning inward. This can be accomplished by placing the therapist's feet around the patient's involved ankle, thus providing additional support. This type of positioning also provides additional support to the entire involved lower extremity. Intervention 11.30 shows a clinician blocking the patient's ankle to prevent instability.

Establishing knee control. Inadequate knee control impedes the patient's ability to stand and to ambulate. The patient's knee may buckle when the joint is required to accept weight. This condition is often caused by weakness in the quadriceps. Clinically, when individuals with quadriceps weakness stand up, they immediately assume a crouched or flexed posture. Quadriceps weakness or inefficient gastrocnemius-soleus function can lead to strong knee hyperextension or genu recurvatum during standing. Patients who demonstrate this condition lock their knees into extension to maintain stability. Several explanations for this phenomenon have been suggested. Decreased proprioceptive input from the

joint may cause the patient to hyperextend the knee joint in an attempt to find a stable point as maximum input is received at the joint's end range or closed-pack position. Overactive or spastic quadriceps, a lack of balance between strength of the hamstrings and quadriceps, and ankle plantar flexion contractures have also been cited as reasons for knee hyperextension (Webster and Darter, 2019). As a consequence, knee instability results. To control these deviations, appropriate manual (tactile) cues around the knee must be used. Pressure on the anterior shin may be needed when buckling is present. The therapist may actually have to assist the knee joint into extension, as illustrated in Intervention 11.31. In contrast, manual cues applied to the posterior knee may be required in the presence of knee hyperextension. The clinician may need to prevent the knee from extending to a completely locked position. Continued knee hyperextension can cause long-term ligamentous and capsular problems, and therefore should be avoided.

INTERVENTION 11.27   Sit-to-Stand Using the Uninvolved Upper Extremity

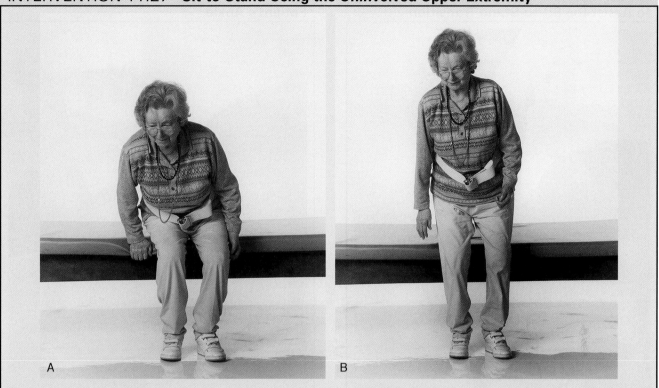

Using the uninvolved upper extremity to assist with coming to stand. Note the increased weight-bearing on the uninvolved side and the associated asymmetry.

INTERVENTION 11.28   Prepositioning the Patient's Involved Upper Extremity

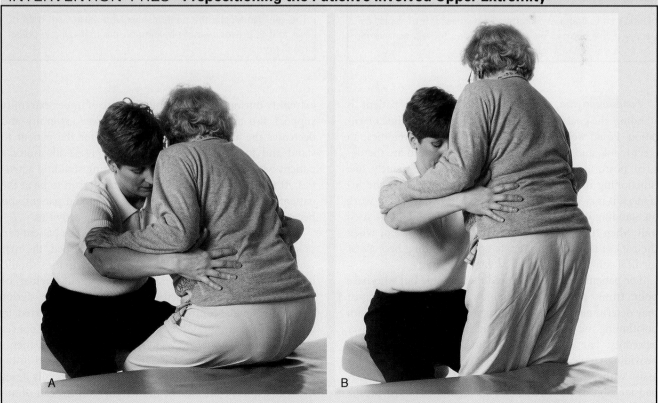

It is necessary to preposition and protect the patient's involved upper extremity during movement transitions to prevent injury to the shoulder.

INTERVENTION 11.29 Using Tactile Cues to Assist the Sit-to-Stand Transition

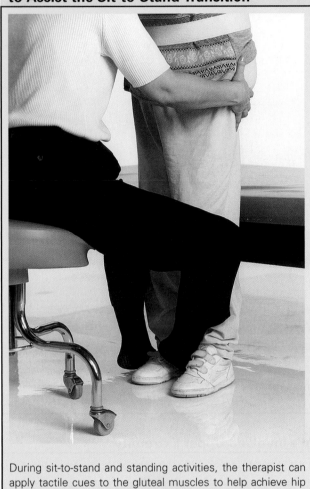

During sit-to-stand and standing activities, the therapist can apply tactile cues to the gluteal muscles to help achieve hip extension and an upright posture.

INTERVENTION 11.30 Blocking the Patient's Ankle

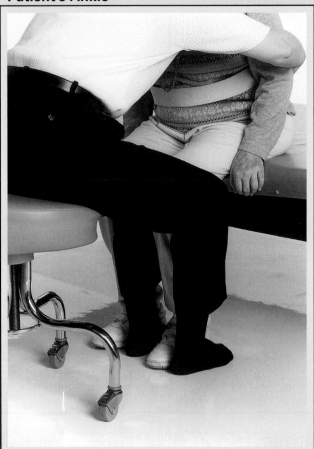

The clinician blocks the patient's involved ankle with both of her feet to prevent weight-bearing on the malleoli and possible injury.

Positioning the standing patient. Once the patient is standing, the goal is to achieve symmetry and midline orientation. Equal weight-bearing on both lower extremities, an erect trunk, and midline orientation of the head are the desired postural outcomes. Patients who are extremely low functioning may require additional assistance. In some instances, it may initially be necessary to have the patient work on standing on the tilt table. The tilt table should be used only when the patient requires maximal assistance or when the patient is unable to tolerate upright standing because of medical complications or physiologic instability.

For patients who do not need the tilt table but who have poor trunk and lower extremity control, the therapist may determine that a second person is needed to assist with positioning the patient's trunk and involved upper or lower extremity. The support person can be behind the patient, providing tactile cues for trunk extension. The person may assist with positioning of the involved upper extremity. A bedside table or an ARJO walker are often used to provide the upper extremities with a weight-bearing surface. Increased proprioceptive input is received through the involved upper extremity during weight-bearing. The use of upper extremity support also assists in unloading the lower extremity and decreases the amount of control needed for the patient to stand and to bear weight. Intervention 11.32 illustrates a patient who is using a bedside table during standing activities. At times, it is helpful for the second person to be at the patient's side. Much depends on the individual patient and her response to standing and weight-bearing activities.

Early standing activities: weight shifting. The patient can practice standing activities from the patient's bed, the mat table, or the parallel bars. Early standing activities should incorporate weight shifts (moving the patient's center of gravity) to the right and left and in anterior and posterior directions. Small, controlled weight shifts are preferred to those that are extreme. Observation of the patient's responses to these early attempts at weight shifting is essential. Patients are often reluctant to shift weight onto the involved lower extremity. To avoid weight shifting, the patient laterally flexes the trunk toward the side of the weight shift instead of accepting weight onto the lower extremity and elongating the trunk.

INTERVENTION 11.31 Using Tactile Cues to Promote Knee Extension

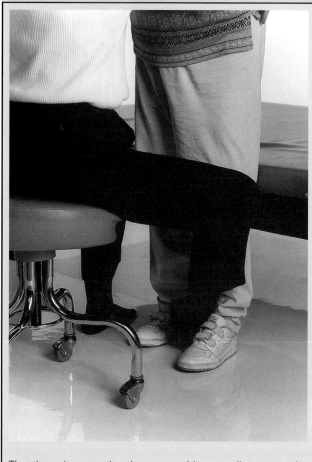

The therapist uses her leg to provide a tactile cue to the patient's shin. This cue is used to promote knee extension in the involved lower extremity.

INTERVENTION 11.32 Using a Bedside Table During Standing Activities

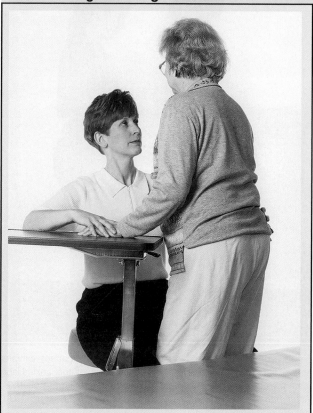

A bedside table can be used during standing activities to support the involved upper extremity. A tactile cue can be applied to maintain the wrist in a neutral to slightly extended position with the fingers extended.

The clinician must monitor the position of the patient's hip, knee, and ankle during all standing activities. Achievement of hip extension with the patient's pelvis in a neutral or slightly anterior position is desired. As stated previously, tactile cues applied to the gluteus maximus may be necessary to assist the patient with hip extension. If the patient is experiencing difficulty with knee control, the therapist can address this problem by having the patient slowly bend and straighten the involved knee. The PT/PTA may have to guide the knee into flexion and then extension manually. The patient should gauge the amount of muscle force generated during this task. Frequently, patients exaggerate knee extension by quickly snapping the knee back into an extended position. Once the patient is able to control this movement, she should practice relaxing the knee into flexion followed by controlled knee extension without producing knee hyperextension or genu recurvatum. Active achievement of the last 10 to 15 degrees of extension is often most difficult for the patient. Clinicians often use terminal knee extension exercises to assist with this control, although current evidence would suggest that patients must practice activities in a functional, task-specific manner and in the appropriate environmental context versus performing components of functional movements (Shumway-Cook and Woollacott, 2017). Therefore, if the patient needs to achieve the final few degrees of knee extension in standing or walking, the patient should practice this component of the movement in an upright standing position or during locomotor activities.

It should be noted that treatment time spent in standing weight shifting activities should be limited. If the patient's goal is to walk independently, ambulation must be repeated and practiced in all environmental contexts.

Assessing balance responses. As the patient continues to perform weight shifting activities, the therapist should observe if the patient has appropriate standing balance responses. Ankle dorsiflexion should be elicited as the patient's body mass is shifted posteriorly. Fig. 11.8 shows an ankle strategy. This motor response normally occurs as a balance strategy in standing. If the patient's balance is disrupted too much, the patient will exhibit a hip or stepping strategy. Movement of the hip occurs to realign the patient. A stepping strategy is used if the patient's balance is displaced too far, and a step is taken to prevent the patient from falling. Many

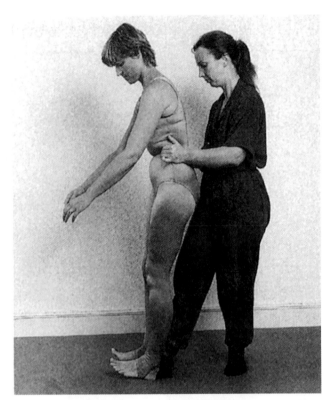

Fig. 11.8 A typical person moved backward. The patient exhibits an equilibrium response. Note the dorsiflexion of the ankles and toes; the arms move forward, as well as the head. (From Bobath B: *Adult hemiplegia: evaluation and treatment,* ed 3, Boston, 1990, Butterworth-Heinemann.)

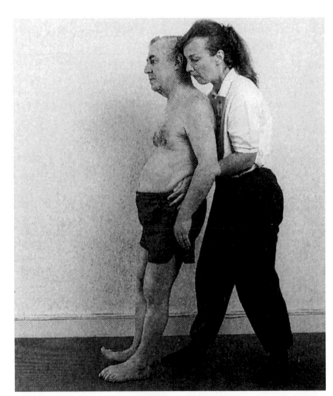

Fig. 11.9 Moving a patient backward. Note the active dorsiflexion of the uninvolved right foot (normal balance reaction) and its absence in the affected foot. (From Bobath B: *Adult hemiplegia: evaluation and treatment,* ed 3, Boston, 1990, Butterworth-Heinemann.)

patients who have sustained strokes lack the ability to elicit these appropriate balance responses in standing secondary to muscle weakness and the inability to time muscle responses. This problem is illustrated in Fig. 11.9. The patient's ability to perform these strategies (ankle, hip, stepping) should be noted, especially if the patient is working on ambulation skills.

Standing Progression (Walking): Position of the Therapist in Relation to the Patient

Once the patient is able to maintain an upright position and accept weight on the lower extremities, it is time to progress the patient to stepping. Because walking is the primary goal for many of our patients and it is the treatment intervention in which patients most wish to participate, walking should be practiced and encouraged during therapy. Although 80% to 90% of patients progress to independent ambulation after their stroke, approximately 80% present with gait defects including decreased gait speed and efficiency and postural instability and asymmetry (Hornby et al., 2011). Practice guidelines related to gait training have changed. Therapists used to think that patients needed to possess adequate trunk and lower extremity control for ambulation. However, with the research available regarding task-specific training and body-weight support treadmill ambulation, therapists are now initiating gait training activities with patients who possess limited balance and lower extremity motor control.

The clinician can position herself in several different places during standing activities with a patient. One can sit or stand in front of the patient and can control the patient at the hips. Standing on the patient's hemiplegic side is also an option. This method of guarding can be of benefit if the patient requires tactile cues at the pelvis or posterior hip area, or if the patient is demonstrating improved control of the involved lower extremity and requires only tactile cueing distally. In patients with pusher syndrome, standing on the patient's involved side can promote excessive weight shifting to that extremity and should be avoided; the clinician should position herself on the patient's uninvolved side in an effort to increase weight-bearing to that side.

Advancing the uninvolved lower extremity. Initially, patients should be taught to step forward with the uninvolved lower extremity, as shown in Intervention 11.33. The advantage to this sequence is that it requires the patient to bear weight exclusively on the involved leg, thus promoting single-limb support (weight-bearing). Many patients take a small step with the uninvolved leg or simply slide the foot forward along the floor in an effort to make this task easier. Both instances decrease the amount of time spent in unilateral limb support on the involved lower extremity. Although patients are able to ambulate in such fashion, the continuance of this pattern can lead to the development of postural deviations and increased lower extremity tone. To achieve a more normal gait pattern, the patient must be able to maintain single-limb support on the involved side during stance to allow the

INTERVENTION 11.33   Pregait Activities

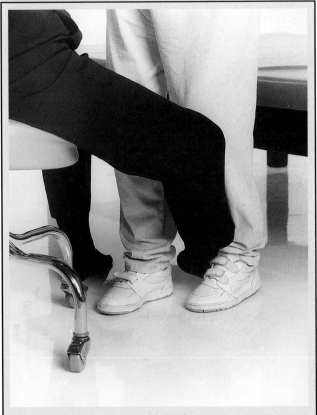

In standing, the patient initially steps forward with the uninvolved lower extremity. This facilitates single limb weight-bearing on the involved leg as the patient steps. The clinician blocks the patient's involved lower extremity as needed to prevent knee buckling.

other leg to take a normal-sized step. Single-limb support is also required for other functional activities, such as negotiation of curbs and stairs.

Advancing the involved lower extremity. Often, a portion of the patient's treatment session is devoted to practicing forward stepping. Once the patient is able to advance the uninvolved leg forward and to maintain weight on it, the patient is progressed to advancing the involved lower extremity. Patients often have difficulty in initiating hip flexion for lower extremity advancement. As previously stated, the extension synergy pattern is frequently present in the involved lower extremity and becomes evident as the patient tries to take a step forward. Instead of using hip flexion to advance the leg forward, the patient uses hip circumduction (hip abduction with internal rotation). Pelvic retraction frequently accompanies this movement pattern. Knee extension and ankle plantar flexion, also part of the extension synergy, can be evident. Consequently, as the patient moves the involved leg forward, the extremity advances as an extended unit. This extension limits the patient's ability to initiate knee flexion, which is needed for the swing phase of the gait cycle, and ankle dorsiflexion, which is necessary for heel strike. Strong

extension in the lower extremity results in decreased weight-bearing on the involved lower extremity during stance. Because of the presence of abnormal tone and the strong desire of many patients to walk, we frequently see patients who ambulate in this fashion. Patients should be discouraged from walking like this if at all possible. Continued substitution of hip circumduction for true hip flexion can cause the patient to relearn an abnormal and inefficient movement pattern. Concomitantly, abnormal stresses are placed on the involved joints, and it becomes increasingly difficult to change or replace the abnormal pattern with a more normal one. Ambulation performed in this way also reinforces the patient's lower extremity spasticity.

Positioning the pelvis. To assist the patient in initiating hip flexion, the following techniques can be employed. Before providing any tactile cues, the PT/PTA must determine the position of the patient's pelvis. The clinician should note the relative position of the patient's pelvis in terms of pelvic tilt and observe whether the pelvis is in a retracted position. If the patient's pelvis is retracted or in an elevated or hiked position, provide a downward and slightly forward tactile cue on the patient's pelvis to restore proper pelvic alignment. It may also be necessary to apply a tactile cue on the patient's posterior buttocks to assist the pelvis into a more neutral pelvic tilt. Often, the patient can be asked to flex (bend) the involved knee to assist in bringing the pelvis to a better position.

Advancing the involved lower extremity forward. Once the pelvis is in proper alignment, the patient is asked to slide the involved foot forward. If the patient is unable to initiate this movement, the therapist may need to help the patient manually. This technique is demonstrated in Intervention 11.34. Sliding the foot forward is easier than having the patient attempt to lift the involved limb off the floor to advance it. Increased effort and possible patient frustration can increase abnormal tone. At times, it may be difficult to slide the involved foot forward because of the friction created between the patient's shoe and the floor. Patients can be requested to take their shoes off, or a pillowcase or small towel can be placed under the patient's foot to make it easier to advance. A piece of stockinet can also be placed on the toe of the patient's shoe to reduce friction. The patient should practice bringing the foot forward and backward several times. One can make this activity easier for the patient by physically moving the towel or pillowcase for the patient. Again, tactile cues applied at the posterior or lateral hip and pelvis are beneficial. Maintaining the involved knee in slight flexion decreases the likelihood that the patient will initiate lower extremity advancement with hip hiking or circumduction.

Backward stepping. Stepping backward should also be practiced. When asking the patient to step backward, the therapist should note the position of the patient's hip and pelvis. Often, the patient performs hip extension with hiking and retraction. The patient should be encouraged to advance the lower extremity backward followed by hip extension.

Putting it all together. Once the patient is able to move the involved leg forward and back with fairly good success, the

INTERVENTION 11.34   **Advancing the Involved Leg Forward**

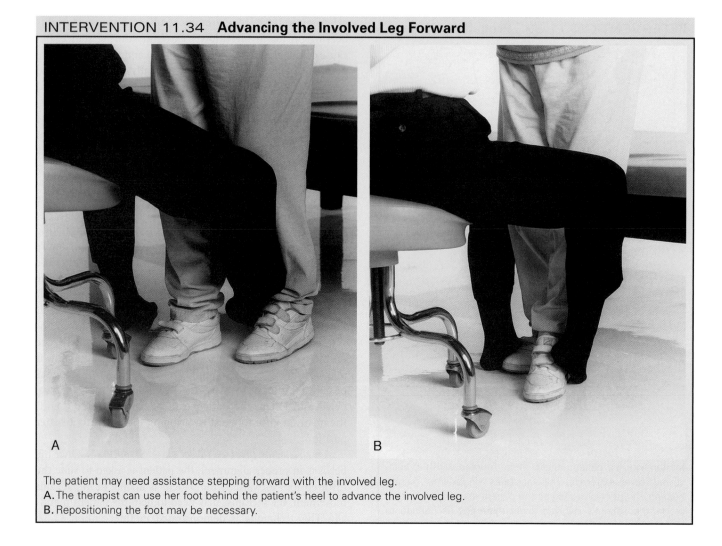

The patient may need assistance stepping forward with the involved leg.
A. The therapist can use her foot behind the patient's heel to advance the involved leg.
B. Repositioning the foot may be necessary.

patient is progressed to putting several steps together. The patient is instructed to step forward first with the uninvolved lower extremity in preparation for toe-off and the swing phase of the gait cycle. Overground locomotor training can begin once the patient is able to take several steps with both lower extremities. Intervention 11.35 illustrates a patient who is ambulating several steps. Table 11.8 provides a review of the normal gait training progression.

Normal components of gait. When assessing the patient's movements during the initial stages of ambulation training, the clinician should note the following movement components: (1) diagonal weight shift to the uninvolved side should occur during advancement of the involved lower extremity; (2) accompanied by this shift is trunk elongation; and (3) the patient needs to flex the involved knee and advance the hip forward. Many patients have a difficult time with this specific movement combination. The ability to flex the knee with the hip in a relatively neutral or extended position, coupled with adequate ankle dorsiflexion to prevent toe drag, is extremely difficult. If one thinks in terms of the stages of recovery, to walk with a normal gait pattern requires that the patient combine different components of various synergy patterns.

Patients who lack the ability to flex the knee and to dorsiflex the foot for swing tend to exaggerate the weight shift to the uninvolved side in an effort to shorten the extremity so that the foot can clear the floor. It may be necessary for the clinician to assist the patient with lower extremity advancement. A towel placed under the patient's foot or manual cues applied to the posterior thigh can be used to advance the extremity forward. The PT/PTA may also need to guide the patient's weight shifts during this time. As stated previously, many patients are unable to gauge the degree of movement during early weight shifting activities appropriately. The patient may need tactile cues at the hip or trunk to promote the proper postural response.

Turning around. While practicing putting several steps together to walk forward, the patient should also learn to turn around. Turning toward the involved side is usually easier. Instead of having the patient think about picking up the involved foot and taking a step, ask the patient to move the involved heel toward the midline. When the patient moves the heel inward, the toes are automatically moved outward and are ready for the directional change. From this position, the patient can easily step with the uninvolved lower extremity. It may be necessary for the patient to repeat this sequence

INTERVENTION 11.35 Assisting Ambulation

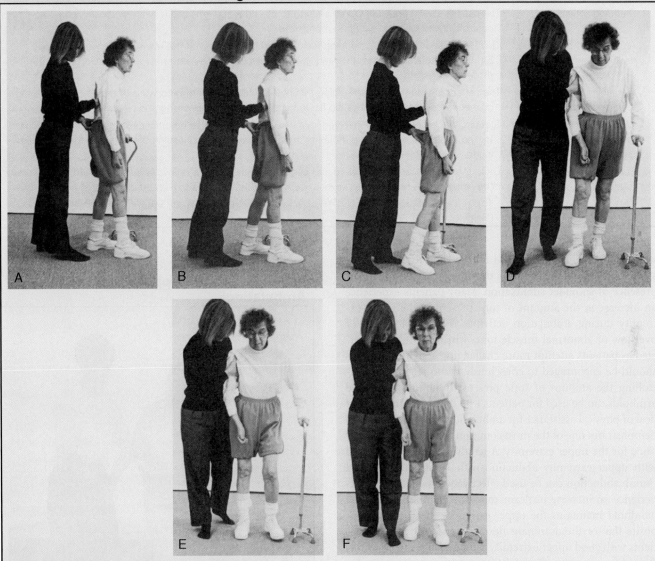

A. The clinician uses an axillary grip with her right arm and lifts the patient's upper trunk up and back. The patient was previously trained to use a quad cane. As the patient gains control, a straight cane can be introduced.

B. The clinician uses her left hand to assist the patient to initiate the movements from her legs in right step stance. It is important to teach the patient how to shift weight over both legs without excessive leaning onto the quad cane.

C. As the patient practices the same movements in left step stance, she cannot keep her right heel on the floor because of overshifting to the cane, insufficient hip extension range and control, or insufficient ankle dorsiflexion range. Forward and backward weight shifting movements are practiced repeatedly in the right and left step stance positions.

D. The clinician's right hand uses an axillary grip to support the upper trunk while her left hand is on the posterolateral side of the patient's left rib cage.

E. The clinician reminds the patient to keep her upper trunk extended as she shifts her trunk and hip forward. Note how the clinician's feet step in parallel with the patient's.

F. The clinician must be careful to time her corrections and assistance to the patient's movement initiation patterns.

(From Ryerson S, Levit K: *Functional movement reeducation: a contemporary model for stroke rehabilitation,* New York, 1997, Churchill Livingstone.)

several times to complete the turn. The clinician must carefully observe the patient's performance of this activity. Frequently, the patient attempts to turn by twisting the lower extremity, a movement that can result in injury to the knee and ankle if not prohibited.

Upper extremity positioning during ambulation. Care must always be given to the position of the patient's upper extremity during gait training activities. The involved arm can be prepositioned on the clinician's upper extremity, on a bedside table, in the patient's pocket, or in an appropriate

TABLE 11.8 Ambulation Progression

1. Standing activities	The patient should practice weight shifting to the right and left, and forward and backward. Knee control activities should also be emphasized.
2. Advancing the uninvolved lower extremity	The patient should practice stepping forward and backward with the uninvolved lower extremity. Emphasis should be on weight-bearing on the involved lower extremity and achievement of the proper step length.
3. Advancing the involved lower extremity	The patient should practice advancing the involved lower extremity forward. A tactile cue at the hip may be necessary to promote hip flexion and to decrease hip hiking and circumduction.
4. Stepping back with the involved lower extremity	Stepping backward with the involved lower extremity must also be practiced. The tendency again is for the patient to hike the hip. Patients must concentrate on releasing the extensor tone and allowing for hip and knee flexion.
5. Putting several steps together	Once the patient can step forward and backward with both the uninvolved and involved extremities, the patient must begin to put several steps together. Emphasis must be placed on advancing the involved lower extremity during swing and appropriate diagonal weight shifts during the stance phase of the gait cycle.

sling. The patient's arm should not be allowed to hang unsupported with gravity pulling down on it, especially in the presence of shoulder subluxation. Many patients experience an increase in the amount of tone present in the upper extremity during ambulation activities. This is the result of overflow of abnormal muscle tone, which is often exaggerated as patients attempt more challenging activities. Patients should be encouraged to consciously try to relax, thus controlling the amount of tone present. Inhibiting hand and armholds can be used for patients who do not require a great deal of physical assistance for ambulation. Intervention 11.36 demonstrates one of the most common tone-inhibiting positions for the upper extremity. A handshake grasp combined with upper extremity abduction with wrist extension and thumb abduction can be used effectively in patients who experience an increase in flexor tone during ambulation. The handhold maintains the upper extremity in a position opposite that of the dominant flexor synergy pattern. For patients with good upper extremity motor return, interventions should focus on the return of reciprocal arm swing.

Observational gait analysis. As previously mentioned, several common gait deviations are seen in patients with hemiplegia. For the purposes of our discussion here, possible gait deviations that may develop are addressed by each individual joint and are summarized in Table 11.9.

Ambulation/Locomotor Training

Selection of an Assistive Device

For the patient who needs additional postural and balance support, an assistive device may be appropriate to consider. This decision should be based on the patient's impairments including cognitive abilities and should be discussed with the patient and the patient's family (if appropriate). Individual differences and preferences do exist regarding which assistive device may be best for the patient.

Generally, walkers are not appropriate for patients who have sustained a stroke because patients frequently lack the hand and upper extremity function needed to use the walker safely and effectively. If the patient does possess functional use of the involved hand, a rolling walker may be prescribed for patients who require more support.

INTERVENTION 11.36 Inhibiting the Patient's Involved Upper Extremity While Ambulating

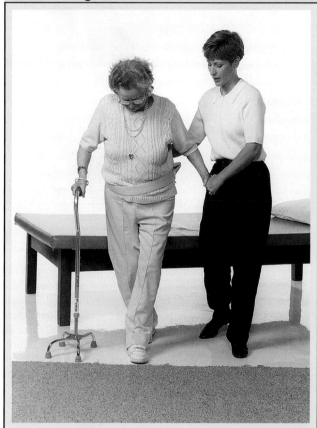

Ambulating the patient while inhibiting increased tone in the involved upper extremity. Shoulder abduction and external rotation combined with elbow extension and wrist and finger extension are desired.

Clinicians may also recommend some type of cane for the patient that requires less balance support. Hemiwalkers (walk-canes), wide-base and narrow-base quad canes, and straight (single-point) canes are the most popular assistive devices. The wider the base of the cane, the more support it

TABLE 11.9 Common Gait Deviations Seen in Patients With Stroke

Deviation	Possible Causes
Hip	
Retraction	Increased lower extremity muscle tone
Hiking	Inadequate hip and knee flexion, increased tone in the trunk and lower extremity
Circumduction	Increased extensor tone, inadequate hip and knee flexion, increased plantar flexion in the ankle or foot drop
Inadequate hip flexion	Increased extensor tone, flaccid lower extremity
Knee	
Decreased knee flexion during swing	Increased lower extremity extensor tone, weak hip flexion
Excessive flexion during stance	Weakness or flaccidity in the lower extremity, increased flexor tone in the lower extremity, weak ankle plantar flexors
Hyperextension during stance	Hip retraction, increased extensor tone in the lower extremity, weakness in the gluteus maximus, hamstrings, or quadriceps
Instability during stance	Increased lower extremity flexor tone, flaccidity
Ankle	
Foot drop	Increased extensor tone, flaccidity
Ankle inversion or eversion	Increased tone in specific muscle groups, flaccidity
Toe clawing	Increased flexor tone in the toe muscles

offers. Unfortunately, some of the wider-base canes are not as functional in the patient's home. For example, if a person lives in a small home or trailer, a hemiwalker may be difficult to maneuver in areas with limited space. In addition, hemiwalkers cannot be used on stairs. Wide-base quad canes are a little smaller than hemiwalkers, but they are still not as easy to use on steps because they often need to be turned sideways to fit onto a step. Narrow-base quad canes and straight (single-point) canes usually offer the most flexibility in the patient's home and can be easily used in the community.

Some PTs will suggest starting the patient with a more stable cane that provides greater support, and then decreasing the support as the patient progresses. That is certainly an option, but one must recognize that once a patient has trained with a device, it is often difficult to advance the patient to the next, less stable one because of the patient's fear of falling and overreliance on the initial device. Many clinicians therefore challenge the patient early on by providing less support initially and transitioning to a different device if the patient requires additional support. Canes should be of adequate height to allow the patient's elbow to bend approximately 20 to 30 degrees when the patient has her hand on the handgrip. It is important to know whether a patient is going to purchase an assistive device for home use because a physician's order is necessary for reimbursement.

Any equipment that may be needed for the patient at home should be ordered so that it can be delivered and properly adjusted before the patient leaves the rehabilitation facility. This can create a challenge for the PT and PTA because it is sometimes difficult to know how much a patient will progress and what the long-term needs might be.

Ambulation Training With Assistive Devices

Instructional demonstration of proper cane usage should occur prior to introduction of the device. Patients will sometimes experience difficulties learning the correct gait sequence once the assistive device is introduced. The patient needs to be able to maintain a stable postural base at the pelvis and trunk to initiate more distal movement. Frequently, a patient masters a more general skill, such as standing and weight shifting, but when asked to move from that position or a greater challenge is applied, the patient regresses and seems to lose the basic postural components.

If the patient is having difficulty with standing or gait activities or if the clinician finds it difficult to control the patient, other types of assistive devices can be used. At times, having the patient stand with an object in front of her can be helpful. For example, some clinicians use a bedside table placed on the side of the patient to allow the patient to bear weight on the upper extremity during ambulation training. This technique can be beneficial if the patient requires more external trunk control or support or if she needs proper positioning of the involved upper extremity. Grocery carts and ARJO walkers offer the same benefits. The patient can position her upper extremities on the handle of the cart or walker and then push it. The therapist can stand behind the patient and offer tactile cues and feedback to assist with lower extremity advancement and single-limb support. For some patients, ambulation training may be best practiced in the parallel bars, at a hemirail, or on a treadmill with body-weight support. All of these pieces of therapeutic equipment provide the patient with upper extremity support. Frequently, decisions related to what equipment should be utilized to assist the patient with gait are determined by what is available in the rehabilitation department or clinic. Progressing the patient to overground ambulation with the most appropriate assistive device to allow functional, independent gait remains the goal of our interventions.

Ambulation progression with a cane. The proper progression when using an assistive device for ambulation is as follows: (1) the patient advances the uninvolved lower extremity first; (2) then advancement of the cane with the uninvolved hand; and finally (3) the involved lower extremity moves forward. Manual assistance at the hip or posterior knee may be necessary to help the patient advance the involved lower extremity. The clinician can also advance the patient's involved lower extremity with her own leg. The patient must be instructed to limit how far forward she advances the cane. On average, a distance of 18 inches in front of the lower extremities is adequate. The patient may need assistance with the diagonal weight shift to allow for the swing phase of the gait cycle. The patient is encouraged to maintain proper postural alignment during ambulation by actively contracting the trunk extensors and the abdominals.

As discussed previously, care must be exercised with the placement of the involved upper extremity during ambulation activities. A permanent sling or a temporary one made from an elastic band, placement of the patient's hand in a pocket, the use of a bedside table, or tactile support provided by the therapist can support the patient's arm during upright activities.

The patient may have more difficulty with ambulation activities once the assistive device is introduced. This is not uncommon because the cane offers more of a challenge for the patient. Weight shifting during the stance phase of the gait cycle and maintaining the correct sequence with the device can be difficult. The ambulation progression with the cane is identical to the one the patient used when beginning ambulation activities from the mat or in the parallel bars. With repetition, the patient's abilities in this area should improve.

Cane use and asymmetry. A common concern expressed by therapists after issuing a cane to a patient is the tendency toward body asymmetry, which the cane promotes. Having the cane in the patient's uninvolved hand promotes weight-bearing on that side and often makes it difficult for the patient to shift weight toward and adequately elongate the trunk on the hemiparetic side. Inadequate weight shifting, coupled with the patient's asymmetric performance of a sit-to-stand transition, will accentuate previously discussed problems with equal weight-bearing on lower extremities. This point is illustrated in Fig. 11.10. The goal should be the achievement of symmetry and bilateral weight-bearing on both lower extremities during all upright movement transitions.

Ambulation Outcomes

An individual's ability to ambulate is a primary factor used in the determination of the appropriate discharge destination and determines whether a patient can return to social and vocational function (Hornby et al., 2011). Additionally, walking speed can be used to predict the level of disability.

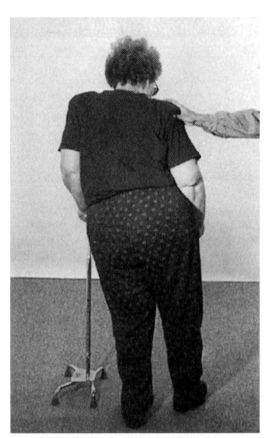

Fig. 11.10 Use of the quad cane during ambulation contributes to asymmetry in the trunk and poor weight shift to the hemiplegic side. The clinician's hand is guarding the patient. (From Ryerson S, Levit K: *Functional movement reeducation: a contemporary model for stroke rehabilitation*, New York, 1997, Churchill Livingstone.)

A walking speed of 0.8 m/sec or greater allows an individual to ambulate in the community, whereas a speed of less than 0.4 m/sec will limit a person to ambulation in the home (Duncan et al., 2011; Schmid et al., 2007).

It is important for the PT to discuss the benefits of ambulation/locomotor training with the patient, as we know repetition and practice are essential for motor learning and neuroplasticity. Current evidence suggests that the average number of steps performed during a typical physical therapy treatment session is approximately 300 to 800, whereas it is also recognized that thousands of steps are needed to induce neuroplasticity. Additionally, data suggest that early gait-training programs foster improvements in both walking and nonwalking tasks (Hornby et al., 2011). The primary PT must determine what type of interventions and at what intensities these tasks should be performed to provide the patient with the most functional outcomes possible.

Walking on Different Surfaces

The patient should practice overground ambulation on standard flooring. This activity is most often accomplished in the physical therapy gym or a treadmill. The patient should, however, quickly progress to ambulating on carpeting and other types of floor coverings because these are much more prevalent in home environments. Once the patient has fair dynamic balance during gait and can advance the involved leg forward, the patient should begin ambulation outside on different types of terrain. Walking on sidewalks, grass, and gravel is beneficial to the patient as the patient begins reentry into the community. Eventually, the patient will need to be able to walk in a crowded mall or to walk while negotiating environmental barriers.

Pusher Syndrome

As described earlier in this chapter, some patients may exhibit pusher syndrome. The previously described treatment interventions are appropriate for patients with this condition. Specific activities that should be practiced include weight-bearing on the involved lower extremity, provision of appropriate tactile and proprioceptive input, midline retraining in both sitting and standing positions with the use of visual cues or a visual aid such as the therapist's arm positioned in a vertical position, and the incorporation of the hands during activity performance (Karnath and Broetz, 2003). The use of fixed resistance on the patient's uninvolved side, such as that given by the clinician's body or a table, can provide the patient with the sensory feedback needed to allow him or her to correct alignment and to relearn appropriate movement strategies (Davies, 1985). During gait-training activities, the therapist can lower the height of the assistive device to encourage weight-bearing on the uninvolved side.

Orthoses

The patient may reach a plateau at any stage and may be left with a variety of motor capabilities. Recovery usually begins proximally and then progresses more distally. Thus for many patients, the hand and the ankle do not regain normal function. Decreased or absent ankle dorsiflexion or increased tone in the plantar flexors can make ambulation activities difficult for the patient. Gait deviations emerge as the patient attempts to clear the foot and prevent the toes from dragging. If the patient is not able to activate the anterior tibialis for heel strike and to maintain the foot in relative dorsiflexion for the swing phase of the gait cycle, some type of orthosis may be needed to clear the foot.

PTs have varying views on the use of orthoses. Some PTs recommend orthoses for all patients, others may be more selective, and still others may not want to recommend orthoses at all, owing to concerns regarding the inability to strengthen weak muscles in a locked brace. One of the simplest ways to assess whether the patient may benefit from some type of orthosis is to ace wrap the foot in dorsiflexion and eversion. The clinician applies the ace wrap over the patient's shoe. This provides support to the foot and a more neutral ankle position on which to practice ambulation.

Various types of custom-made orthoses, shoe inserts, and wedges are available. What is important to remember, however, is that orthoses can be beneficial pieces of adaptive equipment for our patients. A discussion with the patient regarding ambulation goals and potential benefits of orthotic prescription is helpful. If the opportunity exists for the patient to try a training orthosis in the clinic, it is advisable to do so. Information obtained can help inform decisions regarding the best orthotic option for the patient.

Prefabricated ankle-foot orthoses. For the patient who has sustained a stroke, the ankle-foot orthosis (AFO) is the orthosis or brace most frequently prescribed. Patients may begin early ambulation tasks with a plastic prefabricated orthosis found in the clinic or physical therapy gym. These plastic training orthoses are relatively inexpensive and serve to maintain the patient's ankle and foot in a neutral or slightly dorsiflexed position to prevent ankle plantar flexion during initial stance and toe clearance during the swing phase of the gait cycle. Prefabricated AFOs normally come in small, medium, large, and extra-large sizes, and are made for either the right or left lower extremity. The patient dons the orthosis, and then the shoe is applied. The positioning of the patient's foot in the orthosis allows the patient to ambulate without dragging the toes and allows the patient to have some degree of heel strike. However, movement of the tibia over the fixed foot is difficult and may affect the patient's ability to perform a sit-to-stand transfer. A new prefabricated orthosis, the OTS carbon fiber AFO, is available and some provide more of a custom fit (Fig. 11.11). Those with ground-reaction design have been found to assist with knee stability (Hou et al., 2019). AFOs are excellent training tools for patients and use of the orthosis during treatment provides potential information regarding how the patient might ambulate if there were improved control of the ankle.

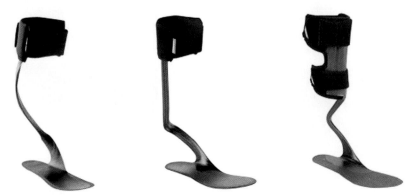

Fig. 11.11 Allard ToeOff OTS carbon ankle-foot orthosis. (From Webster JB, Murphy DP: *Atlas of orthoses and assistive devices,* ed 5, Philadelphia, 2019, Elsevier.)

Posterior leaf splints. A posterior leaf splint is a plastic orthosis that controls ankle movement by limiting dorsiflexion and plantar flexion. During the stance phase of the gait cycle, the posterior portion of the orthosis becomes slightly bent. As the patient advances the lower limb forward, the orthosis recoils and helps lift the foot to prevent foot drop. Fig. 11.12 provides an example of a posterior leaf splint.

Checking for skin irritation. Because some AFOs are prefabricated, they do not fit the unique bony and soft-tissue structures of each patient's lower extremity. Thus areas of redness may develop, and the potential for pressure areas must be considered. This problem can be compounded by a patient's decreased or absent sensation. It is recommended that when a patient first starts to use an orthosis or brace, wearing times should be limited. Initially, a patient may wear the orthosis for 10 to 15 minutes or for one walk with the clinician. The PT/PTA should then remove the orthosis and check the patient's skin for any areas of redness. As the patient begins to accommodate and tolerate the orthosis, wearing times can be increased. Patients should be instructed to visually inspect their feet frequently. Skin checks are extremely important for patients with decreased sensation secondary to their stroke or who exhibit complications of diabetes or impaired circulation to prevent the development of pressure ulcers. If the patient is unable to remove the orthosis independently, a caregiver should be instructed to assist.

Customized ankle-foot orthoses. In addition to prefabricated plastic AFOs, custom-fabricated solid AFOs are also available. These types of orthoses must be made by an orthotist. An orthotist is a health care provider who specializes in the design, fabrication, and patient fitting of orthoses and braces. The orthotist frequently makes a cast of the patient's foot, and then fabricates the orthosis from this model. The orthosis is often set in a neutral or slightly dorsiflexed position (Fig. 11.13). Custom-fabricated orthoses usually fit patients well; however, several problems exist. One disadvantage to this type of orthosis is the cost. Custom-fabricated orthoses are expensive. In some situations, the cost may be prohibitive. In addition, depending on the patient's stage in the recovery process, an orthosis ordered for a patient today may not be what the patient will need at discharge or in 6 months. Therapists often wait to order a custom-made orthosis until later in the patient's rehabilitation stay or when the patient begins outpatient services to ensure that the most appropriate device is fabricated. This is becoming more of a challenge, however, as lengths of stay in rehabilitation are becoming shorter.

Articulated ankle-foot orthoses. Other types of custom-made orthoses exist. Orthoses with articulated ankle joints may also be prescribed for the patient. These types of orthoses offer the clinician and the orthotist the opportunity to vary the degree of ankle joint motion available to the individual patient. The orthosis can be locked in a position of slight dorsiflexion for the patient who has difficulty initiating heel strike. An orthosis positioned in dorsiflexion assists the patient who has a tendency to hyperextend the knee. The dorsiflexed position of the ankle causes the knee to move into slight flexion. Articulated orthoses offer the clinician flexibility in choosing the position of the ankle. Fig. 11.14 depicts an articulated AFO.

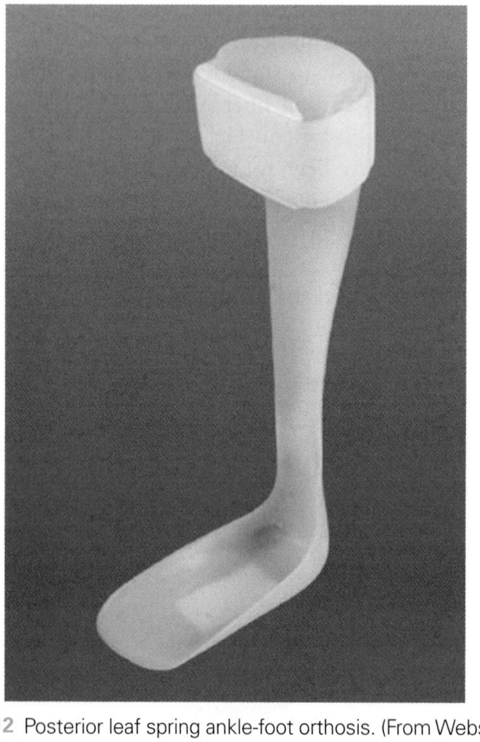

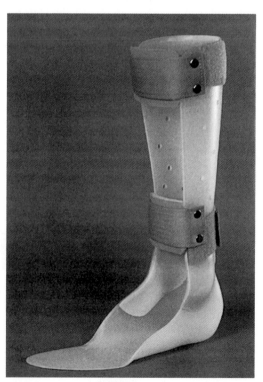

Fig. 11.12 Posterior leaf spring ankle-foot orthosis. (From Webster JB, Murphy DP: *Atlas of orthoses and assistive devices*, ed 5, Philadelphia, 2019, Elsevier.)

Fig. 11.13 The rigid polypropylene ankle-foot orthosis is capable of providing tibial control in stance. (From Nawoczenski DA, Epler ME: *Orthotics in functional rehabilitation of lower limb*, Philadelphia, 1997, WB Saunders.)

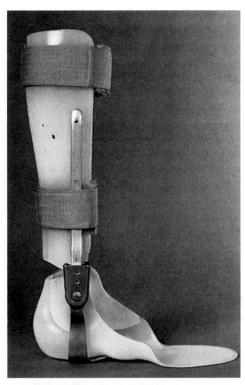

Fig. 11.14 A rigid polypropylene ankle-foot orthosis shell can be modified to incorporate a double-adjustable ankle joint for improved versatility in patient management. (From Nawoczenski DA, Epler ME: *Orthotics in functional rehabilitation of lower limb*, Philadelphia, 1997, WB Saunders.)

As stated previously, the ankle can be locked; however, most clinicians will adjust the orthosis individually to meet the patient's needs. If the patient has weak or absent dorsiflexors, a posterior stop can be used to limit the patient's ability to plantar flex. Alternatively, an anterior stop may be used if the patient has marked weakness in the plantar flexors or if the anterior tibialis is hyperactive.

Articulated orthoses have several advantages. For example, the orthosis can be adjusted and changed at various times during the patient's recovery, especially during the first 6 months when recovery is greatest. Initially, when the involved ankle is weak, the ankle joint can be locked to provide greater stability. As the patient progresses and can initiate more active movement, the ankle joint can be adjusted to allow the patient greater opportunity to initiate as much dorsiflexion as possible. The orthosis can, however, be adjusted to limit plantar flexion. This type of positioning encourages the patient's active attempts at dorsiflexion for heel strike, but also provides passive positioning when the patient is fatigued. If a patient is placed in an orthosis that does not allow active movement, the patient may lose the ability to strengthen weak muscle groups.

The reader is advised to work with the orthotist on their team to identify the most appropriate bracing options for their patients. The design and the materials used in fabrication of the brace can assist in controlling increased tone, muscle weakness, and contractures that may be present.

Knee-ankle-foot orthoses. Clinicians have long had reservations regarding prescribing knee-ankle-foot orthoses (KAFOs) for their patients with stroke. The main reasons for this have been the need to maintain the knee in a locked position during gait, and the increased energy demands that ambulation with KAFOs entails (Hou et al., 2019). Improvements in orthotic design have resulted in newer KAFOs that provide stability during stance but allow for knee flexion during swing. The braces can be prescribed early in the patient's rehabilitation to provide improved postural alignment and weight-bearing on the involved lower extremity. These braces can be modified to AFOs as the patient recovers and gains increased control of lower extremity musculature (Hou et al., 2019). Fig. 11.15 shows a stance control KAFO.

Electrical stimulation as an orthotic. Electrical stimulation applied to the common peroneal nerve and anterior tibialis muscle can serve as an effective orthosis for some patients. Commercially available electrical stimulation units (WalkAide by Innovative Neurotronics, ACP Accelerated Care Products, Reno, NV and L300 by Bioness, Valencia, CA) are available and may be recommended for those patients who lack active dorsiflexion during the swing phase of the gait cycle (Hou et al., 2019; Teasell and Hussein, 2016b). A patient wears a small electrical stimulation unit on the upper calf and a heel switch is placed in the shoe. As the patient lifts the lower extremity for swing, stimulation is applied producing dorsiflexion of the ankle. When the heel comes in contact with the ground, the stimulation is terminated (Senelick, 2011). Therefore the devices do not provide any assistance

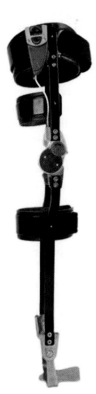

Fig. 11.15 Fillauer SP2 stance control knee-ankle-foot orthosis. (From Webster JB, Murphy DP: *Atlas of orthoses and assistive devices,* ed 5, Philadelphia, 2019, Elsevier.)

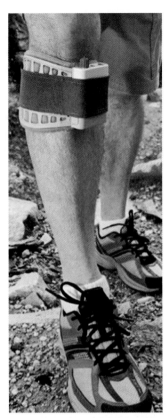

Fig. 11.16 Walk-Aide (Innovative Neurotronics, Reno, NV), a peroneal nerve stimulator cuff with an integrated tilt sensor worn below the knee. (From Webster JB, Murphy DP: *Atlas of orthoses and assistive devices,* ed 5, Philadelphia, 2019, Elsevier.)

with gait deviations during the stance phase of the gait cycle (Hou et al., 2019). Fig. 11.16 illustrates a patient using an electrical stimulation unit to promote ankle dorsiflexion.

Research suggests that use of an AFO after a stroke can provide a number of benefits including improvements in biomechanics, balance, speed, and cadence. Further studies are needed to identify the most appropriate types of orthoses and to better characterize the biomechanics of gait in individuals who have experienced a stroke (Hou et al., 2019).

The Developmental Sequence

Performance of postures and movement transitions that make up the developmental sequence may be included in the plan of care. Having the patient practice transitional movements between postures is not only therapeutic but also functional. Moving from a prone on elbows to a four-point (quadruped) position, from quadruped to tall-kneeling, from tall-kneeling to half-kneeling, and from half-kneeling to standing are used in many ADLs. Practicing these movement transitions independently or with assistance depends on the patient's motor control, balance, cardiopulmonary function, and goals. Because adults do not perform all the postures within the sequence on a daily basis, it is not necessary for every patient to practice all components of the developmental sequence.

Kneeling and half-kneeling positions are, however, important for patients to practice in the clinic. They are the transition positions that patients need to perform if they fall and must get up from the floor. Often, anxiety and apprehension result after a fall at home. By practicing transfers to and from the floor, the patient and family should feel comfortable with the steps necessary should a fall occur once the patient is discharged from the health care facility.

> **CAUTION** The patient must be carefully monitored during the performance of the developmental sequence. During the more difficult and challenging positions, the patient must be observed for signs of fatigue or cardiac compromise. Shortness of breath, diaphoresis, and increased heart rate or blood pressure are signs that the activity may be too difficult for the patient. Thus the selection of some of the more challenging positions, such as the four-point, tall-kneeling, and half-kneeling positions, must be carefully considered.

Prone Activities

The prone position is an extremely difficult position for many older patients to achieve, especially in the presence of arthritic and cardiopulmonary changes. If the patient is able to tolerate the prone position, several activities can be practiced. In a completely prone position, the patient can work on knee flexion and hip extension with the knees bent. Many patients have difficulty in initiating antigravity knee flexion with the hip maintained in a neutral position secondary to decreased control of the hamstrings. The patient tends to flex the hips at the same time the knees are flexed. Hip extension with the knee bent requires that the patient be able to activate the gluteus maximus with minimal assistance from the hamstrings. Careful monitoring of the patient's performance is necessary because substitution is extremely common.

If the patient can tolerate it, prone on elbows is another excellent position for treatment because the patient bears weight through the elbows and into the shoulders. Use of the PNF techniques of alternating isometrics and rhythmic stabilization applied to the shoulders aids in developing proximal control. If the patient has difficulty in maintaining the hand in a relaxed position, a hand or short arm air splint can be applied to keep the wrist in a relatively neutral position with the fingers extended.

Transition From Prone on Elbows to Four-Point

The transition to a four-point or quadruped position from prone on elbows requires that the patient be able to maintain the involved upper extremity in extension and accept weight on it. Because the four-point position is more challenging, only those patients without medical complications and with moderately intact trunk control should attempt this position. It is often easy for the clinician to stand or kneel behind the patient holding on to the patient's waist. The therapist can then direct the patient's weight back toward the feet. As the patient does this, she should be instructed to straighten the arms. If the patient lacks the necessary control in the triceps to maintain adequate elbow extension, a long arm air splint can be used. As stated previously, it is desirable to have the patient bear weight on extended arms with the wrists and fingers extended and the thumb abducted. If the patient is unable to achieve this resting posture actively or passively, allow the patient's fingers to stay in a flexed position. The patient's fingers should not be pulled into extension because it may cause joint subluxation.

Four-point activities. Once in a quadruped position, the patient works on maintenance of the position. Forward, backward, medial, and lateral weight shifts are performed but should be practiced with control and should not be excessive. Alternating isometrics and rhythmic stabilization techniques can again be applied to the patient's shoulder or pelvic region, as depicted in Intervention 11.37, *A*. For the patient with advanced motor control, unilateral upper and lower extremity lifting and reaching exercises can be attempted, as shown in Intervention 11.37, *B*. The PT/PTA needs to monitor the patient's response carefully during performance of these activities. Exaggerated weight shifts to the involved or uninvolved sides may occur or collapse of the involved upper extremity may occur in the presence of triceps weakness.

Creeping. Creeping on hands and knees, better known to much of the lay population as crawling, may also be practiced during the patient's treatment sessions. Creeping provides the patient with the opportunity to practice reciprocal upper extremity and lower extremity activities while maintaining support on the opposite limbs. The patient should move one upper extremity, followed by the opposite lower extremity, then the contralateral upper extremity, followed by the remaining leg. Reciprocal movement of the extremities during creeping is closely related to the movement skills necessary for ambulation. Creeping is also a very good activity to practice in the clinic because patients often need to be able to move in this fashion when they fall at home. The patient can creep to a piece of furniture and transfer back to an upright position. To make creeping more difficult, resistance can be applied at the patient's pelvis or hips, as illustrated in Intervention 11.37, *C*.

Transition From Four-Point to Tall-Kneeling

From a four-point position, the patient can make the transition to tall-kneeling. The patient should shift weight posteriorly and then extend the trunk to assume the upright position. The therapist may need to provide the patient with assistance at the upper trunk (anterior shoulders) to achieve a complete upright position. Patients who have gluteal and trunk extensor weakness may push on their thighs in an effort to assist with knee extension. To achieve and maintain a tall-kneeling position, the patient must possess adequate balance and muscular control of the trunk. If the patient appears unstable in the tall-kneeling position, a small table or a roll can be placed in front of the patient to assist with balance. By providing additional trunk support through upper extremity weight-bearing, the patient may feel more secure, and balance may be improved.

Physical observations. The clinician must diligently observe the patient's position in tall kneeling. Patients often have difficulty in maintaining the pelvis in a neutral or

INTERVENTION 11.37   Activities in Four Point

A. Holding—alternating isometrics and rhythmic stabilization.
B. Upper extremity reaching.
C. Creeping—resisted.

slightly anterior position. As in sitting, the patient's hips should be in line with the shoulders. The patient should bear weight equally on both lower extremities. Frequently, patients have an excessive anterior pelvic tilt and truncal asymmetries. It may be necessary to begin with posture correction before advancing the patient to specific exercises in the tall-kneeling position.

Tall-Kneeling Activities

Alternating isometrics and rhythmic stabilization techniques can be applied at the patient's shoulder and pelvic girdles while the patient is in the tall-kneeling position. Intervention 11.38, *A* illustrates these techniques. These techniques assist in the development of proximal stability and can foster improvements in balance and coordination. Upper extremity PNF patterns can be performed, including the D$_1$ and D$_2$ diagonal patterns and lifts and chops, as demonstrated in Chapter 10. The benefit of performing the bilateral lifting and chopping patterns is that they incorporate a greater amount of trunk movement,

specifically flexion and rotation. Functional activities, such as gardening and house cleaning, can also be simulated in this position.

Another activity that can be performed in this position is tall-kneeling to heel sitting. In this exercise, the patient moves from a tall-kneeling position to one of sitting on the heels, as illustrated in Intervention 11.37, *C*. This exercise allows the patient to work on eccentric control of the quadriceps, a skill needed for many functional activities, including stand-to-sit transitions and stair negotiation. The patient can also perform forward and backward knee walking while in tall-kneeling. The clinician should observe the quality of the patient's lower extremity movement during knee walking. The lower extremity, specifically the

Intervention 11.38   Tall-Kneeling Activities

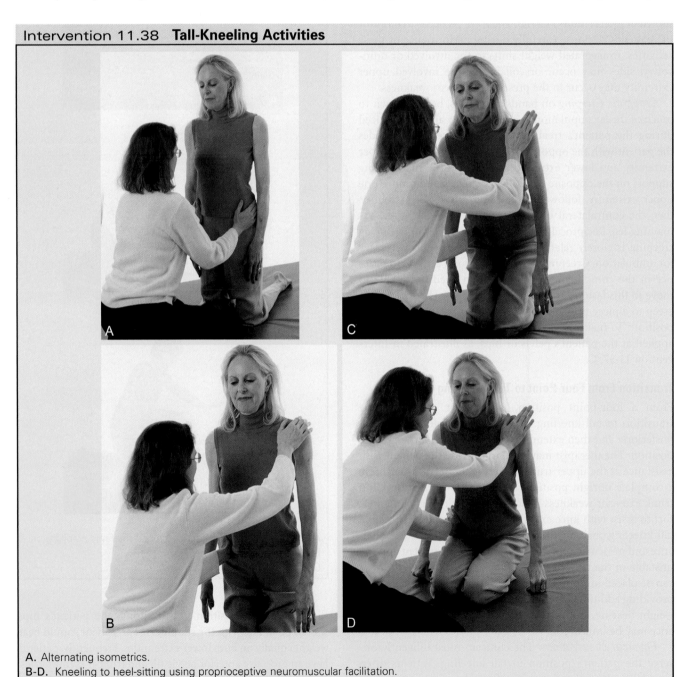

A. Alternating isometrics.
B-D. Kneeling to heel-sitting using proprioceptive neuromuscular facilitation.

hip, should advance in flexion. Hip hiking or circumduction should not be encouraged.

> **SPECIAL NOTE** During the patient's performance of all these developmental postures, the therapist must guard the patient appropriately. Because the patient's balance is challenged, it is possible that the patient may experience a loss of balance and fall.

Transition From Tall-Kneeling to Half-Kneeling

The transition from kneeling to half-kneeling is difficult for many patients. To initiate the transition, the patient must be able to perform a controlled weight shift to one side with elongation of the trunk on the weight-bearing side. The trunk on the side that will move forward to assume the half-kneeling, foot-flat position must shorten. Rotation of the trunk opposite of the weight shift must also occur. The hip on the moving side must hike and slightly abduct. The

moving knee must remain flexed as the patient brings the leg forward. The patient must also keep the foot in a neutral to slightly dorsiflexed position to clear the foot from the floor as the patient brings the leg forward. Adequate ankle range of motion is necessary to maintain the foot on the floor or mat with good contact. Often, patients need physical assistance advancing the lower extremity to assume this challenging position. Half-kneeling with the stronger, uninvolved leg forward is often easier for the patient to achieve initially.

Half-Kneeling Activities

The patient should work on maintaining a half-kneeling position. The patient may sway from side to side while attempting to maintain her center of gravity over the base of support. Asymmetric weight-bearing may also be observed. If the patient is having difficulty in maintaining the position, a Swiss ball can be placed under the hips, as shown in Intervention 11.39, *A*. Active control of hip extension can be practiced in the half-kneeling position. The patient can work on shifting the

---

INTERVENTION 11.39 Half-Kneeling Activities

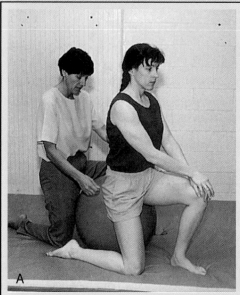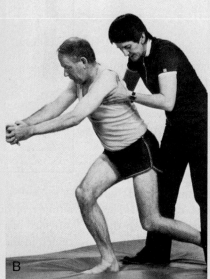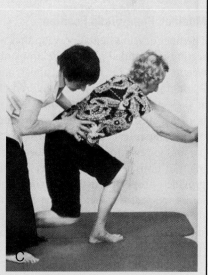

A. Half-kneeling on a Swiss ball: active-assistive movements. Standing up from half-kneeling.
  1. From sitting on a Swiss ball, the therapist assists the patient into half-kneeling.
  2. The therapist instructs the patient to put both hands on the knee flexed forward.
  3. Using manual contact on the pelvis, the therapist provides a diagonally forward and upward weight shift over the forward foot.
  4. Therapist and patient end in standing.
B. The therapist facilitates the transition from half-kneeling to standing (left hemiplegia).
  1. The therapist instructs the patient to clasp hands together while in half-kneeling.
  2. While standing, the therapist uses manual contacts on the axillae and provides a diagonally forward and upward weight shift.
  3. The patient comes to stand over the forward foot.
C. Facilitation of half-kneeling from standing using the pelvis (right hemiplegia).
  1. The therapist instructs the patient to clasp hands while standing.
  2. The therapist assists the patient to bring one leg behind the other in preparation for half-kneeling.
  3. The therapist uses manual contacts on the pelvis to lower the patient into a half-kneeling position.
  Note: Half-kneeling with the stronger, uninvolved leg forward is often easier for the patient to achieve. As the patient gains strength and motor control, half-kneeling with the involved leg forward may be used as a progression of the intervention.

(A, from O'Sullivan SB, Schmitz TJ: *Physical rehabilitation laboratory manual: focus on functional training*, Philadelphia, 1999, FA Davis; B and C, from Davies PM: *Steps to follow: a guide to the treatment of adult hemiplegia*, New York, 1985, Springer Verlag.)

weight forward and backward over the fixed front foot while reaching for an object. As with the other developmental positions previously described, once the patient is in half-kneeling, the PNF techniques of alternating isometrics and rhythmic stabilization can be applied to promote stability and balance control. Active upper extremity exercises and PNF chops and lifts can be performed in this position. Over time, the patient should practice half-kneeling with both the uninvolved and involved lower extremities forward. The transition to and from the position is also important to master. Once the patient is able to maintain the position independently and also able to move in and out of the position, the patient should progress to standing. Initially, the patient may need help from the therapist or from a piece of equipment/furniture or the wall, as depicted in Intervention 11.39, *B* and *C*. To complete the ascent to upright, the patient must be able to perform a forward weight shift over the fixed front foot. This prerequisite demands the necessary postural control and range of motion at the ankle. As the patient assumes more active control of the transition from half-kneeling to standing, the clinician should decrease her support and assistance. For the patient with greater motor control, this activity can be manually resisted with pressure applied to the patient's hips and pelvis.

Modified Plantigrade Position

The final developmental position that we will discuss in this section is modified plantigrade. In plantigrade, the patient is weight-bearing on both the upper and lower extremities. Plantigrade is a position that children often experiment with as they attempt upright standing. It is not, however, a position that most adults achieve with much regularity. It does offer therapeutic benefits to patients because it allows for upper and lower extremity weight-bearing in a modified standing position. Upper and lower extremity weight-bearing provides proprioceptive input into the shoulder and hip joints, respectively, and assists with tone reduction. The therapist may also want to approximate down through the shoulders or pelvis when the patient is in this position, to increase sensory awareness and motor recruitment.

In plantigrade, the patient can work on rocking forward, backward, and to the sides. These activities can be performed actively at first, and, with practice, the clinician can resist the exercise. Alternating isometrics can once again be used to promote stability. Intervention 11.40 illustrates this activity. Lower extremity progressions can be initiated when the patient is in this position, including forward and backward stepping. Knee control activities such as knee flexion, extension, and mini squats can also be practiced. The patient can also perform functional activities in this position, including self-care and homemaking activities.

MIDRECOVERY TO LATE RECOVERY

Depending on the patient's injury, recovery stage, age, and insurance status, the next phase of the patient's rehabilitation may be termed *midrecovery* to *late recovery*. The therapist's involvement with the patient at this stage can occur in a

INTERVENTION 11.40 Modified Plantigrade Activities

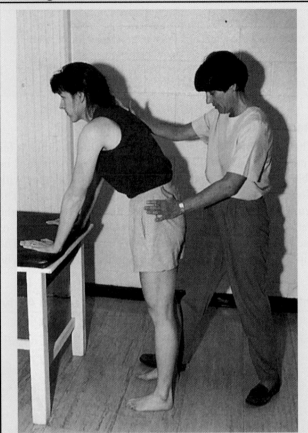

Modified plantigrade position: alternating isometrics. (From O'Sullivan SB, Schmitz TJ: *Physical rehabilitation laboratory manual: focus on functional training*, Philadelphia, 1999, FA Davis.)

number of different practice settings. The services may be provided in a skilled care or subacute unit, in a rehabilitation center, in the patient's home, or in an outpatient clinic. Regardless of the treatment setting, the primary goals for the patient still focus on the achievement of functional mobility and participation in meaningful life roles. Mat activities may continue, but the types of exercises selected should be more challenging and the time spent in a supine position should be limited. Patients should be encouraged to perform their mat exercises as part of an independent exercise program. The emphasis of the patient's treatment sessions should be on a task-oriented approach. This approach recognizes that patients learn best by actively practicing tasks in a functional context rather than practicing component parts of normal movement patterns. Adapting to environmental changes and the patient's ability to complete tasks using a variety of movement strategies must be prioritized during this stage of recovery (Shumway-Cook and Woollacott, 2017).

It is important to remember that the primary PT will need to continue to reexamine the patient and revise the plan of care as needed as the patient transitions to different settings and as goals are achieved.

INTERVENTION 11.41 **Stair Climbing**

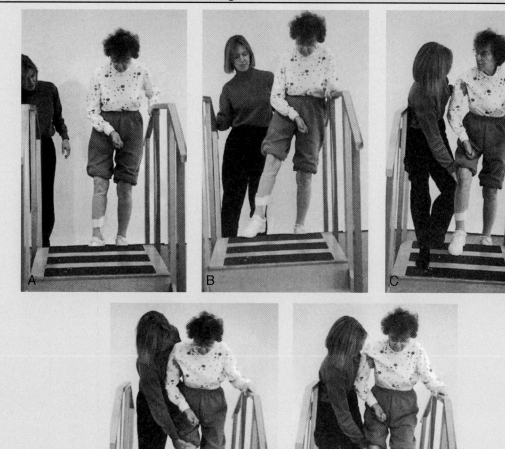

A and B. The patient with right hemiplegia initiates lifting the leg onto a step. She initiates the pattern with pelvic elevation and a strong overshift of her trunk to the left as she circumducts and lifts her leg with knee extension.

C. The clinician uses her left hand in an axillary grip to correct trunk alignment and uses her right hand to help the patient learn to lift her right leg with hip and knee flexion.

D and E. The clinician uses her right hand on the distal femur to teach the patient to move forward over her extending right leg. The clinician's left hand moves the trunk forward and upward as the leg extends and the patient lifts her left leg upward. The patient does not overshift and relies on her left arm as the clinician helps her to learn to use her right leg.

(From Ryerson S, Levit K: *Functional movement reeducation: a contemporary model for stroke rehabilitation,* New York, 1997, Churchill Livingstone.)

Negotiation of Environmental Barriers

Activities that address the negotiation of environmental barriers, including stairs, curbs, and ramps, should also be practiced as the patient is able to tolerate.

Stairs

Patients should be instructed in the following sequence when learning to negotiate stairs.

A patient who is using a handrail should lead with the stronger uninvolved foot when ascending the stairs. The involved foot follows. This sequence continues until the patient has negotiated all the steps. Intervention 11.41 illustrates a patient who is walking up the stairs. The PT/PTA must guard the patient carefully to avoid loss of balance or a fall. Clinicians may find it safer and easier to guard the patient from behind during stair ascent.

When descending the stairs with a handrail, the patient needs to lead with the involved foot. Intervention 11.42 shows a patient going down the steps. The therapist observes the response of the involved lower extremity as it begins to accept

INTERVENTION 11.42 Descending Stairs

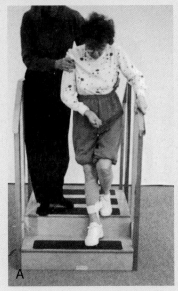
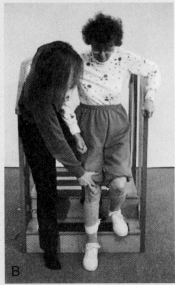
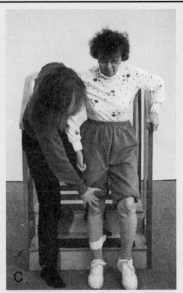

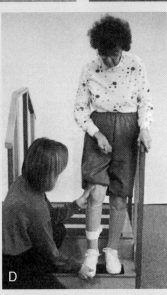
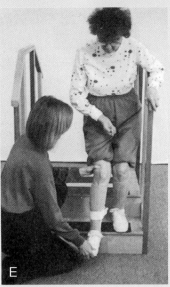

A. The patient leads with her right leg. The right leg is adducting as it reaches to the step. This leg adduction contributes to the feeling of "falling" to the hemiplegic side.

B and C. The clinician uses her left hand in an axillary grip to support the patient's trunk and pelvis. She reminds the patient to keep the upper trunk extended over the pelvis as the right foot reaches to the floor and the left foot steps down.

D and E. The clinician lets the patient control the trunk as she reeducates the forward movement pattern of the right leg.

(From Ryerson S, Levit K: *Functional movement reeducation: a contemporary model for stroke rehabilitation,* New York, 1997, Churchill Livingstone.)

weight. The patient must possess ample lower-extremity control to maintain the leg in relative extension during lowering of the involved lower extremity. As previously stated, the extension synergy pattern is common in many patients with strokes. This extension pattern may cause the involved lower extremity to stay extended during stair climbing. When the patient is descending the stairs, the clinician will want to guard the patient from the front. It may also be necessary for the PT/PTA to provide manual cues at the patient's knee. Prevention of genu recurvatum on descent should be encouraged by maintaining the involved knee in slight flexion.

> **CAUTION** A safety belt should always be used during stair training. Patients should initially be instructed to ascend and descend stairs one step at a time. As the patient progresses, a step over step sequence can be utilized.

Stair climbing with a cane. If the patient is going to use an assistive device on the stairs, the sequence will be the same. When going up the stairs, the patient leads with the uninvolved foot, followed by the involved leg, and then the cane. The sequence for going down the stairs is to have the patient lower the cane and the involved lower extremity at the same time if possible and then lower the uninvolved leg.

> **SPECIAL NOTE** Depending on the type of cane selected for the patient, the cane may or may not fit on the step. Straight canes and narrow-base quad canes can be used without modification. A wide-base quad cane must be turned sideways to fit safely on the step. Hemiwalkers cannot be used on steps safely. Patients should be encouraged to negotiate 12 steps (a flight) if possible, as this number is used in the FIM and Quality Indicators scoring and represents community independence. When practicing stair climbing, it is important to note if an assistive device or handrails are used during activity performance.

Curbs and Ramps

Negotiation of a curb is similar to that of a single step. Ramps can be a challenge, based on their degree of incline or grade.

Family Participation

Family members should practice the skills needed to assist the patient at home and should be responsible for return demonstrations in the clinic. Encourage family members to take an active role in practicing these activities. Family members may tell you that they feel confident with the activity simply after observing it. It is optimal for both the patient and the patient's family to practice these tasks with a skilled therapist present. These practice sessions allow the clinician to provide feedback on technique performance and to identify potential challenges that the patient and the caregiver may experience in the home setting.

Promotion of Upper Extremity Function

Frequently, at this point in the recovery process, the patient is trying to gain control of the distal joint components. The ability to abduct the shoulder, extend the wrist, and to release a mass grasp are considered early positive indicators for improved upper extremity and hand function (Edwardson, 2019). It has been shown that patients who demonstrate some shoulder abduction and finger extension by the second day after their stroke have a 98% probability of achieving some degree of hand function within 6 months (Teasell and Hussein, 2016b). Exercises and functional activities that stress upper extremity range of motion should be included in the patient's plan of care. Depending on the level of motor return in the hand, the patient may be able to complete fine motor activities (grasp, release, opposition, manipulation of objects). Dressing, bathing, and grooming tasks are frequently used to improve hand coordination because of the large degree of fine motor control necessary to complete these activities. In addition, ADLs are functionally oriented. Determining if the patient has any hobbies or areas of interest helps in identifying additional treatment interventions. If the therapist can select tasks that are meaningful and have functional relevance, patient compliance is improved. Cooking, gardening, writing, computer work, manipulation of coins, and crafts are just a few examples of the types of activities

that may promote fine motor control and dexterity in the upper extremity. The patient should be encouraged to use the involved upper extremity as much as possible. If the involved arm lacks the necessary motor control to complete fine motor tasks, it should be positioned in weight-bearing or be used as an assist/stabilizer during activity performance.

The use of neuromuscular electrical stimulation may also be prescribed for the patient with limited hand function. Electrodes applied to the wrist and finger extensors can assist with hand opening. Newer approaches to the administration of neuromuscular electrical stimulation, such as contralaterally controlled electrical stimulation, require that the patient wear a glove on the uninvolved hand while stimulation is applied to the involved finger and thumb extensors. The patient is thus able to actively control the intensity of the stimulation applied to the hand and can practice using the involved upper extremity in task-specific activities (Knutson et al., 2019).

Strengthening Exercises for the Lower Extremity

Exercises designed to enhance lower extremity function can also be performed. Again, the selection of different treatment interventions will depend on the patient's level of motor return. Once the patient is up and ambulating, supine exercises should be limited, if not discontinued, and more challenging closed chain activities should be used for strengthening and training purposes. To continue to improve hip and knee control, the patient can transfer to a high-low mat table. With the height of the table raised and the involved lower extremity weight-bearing on the floor, the patient can work on hip and knee extension from this position. In a supported standing position, the patient can perform the following exercises: standing hip abduction on both the involved and uninvolved sides; hip extension with the knee straight; hip flexion or marching; and knee flexion with the hip in a neutral or slightly extended position. Other advanced exercises include mini squats, resisted gait, pushing or carrying an object, lunges, and ambulation with lower extremity weights. The benefits of these exercises are that they activate the lower extremity musculature in ways directly opposite the normal lower extremity synergy patterns, while also promoting unilateral weight-bearing, balance, and coordination skills.

Strengthening Exercises for the Ankle

Exercises that address range of motion of the involved ankle should also be included. Patients who are experiencing difficulties in achieving active ankle dorsiflexion can place a rolling pin under the foot and work on moving the rolling pin back and forth. This maneuver can be performed when the patient is either in sitting or standing. If the patient has relatively good active dorsiflexion and plantar flexion, she can work on tapping the foot, drawing a circle or alphabet on the floor, or kicking a small ball forward. Additional activities that can be performed include heel raises with the knee in slight flexion, active ankle eversion, or resistive exercises with an elastic band. Patients can also work on active ankle exercises while standing on a tilt board, BOSU ball (BOSU,

Ashland, OH), or BAPS (Biomechanical Ankle Platform System, Adrian, MI) board.

Coordination Exercises

Exercises targeted at improving coordination of the upper and lower extremities should also be performed. Standard coordination tests performed when the patient is sitting include finger to nose, the patient's finger to the therapist's finger, alternating nose to finger, finger opposition, and bilateral pronation and supination activities. Lower extremity coordination exercises include alternating heel to knee and heel to toe, toe to examiner's finger, and heel to shin. The incorporation of these exercises into the patient's treatment plan depends on the degree of motor return in the upper and lower extremities.

Balance Exercises

Balance and coordination exercises can be performed with the patient in a standing position. Examples of exercises that can be performed to improve a patient's static balance include standing with both feet together with a narrow base of support; tandem standing, which is standing with one foot directly in front of the other; and standing on one foot.

Additionally, the patient's balance strategies should be observed by displacing the patient's center of gravity unexpectedly. As described previously, the PT/PTA should observe the presence of appropriate ankle, hip, and stepping strategies. Balance responses are normal reactions to perturbation or a sudden change in the patient's center of gravity as it relates to the patient's base of support. Patients who do not possess adequate dorsiflexion may not be able to initiate or perform the ankle strategy. Patients with limited ability to activate lower extremity musculature may not be able to use hip and protective stepping responses to prevent falls when their balance is disturbed.

There are many balance and mobility assessment tools that may be administered to the patient following a stroke. The Berg Balance Scale is one such tool that measures balance in older adults including those that have sustained a stroke and is part of the Core Set of Outcome Measures (Moore et al., 2018). The maximum score is 56 and a score less than 45 indicates that the individual is at risk for falling. Other assessment tools that evaluate mobility and are used clinically in the rehabilitation setting include the Timed Up and Go Test and the 6 Minute Walk Test, both of which assess mobility and gait and are used in determining the patient's functional capacity (Teasell and Hussein, 2016b). The Functional Gait Assessment, another one of the tools in the Core Set of Outcomes Measures, should also be administered to assess balance during ambulation (Moore et al., 2018). Clinicians are encouraged to review the following websites for additional information regarding the administration of various balance assessment instruments for patients poststroke: www.rehabmeasures.org and www.ebrsr.com.

Dynamic Balance Activities

Other examples of activities that can be performed to challenge the patient's dynamic balance include walking on uneven surfaces, tandem walking, walking on a balance beam, side stepping, walking backward, braiding (walking sideways, crossing one foot over the other), throwing and catching a small ball, batting a balloon, and marching in place. All are useful activities for the patient to perform if the goal is to improve the patient's ability to maintain a balanced postural base while moving the lower extremities and, in the case of throwing and catching, while the upper extremities are also moving.

Additional activities that can be performed include walking activities in which the patient is asked to change speed or direction. Abrupt stopping and starting, walking in a circle, walking over and around objects as in an obstacle course, walking while carrying an object, or having the patient walk on heels or toes will challenge the patient's dynamic balance and coordination.

A systematic review and meta-analysis conducted by van Duijnhoven et al. (2016) demonstrated that balance in patients with chronic stroke could be improved through exercise, specifically balance, functional weight shifting, and gait training activities. The gait training studies that reported improvements in balance all incorporated additional challenges during walking including virtual reality (VR), head movements, and did not include treadmill training with or without body-weight support as part of the intervention (van Duijnhoven et al., 2016).

Dual-Task Training

Clinicians are encouraged to perform dual-task training if the patient is able to tolerate. These tasks incorporate concurrent performance of motor and cognitive tasks and require the patient's attention while engaged in a balance or mobility activity (Allison and Fuller, 2013). Examples of balance related dual-task training include throwing or catching a ball or shooting a basketball while standing on a foam pad. Other cognitive challenges include word association, math calculations, or reciting a sequence of numbers. Dual-task locomotor training is an important area of research for individuals poststroke due to residual patient deficits. During training, patients can be asked to focus on the gait task, the cognitive task, or they can alternate between the two. Evidence suggests that gait speed can increase under dual-task training conditions (Shumway-Cook and Woollacott, 2017). These tasks also simulate normal everyday activities and assist the patient and the clinician in recognizing the cognitive and motor aspects of activity performance.

Advanced Balance Exercises

For patients who need even more challenging activities, the therapist can remove the patient's visual feedback and have the patient stand on a level surface with eyes closed. A patient who is able to do this can be progressed to standing on different types of surfaces (foam) with eyes open and then with eyes closed. It is extremely important to guard the patient closely during advanced balance activities, although the clinician must gauge the amount of assist provided. If too much physical support is provided, the patient will rely on the assistance and will not make the necessary postural modifications to maintain and improve balance.

Dynamic Sitting and Standing Balance Exercises Using Movable Surfaces

Movable surfaces provide another means of working on the patient's sitting and standing dynamic balance. Swiss (therapeutic) balls, BOSU balls, and tilt boards can be used effectively for the patient who needs to continue to work on dynamic balance and core stability.

Swiss ball. When the Swiss ball is used, the right-sized ball must be selected for the patient. The patient should be able to sit on the ball and have both feet touch the floor. In addition, the hips, knees, and ankles should be at a 90-90-90 position. Intervention 11.43 illustrates the use of the Swiss ball during treatment. The patient can be assisted to the ball and can work on the achievement of an upright erect posture. The ability to achieve proper posture requires that the patient actively contract the abdominal muscles to keep the shoulders in line with the hips. In addition, the patient must keep the knees over the feet. Some of the first exercises that should be performed on the ball are those that address pelvic mobility. While sitting on the ball, the patient can isolate anterior and posterior pelvic tilts and lateral tilts to the right and left. The lateral shifts assist the patient with the ability to elongate the trunk on the weight-bearing side and shorten it on the opposite side. Once the patient is able to maintain balance on the ball while moving the pelvis, the patient can be progressed to adding movements of the limbs. While sitting on the ball, the patient can perform the following exercises: reciprocal arm movements of the upper extremities; marching in place; and unilateral knee extension. As her balance improves, the patient can perform PNF chops and lifts or trunk rotation exercises.

The ball, as a movable surface, provides the patient with some uncertainty in terms of stability. A sudden movement of the ball requires the patient to be able to make a quick, unanticipated postural response to realign the center of gravity in relation to the base of support. Many patients lack the ability to adjust their postural responses in this way. As stated previously, it is necessary to guard the patient carefully while on the ball. Only those patients who already exhibit a certain degree of trunk control should attempt these activities.

Tilt boards. Tilt boards offer another type of movable surface for our patients. Therapists often use boards on which the adult patient can stand to work on postural reactions. As with the ball, selection of a tilt board as part of the treatment plan requires that the patient possess a certain amount of trunk and extremity control in addition to fairly good dynamic balance. A patient who requires an assistive device for ambulation would not be an appropriate candidate for standing tilt board activities. It is often beneficial to first demonstrate for the patient what the clinician wants the patient to do on the board. The patient needs to be advised that the board will move as she tries to position herself on it. The patient should be assisted onto the board. Standing in front of the patient and allowing her to hold on to your hands is often easiest. At times, it may be necessary to have someone else hold the board as the patient steps up onto it. Once on the board, the patient must accommodate to the movable surface, as illustrated in Fig. 11.17. A slight shift in the patient's weight from one side to the next causes the board to move. Initially, maintaining the board in a balanced position is difficult. In an attempt to improve stability, the patient often locks the knees into extension, so she does not have to concentrate on knee control in addition to maintaining balance on the board. If one observes compensatory strategy, it may indicate that the activity is too difficult for the patient.

During the patient's acclimation to the tilt board, the therapist should continue to hold on to the patient's arms for balance support. Once the patient is relatively stable and safe on the board, the PT/PTA can help the patient with small weight shifts to the right and left. Through manual contacts, the therapist is able to grade the excursion of the patient's weight shift.

Observations. When the patient shifts the weight to the right, the patient should exhibit elongation of the trunk on the right with trunk and head righting. Intervention 11.44 shows a patient on a tilt board. The position of the patient's lower extremities should also be noted, in addition to the position of the upper extremities. On occasion, the patient will overcompensate with the upper extremities if she believes that balance is being compromised. Extension and abduction of the upward side with protective extension on the opposite (downward) side may be evident. As the patient becomes more comfortable on the board, she can begin to shift weight actively to the right and

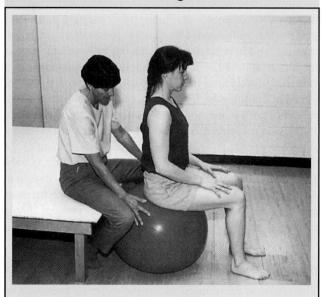

INTERVENTION Sitting on a Swiss Ball

The patient should be able to sit on the ball and have both feet touch the floor. Hips, knees, and ankles should be at a 90-90-90 position. The patient should first work on maintaining an upright erect posture on the ball before progressing to other exercises such as pelvic mobility and movement of the limbs.

(From O'Sullivan SB, Schmitz TJ: *Physical rehabilitation laboratory manual: focus on functional training*, Philadelphia, 1999, FA Davis.)

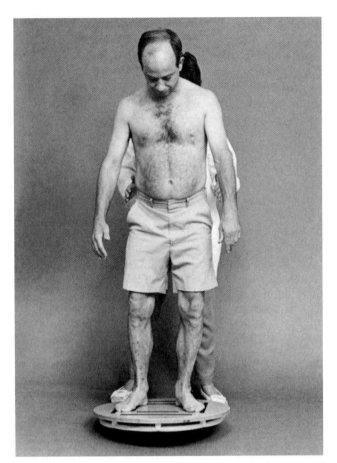

Fig. 11.17 A patient can increase speed amplitude and the type of balance responses on an adjustable tilt board. (From Duncan PW, Badke MB: *Stroke rehabilitation: recovery of motor control*, Chicago, 1987, Year Book.)

left. The patient needs to possess adequate control of the weight shift. Often, the patient limits the shift to the involved side because of anxiety associated with having all the weight on her involved lower extremity. The patient can also work on trying to maintain the board in a neutral position with equal weight on both lower extremities.

Anterior and posterior weight shifts on the tilt board. The position of the board can also be changed to allow the patient to work on anterior and posterior weight shifts. The patient again needs to be assisted onto the board. The advantage of this board position is that it allows the patient to work on active ankle dorsiflexion and plantar flexion. As the board moves in a posterior direction, the patient is dorsiflexing both ankles. For patients who have difficulties with active dorsiflexion or performance of the ankle strategy for balance control, this exercise can be effective. Selection of a tilt board requires that the patient possess a fairly high level of motor function and is simply in need of refinement of ankle movements and postural responses.

For those patients who are discharged to home after completing their rehabilitation, dynamic balance deficits have been identified as a strong predictor of falls in this group (Lubetzky-Vilnai and Kartin, 2010). As stated earlier, research supports the use of balance training for these individuals. The systematic review conducted by van Duijnhoven (2016) found that

patients in the chronic phase after stroke who engaged in repetitive static standing exercises, reaching tasks, sit-to-stand transitions, walking, stair climbing, and altering their base of support during activity performance were able to improve their balance performance (van Duijnhoven et al., 2016).

Management of Abnormal Tone

The presence of abnormal tone may become apparent during the patient's recovery. Spasticity and the dominance of the synergy patterns can interfere with the patient's attempts at active movement. Although, at present, no surgical, pharmacologic, or physical therapy interventions can permanently eliminate increased tone, PTs and PTAs can intervene to make the tone more manageable for a short period of time. Our goal is to decrease the abnormal tone long enough for the patient to perform an active movement or functional task. This allows the patient the opportunity to move with increased ease and to have a more "normal sensory experience." Abnormal movement patterns develop in response to the abnormal sensory feedback perceived. Thus abnormal movement patterns are reinforced each time the patient moves.

As mentioned earlier, positioning the patient in the antispasm patterns described can assist in decreasing the abnormal tone that may develop. Rhythmic rotation applied with steady passive movement, such as that applied with lower trunk rotation or rhythmic rotation of the extremities, is beneficial. Rotational exercises followed by activities that incorporate weight-bearing can be extremely beneficial in providing the patient with a more normal postural base. Weight-bearing through the upper or lower extremities is an excellent treatment modality for tone reduction. Other activities that can be administered to assist in managing the patient's abnormal tone include PNF diagonals (including the chopping and lifting patterns), tapping and vibration to the weaker antagonist muscles, tendon pressure applied directly to the spastic muscle tendon, air splints, the prolonged application of ice, functional electrical stimulation, and biofeedback. Any of these treatment interventions may be beneficial to the patient. Often, it is necessary to try one and then grade the patient's response to the sensory intervention applied. Again, it is not sufficient simply to apply a tone-reducing modality. The patient's tone should be decreased through a therapeutic modality, but the patient must then be provided with a movement transition or functional task that allows the patient to experience more normal sensory feedback while moving. This concept should ultimately reinforce the desired movement and, one hopes, should lead to improved function.

Current Treatment Approaches

The reader is encouraged to review materials presented in Chapters 2 and 3 regarding principles of neuroplasticity and motor learning and their relationship to treatment planning. This will provide a framework for discussion of the following interventions. CIMT is an intervention designed to reduce the effects of learned nonuse. Learned nonuse develops as the patient attempts to move the involved side and is unsuccessful. The patient may experience failure and frustration after unsuccessful movement attempts. Consequently, the patient

INTERVENTION 11.44   Using a Tilt Board

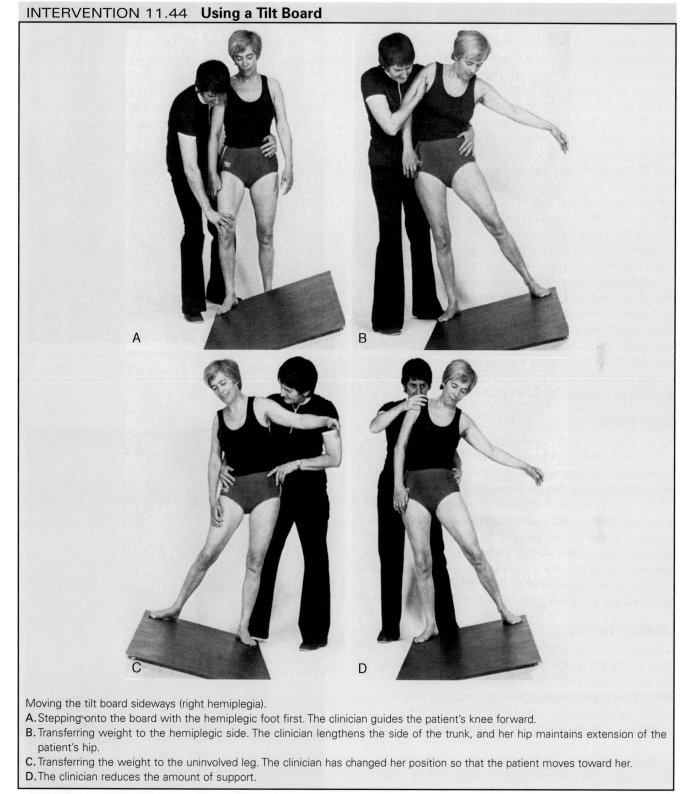

Moving the tilt board sideways (right hemiplegia).

A. Stepping onto the board with the hemiplegic foot first. The clinician guides the patient's knee forward.

B. Transferring weight to the hemiplegic side. The clinician lengthens the side of the trunk, and her hip maintains extension of the patient's hip.

C. Transferring the weight to the uninvolved leg. The clinician has changed her position so that the patient moves toward her.

D. The clinician reduces the amount of support.

(From Davies PM: *Steps to follow: a guide to the treatment of adult hemiplegia,* New York, 1985, Springer Verlag.)

begins to compensate for these experiences by using the uninvolved extremity to complete functional tasks. Over time, the patient learns to disregard and not use the involved extremity (Bonifer and Anderson, 2003).

CIMT is a treatment approach based on neuroscience and behavioral techniques. There are three components to CIMT including: (1) repetitive, task-specific training of the involved extremity for 2 to 3 weeks; (2) required use of the involved extremity during waking hours (restraining the involved extremity is sometimes required); and (3) use of behavioral strategies to allow transference of improvements made in the clinic to the patient's home environment (Taub and Uswatt,

2006). When using CIMT in a clinical setting, the patient's uninvolved upper extremity is restrained or immobilized in a mitt or glove. This forces the patient to use the involved upper extremity repetitively for the completion of functional tasks (Liepert, 2000). Sessions with a physical or occupational therapist are typically 6 to 7 hours a day and include verbal and tactile cues as well as hand-over-hand assistance to perform desired tasks. Patients are also responsible for keeping a journal regarding their performance. Most research studies have as inclusion criteria that subjects must demonstrate at least 10 degrees of finger and 20 degrees of active wrist extension. Positive results have been reported for those patients with mild to moderate deficits (Umphred et al., 2013; Taub and Uswatt, 2006). Use of CIMT does provide challenges to both the patient and the clinician. The intervention is extremely time and labor intensive, and patient adherence to the intensity and practice schedule can be problematic.

A systematic review and meta-analysis conducted by Etoom et al. (2016) indicated that CIMT was not superior to other conventional interventions. However, in another systematic review conducted by Wattchow et al. (2018) it was reported that positive effects on upper extremity function were achieved with CIMT and task-specific training. Additional research regarding the optimal dose and time to initiate this intervention must still be explored (Wattchow et al., 2018).

Mirror Therapy

Mirror therapy is another intervention that may be used in patients with stroke. Patients sit or stand with a mirror placed in the patient's midsagittal plane and perform movements with their uninvolved upper or lower extremity. While watching the reflection in the mirror, it appears that the involved extremity is moving. Mirror visual feedback can be combined with task-specific training, mental imagery, or electrical stimulation. Evidence suggests that mirror therapy can improve motor function and the patient's ability to perform ADLs, as well as decrease shoulder pain (Deutsch and O'Sullivan, 2019; Shumway-Cook and Woollacott, 2017; Teasell and Hussein, 2016b).

Locomotor Training

Locomotor training is an important component of the treatment plan for a patient poststroke, as improved walking is one of the most commonly reported goals (Mulroy et al., 2010). Body-weight support treadmill training (BWSTT) is an effective intervention in the treatment of gait disturbances in patients with stroke (Fig. 11.18). Individuals, even those unable to stand independently, are able to practice stepping in a safe environment (Hornby et al., 2011). With BWSTT, a percentage of the patient's weight is supported by an overhead harness while the patient is walking on a treadmill. For individuals that walk at speeds less than 0.2 m/s, it is beneficial to provide body-weight support, and the recommended unweighting is 40% or less to ensure loading and muscle activation patterns similar to normal walking (Visintin et al., 1998). During BWSTT, clinicians can help stabilize the patient's pelvis and assist with lower extremity advancement as the treadmill moves (Fig. 11.19).

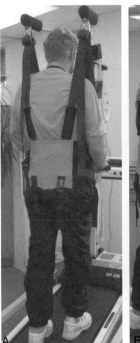
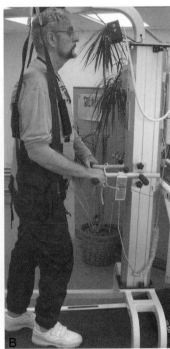

Fig. 11.18 (A and **B)** Client with right hemiplegia walking on a treadmill with partial body-weight support. (From Umphred DA, Lazaro RT, Rollere ML, Burton GU: *Neurological rehabilitation,* ed 6, St. Louis, 2013, Elsevier, p. 744).

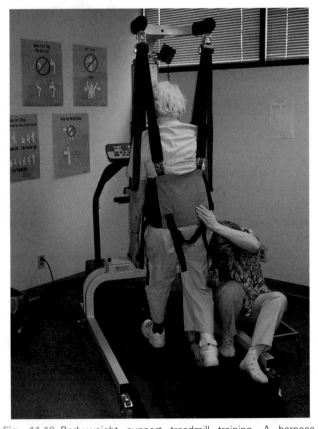

Fig. 11.19 Body-weight support treadmill training. A harness, mounted overhead, supports part of the person's weight while the individual walks on a treadmill with a therapist assisting movements of the paretic lower limb. (From Lundy-Ekman: *Neuroscience fundamentals for rehabilitation,* ed 5, St. Louis, 2018, Elsevier.)

However, evidence is emerging that suggests offering body-weight support to individuals in the chronic stages (more than 6 months) poststroke who are ambulatory may not be beneficial (Combs-Miller et al., 2014; Middleton et al., 2014; Suputtitada et al., 2004). This evidence suggests that individuals who are able to walk should do so without additional support from the harness.

Other robotic systems are available that provide similar gait opportunities for the patient but require less assistance from clinicians. Studies performed to evaluate the effectiveness of this intervention have demonstrated improvements in gait velocity, endurance, and balance (Fulk, 2004; Hornby et al., 2011). There is some conflicting evidence regarding the effectiveness of body-weight support treadmill ambulation in comparison with typical physical therapy interventions. In the LEAPS trial, a randomized control study, BWSTT did not result in superior gait outcomes when compared with in-home physical therapy services, which consisted of range of motion, flexibility, and strengthening exercises, balance and coordination activities, and encouragement of the patient to walk daily (Duncan et al., 2011). However, exercise intensity in this study was very low with participant heart rates limited to less than 110 and Rates of Perceived Exertion (RPE) of less than 13, which likely contributed to the outcomes (Hornby et al., 2011). Despite this conflicting information, many therapists support the use of BWSTT in improving gait performance, specifically gait speed and walking endurance, especially when compared with more traditional physical therapy interventions (Mehrholz and Elsner, 2017). Additionally, BWSTT supports the premise of task-specific interventions (Teasell and Hussein, 2016b; Mulroy et al., 2010). Further research is needed to identify specific frequencies, intensities, duration, and the use of upper extremity support during treadmill training (Mehrholz and Elsner, 2017).

Robotic Walking

Robotic (electromechanical) assisted locomotor training is also used to improve walking capabilities after stroke. In a Cochrane review conducted by Mehrholz et al. (2017), it was found that patients who received robotic-assisted gait training in combination with physical therapy were more likely to achieve independent ambulation than those that did not receive this intervention. Individuals who participated in robotic-assisted locomotion in the first 3 months after injury or were nonambulatory initially achieved the greatest benefit. Additional research is needed, as there were variations between the trials with respect to duration and frequency of treatment, the use of electrical stimulation, and the ambulatory status of participants as some subjects were able to walk independently prior to the start of the study (Mehrholz et al., 2017).

High Intensity Gait Training

Emerging evidence over the past several decades has suggested that the amount, intensity, and variability of task-specific practice may be important contributors to the recovery of specific motor skills, such as walking, in individuals

poststroke (Kleim and Jones, 2008; Langhammer and Stanghelle, 2000; Wolf et al., 2006). High intensity gait training can be defined as walking interventions, both on the treadmill and overground, with graded and specific challenges to promote skill acquisition, while achieving specific cardiovascular intensities. The following paragraphs aim to provide an overview of these training parameters with the understanding that more evidence is emerging to guide implementation in the clinical setting.

Specificity/amount. Learning or skill acquisition (as opposed to mere use) seems to be a critical component in producing significant changes in the patterns of neural connectivity in both healthy and damaged brains (Kleim and Jones, 2008). For recovery of locomotor function poststroke, previous studies have suggested that large amounts of task-specific (i.e., walking) practice may be more effective than traditional, impairment-based interventions (Wolf et al., 2006; Van Peppen et al., 2004; Hornby et al., 2011). Task-specific gait training can take place on a treadmill or overground, with or without body-weight support, and with or without therapist assistance, in an effort to maximize stepping practice. Although previous studies have emphasized the provision of specific types or amount of assistance, more recent data suggest that aiding only as much as needed to perform stepping is likely sufficient (Hornby et al., 2011, 2016). The amount of practice is typically estimated as the amount or duration of sessions, or can be measured more objectively by the number of steps provided (Moore et al., 2010). In both animal and human studies, greater amounts of stepping practice appear to result in more favorable outcomes. For example, walking practice on a treadmill can provide up to 4000 steps within a 1-hour session, and is focused entirely on stepping practice (Moore et al., 2010; Cha et al., 2007; De Leon et al., 1998). Conversely, observational studies have reported that conventional therapy sessions poststroke generally provide a fraction of the amount of stepping, ranging from 250-900 steps/session (Lang et al., 2007, 2009). Selected studies have indicated that the amount of practice provided may be related to the amount of improvements in walking speed, distance, and daily stepping activity in the community (Moore et al., 2010).

Intensity. Intensity is defined as the amount of work per unit time, or power output, with higher intensity interventions resulting in greater walking outcomes (Holleran et al., 2015; Globas et al., 2012). The benefits of higher versus lower intensity practice may be due in part to greater neuromuscular demands, which can facilitate generation and release of neurotrophic processes that may facilitate plastic changes that may underlie improved function (Jacobs and Fornal, 1999; Baker-Herman et al., 2004; Chau et al., 1998; Fong et al., 2005). Intensity is typically measured using cardiovascular parameters, specifically heart rate responses, given the difficulty of estimating neuromuscular demands during exercise interventions. Targeted ranges during high intensity gait training are 70% to 80% of heart rate reserve and patient-reported Ratings of Perceived Exertion at 15 to 18 (Moore and Hornby, 2018). Conversely, observational studies in humans have shown that conventional therapy sessions poststroke are delivered at very low cardiovascular intensities, with less than 3 mins/session spent at heart rate intensities that exceed 60% of maximum heart rate. This intensity is insufficient to drive a cardiovascular response to induce a training effect (Mackay-Lyons and Makrides, 2002).

Variability/error. Finally, the incorporation of variability during walking tasks has been shown to be an important parameter in the recovery of walking poststroke. Variable practice can result in increased rate or magnitude of errors (e.g., mistakes), which ultimately results in optimal motor learning and skill acquisition. Training scenarios in which individuals poststroke are allowed to make errors while being challenged to maintain stepping in a variety of contexts may be more effective than interventions with less variability (Hornby et al., 2016; Moore and Hornby, 2018; Holleran et al., 2014; Hornby et al., 2015). An example of a walking intervention with high variability is the incorporation of an obstacle course in which an individual is challenged to walk in multiple directions and negotiate several obstacles on a variety of surfaces. In contrast, an example of a walking intervention with low variability is treadmill walking at a constant speed in a forward direction.

Summary

Given the current evidence supporting the important contribution of each of these training parameters to walking recovery poststroke, gait-prioritized treatment sessions should be structured with consideration for the amount, intensity, and variability of stepping practice that will be provided by the selected intervention. Future studies will need to continue to investigate how each of these training parameters should be ideally incorporated, manipulated, and prioritized during rehabilitation to promote the recovery of walking and facilitate optimal locomotor outcomes for this patient population.

Virtual Reality

An area of treatment that is developing is the use of VR and video gaming to improve upper limb function, balance, and gait abilities. VR systems can challenge a patient's gait abilities by projecting visual images on a screen in front of a treadmill or on a treadmill belt, on the ground, or on a balance beam. Patients are required to modify their balance and gait to adapt to the virtual object presented. Examples include stepping over objects, avoiding obstacles, kicking a ball, speeding up, slowing down, and tandem walking. VR provides the patient with the opportunity for repetitive, task-specific practice and adds the benefit of incorporating variability, which fosters a patient's ability "to adapt to novel situations," thereby promoting motor learning (de Rooij et al., 2016). Improvements in gait speed, Berg Balance scores, and the Timed Up and Go were reported with use of this intervention (de Rooij et al., 2016; Shumway-Cook and Woollacott, 2017).

VR training for the upper extremity often includes practice of ADLs and other activities performed on a daily basis. The following results were reported for the upper extremity in a Cochrane review (2018) published in the journal *Stroke* (Laver et al., 2018). When VR outcomes were compared with those achieved through conventional therapy, there was not a statistically significant difference. However, when VR was used as an adjunct to standard therapy, there was a statistically significant difference in ADL outcome. It is, however, important to note that those subjects who received VR as a treatment supplement received an increased amount or dose of therapy, which may have impacted their improved outcomes (Laver et al., 2018).

> **SPECIAL NOTE** When designing the patient's treatment plan and selecting interventions to perform, therapists must always consider the patient's goals and task-specific training principles for inclusion.

Preparation for Discharge

Depending on the patient's recovery and home situation (including family support), the PT and PTA will need to plan for the patient's discharge to home or another type of health care facility. This planning should begin during the initial examination and continue throughout the patient's episode of care.

Assessing the Patient's Home Environment

During the initial examination, the primary PT needs to ask questions regarding the patient's home environment. Factors that must be considered when addressing discharge include the type of dwelling in which the patient resides, whether it is an apartment (with steps or an elevator), a house, a trailer, or another type of structure. Asking patients or their significant others whether they rent or own their home is also important because renting may preclude the family from making any permanent structural changes. The entrance to the home should also be assessed. The number, height, and condition of the steps, the presence or absence of a handrail or landing area, proximity to the driveway or parking lot, and the direction in which the front door opens will help in planning for the patient's safe return to the home environment.

The following is a list of general considerations for exterior accessibility. These guidelines are provided to assist clinicians in suggesting environmental modifications to their patients' existing dwellings.

1. Steps should not be higher than 7 inches or deeper than 11 inches.
2. Handrails should measure between 34 to 38 inches maximum in height.
3. One handrail should extend a minimum of 12 inches beyond the foot and top of the stairs.
4. If a ramp is needed, the recommended grade for wheelchairs is 12 inches of ramp for every inch of threshold height.
5. Ramps should be a minimum of 36 inches wide and should be covered with a nonslip surface.
6. A door width of 32 to 34 inches is acceptable and accommodates most wheelchairs.
7. Raised doorway thresholds should be removed.
8. Additional space and equipment considerations are required for patients who are obese (Schmitz, 2019).

Much of the information pertaining to the patient's home may be provided by the family. Many facilities use a checklist that a family member can complete regarding the home and its accessibility. In some cases, it may be necessary for the rehabilitation team to go out and perform a home assessment. This assessment may be conducted by the primary PT, the PTA, the occupational therapist, or a combination of these team members. Family members are often included in these assessments, so information regarding home modifications or equipment needs can be provided.

Other information that is needed regarding the patient's home includes interior accessibility, specifically in the areas of the bedroom and bathroom. The amount of space needed by the patient for negotiation depends on her ambulatory status. Wheelchairs require space for turning and also for positioning of the chair near furniture for transfers. In the patient's bedroom, the therapist will want to note the type of bed, whether space is adequate for transfers, the location of a nightstand or bedside table, and the need for a bedside commode or urinal. The width of the bathroom door also needs to be assessed because frequently these entrances are narrower than other interior door frames. An elevated toilet seat and grab bars may be necessary to ensure the patient's safety when toileting. Talking with the patient and primary caregiver provides information on the bathing patterns of the patient. A tub bench or shower chair in addition to a hand spray attachment may be suggested.

Other considerations for interior accessibility include the type of carpeting. Low, dense-pile carpets are recommended because they tend to be the easiest on which to ambulate or over which to propel a wheelchair. All throw rugs should be removed because they create a safety hazard for the patient who is ambulatory. The design of the kitchen should also be observed. Counter heights and handles on cabinets should be noted. Frequently used items should be moved to lower cabinets to allow for easier reach.

The rehabilitation team will also want to question the patient about her primary means of transportation at discharge. This information helps in identifying the most appropriate car transfer to practice and aids in planning follow-up care for the patient. Car transfers with and without the patient's family should be practiced before discharge. In addition, family members should be instructed in safe techniques for loading and unloading the wheelchair from their vehicle.

Further recommendations for rehabilitation services should be made before the patient's discharge from the health care facility. The primary PT needs to reexamine the patient and, with input from the PTA, suggest equipment and additional physical therapy needs to the patient's physician. Properly planning for the patient's discharge facilitates the patient's transition from the rehabilitation setting to the home and the community.

The development of the patient's home exercise program is also an important component of the discharge planning process. As with other patients who are being discharged from physical therapy services, identification of three to four critical exercises or activities is necessary to maintain patient function and prevent the development of secondary complications. It is also important to note, however, that the patient's performance of a home exercise program is not sufficient to maintain the patient's overall health status.

Exercise Training

In 2004, the American Heart Association released exercise recommendations for individuals poststroke, which recognize the benefits of physical fitness programs and aerobic exercise. The American College of Sports Medicine, fourth edition (Gordon et al., 2016), and the US Department of Health and Human Services (2018) have published exercise guidelines for individuals with chronic conditions, including those with stroke. Every person should perform a minimum of 150 minutes of moderate-intensity physical activity weekly, or if that is too difficult, 150 minutes of light-intensity activity and 2 days of general strengthening and flexibility exercises. Additionally, individuals at risk for fall may benefit from balance training (US Department of Health and Human Services, 2018; Macko, 2016). Resistive exercises, which target the major muscle groups, should be a component of the strengthening program, with 10 to 15 repetitions of each exercise performed 2 to 3 days per week (US Department of Health and Human Services, 2018; Macko, 2016; Gordon et al., 2004). Progressive resistive exercises have been shown to increase strength in hemiparetic muscles without increasing spasticity; however there is mixed evidence regarding strength training and its impact on stroke outcomes including gait (Teasell and Hussein, 2016b). Flexibility exercises and strength training including yoga and tai chi have been found to improve balance, quality of life, and an individual's fear of falling (Billinger et al., 2014).

As clinicians, we must recognize the importance of incorporating physical fitness into our patients' home programs in an effort to improve poststroke outcomes and reduce the risk of future cardiovascular events (Tang and Eng, 2014). Exercise training decreases blood pressure, improves cholesterol levels, and improves body composition by increasing fat-free muscle mass. Furthermore, evidence suggests that moderate-intensity exercise can improve insulin sensitivity and glucose tolerance; increases cerebral artery dilation; and can improve walking speed, endurance, and balance (Macko, 2016; Tang and Eng, 2014; Billinger et al., 2012; Gordon et al., 2016).

> **CAUTION** Graded exercise testing and physician clearance is dependent on the planned intensity and the goals of the exercise sessions. Individuals who want to start a low-intensity exercise program do not normally need to complete a formal exercise test, as the intensity involved is similar to that of a typical physical therapy session or the completion of daily activities. Patients should, however, receive medical clearance from a health care provider to ensure the patient's safety (Macko, 2016). It has, however, been recommended that individuals poststroke complete a graded exercise test before they begin their participation in a fitness program (Billinger et al., 2014).

The physical therapy management of the patient with a stroke has evolved from one based on neurophysiologic approaches to one that now addresses motor learning and the brain's capacity to change and adapt after injury. Because of changes in reimbursement and our health care system, it has become essential that the primary PT is diligent in the development of a plan of care that has the potential to provide the patient with the best possible functional outcome. At all times, the clinician must keep the patient actively engaged in the activity performance and consider the task itself, the intensity of the training, the feedback provided, and the structure of the practice session. When these factors are included in the planning and implementation of the treatment session, the clinician has provided the patient with the very best evidence-based care possible.

CHAPTER SUMMARY

Adults who have experienced a stroke constitute a significant number of the patients treated in physical therapy. Based on the type and extent of the initial insult, patients present with a multitude of different impairments, and the extent of these problems can be highly variable. Different treatment interventions are presented in this chapter to assist patients in improving their volitional motor control and functional abilities. As PTs and PTAs working with these patients, the primary goal of our interventions is to improve patients' abilities to perform meaningful functional activities and thus improve their quality of life.

REVIEW QUESTIONS

1. Describe the major impairments seen in patients who have had strokes (cardiovascular accidents).
2. What are risk factors for the development of a stroke?
3. Describe the upper extremity and lower extremity flexion and extension synergy patterns.
4. Discuss the benefits of patient positioning.
5. The acute care physical therapy management of a patient who has had a stroke should include what type of interventions?
6. What are appropriate physical therapy interventions to be performed with the patient in sitting?
7. Describe the gait training sequence for patients after an acute stroke.
8. Name four advanced dynamic standing balance exercises.
9. What environmental factors must be considered when preparing the patient for discharge to home?
10. Discuss the benefits of body-weight support treadmill ambulation.
11. Describe how principles of neuroplasticity can be incorporated into the treatment plans of patients with strokes?

CASE STUDIES REHABILITATION UNIT INITIAL EXAMINATION AND EVALUATION

History
Chart Review
Patient is a 67-year-old male who is a retired accountant. He came to the emergency department 3 days ago for vomiting in what his wife thought was an allergic response to shellfish, but Benadryl was ineffective. Patient was then admitted to the hospital. An initial computed tomography scan showed no evidence of significant mass and normal-sized ventricles. Computed tomography scan today revealed an abnormality in the left parietal lobe compatible with ischemic infarction in the distribution of the left middle cerebral artery. Past medical history includes hypertension, hyperlipidemia, and occasional low-back pain. Patient is currently taking atenolol 25 mg qd, simvastatin 20 mg qd, and a baby aspirin. Blood test at admission revealed normal blood urea nitrogen, electrolytes, and blood gases. Lumbar puncture was negative; electrocardiogram showed an old nonsymptomatic infarct. Admitting diagnosis: Patient is now being admitted to inpatient rehabilitation unit 3 days post–left cerebrovascular accident (stroke) of the middle cerebral artery distribution with resultant right hemiparesis; in addition, patient exhibits mild chronic obstructive lung disease and mild emphysema.

Physical therapy order for examination and treatment received.

Subjective
Patient is unable to communicate verbally. He can communicate by nodding or shaking his head to indicate yes or no. A social history was obtained from his wife during the initial examination. Patient lives with his wife, who is in good health, in a one-story house. The house has two steps without a railing at the entry. There are carpeted, tiled, and hardwood floors; the shower does not have grab bars or a shower seat. Patient has two daughters, who both live out of town. Patient's goal is to return home and to be walking and be able to communicate; these are his wife's goals as well. Wife states that they have neighbors and friends who will help her take care of her husband. Patient has been sleeping a lot since admission, but before the stroke, he and his wife liked to walk for exercise, camped, visited their daughters, and golfed. Patient was in good health before the stroke. Patient nodded yes when asked for consent to perform therapy; wife also agrees to her husband's participation in therapy.

Objective
Appearance, Rest Posture, and Equipment
Patient is supine in bed on a pressure-relieving mattress. His right shoulder is internally rotated and adducted; right elbow is in maximum flexion, and right wrist and fingers are also flexed. His right hip is extended, adducted, and internally rotated; right knee is extended, and right ankle is in plantar flexion and inversion. The left extremities are resting at the patient's side. Patient has a catheter.

Systems Review
Communication/Cognition: Patient is unable to communicate verbally except for one-word answers, such as yes and no. Is

CASE STUDIES REHABILITATION UNIT INITIAL EXAMINATION AND EVALUATION—cont'd

reliable with yes/no questions via head nods. Is alert and oriented x3.

Cardiovascular/Pulmonary: Blood pressure = 114/71 mm Hg; heart rate = 58 bpm; RR = 11 breaths/min using 2-chest 2-diaphragm breathing pattern. Minimal edema noted in right ankle.

Integumentary: Both upper extremities (UEs) and lower extremities (LEs) are not impaired.

Musculoskeletal: Left (L) UE and LE gross range of motion (ROM)—not impaired; right (R) UE and LE gross ROM—impaired; (L) UE and LE gross strength—not impaired; (R) UE and LE strength—impaired.

Neuromuscular: Gait and transfers are impaired; balance is impaired; motor function: (R) UE and LE are impaired; (L) UE and LE are not impaired.

Learning Preferences: Learning barriers caused by inability to expressively communicate; education needs include safety and precautions, activities of daily living (ADLs), and functional mobility training.

Tests and Measures

Anthropometrics: Height 5 feet 11 inches, weight 180 lbs., body mass index 25 (20 to 24 is normal).

Arousal, Attention, Cognition: Patient is alert and awake. He often loses focus but regains attention when his name is called. Patient able to respond to one-step commands consistently.

Cranial Nerve Integrity: Both pupils have direct and consensual responses to light. Peripheral vision is within functional limits (WFL). Horizontal, vertical, and diagonal smooth pursuit and tracking are WFL and symmetric in both eyes. Facial sensation is present. Facial movement is unimpaired. The uvula and tongue are in midline.

Joint Integrity and Mobility: Right (R) UE active movement is limited to one-quarter of flexion and extension synergies. Passive ROM is WFL in the (R) UE but rhythmic rotation is used to relax (R) UE; (R) LE is able to actively move through one-half of the flexion synergy with assist. Right LE actively moves back into full extension synergy from flexion synergy. No other active movements are possible. Passive ROM of (R) LE is WFL. (L) UE and LE active ROM is WFL bilaterally.

Reflex Integrity: Deep tendon reflexes 3 + (R) biceps, brachioradialis, patellar, and Achilles. All deep tendon reflexes 2 + on (L). Babinski present on (R); absent on (L). No associated or primitive reflexes are present. Moderate increased tone in (R) shoulder internal rotators and adductors; (R) biceps; (R) wrist and finger flexors; minimal increase in tone in (R) hip adductors, internal rotators, and extensors; (R) knee extensors; and (R) ankle plantar flexors and invertors also present with a minimal increase in muscle tone.

Motor Function: Bridging is performed asymmetrically, and patient's right pelvis is retracted, posteriorly tilted, and rotated to the right. Bridging improves with approximation at knees through heels and manual tapping on right gluteus maximus.

Posture: In supine, patient's head is turned to the right with UEs and LEs positioned as described previously. In sitting, patient leans to the left and has a forward head, rounded shoulders, increased thoracic kyphosis, and posterior pelvic tilt; right foot is placed in front of left with heel off floor. Patient uses the left upper extremity to support self in sitting.

Neuromotor Development: Patient demonstrates head righting bilaterally. Trunk righting is delayed on the right but present on the left. Protective reactions are absent on the right.

Sensory Integrity: Light touch sensation is intact on the left. Light touch sensation is impaired on the dorsum and palm of the right hand; the dorsum, heel, and ball of the foot; and the lower one-third of the right LE. Proprioception is impaired distally in right wrist, fingers, ankle, and toes.

Pain: Patient does not report any pain verbally or through facial grimacing. A pain scale is not administered.

Range of Motion: Right UE demonstrates little active movement from initial resting position. Patient moves his right UE back into shoulder internal rotation and adduction, elbow flexion, and wrist and finger flexion once placed in recovery position. Right LE hip, knee flexors, ankle dorsiflexors, and trunk musculature are weak, with difficulty in muscle recruitment causing decreased ability to initiate movement.

Bed Mobility: Patient rolls to left and right from hook-lying position with minimal assist of 1 to provide approximation through the right knee toward the ankle. Patient has been instructed in interlacing fingers together and holding hands in midline during rolling. He requires minimal assist of 1 to scoot, with manual cues given on opposite hip and shoulder to assist with weight shifting and moving pelvis in bed.

Transfers: Supine-to-sit: moderate assist of 1 to move right LE on and off bed and guide shoulders. Sit-to-stand: moderate assist of 1 to keep feet apart and block right knee.

Stand-Pivot Transfer: Maximal assist of 1. Patient's right knee buckles two times when three steps are taken to turn and sit. He also requires verbal and manual cues to stand upright because of a posterior lean.

Sitting Balance: Patient leans to the left unless the right UE is extended in weight-bearing. Once patient supports himself using both UEs, he requires only stand-by assist (SBA) to remain upright. However, he is unable to weight shift and take any outside perturbations without losing his balance. Patient closes eyes in sitting, and this causes him to sway significantly.

Standing Balance: Patient leans to the left and needs moderate assist of 1 to remain upright. He requires manual assist to keep his right knee from collapsing. He also tends to shift his center of mass posteriorly, which causes him to lean backward in an unsafe upright position. Verbal and tactile cues are applied to the buttocks to assist with hip extension and to promote upright standing.

Gait/Locomotion: Patient able to ambulate 5 feet x 1 with maximal assist of 1 on level surfaces. Patient requires tactile cue at right hip to decrease hiking and to assist with advancement. Manual cues are also needed to assist with right knee extension and to initiate weight shifts. Stairs not assessed to this date secondary to patient's status.

Wheelchair Mobility: Patient is able to propel self 20 feet in wheelchair using his left extremities with moderate assist of 1.

Self-Care: Patient is dependent in grooming activities with his right UE because he lacks voluntary movement. He is also unable to dress, tie his shoes, and bathe because of insufficient sitting and standing balance.

Assessment/Evaluation

Patient is a 67-year-old man who is 3 days post–left stroke of the middle cerebral artery distribution with right hemiparesis

Continued

CASE STUDIES REHABILITATION UNIT INITIAL EXAMINATION AND EVALUATION—cont'd

and sensory deficits. Patient able to complete 45-minute initial examination without changes in physiologic measures although appears lethargic and slightly fatigued.

Functional Independence Measure: Bed transfers, 2; wheelchair transfers, 2; walk/wheelchair, 1; stairs, not assessed.

Brunnstrom stages: right UE—level 3; right LE—level 3.

Problem List
1. Decreased voluntary movement of right UE and LE.
2. Decreased functional mobility (bed mobility, transfers, and gait).
3. Decreased balance in sitting and standing.
4. Decreased sensory awareness of right UE and LE.
5. Decreased ability to perform self-care activities.
6. Decreased ability to verbally communicate.
7. Patient and family lack understanding of the rehabilitation process.
8. Patient unable to participate in leisure time activities.

Diagnosis: Patient shows neuromuscular impairments with impaired motor function and sensory integrity associated with nonprogressive disorders of the central nervous system acquired in adulthood.

Prognosis: Patient will demonstrate optimal motor function, sensory integrity, and the highest level of functioning in home, community, and leisure environments within the context of the impairments, functional limitations, and disability. Number of physical therapy visits in rehabilitation is up to 60 visits. Patient's rehabilitation potential for stated goals is good secondary to his level of motor return in right LE and family support.

Short-Term Goals (to be Achieved by 1 Week)
1. Patient will segmentally roll to the right and left with minimal assist of 1.
2. Patient will transfer from supine to sitting with minimal assist.
3. Patient will transfer from sitting to standing with minimal assist of 1.
4. Patient will perform a stand-pivot transfer with moderate assist of 1.
5. Patient will sit on edge of the mat or bed with SBA and a neutral pelvis and erect posture, while performing ADLs with the left UE.
6. Patient will actively move right arm to mouth to feed himself.
7. Patient will independently propel himself in wheelchair to therapies.
8. Patient will ambulate 20 feet with moderate assist of 1 with assistive device on level surfaces.

Long-Term Goals (to be Achieved by 3 Weeks)
1. Patient will be independent in rolling to the right and left.
2. Patient will be independent in supine to sitting.
3. Patient will be independent with sit-to-stand transfers.
4. Patient will perform stand-pivot transfer with stand by assist of 1.
5. Patient will sit independently to don and doff shoes and put on pants independently.
6. Patient will stand for 5 minutes with arms supported on counter/sink/etc, with SBA of 1 while performing self-care.
7. Patient will actively move right UE above head with appropriate mechanics to dress himself and perform self-care tasks.
8. Patient will ambulate at least 150 feet with least restrictive assistive device at modified independent level on level surfaces.
9. Patient will ascend/descend 12 steps with stand-by assistance for safety.
10. Family will demonstrate an understanding of correct techniques to assist patient with transfers and gait.
11. Patient will perform home exercise and aerobic training program independently.

Plan
Treatment Schedule: The physical therapist (PT) and physical therapist assistant (PTA) will see the patient twice a day, Monday through Saturday, for 45-minute treatment sessions for the next 3 weeks. This plan was discussed with the patient and his wife and was agreed on. Treatment sessions will focus on positioning, early shoulder and hip care, functional mobility training, intensive gait/locomotor training, patient/family education, and discharge planning. The PT will reexamine the patient and make necessary changes to the plan as needed in 1 week. Anticipated discharge from inpatient rehabilitation is after 3 weeks.

Coordination, Communication, and Documentation: The PT and PTA will communicate with patient, wife, physician, speech pathologist, and occupational therapist on a regular basis. In addition, the PT will communicate about discharge date, findings from this examination, necessary assistive devices for home, and continued therapy or services after discharge. Outcomes of rehabilitation will be documented on a weekly basis.

Interventions:
Patient/Client Instruction: Patient and his family will receive verbal and written instructions for the home exercise program. Patient and his family will be instructed in transfer and gait techniques. Education regarding the patient's condition and the prevention of secondary complications will be provided to the patient and his wife. A home assessment is recommended before discharge.

Integumentary Protection Techniques:
1. Positioning:
   a. Side-lying on affected side with right UE and LE in recovery position to increase right side awareness and decrease the dominance of the synergy patterns.
   b. Supine and side-lying on left side with right UE and LE in recovery position to decrease tone.

Therapeutic Exercise:
1. Early shoulder and hip care:
   a. Side-lying scapular protraction to promote scapular mobility and normal scapular rhythm: (1) begin with the clinician's hand on scapula and upper arm and apply approximation through the shoulder joint; (2) as patient gains control, the manual contacts will move farther distally until the right arm is supported by a pillow and the clinician is applying approximation through the right palm.
   b. Double-arm elevation in supine to increase ROM in right UE: (1) left hand will grasp right hand interlocking fingers and the right thumb on top of left; (2) left arm will assist the right in moving the UEs overhead; (3) progress this to active-assisted ROM and, finally, active ROM.

CASE STUDIES REHABILITATION UNIT INITIAL EXAMINATION AND EVALUATION—cont'd

c. Bridging: (1) approximation is given through knees to promote heel weight-bearing, may use sheet to promote symmetrical pelvic motions progressing to bridging with agonist reversals, alternating isometrics, and rhythmic stabilization for core stability to assist with sitting and standing balance; (2) start hip extension over mat: initially have right hip in flexion and progress to starting with the hip in neutral to increase hip extensor strength, thus increasing step length; (3) supine with ball under feet and knees: trunk rotations, posterior pelvic tilt and anterior pelvic tilt to promote trunk-pelvic-hip control to increase sitting and standing balance; (4) proprioceptive neuromuscular facilitation chops and lifts in sitting.

d. Bridging with manual contacts on right gluteus maximus to facilitate symmetrical pelvic motions and approximation at knee to promote weight-bearing through heel.

2. ROM and strengthening exercises:

a. Air splint on right UE: (1) in sitting, have patient bear weight on right UE and reach across body to facilitate proprioception and inhibit flexion synergy; (2) have left UE reach across body for objects (glass, food, clothes, etc.). Have patient attempt reaching for objects with the right UE; provide manual contacts at the scapula to promote scapular abduction and upward rotation.

b. Instruct patient in self-ROM to the right UE and right LE. Perform stretching to the right wrist and fingers and right ankle to prevent contracture development.

c. Place a mirror in front of the patient in sitting and standing to encourage an upright symmetrical posture, as well as movement of the right UE and LE.

Motor Function Training

a. Practice supine-to-sit transfers using diagonals to activate trunk and abdominals.

b. Practice sit-to-stand transfers, beginning at higher surfaces and progressing to lower surfaces to activate quads in different angles and enhance timing of muscle recruitment. Also practice sit-to-stand transfers from different surfaces.

c. Lateral weight shifts in sitting to assist with scooting to edge of mat in preparation for transfers.

d. Sitting with neutral pelvis and erect posture statically, sitting on a foam surface and maintaining sitting balance.

e. Dynamic sitting balance activities: weight shifts, reaching outside limits of stability, reaching to the floor (as in putting on and removing shoes) so patient can become independent in ADLs while maintaining neutral pelvis and erect trunk.

f. Static and dynamic standing balance activities: begin with weight shifts in standing, progressing to forward and back stepping with both LEs, standing on foam and maintaining an upright position, tandem standing, standing on one foot, step-ups, side stepping, mini squats, maneuvering around obstacles; progress to holding and swinging a golf club.

g. Modified plantigrade to promote weight-bearing through UEs with neutral hip and knee flexion to promote strength and control for swing phase of gait. Practice performance of ADLs and meal preparation in the position.

h. Negotiation of wheelchair on level surfaces; instruction in operation of wheelchair parts.

i. Transfer to the floor: transitions from prone on elbows, four-point, tall-kneeling, half-kneeling to standing.

j. Gait training: initiate body-weight support treadmill ambulation 1 time a day for 45 minutes. Also initiate overground ambulation with assistive device and manual assist. Challenge patient with obstacles, weight the LEs, introduce different environmental terrains. Begin stair climbing as the patient is able to tolerate.

k. Dual-task training: Practice carrying an object while walking, encourage verbalizations during standing and walking tasks.

Family Training:

a. Schedule family training days.

b. Work with family on positioning, transfers, car transfers, and ambulation.

c. Educate family regarding the patient's condition, potential complications, barriers to recovery, need for architectural modifications, safety concerns, and probability of long-term sequelae.

Discharge Planning:

a. Perform a home assessment if indicated.

b. Secure necessary medical equipment, including assistive device, tub bench, and elevated toilet seat.

c. Teach patient and family home exercise program including strengthening exercises and aerobic conditioning program.

d. Refer patient to outpatient services and provide resources regarding social support.

Questions to Think About

- What type of specific strengthening exercises should be included in the patient's plan of care?
- How can aerobic conditioning be included in the patient's treatment program?
- What types of activities or exercises would be included as part of the patient's home exercise program?

REFERENCES

Abe H, Kondo T, Oouchida Y, et al.: Prevalence and length of recovery of pusher syndrome based on cerebral hemisphere lesion in patients with acute stroke, *Stroke* 43:1654–1656, 2012.

Academy of Neurologic Physical Therapy: *StrokEDGE II outcome measures student*, 2018. Available at: http://neuropt.org/docs/default-source/edge-documents/strokedge-ii-student.pdf?sfvrsn.17fc5443_2. Accessed June 20, 2018.

Allison LK, Fuller K: Balance and vestibular dysfunction. In Umphred DA, Lazaro RT, Roller ML, Burton GU, editors: *Neurological rehabilitation*, ed 6, St. Louis, MO, 2013, Elsevier, pp 653–709.

American Heart Association, American Stroke Association: *FACTS: Preventable. Treatable. Beatable. Stroke in the U.S.*, 2017. Available at: heart.org/idc/groups/heart-public/@wcm/@adv/documents/downloadable/ucm_305054.pdf. Accessed July 9, 2019.

American Physical Therapy Association: *Direction and supervision of the physical therapist assistant, HOD 06-18-28-35*, Alexandria, VA, 2018, American Physical Therapy Association.

American Stroke Association: *About stroke*, Dallas, TX, 2020. Available at: www.stroke.org/en/about-stroke. Accessed January 7, 2020.

Baker-Herman TL, Fuller DD, Bavis RW, et al.: BDNF is necessary and sufficient for spinal respiratory plasticity following intermittent hypoxia, *Nat Neurosci* 7:48–55, 2004.

Baldrige RB: Functional assessment of measurements, *Neurol Rep* 17:3–10, 1993.

Billinger SA, Arena R, Bernhardt J, et al.: Physical activity and exercise recommendations for stroke survivors: a statement for healthcare professionals from the American Heart Association/American Stroke Association, *Stroke* 45:2532–2553, 2014.

Billinger SA, Mattlage AE, Ashenden AL, et al.: Aerobic exercise in subacute stroke improves cardiovascular health and physical performance, *JNPT* 36:159–165, 2012.

Bobath B: *Adult hemiplegia: evaluation and treatment*, ed 3, Oxford, UK, 1990, Butterworth-Heinemann, pp 9–66.

Bohannon RW, Smith MB: Interrater reliability of a modified Ashworth scale of muscle spasticity, *Phys Ther* 67:206–207, 1987.

Bonifer NM, Anderson KM: Application of constraint-induced movement therapy on an individual with severe chronic upper-extremity hemiplegia, *Phys Ther* 83:384–398, 2003.

Centers for Disease Control and Prevention: *Preventing stroke: healthy living*, 2018b. Available at: www.cdc.gov/stroke/healthy_living.htm. Accessed June 14, 2019.

Centers for Disease Control and Prevention: *Family history and other characteristics that increase risk for stroke*, 2018c. Available at: www.cdc.gov/stroke/family_history.htm. Accessed June 14, 2019.

Centers for Disease Control and Prevention: *Know the signs and symptoms of a stroke*, 2018a. Available at: www.cdc.gov/dhdsp/data_statistics/fact_sheets/fs_strokesigns.htm. Accessed June 14, 2019.

Centers for Disease Control and Prevention: *Stroke facts*, 2017a. Available at: www.cdc.gov/stroke/facts.htm. Accessed June 14, 2019.

Centers for Disease Control and Prevention: *Progress has stalled in US stroke death rates after decades of decline*, 2017b. Available at: www.cdc.gov/media/releases/2017/p0906-vs-stroke.html. Accessed July 14, 2019.

Centers for Medicare and Medicaid Services: Quality Initiatives General Information, 2019a. Available at: www.cms.gov/Medicare/Quality-Initiatives-Patient-Assessment-Instruments/Quality-InitiativesGenInfo. Accessed January 20, 2020.

Centers for Medicare and Medicaid Services: Inpatient Rehabilitation Facility Patient Assessment Instrument, 2019b. Available at: www.cms.gov/Medicare/Quality-Initiatives-Patient-Assessment-Instruments/IRF-Quality-Reporting/Downloads/Proposed-IRF-PAI-Version-30-Effective-October-1-2019-FY2020.pdf. Accessed January 20, 2020.

Cha J, Heng C, Reinkensmeyer DJ, et al.: Locomotor ability in spinal rats is dependent on the amount of activity imposed on the hindlimbs during treadmill training, *J Neurotrauma* 24:1000–1012, 2007.

Chau C, Barbeau H, Rossignol S: Early locomotor training with clonidine in spinal cats, *J Neurophysiol* 79:392–409, 1998.

Combs-Miller SA, Kalpathi Parameswaran A, Colburn D, et al.: Body weight-supported treadmill training vs. overground walking training for persons with chronic stroke: a pilot randomized controlled trial, *Clin Rehabil* 28:873–884, 2014.

Craik RL: Abnormalities of motor behavior. In *Contemporary management of motor control problems [Proceedings of the II STEP Conference]*. Alexandria, VA, 1991, Foundation for Physical Therapy, pp 155–164.

Cumming TB, Thrift AG, Collier JM, et al.: Very early mobilization after stroke fast tracks return to walking: further results from the Phase II AVERT randomized control trial, *Stroke* 42:153–158, 2011.

Davies PM: *Steps to follow: a guide to the treatment of adult hemiplegia*, Berlin, 1985, Springer Verlag, pp 266–284.

Denissen S, Staring W, Kunkel D, et al: Interventions for preventing falls in people after stroke. Cochrane Database Syst Rev 2019, Issue 10. Art. No.: CD008728. DOI:10.1002/14651858.CD008728.pub3.

De Leon RD, Hodgson JA, Roy RR, Edgerton VR: Locomotor capacity attributable to step training versus spontaneous recovery after spinalization in adult cats, *J Neurophysiol* 79:1329–1340, 1998.

De Rooij IJM, van de Port IGL, Meijer JWG: Effect of virtual reality training on balance and gait ability in patients with stroke: systematic review and meta-analysis, *Phys Ther* 96(12):1905–1918, 2016.

Deutsch JE, O'Sullivan SB: Stroke. In O'Sullivan SB, Schmitz TJ, Fulk GD, editors: *Physical rehabilitation*, ed 6, Philadelphia, PA, 2019, FA Davis, pp 592–661.

Dieruf K, Poole JL, Gregory C, Rodriguez EJ, Spizman C: Comparative effectiveness of the GivMohr sling in subjects with flaccid upper limbs on subluxation through radiographic analysis, *Arch Phys Med Rehabil* 86:2324–2329, 2005.

Duncan PW, Badke MB: Measurement of motor performance and functional abilities following stroke. In Duncan PW, Badke MB, editors: *Stroke rehabilitation: the recovery of motor control*, Chicago, IL, 1987, Year Book, pp 199–221.

Duncan PW, Sullivan KJ, Behrman A, et al.: Body-weight support treadmill rehabilitation after stroke, *N Engl J Med* 354:2026–2036, 2011.

Edwardson MA: *Ischemic stroke prognosis in adults*, 2019, UpToDate. Available at: www.uptodate.com/contents/ischemic-stroke-prognosis-in-adults. Accessed July 11, 2019.

Etoom M, Hawamdeh M, Hawamdeh Z, et al.: Constraint-induced movement therapy as a rehabilitation intervention for upper extremity in stroke patients: systematic review and meta-analysis, *Int J Rehabil Res* 39(3):197–210, 2016.

Fong AJ, Cai LL, Otoshi CK, et al.: Spinal cord-transected mice learn to step in response to quipazine treatment and robotic training, *J Neurosci* 25:11738–11747, 2005.

Fulk GD: Locomotor training with body-weight support after stroke: the effects of different training parameters, *JNPT* 28:20–28, 2004.

Fuller KS: Stroke. In Goodman CC, Fuller KS, editors: *Pathology implications for the physical therapist*, ed 4, St. Louis, MO, 2015, Elsevier, pp 1507–1534.

Globas C, Becker C, Cerny J, et al.: Chronic stroke survivors benefit from high-intensity aerobic treadmill exercise: a randomized control trial, *Neurorehabil Neural Repair* 26(1):85–95, 2012.

Gordon NF, Gulanick M, Costa F, et al.: Physical activity and exercise recommendations for stroke survivors, *Circulation* 109:2031–2041, 2004.

Gordon BT, Durstine JL, Painter DL, Moore GE: In Moore GE, Durstine JL, Painter PL, editors. *ACSM's exercise management for persons with chronic diseases and disabilities*, Champaign, IL, 2016, Human Kinetics, pp 15–32.

Holleran CL, Rodriguez KS, Echauz A, Leech KA, Hornby TG: Potential contributions of training intensity on locomotor performance in individuals with chronic stroke, *JNPT* 39:95–102, 2015.

Holleran CL, Straube DD, Kinnaird CR, Leddy AL, Hornby TG: Feasibility and potential efficacy of high-intensity stepping training in variable contexts in subacute and chronic stroke, *Neurorehabil Neural Repair* 28(7):643–651, 2014.

Hornby TG, Holleran CL, Hennessy PW, et al.: Variable intensive early walking poststroke (views): a randomized controlled trial, *Neurorehabil Neural Repair* 2015.

Hornby TG, Moore JL, Lovell L, Roth EJ: Influence of skill and exercise training parameters on locomotor recovery during stroke rehabilitation, *Curr Opin Neurol* 29(6):677–683, 2016.

Hornby TG, Straube DS, Kinnaird CR, et al.: Importance of specificity, amount, and intensity of locomotor training to improve ambulatory function in patients poststroke, *Top Stroke Rehabil* 18:293–307, 2011.

Hou J, Forston BD, Lovegreen W, Fox JR: Lower limb orthoses for persons who have had a stroke. In Webster JB, Murphy DP, editors: *Atlas of orthoses and assistive devices*, ed 5, Philadelphia, PA, 2019, Elsevier, pp 289–295.

Jacobs BL, Fornal CA: Activity of serotonergic neurons in behaving animals, *Neuropsychopharmacology* 21:9S–15S, 1999.

Johnstone M: *Restoration of normal movement after stroke*, New York, 1995, Churchill Livingstone, pp 49–74.

Karnath HO, Broetz D: Understanding and treating pusher syndrome, *Phys Ther* 83:1119–1125, 2003.

Kleim JA, Jones TA: Principles of experience dependent neural plasticity: implications for rehabilitation after brain damage, *J Speech Lang Hear Res* 51:S225–S239, 2008.

Knutson JS, Makowski NS, Kilgore KL, Chae J: Neuromuscular electrical stimulation applications. In Webster JB, Murphy DP, editors: *Atlas of orthoses and assistive devices*, ed 5, Philadelphia, PA, 2019, Elsevier, pp 432–437.

Kollen BJ, Lennon S, Lyons B, et al.: The effectiveness of the Bobath concept in stroke rehabilitation, *Stroke* 40:e89–e87, 2009.

Lang CE, Macdonald JR, Reisman DS, et al.: Observation of amounts of movement practice provided during stroke rehabilitation, *Arch Phys Med Rehabil* 90:1692–1698, 2009.

Lang C, Macdonald J, Gnip C: Counting repetitions: an observational study of outpatient therapy for people with hemiparesis post-stroke, *JNPT* 31:3–11, 2007.

Langhammer B, Stanghelle JK: Bobath or motor relearning programme? A comparison of two different approaches of physiotherapy in stroke rehabilitation: a randomized controlled study, *Clin Rehabil* 14:361–369, 2000.

Laver KE, Lange B, George S, et al.: Virtual reality for stroke rehabilitation, *Stroke* 49:e160–e161, 2018.

Liepert L, Bauder H, Miltner HR, et al.: Stroke rehabilitation constraint-induced movement therapy, *Stroke* 31:1210–1216, 2000.

Light KE: Clients with spasticity: to strengthen or not to strengthen, *Neurol Rep* 15:63–64, 1991.

Lubetzky-Vilnai A, Kartin D: The effect of balance training on balance performance in individuals poststroke: a systematic review, *JNPT* 34:127–137, 2010.

Lundy-Ekman L: *Neuroscience fundamentals for rehabilitation*, ed 5, St. Louis, MO, 2018, Elsevier, pp 284–285.

MacKay-Lyons MJ, Makrides L: Cardiovascular stress during a contemporary stroke rehabilitation program: is the intensity adequate to induce a training effect? *Arch Phys Med Rehabil* 83:1378–1383, 2002.

Macko R: Stroke, brain trauma, and spinal cord injuries. In Moore GE, Durstine JL, Painter PL, editors: *ACSM's exercise management for persons with chronic diseases and disabilities*, Champaign, IL, 2016, Human Kinetics, pp 237–247.

Maitland GD: *Peripheral manipulation*, ed 2, Boston, MA, 1977, Butterworths, pp 3–31.

Mehrholz J, Thomas S, Werner C, et al.: Electromechanical-assisted training for walking after stroke, *Cochrane Database Syst Rev* May 2017. Available at: www.cochranelibrary.com/cdsr/doi/10.1002/14651858.CD006185.pub4/full. Accessed June 21, 2019.

Mehrholz J, Elsner TS: Treadmill training and body weight support for walking after stroke, *Cochrane Database Syst Rev* (8):CD002840, 2017. doi:10.1002/14651858.CD002840.pub4. Accessed July 28, 2019.

Middleton A, Merlo-Rains A, Peters DM, et al.: Body weight-supported treadmill training is no better than overground training for individuals with chronic stroke: a randomized controlled trial, *Top Stroke Rehabil* 21:462–476, 2014.

Moore JL, Hornby TG: *Walk the walk: high-intensity gait training in stroke rehabilitation*, October 2018, Educational Course, Institute for Knowledge Translation.

Moore JL, Potter K, Blankshain K, et al.: A core set of outcome measures for adults with neurologic conditions undergoing rehabilitation: a clinical practice guideline, *JNPT* 42:174–220, 2018.

Moore JL, Roth EJ, Killian C, Hornby TG: Locomotor training improves daily stepping activity and gait efficiency in individuals poststroke who have reached a "plateau" in recovery, *Stroke* 41:129–135, 2010.

Mulroy SJ, Klassen T, Gronley JK, et al.: Gait parameters associated with responsiveness to treadmill training with body-weight support after stroke: an exploratory study, *Phys Ther* 90:209–223, 2010.

National Aphasia Association. *Aphasia fact sheet*, 2019. Available at: www.aphasia.org/aphasia-resources/aphasia-factsheet. Accessed July 13, 2019.

National Stroke Association: Rehab therapy after a stroke, Centennial, CO, 2019b. Available at: www.stroke.org/en/life-after-stroke/stroke-rehab/rehab-therapy-after-a-stroke. Accessed July 23, 2019.

National Stroke Association: *What is TIA?* Centennial, CO, 2019a. Available at: https://www.stroke.org/understand-stroke/what-is-stroke/what-is-tia/. Accessed June 14, 2019.

Ostrosky KM: Facilitation vs motor control, *Clin Manag* 10:34–40, 1990.

Rehabilitation Measures Database: *Ashworth scale/modified Ashworth scale*, 2016a. Available at: www.sralab.org/rehabilitation-measures. Accessed July 11, 2019.

Rehabilitation Measures Database: *Fugl-Meyer assessment of motor recovery after stroke*, 2016b. Available at: www.sralab.org/rehabilitation-measures. Accessed July 13, 2019.

Rehabilitation Measures Database: *Functional independence measure*, 2015. Available at: www.rehabmeasures.org/lists/rehabmeasures/dispform.aspxID889. Accessed July 11, 2019.

Roller M: The pusher syndrome, *JNPT* 28:29–34, 2004.

Roth EJ, Harvey RL: Rehabilitation of stroke syndromes. In Braddom RL, editor: *Physical medicine and rehabilitation*, Philadelphia, PA, 1996, WB Saunders, pp 1053–1087.

Ryerson SD: Movement dysfunction associated with hemiplegia. In Umphred DA, Burton GU, Lazaro RT, Roller ML, editors: *Neurological rehabilitation*, ed 6, St. Louis, MO, 2013, Elsevier, pp 711–751.

Sawner KA, LaVigne JM: *Brunnstrom's movement therapy in hemiplegia*, ed 2, Philadelphia, PA, 1992, JB Lippincott, pp 41–65.

Schmid A, Duncan PW, Studenski S, et al.: Improvements in speed-based gait classifications are meaningful, *Stroke* 38:2096–2100, 2007.

Schmitz TJ: Examination and modification of the environment. In O'Sullivan SB, Schmitz TJ, Fulk GD, editors: *Physical rehabilitation*, ed 7, Philadelphia, 2019, FA Davis, pp 316–360.

Shumway-Cook A, Woollacott MH: *Motor control: translating research into clinical practice*, ed 5, Philadelphia, PA, 2017, Wolters Kluwer, pp 16–18, 407–461.

Senelick RC: Technological advances in stroke rehabilitation: high tech marries high touch, *US Neurol* 6(2):102–104, 2011.

Suputtitada A, Yooktanan P, Rarerng-Ying T: Effect of partial body weight support treadmill training in chronic stroke patients, *J Med Assoc Thai* 87(Suppl 2):S107–S111, 2004.

Tang A, Eng JJ: Physical fitness training after stroke, *Phys Ther* 94:9–13, 2014.

Taub E, Uswatt G: Constraint-induced movement therapy: answers and questions after two decades of research, *NeuroRehabilitation* 21:93–95, 2006.

Teasell R, Hussein N: Brain reorganization, recovery, and organized care. In *Stroke rehabilitation clinician handbook*, 2016a, Heart and Stroke Foundation, Canadian Partnership for Stroke Recovery. Available at: www.ebrsr.com. Accessed July 26, 2019.

Teasell R, Hussein N: Motor Rehabilitation 4A. Lower extremity and mobility and 4B Rehab of hemiplegic upper extremity post stroke. In *Stroke rehabilitation clinician handbook*, 2016b, Heart and Stroke Foundation, Canadian Partnership for Stroke Recovery. Available at: www.ebrsr.com. Accessed July 26, 2019.

United States Department of Health and Human Services: *Physical activity guidelines for americans*, ed 2, Washington, DC, 2018, pp 78–86.

Umphred DA, Bly NN, Lazaro RT, Roller M: Interventions for clients with movement limitations. In Umphred DA, Lazaro RT, Roller ML, Burton GU, editors: *Neurological rehabilitation*, ed 6, St. Louis, MO, 2013, Elsevier, 191–249.

Uniform Data System for Medical Rehabilitation: *The FIM® instrument: its background, structure, and usefulness*, Buffalo, 2012, UDS. Available at: http://www.udsmr.org/Documents/The_FIM_Instrument_Background_Structure_and_Usefulness.pdf. Updated July 8, 2014. Accessed September 14, 2014.

Van Peppen RP, Kwakkel G, Wood-Dauphinee S, et al.: The impact of physical therapy on functional outcomes after stroke: what's the evidence? *Clin Rehabil* 18:833–862, 2004.

Van Duijnhoven HJ, Heeren A, Peters MA, et al.: Effects of exercise therapy on balance capacity in chronic stroke: systematic review and meta-analysis, *Stroke* 47:2603–2610, 2016.

Visintin M, Barbeau H, Korner-Bitensky N, Mayo N: A new approach to retrain gait in stroke patients through body weight support and treadmill stimulation, *Stroke* 29:1122–1128, 1998.

Watchie J: Cardiopulmonary implications of specific diseases. In Hillegass EA, Sadowsky HS, editors: *Essentials of cardiopulmonary physical therapy*, Philadelphia, PA, 1994, WB Saunders, pp 285–323.

Wattchow KA, McDonnell MN, Hillier SL: Rehabilitation interventions for upper limb function in the first four weeks following stroke: a systematic review and meta-analysis of the evidence, *Arch Phys Med Rehabil* 99(2):367–382, 2018.

Webster JB, Darter BJ: Principles of normal and pathologic gait. In Webster JB, Murphy DP, editors: *Atlas of orthoses and assistive devices*, ed 5, Philadelphia, PA, 2019, Elsevier, pp 49–62.

Whiteside A: Clinical goals and application of NDT facilitation, *NDTA Netw* 2–14, Sept–Oct 1997.

Wolf SL, Winstein CJ, Miller JP, et al.: Effect of constraint-induced movement therapy on upper extremity function 3 to 9 months after stroke: the EXCITE randomized clinical trial, *JAMA* 296:2095–2104, 2006.

12

Traumatic Brain Injuries

Mary Kessler and Jordana Lockwich

OBJECTIVES

After reading this chapter, the student will be able to:

1. Identify causes and mechanisms of traumatic brain injuries.
2. List secondary complications associated with traumatic brain injuries.
3. Explain specific treatment interventions to facilitate functional movement.
4. Discuss strategies that will improve cognitive deficits.
5. Select outcome measures to track recovery and progress in patients with traumatic brain injury.

INTRODUCTION

The Brain Injury Association of America defines traumatic brain injury (TBI) as "an alteration in brain function, or other evidence of brain pathology caused by an external force" (Brain Injury Association of America [BIA], 2019). Effects of TBI include impairments in motor function, cognitive abilities, movement and sensory deficits, and disruptions in behavioral responses and emotions. These impairments may be either temporary or permanent and not only affect the individual but also the individual's family (Centers for Disease Control and Prevention [CDC], 2014).

More than 3.5 million adults and children sustain a brain injury annually. Of that number, approximately 2.2 million Americans are treated for their injuries. And, of that number, 280,000 individuals are admitted to the hospital with a diagnosis of mild to moderate TBI; 80,000 incur a TBI with a significant loss of function, including the onset of long-term disability; and more than 56,000 people die as a result of their injury (BAI, 2019; CDC, 2014). Because TBI may result in lifetime impairments of an individual's physical, cognitive, and psychosocial functioning, TBI is considered a condition of major public health significance (CDC, 2014).

The economic impact of TBI is also significant. The estimated cost for direct and indirect medical costs was $76.5 billion in 2010 (CDC, 2014). Cost for acute-care hospitalization and rehabilitation is $9 to $10 billion annually. Average lifetime expenses associated with caring for someone with TBI range from $600,000 to $1,875,000. These figures may, however, underestimate the total costs to families and society because they do not include lost wages and the costs associated with social service programs (CDC, 2014).

The most common cause of TBI is falls (40.5%); followed by unknown/other (19%); being struck by an object (15.5%); motor vehicle accidents (MVA) (14.3%); and assaults (10.7%)

(BAI, 2019). Men are more frequently affected than women at a ratio of 2:1. The incidence of TBI peaks at three different age ranges: 1 to 2 years, 15 to 24 years, and the elderly (those over 75 years of age) (CDC, 2014). Child abuse, including shaken baby syndrome; falls; automobile accidents; and bicycle accidents are the primary causes of brain injury in children. The risk of severe brain injury in children can be reduced by 88% if children wear bicycle helmets (McCulloch and Fuller, 2015).

It is difficult to predict an individual's outcome after TBI. Several factors have been identified that may contribute to the person's outcome after brain injury. These include (1) the amount of immediate damage from the impact or insult; (2) low initial scores on the Glasgow Coma Scale, especially in the eye opening and motor response categories; (3) the cumulative effects of secondary brain damage; (4) the individual's premorbid cognitive characteristics, such as intellect, level of education, and memory; (5) the presence or absence of substance abuse; (6) age of the individual at the onset of injury; and (7) the individual's preinjury personality, including the quality of interpersonal relationships and work history (Fulk and Nirider, 2019; Osterman et al., 2018; Winkler, 2013).

CLASSIFICATIONS OF BRAIN INJURIES

Open and Closed Injuries

The two major classifications of brain injuries are open and closed injuries. *Open injuries* result from penetrating types of wounds. such as those received from a gunshot, knife, or other sharp objects. The skull can be either fractured or displaced. The damage to the brain appears to follow the path of the object's entry and exit, thus resulting in more focal deficits. Furthermore, with an open injury, the meninges are compromised, and the risk of infection is increased as bony fragments, hair, and skin penetrate brain tissue. A *closed or intracranial injury* is the second type of injury, and several subtypes are recognized. An individual is said to have sustained a closed injury when there is an impact to the head, but the skull does not fracture or displace. Neural (brain) tissue is damaged and the dura remains intact.

Subtypes of Traumatic Brain Injuries

Concussion

A concussion, the most common type of TBI, can result from either an open or closed injury. A concussion is defined as a "trauma that induces an alteration in mental status (physical and cognitive abilities) that may or may not involve a loss of consciousness" (BIA, 2019). Symptoms of a concussion include dizziness, disorientation, blurred vision, difficulty in concentrating, alterations in sleep patterns, nausea, headache, and a loss of balance (BIA, 2019). The individual can have retrograde (before the injury) or anterograde (posttraumatic) amnesia. Retrograde amnesia is characterized by a loss of memory of the events before the injury, whereas in posttraumatic amnesia, individuals are unable to learn new information. The duration of posttraumatic amnesia (PTA) is considered a clinical indicator of the severity of the injury (McCulloch and Fuller, 2015). A recent study showed that the duration of PTA may be a better predictor of outcome than Glasgow Coma Scale (GCS) score or time to follow commands (Perrin et al., 2015). With a concussion, there is no structural damage to the brain tissue; however, because of the shearing forces, the synapses are disrupted.

Three different grades of concussion have been identified. In a grade 1 concussion, the person is confused and dazed, and experiences difficulty in following directions and thinking clearly, but the individual remains conscious. Symptoms resolve within 15 minutes. Grade 2 concussions are characterized by consciousness, although the person develops amnesia, and the symptoms last longer than 15 minutes. Persons with grade 3 concussions are unconscious for several seconds or minutes and there is an observable change in the individual's physical, cognitive, or behavioral function. Concussions represent a significant health concern for the public as it is "estimated that 1.6 to 3.8 million sport- and recreation-related brain injuries" occur each year (Borich et al., 2013). For most individuals who sustain a concussion, a full recovery is possible (BIA, 2019). Concussion management, including return to sport, is a significant issue for medical professionals and has been a popular point of discussion in the media. Physical and cognitive rest followed by a gradual return of activity is recommended (Borich et al., 2013). The American Physical Therapy Association (APTA, 2013) has endorsed legislation and practice guidelines related to the risks for concussion, assessment standardization, and return to play guidelines. Athletes should not return to sport until they are symptom-free and without medications (Giza et al., 2013).

Contusion

A contusion is another type of intracranial injury. With a *contusion*, bruising on the surface of the brain is sustained at the time of impact. Small blood vessels on the surface of the brain hemorrhage and lead to the condition. A contusion that occurs on the same side of the brain as the impact is called a *coup lesion*. Surface hemorrhages that occur on the opposite side of the trauma as a result of deceleration are called *contrecoup lesions*. The acceleration associated with contrecoup injuries can cause further vessel occlusion and edema formation. Fig. 12.1 depicts both a coup injury and a contrecoup injury.

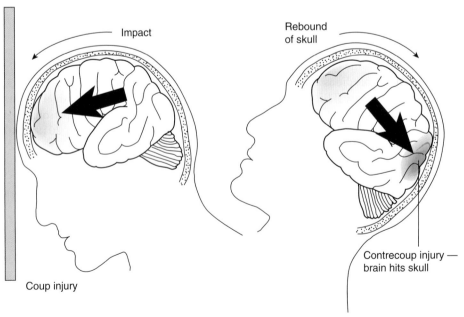

Impact

Rebound of skull

Contrecoup injury — brain hits skull

Coup injury

Fig. 12.1 Types of contusions: coup and contrecoup. (Modified from Gould BE: *Pathophysiology for the health-related professions*, Philadelphia, 1997, Saunders.)

Damage to brain tissue may take several forms. The extent of the injury depends on the nature of the insult and the type and amount of force that impacts the head. In individuals with open wounds, local brain damage occurs at the site of impact. Secondary brain damage can occur as a consequence of lacerations to cerebral tissue, as is frequently seen with skull fractures. Acceleration and deceleration forces can produce coup or contrecoup injury. Polar brain damage can occur as the brain moves forward within the skull. The frontal and temporal lobes are most frequently affected. High-velocity and rotational injuries can cause diffuse axonal injury because the brain tissue accelerates and decelerates within the skull. Subcortical axons can shear and become disrupted within the myelin sheath (BIA, 2019). Calcium enters the cell further propagating axonal injury (Lundy-Ekman, 2018). This diffuse axonal injury can disconnect the brain stem activating centers from the cerebral hemispheres (Bontke et al., 1992). Areas most susceptible to this type of injury include the corpus callosum, basal ganglia, periventricular white matter, and superior cerebellar peduncles (Lundy-Ekman, 2018). The amount of white matter loss determines the outcome in TBI (Lundy-Ekman, 2018).

Hematomas

Vascular hemorrhage with *hematoma* formation is another type of closed head injury. Two specific types of hematomas are worthy of notation. *Epidural hematomas* form between the dura mater and the skull (Fig. 12.2, *A*). These types of injuries are frequently seen after a blow to the side of the head or severe trauma from a motor vehicle accident. Rupture of the middle meningeal artery within the temporal fossa can cause epidural hematomas. Clinically, the individual has a period of unconsciousness and then becomes alert and lucid. As blood continues to leak from the ruptured vessel, the hematoma enlarges. This is followed by rapid deterioration of the person's condition. Immediate surgical intervention consisting of craniotomy and hematoma evacuation is necessary to save the individual's life or to prevent further deterioration of his or her condition.

A *subdural hematoma,* on the other hand, is an acute venous hemorrhage that results because of rupture to the cortical bridging veins. This hematoma develops between the dura and the arachnoid. Blood leaking from the venous system accumulates more slowly, generally over a period of several hours to a week. An injury of this type is often seen in older adults after a fall with a blow to the head. The symptoms fluctuate and can resemble those seen in individuals with stroke. The individual can experience decreased consciousness, ipsilateral pupil dilation, and contralateral hemiparesis. Smaller clots may be reabsorbed by the body, whereas larger hematomas may require surgical removal. Fig. 12.2, *B* shows the location of a subdural hematoma.

Anoxic Injuries

Brain tissue demands a constant flow of blood to maintain proper oxygen saturation levels and metabolic functions (Hubert and VanMeter, 2018). When the brain is deprived of oxygen for a period of time this can result in an anoxic injury.

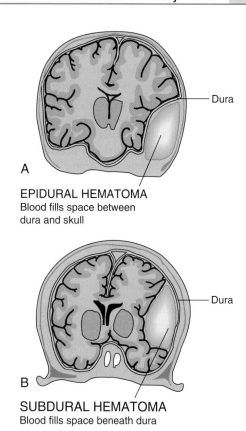

EPIDURAL HEMATOMA
Blood fills space between dura and skull

SUBDURAL HEMATOMA
Blood fills space beneath dura

Fig. 12.2 **Types of hematomas.** (Modified from Gould BE: *Pathophysiology for the health-related professions*, Philadelphia, 1997, Saunders.)

Anoxic injuries are most frequently caused by cardiac arrest. These types of injuries typically cause diffuse damage within brain tissue. However, some areas such as neurons in the hippocampus (an area involved in memory storage), the cerebellum, and the basal ganglia, have been shown to be more vulnerable to local damage. This explains the prevalence of amnesia and movement disorders in this patient population (Bontke and Boake, 1996; Jennett and Teasdale, 1981).

Diffuse Axonal Injuries

The skull is a rigid structure that can cause damage to brain tissue while still remaining intact. Subsequent high velocity trauma that causes a strong rotational and translational force to brain tissue against the skull can result in a *diffuse axonal injury* (Frati et al., 2017). *Diffuse axonal injuries* produce multiple brain tissue microtears as a result of the shearing movement of the brain against the rigid structure of the skull. This often results in widespread, diffuse damage of both mechanical stress as well as the systematic effects owing to the cascade of swelling that follows. Diffuse axonal injuries often cause cognitive physical and behavioral changes that compromise recovery.

Locked-in Syndrome, Acquired Brain Injuries, and Second Impact Syndrome

Additional categories of brain injuries also need to be understood. *Locked-in syndrome* is a rare neurologic disorder that can result after a TBI. The condition is characterized by complete paralysis of all voluntary muscles except those that control eye movements. The individual remains conscious and possesses cognitive function, but is unable to move. The prognosis for this condition is poor. *Acquired brain injuries* are those that are not hereditary, congenital, degenerative, or induced by trauma at birth. Causes of acquired brain injuries may include airway obstruction, near-drowning, myocardial infarction, stroke, exposure to toxins, and electrical shock or lightning strike. *Sudden impact syndrome* is also known as recurrent traumatic brain injury. This syndrome occurs when an individual receives a second injury before the symptoms of a first injury have resolved and typically involves a young athlete who returns to sport prematurely. In these cases, one is more likely to see edema and diffuse damage (BIA, 2012).

SECONDARY PROBLEMS

Individuals who sustain a TBI may also sustain secondary cerebral damage as a result of the brain's response to the initial injury. Often these secondary complications are more detrimental than the primary injury and need to be managed appropriately. This damage can occur within an hour of the initial injury or several months later. The following is a discussion of common secondary problems that may affect the patient's outcome.

Increased Intracranial Pressure

Increased intracranial pressure (ICP) is a common finding after a traumatic brain injury. Patients with serious injuries have a significant risk for developing increased ICP owing to metabolic changes (Kinoshita, 2016). The adult skull is rigid and does not expand to accommodate increasing volumes of fluid secondary to edema formation or hemorrhage. The result is an increase in pressure that can lead to compression of brain tissue, decreased perfusion of blood in brain tissues, and possible herniation. Normal ICP is approximately 5 to 10 mm Hg. Pressures greater than 20 mm Hg are considered abnormal and can result in neurologic and cardiovascular changes. Activities that may increase a patient's ICP include cervical flexion, the performance of percussion and vibration techniques, and coughing. Signs and symptoms of increased ICP include: (1) decreased responsiveness; (2) impaired consciousness; (3) severe headache; (4) vomiting; (5) irritability; (6) papilledema; and (7) changes in vital signs, including increased blood pressure and decreased heart rate (Hubert and VanMeter, 2018). If a patient is going to develop increased ICP, it will normally occur within the first week after the injury. However, it is important for all clinicians to recognize the signs and symptoms of this condition because patients can develop it months or weeks after initial injuries. Treatment of increased ICP includes careful monitoring, and judicious use of pharmacologic agents such as mannitol. Mannitol is a diuretic that if used inappropriately can cause intravascular dehydration (Kinoshita, 2016). Hyperventilation has been used to decrease ICP in this population (Ghajar, et al., 1993), but again, excessive hyperventilation can be problematic.

Seizures

Approximately 25% of patients with contusions and 50% of patients with penetrating open injuries develop seizure activity immediately (National Institute of Neurological Disorders and Stroke [NINDS], 2015; Winkler, 2013). Seizures are defined as "discrete clinical events reflecting temporary, physiologic brain dysfunction, characterized by excessive hypersynchronous cortical neuron discharge" (Hammond and McDeavitt, 1999). Events that may trigger a seizure include stress, poor nutrition, electrolyte imbalance, missed medications or drug use, flickering lights, infection, lack of sleep, fever, anger, worry, and fear (Fuller, 2015). Certain physical therapy interventions are also contraindicated in patients with a history of seizure activity. Vestibular stimulation techniques, such as fast spinning, and irregular movements with sudden acceleration and deceleration components should be avoided. If a patient should have a seizure during treatment, the assistant should transfer the patient to the floor to avoid possible injury. Observation of the patient of physical signs, respiratory status, and the duration of the seizure is important (Fuller, 2015). Notification of the patient's physician and primary nurse is necessary. Patients who remain unconscious after the seizure should be positioned on their side to prevent possible aspiration. Medications are prescribed according to the type of seizure activity demonstrated by the patient. Common medications given to control seizure activity include phenytoin (Dilantin) and phenobarbital (Luminal). Phenytoin should be given for 1 to 2 weeks after the injury as a prophylactic measure for patients with severe injuries to decrease the risk of posttraumatic seizure disorder (Fulk and Nirider, 2019; Fuller, 2015). Arousal, memory, and cognition are decreased due to the sedative side effects of medication. In addition ataxia, dysarthria, double vision, and hepatotoxicity can occur. Newer drugs, such as lacosamide (Vimpat), gabapentin (Neurontin), and pregabalin (Lyrica), have fewer drug interactions (Fuller, 2015). An important consideration for physical therapists (PTs) and physical therapist assistants (PTAs) is that relatively small changes in a patient's level of arousal or awareness may affect the patient's ability to respond to the environment.

Heterotopic Ossification

Heterotopic ossification (HO) is abnormal bone formation in soft tissues and muscles surrounding joints that can occur after TBI. The origin of this problem is unknown; however, this condition is noted after brain or spinal cord injury. A common denominator in all cases of heterotopic ossification is prolonged immobilization. The incidence of this condition in patients with TBI has previously been reported to be between 11% and 76% (Hammond and McDeavitt, 1999; Varghese, 1992). Blast injuries affect many body systems because of the massive amount of injury to soft tissues (Hoyt et al., 2018). A higher incidence of HO has been documented in combat veterans (Eisenstein et al., 2018). Patients can present with loss of range of motion, pain on movement, localized swelling, and erythema. If therapists suspect that a patient is developing this condition, they should notify the physician of the symptoms. A definitive diagnosis is made with a computerized tomography (CT) scan. Common joints affected include the hips, knees, shoulders, and elbows. In patients with TBI, the hip is the most common joint affected. No effective method is available to treat HO once it has developed, which has led to controversy regarding continuation of physical therapy after diagnosis of the condition. Most experts do agree that range-of-motion exercises should continue to prevent possible ankylosis and that positioning, splinting, and managing abnormal muscle tone can be helpful (Fulk et al., 2019). The most commonly used drugs to prophylactically treat HO are nonsteroidal anti-inflammatory agents (NSAIDs) (Łęgosz et al., 2018).

Paroxysmal Sympathetic Hyperactivity (PSH)

Paroxysmal sympathetic hyperactivity (PSH), commonly referred to as brain storming, is a consequence of severe traumatic brain injury that is associated with poorer outcomes. These episodes are thought to be caused by a disconnection between the parasympathetic and sympathetic nervous system. Individuals are left in an excitatory state and present with tachycardia, arterial hypertension, tachypnea, hyperthermia, diaphoresis, episodic agitation, and decerebrate posturing (Meyfroidt et al., 2017). Therapeutic strategies to treat a PSH episode include avoiding provoking external stimuli, decreasing the sympathetic nervous outflow with pharmacology agents, and addressing the secondary effects that result from the episode (Meyfroidt et al., 2017). PSH can lead to poorer outcomes, including prolonged hospital length of stays, reduced GCS scores, and higher risks for infection and ventilator support. Clinicians need to be aware of the common presentation of PSH so it can be reported and managed immediately.

Cerebral Spinal Fluid Leak

Cerebral spinal fluid leaks can occur as a result of high impact traumatic injuries, periods of increased intracranial pressure, the presence of skull fractures, and can be also be spontaneous. Common signs and symptoms include clear drainage from the nose or ear, severe headache, changes in vision or hearing, as well as a dramatic difference in functional presentations. Immediate bed rest is initiated when this is present, and surgery is scheduled for an endoscopic repair that often has a high success rate (Anstead, 2014).

Other Secondary Complications

Clinicians treating individuals with traumatic brain injury need to be aware of other possible secondary complications that can occur. Owing to the severity of the injury, patients do not have opportunities for mobility early in recovery. This can put patients at risk for developing both deep vein thrombosis and pulmonary embolism. Signs and symptoms, such as shortness of breath, chest pain, redness or swelling, pain, and changes in functional mobility, should be monitored closely owing to these unforeseen possibilities. Patients

with traumatic brain injury may not be able to communicate the symptoms of secondary complications; therefore, it is important for the clinician to check closely for the signs and to advocate for medical care, if needed.

PATIENT EXAMINATION AND EVALUATION

Glasgow Coma Scale

A patient who is brought to the emergency room following a TBI is evaluated to determine the extent of injury. The Glasgow Coma Scale is used to assess the individual's level of arousal and function of the cerebral cortex. The scale specifically evaluates the patient's eye opening, best motor response, and best verbal response (Teasdale and Jennett, 1974) (Table 12.1). Scores for this assessment can range from 3 to 15, with higher scores indicating less severe brain damage and a better chance of survival. Individuals who are admitted through the emergency room with scores of 3 or 4 often do not survive. A score of 8 or less indicates that the patient is in a coma and has sustained a severe brain injury (Winkler, 2013). "It has been repeatedly demonstrated that the depth and duration of unconsciousness, as indexed by the GCS score, is the single most powerful predictor of outcome from TBI" (Bontke and Boake, 1996).

TABLE 12.1 Glasgow Coma Scale[a]

Eye Opening	Score
Spontaneous: Opening before stimulus	4
To sound: After spoken or shouted request	3
To pressure: Fingertip stimulus	2
None: No response at any time	1
Closed by local factor	Not testable
Motor Response	**Score**
Obeys verbal command; 2-part request	6
Localized; brings hands above clavicle to stimulus	5
Normal withdrawal flexion; bends arm rapidly	4
Decorticate posturing; abnormal flexion	3
Decerebrate posturing; extends arm at elbow	2
No response; no movement in arms and legs	1
Paralyzed or other limiting factor	Not testable
Verbal Response	**Score**
Oriented; correctly gives name, place, date	5
Confused; not oriented but communicated coherently	4
Words: Intelligible single words	3
Sounds: Incomprehensible (moans, groans)	2
None; no audible response	1
Factor interfering with communication	Not testable

[a]Overall score equals the sum of eye opening and motor response and verbal response.
(Modified from Royal College of Physicians and Surgeons of Glasgow. https://www.glasgowcomascale.org/)

Classifying the Severity of Traumatic Brain Injury

Traumatic brain injury is classified as mild, moderate, or severe. An individual with mild TBI has a GCS of 13 or higher, a loss of consciousness lasting less than 20 minutes, and a normal CT scan. Individuals with mild TBI are awake on their arrival to the acute-care facility, but may be dazed, confused, and complaining of headache and fatigue. An individual with a moderate TBI has a GCS score of 9 to 12. On admission to the hospital, the individual is confused and unable to answer questions appropriately. Many individuals with moderate TBIs have permanent physical, cognitive, and behavioral deficits. A severe TBI corresponds to a score of 3 to 8 and indicates that the individual is in a coma. Most people with severe TBIs have permanent functional and cognitive impairments (Bontke and Boake, 1996).

PATIENT PROBLEM AREAS

The clinical manifestations of TBI vary, secondary to the diffuse neuronal damage that may occur. Common problems seen in this patient population include: (1) decreased level of consciousness; (2) cognitive impairments; (3) motor or movement disorders; (4) sensory problems; (5) communication deficits; (6) behavioral changes; and (7) associated problems.

Decreased Level of Consciousness

A decreased or altered level of arousal or consciousness is frequently seen in individuals who have sustained a TBI. *Arousal* is a primitive state of being awake or alert. The reticular activating system is responsible for an individual's level of arousal. *Awareness* implies that an individual is conscious of internal and external environmental stimuli. *Consciousness* is the state of being aware. The term *coma* is described as a decreased level of awareness. A coma is a state of unconsciousness in which the patient is neither aroused nor responsive to the internal or external environments (NINDS, 2015).

When patients are in a coma, their eyes remain closed; they are unable to initiate voluntary activity; and their sleep and wake cycles cannot be distinguished on an electroencephalogram. Coma, by definition, does not last longer than 3 to 4 weeks as sleep-wake cycles return, and there is restoration of brainstem functions, such as respiration, digestion, and blood pressure control. A person who demonstrates a return of brainstem reflexes and sleep-wake cycles yet remains unconscious is said to be in a vegetative state (van Erp et al., 2014). An individual at this stage may experience periods of arousal and may demonstrate spontaneous eye opening without tracking. General responses to pain, such as increased heart or respiration rates, sweating, or abnormal posturing, may be evident. The individual remains unaware of the external environment or internal needs (NINDS, 2015). A *persistent vegetative state* is the term used to identify a person who has been in a vegetative state for 30 days or longer. Adults generally have a 50% chance of regaining consciousness after being in a persistent

vegetative state (NINDS, 2015). Patients are able to localize to noxious stimuli or sounds and may be able to visually fix on an object (Fulk and Nirider, 2019).

Other terms are also used to define unresponsiveness. *Stupor* is a condition of general unresponsiveness in which the patient is able to be aroused only after significant sensory stimulation. *Obtundity* is evident in people who sleep a great deal of the time. When these individuals are aroused, they demonstrate disinterest in the environment and are slow to respond to sensory stimulation. *Delirium* is categorized by disorientation, fear, and misperception of sensory stimuli. Patients at this stage can be agitated, loud, and socially inappropriate. *Clouding of consciousness* is a state in which the person is confused, distracted, and has poor memory (Winkler, 2013). Once an individual regains awareness of self and the surrounding environment, she is now described as being in a *minimally conscious state*. Localized motor responses now occur when a sensory stimulus is presented (Gosseries et al., 2011). The minimally conscious state may also include periods of arousal throughout the day, comprehension of simple sounds, manipulation of objects, and early forms of communication. Individuals at this stage should be engaged with the environment as much as possible in order to improve the ability to follow commands, and to perform basic activities of daily living and functional mobility tasks.

Recovery of consciousness is a gradual process whereby individuals demonstrate improvements in orientation and recent memory. Progress through the stages is variable, and patients may plateau at any stage.

Cognitive Deficits

In addition to deficits in arousal and responsiveness, many individuals with TBIs also experience cognitive deficits. Cognitive dysfunction can include disorientation, poor attention span, loss of memory, loss of executive functions (including poor planning and organizational skills, recognizing errors, problem solving, and abstract thinking), and an inability to control emotional responses. The severity of an individual's cognitive deficits greatly impacts the ability to learn new skills, an ability that is an integral part of the rehabilitation process (Vakil, 2005; Vakil and Lev-Ran Galon, 2014). The following is a case example that illustrates this point.

A patient receiving physical therapy services in an inpatient rehabilitation center was able to ambulate independently without an assistive device to negotiate environmental barriers and to perform complex fine-motor tasks. The patient was not, however, able to remember his name, he could not identify family members, and he was not oriented to time or place. The patient would often become confused by the external environment and would fill in gaps in his memory with inappropriate words or fabricated stories—an incident also known as *confabulation*. This patient's cognitive deficits were much more problematic to his overall functional independence and safety than were his physical limitations. Intervention strategies to address these impairments are discussed later in this chapter.

Motor Deficits

A second major area affected in individuals with TBI is motor function. When a patient is unconscious, mobility is impaired. The patient is not able to initiate active movements. Abnormal postures are also frequently seen as a consequence of brainstem injury. The two most prevalent abnormal postures exhibited are decerebrate and decorticate rigidity. In *decerebrate rigidity,* the patient's lower extremities are in extension. The hips are adducted and internally rotated, the knees are extended, the ankles are plantar flexed, and the feet are supinated. The upper extremities are internally rotated and extended at the shoulders, extended at the elbows, pronated at the forearms, and flexed at the wrists and fingers. Thumbs may be entrapped within the palm of the hand. Decerebrate rigidity results from severing of the neuroaxis in the midbrain region. The vestibular nuclei provide the source of the extensor tone. *Decorticate rigidity* appears as upper extremity flexion with adduction and internal rotation of the shoulders, flexion of the elbows, pronation of the forearms, flexion of the wrists, and extension of the lower extremities. Decorticate posturing results from dysfunction above the level of the red nucleus, specifically between the basal nuclei and the thalamus. Patients with significant injuries can be dominated by either abnormal pattern. Challenges arise when the patient is unable to deviate from the posture, and voluntary active movement is not possible.

In addition to the presence of abnormal postures, individuals who have sustained a TBI can present with other types of motor disorders. Individuals can demonstrate generalized weakness and difficulty initiating movement, as well as disorders of muscle tone. The reemergence of primitive and tonic reflexes without voluntary motor control can also affect the patient's ability to move into and out of different positions. The presence of the tonic labyrinthine reflex, asymmetrical tonic neck reflex, symmetrical tonic neck reflex, positive support reflex, and flexor withdrawal reflex can inhibit the patient's ability to initiate active movement. Motor sequencing, ataxia, incoordination, and decreased static and dynamic balance may also interfere with the patient's ability to perform functional movements.

Sensory Deficits

Sensory deficits are also apparent in a person with TBI. The sense of smell may be lost or impaired secondary to damage of the cribriform plate or anterior fossa fracture. Up to 66% of those with a TBI experience loss of smell, which can result in an enduring impairment (Drummond et al., 2017). Perceptions of cutaneous (tactile and kinesthetic) sensations can be impaired or absent. In addition, individuals may experience visual, perceptual, and proprioceptive deficits, depending on the area of the brain that was affected.

Communication Deficits

The ability to communicate is often initially lost or severely impaired in the patient with TBI. A decreased awareness of the environment can limit opportunities for interaction. Patients with severe motor deficits may not be able to initiate communication because of abnormal tone or posturing. Mechanisms other than verbal communication must be explored. Eye blinks, head nods, or finger movements may be the only available options to establish yes or no responsiveness. PTs and PTAs often discover that the patient's first successful attempts at communication occur during the physical therapy treatment session. The inhibitory techniques used to manage abnormal tone and to facilitate normal movement patterns may allow the patient to initiate a motion or verbal response that can serve as a means for communicating basic needs.

Behavioral Deficits

Behavioral problems can also become evident after TBI. These deficits are frequently the most enduring and socially disabling. Patients can be debilitated by changes in their personalities and temperaments. Patients can exhibit neuroses, psychoses, sexual disinhibition, apathy, irritability, lability, aggression, and low frustration tolerance. These personality changes can be challenging for the rehabilitation professionals, as well as for caregivers and family members. The clinician should consult with the patient's neuropsychologist who can develop and suggest appropriate strategies to use to address the patient's behavioral issues.

Associated Problems

A final area that must be mentioned in this population is that of associated problems that individuals may experience. Approximately 40% of individuals with TBI will have other injuries (Campbell, 2000). Serious medical complications, as well as orthopedic injuries, can occur during the traumatic event leading to the actual brain injury. A person who has sustained a TBI may also present with fractures, lacerations, and even spinal cord injury. These associated problems affect the individual's care and can make rehabilitation even more challenging.

PHYSICAL THERAPY INTERVENTION: ACUTE CARE

The physical therapy care of the patient with a TBI should begin in the acute care setting as soon as the patient is medically stable. Early goals of intervention should include (1) increasing the patient's level of arousal; (2) preventing the development of secondary impairments; (3) improving patient function; and (4) providing the patient and the patient's family with education regarding the injury. The patient's length of stay in the acute-care facility may be short, especially if the patient does not experience any medical complications. Average lengths of acute-care hospitalization may be less than two weeks.

Positioning

One of the most important early treatment interventions that must be addressed is patient positioning. This is imperative because patients with TBI can exhibit abnormal tone and postures. Supine is the position in which many of these

INTERVENTION 12.1   Side-Lying Positioning

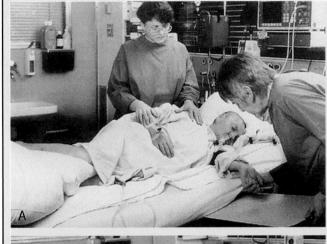

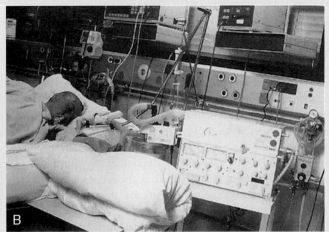

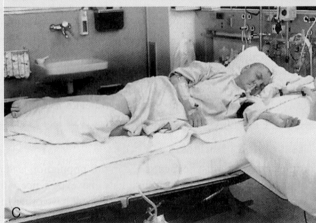

A. One end of the footboard is beneath the mattress.
B. A rolled pillow supports the extended arm.
C. The arm is well-supported in the corrected position.

(Modified from Davies PM: *Starting again: early rehabilitation after traumatic brain injury or other severe brain lesion*, New York, 1994, Springer-Verlag.)

patients are placed because it facilitates performance of both nursing and self-care tasks. Supine is also the position in which the greatest impact of the tonic labyrinthine reflexes and the dominance of extensor tone may be evident. Interventions 12.1 and 12.2 provide positioning examples. Side-lying and semiprone positions are more desirable positions because the influence of the tonic labyrinthine reflex is reduced. Care must be taken when positioning these patients because of the potential for respiratory complications. Often, patients with TBI may be receiving mechanical ventilation or have tracheostomies. The patient can be positioned in prone by placing a pillow or a wedge under the chest and forehead. This position maintains the patient's airway. Positioning the upper extremities in slight abduction and external rotation while the patient is in prone or supine position also exerts an inhibitory influence on abnormal muscle tone (Davies, 1994).

The clinician should position the patient out of the decerebrate or decorticate posture. The nursing staff as well as the patient's family must be educated on the ways in which the

INTERVENTION 12.2   Prone Positioning

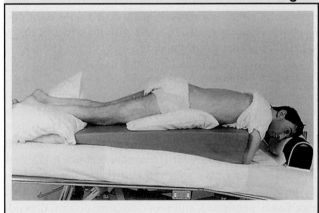

Despite severe contractures, this patient is able to lie prone with the help of different supports.

(Modified from Davies PM: *Starting again: early rehabilitation after traumatic brain injury or other severe brain lesion*, New York, 1994, Springer-Verlag.)

patient should be positioned. Firm towels, small bolsters, or half-rolls should be used to assist the patient in maintaining the optimal position. Pillows and other soft objects should be avoided because they provide the patient with something to push against, which may elicit a stretch reflex and exacerbate abnormal posturing.

The abnormal muscle tone present in these patients can be significant. Contractures can develop quickly, especially in the elbow and ankle. Proper positioning, accompanied by range-of-motion exercises and static splinting, can alleviate these potentially limiting complications.

Activities Aimed at Increasing Patient Awareness

During this acute stage of recovery, activities targeted at increasing the patient's level of awareness are employed. These activities are important even for patients who are in a coma. Even though a patient may not be able to respond verbally or motorically, it should not be assumed that the patient is unable to hear or understand the information that is being provided. In fact, clinicians should assume that the patient can hear and understand all that is being said. All members of the rehabilitation team should be orienting the patient to his or her name, the facility in which he or she is currently residing, and why the patient is receiving medical intervention. The rehabilitation team often develops a script outlining pertinent orientation information about the patient so there is consistency in interactions between team members and the patient. Referring to subjects that are familiar to the patient within treatment sessions and conversations is beneficial. As clinicians work with the patient, it is imperative that they explain what they are doing at all times. Communicating with the patient in a respectful and personal manner demonstrates the core values of our profession to the patient and family.

Movement Transitions

Changing the position of the patient in a coma can produce an alerting response. Moving the person into an upright position may improve the patient's ability to respond to sensory information. Even if it requires more than one person to move the patient into a more upright position, the change in orientation may produce environmental awareness. Rotational movement of the limbs and trunk can decrease tone and allow for greater ease in positioning over a wedge as seen in Intervention 12.2. Distribution of tone may be affected by positional changes.

Muscle spasticity is a major physical complication following TBI. In a 2017 systematic review, Synnot et al. assessed pharmacologic (Baclofen and Botox) and nonpharmacologic interventions (physical therapy, casting, splints, tilt table standing, and electrical stimulation). Owing to limited evidence and low quality studies, no conclusions could be drawn from their review. The patients with TBI in the studies reviewed were a subset of a larger group with other neurologic disorders.

Sensory Stimulation

The use of sensory stimulation for patients in a coma continues to be under review. A Cochrane review showed no reliable evidence to support or dispute the use of sensory stimulation in the facilitation of a person's level of arousal (Lombardi et al., 2002). In the past, the rationale for the use of sensory modalities was to increase the patient's level of arousal and responsiveness and to facilitate the patient's emergence from coma (Bontke et al., 1992). Padilla and Domina's 2016 systematic review of the effectiveness of sensory stimulation concluded that strong evidence exists to support that multimodal sensory stimulation improves arousal and outcomes. Sensory stimulation does play a significant role in assisting the rehabilitation team in the *assessment* of the patient's level of arousal and ability to perceive and attend to stimuli in the environment (Bontke et al., 1992). Auditory, olfactory, tactile, kinesthetic, vestibular, and oral stimuli can be administered for assessment and intervention purposes. Pairing multimodal stimulation with action initiation cues may improve localizing or tracking a stimulus (Padilla and Domina, 2016).

When providing sensory information to the patient who is unresponsive, it is best to limit the time of exposure. Brief periods of stimulation are best. Overstimulation can agitate the patient and may cause increased fatigue. It is also important to monitor responses to sensory stimulation when the patient is most aroused. Therapists are more likely to see a response from the patient after assisting with range-of-motion exercises, movement transitions, or transfers. Only one sensory stimulus should be administered at a time. If the therapist is using tactile stimuli, no other sensory input should be provided. When multiple inputs are administered, it is not possible to determine what stimuli elicited the patient's response. Patients must also be given adequate time to respond once the stimulus has been presented. Response times can be greatly increased in patients who have sustained a TBI (Krus, 1988).

Patients' responses to the different sensory modalities administered must be observed. The rehabilitation team hopes that one type of stimulus will be effective in eliciting a response. Examples of various patient responses include changes in heart rate, blood pressure, or respiration rate; diaphoresis; increases or decreases in muscle tone; head turning; eye movements; grimacing; or vocalizations. Small vials of different scents, such as coffee, peppermint, or ammonia, can be passed under the patient's nose. Tactile stimuli, such as different textures (cotton, paintbrushes, sandpaper), can be applied to areas of the patient's skin. Noxious stimuli are only used if the patient is not responding to other forms of stimulation. Pressure on the patient's nail bed, sticking the patient with a pin, or pinching the patient's skin slightly may elicit a pain response. Brightly colored objects, familiar pictures, or objects presented to the patient can provide visual stimulation. Ice, mouth swabs, and tongue depressors can provide oral stimulation. Finally, range-of-motion exercises and position changes can be performed to assess the patient's response to kinesthetic input. Once a response to a specific stimulus is observed, team members can monitor the consistency of the response over time to record trends and patient improvements.

The clinician's voice can also be used as a tool to influence the patient's response. For patients who are in a heightened state of awareness, the use of a soft tone of voice may calm the patient. On the contrary, for patients who are lethargic, the use of the patient's name followed by a brief, concise command in a loud voice may be used to arouse the patient.

Cognitive Functioning

The Rancho Los Amigos Scale of Cognitive Functioning is a tool used to measure and describe the patient's level of cognitive function. Table 12.2 highlights major patient responses and suggests interventions for individuals in each of the categories. The levels start with the patient at level I. Patients at this level do not respond to any type of stimuli, whereas individuals at level VIII are alert, oriented, and able to function independently within the community. Although this scale would appear to be an easy way to classify patients and their recoveries, some individuals may exhibit behaviors or responses from more than one category as they transition between stages. Furthermore, not every patient will progress through each of the stages and some patients may plateau at a given level. Despite these challenges, the scale remains an excellent means to classify an individual's cognitive functioning. It is important to remember that the Rancho Scale does not address the patient's physical capabilities.

Patient responses may be generalized or localized. Generalized responses are inconsistent and nonpurposeful. They can be physiologic changes, including fluctuations in respiration rates, sweating, skin color changes, or goose bumps. Generalized responses may also present as gross body movements, including changes in the amount of extremity movement, increased tone or abnormal posturing, or withdrawal from the stimulus. Vocalizations or increased oral movements are also characteristic of generalized patient responses. Patients exhibiting generalized responses frequently respond in a similar manner regardless of the stimulus applied. Patients with the ability to localize sensory responses will react specifically to the stimulus applied. Patients demonstrating this type of sensory processing may be able to follow simple one-step commands; however, responses are frequently delayed and are not consistently completed. An example of this is when the therapist touches the patient's right shoulder and asks the patient to do the same; after a short delay, the patient may reach and touch his or her right upper arm.

Patient and Family Education

Patient and family education is an important component of our physical therapy interventions. TBI is devastating to an individual's family and friends as well as to the individual. Initially, most families are overwhelmed and may not know how to react to the patient. It is important for PTs and PTAs to provide the family with support and accurate information. Family members must be educated about changes in the patient's appearance and cognitive and physical functioning.

Although this information may be initially shared with the family in the acute-care setting, it will need to be reinforced and continually updated as the patient is transferred to new facilities. Expectations for each stage and possible progress must be addressed. As soon as possible, family members should be encouraged to participate in the patient's care.

PHYSICAL THERAPY INTERVENTIONS DURING INPATIENT REHABILITATION

Once the patient is medically stable, the patient will most likely be transferred to an inpatient rehabilitation setting if further intensive intervention is required. Primary patient problems at this stage are as follows: (1) decreased range of motion and the potential for contractures; (2) increased muscle tone and abnormal posturing; (3) decreased awareness and responsiveness to the environment; (4) the presence of primitive tonic reflexes; (5) decreased functional mobility and tolerance to upright; (6) decreased endurance; (7) decreased sensory awareness; (8) an impaired or absent communication system; and (9) decreased knowledge of present condition.

Positioning

Proper positioning continues to be an important component of care during rehabilitation. As discussed in the section on acute-care interventions, positioning warrants much attention by all health care providers. The patient's position should be changed every 2 hours to prevent skin breakdown or the development of pneumonia. Proper positioning depends on the patient's resting posture, abnormal muscle tone, and the presence of any primitive reflexes. Side-lying and prone positions are the two most desirable positions. As the patient becomes medically stable, sitting in a wheelchair and acclimation to an upright position become important. Sitting orients the patient to a different position and assists with endurance and bronchial hygiene. For patients who are functioning at a low level and who do not possess head and trunk control, a tilt-in-space wheelchair may be necessary. A tilt-in-space wheelchair differs from a reclining wheelchair by allowing the trunk to recline while maintaining 90-degree angles at the hips, knees, and ankles. The tilt-in-space feature is beneficial because it assists in positioning the trunk and in maintaining proper alignment, and it allows for a change in the environment and the kinesthetic input the patient receives. A drawback to this type of wheelchair and seating system is that it changes the patient's visual field. Gaze is directed upward, thus making it difficult for the patient to see individuals and objects in his or her environment.

Standard wheelchairs may be satisfactory for the individual with fair trunk and head control. Lap trays securely fastened to the chair support the patient's upper extremities and help in maintaining proper sitting alignment. Intervention 12.3 provides an example of a patient positioned in a standard wheelchair. The patient must be carefully monitored when sitting activities are initiated. Complications that result from immobility and prolonged supine positioning can become

TABLE 12.2 Levels of Cognitive Functioning

Rancho Level	Patient Presentation	Therapy Implications
Low-Level TBI (Rancho 1,2,3)		
I Coma/No Response	Complete absence of observable change in behavior when presented visual, auditory, tactile, proprioceptive, vestibular, or painful stimuli No sleep/wake cycles, all behaviors reflexive, no evidence of eyes opening (spontaneous or stimulus induced)	PROM and flexibility Positioning with emphasis on arousal Use of splints and braces to prevent contractures Monitor emerging changes with CRS-R
II Vegetative State/ Generalized Response	Demonstrates generalized reflex response to painful stimuli Responds to repeated auditory stimuli with increased or decreased activity Responds to external stimuli with physiologic changes generalized, gross body movement, and/or non-purposeful vocalization Responses noted above may be the same regardless of type and location of stimulation Responses may be significantly delayed	Out of bed activity Ongoing positioning considerations in wheelchair and bed Transfer training with health care team 1–2 step command following activities Develop consistent communication system PROM/AAROM/AROM when possible
III Minimally Conscious State/ Localized Response	Demonstrates withdrawal or vocalization to painful stimuli Turns toward or away from auditory stimuli Blinks when strong light crosses visual field Follows moving object passed within visual field Responds to discomfort by pulling tubes or restraints Responds inconsistently to simple commands Responses directly related to type of stimulus May respond to some persons (especially family and friends), but not to others	Consistent environment and schedule Activities that work on tracking Object manipulation tasks Ongoing orientation Allow for extra time to respond Low stimulation environment Engage in familiar activities
Mid-Level TBI (Rancho 4,5,6)		
IV Agitated/ Confused	Alert and in heightened state of activity Purposeful attempts to remove restraints or tubes or crawl out of bed May perform motor activities, such as sitting, reaching and walking, but without any apparent purpose or upon another's request Very brief and usually non-purposeful moments of sustained alternatives and divided attention Absent short-term memory May cry out or scream out of proportion to stimulus even after its removal May exhibit aggressive or flight behavior Mood may swing from euphoric to hostile with no apparent relationship to environmental events Unable to cooperate with treatment efforts Verbalizations are frequently incoherent and/or inappropriate to activity or environment	Low stimulation environment Keep sessions structured and short Increase participation in familiar activities Facilitate goal directed behaviors Reorient and redirect every interaction Manage emerging challenging behaviors Implement consistent behavior plans to improve consistency by health care team
V Confused/ Inappropriate	Alert, not agitated but may wander randomly or with a vague intention of going home May become agitated in response to external stimulation, and/or lack of environmental structure Not oriented to person, place, or time Frequent brief periods, non-purposeful sustained attention Severely impaired recent memory, with confusion of past and present in reaction to ongoing activity Absent goal-directed, problem-solving, self-monitoring behavior Often demonstrates inappropriate use of objects without external direction May be able to perform previously learned tasks when structured and cues provided Unable to learn new information Able to respond appropriately to simple commands, fairly consistently with external structures and cues	Reinforce positive behaviors Redirect away from inappropriate behaviors Provide positive feedback Maintain consistency within health care team and anyone that is interacting with patient Monitor for signs of agitation Control environment when needed (low stimulation if patient demonstrates agitation) Keep consistent schedule with consistent team to help with memory and reduce episodes of agitation

Continued

TABLE 12.2 Levels of Cognitive Functioning—cont'd

Rancho Level	Patient Presentation	Therapy Implications
	Responses to simple commands without external structure are random and non-purposeful in relation to command Able to converse on a social, automatic level for brief periods of time when provided external structure and cues Verbalizations about present events become inappropriate and confabulatory when external structure and cues are not provided	
VI Confused/ Appropriate	Inconsistently oriented to person, time, and place Able to attend to highly familiar tasks in non-distracting environment for 30 minutes with moderate redirection Remote memory has more depth and detail than recent memory Vague recognition of some staff Able to use assistive memory aide with maximum assistance Emerging awareness of appropriate response to self, family, and basic needs Moderate assist to problem solve barriers to task completion Supervised for old learning (e.g., self-care) Shows carryover for relearned familiar tasks (e.g., self-care) Maximum assistance for new learning with little or no carryover Unaware of impairments, disabilities, and safety risks Consistently follows simple directions Verbal expressions are appropriate in highly familiar and structured situations	Consistency is key Repetition Positive feedback Redirection from inappropriate actions

High-Level TBI (7,8)

Rancho Level	Patient Presentation	Therapy Implications
VII Automatic/ Appropriate	Consistently oriented to person and place within highly familiar environments Moderate assistance for orientation to time Able to attend to highly familiar tasks in a non-distracting environment for at least 30 minutes with minimal assist to complete tasks Minimal supervision for new learning Demonstrates carryover of new learning Initiates and carries out steps to complete familiar personal and household routine but has shallow recall of what he/she has been doing Able to monitor accuracy and completeness of each step in routine personal and household ADLs and modify plan with minimal assistance Superficial awareness of his/her condition but unaware of specific impairments and disabilities and the limits they place on his/her ability to safely, accurately and completely carry out his/her household, community, work, and leisure ADLs Minimal supervision for safety in routine home and community activities Unrealistic planning for the future Unable to think about consequences of a decision or action Overestimates abilities Unaware of others' needs and feelings Oppositional/uncooperative Unable to recognize inappropriate social interaction behavior	Challenge in unfamiliar environments Goal directed sessions led by patient input High stimulation environments Allow for problem solving Motivate the patient Interventions for patient to sequence activities Provide verbal cues for correct only when desired response is wrong Allow for extra time to process higher level activities Implement use of memory aides (such as technology applications, planners) Ask for clarification of activities to fully check if the patient understands the information Maintain safety at all times Monitor for signs of resistance if deficits are addressed and patient still demonstrates poor awareness
VIII Purposeful/ Appropriate	Consistently oriented to person, place, and time Independently attends to and completes familiar tasks for 1 hour in distracting environments Able to recall and integrate past and recent events Uses assistive memory devices to recall daily schedule, to-do lists and record critical information for later use with stand-by assistance	Increase independence with functional activities Community outings and activities Decrease cues and assistance as able engagements in different environments

TABLE 12.2 Levels of Cognitive Functioning—cont'd

Rancho Level	Patient Presentation	Therapy Implications
	Initiates and carries out steps to complete familiar personal, household, community, work, and leisure routines with stand-by assistance and can modify the plan when needed with minimal assistance	Promote new learning and problem solving
		Opportunities to try and fail
	Requires no assistance once new tasks/activities are learned	Increase individuals responsibility for actions and goals
	Aware of and acknowledges impairments and disabilities when they interfere with task completion but requires stand-by assistance to take appropriate corrective action	Challenge balance in different environments
	Thinks about consequences of a decision or action with minimal assistance	
	Overestimates or underestimates abilities	
	Acknowledges others' needs and feelings and responds appropriately with minimal assistance	
	Depressed	
	Irritable	
	Low frustration tolerance/easily angered	
	Argumentative	
	Self-centered	
	Uncharacteristically dependent/independent	
	Able to recognize and acknowledge inappropriate social interaction behavior while it is occurring and takes corrective action with minimal assistance	

ADLs, Activities of daily living; *CRS-R*, Coma Recovery Scale-Revised: *PROM*, premature rupture of membranes.
(Modified from Rancho Los Amigos: Revised Assessment Scales. Original scale authored by Chris Hagen, PhD, Danese Malkmus, MA, and Patricia Durham, MA. Communication Disorders Service, Rancho Los Amigos Hospital, 1972. Most recent revised scale in 1997 by Chris Hagen.)

INTERVENTION 12.3 Wheelchair Positioning

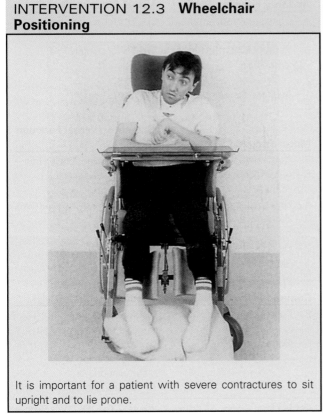

It is important for a patient with severe contractures to sit upright and to lie prone.

(Modified from Davies PM: *Starting again: early rehabilitation after traumatic brain injury or other severe brain lesion*, New York, 1994, Springer-Verlag.)

evident, including orthostatic hypotension and fatigue. In addition, the patient's skin condition must be carefully monitored to avoid any chance of pressure areas or skin breakdown. When attempting to position the patient, the therapist must remember the basic positioning concepts discussed in Chapter 11. Positioning begins by placing the patient's proximal body areas, including the pelvis and the shoulder girdle, in correct alignment. From there, the therapist can work more distally. Intervening at the more proximal joints initially will help to influence tone more distally. Poor positioning in the wheelchair or bed can lead to the development of contractures and an increase in abnormal muscle tone.

Wheelchair Propulsion

Once the patient is able to tolerate sitting in the wheelchair, self-propulsion activities can be initiated. Initially, the clinician may need to help the patient with hand-over-hand or guided practice. As the patient becomes more proficient, the goal will be for the patient to propel the wheelchair independently and to negotiate safely around the facility.

Range of Motion

Range-of-motion exercises are also important during the early stages of rehabilitation to minimize the likelihood of contracture formation. Because most patients with TBI have extensive problems, it is necessary to be as efficient as possible with our interventions. Stretching of individual joints is time-intensive and may have limited short-term benefits. Instead, greater therapeutic benefits can often be achieved through the use of different developmental postures and positions to increase patient flexibility. For example, positioning a patient in prone or tall kneeling can be used to stretch the hip flexors; quadruped and sitting can be used to stretch the gluteals and quadriceps; and standing on a tilt table or approximation directed down through the knee when the foot is weight bearing can assist with stretching the gastrocnemius and soleus. It may, however, be necessary to spend dedicated treatment time to manually stretch the hamstrings and the heel cords more aggressively.

Whenever functional positions or developmental postures will meet the same goal as static stretching, they should be employed. Patients who have developed deformities or contractures as a result of abnormal tone and posturing may require more intensive stretching. A more effective intervention for these individuals may be static splinting or serial casting. A plaster cast is applied to the joint with the range-of-motion limitation or contracture and is left on for 7 to 10 days. Thus, a prolonged stretch is applied to the joint and soft tissues. The goal is to decrease the contracture through subsequent castings and stretching. More than one cast may need to be applied to achieve the desired results, but casting is considered best practice (Mortenson and Eng, 2003). Ultimately, the final cast should be bivalved as it is removed so it can become a permanent splint for the patient. Areas that respond well to serial casting include the ankle, knee, elbow, and wrist. Clinicians working with patients who have been casted need to monitor the patient's response to the cast because the patient may not be able to verbalize pain or discomfort. Skin discoloration of the toes or fingers may indicate that the cast is too tight. Casts that are applied too loosely may slip down. It is not uncommon to find that a patient may have worked the cast off completely. A detailed description of the application of serial casts is beyond the scope of this text (Davies, 1994).

As stated earlier, it is important to explain to the patient what is being done even if the patient appears to be unresponsive. Orienting the patient to the surroundings and the circumstances regarding admission to the facility may be beneficial in increasing awareness levels. Many brain injury rehabilitation teams develop patient scripts that assist in orienting the patient to the environment. Strategies to manage some of the other cognitive deficits demonstrated by this population are discussed later in this chapter.

Improving Awareness

Increasing awareness of self and the environment is another important aspect of the patient's plan of care. Enhancing a patient's awareness is most often accomplished through the administration of various sensory stimuli. The Coma Recovery Scale-Revised can be administered to the patient and the results used to assist in identifying or categorizing the patient's responses to stimuli.

Coma Recovery Scale-Revised (CRS-R)

Disorders of consciousness include individuals who are present in a coma, a vegetative state, or a minimally conscious state. Specifics of these low-level injuries will be discussed

later in the chapter. The CRS-R (Giacino et al, 2004) can be utilized with patients who exhibit disorders of consciousness to track meaningful progress. The scale consists of 25 items arranged in a hierarchy with 6 subscales, including auditory, visual, motor, oromotor/verbal, arousal, and communication (Table 12.3). Points are scored for the presence or absence of the desired motor behavior after a sensory stimulus is presented. The maximum score is 24. Higher scores indicate cognitively mediated behaviors. Lower scores indicate reflexive activity. The CRS-R can be used to assist with differential diagnosis, prognostic assessment, and treatment planning in individuals with disorders of consciousness (Giacino et al, 2004). The tool can pick up the small yet meaningful changes that are not detected with standard inpatient rehabilitation outcomes, such as the functional independence measure (FIM). Detecting changes early in recovery can allow for use of targeted treatment strategies to improve function. The CRS-R is a comprehensive tool that tracks behaviors that may demonstrate emergence from an alerted state of consciousness. This tool should also be taught to caregivers in order to track emergence in all stages of recovery. Furthermore, utilization of this tool across the continuum of care improves communication among all health care providers and better addresses the needs of the individual.

TABLE 12.3 Coma Recovery Scale-Revised	
Auditory Function Scale	**Visual Function Scale**
4 – Consistent movement to command	5 – Object recognition
3 – Reproducible movement to command	4 – Object localization
2 – Localization to sound	3 – Visual pursuit
1 – Auditory startle	2 – Fixation
0 – None	1 – Visual startle
	0 – None
Motor Function Scale	**Oromotor/Verbal Function Scale**
6 – Functional object use	3 – Intelligible verbalization
5 – Automatic motor response	2 – Vocalization/oral movement
4 – Object manipulation	1 – Oral reflexive movement
3 – Localization to noxious stimulation	0 – None
2 – Flexion withdrawal	
1 – Abnormal posturing	
0 – None/flaccid	
Communication scale	**Arousal Scale**
2 – Functional	3 – Attention
1 – Nonfunctional	2 – Eye opening without stimulation
0 – None	1 – Eye opening with stimulation
	0 – Unarousable

(Modified from Giacino JT, Kalmar K, Whyte J: The JFK Coma Recovery Scale-Revised: measurement characteristics and diagnostic utility, *Arch Phys Med Rehabil*, 85(12):2020–2029, 2004. Retrieved from https://www.ncbi.nlm.nih.gov/pubmed/15605342.)

Family Education

The physical therapist and physical therapist assistant must educate the patient's family on ways to orient the patient and increase her self and environmental awareness. Specifically, for patients with a disorder of consciousness, families should be trained and educated on the coma recovery scale revised (CRS-R) to allow for consistent communication and intervention. As patients recover, families should bring in favorite pictures, music, or other items to help promote arousal and emergence. However, family members should be cautioned against overstimulation because once the patient begins to emerge there is a greater risk that stimulation may produce agitation. In an effort to wake the patient, families often play music or leave the patient's television on for extended periods. Few of us listen to music or watch television 24 hours a day. It is important to vary the amounts and intensities of the stimuli provided so the patient does not habituate to the sensory modality.

Family members should also be instructed in patient positioning and passive range-of-motion exercises. As the patient progresses, families can assist with bed mobility, transfers, wheelchair propulsion, and self-care activities. It is important to instruct family members in proper body mechanics when moving the patient to avoid injury. The team must also provide the family with education regarding the patient's cognitive recovery. Providing the family with an understanding of why the patient may be acting or responding in a given way coupled with strategies the family can employ to deal with the exhibited behavior is important. As the team prepares for the patient's eventual discharge, families should be provided with information on the support services that are available to them.

Functional Mobility Training

Functional mobility tasks are another important aspect of intervention. Often, patients are dependent in all aspects of mobility. Early on, it may be necessary for the PT or PTA to cotreat the patient with another member of the rehabilitation team. When patients have an extremely low functional level, it can be helpful to have two sets of hands available. However, in this current climate of cost containment, clinicians must use resources efficiently. For example, it may be more cost-effective for the assistant and the rehabilitation aide to treat the patient as compared with the physical and occupational therapists. The patient's status, level of acuity, and the interventions to be provided must be considered before these types of patient care decisions are made.

Frequently, therapists need to spend some time inhibiting abnormal tone or postures so functional activities can be attempted. Methods to inhibit abnormal tone, which are discussed in Chapter 11, include prolonged stretch, weight bearing, approximation, slow rhythmic rotation, and tendon pressure. These techniques work effectively with this patient population as well. Total body postures and positions, such as upper and lower trunk rotation, sitting, prone, and standing, are also effective in decreasing abnormal tone. Slow vestibular stimulation, including rocking in a sitting or side-lying position, and neutral warmth can be effective in decreasing abnormal tone or promoting a more relaxed state in a patient who is agitated or highly aroused (O'Sullivan, 2014). As stated in Chapter 11, once the abnormal muscle tone has been decreased, normal movement patterns and task-specific training must be encouraged to promote motor relearning.

Individuals who have sustained a severe TBI lack postural and motor control. They are unable to initiate voluntary movement, are dominated by abnormal muscle tone and reflex activity, and exhibit difficulty in dissociating extremity movements from the trunk. In addition, these patients often are unable to perform automatic postural adjustments. Consequently, an early emphasis in the patient's physical therapy plan of care must be on the development of postural control. Head and trunk control must be developed before the patient can hope to have control over the distal extremities. The principles discussed in Chapter 11 regarding the development of functional movements are also applicable to this patient population. Therapeutic interventions performed with the patient in prone or prone over a wedge or bolster may provide excellent opportunities to address head and trunk control. These positions require that the patient work the cervical extensors against gravity and also provide inhibition to the supine tonic labyrinthine reflex. The prone position facilitates increased flexor tone in patients with the presence of this reflex. Patients who have significant extensor tone can also be positioned in prone over a ball. Although transferring and maintaining the patient's position on the ball is challenging, the activity has a profound effect on reducing abnormal tone. Once the patient is on the ball, a gentle rocking can be performed to decrease the effects of abnormal tone even further. This position is contraindicated in patients with seizure disorders and increased ICP. Moreover, all patients should be carefully monitored during prone activities to ensure adequacy of ventilation.

Repetitive practice of well-learned and automatic activities is beneficial and promotes motor learning. Often, patients have difficulty in learning new motor tasks, but they respond well to activities they have performed thousands of times before. Selection of common, daily activities, such as washing the face, brushing the teeth, combing the hair, and walking, often result in active movement attempts by the patient because they are meaningful and have been performed thousands of times. During the performance of these tasks, the PT or PTA may see active movement attempts by the patient. Hand-over-hand or therapeutic guiding techniques, in which the therapist guides the patient's own extremity or body movements, are effective. The patient receives proprioceptive and kinesthetic feedback as he or she performs a functional movement pattern (Davies, 1994). Intervention 12.4 shows examples of a family member assisting a patient with hand-over-hand techniques.

Vision is a valuable sensory modality that can be used during treatment. Activities that incorporate visual tracking or maintain visual contact with an object assist with the development of head control. For example, if the patient is in a sitting position and is unable to maintain the head in an erect

INTERVENTION 12.4 **Hand-Over-Hand Guiding (Face Washing)**

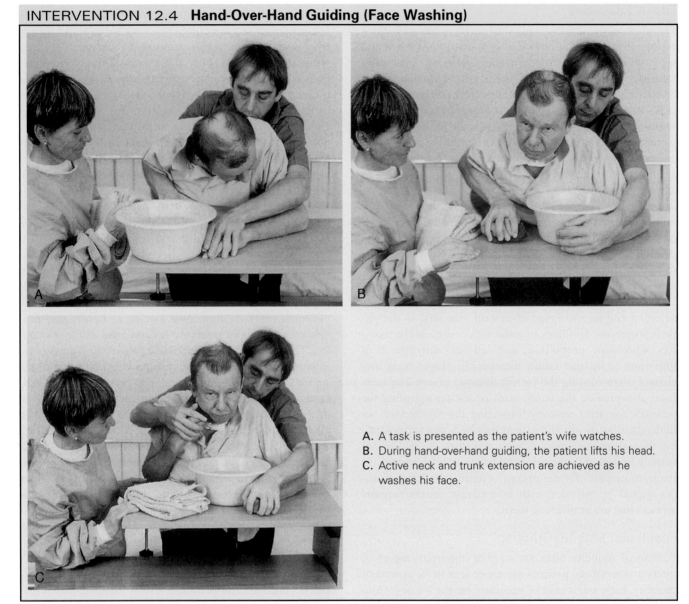

A. A task is presented as the patient's wife watches.
B. During hand-over-hand guiding, the patient lifts his head.
C. Active neck and trunk extension are achieved as he washes his face.

(Modified from Davies PM: *Starting again: early rehabilitation after traumatic brain injury or other severe brain lesion*, New York, 1994, Springer-Verlag.)

position, the patient can be encouraged to maintain eye contact with the therapist or to look at a specific object. Vision can also be used to guide a patient's movement, as with rolling or turning.

Sitting Activities

Sitting is an important position to emphasize during treatment. Sitting can increase arousal and it also provides a challenge to the patient's postural alignment and righting and equilibrium responses. Transferring the patient from supine to sitting can be accomplished in the same ways as discussed in Chapter 11. Intervention 12.5 shows a progression to sitting. Patients with a low functional level may require assistance from two individuals, one who is responsible for the head and upper trunk and one who transfers the lower trunk and legs. Changes in the patient's level of awareness and muscle tone should be noted during the change in position. Patients who exhibit strong extensor tone and posturing may become flexed and hypotonic once they are upright.

Once the patient is sitting upright on the side of the mat table, the goal for the activity is the patient's achievement of a neutral pelvic position with an erect trunk and head. Frequently it is necessary to use two individuals during sitting activities because of abnormal tone in the patient's trunk.

INTERVENTION 12.5 Supine-to-Sit Transfer

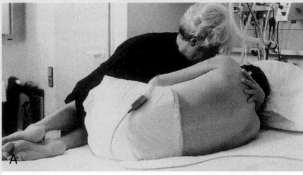

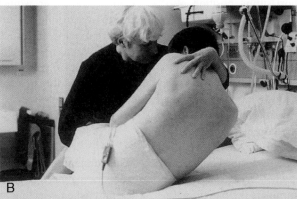

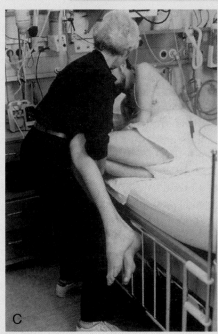

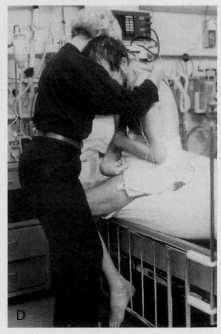

A. The therapist's arm is around the patient's flexed knees; her other arm is beneath his neck.
B. His legs are brought over the side of the bed and are maintained in flexion.
C. His trunk is lifted toward the vertical.
D. His knees are prevented from sliding forward while supporting his head and trunk.

(Modified from Davies PM: *Starting again: early rehabilitation after traumatic brain injury or other severe brain lesion*, New York, 1994, Springer-Verlag.)

One person can assist the patient with trunk and head control from behind while the other therapist, facing the patient, works on the position of the patient's pelvis, the position of the upper and lower extremities, and general awareness. Supporting the upper extremities on a large ball in the patient's lap can be beneficial for the patient with poor trunk control or hypotonia. The ball assists the therapist in maintaining trunk stabilization and may provide a sensation of support for the patient. Gentle anterior and posterior weight shifts can also be performed with the patient in this position. The weight shifts provide a mechanism to assess the patient's postural responses and also serve to increase awareness through kinesthetic input. Trunk flexion performed in the short-sitting position also maintains range of motion. Intervention 12.6 depicts this activity.

Other sitting activities can also be employed. Weight bearing on the upper extremities decreases abnormal muscle tone and also promotes proximal joint stability. As the patient progresses, reaching activities, throwing and catching tasks, and the performance of activities of daily living, such as donning socks and shoes, can be completed when the patient is in a sitting position. Intervention 12.7 shows examples of upper extremity activities performed with the patient in a sitting position.

Care must be taken not to over-stimulate the patient with multiple sensory and verbal cues. Only one person should speak to the patient at a time. To maximize the patient's understanding of verbal information, the therapist facing the patient should be designated as the person to interact with him or her. This approach minimizes the likelihood that the patient will receive verbal information from multiple sources. In addition, instructions given should be brief, direct, and stated in simple terms.

Transfers

The techniques used to transfer the patient with hemiplegia discussed in Chapter 11 can be used for the patient with TBI. A sit-pivot transfer is recommended for patients who have low functioning and lack trunk control. Intervention 12.8 shows a therapist assisting a patient with a sit-pivot transfer. As the patient progresses, stand-pivot transfers to both the right and left sides should be attempted.

Standing Activities

Standing is another excellent position that can provide opportunities for the completion of functional tasks while promoting weight bearing and sensory input. If the patient has low functional capabilities, the tilt table may need to be used initially to provide necessary stabilization to maintain a standing posture. Patients can be transferred to a tilt table or a standing frame and acclimated to an upright position. Activities that increase awareness and cognition can be performed while the patient is standing on the tilt table. Administering different sensory modalities through the use of the Coma/Near Coma (CNC) scale can be easily accomplished while the patient is on the tilt table. The upright posture may also serve to increase the patient's level of alertness. Performance of

simple activities of daily living, such as face washing or teeth brushing, is also possible. During early standing activities, it is important to monitor the patient's vital signs to assess the patient's physiologic status.

As the patient progresses, standing activities at the bedside or mat table can be instituted with appropriate assistance. (See Chapter 11 for specific techniques.) Bedside tables, grocery carts, or high-low mat tables can be used for upper-extremity support when upright gait activities are initiated. Depending on the gait training philosophy of the facility, body-weight support treadmill training (BWSTT) may also be used to promote task-specific locomotor training. Some evidence, however, would suggest that BWSTT is not superior to overground locomotor training in improving gait and balance in patients with TBI. Additional research studies are needed regarding the effectiveness of interventions for the TBI population (Bland et al., 2011). Intervention 12.9 demonstrates standing of a patient who is unconscious. Intervention 12.10 demonstrates various examples of assisting the patient with standing.

Treatment Planning

When designing the plan of care, the primary PT should consider the patient's cognitive status and the stages of motor learning when selecting appropriate treatment interventions. Practice of motor tasks, which can cause patient fatigue, should be interspersed with rest periods. Extrinsic feedback is beneficial in the early stages to assist patients in activity performance. The focus of interventions may encompass either a *compensatory* or *restorative* approach. Compensation, as the term implies, means teaching the patient a skill using alternative means and strategies. When implementing the restorative approach, the therapist attempts to restore normal functional movements through the processes of task-specific training and the principles of neuroplasticity. Examples of activities that are directed at the restorative approach include constraint-induced therapies and BWSTT (Fulk and Nirider, 2019). (See Chapter 11 for additional treatment interventions.)

The Physical Environment

Careful attention to the physical environment must be made when working with this patient population. Patients who have sustained a TBI often have exaggerated responses to sensory stimuli in the environment. The lighting, noise level, and number of individuals present must be assessed. Think about the amount of activity that takes place in a typical physical therapy gym. Many people are present, and there is a great deal of auditory stimulation from people talking, background music, and public address systems. Frequently, patients with TBIs cannot filter out extraneous stimuli in the environment. Too much sensory stimuli can over-stimulate the patient and lead to confusion or an adverse behavioral response (Persel and Persel, 1995). Patients may become more agitated, aggressive, or distracted in this type of environment. Many facilities have smaller private treatment areas for these patients. In addition, physical performance is often adversely affected when cognitive stress is increased

INTERVENTION 12.6 Trunk Flexion in Sitting

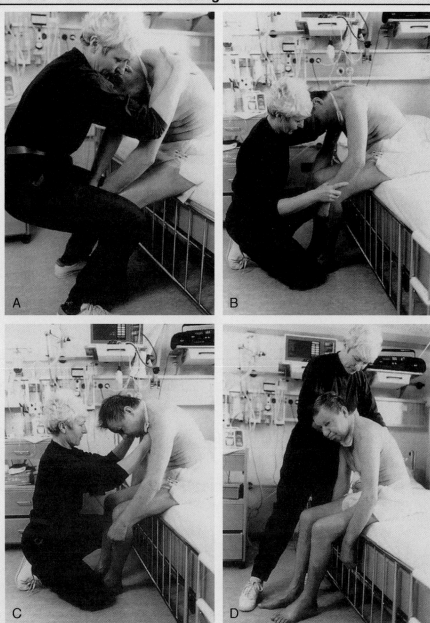

A. The patient is bending the trunk forward with the therapist blocking his knees.
B. The patient's hands reach for the feet.
C. The patient is being assisted to return to an upright position.
D. The patient is assisted for the extension of the thoracic spine.

(Adapted from Davies PM: Starting again: early rehabilitation after traumatic brain injury or other severe brain lesion, New York, 1994, Springer-Verlag.)

(Abd-Elfattah et al., 2015). Cognitive fatigue is associated with decreased muscle and proprioceptive function which is definitely present in patients with TBI.

Structure is also important to the patient with TBI. A daily schedule, a consistent treatment team, and the establishment of some level of routine within the treatment sessions will assist the patient in adjusting to his or her injury and the rehabilitation environment. In addition, repetition and practice are needed for learning new information and tasks.

Integration of Physical and Cognitive Task Components in Treatment

Often, one of the most challenging aspects of treating patients with TBIs is the integration of the physical and cognitive components of a task. The cognitive deficits frequently are the more debilitating and difficult to treat. PTs and PTAs are adept with treatment interventions that address the patient's physical limitations; however, they often have more challenges with the patient's cognitive deficits and designing

INTERVENTION 12.7 Sitting Activities

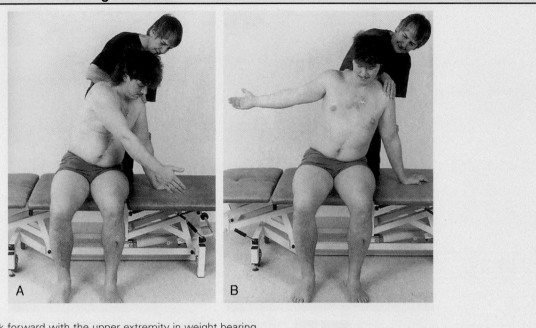

A. Rotating the trunk forward with the upper extremity in weight bearing.
B. Trunk rotated back with the contralateral arm abducted.

(Modified from Davies PM: *Starting again: early rehabilitation after traumatic brain injury or other severe brain lesion*, New York, 1994, Springer-Verlag.)

INTERVENTION 12.8 Sit-Pivot Transfer

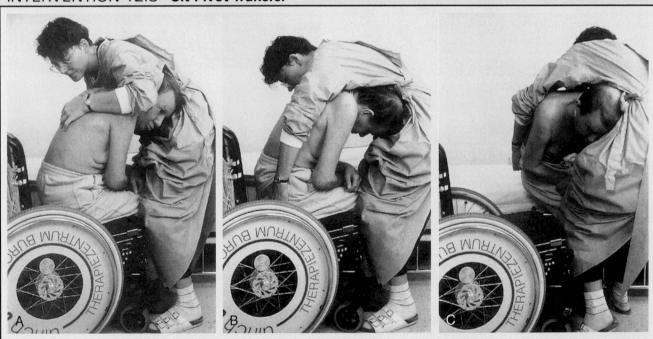

Transferring the patient with his trunk flexed forward.
A. The therapist flexes the patient's trunk and supports his head against her side.
B. She puts one hand under each trochanter.
C. Pressing her knees against his, she lifts and turns his buttocks onto the bed.

(Modified from Davies PM: *Starting again: early rehabilitation after traumatic brain injury or other severe brain lesion*, New York, 1994, Springer-Verlag.)

INTERVENTION 12.9 Standing the Patient Who Is Unconscious

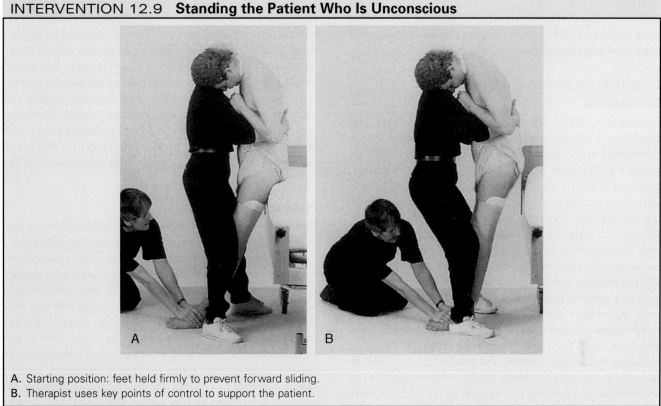

A. Starting position: feet held firmly to prevent forward sliding.
B. Therapist uses key points of control to support the patient.

(Modified from Davies PM: *Starting again: early rehabilitation after traumatic brain injury or other severe brain lesion*, New York, 1994, Springer-Verlag.)

INTERVENTION 12.10 Supporting the Patient in Standing

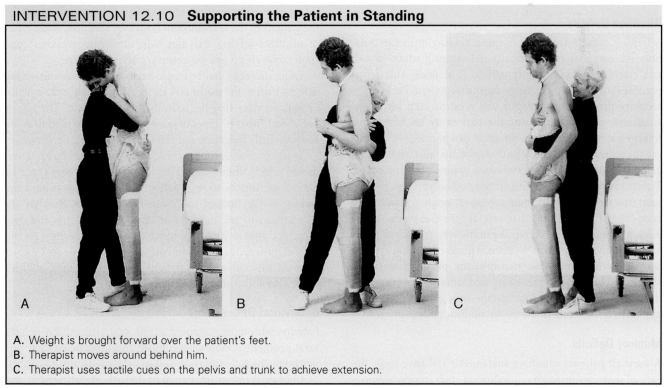

A. Weight is brought forward over the patient's feet.
B. Therapist moves around behind him.
C. Therapist uses tactile cues on the pelvis and trunk to achieve extension.

(Modified from Davies PM: *Starting again: early rehabilitation after traumatic brain injury or other severe brain lesion*, New York, 1994, Springer-Verlag.)

interventions that are at an appropriate intensity to address both the physical and cognitive challenges. The following is to be used as a guide in addressing the various cognitive and behavioral impairments seen in these patients.

Cognitive and Behavioral Impairments

Disorientation

Patients with TBI are often disoriented to place or time. Frequently, you will see caregivers quizzing the patient who is disoriented in the hope that eventually the patient will respond with the right answer. A better approach to this impairment is to provide the patient with correct information during the treatment session. In essence, the therapist fills in the missing information for the patient. As stated previously, the use of a script or a calendar can be effective in dealing with disorientation. If the patient's level of orientation does not improve, strategies that will allow the patient to retrieve the information independently from some type of source, such as a memory book, will need to be employed. The contents of memory books vary. Photographs of the patient, family members, and caregivers, along with calendars, daily schedules, and pertinent information about the patient including name, age, address, and medical history may be included in the patient's book. As the patient improves, responsibility for recording information in the memory book can be shifted to the patient. This provides an excellent means for family members to see what the patient is doing in therapy. Additionally, patient's photographs, videos, and audiotaping are other means used to document changes in the patient's performance.

Attention Deficits

Attention deficits are also a frequent finding in this population. Patients may have difficulty maintaining attention to a task even for periods as short as 10 to 15 seconds. This deficit becomes a significant challenge during treatment. Early in the recovery process, the therapist will need to keep verbal instructions simple. Addressing the patient by his first name followed by a concise verbal direction can be effective in gaining the patient's attention. The therapist may also wish to have a number of different interventions planned and prepared. Treatment will be implemented more efficiently, and the patient may be successfully redirected to an original activity at a later time, if the therapist has several activities ready. As the patient progresses, the therapist can use a stopwatch or timer to encourage the patient to remain focused during specific activity performance. For example, the patient can ride a stationary bike for a predetermined amount of time and the therapist can try to increase the time each session. This approach is an excellent means to monitor patient progress.

Memory Deficits

Almost all patients who have sustained a TBI have some degree of memory impairment following their injury. Memory is an active process that organizes information so that it can be remembered and associated with similar items and events already stored (Bleiberg, 2009). Explicit memory deficits are well documented in patients with TBI (Zec et al., 2001). Procedural learning and memory ("how to" knowledge) appears to be relatively preserved (Vakil and Lev-Ran Galon, 2014). As already discussed, the use of a day planner, cell phone, computer, or memory book may be recommended. Computerized schedule books, watches, and electronic paging systems are available. These devices sound alarms to remind patients of important times and events. Those patients with residual memory deficits must be instructed in the use of compensatory strategies to assist with functioning in the community.

Problem-Solving Deficits

Problem-solving deficits may also be apparent. Patients may demonstrate difficulties organizing and sequencing information to solve everyday problems. They may possess poor judgment or difficulties with abstract thinking. Consequently, it may not be appropriate to use humor during a treatment session because humor is an abstract concept and may only confuse the patient. Asking the patient to pretend to complete an activity is also not advised. Therapists often design activities for the patient to practice without the necessary tools or environmental setup. Far greater therapeutic benefits can be achieved by creating a more realistic activity. For example, if the patient likes to garden, the use of pots, potting soil, and gardening tools is an excellent way to have the patient plan and execute a task. Safety issues are also a primary concern. Patients may not recognize their own impairments or understand the significance of a hot stove or a stranger at the front door. Creation of situations that require attention to safety within the confines of the rehabilitation unit can assist the patient in the transition to home. In addition, these types of problem-solving activities help to identify whether constant supervision will be necessary after discharge.

Other strategies may be employed to address problem-solving deficits, such as the use of task cards that organize and sequence various activities that the individual is to perform. The use of "why" and "what if" types of questions can also be used to assess an individual's judgment and ability to solve simple challenges.

Difficulties with topographic orientation may be apparent in some individuals with TBIs. Patients with these types of deficits are unable to negotiate or find their way around the facility. Route-finding tasks can be employed. Patients are encouraged to use markers or cues, such as signs and pictures, for guidance as they move through the facility. As the patient progresses, obstacle courses and mazes can be constructed to challenge the patient's problem-solving abilities while also addressing dynamic balance.

Behavioral Deficits

Patients who have sustained a TBI may also exhibit behavioral problems. Some of the more common behavioral impairments include agitation and irritability, decreased control of emotional responses, denial of deficits, impulsiveness, and a lack of inhibition (Kim, 2002). Considering the physiologic cause of these behavioral problems may allow therapists to treat these patients more effectively. Agitation and irritability may be caused or heightened by the patient's level of disorientation, by the patient's fatigue, or because the demands of the activity are too great for the patient. If you can imagine for a moment what it would be like to have little or no memory, not to recognize family and friends, and perhaps to have some significant physical limitations, you may be better able to see why someone with a TBI may be agitated and irritable. Following a consistent schedule, environmental structure, and keeping the patient occupied can assist in managing the patient's disorientation. Limited use of television is also recommended. Patients can become easily confused by the events they see within the context of a television program and may have difficulty in distinguishing the television programming from reality.

For patients who are overreacting or exhibiting poor emotional control, the therapist or assistant may elect to ignore the behavior, reinforce positive behaviors, or communicate to the patient the inappropriateness of his or her actions. Having the therapist provide appropriate positive alternatives is also advisable because patients often are unable to select appropriate responses on their own. Sometimes, offering the patient a choice between two activities assists in redirecting inappropriate responses and allows the patient some control over the situation.

The use of group treatment activities may be of benefit for remediation of some behavioral and cognitive issues. Peer support, appropriate modeling of behaviors by others, and pressure to conform can assist patients in the recognition of their deficits.

Aggressive Behavior

An area of concern for some clinicians working with this patient population is the aggressive and combative behavior that can sometimes be exhibited. Because of this possibility, many rehabilitation facilities require staff members to attend certified programs in crisis intervention. You should receive specialized training to assist with techniques that will keep both the patient and yourself safe when dealing with aggressive behaviors. The Rancho Los Amigos Scale of Cognitive Functioning discusses possible patient responses at the confused-agitated level. Although aggressive and combative behaviors can occur, these are not the norm. The goal is to assist the patient in the development of self-controlling behaviors. Assisting the patient in the ability to deal with stressful and anxiety-producing situations is the first step in managing behavior.

Agitated Behavior Scale

The agitated behavior scale (ABS) was developed to assess the nature and extent of agitation during the acute phase or recovery after TBI. The scale consists of 14 behaviors that are rated primarily based on observation of the individual. The challenging behaviors are scored on a 1 to 4 scale (Table 12.4). Scoring depends on the presence or absence of the behavior and how much redirection is needed to decrease the behavior. The ABS scale allows for serial assessment to track behaviors after TBI as well as a means to provide objective feedback and communication for patients in an agitated state.

TABLE 12.4 Agitated Behavior Scale

14 Challenging Traumatic Brain Injury Behaviors

1. Short attention span, easy distractibility, inability to concentrate
2. Impulsive, impatient, low tolerance for pain or frustration
3. Uncooperative, resistant to care, demanding
4. Violent and/or threatening violence toward people or property
5. Explosive and/or unpredictable anger
6. Rocking, rubbing, moaning, or other self-stimulating behavior
7. Pulling at tubes, restraints, and so forth
8. Wandering from treatment areas
9. Restlessness, pacing, excessive movement
10. Repetitive behaviors, motor and/or verbal
11. Rapid, loud, or excessive talking
12. Sudden changes of mood
13. Easily initiated or excessive crying and/or laughter
14. Self-abusiveness, physical and/or verbal

Scoring of Challenging Behaviors

1 = Absent: the behavior is not present.

2 = Present to a slight degree: the behavior is present, but does not prevent the conduct of other, contextually appropriate behavior. (The individual may redirect spontaneously, or the continuation of the agitated behavior does not disrupt appropriate behavior.)

3 = Present to a moderate degree: the individual needs to be redirected from an agitated to an appropriate behavior, and benefits from such cueing.

4 = Present to an extreme degree: the individual is not able to engage in appropriate behavior owing to the interference of the agitated behavior, even when external cueing or redirection is provided.

(Modified from Rehabilitation Measures Database. Available at: *srlab.org.* Shirley Ryan Ability Lab, 2019.)

Patients with TBI often have difficulty in dealing with both internal and external environmental stressors. Behavioral changes including physical aggression can occur as patients become afraid, feel threatened, or are fatigued. If a patient is unable to manage stress and frustration successfully, a crisis situation can develop. During a crisis, the sympathetic nervous system responds, and certain physical and cognitive changes occur. Heart rate, blood pressure, and respiration rate increase, whereas cognitive skills become depressed. Communication skills, reasoning, and judgment become impaired. Thus, it is important for the PT and PTA to recognize how to assist the patient in dealing with stressors and to prevent a crisis from occurring. Several different models of crisis and behavior management have been developed. Many facilities provide crisis training programs for staff involved in the care of patients with TBIs. Individuals who work with this population should attend one of these courses.

Initially, if a patient becomes anxious and overstimulated, it is a good idea to be supportive and attempt to remove the stimulus. If the patient becomes frustrated during activity performance, assess the demands of the activity and if they are too great, decrease them. Sometimes it is not possible for the clinician to identify the triggering event or source of irritation to the patient. As the patient becomes anxious or distressed, the therapist may notice changes in the patient's tone of voice or other physical changes, including pacing, tapping of the feet, or wringing of the hands. If such changes occur, it is advisable to remove the patient from the area, continue to offer emotional support, and redirect the patient to another task. Allowing an outlet for the patient's increased energy may assist in calming the patient. Reorientation may also prove beneficial because disorientation is often the underlying factor in severe behavior disturbances (Campbell, 2000).

If these interventions do not help the patient relax, the situation can escalate to a full crisis. During a crisis, a patient can lose control over verbal and physical responses and may exhibit destructive and assaulting behaviors. The patient can be dangerous to self and to others. Often, when this situation occurs, the health care provider becomes extremely anxious as well. If the PT and PTA do not remain calm, they, too, can escalate to a sympathetic state. If you become involved in such an incident and notice yourself becoming excessively stressed, remove yourself from the situation. Once the patient is in a crisis, your role should be to protect the patient from harming self or others. The episode will need to run its course. If possible, limit the audience. As the patient recovers from the event, the clinician will again need to provide emotional support. Reestablishing a therapeutic rapport with the patient is advisable. The patient will eventually return to his or her baseline behavioral state. Once the patient has moved through all the stages of crisis, the patient and the health care provider who intervened will develop postcrisis drain or depression. This can last for several hours after the initial episode and manifests itself as exhaustion and withdrawal. It is best to allow the patient to rest following this experience. Once the patient has returned to a resting state, the clinician will want to reflect with the patient about the incident and what transpired. Questioning the patient about the event, object, or individual who triggered the episode is valuable. Reassuring the patient that the therapist is there to offer support and care for the patient is also important. If the rehabilitation team is able to identify the stressful object or trigger, methods to minimize the patient's response can be employed.

All members of the rehabilitation team should remember that patients who exhibit agitation or aggressive behaviors are demonstrating the need for structure and control over their environments. A health care provider has no reason to take the event personally. Internalizing the event can affect the patient–therapist relationship and may ultimately affect the care that is provided.

Motor Deficits and Interventions

Much time has been spent discussing the cognitive aspects of treatment for the patient with TBI. Many of the physical interventions previously discussed for patients following a stroke are appropriate for this patient population as well. The movement transitions presented, as well as the interventions used to facilitate functional movements, can be used.

Students and experienced clinicians alike often report that the most challenging patients are those who have good motor skills, but significant cognitive deficits. A review of

interventions for patients who are functioning at a high physical level is now provided. High-level balance activities are challenging for these patients. Patients must maintain postural stability while performing selective movement patterns and attending to a cognitive task. Movable surfaces, such as balls, bolsters, tilt boards, or balance systems, can be used. Exercises that can be performed on the ball include the following:

1. Maintaining balance
2. Raising arms overhead
3. Performing proprioceptive neuromuscular facilitation diagonal patterns
4. Rotating or laterally bending the trunk
5. Reciprocally moving the arms
6. Performing anterior and posterior pelvic tilts
7. Marching or knee extension exercises
8. Bouncing in a circle
9. Practicing more difficult exercises, including moving from sitting to supine and from sitting to prone on the ball can also be practiced.

Bolsters are used for static positioning or to provide the patient with a movable surface. Patients can straddle the bolster and can practice weight shifting and coming to stand. Tilt boards can be used to practice weight shifting and equilibrium responses. Patients can either sit or stand on the tilt board, depending on their motor abilities. Other activities that challenge the patient's static and dynamic balance include one-foot standing, heel-toe walking, walking on a balance beam, turning, abrupt stopping and starting, braiding (walking sideways, crossing one foot over the other), walking over and around obstacles, carrying objects during ambulation, negotiating environmental barriers, jumping, and skipping.

The sensory components of an activity can also be modified to make the activity more challenging for the patient. Lighting can be changed. Patients can be asked to work on foam or floor mats, or they can take their shoes and socks off to change the proprioceptive input received through the feet. Patients can also progress from working in a quiet environment to working in one that is noisier and more congested, although the focus remains on the patient's ability to complete the motor task presented.

Performing cardiovascular and aerobic conditioning activities are good exercises for patients with good motor abilities. Walking on a treadmill, cycling, swimming, and performing an aerobics program are all useful activities to improve cardiovascular responses and to challenge the patient's coordination. As stated previously, many patients who have sustained a TBI are deconditioned, and aerobic exercise is a good way to improve the patient's level of cardiovascular fitness. Exercise can also be used for stress management. Following the 2008 Physical Activity Guidelines for Adults with Disabilities is recommended when designing an exercise program for the patient. A hundred and fifty minutes of exercise of moderate intensity per week coupled with a general strengthening program two times a week is recommended (Gordon et al., 2016; U.S. Department of Health and Human Services, 2008).

Dual Task Training

Dual task training, which consists of performance of cognitive and motor tasks simultaneously, has been shown to be beneficial for patients with TBI (Fritz and Basso, 2013). Patients can practice ambulation skills while engaging in a conversation or performing simple mathematical calculations, or they might attempt walking on a treadmill and reading. Difficulty completing or an inability to perform dual tasks has been associated with safety concerns for the patient (Scherer et al., 2013). Damiano et al. (2016) investigated the effects of a novel rehabilitation strategy in a small group of ambulatory adults with chronic TBI. The subjects participated in an 8-week intensive daily program using a rapid-resisted elliptical trainer. Balance reaction times improved and were correlated with improvements on the High-Level Mobility Assessment Tool. Reaction time has been associated with cognitive function after brain injury (Brogolio et al., 2009).

Korman et al. (2018) used a finger opposition sequencing task to study procedural learning in 10 hospitalized patients with a subacute phase of moderate to severe TBI and compared their performance with a healthy control group. The treatment group was found to exhibit the same three phases of skill learning as the healthy control group except that the time course was atypical. The rate slowed in the TBI group in the second week when training intensified. This may have been owing to cognitive fatigue. The treated TBI group was able to demonstrate procedural learning albeit at a slower rate than healthy controls. Initial FIM scores were correlated to gains made at the end of the study. These gains were retained. The researchers recommend optimizing practice schedules to take advantage of the potential for long-term plasticity.

The patient's plan of care should be composed of activities that include both physical and cognitive challenges. Throwing and catching, maneuvering through an obstacle course, and following a map allow for the performance of high-level motor and cognitive tasks. Balance activities previously mentioned can also be performed, and an additional cognitive component, such as counting the repetitions, can be incorporated. Decreasing the amount of structure or cueing provided or increasing the complexity of the task are ways in which the assistant can challenge the patient's cognitive abilities. Some facilities have access to simulated city environments (Easy Street). A grocery store, bank, fast-food counter, and environmental barriers one would encounter in the community are represented and available for patient practice. Community outings are another therapeutic way to work on physical and cognitive tasks. Many facilities arrange outings for patients at various stages in their rehabilitation. Trips to a restaurant, the zoo, or a bowling alley are common examples of community trips. On these trips, patients are encouraged to practice the skills they have been working on in therapy. The benefit of these outings is that therapists are there to assist the patients and can assess areas in which the patients may have difficulty once they are discharged to home.

DISCHARGE PLANNING

Prior to discharge, it is important to provide opportunities for the patient to experience therapy services outside the typical hospital setting to incorporate community-based environments. This may include, but not be limited to, trials outside the unit in which the patient currently resides and community outings outside the hospital, such as trips to a restaurant or even crossing a busy street. These opportunities will provide the patient with the chance to practice skills that will be needed at discharge as well as give the clinician a chance to implement strategies to ease discharge. Discharge planning is an important component of treatment for the patient with TBI. Decisions must be made about the most appropriate discharge destination. It would be unrealistic to assume that all patients will make a full recovery and resume all previous aspects of their lives. Many patients require follow-up care ranging from supervision in the home to placement in an extended-care or residential facility. Planning for the patient's discharge should include the patient, the family, and appropriate members of the rehabilitation team. Patient-centered care with strong family support is needed to assure that all needs and wants are met at discharge. Procurement of adaptive equipment, environmental modifications required at the patient's home, and home health care services should be arranged before the patient's discharge from the facility secondary to lingering physical and cognitive deficits that can cause safety concerns. Some patients may require additional services following their discharge from rehabilitation. Comprehensive outpatient physical therapy services, day treatment programs, and residential programs that address community reentry may continue to be needed to improve the patient's physical, cognitive, and behavioral limitations.

CHAPTER SUMMARY

Traumatic brain injury is a public health issue that affects all ages. It is a progressive and chronic disorder that results in lifetime consequences. The heterogeneous nature of TBI makes it difficult for research to draw definitive conclusions about the effectiveness of interventions. Treating a patient with TBI can be extremely challenging and rewarding. Patients who have experienced a traumatic brain injury may present in a multitude of ways that vary from coma and no voluntary movement to high motor function with significant cognitive deficits. Family- and patient-centered care is crucial for successful outcomes. Family education provides accurate information about the person's physical and behavioral status. For many physical therapists and physical therapist assistants, the cognitive component of intervention is most difficult. To provide patients with the highest quality care possible, the clinician must be able to address motor and cognitive issues simultaneously. Creative interventions that integrate physical and cognitive tasks coupled with principles of motor learning and task-specific training will provide our patients with the most effective care possible to improve their functional abilities and, hopefully, resume their previous lifestyles.

REVIEW QUESTIONS

1. Describe the clinical manifestations of a subdural hematoma.

2. What are some signs and symptoms of increased intracranial pressure (ICP)?

3. Differentiate between a patient in a coma and a patient in a persistent vegetative state.

4. List four goals of acute physical therapy intervention for the patient with a traumatic brain injury (TBI).

5. Define the eight stages within the Rancho Los Amigos Scale of Cognitive Functioning.

6. Discuss the benefits of hand-over-hand modeling for patients with decreased cognitive functioning.

7. How may the physical environment affect the patient's response to intervention?

8. A patient is exhibiting significant disorientation and attention deficits. How could the physical therapist assistant (PTA) intervene to assist the patient in therapy?

9. A patient becomes easily agitated and frustrated during therapy. At times, he or she can escalate into a full crisis. What can the PTA do to minimize these episodes? What should the PTA do if a crisis situation occurs?

10. A patient who has had a TBI possesses good motor skills. She is able to walk independently without an assistive device and is able to transfer independently. The patient does exhibit occasional losses of balance. The patient's cognitive abilities are more seriously impaired. She is disoriented and has memory deficits. Identify four treatment activities for this patient that incorporate physical and cognitive components.

CASE STUDIES REHABILITATION UNIT INITIAL EXAMINATION AND EVALUATION

History

Chart Review

Patient is a 25-year-old divorced male from Indiana. Patient works full-time as a self-employed contractor. He was transferred to University Hospital from a small rural hospital following a motor vehicle accident (MVA). Patient was unconscious at the scene and remained so to the time of arrival in the ER. His head CT showed evidence of considerable scalp hematoma involving the left parietal area, and a minimal hematoma in the right parietotemporal area. The CT was positive for depressed fracture left midparietal bone with no significant intracranial abnormality noted. Skull x-ray was positive for left parietal bone fracture. Chest x-ray showed mild prominence superior mediastinum, and localized pleural thickening along the left lateral chest wall, possibly related to nondisplaced rib fracture. Patient was placed on volume ventilator. One week later, the tracheostomy was capped after he was weaned off the ventilator. Patient is currently taking Tegretol, Zanaflex, and Ativan.

Physical therapy (PT) order for examination and treatment received.

Subjective

Patient is unable to respond and no family members were present at the time of the initial examination to provide information. Chart review was referred to for information. Not able to receive informed consent for examination.

Objective

Appearance/Rest Posture/Equipment: Patient is supine in hospital bed with midline head position; decerebrate posturing with wrist and fingers flexed, shoulders internally rotated and adducted, lower extremities adducted and extended. Patient is wearing low top tennis shoes. The tracheostomy is plugged; catheter and intravenous lines in place.

Systems Review

Cognition/Communication: Patient is moaning, no other verbalizations

Cardiovascular/Pulmonary: BP = 135/80 mm Hg; HR = 140 bpm; RR = rapid at 40 bpm

Integumentary: Ecchymosis about the left ear, lacerations on the scalp

Musculoskeletal: Impaired bilaterally

Neuromuscular: Nonpurposeful movement in left upper extremity shown once. Trace volitional movement in bilateral upper and lower extremities. Gait, locomotion, and balance impaired.

Psychosocial: Patient has a fair support system: family (parents) and friends.

Tests and Measures

Anthropometrics: Height 6'3", Weight 180 lbs, BMI 22 (20–24 is normal).

Arousal, Attention, Cognition: Patient is able to open his eyes without stimulation. He is not oriented to person, place, or time. He uses nonverbal, nonfunctional vocalization (moans and groans). He is able to withdraw from stimuli when a noxious stimulus is presented. He is able to follow one-step commands inconsistently. He orients toward sound, opens eyes in response to command, and displays partial localization to light flashes inconsistently. Patient demonstrates blinks in response to threat consistently. He is partially able to track pictures of family members inconsistently. He is able to reach for a familiar object, but loses it quickly and unable to use it functionally.

Cranial Nerve Integrity: Patient squints with his eyes in response to light. He withdraws from noxious scent with grimacing 3/3 times.

Range of Motion: Passive range of motion in the upper extremities is within functional limits after inhibition; hip flexion is 90 degrees bilaterally, and both ankles lack 5 degrees from neutral. Active hip and knee flexion and elbow flexion to 30 degrees bilaterally.

Reflex Integrity: Bilateral patellar, biceps, ankle DTRs 3 +; Babinski present bilaterally. Asymmetric tonic neck reflex is present to R. Marked increase seen in tone in hip extensors and gastrocnemius soleus. A slight increase in tone of the hip internal rotators, hip adductors, triceps, forearm, and finger flexors is noted bilaterally during passive range of motion. Tone decreases with rhythmic rotation of the limb(s) or trunk. Extensor tone increases in the lower extremities when patient transferred into sitting.

Motor Function: Rolls to right and left with maximal assist of 1. Transfers from side-lying to sitting with maximal assist of 1; increased extensor tone in the lower extremities. Transfers from sit to supine with maximal assist of 1.

CASE STUDIES REHABILITATION UNIT INITIAL EXAMINATION AND EVALUATION—cont'd

Posture: Patient's head is in midline. He demonstrates extension posture in supine: bilateral shoulder adduction, elevation and internal rotation, elbow extension, finger and wrist flexion. He also demonstrates hip extension, adduction, and internal rotation; knee extension, and ankle plantar flexion bilaterally. In supported sitting, patient demonstrates rounded shoulders, flexed head and neck, thoracic kyphosis, both upper extremities extended at sides, and lower extremities are in extension.

Muscle Performance: Not assessed because of patient's inability to follow complex commands.

Neuromotor Development: Patient's swallowing is facilitated by stroking downward on the anterior neck. No head or trunk righting is noted; protective reactions are not absent.

Gait, Locomotion, Balance: Patient shows fair sitting balance. Needs mod assist 1 to maintain head and trunk in midline. Patient stood at bedside for approximately 1 minute with maximal assist of 2 and requires assist to maintain hips in extension and an erect trunk. Gait not assessed.

Sensory Integrity: Unable to assess accurately because of the patient's inability to respond, although patient does respond inconsistently to pain and tactile stimulation.

Self-Care: Patient is dependent for all care.

Assessment/Evaluation

Patient is a 25-year-old man who sustained a traumatic brain injury as a result of an MVA. He is assessed to be at a level II/III of cognitive function on the Rancho Scale, based on inconsistent responses to sensory stimuli and verbal commands. Patient also demonstrates limited active movement and decerebrate posturing.

Glasgow Coma Scale is eye opening 4; motor response 4; verbal response 2; 11 total

Coma Recovery Scale Revised Score: 10 (Vegetative state with emerging behaviors of a minimally conscious state)

FIM: Transfers 1, locomotion 1

Problem List

1. Dependent in functional mobility
2. Lacks head control in sitting
3. Poor head and trunk control in sitting and standing
4. Lacks ability to communicate
5. Decreased awareness and inconsistent responses to sensory stimuli
6. Decreased volitional movement

Diagnosis: Patient demonstrates impaired arousal, range of motion, and motor control associated with coma. Rancho Scale level of cognitive function is II/III.

Prognosis: Over the course of 3 months, the patient will demonstrate optimal arousal, range of motion, and motor control and the minimization of secondary impairments. Potential to reach rehab goals is fair secondary to the patient's decreased cognitive abilities and motor deficits.

Short-Term Goals (to be Achieved by 2 Weeks)

1. Patient will roll to both sides in bed with minimal assist of 1 while demonstrating dissociation of trunk and pelvis.
2. Patient will transfer supine to sit with minimal assist of 1 and sit to stand with moderate assist of 1.
3. Patient will demonstrate head control in sitting for 5 minutes while performing self-care activities.

4. Patient will consistently respond to one-step commands three of four times.
5. Patient will be able to communicate wants and needs via actions, such as eye blinks or hand squeezes, 75% of the time.
6. Patient will initiate upper extremity movement bilaterally to perform self-care activities in sitting with minimal assist of 1 using hand-over-hand technique.

Long-Term Goals (to Be Achieved By 4 Weeks)

1. Patient will be independent in bed mobility and transfers to improve basic activities of daily living at home.
2. Patient will ambulate 150 feet with a rolling walker and minimal assist of 1 to improve household ambulation for future mobility.
3. Patient will consistently be able to communicate basic wants and needs 100% of the time to improve communication with friends and family.
4. Patient will ascend/descend 12 stairs with supervision and one handrail to access community safely.
5. Patient will return to home with supervision assist to improve safety in home environment.
6. Patient will perform a car transfer with supervision assist to improve mobility for outside appointments and community engagement.
7. Patient will perform home exercise program (HEP) independently to maintain strength and range of motion for mobility after discharge.
8. Family will demonstrate independence in all functional mobility tasks (transfers, ambulation, stairs) in order to improve patient safety with discharge home.

Plan

Treatment Schedule: The physical therapist (PT) and physical therapist assistant (PTA) will see the patient BID 5 days a week and once on Saturday and Sunday for 60-minute treatment sessions. Occupational therapy will be consulted regarding possible co-treatment. Treatment sessions are to include increasing the patient's level of awareness, positioning, functional mobility training (including body-weight support treadmill training and patient and family education), and discharge planning. Patient will be reassessed weekly.

Coordination, Communication, and Documentation: The PT and PTA will communicate with the patient and with his family on a regular basis as much as possible. The PT will communicate with the rehabilitation team. Outcomes of rehabilitation will be documented on a weekly basis.

Patient/Client Instruction: Patient's parents will be educated in proper transfer and functional mobility interventions. Education regarding the patient's condition and the prevention of secondary complications will be provided to the family. The family will participate in family training to learn to assist the patient with activities of daily living, transfers, and functional mobility. Instruction in a HEP will occur before discharge.

Interventions

1. Communication:
   a. A communication system of actions, such as eye blinks or hand squeezes, will be developed in order for the patient to communicate yes-no responses with visitors and the rehabilitation team.

Continued

CASE STUDIES REHABILITATION UNIT INITIAL EXAMINATION AND EVALUATION—cont'd

2. Cognitive retraining:
   a. A memory book will be developed, which will include pictures, pastimes, interests, and a daily schedule of therapy sessions, meals, medical interventions, and sleep.
   b. The book will be used in conjunction with other interventions to help orient the patient.
   c. A structured environment will be maintained at all times until the patient becomes less confused and can tolerate less structure.
   d. Patient will be treated in a quiet environment with minimal distractions until he can tolerate one in which there are more distractions.
   e. Orientation of person, place, current events, and time will be performed frequently throughout the treatment session.

3. Positioning:
   a. Patient will be positioned in side-lying (to both sides) to prevent the influence of the right asymmetric tonic neck reflex.
   b. To decrease the effects of the decerebrate posture, the patient will be positioned in supine with his upper extremities flexed over his head with his hands weight bearing flat on the bed and his lower extremities flexed with a roll under his knees; prone positioning over a wedge will also be used.
   c. Rhythmic rotation to the upper and lower extremities and trunk will be used to decrease rigidity to allow positioning and movement transitions.
   d. Bottoms-up position will be attained with the therapist providing reciprocal rhythmic rotation of the lower and upper extremities to promote dissociation of the upper and lower trunk to decrease the decerebrate posture.

4. Functional mobility training:
   a. Assisted rolling to both sides with progression from maximal assist of 1 → moderate assist of 1 → minimal assist of 1 → standby assist of 1 as patient is able.
   b. Practice of supine ←→ sit and sit ←→ stand transfers with maximal assist of 1-2 → moderate assist of 1 → minimal assist of 1 as patient progresses.
   c. Sitting on the edge of the bed or mat with both upper extremities flexed and weight bearing on a table at lap height with therapist supporting head, attending to memory book, and completion of upper extremity activities.
   d. Patient will be transferred to a tilt-in-space wheelchair, will transition to a regular wheelchair as the patient is able to tolerate.
   e. Hand-over-hand techniques to promote self-care activities or upper extremity PNF techniques will be used with the patient in this position with one hand support.
   f. Washing of the face will be performed to increase sensory awareness to the face.
   g. Patient can also look at the memory book while in this position.
   h. Patient will be placed prone over a bolster (lengthwise) with upper and lower extremities bearing weight.
   i. In prone on elbows, patient will perform weight shifts to the right and left to increase proprioceptive input.
   j. Facilitation techniques, including tapping to the posterior cervical muscles, will be performed to facilitate head and neck extension; these will be decreased as the patient is able to control his head posture.
   k. Patient can use the memory book in prone position for orientation.
   l. Transition from prone on elbows to quadruped and tall-kneeling to increase patient's awareness, to lower extremity flexibility, and to increase tolerance to a more upright position.
   m. Patient will be placed in a plantigrade position with upper extremities over a bolster and lower extremities in a step stance; weight shifts will be performed in all directions to increase proprioceptive information, facilitate postural reactions, and prepare for ambulation.
   n. Patient will use the memory book or other cognitive challenges in conjunction with plantigrade position.
   o. Patient will participate in BWSTT for 20 to 30 minutes each day, will progress to overground ambulation as the patient tolerates.
   p. Patient will practice gait activities with a rolling walker with maximal assist of 1 to 2 → moderate assist of 1 → minimal assist of 1 → standby assist of 1 as he progresses.
   q. Patient will be asked to walk toward an object or place of interest; orientation will be incorporated in this exercise by having the patient walk to get a newspaper or objects he may need in the home.
   r. As patient progresses, simulated shopping may be included with gait activities.
   s. Patient will be asked to make a list of items or remember a list given to him verbally to make the task more cognitively challenging.

5. Dynamic balance activities:
   a. In a standing position, the patient will shoot baskets and count baskets made.
   b. Patient will carry objects while ambulating.

6. Discharge planning:
   a. Patient will be discharged to home with supervision by caregiver.
   b. A home assessment will be performed if needed.
   c. Equipment will be secured as necessary.
   d. If a proper caregiver cannot be obtained for discharge to home, the patient will be discharged to assisted-living facility.
   e. Vocational rehabilitation will be contacted.

Questions To Think About

- How can the therapists facilitate the performance of functional activities?
- What other therapeutic interventions can be used to help the patient with motor learning?
- How can aerobic conditioning be included in the patient's treatment program?
- What types of activities or exercises would be included as part of the patient's home exercise program?

REFERENCES

Abd-Elfattah HM, Abdelazeim FH, Elshennawy S: Physical and cognitive consequences of fatigue: a review, *J Adv Res* 6:351–358, 2015.

American Physical Therapy Association: *Position paper: protecting student athletes from concussions act of 2013 (HR 3530)*, 2013. Available at: www.apta.org/PolicyResources/PositionPapers/ConcussionsStudentAthletes. Accessed November 3, 2014.

Anstead A: Cerebral spinal fluid leak repair, *Oper Tech Otolaryngol* 25:187–193, 2014.

Bland DC, Zampieri-Gallagher C, Damiano DL: Effectiveness of physical therapy for improving gait and balance in ambulatory individuals with traumatic brain injury: a systematic review of the literature, *Brain Inj* 25:664–679, 2011.

Bleiberg J: *The road to rehabilitation. Part 3. Guideposts to recognition: cognition, memory, and brain injury*, Vienna, VA, 2009, Brain Injury Association of America.

Bontke CF, Baize CM, Boake C: Coma management and sensory stimulation, *Phys Med Rehabil Clin N Am* 3:259–272, 1992.

Bontke CF, Boake C: Principles of brain injury rehabilitation. In Braddom RL, editor: *Physical medicine and rehabilitation*, Philadelphia, PA, 1996, Saunders, pp 1027–1051.

Borich MR, Cheung KL, Jones P, et al.: Concussion: current concepts in diagnosis and management, *JNPT* 37:133–139, 2013.

Brain Injury Association of America: *Brain injury facts and statistics*, Vienna, VA, 2019. Available at: www.biausa.org. Accessed June 6, 2019.

Brogolio SP, Sosnoff JJ, Ferrara MS: The relationship of athlete-reported concussion symptoms and objective measures of neurocognitive function and postural control, *Clin J Sport Med* 19:377–382, 2009.

Campbell M: *Rehabilitation for traumatic brain injury physical therapy practice in context*, London, 2000, Churchill Livingstone, pp 17–45.

Centers for Disease Control and Prevention: *Traumatic brain injury in the United States: fact sheet*, Updated February 2014. Available at: www.cdc.gov/traumaticbraininjury/get_the_facts.html. Accessed June 6, 2019.

Damiano DL, Zampieri C, Ge J, Acevedo A, Dsurney J: Effects of a rapid-resisted elliptical training program on motor, cognitive and neurobehavioral functioning in adults with chronic traumatic brain injury, *Exp Brain Res* 234(8):2245–2252, 2016.

Davies PM: *Starting again: early rehabilitation after traumatic brain injury or other severe brain lesion*, New York, 1994, Springer-Verlag, pp 23–44, 65–68, 86–88, 316–352, 361–364.

Drummond M, Douglas J, Olver J: "I really hope it comes back"—olfactory impairment following traumatic brain injury: a longitudinal study, *NeuroRehabilitation* 41(1):241–248, 2017.

Eisenstein N, Stapley S, Grover L: Post-traumatic heterotopic ossification: an old problem in need of new solutions, *J Orthop Res* 36:1061–1068, 2018.

Frati A, Cerretani D, Fiaschi AI, et al.: Diffuse axonal injury and oxidative stress: a comprehensive review, *Int J Mol Sci* 18(12):E2600, 2017. doi:10.3390/ijms18122600.

Fritz NE, Basso DM: Dual-task training for balance and mobility in a person with severe traumatic brain injury: a case study, *J Neurol Phys Ther* 37:37–43, 2013.

Fulk GD, Bouden, Behrman A: Spinal cord injury. In O'Sullivan SB, Schmitz TJ, Fulk GD, editors: *Physical rehabilitation*, ed 7, Philadelphia, 2019, FA Davis, pp 855–917.

Fulk GD, Nirider CD: Traumatic brain injury. In O'Sullivan SB, Schmitz TJ, Fulk GD, editors: *Physical rehabilitation*, ed 7, Philadelphia, 2019, FA Davis, pp 817–854.

Fuller KS: Seizures and epilepsy. In Goodman CC, Fuller KS, editors: *Pathology implications for the physical therapist*, ed 4, St. Louis, 2015, Elsevier, pp 1591–1605.

Ghajar JB, Hariri RJ, Patterson RH: Improved outcome from traumatic coma using only ventricular CSF drainage for ICP control, *Adv Neurosurg* 21:173–177, 1993.

Giacino JT, Kalmar K, Whyte J: The JFK Coma Recovery Scale-Revised: measurement characteristics and diagnostic utility, *Arch Phys Med Rehabil* 85(12):2020–2029, 2004.

Giza CC, Kutcher JS, Ashwal S, et al.: *Summary of evidence-based guidelines update: evaluation and management of concussion in sports; report of the Guideline Development Subcommittee of the American Academy of Neurology*, Published July 2013. Available at: https://www.ptnow.org/clinical-practice-guideline-detail/summary-of-evidencebased-guideline-update-evaluati. Accessed April 2015.

Gordon BT, Durstine JL, Painter PL, Moore GF: Basic physical activity and exercise recommendations for person with chronic conditions. In Moore GF, Durstine JL, Painter PL, editors: *ACSM's exercise management for persons with chronic diseases and disabilities*, ed 4, Champaign, IL, 2016, Human Kinetics, pp 15–32.

Gosseries O, Vanhaudenhuyse A, Bruno A, et al.: Disorders of consciousness: coma, vegetative, minimally conscious state. In Cvetkovic, D, Cosic I, editors: *States of consciousness: experimental insights into meditation, waking, sleep, and dreams*, Berlin, 2011, Springer-Verlag, pp 29–54.

Hammond FM, McDeavitt JT: Medical and orthopedic complications. In Rosenthal M, Griffith ER, Kreutzer JS, et al., editors: *Rehabilitation of the adult and child with traumatic brain injury*, ed 3, Philadelphia, 1999, FA Davis, pp 53–73.

Hoyt BW, Pavey GJ, Potter BK, Forsberg JA: Heterotopic ossification and lessons learned from fifteen years at war: a review of therapy, novel research, and future directions for military and civilian orthopaedic trauma, *Bone* 109:3–11, 2018.

Hubert RJ, VanMeter KC: *Gould's pathophysiology for the health professions*, ed 6, St. Louis, 2018, Elsevier, pp 354–358.

Jennett B, Teasdale G: *Management of head injuries*, Philadelphia, 1981, FA Davis, pp 122–131.

Kim E: Agitation, aggression, and disinhibition syndromes after traumatic brain injury, *NeuroRehabilitation* 17:297–310, 2002.

Kinoshita K: Traumatic brain injury: pathophysiology for neurocritical care, *J Intensive Care* 4:29, 2016. doi:10.1186/s40560-016-0138-3.

Korman M, Shaklai S, Cisamariu K, et al.: Atypical within-session motor procedural learning after traumatic brain injury but well-preserved between-session procedural memory consolidation, *Front Hum Neurosci* 12:10, 2018. doi:10.3389/fnhum.2018.00010.

Krus LH: Cognitive and behavioral skills retraining of the brain-injured patient, *Clin Manage* 8:24–31, 1988.

Łęgosz P, Drela K, Pulik Ł, Sarzyńska S, Małdyk P: Challenges of heterotopic ossification-molecular background and current treatment strategies, *Clin Exp Pharmacol Physiol* 45(12):1229–1235, 2018. doi:10.1111/1440-1681.13025.

Lombardi F, Taricco M, De Tanti A, Telaro E, Liberati A: Sensory stimulation for brain injured individuals in coma or vegetative state, *Cochrane Database Syst Rev* (2):CD001427, 2002.

Lundy-Ekman L: *Neuroscience: fundamentals for rehabilitation*, ed 5, St. Louis, 2018, Elsevier, pp 534–535.

McCulloch K, Fuller KS: Traumatic brain injury. In Goodman CC, Fuller KS, editors: *Pathology implications for the physical therapist*, ed 4, St. Louis, 2015, Elsevier, pp 1535–1555.

Meyfroidt G, Baguley IJ, Menon DK: Paroxysmal sympathetic hyperactivity: the storm after acute brain injury, *Lancet Neurol* 16(9):721–729, 2017.

Mortenson PA, Eng JJ: Use of casts in the management of joint mobility and hypertonia following brain injury in adults: a systematic review, *Phys Ther* 83:648–658, 2003.

National Institute of Neurological Disorders and Stroke: *Traumatic brain injury: hope through research*, Published September 20, 2015. Available at: www.ninds.nih.gov/Disorders/patient-caregiver-education/hope-through-research/traumatic-brain-injury-hope-through. Accessed December 17, 2019.

O'Sullivan SB: Strategies to improve motor control and motor learning. In O'Sullivan SB, Schmitz TJ, Fulk GD, editors: *Physical rehabilitation*, ed 6, Philadelphia, 2014, FA Davis, pp 393–443.

Ostermann RC, Joestl J, Tiefenboeck TM, et al.: Risk factors predicting prognosis and outcome of elderly patients with isolated traumatic brain injury, *J Orthop Surg Res* 13(1):277, 2018. doi:10.1186/s13018-018-0975-y.

Padilla R, Domina A: Effectiveness of sensory stimulation to improve arousal and alertness of people in a coma or persistent vegetative state after traumatic brain injury: a systematic review, *Am J Occup Ther* 70(3):7003180030p1-8, 2016. doi:10.5014/ajot.2016.021022.

Perrin PB, Niemeier JP, Mougeot JL, et al.: Measures of injury severity and prediction of acute traumatic brain injury outcomes, *J Head Trauma Rehabil* 30(2):136–142, 2015.

Persel CS, Persel CH: The use of applied behavior analysis in traumatic brain injury rehabilitation. In Ashley MJ, Krych DK, editors: *Traumatic brain injury rehabilitation*, Boca Raton, FL, 1995, CRC Press, pp 231–273.

Scherer MR, Weightman MM, Radomski MV, Davidson LF, McCulloch KL: Returning service members to duty following mild TBI: exploring the use of dual-task and multi-task assessment methods, *Phys Ther* 93:1254–1267, 2013.

Synnot A, Chau M, Pitt V, et al.: Interventions for managing skeletal muscle spasticity following traumatic brain injury, *Cochrane Database Sys Rev* 11:CD008929, 2017. doi:10.1002/14651858.CD008929.pub2.

Teasdale G, Jennett B: Assessment of coma and impaired consciousness: a practical scale, *Lancet* 2(7872):81–84, 1974.

U.S. Department of Health and Human Services: *2008 Physical Activity Guidelines for Americans*. Available at: www.health.gov/paguidelines/guidelines. Accessed October 2, 2014.

Vakil E: The effect of moderate to severe traumatic brain injury (TBI) on different aspects of memory: a selective review, *J Clin Exp Neuropsychol* 27(8):977–1021, 2005.

Vakil E, Lev-Ran Galon C: Baseline performance and learning rate of conceptual and perceptual skill-learning tasks: the effect of moderate to severe traumatic brain injury, *J Clin Exp Neuropsychol* 36:447–454, 2014.

Van Erp WS, Lavrijsen JC, van de Laar FA, et al.: The vegetative state/unresponsive wakefulness syndrome: a systematic review of prevalence studies, *Eur J Neurol* 21(11):1361–1368, 2014.

Varghese G: Heterotopic ossification, *Phys Med Rehabil Clin N Am* 3:407–415, 1992.

Winkler PA: Traumatic brain injury. In Umphred DA, Lazaro RT, Roller ML, Burton GU, editors: *Neurological rehabilitation*, ed 6, St. Louis, 2013, Elsevier, pp 753–790.

Zec RF, Zellers D, Belman J, et al.: Long-term consequences of severe closed head injury on episodic memory, *J Clin Exp Neuropsychol* 23:671–691, 2001.

13

Spinal Cord Injuries

OBJECTIVES

After reading this chapter, the student will be able to:

1. Discuss the causes, clinical manifestations, and possible complications of spinal cord injury.
2. Differentiate between complete and incomplete types of spinal cord injuries.
3. Discuss the various levels of spinal cord injury.
4. Relate segmental level of muscle innervation to level of function in the patient with a spinal cord injury.
5. Instruct patients with spinal cord injuries in pulmonary exercises, strengthening exercises, and mat and transfer activities.
6. Identify differences between a compensatory and recovery approach to patient care.
7. Teach gait/locomotor training and wheelchair mobility interventions to the patient, as appropriate.

INTRODUCTION

An estimated 17,730 new cases of spinal cord injury (SCI) occur annually. Within the United States, currently more than 291,000 people are living with SCIs (National Spinal Cord Injury Statistical Center, 2019). SCIs are most likely to occur in young adults between the ages of 16 and 30 years. However, as the population in the United States continues to age, the average age at time of injury has also increased to 43 years. Approximately 78% of the individuals with SCIs are male (National Spinal Cord Injury Statistical Center, 2019). The etiology of SCIs continues to change. Previously, motor vehicle accidents and sporting activities were identified as the most likely causes of these injuries. More recent statistics suggest that motor vehicle accidents (39.3%), falls (31.8%), acts of violence (13.5%), sports and recreation related injuries (8.0%), and medical and surgical complications (4.3%) are the most common causes of SCIs in the United States (National Spinal Cord Injury Statistical Center, 2019).

Life expectancies for individuals with SCIs are still below those without SCI, and there has not been an improvement in this statistic since the 1980s. Individuals with SCIs can experience a lifetime of disability and life-threatening medical complications. Potential causes of death that significantly affect life expectancy include pneumonia and septicemia. The cost of medical care for these individuals is in the billions of dollars. Lifetime medical expenses for individuals with high cervical injuries are approximately $5 million, and $2.5 million for individuals with paraplegia. These figures can exceed the maximum insurance benefit allowed by many insurance policies. In addition to the direct costs of medical care, there are indirect costs associated with lost wages, employee benefits, and productivity—costs that can average $76,327 a year (National Spinal Cord Injury Statistical Center, 2019).

ETIOLOGY

To understand the etiology of SCIs, it is necessary to review the anatomy of the region. There are 31 pairs of spinal nerves within the peripheral nervous system. There are eight pairs of spinal nerves in the cervical region. The first seven pairs exit above the first seven cervical vertebrae. Spinal nerve C8 exits between C7 and T1, because there is no eighth cervical vertebra. The remaining spinal nerve roots exit below the corresponding bony vertebrae. This holds true through L1. At this point, the spinal cord becomes a mass of nerve roots known as the *cauda equina*. Fig. 13.1 illustrates segmental and vertebral levels.

Certain areas of the spinal column are more susceptible to injury than others. In the cervical spine, the spinal segments of C1, C2, and C5 through C7 are often injured, and in the thoracolumbar area, T12 through L2 are most often affected. The biomechanics of the vertebral column accentuates this situation. Movement (rotation) is greatest at these segments and leads to instability within the regions. In addition, the spinal cord is larger in these areas because of the large number of nerve cell bodies, which are located here. Fig. 13.2 illustrates this configuration.

NAMING THE LEVEL OF INJURY

To name the level of an individual's injury, the health care professional first identifies the vertebral or bony spine segment involved. For example, cervical injuries are designated with C, thoracic injuries with T, and lumbar injuries with L. This designation is followed by the last spinal nerve root segment in which innervation is present. Therefore, if a patient has an injury in the cervical region and has innervation of the biceps, the lesion would be classified as a C5 injury. Medical personnel have used the following terms to describe the extent

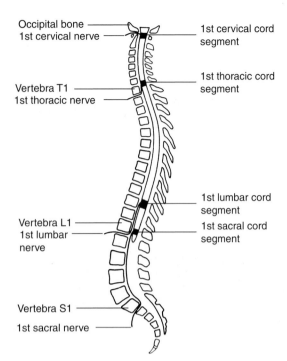

Fig. 13.1 Segmental and Vertebral Levels Compared. Spinal nerves 1 to 7 emerge above the corresponding vertebrae, and the remaining spinal nerves emerge below them. (From Fitzgerald MJT: *Neuroanatomy: basic and clinical, clinical neuroanatomy and related neuroscience*, ed 4, London, 2002, WB Saunders.)

of involvement a patient may be experiencing. Individuals with injuries to the cervical region of the spine are classified as having *tetraplegia,* which is the preferred term. Tetraplegia encompasses impairments to the upper extremities, lower extremities, trunk, and pelvic organs. Injuries involving the thoracic spine can produce *paraplegia.* With paraplegia upper extremity function is spared, but there are varying degrees of lower extremity, trunk, and pelvic organ involvement. Injuries to the spinal roots at L1 or below are called cauda equina injuries (Lundy-Ekman, 2018; Burns et al., 2012).

The American Spinal Injury Association (ASIA) has developed a classification system to assist clinicians with a standard mechanism to document a patient's sensory and motor function after an SCI. The International Standards for Neurological Classification of Spinal Cord Injury (ISNCSCI) allows health care providers to determine the level and severity of a patient's injury objectively, assists in the determination of the patient's prognosis, and promotes improved consistency in the communication among the health care team (ASIA, 2019; Fulk et al., 2019). Fig. 13.3 is a reprint of the assessment tool.

The *neurologic level* is defined as the "most caudal segment of the cord with intact sensation and antigravity (3 or more) muscle function strength, provided that there is normal (intact) sensory and motor function rostrally respectively" (ASIA, 2019). The neurologic level is determined by testing key dermatomes (sensory areas) and myotomes (muscles) in a supine position. A patient's sensory level is determined by assessing both light touch and pinprick sensation bilaterally in the extremities and trunk (ASIA, 2019).

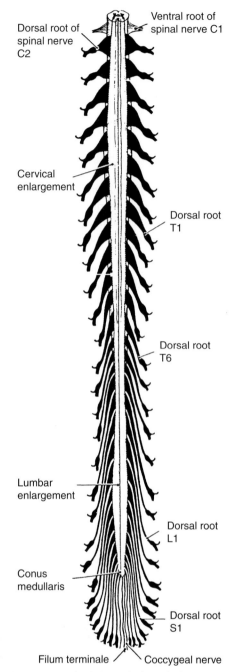

Fig. 13.2 Posterior view of the spinal cord showing the attached dorsal roots and spinal ganglia. (From Carpenter MB, Sutin J: *Human neuroanatomy*, ed 8, Baltimore, 1983, Williams & Wilkins.)

The motor level for the right and left sides is defined as the lowest key muscle with a manual muscle testing grade of fair (3/5), provided that the key muscles above this level have intact (normal, 5/5) strength. ASIA has chosen these muscles because they are consistently innervated by the designated segments of the spinal cord and are easily tested in a clinical setting (ASIA, 2019). Table 13.1 lists the ASIA key muscles for the upper and lower extremities. For example, the elbow extensors (C7) are a key muscle group. Patients with C7 innervation have the potential to transfer independently without a sliding board because of their

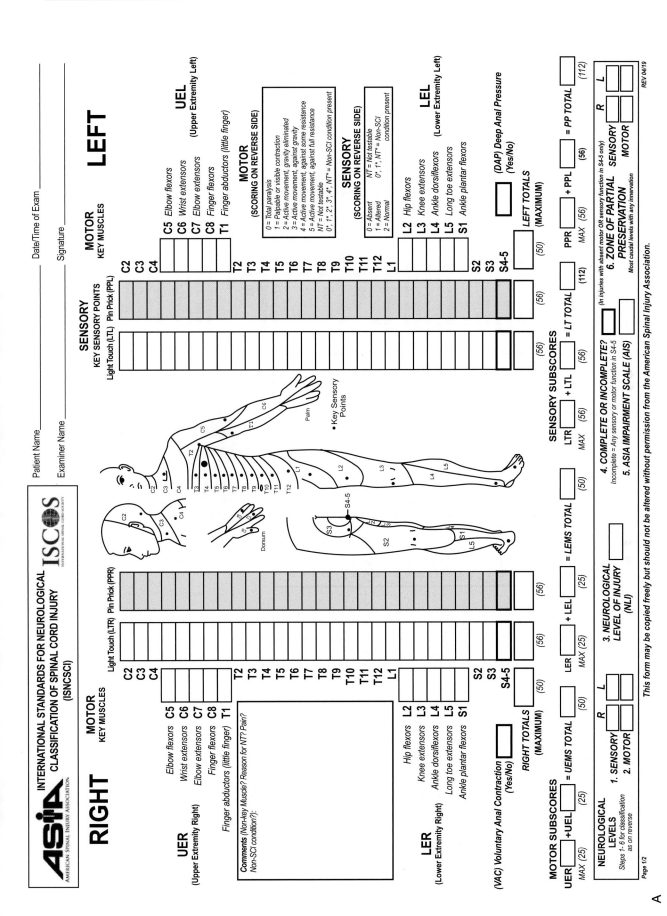

Fig. 13.3 ASIA Standard Neurological Classification of Spinal Cord Injury. (From American Spinal Injury Association: *International standards for neurological classification of spinal cord injury, revised*. Richmond, VA, 2019, American Spinal Injury Association. Available at: https://asia-spinalinjury.org/international-standards-neurological-classification-sci-isncsci-worksheet/.)

Muscle Function Grading

0 = Total paralysis

1 = Palpable or visible contraction

2 = Active movement, full range of motion (ROM) with gravity eliminated

3 = Active movement, full ROM against gravity

4 = Active movement, full ROM against gravity and moderate resistance in a muscle specific position

5 = (Normal) active movement, full ROM against gravity and full resistance in a functional muscle position expected from an otherwise unimpaired person

NT = Not testable (i.e. due to immobilization, severe pain such that the patient cannot be graded, amputation of limb, or contracture of > 50% of the normal ROM)

0*, 1*, 2*, 3*, 4*, NT* = Non-SCI condition present [a]

Sensory Grading

0 = Absent   1 = Altered, either decreased/impaired sensation or hypersensitivity

2 = Normal   NT = Not testable

0*, 1*, NT* = Non-SCI condition present [a]

[a] Note: Abnormal motor and sensory scores should be tagged with a '*' to indicate an impairment due to a non-SCI condition. The non-SCI condition should be explained in the comments box together with information about how the score is rated for classification purposes (at least normal / not normal for classification).

When to Test Non-Key Muscles:

In a patient with an apparent AIS B classification, non-key muscle functions more than 3 levels below the motor level on each side should be tested to most accurately classify the injury (differentiate between AIS B and C).

Movement	Root level
Shoulder: Flexion, extension, abduction, adduction, internal and external rotation **Elbow:** Supination	C5
Elbow: Pronation **Wrist:** Flexion	C6
Finger: Flexion at proximal joint, extension **Thumb:** Flexion, extension and abduction in plane of thumb	C7
Finger: Flexion at MCP joint **Thumb:** Opposition, adduction and abduction perpendicular to palm	C8
Finger: Abduction of the index finger	T1
Hip: Adduction	L2
Hip: External rotation	L3
Hip: Extension, abduction, internal rotation **Knee:** Flexion **Ankle:** Inversion and eversion **Toe:** MP and IP extension	L4
Hallux and Toe: DIP and PIP flexion and abduction	L5
Hallux: Adduction	S1

ASIA Impairment Scale (AIS)

A = Complete. No sensory or motor function is preserved in the sacral segments S4-5.

B = Sensory Incomplete. Sensory but not motor function is preserved below the neurological level and includes the sacral segments S4-5 (light touch or pin prick at S4-5 or deep anal pressure) AND no motor function is preserved more than three levels below the motor level on either side of the body.

C = Motor Incomplete. Motor function is preserved at the most caudal sacral segments for voluntary anal contraction (VAC) OR the patient meets the criteria for sensory incomplete status (sensory function preserved at the most caudal sacral segments S4-5 by LT, PP or DAP), and has some sparing of motor function more than three levels below the ipsilateral motor level on either side of the body.
(This includes key or non-key muscle functions to determine motor incomplete status.) For AIS C – less than half of key muscle functions below the single NLI have a muscle grade ≥ 3.

D = Motor Incomplete. Motor incomplete status as defined above, with at least half (half or more) of key muscle functions below the single NLI having a muscle grade ≥ 3.

E = Normal. If sensation and motor function as tested with the ISNCSCI are graded as normal in all segments, and the patient had prior deficits, then the AIS grade is E. Someone without an initial SCI does not receive an AIS grade.

Using ND: To document the sensory, motor and NLI levels, the ASIA Impairment Scale grade, and/or the zone of partial preservation (ZPP) when they are unable to be determined based on the examination results.

Steps in Classification

The following order is recommended for determining the classification of individuals with SCI.

1. Determine sensory levels for right and left sides.
The sensory level is the most caudal, intact dermatome for both pin prick and light touch sensation.

2. Determine motor levels for right and left sides.
Defined by the lowest key muscle function that has a grade of at least 3 (on supine testing), providing the key muscle functions represented by segments above that level are judged to be intact (graded as a 5).
Note: in regions where there is no myotome to test, the motor level is presumed to be the same as the sensory level, if testable motor function above that level is also normal.

3. Determine the neurological level of injury (NLI).
This refers to the most caudal segment of the cord with intact sensation and antigravity (3 or more) muscle function strength, provided that there is normal (intact) sensory and motor function rostrally respectively.
The NLI is the most cephalad of the sensory and motor levels determined in steps 1 and 2.

4. Determine whether the injury is Complete or Incomplete.
(i.e. absence or presence of sacral sparing)
If voluntary anal contraction = **No** AND all S4-5 sensory scores = 0 AND deep anal pressure = **No**, then injury is **Complete.**
Otherwise, injury is **Incomplete.**

5. Determine ASIA Impairment Scale (AIS) Grade.
Is injury Complete? If YES, AIS=A

NO ↓

Is injury Motor Complete? If YES, AIS=B

NO ↓   (No=voluntary anal contraction OR motor function more than three levels below the motor level on a given side, if the patient has sensory incomplete classification)

Are at least half (half or more) of the key muscles below the neurological level of injury graded 3 or better?

NO ↓   YES ↓

AIS=C   AIS=D

If sensation and motor function is normal in all segments, AIS=E
Note: AIS E is used in follow-up testing when an individual with a documented SCI has recovered normal function. If at initial testing no deficits are found, the individual is neurologically intact and the ASIA Impairment Scale does not apply.

6. Determine the zone of partial preservation (ZPP).
The ZPP is used only in injuries with absent motor (no VAC) OR sensory function (no DAP, no LT and no PP sensation) in the lowest sacral segments S4-5, and refers to those dermatomes and myotomes caudal to the sensory and motor levels that remain partially innervated. With sacral sparing of sensory function, the sensory ZPP is not applicable and therefore "NA" is recorded in the block of the worksheet. Accordingly, if VAC is present, the motor ZPP is not applicable and is noted as "NA".

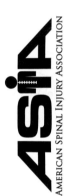

AMERICAN SPINAL INJURY ASSOCIATION

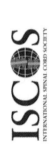

INTERNATIONAL STANDARDS FOR NEUROLOGICAL CLASSIFICATION OF SPINAL CORD INJURY

INTERNATIONAL SPINAL CORD SOCIETY

Page 2/2

Fig. 13.3, cont'd

B

TABLE 13.1 ASIA Identification of Key Muscles That Can Provide Greatest Functional Improvements

Level	Key Muscles
C5	Elbow flexors
C6	Wrist extensors
C7	Elbow extensors
C8	Finger flexors
T1	Finger abductors
L2	Hip flexors
L3	Knee extensors
L4	Ankle dorsiflexors
L5	Big toe extensors
S1	Ankle plantar flexors

Data from American Spinal Cord Injury Association: *International standards for neurological classification of spinal cord injury, revised*, Richmond, VA, 2019, American Spinal Injury Association.

ability to extend the elbow and perform a lateral push-up. The ASIA standards also recognize that muscles are innervated by more than one spinal cord segment. Thus, assigning one muscle or group to represent a single spinal nerve is not appropriate and leads to over simplification. Muscle innervation by one spinal nerve in the absence of additional innervation will result in muscle weakness (Burns et al., 2012). In areas where no specific myotomes exist to test, the motor level is presumed to correspond to the sensory level if the muscles above that level are judged to have normal strength (ASIA, 2019).

MECHANISMS OF INJURY

Traumatic impact is a common cause of SCI. Traumatic injuries are often caused by compression, penetrating injury, and hyperextension or hyperflexion forces. The resultant injury to the spinal cord can be temporary or permanent. Associated injuries to the vertebral bodies may also lead to spinal cord damage.

Vertebral subluxation (separation of the vertebral bodies), compression fractures, and fracture-dislocations can further damage the spinal cord by encroachment or additional compression of the spinal cord. Severe injuries to the vertebral column can also result in partial or complete transection of the spinal cord.

Cervical Flexion and Rotation Injuries

In the cervical region, the most common type of injury is one that involves flexion and rotation. With this type of force, the posterior spinal ligaments rupture, and the uppermost vertebra is displaced over the one below it. Rupture of the intervertebral disc and, in severe cases, the anterior longitudinal ligament can also occur. Transection of the spinal cord is often associated with this type of injury. Rear-end motor vehicle accidents frequently produce flexion and rotation injuries. Fig. 13.4, *A* provides an example of a flexion and rotation mechanism of injury.

Cervical Hyperflexion Injuries

A pure hyperflexion force causes an anterior compression fracture of the vertebral body with stretching of the posterior longitudinal ligaments. The ligaments remain intact, however. The force sustained by the bony structures leads to a wedge-type fracture of the vertebral bodies. This type of injury frequently severs the anterior spinal artery and results in an incomplete anterior cord syndrome. A head-on collision or a blow to the back of the head is a cause of this type of injury. Fig. 13.4, *B* depicts an example.

Cervical Hyperextension Injuries

Hyperextension injuries are common in the older adult as a result of a fall. The individual's chin often strikes a stationary object, and this leads to neck hyperextension. The force ruptures the anterior longitudinal ligament and compresses and ruptures the intervertebral disc. The spinal cord can become compressed between the ligamentum flavum and the vertebral body, with a resulting central cord type of injury. Fig. 13.4, *C* shows an example.

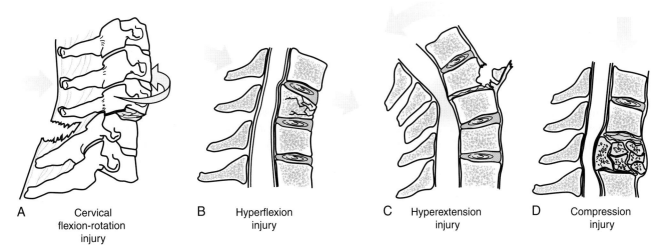

A Cervical flexion-rotation injury   **B** Hyperflexion injury   **C** Hyperextension injury   **D** Compression injury

Fig. 13.4 A–D, Types of spinal cord injuries.

Compression Injuries

Vertical compressive forces can also injure the spine. Diving accidents cause injuries that are a combination of compression and flexion forces. Falls from elevated surfaces can also produce this type of injury. With vertical compression, one sees fracture of the vertebral end plates and movement of the nucleus pulposus into the vertebral body. Bone fragments can be produced and displaced outward. The longitudinal ligaments are stretched but remain intact (see Fig. 13.4, *D*).

Compression injuries caused by the effects of osteoporosis, osteoarthritis, or rheumatoid arthritis can also produce an SCI in the older adult. A discussion of the pathologic processes that lead to these conditions is beyond the scope of this text.

MEDICAL INTERVENTION

Following an acute SCI, the patient should be immobilized and transferred to a trauma center. Proper management during the acute care phase of the injury can make a significant difference in the patient's long-term functional outcome. Monitoring the patient's respiratory and neurologic function is critical during this period. New pharmacologic interventions are under investigation to limit cell death at the site of injury and promote tissue sparing. Current guidelines discourage the administration of steroids after injury because there is limited evidence of benefit in the clinical setting and reports also indicate "high dose steroids are associated with harmful adverse effects" (Tefertiller et al., 2015).

Once the patient is medically stable, a primary concern of the physician is stabilization of the spine to prevent further spinal cord or nerve root damage. Surgery is indicated in the following situations: (1) to restore the alignment of bony vertebral structures; (2) to decompress neural tissue; (3) to stabilize the spine by fusion or instrumentation; (4) to minimize deformities; and (5) to allow the individual earlier opportunities for mobilization (Somers, 2010).

Several different stabilization procedures are available to the surgeon. Skeletal traction may be used on an interim basis while the patient's medical condition is fragile. Traction can reduce the overlapping of fracture fragments and can assist with spinal alignment. Once the patient is medically stable, the physician may schedule the patient for surgery. During surgery, fusion of the fracture fragments is performed. Bone grafting from the iliac crests, combined with placement of internal fixation devices, is often employed during this procedure. In some situations, surgery is not indicated, and external fixation with a halo jacket, a hard cervical collar, or a rigid body jacket may be all that is needed to stabilize the involved spinal segments. Bony fusion is usually complete in 6 to 8 weeks. Fig. 13.5 shows various types of spinal orthoses.

PATHOLOGIC CHANGES THAT OCCUR FOLLOWING INJURY

The changes that occur after spinal cord injury can be divided into two distinct phases: firstly, the *primary injury* phase, which occurs immediately after the injury and includes the structural damage that is sustained with the injury. The *secondary injury* phase includes the cascade of pathophysiologic events that are initiated shortly after the injury occurs.

Following spinal cord injury, ischemia, hypoxia, edema, and biochemical changes will cause cell death (necrosis) and excitotoxic damage (Tefertiller et al., 2015). Electrolyte changes, including increased levels of intracellular calcium, increased potassium in the extracellular spaces, and increased sodium permeability, will be evident. Calcium entrance into the neuronal cell activates various cellular processes that can lead to cell death. Accumulation of excitatory neurotransmitters, prostaglandin, and free radical production as well as lipid oxidation can cause additional ischemia, edema, "membrane destruction, cell death, and eventually permanent neurologic deficits" (Tefertiller et al., 2015).

Ischemia or decreased blood flow and microhemorrhage into the gray matter of the spinal cord occur after the injury. Neuronal cell death ensues as hypoxia and ischemia deprive the spinal cord of needed oxygen and nutrients. Macrophages proliferate and digest the necrotic tissue forming fat. There is necrosis of the axons that were damaged by the actual injury. Edema develops at the injury site and can spread within the spinal cord as permeability of blood vessels and axonal edema develop. The myelin sheaths begin to disintegrate secondary to direct injury to the oligodendroglial cells. The immune system appears to release nerve growth factor, which can be protective to some cells but toxic to others within the spinal cord. Eventually, a scar forms around the injury site. This scar serves as barrier to axonal regeneration (Tefertiller et al., 2015).

It is extremely important to monitor the patient's level of injury for the first 24 to 48 hours. The injury may ascend one or two levels because of vascular changes. If loss of function is apparent more than two spinal cord segments above the initial level of the injury, it may mean that the spinal cord was damaged in more than one place. Immediate notification of the patient's primary nurse and physician is necessary.

Immediately after an SCI, the patient exhibits spinal shock. The condition results from interruption of the pathways between higher cortical centers and the spinal cord. *Spinal shock* is characterized by a period of flaccidity, areflexia, loss of bowel and bladder function, and autonomic deficits, including decreased arterial blood pressure and poor temperature regulation below the level of the injury (Lundy-Ekman, 2018). Spinal shock normally lasts for approximately 24 to 48 hours; however, certain sources state that it may last up to several weeks. Because of suppressed reflex activity, one cannot accurately assess the patient's level of injury during spinal shock. As spinal shock resolves, reflex activity below the level of the lesion will return; if motor and sensory tracts have been salvaged, function in these areas will also be evident.

TYPES OF LESIONS

Spinal cord injuries are classified into two primary types: complete and incomplete. The ASIA Impairment Scale (AIS) uses information obtained from motor and sensory testing as

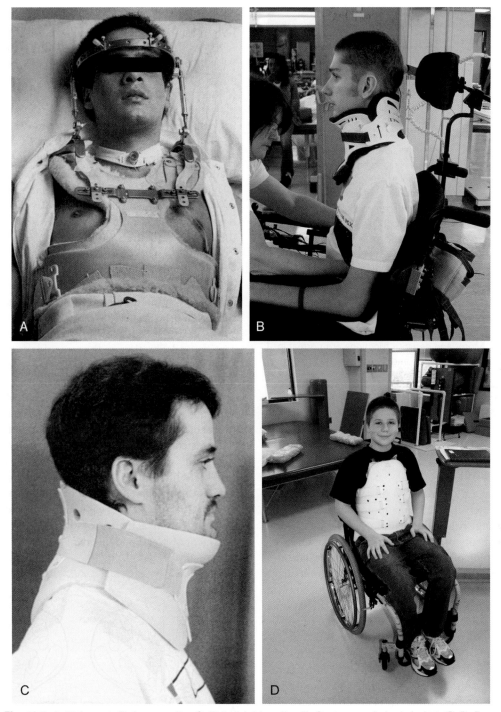

Fig. 13.5 **A,** Halo vest. **B,** Aspen collar. **C,** Philadelphia collar. **D,** Custom-made body jacket. (**B–D,** From Umphred DA, editor: *Umphred's neurological rehabilitation*, ed 6, St. Louis, 2013, Elsevier, pp 464, 466.)

well as the presence of anal sensation and voluntary anal contraction to classify patients as having complete or incomplete injuries (Tefertiller et al., 2015). The AIS is summarized in Table 13.2.

Complete Injuries

If an injury is complete, sensory and motor function will be absent below the level of the injury and in the lowest sacral segments of S4 and S5. *Complete injuries* are most often the result

of complete spinal cord transection, spinal cord compression, or vascular impairment. Approximately 12.3% of individuals have complete tetraplegia whereas 19.6% of all patients have complete paraplegia (National Spinal Cord Injury Statistical Center, 2019). It is possible that an individual with a complete injury may have partial innervation of motor or sensory function in up to three segments below the injury site. The most caudal segment with some sensory or motor function (or both) is defined as the *Zone of Partial Preservation* (ASIA, 2019).

TABLE 13.2   ASIA Impairment Scale

Grade	Impairment
A = Complete	No motor or sensory function is preserved in the sacral segments S4–S5.
B = Sensory Incomplete	Sensory, but not motor, function is preserved below the neurologic level and includes the sacral segments S4–S5, and no motor is preserved more than three levels below the motor level on either side of the body.
C = Motor Incomplete	Motor function is preserved below the neurologic level for voluntary anal contraction or the patient meets criteria for sensory incomplete. Some sparring of motor function more than 3 levels below the ipsilateral motor level on the right or left. For AIS C, less than half of key muscles have a grade greater than 3/5.
D = Motor Incomplete	Motor function is preserved below the neurologic level, and at least half of key muscle functions below the neurologic level have a muscle grade of 3 or greater.
E = Normal	Motor and sensory functions are normal in all segments, and the patient had prior deficits.

From American Spinal Cord Injury Association: *International standards for neurological classification of spinal cord injury, revised*, Richmond, VA, 2019, American Spinal Injury Association.

Incomplete Injuries

Incomplete injuries are described as those injuries in which there is partial preservation of some motor or sensory function (sacral sparing) below the neurologic level and in the lowest sacral segments of S4 and S5. Perianal sensation or voluntary contraction of the external anal sphincter indicates an incomplete injury (Burns et al., 2012). Investigators have estimated that more than 47.6% of patients have incomplete tetraplegia and 19.9% have incomplete paraplegia (National Spinal Cord Injury Statistical Center, 2019).

Updated standards for the classification of SCI were released by ASIA in 2019. Within those guidelines is a revised definition for the Zone of Partial Preservation *(ZPP)*. Therapists should now record ZPPs for patients with complete as well as incomplete injuries. "Motor ZPPs are now defined and should be documented in all cases including patients with absent voluntary anal contractions. The sensory ZPP on a given side is defined in the absence of sensory function in S4-5 on this side as long as deep anal pressure is not present" (ASIA, 2019).

The clinical picture of incomplete injuries is highly variable and unpredictable. The area of the spinal cord damaged and the number of spinal cord tracts that remain intact dictate the amount of motor and sensory functions preserved. Several clinical findings help to confirm a diagnosis of an incomplete injury. Sacral sparing is one such finding. Because the sacral tracts run most medially within the spinal cord, they are often salvaged. Patients with sacral sparing may have perianal sensation and/or the ability to have voluntary control over the rectal sphincter muscle. These spared motor and sensory functions can be of great functional benefit to the patient because they may provide for normal bowel, bladder, and sexual activities.

Another clinical finding observed in patients with incomplete injuries is *abnormal tone* or *muscle spasticity*. Resistance to passive stretching, clonus, increased deep tendon reflexes, and muscle spasms may be present. Decreased inhibition from descending supraspinal pathways, loss of sensory information associated with weight bearing, "loss of descending facilitation of afferents from Golgi tendon organs," sprouting of synaptic terminals, and increased responsiveness to neurons distal to the injury may be possible explanations for these findings (Somers, 2010).

Brown-Séquard Syndrome

Brown-Séquard syndrome results from an injury involving half of the spinal cord (Fig. 13.6, *A*). Penetrating injuries, such as injuries sustained from gunshot or stab wounds, are common causes. The patient loses motor function, proprioception, and vibration on the same side as the injury because the fibers within the corticospinal tract and dorsal columns do not cross at the spinal cord level. Pain and temperature sensations are absent on the opposite side of the injury a few segments lower. The reason for the loss of pain and temperature sensations in this distribution is that the lateral spinothalamic tract ascends several spinal segments on the same side of the spinal cord before it crosses to the contralateral side (Tefertiller et al., 2015). Light touch sensation may or may not be preserved in these patients. Prognosis for recovery with this type of injury is good. Many individuals become independent in activities of daily living (ADLs) and are continent of bowel and bladder.

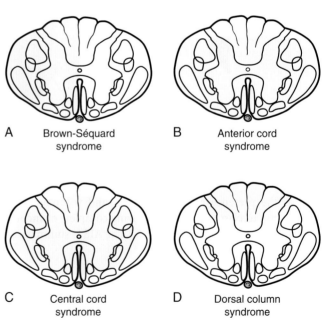

A   Brown-Séquard syndrome   B   Anterior cord syndrome

C   Central cord syndrome   D   Dorsal column syndrome

Fig. 13.6 **A–D,** Types of incomplete spinal cord injuries.

Anterior Cord Syndrome

Anterior cord syndrome results from a flexion injury to the cervical spine in which a fracture-dislocation of the cervical vertebrae occurs. The anterior spinal cord or anterior spinal artery may be damaged (see Fig. 13.6, *B*). The patient loses motor, pain, and temperature sensations bilaterally below the level of the injury as a result of injury to the corticospinal and spinothalamic tracts. The posterior (dorsal) columns remain intact, and therefore the patient retains the ability to perceive position sense and vibration below the injury. The prognosis for functional return is limited because all voluntary motor function is lost.

Central Cord Syndrome

Central cord syndrome, another type of incomplete injury, is the one most common. This type of SCI results from progressive stenosis or compression that is a consequence of hyperextension injuries. Bleeding into the central gray matter causes damage to the spinal cord (see Fig. 13.6, *C*). Characteristically, the upper extremities are more severely involved than the lower extremities. This is because the cervical tracts are located more centrally in the gray matter. Injury to the central spinal cord damages three different motor and sensory tracts: the spinothalamic tract, the corticospinal tract, and the dorsal column. Sensory deficits tend to be variable. Bowel, bladder, and sexual functions are preserved if the sacral portions of the tracts are spared. Ambulation is possible for many patients. Functional independence in ADLs depends on the amount of upper extremity innervation the patient regains.

Dorsal Column Syndrome

Dorsal column syndrome or *posterior cord syndrome* is a rare incomplete injury that results from damage to the posterior spinal artery by a tumor or vascular infarct (see Fig. 13.6, *D*). A patient with this type of injury loses the ability to perceive proprioception and vibration. The ability to move and to perceive pain remains intact.

Cauda Equina Injuries

A *cauda equina injury* usually occurs after the patient sustains a direct trauma from a fracture-dislocation below the L1 vertebrae. This type of injury often results in an incomplete lower motor neuron lesion. Flaccidity, areflexia, and loss of bowel and bladder function are the common clinical manifestations. Regeneration of the involved peripheral nerve root is possible, but it depends on the extent of initial damage.

Conus Medullaris Syndrome

Patients with injuries to the *conus medullaris* present with back pain, flaccid paralysis, and areflexic bowel and bladder function. Sacral sensation is also decreased.

Table 13.3 summarizes the causes and clinical findings seen in patients with incomplete injuries.

Root Escape

Damage to the nerve root within the vertebral foramen can lead to a peripheral nerve injury. *Root escape* is the term used

TABLE 13.3 Types of Incomplete Spinal Cord Injuries

Type	Cause	Findings
Brown-Séquard syndrome	Penetrating injury: gunshot or stab wounds	Loss of motor function, proprioception, and vibration on the same side as the injury Pain and temperature lost on the opposite side
Anterior cord syndrome	Flexion injury with fracture-dislocation of the cervical vertebrae	Loss of motor, pain, and temperature sensation bilaterally below the level of the injury Position and vibration sense intact
Central cord syndrome	Progressive stenosis or hyperextension injuries	Damage to all three tracts Upper extremities more involved than lower Sensory deficits variable
Dorsal column or posterior cord syndrome	Compression of the posterior spinal artery by tumor or vascular infarction	Loss of proprioception and vibration bilaterally
Cauda equina injuries	Direct trauma from a fracture-dislocation below L1	Peripheral nerve injury; flaccidity, areflexia, loss of bowel and bladder function
Conus medullaris syndrome	Damage to the sacral aspect of the spinal cord and the lumbar nerve roots	Upper and lower motor neuron injury Sacral reflexes remain intact in some individuals

to describe the preservation or return of motor or sensory function in various nerve roots at or near the site of injury. Therefore, a patient may experience some improved function or a return of function in the muscles innervated by the peripheral nerve several months after the initial injury. This increased motor or sensory return should not, however, be mistaken for return of spinal cord function.

CLINICAL MANIFESTATIONS OF SPINAL CORD INJURIES

The clinical picture of a patient who has experienced an SCI is variable. Much depends on the level of the injury and the muscle and sensory functions that remain. In addition, one must consider whether the injury is complete or incomplete. In general, the following signs or symptoms may be present in an individual who has sustained an SCI: (1) motor paralysis or paresis below the level of the injury or lesion; (2) sensory loss (sensory function may remain intact two spinal cord segments below the level of the injury); (3) cardiopulmonary dysfunction; (4) impaired temperature control; (5) spasticity; (6) bladder and bowel dysfunction; and (7) sexual dysfunction.

RESOLUTION OF SPINAL SHOCK

Reflex activity below the injury resumes after spinal shock subsides. The earliest reflexes that return are the sacral level reflexes. As a result, reflexive bowel and bladder function may return. Flexor withdrawal responses may also become apparent. Initially, these reflexes are evoked by a noxious stimulus and, as recovery progresses, they may be evoked by other, less noxious means. As time goes on, upper or lower extremity spasticity can develop in muscle groups that lack innervation. Additional muscle tightness and shortening become evident as a result of static positioning and muscle imbalances. For example, tightness in the hip flexors can develop as the patient spends increased amounts of time sitting upright in a wheelchair.

COMPLICATIONS

Multiple complications can result following an SCI. Careful prevention of possible secondary complications can improve a patient's rehabilitation potential and quality of life.

Pressure Ulcers

One of the most common complications seen after an SCI is the development of *pressure ulcers*. Pressure areas develop over bony prominences in response to the patient's inability to perceive the need to shift weight or relieve pressure. Additionally, changes in collagen degradation and decreased peripheral blood flow make the skin more vulnerable to injury (Somers, 2010). Patients with poor nutrition, complete injuries, those who smoke, and those who do not follow their self-care and skin care programs are more susceptible to develop pressure ulcers (Tefertiller et al., 2015). The treatment of open wounds that develop as a consequence of excessive pressure is a common cause for re-hospitalization (National Spinal Cord Injury Statistical Center, 2019). For health care professionals, prevention of pressure ulcers is of the utmost importance. Patients must be instructed in pressure relief techniques, or family members and caregivers must be taught how to assist the patient with weight-shifting activities. Patients should be instructed to perform 1 minute of pressure relief for every 15 to 30 minutes of sitting (Monroy, 2017; Somers and Bruce, 2014). Patients who are able should perform skin inspection independently with the use of a handheld mirror. Patients who require physical assistance with skin inspection should be advised to instruct others in the performance of this activity. Protective padding can also be applied during the performance of functional activities to decrease sheer forces and the possibility of trauma. Equipment, including specialized beds, mattresses, custom wheelchairs, cushions, and lower extremity splints and padding, may be necessary to provide patients with some pressure-reducing capacities.

Autonomic Dysreflexia

Autonomic dysreflexia occurs in patients with injuries above T6. This pathologic autonomic reflex is caused by sympathetic nervous system instability. All sympathetic outflow occurs below the T6 level. Consequently, in cervical and upper thoracic injuries, descending excitatory and inhibitory input from the medulla to sympathetic neurons is lost. Autonomic responses are discharged as a result of a noxious sensory stimulus applied below the level of the lesion. This noxious sensory input causes autonomic stimulation, vasoconstriction, and a rapid and massive rise in the patient's blood pressure. Normally, an increase in an individual's blood pressure would stimulate the baroreceptors in the carotid sinus and aorta and would cause an adjustment in peripheral vascular resistance, thereby lowering the patient's blood pressure. Because of the patient's condition, impulses are unable to travel below the level of the injury to decrease the patient's blood pressure. Thus, hypertension persists unless the noxious stimulus is removed or the patient receives medical intervention. This condition can cause life-threatening complications, including renal failure, seizures, subarachnoid hemorrhage, and even death, if left untreated. Common causes of autonomic dysreflexia include bladder or bowel distention, bowel impaction, disruption of the patient's catheter, urinary tract infections, noxious cutaneous stimulation, pressure sores, kidney malfunction, environmental temperature changes, and a passive stretch applied to the patient's hip (Lundy-Ekman, 2018; Somers, 2010).

Symptoms of autonomic dysreflexia include significant hypertension, severe and pounding headache, bradycardia, vasoconstriction below the level of the lesion, vasodilation (flushing) and profuse sweating above the level of the injury, constricted pupils, goose bumps (piloerection), blurred vision, and a runny nose. Immediate recognition and treatment of these signs or symptoms is essential. The first thing to do is to look for the likely source of noxious stimulation. Often, the patient's catheter is kinked or the catheter bag may need emptying. If the source of the problem cannot be identified immediately, try to lower the patient's blood pressure by sitting or standing the patient. Monitoring of the patient's vital signs is necessary. Application of a nitroglycerin patch, a potent vasodilator, or administration of antihypertensive drugs can assist in lowering the patient's blood pressure in the acute phase (Fulk et al., 2019). The patient's primary nurse and physician must be notified as soon as possible. Prevention of recurrent episodes and patient and family education are critical. Medications or surgical intervention may be needed to assist the patient in the regulation of this condition.

Orthostatic (Postural) Hypotension

Another possible complication is *orthostatic (postural) hypotension,* which is defined as a 20 mm Hg or greater decrease in systolic blood pressure or a 10 mm Hg decrease in diastolic blood pressure (Lundy-Ekman, 2018). Patients who have experienced an SCI often develop low blood pressure. Lack of an efficient skeletal muscle pump, combined with an absent vasoresponse in the lower extremities, leads to venous pooling. Consequently, the amount of blood circulating in the body is decreased, thereby precipitating decreases in stroke volume and cardiac output. Postural hypotension can develop when patients are transferred to sitting, when they are placed in upright standing, or during exercise. Thus, careful monitoring of blood pressure responses must occur during treatment activities. The application of an abdominal binder before beginning upright activities promotes venous return by minimizing the drops in intraabdominal pressure that can occur when the patient's position is changed. In addition, elastic stockings may be worn to prevent venous pooling in the lower extremities (Lundy-Ekman, 2018). Medications (vasopressors or mineralocorticoids) increase the patient's blood pressure and increasing fluid intake in the presence of hypovolemia may be prescribed to manage this condition (Somers and Bruce, 2014).

Pain

Pain is a common problem seen in patients after spinal cord injury. It has been reported that 26% to 96% of all individuals with an SCI experience chronic pain (Fulk et al., 2019). Pain can limit the patient's ability to participate in rehabilitation and may have negative consequences on one's ability to perform ADLs, sleep, and one's overall quality of life. Two types of pain have been identified: nociceptive and neuropathic. Nociceptive pain is associated with musculoskeletal structures (i.e., muscles, bones, tendons) and can develop as a result of the initial injury, inflammation, poor handling and positioning, or muscle spasm. Over time, the patient with an SCI can develop musculoskeletal pain and overuse pain syndromes, especially in the upper extremity. Common conditions seen include rotator cuff tears, shoulder impingement, lateral epicondylitis, carpal tunnel syndrome, and tendonitis of the wrist. These overuse injuries develop as a result of repetitive upper extremity movements and weight-bearing conditions needed to complete functional tasks, including wheelchair propulsion, transfers, and pressure relief (Somers, 2010; Fulk et al., 2019).

Neuropathic pain develops as a consequence of injury to the central and or peripheral nervous system and can occur at, above, or below the level of the initial injury. Neuropathic pain above the injury site is often caused by damage to a peripheral nerve from compression or entrapment. The nature of the pain can be variable and may be constant or intermittent, and can be sharp, shooting, or burning in nature. Treatment of neuropathic pain is challenging for health care practitioners. Medical interventions include patient education about the nature of the pain and pharmacologic management. The physician may prescribe acetaminophen or other nonsteroidal anti-inflammatory drugs, including ibuprofen (Motrin), naproxen (Naprosyn), and indomethacin (Indocin); anticonvulsants such as gabapentin (Neurontin), pregabalin (Lyrica), and valproic acid (Depakote); the antidepressant amitriptyline (Elavil); and analgesics (tramadol). Psychological pain management techniques, transcutaneous electrical nerve stimulation, acupuncture, and mental imagery may also be helpful in the management of chronic pain (Fulk et al., 2019; Tefertiller et al., 2015; Somers, 2010).

Contractures

Patients tend to develop flexion *contractures* as a result of the flexor reflex activity that develops after the injury and also as a consequence of prolonged sitting. Muscle imbalances around a joint may also predispose an individual to contracture formation. Prevention of contractures is important to maintain maximal function. Patients should be instructed in a good stretching program that they can perform independently or with the assistance of a family member or caregiver. In addition, all patients should be encouraged to perform a regular prone positioning program. Patients should spend at least 20 minutes each day on their stomachs to stretch the hip flexors. The prone position also relieves pressure on the ischial tuberosities and can provide aeration to the buttocks.

Heterotopic Ossification

Heterotopic ossification (HO) is another potential secondary complication. Bone forms in the soft tissues below the level of the injury. Usually heterotopic bone develops adjacent to a large lower extremity joint, such as the hip or knee. The etiology of heterotopic ossificans continues to be investigated, although spasticity, trauma, complete spinal cord injury, and urinary tract infection are thought to contribute to its development. Clinical signs of heterotopic ossification include range-of-motion limitations, swelling, warmth, and pain; fever may or may not be present. The management of this condition entails prevention and interventions administered once HO has developed. Nonsteroidal anti-inflammatories and localized low-dose irradiation applied as soon as possible is the standard preventative treatment for HO development (Legosz et al., 2018). In patients with HO, range-of-motion exercises and pharmacologic interventions are recommended. Surgical resection is performed when there is a significant limitation (Fulk et al., 2019; Somers, 2010). New potential therapies are under investigation that target the pathologic development of the condition Łegosz et al., 2018).

Deep Vein Thrombosis

The development of a *deep vein thrombosis* or *venous thromboembolism* is a common and life-threatening complication. The risk appears to be greatest during the acute-care phase. Because patients are often immobile and are medically fragile during this period, it is recommended that they receive low-molecular-weight-heparin to prevent blood clotting. The application of pneumatic compression devices (sequential compression devices) with or without compression stockings should be applied to the lower extremities as soon as possible to reduce venous stasis (Consortium for Spinal Cord Medicine, 2016). Surgical implantation of a temporary vena cava filter may be necessary in patients who are unable to tolerate anticoagulation to decrease the risk of pulmonary embolus. Regularly scheduled turning programs and early mobilization, including sitting up in bed and transferring to a wheelchair, are important to prevent venous pooling. In individuals with limited mobility, anticoagulant thromboprophylaxis is recommended for at least eight weeks after injury. During rehabilitation, low-molecular-weight-heparin or warfarin should be prescribed (Consortium for Spinal Cord Medicine, 2016).

Osteoporosis

Osteoporosis can be seen after SCIs because of changes in calcium metabolism. Although the exact etiology is not clear, decreased opportunities for weight bearing and limited muscle activity are thought to contribute to decreased bone density. The reduction in bone mass also places patients at an increased risk for fractures, with an incidence as high as 46% of all patients experiencing a pathologic fracture (Somers, 2010). Early mobilization, therapeutic standing, use of functional electric stimulation, administration of calcium supplements, and good dietary management can minimize the development of these potential complications (Fulk et al., 2019).

Respiratory Compromise

Serious and sometimes life-threatening complications can develop as a result of a patient's decreased respiratory capabilities. These complications develop in response to decreased innervation of the muscles of respiration and immobility. The diaphragm, innervated by cervical nerve roots C3 through C5, is the primary muscle of inspiration. Therefore, patients with high cervical injuries may lose the ability to breathe on their own, secondary to paralysis or weakness of the diaphragm muscle. The external intercostal muscles assist with inspiration and are innervated segmentally starting at T1. They act to lift the ribs and increase the dimension of the thoracic cavity. Patients with paraplegia below T12 have innervation of the external intercostals and should be able to exhibit a normal breathing pattern using the chest and diaphragm equally. This is often described as a *two-chest two-diaphragm breathing pattern* (Wetzel, 1985). The abdominals are the other important muscle group needed for respiration. The upper abdominal muscles are innervated by T7 through T9, and spinal segments T9 through T12 innervate the lower abdominals. The abdominals are activated when the patient attempts forceful expiration, such as coughing. Patients who are unable to generate an adequate amount of muscle force to cough will be susceptible to accumulation of bronchial secretions. This can lead to pneumonia, atelectasis, and respiratory compromise in many individuals. Weakness in the muscles of respiration can also lead to a decreased inspiratory effort and impairment of the patient's ability to tolerate exercise—a factor that ultimately affects endurance for functional activities.

Multiple interventions are used to minimize the effects of impaired respiratory function. These include early acclimation to the upright position, abdominal corsets and binders to assist with positioning of the abdominal contents, assisted cough techniques taught to the patient and caregivers, diaphragmatic strengthening, and incentive spirometry techniques. A more in-depth discussion of these techniques occurs in the treatment section of this chapter.

Bladder and Bowel Dysfunction

Bladder and bowel dysfunction may be considered a clinical finding or a complication of SCI. Patients with SCIs often experience difficulties with this area of function, and urinary tract infections are a major cause of mortality in individuals with SCIs (Fulk et al., 2019; Tefertiller et al., 2015). The lower sacral segments innervate the bladder, specifically S2 through S4. During the period of spinal shock, the bladder is flaccid or areflexic. Once spinal shock resolves, two possible situations can prevail, depending on the location of the injury. If the patient's injury is above S2, the sacral reflex arc remains intact, and the patient is said to have a *hyperreflexic* or *spastic bladder* with reduced capacity.

In this condition, the bladder empties reflexively when the pressure inside it reaches a certain level. Patients can apply specific cutaneous stimulation techniques to the suprapubic region to assist with bladder emptying. If the patient's injury is to the cauda equina or the conus medullaris, the patient is said to have an *areflexive* or *flaccid bladder*. The sacral reflex arc is not intact, and thus the bladder remains flaccid, requiring manual emptying at predetermined time periods (Fulk et al., 2019).

Bladder-training programs are important components of the patient's rehabilitation program. Intermittent catheterization, timed voiding programs, and manual stimulation can be used to empty the bladder and allow the patient to be catheter-free. Residual volumes of urine must be monitored to aid in the prevention of urinary tract infections (Fulk et al., 2019).

Bowel dysfunction, a major concern for many patients, can have an impact on one's involvement in social activities and how one perceives her overall quality of life. In patients with injuries above S2, the patient will have a spastic or reflex bowel. Reflexive emptying of stool will occur once the rectum is full. In injuries at S2 to S4, patients have a flaccid or areflexive bowel and, as such, the bowels do not empty reflexively, leading to possible impaction or incontinence (Fulk et al., 2019).

The establishment of a regular bowel program is also part of the patient's comprehensive plan of care. Patients are often placed on a regular schedule of bowel evacuation. High-fiber diets, adequate intake of fluids, use of stool softeners, and manual stimulation or evacuation may be suggested to assist the patient in the establishment of a bowel program (Fulk et al., 2019).

The rehabilitation team needs to be aware of the patient's schedule for bladder and bowel training. Therapies should not be scheduled during times designated for these activities.

Sexual Dysfunction

A common concern expressed by patients following an SCI is the impact the injury will have on sexual relationships. As stated previously, physical function depends on the patient's motor level. Males with upper motor neuron injuries have the potential for reflex erections (ones that occur in response to external stimulation) if the sacral reflex arc remains intact. Psychogenic erections are not possible and genital sensation is absent. The ability to ejaculate is limited for patients with both upper and lower motor neuron injuries. Therefore, men experience significant challenges with fertility (Lundy-Ekman, 2018).

Advances in medications, topical agents, and mechanical devices are available to improve erectile function. Women with SCIs continue to experience menstruation and thus are able to become pregnant. Women who do become pregnant and are ready to deliver are often hospitalized as a precautionary measure, because they may not be able to feel the start of labor contractions. Cesarean deliveries are frequently performed owing to the patient's impaired sensory function and lack of volitional muscle control (Fulk et al., 2019; Lundy-Ekman, 2018).

Physical therapists (PTs) and physical therapist assistants (PTAs) must be comfortable discussing this information with their patients. Because of the time we spend working with our patients, questions related to sexual activity may be directed to us. We must answer questions honestly and accurately. If you do not feel comfortable fielding these types of questions, you need to refer the patient to someone who can.

Spasticity

Spasticity is a common sequela of SCI. The prevalence of spasticity is higher in patients with cervical and incomplete injuries, specifically those classified as ASI B and C. Approximately 65% to 78% of the SCI population present with some degree of spasticity (Model Systems Knowledge Translation Center, 2019; Somers, 2010). Research suggests that increased tone is the result of residual influence of supraspinal centers (cortex, red nucleus, reticular system, and vestibular nuclei) on the spinal cord and ineffective modulation of spinal pathways (Craik, 1991). Spasticity may also be greater in patients who have experienced significant and multiple complications. Investigators have also shown that noxious stimuli tend to exacerbate abnormal muscle tone. In most instances, PTs and PTAs focus treatment on ways to decrease or minimize the effects of abnormal muscle tone. However, in some instances, an increase in muscle tone can be advantageous to the patient. Spasticity can help maintain muscle bulk, prevent atrophy, and assist in the maintenance of circulation. Spasticity can also assist the patient in performing functional activities, including transfers, basic bed mobility, and standing, when the patient has adequate innervation and sufficient trunk control. In addition, spasticity can provide increased tone to the anal sphincter, tone that may aid the patient in performing a bowel program.

The management of spasticity can be challenging. At this time, no treatment is available that completely ameliorates the effects of abnormal tone. Physicians may recommend a multitude of interventions to help the patient. Elimination of the stimuli or factors that contribute to increased sensory input is beneficial. Physical therapy interventions may include positioning, static stretching, weight bearing, cryotherapy, aquatics, and functional electrical stimulation. These different treatment interventions are discussed in more depth in the treatment section of this chapter.

Pharmacologic interventions may be necessary for some patients with significant abnormal tone. Baclofen is commonly prescribed for patients with spasticity. It restricts excitatory neurotransmitters and also inhibits mono- and polysynaptic spinal reflexes. Adverse responses include general muscle relaxation, fatigue, and sedation. Hepatotoxicity may develop and thus liver function must be monitored. Given its penetration across the blood–brain barrier, efficacy is limited when lower doses are prescribed. Clonidine "inhibits afferent sensory transmission below the level of the injury, decreasing spasticity" (Chang et al., 2013). Its use has become more limited secondary to variable outcomes and side effects, including drowsiness, bradycardia, and hypotension. Benzodiazepines (Diazepam) are anticonvulsants, which decrease CNS activity. Diazepam acts primarily on flexor reflexes, but can decrease extensor tone if administered in higher doses. One of the other benefits of this drug is that it induces sedation, which does assist patients in their ability to sleep without interruptions. Gabapentin is often prescribed as a treatment adjunct and is frequently administered to patients with neuropathic pain and spasticity. Dantrolene sodium is an oral spasticity drug that works peripherally on the muscles themselves by inhibiting calcium release. Because it targets all muscles, the use of this medication can lead to generalized muscle weakness. Liver failure has also been reported (Chang et al., 2013; Somers, 2010; Katz, 1988, 1994; Scelza and Shatzer, 2003; Yarkony and Chen, 1996).

Intrathecal baclofen pumps and *botulism injections* are other forms of treatment for spasticity. With an intrathecal pump, a pump and small catheter are implanted subcutaneously into the patient's abdominal wall. Baclofen is then delivered directly into the spinal canal, thereby reducing the dosage needed and some of the side effects. Baclofen has been found to be more effective in reducing tone in the lower extremities compared with the upper extremities because of catheter placement (Chang et al., 2013; Katz, 1988; Scelza and Shatzer, 2003). Botulinum toxin A is injected directly into the spastic muscle. This neurotoxin inhibits the release of acetylcholine at the neuromuscular junction, thereby causing temporary muscle paralysis (3 to 4 months). Botox does not have the same side effects of sedation and generalized fatigue; however, dysphagia can result with injections to the neck and upper extremities (Chang et al., 2013; Cromwell and Paquette, 1996).

Surgical intervention is a final type of management for abnormal tone. Neurectomies, rhizotomies, myelotomies, tenotomies, and nerve and motor point blocks may be administered to assist the patient with management of abnormal tone. *Neurectomy* is the surgical excision of a segment of peripheral nerve. *Rhizotomy* is a surgical procedure in which the dorsal or sensory root of a spinal nerve is resected and is primarily used for pain syndromes. In *myelotomy*, the tracts within the spinal cord are severed. *Tenotomy* is the surgical release of a tendon. Nerve blocks are performed with injectable phenol to destroy the nerve causing spasticity. Owing to potential nerve regeneration and sprouting, the effects of the injection will vary. Phenol injections are often administered to assist with hygiene, gait, and balance. A more detailed description of these procedures is beyond the scope of this text (Chang et al., 2013; Katz, 1988, 1994; Yarkony and Chen, 1996).

FUNCTIONAL OUTCOMES

A patient's functional outcome following an SCI depends on many factors. Age, the type and level of the injury, the motor and sensory function preserved, the patient's general health and preinjury activity level, status before the injury, body build, support systems, financial security, motivation, access to medical and rehabilitation services, and preexisting personality traits—all play a role in the patient's eventual outcome (Somers and Bruce, 2014; Lewthwaite et al., 1994). In patients with motor complete injuries (AIS A), the neurologic level is the most important factor in determining the patient's eventual functional outcome (Somers and Bruce, 2014).

Key Muscles by Segmental Innervation

Before we can begin to talk about functional capabilities in an individual with SCI, we must review key muscles and their actions. The innervation of key muscle groups allows patients to achieve a certain level of functional skill and independence. Table 13.4 highlights key muscles at each spinal level.

Functional Potentials

Each successive motor level provides the patient with the potential for greater function. Strength of a muscle must be at least fair-plus to perform a functional activity (Alvarez, 1985). Table 13.5 provides a review of functional potentials based on the patient's motor innervation and limitations encountered because of decreased muscle strength or range of motion. A description of each level and of the patient's potential for achievement of functional activities is provided. It is important to keep in mind that these functional expectations should serve only as a guide and that individual patient differences must be considered when developing patient goals or the plan of care.

C1 Through C3

A patient with an injury above C4 has limited muscle innervation. Because the diaphragm is only minimally innervated by C3, most patients with injuries at these levels will likely require mechanical ventilation. Some patients with high cervical lesions may, however, be able to tolerate electric stimulation to the phrenic nerve (bilateral diaphragmatic nerve pacing). Stimulation to the phrenic nerve causes the diaphragm to contract, thereby reducing the patient's reliance on mechanical ventilation (Tefertiller et al., 2015; Atrice et al., 2013). Patients with injuries at C1 through C3 require full-time attendants and will be totally dependent in all ADLs, bed mobility, and transfers. A power wheelchair with a reclining feature will be needed to allow for pressure relief and rest (Fig. 13.7). The patient should have adequate breath support or neck range of motion to operate a power wheelchair by a sip-and-puff mechanism or with a chin cup. With a sip-and-puff unit, the patient either sips or blows into a straw mounted in front of his or her face to provide the stimulus for the wheelchair to move. A few patients may be able to use a chin cup. The device requires that the patient have at least

TABLE 13.4 Key Muscles by Segmental Innervation

Spinal Level	Muscles
C1–C2	Facial muscles, partial sternocleidomastoid, capital muscles
C3	Sternocleidomastoid, partial diaphragm, upper trapezius
C4	Diaphragm, partial deltoid, sternocleidomastoid, upper trapezius
C5	Deltoid, biceps, rhomboids, brachioradialis, teres minor, infraspinatus
C6	Extensor carpi radialis, pectoralis major (clavicular portion), teres major, supinator, serratus anterior, weak pronator
C7	Triceps, flexor carpi radialis, latissimus, pronator teres
C8	Flexor carpi ulnaris, extensor carpi ulnaris; patient may have some hand intrinsics
T1–T8	Hand intrinsics, top half of the intercostals, pectoralis major (sternal portion)
T7–T9	Upper abdominals
T9–T12	Lower abdominals
T12	Lower abdominals, weak quadratus lumborum
L2	Iliopsoas, weak sartorius, weak adductors, weak rectus femoris
L3	Sartorius, rectus femoris, adductors
L4	Gluteus medius, tensor fascia latae, hamstrings, tibialis anterior
L5	Weak gluteus maximus, long toe extensors, tibialis posterior
S1	Gluteus maximus, ankle plantar flexors (gastrocnemius, soleus)
S2	Anal sphincter

30 degrees of active cervical motion. Patients with injuries at C1 through C3 may or may not have sufficient active range of motion in the cervical spine.

Advances in technology have improved the capabilities of all patients with SCIs, especially those with injuries at higher levels. Environmental control units that can be operated from the wheelchair allow some patients an increase in control over their home and work environments. These control units can be networked with one's personal computer and can operate appliances, lights, phones, and so forth. Individuals with injuries at this level must be empowered to direct their care through instructions provided to attendants and caregivers. This provides the patient with a certain level of independence and autonomy regarding her situation and care.

C4

A patient with a C4-level injury likely has some innervation of the diaphragm. This has significant functional implications because it means that a patient may not have to depend on a ventilator. The vital capacity of patients with diaphragmatic

TABLE 13.5 Functional Potential for Patients With Spinal Cord Injuries

Level	Muscles	Present Potential	Limitations
Above C4	C1–C2: Facial muscles	Vital capacity 20% to 30% of normal	Dependent on ventilator
	C3: Sternocleidomastoid, upper trapezius	Power recline wheelchair with breath or chin control and portable ventilator Ability to perform pressure relief in wheelchair with power recline feature Full-time attendant required Ability to direct care verbally Use of environmental control units with set-up	Dependent in all ADLs Dependent in bed mobility and transfers
C4	Diaphragm Upper trapezius	Vital capacity 30% to 50% of normal Power wheelchair with mouth stick or chin control 30° of cervical motion needed to drive a wheelchair with a chin control Maximal assistance with bed mobility Independent pressure relief with power reclining wheelchair Full-time attendant required Ability to direct care verbally Use of environmental control units with set-up	No upper extremity innervation Dependent in all ADLs Dependent in bed mobility and transfers
C5	Deltoid Biceps Rhomboids Lateral rotators (teres minor and infraspinatus)	Vital capacity 40% to 60% of normal Power wheelchair with hand controls Manual wheelchair with rim projections Moderate assistance for bed mobility Maximal assistance needed for transfers (sliding board or sit pivot) Independent forward raise for pressure relief with loops attached to the back of the wheelchair Possible independence with some grooming tasks with adaptive equipment (wrist splints) and set-up Attendant needed Use of environmental control units	Has only elbow flexors, prone to elbow flexion contractures Must consider energy and time requirements for activity completion Dependent in bathing and dressing
C6	Extensor carpi radialis Pectoralis major (clavicular portion) Teres major	Vital capacity: 60% to 80% of normal Independent rolling Independent pressure relief via weight shift Independent sliding board transfers possible or patient may require minimal assist Modified independent manual wheelchair propulsion with rim projections Modified independent feeding with adaptive equipment Independent upper extremity dressing Requires assistance for lower extremity dressing Ability to drive automobile with hand controls Vocation outside the home possible Prehension with flexor hinge splint Attendant needed for AM and PM care Assistance needed for commode transfers	No elbow extension or hand function (patient susceptible to contractures)
C7	Triceps Latissimus dorsi Pronator teres	Vital capacity 80% of normal Independent living possible Independent pressure relief via lateral pushup Independent self–range of motion of lower extremities Modified independent transfers, wheelchair propulsion, pressure relief, and upper and lower extremity dressing	No finger muscles Transfers to floor require moderate or maximal assistance Assist needed to right wheelchair Some assistance needed for wheelchair propulsion on ramps and uneven terrain
C8	Flexor carpi ulnaris Extensor carpi ulnaris Hand intrinsics	Same potential as individual at C7 Independent living Negotiation of 2- to 4-inch curbs in wheelchair Wheelies in wheelchair	Some intrinsic hand function Writing, fine-motor coordination activities can be difficult Assistance with floor transfers

Continued

TABLE 13.5 Functional Potential for Patients With Spinal Cord Injuries—cont'd

Level	Muscles	Present Potential	Limitations
T1–T8	Hand intrinsics Top half of intercostals Pectoralis major (sternal portion)	Independent in manual wheelchair propulsion on all levels and surfaces (6-inch curbs) Therapeutic ambulation with orthoses in parallel bars (T6–T8)	No lower abdominal muscle function Minimal assistance to independent with floor transfers and righting wheelchair
T9–T11	Abdominals	Independent wheelchair mobility Therapeutic ambulation with orthoses and assistive devices possible T10 vital capacity 100%	No hip flexor function
T12–L2	Quadratus lumborum	Household ambulation Independent in coming to stand and ambulation with orthoses	No quadriceps function Wheelchair used for community ambulation
L3–below	L3: Iliopsoas and rectus	Community ambulation with orthoses	No gluteus maximus function
L4–L5	Quadriceps, medial hamstrings	Community ambulation; may only need ankle-foot orthoses and canes for ambulation	
S1–S2	S1: plantar flexors, gluteus maximus S2: anal sphincter	Ambulation with articulated ankle-foot orthoses	Loss of bowel and bladder function

ADLs, Activities of daily living.

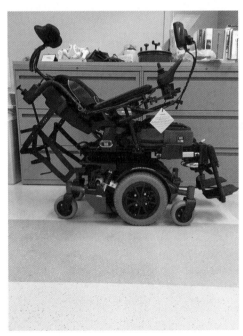

Fig. 13.7 **A** and **B,** Power recline wheelchair. (From Webster JB, Murphy DP, editors: *Atlas of orthoses and assistive* devices, ed 5, Philadelphia, 2019, Elsevier, p 395.)

innervation is still markedly decreased. Individuals at this level should be able to operate a power wheelchair using a chin cup, chin control, or mouth stick. Patients still must have sufficient range of motion to drive a wheelchair with a chin control. Environmental control units may also be prescribed for these patients. Individuals with C4 innervation continue to require full-time attendants because they are completely dependent in all transfers and ADLs. The ability to direct others regarding assistance needed is also important at this level.

C5

Patients with C5 innervation have some functional abilities. A patient with C5 innervation has deltoid, biceps, and rhomboid function. However, even though these muscles are innervated at this level, they may not have normal strength. Each patient has different motor capabilities, and the PT must thoroughly examine muscle function. Because of innervation of these key muscles, a patient with innervation at C5 should be able to flex and abduct the shoulders to 90 degrees, flex the elbows, and adduct the scapulae. The ability to flex and abduct the shoulders means that the patient will be able to raise her arms to assist with rolling and can also bring her hand to the mouth. She cannot, however, extend the elbow because the triceps are not innervated. The patient will be able to operate a power wheelchair with a hand control. A few patients are able to propel a manual wheelchair with rim projections. Although manual wheelchair propulsion may be possible, one must consider the high energy costs associated with this activity. For this reason, power wheelchairs are preferred for patients with innervation at this level.

The individual with C5 innervation may be able to be independent with some self-care activities, but the patient will require setup of the activity by an attendant or a family member. Patients also need to use adaptive equipment, including splints and built-up ADL devices, to perform self-care activities. Fig. 13.8 provides an example of an orthosis used to assist with ADL performance. Our experience has shown that even though patients may be able to

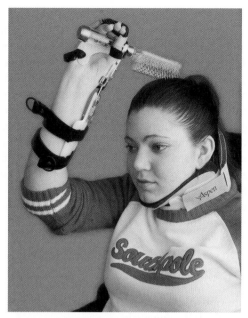

Fig. 13.8 Wrist-driven Flexor Hinge Orthosis. A person with C6 tetraplegia holding a brush with the assistance of a wrist-driven flexor hinge orthosis. (From Webster JB, Murphy DP, editors: *Atlas of orthoses and assistive* devices, ed 5, Philadelphia, 2019, Elsevier, p 159.)

perform a self-care activity independently after setup, the time and energy required to complete the task are often too great to continue performance on a regular basis. Individuals with innervation at the C5 level can provide minimal assistance with sliding board transfers from their wheelchairs and will require assistance for bed mobility. They can perform independent pressure relief by leaning forward in the wheelchair or by looping one of their upper extremities over the push handles on the back of the wheelchair and performing a weight shift. The rhomboids provide limited scapular stabilization for upper extremity self-care activities and for assuming functional positions, such as prone on elbows and long sitting with extended arm support. Driving is possible with a van and adaptive hand controls.

C6

Patients with C6 innervation have some greater functional abilities. Because of innervation of the wrist extensors, the pectoralis major, and the teres major, patients at this level are able to be independent with rolling, feeding, and upper extremity dressing. The patient should be able to propel a manual wheelchair independently with rim projections, and the potential exists for the person to be independent with sliding board transfers. Patients may need assistance in the morning and at night with self-care activities, and some patients need assistance for transfers, especially to the commode. Assistance is also required for lower extremity dressing. The ability to drive a motor vehicle with adaptive controls and gainful employment outside the home is possible for individuals with innervation at this level.

C7

An individual with a C7 injury has the potential for living independently because patients at this level have innervation of the triceps. With triceps strength, the patient can use her upper extremities to lift the body during transfers. In addition, the person will be able to perform a wheelchair push-up for pressure relief. Independence in self-care activities is possible, including upper and lower extremity dressing. A person should become independent in transferring from the wheelchair to the bed or mat, at first with a sliding board and eventually without the use of a board. Additional functional capabilities include independence with pressure relief, self–range of motion to the lower extremities, and operation of a standard motor vehicle with adapted hand controls.

C8

With innervation at C8, a patient can live independently. An individual is able to perform everything that a patient with innervation at a C7 level is able to complete. With the addition of some increased finger control, the patient may also be able to perform wheelies and negotiate 2- to 4-inch curbs in the wheelchair.

T1 Through T9

We look at capabilities of individuals with T1 through T9 innervation as a group. With increased motor return in the thoracic region, the patient demonstrates improved trunk control and breathing capabilities, including the ability to clear secretions because of increasing innervation of the intercostal muscles. Individuals are able to operate a manual wheelchair on all levels and surfaces and should be able to transfer into and out of the wheelchair to the floor. Patients with innervation at the T1 through T9 level may also be candidates for physiologic standing and limited therapeutic ambulation in the parallel bars with physical assistance and orthoses. *Therapeutic ambulation* is defined as walking for the physiologic benefits that standing and weight bearing provide. The section of this chapter on ambulation discusses this concept in greater detail.

T10 Through L2

Patients with innervation at the T10 through L2 level have abilities similar to those mentioned for individuals with T1 through T9 function. Therapeutic ambulation and ambulation in the home with orthoses and assistive devices may be possible, although manual wheelchair propulsion is the typical mode of functional mobility.

L3 Through L5

The quadriceps are partially innervated by L3. The presence of lower extremity innervation improves the patient's capacity for ambulation activities. Patients with innervation at this level should be independent in household ambulation and may become independent in community ambulation at the L3 level. Knee-ankle-foot orthoses or ankle-foot orthoses are necessary. Patients with injuries at the L4 and L5 levels should be independent with all functional activities, including gait.

These individuals can ambulate in the community with some type of orthoses and assistive device.

Outcome Measures

The SCI Edge task force has provided recommendations for entry-level physical therapy educators regarding the outcome measures that students should learn and those that students should be exposed to as part of their training. These measures are frequently administered to patients with SCIs. All students should be able to administer the 6-minute walk, 10-meter walk, ASIA Impairment Scale, Berg Balance Test, the Functional Independence Measure, Handheld Myometry, Manual Muscle Tests, a Numeric Pain Rating Scale, and the Timed Up and Go. Exposure to other outcome measures is also recommended. The recommendations are provided at: www.neuropt.org/docs/sci-edge-/sci-edge-entry-level-recommendations.pdf. Additionally, as discussed in Chapter 12, therapists should administer the Core Set of Outcome Measures as appropriate for adults with SCIs (Moore, et al., 2018).

Rehabilitation Approaches

The physical therapy management of patients after spinal cord injury is at a critical crossroads as research is providing evidence regarding the adult nervous system's plasticity and capacity for reorganization. This has presented physical therapists with a dilemma as to whether treatment should be directed at *compensation* or the *recovery* of function. Compensation is best thought of as a substitution or altered strategy to complete a task, whereas recovery is completing a task using the same or original processes (Shumway-Cook and Woollacott, 2017) (Table 13.6).

TABLE 13.6 Distinguishing the Behavioral and Neural Definitions of Recovery Versus Compensation

	Recovery	Compensation
Neural	Restoring function in neural tissue that was initially lost owing to injury or disease	Residual neural tissue takes over a function lost owing to injury or disease
Behavioral: Body Function *(Impairment)*	Restoring the ability to perform movement in the same manner it was performed prior to injury or disease	Performing movement in a manner different from how it was performed prior to injury or disease
Behavioral: Activity *(Function)*	Restoring the ability to perform a task in exactly the same manner as it was performed prior to injury or disease	Performing a task in a manner different from how it was performed prior to injury or disease

(From Kleim JA: Neural plasticity and neurorehabilitation: teaching the new brain old tricks, *J Commun Disord*, 44:521–528, 2011, Table 1.)

The treatment of individuals with spinal cord injuries has historically centered on compensation strategies in which the patient utilizes intact muscles, substitution, movement strategies (momentum, the head-hips relationship), assistive devices, and bracing to achieve functional movement and independence (Fulk et al., 2019). Our understanding of neuroplasticity and activity-based therapies, such as locomotor training and task-specific practice, is changing our treatment approaches and emphasis during the physical therapy session. As new research is disseminated, the physical therapy management of the patient with a spinal cord injury is likely to change. We will provide the reader with examples of both approaches in order to provide the patient with the most effective treatment options available.

PHYSICAL THERAPY INTERVENTION: ACUTE CARE

The acute-care management of the patient with a SCI is focused on the following goals:
1. Prevention of joint contractures and deformities
2. Improvement of muscle and respiratory function
3. Acclimation of the patient to an upright position
4. Prevention of secondary complications
5. Pain management
6. Patient and family education

The patient's initial physical therapy examination includes information on the patient's respiratory function, muscle strength, muscle tone, reflex activity, skin status, cardiac function, and functional mobility skills. The PT develops a plan of care to address the patient's primary impairments, functional limitations, and activity restrictions. In this early stage, interventions should focus on breathing exercises, selective strengthening and range-of-motion exercises, functional mobility training, activities to improve the patient's tolerance to upright, and patient and family education.

A patient with a cervical or thoracic injury may not immediately undergo surgical stabilization; therefore, the PT may be involved in the care of the patient in the intensive care unit. Prior to the initiation of physical therapy services, patients with spinal instability must be given medical clearance by their physician. Because of the acuity of the patient's condition and the potential for unpredictable patient responses, it is best for the patient to be treated by the PT at this stage. Cotreatments with the PTA or other members of the team may be appropriate.

Breathing Exercises

Exercises performed in the acute stage should emphasize maximizing respiratory function. Much depends on the patient's current level of muscle innervation. For those patients with innervation between C4 and T1, emphasis is on increasing the diaphragm's strength and efficiency. These patients possess diaphragm function and often demonstrate a diaphragmatic breathing pattern. If the diaphragm is weak, use of accessory muscles, such as the sternocleidomastoid and scalenes, may be evident. A good way to assess respiratory function is to observe the epigastric area and to watch for *epigastric rise*, an exaggerated movement of the abdominal area indicates that the diaphragm is working. The clinician can place a hand over this area to determine how much movement is actually occurring, as depicted in Fig. 13.9. If the patient is having difficulty, a quick stretch applied before the diaphragm contracts can help facilitate a response. If the patient is able to move the epigastric area at least two inches, the strength of the diaphragm is said to be fair (Wetzel, 1985). To strengthen this muscle even more, the therapist can apply manual resistance during the inspiratory phase of respiration. If the patient is able to take resistance to the diaphragm during inspiration, the strength of the muscle is considered good. Care must be taken to gauge the amount of manual resistance applied. Early on, patients may experience difficulties in breathing as a consequence of diaphragm weakness. In addition, respiratory muscle fatigue may become evident. Observation of the neck area can provide the clinician with valuable information regarding accessory muscle use. Patients often use accessory muscles extensively when the diaphragm is weak. Visible contraction of the sternocleidomastoids, scalenes, or platysma indicates accessory muscle use.

Glossopharyngeal Breathing

Patients with injuries at the C1 through C3 level and some patients with injuries at C4 require mechanical ventilation. These patients need to be taught a technique to assist their ability to tolerate short periods of breathing while they are off the ventilator. *Glossopharyngeal breathing* is a technique that can be taught to patients with high-level tetraplegia. The patient takes a breath of air and closes the mouth. The patient raises the palate to trap the air. Saying the words "ah" or "oops" accomplishes this. The larynx is then opened as the tongue forces the air through the open larynx and into the lungs. This technique is extremely beneficial if, for some reason, the patient needs to be disconnected from the ventilator

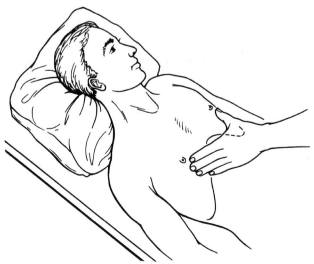

Fig. 13.9 Placement of the hand for diaphragmatic breathing. (From Myers RS: *Saunders manual of physical therapy practice*, Philadelphia, 1995, WB Saunders.)

for a short time because of equipment failure, power outage, showering, or another unforeseeable circumstance. This technique allows the patient to receive adequate breath support until mechanical ventilation can be resumed.

Lateral Expansion

For patients who have some intercostal innervation (T1 through T12), lateral expansion or basilar breathing should be emphasized. Patients are encouraged to take deep breaths as they try to expand the chest wall laterally. Clinicians can place their hands on the patient's lateral chest wall and can palpate the amount of movement present. Manual resistance can eventually be applied as the patient gains strength in the intercostal muscles. Progression to a two-diaphragm, two-chest breathing pattern is desirable if the patient has innervation through T12 (external intercostals).

Incentive Spirometry

Another activity that can be used to improve the function of the pulmonary system is *incentive spirometry* and the use of *inspiratory muscle trainers*. A measurement of vital capacity can be taken with a handheld spirometer. Vital capacity is the maximal amount of air expelled after maximal inhalation. Measurements of the patient's vital capacity can be taken throughout rehabilitation to document changes in ventilation (Wetzel, 1985). Patients can also be instructed to vary their breathing rate and to hold their breath as a means to promote improved respiratory function.

Chest Wall Stretching

Spasticity and muscle tightness within the chest wall can develop. *Manual chest stretching* may be indicated to increase chest expansion. The therapist places one hand under the patient's ribs and the other on top of the chest. The clinician then brings the hands together in a wringing type of motion, moving segmentally up the chest. This procedure, however, is contraindicated in the presence of rib fractures (Wetzel, 1985). Intervention 13.1 illustrates a clinician performing this technique.

Postural Drainage

Postural drainage with percussion and vibration may be necessary to aid in clearing secretions. Many facilities employ respiratory therapists who are responsible for these activities. However, the PT or PTA may be the health care provider responsible for the patient's *bronchial hygiene* (removal of secretions). Postural drainage positions are outlined in Chapter 8.

Physical therapy plays an important role in teaching the patient assisted cough techniques. For patients who lack abdominal innervation, it is imperative to identify ways in which the patient can expel secretions. If the patient is unable to perform these assistive cough techniques independently, a caregiver or a family member should be instructed in the technique. These techniques are discussed in the next section. Maintaining good bronchial hygiene assists in the prevention of secondary complications, such as pneumonia.

INTERVENTION 13.1 Chest Wall Stretching

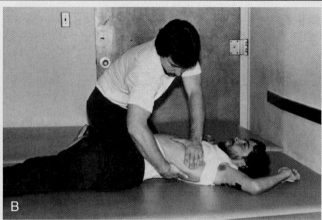

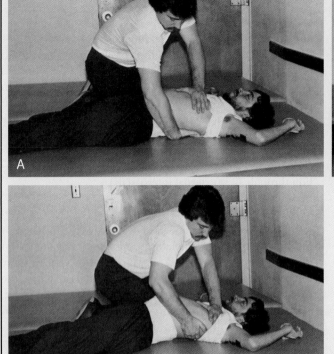

A. Starting position for manual chest stretching with one hand under the patient's ribs and the other on top of the patient's ribs.

B. Ending position of the clinician's hands after applying a wringing motion to the patient's chest for manual stretching.

C. The last hand position after the clinician progresses up the patient's chest for manual chest stretching with the clinician's top hand just inferior to the patient's clavicle.

(From Adkins HV, editor: *Spinal cord injury*, New York, 1985, Churchill Livingstone.)

Coughs

Coughs are classified into three different categories, based on the amount of force the individual is able to generate. *Functional coughs* are those that are strong enough to clear secretions. *Weak functional coughs* produce an adequate amount of force to clear the upper airways. *Nonfunctional coughs* are ineffective in clearing the airways of bronchial secretions (Wetzel, 1985).

Assisted Cough Techniques

Several methods are available to assist patients with the ability to cough. Depending on the patient's medical status, these techniques can be initiated in the acute-care setting or during the early phases of rehabilitation.

Technique 1. The patient inhales two or three times and, on the second or third inhalation, attempts to cough. Intrathoracic pressure increases, which allows the patient to generate a greater force to expel secretions.

Technique 2. The patient places her forearms over the abdomen. As the patient tries to cough, the patient pulls downward with the upper extremities to assist with force production. This can be completed in either a supine or a sitting position. This technique can be modified by having the patient flex forward toward her knees as she attempts to cough. This is illustrated in Intervention 13.2, *A*.

Technique 3. In a prone-on-elbows position, the patient raises her shoulders, extends her neck, and inhales. As the patient coughs, the patient flexes the neck downward and leans onto the elbows.

Technique 4. If the patient is unable to master any of the previously mentioned assistive cough techniques, a caregiver can assist the patient with secretion expulsion. A modified Heimlich maneuver can be performed by placing the caregiver's hands on the patient's abdomen, just below the rib cage, and providing resistance in a downward-and-upward direction as the patient coughs (Intervention 13.2, *B*).

Range of Motion

Range-of-motion exercises are an important component of the early stage of rehabilitation. For patients with tetraplegia, stretching of the shoulders, elbows, wrists, and fingers is essential. Patients immobilized in a halo will be limited in their ability to perform active or passive range of motion of the shoulder. The halo vest sits over the patient's shoulders, thus limiting shoulder flexion and abduction to approximately 90 degrees. The following shoulder ranges of motion are necessary to maximize function in the patient with tetraplegia. Approximately 60 degrees of shoulder extension and 90 degrees of shoulder external rotation are desirable. The patient needs shoulder extension to perform transfers from

INTERVENTION 13.2 Assistive Cough Techniques

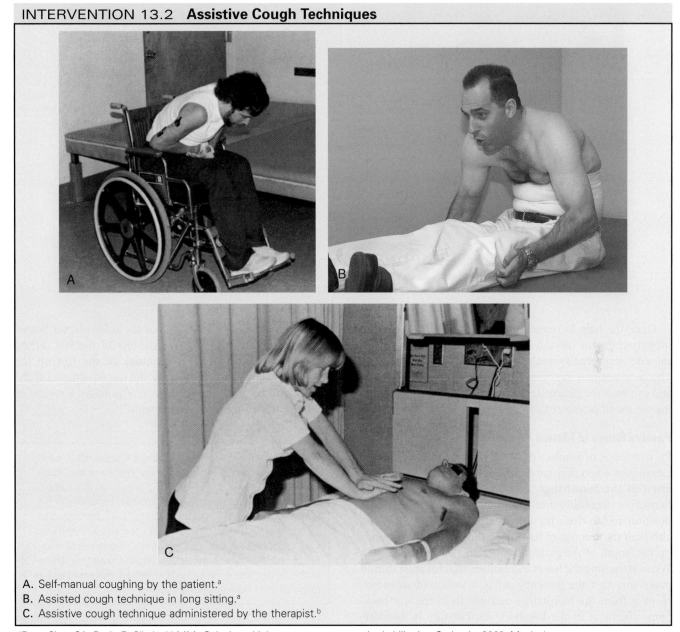

A. Self-manual coughing by the patient.[a]
B. Assisted cough technique in long sitting.[a]
C. Assistive cough technique administered by the therapist.[b]

[a](From Sisto SA, Druin E, Sliwinski MM: *Spinal cord injury: management and rehabilitation*, St. Louis, 2009, Mosby.)
[b](From Adkins HV, editor: *Spinal cord injury*, New York, 1985, Churchill Livingstone.)

supine to the long-sitting position. External rotation of the shoulder is needed so the patient can perform the elbow-locking maneuver to assume a sitting position. Full elbow extension is essential to ensure that the patient is able to use elbow locking for the long-sitting position and for transfers. Patients who lack innervation of the triceps (patients with C5 and C6 tetraplegia) use the elbow-locking mechanism to improve their functional potentials.

Adequate forearm pronation is necessary for feeding. Patients who lack finger function need 90 degrees of wrist extension. When an individual extends the wrist, passive insufficiency causes a subsequent flexing of the finger flexors referred to as *tenodesis* (Fig. 13.10). Tenodesis can be used functionally to allow a patient to grip objects with built-up handles using passive or active wrist extension. As a result of this functional movement, stretching of the extrinsic finger flexors in combination with wrist extension should be avoided. If the finger flexors become overstretched, the patient will lose the ability to achieve a tenodesis grasp. Sitting on the mat with an open hand will overstretch the finger flexors; therefore, the patient should be encouraged to maintain the proximal interphalangeal joints and the distal interphalangeal joints in flexion. Overstretching of the thumb web space should also be avoided, as tightness in the thumb adductors and flexors allows the thumb to oppose the first and second fingers during tenodesis. Patients are then able to use the thumb as a hook for completion of functional activities.

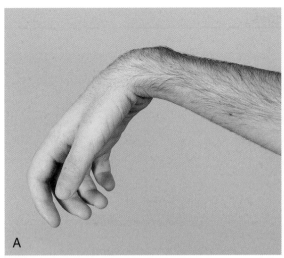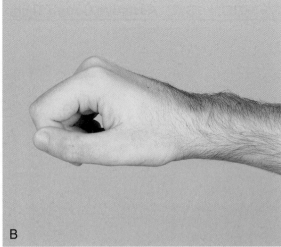

A   B

Fig. 13.10 **Fundamental Principle of Tetraplegia Hand Function. A,** With gravity-assisted WRIST flexion, the fingers and thumb passively open for grasp. **B,** With volitional WRIST extension, the thumb and fingers passively close for grasp. A tenodesis grasp provides hand function for the manipulation of light objects.

Once the halo is removed, clinicians should also avoid overstretching the cervical extensors. Stretching of the cervical extensors predisposes one to forward head posturing. This head position interferes with the patient's sitting balance and can limit the patient's respiratory capabilities by inhibiting the use of accessory muscles.

Passive Range of Motion

Passive range of motion must be performed to the lower extremities when they are flaccid. Special attention must be given to the hamstrings. The desired amount of passive hamstring flexibility needed to maintain a long-sitting position and to dress the lower extremities is 110 degrees, although the amount of hamstring range required depends on the length of the patient's upper and lower extremities. When stretching the lower extremities, the therapist should make sure that the patient's pelvis is stabilized so movement is from the hamstrings and not from the low back. Some tightness in the low-back musculature is desirable because this assists the patient with rolling, transfers, and maintenance of sitting positions. Tightness in the low back also provides the patient with a certain degree of passive trunk stability. In addition, maintenance of a "tight" back and the presence of adequate hamstring flexibility prevents the patient from developing a posterior pelvic tilt that can lead to sacral sitting and pressure areas when sitting in the wheelchair.

Stretching of the hip extensors, flexors, and rotators is necessary because gravity and increased tone may predispose patients to contractures. Hip flexion range of 100 degrees is needed to perform transfers into and out of the wheelchair. The patient needs 45 degrees of hip external rotation for dressing the lower extremities. Early in rehabilitation it may not be possible to position the patient in prone to stretch the hip flexors because of respiratory compromise. The prone position can inhibit the diaphragm's ability to work. However, as soon as the patient can safely maintain this position,

it should be initiated. Stretching of the ankle plantar flexors is necessary to provide passive stability of the feet during transfers, to allow proper positioning of the feet on the wheelchair footrests, and to allow the use of orthoses if the patient will be ambulatory. Table 13.7 provides a review of passive range-of-motion requirements.

> **CAUTION** If the patient's cervical spine is unstable, passive range-of-motion exercises to the shoulders should be limited to 90 degrees of flexion and abduction to avoid possible movement of the cervical vertebrae. Instability in the lumbar spine requires that passive hip flexion be limited to 90 degrees with knee flexion and 60 degrees with the knees straight (Somers, 2010). Passive straight leg raises should be limited to ranges that do not produce movement (lifting of the pelvis). Once the spine is stabilized, more aggressive range-of-motion exercises can begin.

TABLE 13.7 Range-of-Motion Requirements

Movement	Range Needed
Shoulder extension	60°
Shoulder external rotation	90°
Elbow extension	Full elbow extension
Forearm pronation	Full forearm pronation
Forearm supination	Full forearm supination
Wrist extension	90°
Hip flexion	100°
Hip extension	10°
Hip external rotation	45°
Passive straight leg raising	110°
Knee extension	Full knee extension
Ankle dorsiflexion	To neutral

Strengthening Exercises

Strengthening exercises are another essential component of the patient's rehabilitation. During the acute phase, certain muscles must be strengthened cautiously to avoid stress at the fracture site and possible fatigue. Initially, muscles may need to be exercised in a gravity-neutralized (antigravity) position secondary to weakness. Intervention 13.3, *A* and *B*, illustrates triceps strengthening in a gravity-neutralized position. Application of resistance may be contraindicated in the muscles of the scapulae and shoulders in patients with tetraplegia and in the muscles of the hips and trunk in patients with paraplegia, depending on the stability of the fracture site. When the PT is designing the patient's plan of care, exercises that incorporate bilateral upper extremity movements are beneficial.

For example, bilateral upper extremity exercises performed in a straight plane or in proprioceptive neuromuscular facilitation patterns offer the patient many advantages. These types of exercises are often more efficiently performed and reduce the asymmetric forces applied to the spine during upper extremity exercises. Key muscles to be strengthened for patients with tetraplegia include the anterior deltoids, shoulder extensors, and biceps. Key muscles to be emphasized for patients with paraplegia include shoulder depressors, triceps, and latissimus dorsi.

During this early stage of rehabilitation, the clinician may use manual resistance as the primary means of strengthening weakened muscles. In addition, Velcro weights or elastic bands may be used (see Intervention 13.3, *C* and *D*). As the

---

INTERVENTION 13.3 Triceps and Upper Extremity Strengthening

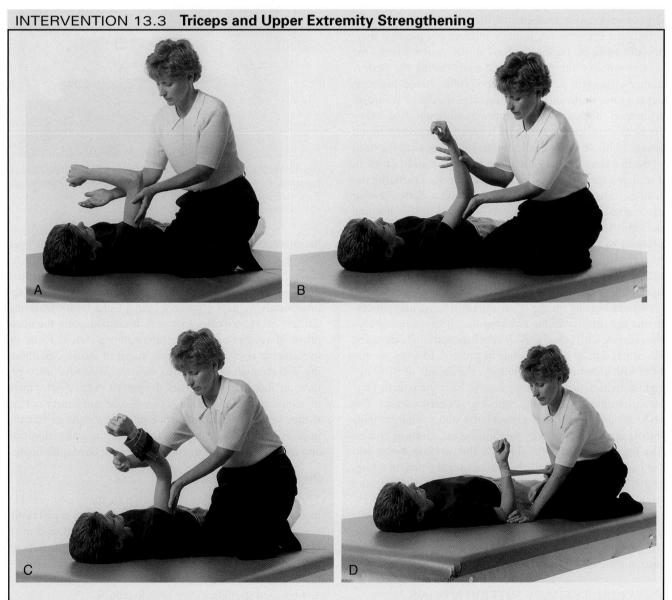

A. and **B.** Triceps strengthening. The patient's forearm must be carefully guarded. Weakness in the upper extremity may cause the patient's hand to flex toward her face.
  C. Using a Velcro weight for additional resistance during triceps strengthening.
  D. Using an elastic band for biceps strengthening.

patient progresses, these items may be left at the patient's bedside to allow the patient the opportunity to exercise at other times during the day. If you do decide to leave one of these items for the patient, make sure that the patient can apply the device independently. Often, when a patient has decreased hand function, using one of these devices can be difficult. Patients with paraplegia can perform more rigorous upper extremity strengthening. Barbells, exercise equipment, free weights, and elastic bands can be utilized for resistive exercise.

Acclimation to Upright

In addition to passive stretching and strengthening exercises, the patient should also begin sitting activities. Because of the initial trauma and secondary medical conditions, the patient may have been immobilized in a supine position for several days or weeks. As a consequence, the patient may experience orthostatic hypotension. Initially, nursing and physical therapy can work on raising the head of the patient's bed. One should monitor the patient's vital signs during the performance of upright activities. Baseline pulse, blood pressure, oxygen saturation, and respiration rates should be recorded. As long as the patient's blood pressure does not drop below 80/50 mm Hg, kidney perfusion is adequate (Finkbeiner and Russo, 1990). If the patient can tolerate sitting with the head of the bed elevated, the patient can be progressed to sitting in a reclining wheelchair with elevating leg rests. Often, the patient is transferred to the wheelchair with a draw sheet or mechanical lift initially. Transfers into and out of hospital beds are often difficult, based on the height of the bed and the presence of a halo. As the patient is better able to tolerate sitting, the time and degree of elevation can be increased. The tilt table can also be used to acclimate the patient to the upright position (Fig. 13.11).

Weight bearing on the lower extremities has many therapeutic benefits, including reducing the effects of osteoporosis, assisting with bowel and bladder function, and decreasing abnormal muscle tone that may be present. To assist the patient with blood pressure regulation during any of these upright activities, it may be necessary to have the patient wear an abdominal binder, elastic stockings, or elastic wraps. The abdominal binder helps support the abdominal contents during upright activities by minimizing the effects of gravity. The top of the binder should cover the two lowest ribs, and the bottom portion should be placed over the patient's anterior superior iliac spines. The binder should be tighter more distally. Elastic wraps or elastic stockings assist the lower extremities with venous return in the absence of skeletal muscle action in the lower extremities. The patient should also be carefully monitored for possible autonomic dysreflexia during these early attempts at upright positioning.

PHYSICAL THERAPY INTERVENTIONS DURING INPATIENT REHABILITATION

Once the patient is medically stable, the patient will likely be transferred to a comprehensive rehabilitation center. Most

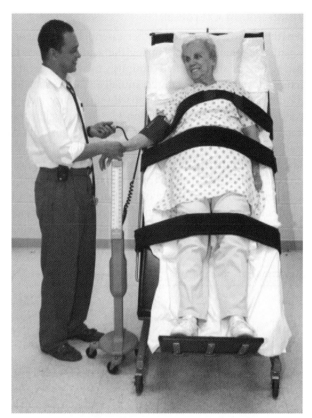

Fig. 13.11 The tilt table is used to help a patient gradually build up tolerance to the upright position. (From Fairchild SL: *Pierson and Fairchild's principles and techniques of patient care*, ed 5, St. Louis, 2013, Elsevier.)

patients spend approximately 11 days in an acute-care center. During the inpatient rehabilitation phase of the patient's recovery, the emphasis is on maximizing functional potential. The average length of stay for inpatient rehabilitation is approximately 31 days (National Spinal Cord Injury Statistical Center, 2019). Activities that were initiated during the acute phase of recovery continue. Interventions should focus on maximizing respiratory function, range of motion, positioning, and strength of innervated muscles. Additional interventions are incorporated to assist the patient in the development of motor control, acquisition of self-care and functional activities, including gait (if appropriate), therapeutic exercises to improve flexibility and overall fitness, patient/family education and training, and recommendations for adaptive equipment.

Physical Therapy Goals

The goals of intervention at this stage are many and variable. Much depends on the patient's level of innervation and resultant muscle capabilities. Additionally, goals developed must incorporate what is important and meaningful to the patient. Examples of goals for this stage of the patient's recovery include the following:

1. Increased strength of key muscle groups
2. Independence in skin inspection and pressure relief
3. Increased passive range of motion of the hamstrings and shoulder extensors
4. Increased vital capacity

5. Increased tolerance to upright positioning in bed and the wheelchair
6. Independence in transfers or independence directing a caregiver
7. Independence in bed and mat mobility or independence directing a caregiver
8. Independence in wheelchair propulsion on level surfaces
9. Independence in the operation of a motor vehicle (if appropriate)
10. Return to home and school or work
11. Independence in a home exercise and fitness program
12. Patient and family education and instruction

Goals regarding ambulation may be appropriate, depending on the patient's motivation, type of injury, and motor level.

Development of the Plan of Care

The primary PT is responsible for developing the patient's plan of care. The treatment interventions selected to achieve patient goals can be separated into two different approaches: *compensatory* and *recovery/activity based* as discussed earlier in this chapter. The compensatory approach is guided by the premise that the patient will learn new motor skills through the use of compensatory strategies, including strengthening intact muscles; using muscle substitution, momentum, and principles, such as the head-hips relationship; and the incorporation of adaptive equipment and environmental modifications. When using the recovery approach to SCI rehabilitation, the focus is on the patient's ability to use normal movement patterns in the acquisition of functional skills. Relearning previous motor skills and limiting the use of compensatory strategies form the basis of the recovery approach. Functional gains can be achieved through the incorporation of either approach exclusively or in combination (Shumway-Cook and Woollacott, 2017; Somers and Bruce, 2014; Somers, 2010).

In addition to mastery of functional skills, the PT will want to promote certain behaviors in the patient. Patients who have sustained SCIs must become active problem solvers. The patient needs to determine how to move using her remaining innervated muscles. The patient also needs to know what to do in emergency situations. For example, the patient must be able to direct someone if she should fall out of the wheelchair and is unable to transfer back into it. During the treatment session, tasks should be broken down into component parts, and the therapist should allow the patient to find solutions to the movement problems presented. Patients should practice the activity in its entirety, but must also work on the steps leading up to the completed activity. An example is practicing the transition from a supine-on-elbows position to long sitting. Patients should also be taught to work in reverse. Once the patient has achieved the desired end position, the patient should practice moving out of that position and back into the start posture.

Patients who have sustained SCIs must also experience success during rehabilitation. Activities to be selected should provide the patient with the opportunity to succeed. These tasks should be interspersed with activities that are challenging and difficult. Treatment activities selected should help the patient to develop a balance of skills between different postures and stages of motor control. The patient does not need to perfect movement in one postural set before attempting something more challenging. Finally, interventions within the plan of care should be varied. Examples of some of the different components of the patient's treatment plan that are possible include pool therapy, mat programs, functional mobility activities, group activities, and strengthening exercises.

Early Treatment Interventions

Mat Activities

Early in treatment, the patient should work on rolling. Learning to do this independently can assist with the prevention of pressure ulcers. As the patient practices rolling, the clinician can also work on the patient's achievement of the prone position. As stated previously, prone is an excellent position for pressure relief and stretching hip flexors. If the patient is wearing a halo, it will often be necessary for the therapist to help the patient with rolling. Prepositioning a wedge under the patient's chest is desirable when the patient is prone. If the patient does not have a halo, rolling can be facilitated in the following way:

Step 1. The patient should flex the head and neck and rotate the head from right to left.

Step 2. Both upper extremities should be extended above the head (in approximately 80 degrees of shoulder flexion). For patients at C5 and C6, care should be taken to limit the amount of shoulder flexion to less than 90 degrees to prevent the elbows from flexing toward the patient's face as triceps innervation is not present. The patient should move the upper extremities together from side to side.

Step 3. With momentum and on the count of three, the patient should flex and turn the head in the direction she wishes to roll while moving the arms in the same direction.

Step 4. To make it easier for the patient, the patient's ankles can be crossed at the start of the activity. This prepositioning allows the patient's lower extremities to move more easily. To roll to the left, you would cross the patient's right ankle over the left. Intervention 13.4 illustrates a patient who is completing the rolling sequence. Cuff weights applied to the patient's wrists can add momentum and facilitate rolling.

Once the patient has rolled from supine to prone, strengthening exercises for the scapular muscles can also be performed. Shoulder extension, shoulder adduction, and shoulder depression with adduction are three common exercises that can be performed to strengthen the scapular stabilizers. Intervention 13.5 shows a patient performing these types of exercises.

Prone

From the prone position, the patient can attempt to assume a prone-on-elbows position. Prone on elbows is a beneficial position because it facilitates head and neck control, as well as requiring proximal stability of the glenohumeral joint and scapular muscles. The patient may need assistance to attain the prone-on-elbows position. The therapist can place her hands under the patient's shoulders anteriorly and lift up (Intervention 13.6, *A*). As the patient's chest is lifted, the PT or PTA should move her

INTERVENTION 13.4 **Rolling from Supine to Prone**

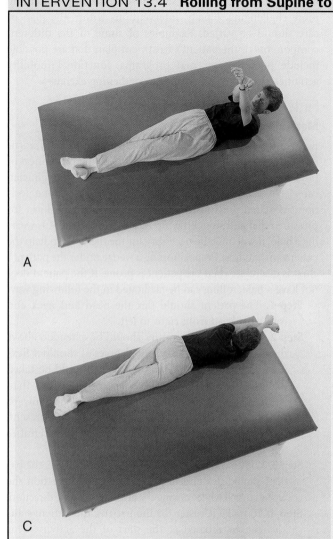

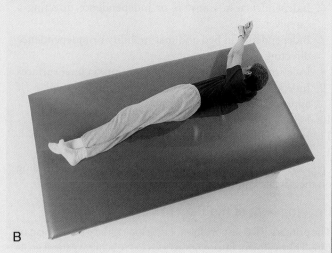

A

B

C

A. Rolling from supine to prone can be facilitated by having the patient flex her head and use upper extremity horizontal adduction for momentum. The upper extremities must remain in less than 90 degrees of shoulder flexion to prevent elbow flexion. The patient's lower extremities should be crossed to unweight the hip to assist with rolling.

B. and C. With momentum and on the count of three, the patient should flex and turn her head in the direction she wishes to roll while throwing her arms in the same direction.

INTERVENTION 13.5 **Scapular Strengthening**

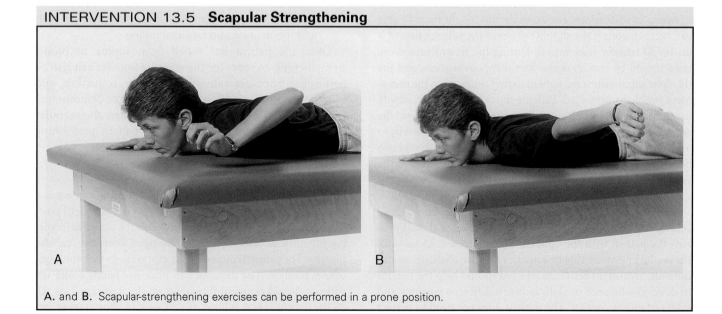

A

B

A. and B. Scapular-strengthening exercises can be performed in a prone position.

INTERVENTION 13.6   Prone to Prone on Elbows

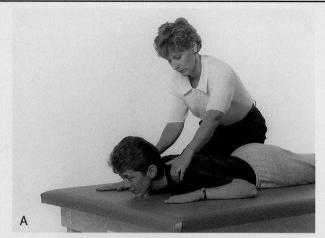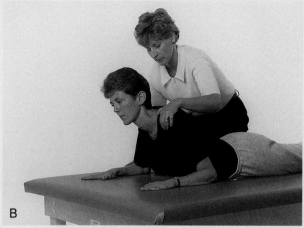

A. The therapist may need to help the patient achieve the prone-on-elbows position.
B. Weight shifting from one side to the other allows the patient to move her elbows into correct alignment.

hands posteriorly to the patient's shoulder or scapular region. If the patient is to attempt achievement of the position independently, the patient should be instructed to place her elbows close to the trunk, hands near her shoulders. The patient is then instructed to push the elbows down into the mat while lifting her head and upper trunk. To position the elbows under the shoulders, the patient needs to shift weight from one side to the other to move the elbows into correct alignment. This is accomplished by movement of the head to the right or the left. The PT or PTA can also facilitate weight shifts in the appropriate direction during these activities (see Intervention 13.6, B).

Prone on Elbows

Before beginning activities in the prone-on-elbows position, the patient needs to assume the correct alignment, as shown in Fig. 13.12. The patient should also try to keep the scapulae slightly adducted and downwardly rotated to counteract the natural tendency to hang on the shoulder ligaments. The therapist may need to provide the patient with manual cues on the scapulae to maintain the correct position. Downward approximation applied through the shoulders or tapping to the rhomboids is often necessary to increase scapular stability. Approximation promotes tonic holding of the muscles. In the prone-on-elbows position, the patient should practice weight shifting to the right, left, forward, and back. The patient should be encouraged to maintain good alignment and to avoid shoulder sagging as she performs exercises in this position.

Once the patient can maintain the position, she can progress to other exercises that will increase proximal control and stability. Alternating isometrics and rhythmic stabilization can be performed. To perform alternating isometrics, the patient should be instructed to hold the desired position as the PT or PTA applies manual resistance to the right or left, forward or backward. Intervention 13.7, A illustrates this exercise.

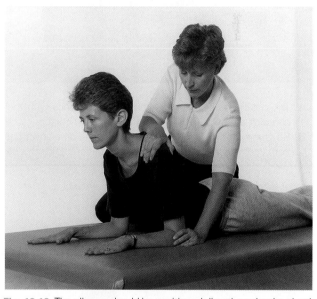

Fig. 13.12 The elbows should be positioned directly under the shoulders when the patient is prone on elbows. The physical therapist assistant is applying a downward force (approximation) through the shoulder to promote tonic holding and stabilization of the shoulder musculature. To preventing overstretching of the finger flexors, the patient's fingers may remain flexed.

With rhythmic stabilization, the patient performs simultaneous isometric contractions of agonist and antagonist patterns as the therapist provides a rotational force. Intervention 13.7, B shows a clinician performing this activity with a patient. Other activities that can be performed in a prone-on-elbows position include lifting one arm, unilateral reaching activities, and serratus strengthening (Intervention 13.8, A). To strengthen the serratus, the patient is instructed to push her elbows down into the mat and to tuck the chin while lifting and rounding the shoulders. For patients with paraplegia, instruction in prone push-ups, as depicted in Intervention 13.8, B, can be provided.

INTERVENTION 13.7 Alternating Isometrics and Rhythmic Stabilization

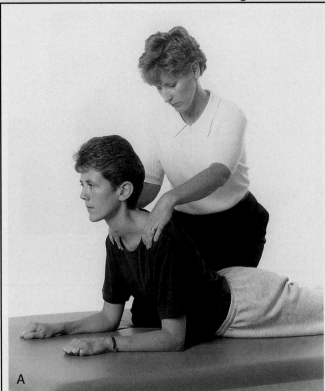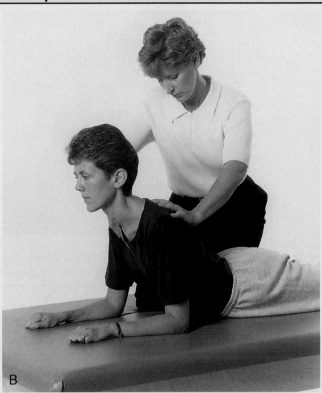

A. The clinician is performing alternating isometrics with the patient in a prone-on-elbows position. Force is applied in a posterior direction as the patient is asked to hold the position.
B. Rhythmic stabilization performed in a prone-on-elbows position. The therapist is applying simultaneous isometric contractions to both agonists and antagonists. As the patient holds the position, a gradual counterrotational force is applied.

INTERVENTION 13.8 Other Scapular-Strengthening Exercises

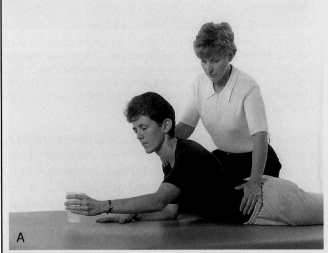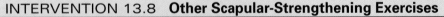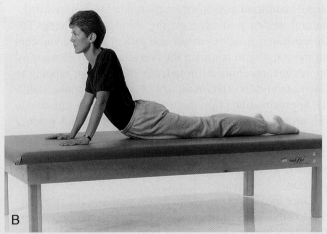

A. The patient reaches for a functional object. The therapist stabilizes the weight-bearing shoulder to prevent collapse.
B. The patient with paraplegia performs a prone press-up.

INTERVENTION 13.9 Supine to Supine on Elbows

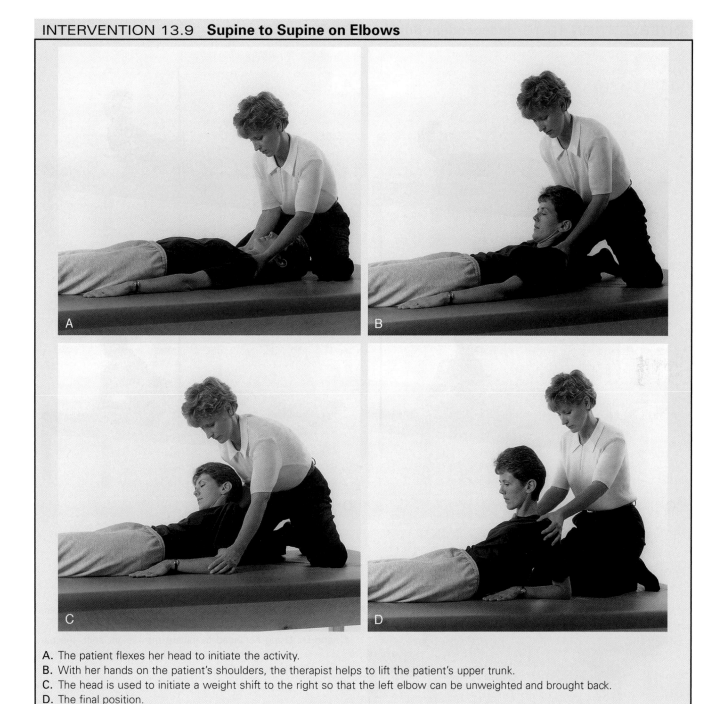

A. The patient flexes her head to initiate the activity.
B. With her hands on the patient's shoulders, the therapist helps to lift the patient's upper trunk.
C. The head is used to initiate a weight shift to the right so that the left elbow can be unweighted and brought back.
D. The final position.

Prone to Supine

From a prone-on-elbows position, the patient can transition back to supine. The patient shifts weight onto one elbow and extends and rotates her head in the same direction. As she does this, the patient "throws" the unweighted upper extremity behind. The momentum created by this maneuver facilitates rolling back to a supine position.

Supine on Elbows

The purpose of the supine-on-elbows position is to assist the patient with bed mobility and to prepare her for the attainment

of long sitting. Patients with innervation at the C5 and C6 levels may need assistance to achieve the supine on elbows position. Intervention 13.9 depicts a clinician helping a patient complete the transition from supine to the supine-on-elbows position. Several different techniques can be used to assist the patient in learning to achieve this position. A pillow or bolster placed under the upper back can assist the patient with this activity. This technique helps acclimate the patient to the position and assists the patient with stretching the anterior shoulder capsule. As the patient is able to assume more independence with the transition from a supine

INTERVENTION 13.10   Independent Supine to Supine on Elbows

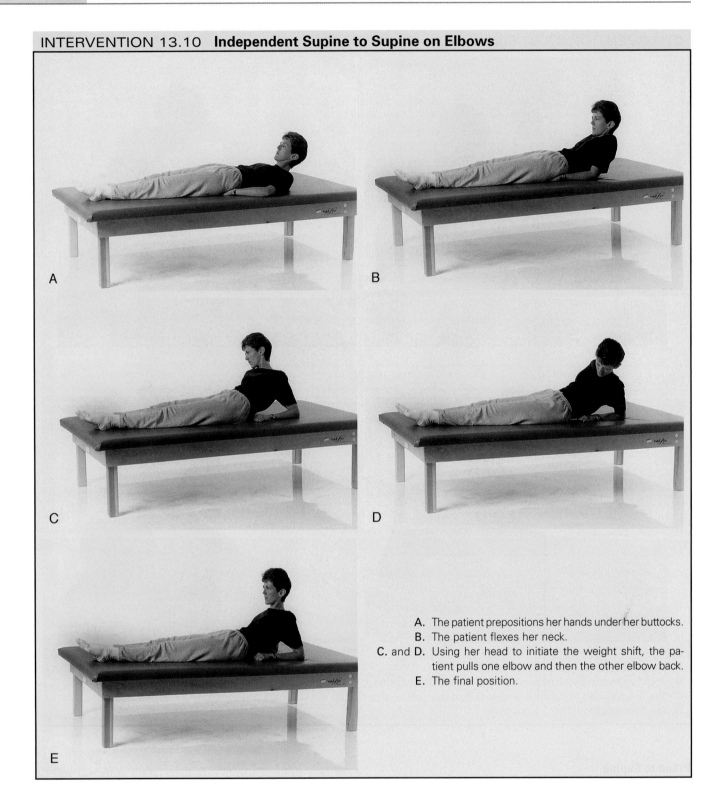

A. The patient prepositions her hands under her buttocks.
B. The patient flexes her neck.
C. and D. Using her head to initiate the weight shift, the patient pulls one elbow and then the other elbow back.
E. The final position.

position to supine on elbows, the PT or PTA can have the patient hook her thumbs into her pockets or belt loops or position the hands under the buttocks. Intervention 13.10 illustrates this approach. As the patient does this, she stabilizes with one arm as she pulls back with the other, using the reverse action of the biceps. The PT or PTA may need to reposition the patient's arms at the end of the movement. Once the patient is in the supine-on-elbows position, work can begin on strengthening the shoulder extensors and scapular adductors. Activities to accomplish this include weight shifting in the position, transitioning back to prone, and progressing to long sitting. Supine pull-ups can also be practiced. While the patient is in a supine position, the clinician holds the patient's supinated forearms in front of the body and has the patient pull up into a modified sit-up position. This exercise helps strengthen both the shoulder flexors and the biceps. From supine on elbows, the patient can roll to prone by shifting weight onto one elbow, looking in the same direction, and reaching across the body with the other upper extremity. This maneuver provides the patient with another option to achieve the prone position.

Long Sitting

Long sitting can also be achieved from a supine-on-elbows position. Long sitting is sitting with both upper and lower extremities extended and is a functional posture for patients with tetraplegia. This position allows patients with C7 innervation a position in which they can perform lower extremity dressing, skin inspection, and self-range of motion. It may be necessary for the therapist to help the patient achieve the position initially. The technique to assume long sitting is as follows:

Step 1. In the supine-on-elbows position, the patient shifts her weight to one side. The patient's head should follow the movement (Intervention 13.11, A and B).

Step 2. With the weight on one elbow, the patient throws her other upper extremity behind the buttocks into shoulder extension and external rotation (see Intervention 13.11, C). Once the hand makes contact with the surface, the

shoulder is quickly elevated and then depressed to maintain the elbow in extension. The elbow is locked biomechanically (see Intervention 13.11, D and E).

Step 3. The patient shifts her weight back to the midline (see Intervention 13.11, E).

Step 4. Once the patient has the elbow locked on one side, she repeats the motion with the other upper extremity (see Intervention 13.11, F and G).

> **SPECIAL NOTE** The fingers should be maintained in flexion (tenodesis) during performance of functional activities to avoid overstretching the finger flexors. Overstretching can lead to the loss of the ability to use wrist extension and flexor finger tightness to hold and manipulate adaptive devices. This is illustrated in Intervention 13.11, F and G.

Initially, the clinician may need to help the patient with the movement and placement of the upper extremities. Patients who lack the necessary range of motion in their shoulders have difficulty in achieving the long-sitting position. As mentioned earlier, patients who have developed elbow flexion contractures are not able to achieve and maintain

INTERVENTION 13.11 Supine on Elbows to the Long-Sitting Position

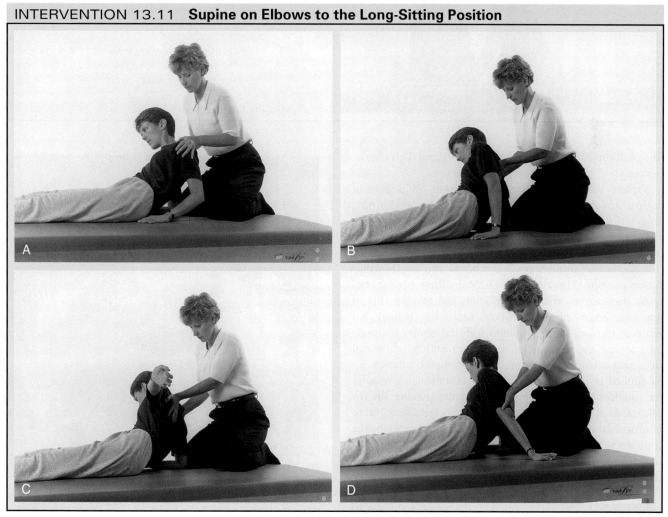

Continued

INTERVENTION 13.11   Supine on Elbows to the Long-Sitting Position—cont'd

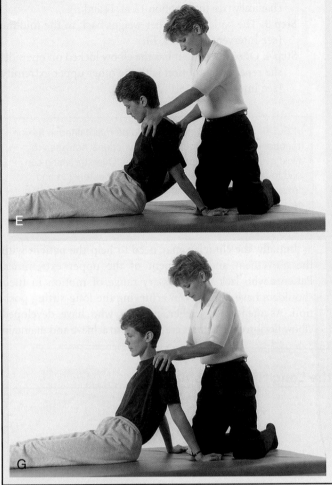

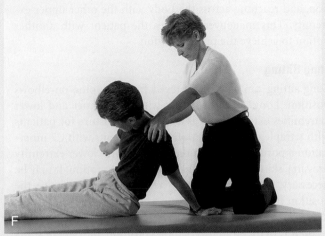

A. and **B.** Supine on her elbows, the patient shifts her weight to one side by moving the head in that direction.

C. With her weight on one elbow, the patient throws her other upper extremity behind her buttocks into extension and external rotation.

D. Once the weight is shifted onto the extremity, the elbow is biomechanically locked into extension because of the bony alignment of the joint when it is positioned in shoulder external rotation and then depressed.

E. The patient shifts her weight back to the midline.

F. Once the patient has the elbow locked on one side, she repeats the motion with the other upper extremity.

G. The final position.

this position because of their inability to extend their elbows passively.

Patients who do not possess at least 90 to 100 degrees of passive straight leg raising should refrain from performing long-sitting activities. Failure to possess adequate hamstring range of motion causes patients to overstretch the low back musculature and ultimately decrease their functional abilities.

Patients with injuries at C7 and below also use the long-sitting position. However, it is easier for these patients because they possess triceps innervation and may be able to maintain active elbow extension. Once the patient has achieved the long-sitting position with the elbows anatomically locked and is comfortable in the position, additional treatment activities can be practiced. Manual resistance can be applied to the shoulders to foster cocontraction around the shoulder joint and to promote scapular stability. Rhythmic stabilization and alternating isometrics are also useful to improve stability. If the patient has triceps innervation, the clinician will want to work with the patient on the ability to sit in a long-sitting position without upper extremity support (Fig. 13.13). The patient moves her hands from behind the hips, to the hips, and finally to forward at the knees. Hamstring range of motion is essential for the patient to be able to

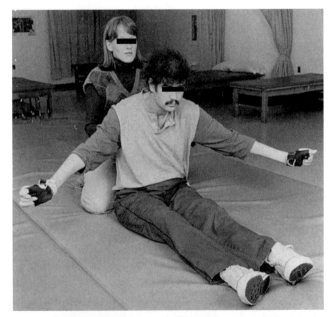

Fig. 13.13 Balance activities should always be emphasized in the long-sitting position to prepare the patient for numerous functional activities. (From Buchanan LE, Nawoczenski DA: *Spinal cord injury and management approaches*, Baltimore, 1987, Williams & Wilkins.)

INTERVENTION 13.12   Push-Up in the Long-Sitting Position

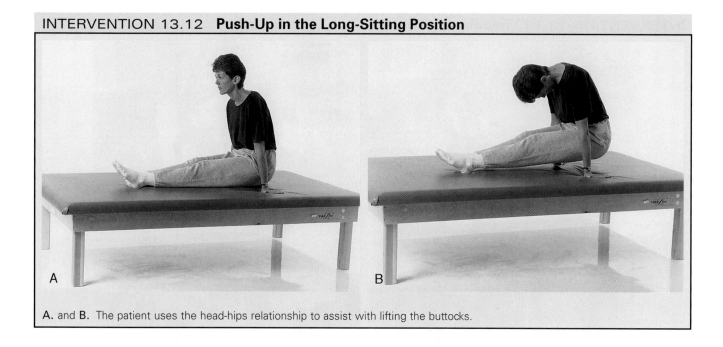

A. and **B.** The patient uses the head-hips relationship to assist with lifting the buttocks.

perform this transition safely. Once the patient can place her hands in front of the hips and close to the knees, she can try maintaining the position with only one hand for support and eventually with no hands. In this position, the patient learns to perform self-range of motion and self-care activities. The clinician guards the patient carefully during the performance of this activity. In addition, the patient's *vital signs* should be monitored to minimize the possibility of orthostatic hypotension or autonomic dysreflexia.

A goal for the patient with triceps function is to do a push-up with the upper extremities in a long-sitting position (Intervention 13.12). This activity usually requires that the patient have at least fair-plus strength in the triceps. To complete the movement, the patient straightens the elbows and depresses the shoulders to lift the buttocks. The patient flexes the head and upper trunk to facilitate a greater rise of the buttocks. Tightness in the low back also allows this to occur. The patient uses this technique *(the head-hips relationship)* to move around on the mat. This strategy is illustrated when a patient moves the head in one direction and the hips move directly opposite (Somers, 2010). Upper extremity push-ups are also used for transfers in and out of the wheelchair and as a means for the patient to perform independent pressure relief. Considered a compensatory strategy, the head-hips relationship assists patients in performing functional activities.

Transfers

Transfers into and out of the wheelchair are important skills for patients with SCIs. Patients with high cervical injuries (C1 through C4 level) are completely dependent in their transfers. A two-person lift, a dependent sit-pivot transfer, or a mechanical lift must be used.

Preparation phase. Before the transfer, the patient and the wheelchair must be positioned in the correct place. The wheelchair should be positioned parallel to the mat or the bed. The brakes must be locked and the wheelchair leg rests removed. A gait belt must be applied to the patient before the therapist begins the activity.

Two-person lift. A two-person lift may be necessary for the patient with high tetraplegia. This type of transfer is illustrated in Intervention 13.13.

Sit-pivot transfer. The technique for a dependent sit-pivot transfer is as follows:

Step 1. The patient must be forward in the wheelchair to perform the transfer safely. The PT or PTA shifts the patient's weight from side to side to move the patient forward. Often, placing one's hands under the patient's buttocks in the area of the ischial tuberosities is the best way to assist the patient with weight shifting. The clinician must monitor the position of the patient's trunk carefully as she performs this maneuver owing to a lack of trunk control necessary to maintain the trunk upright. Once the patient is forward in the wheelchair, the armrest closest to the mat or bed should be removed.

Step 2. The therapist then flexes the patient's trunk over the patient's feet. The clinician brings the patient forward over her hip that is farther away from the wheelchair. This maneuver allows the PT or PTA to be close to the area where most individuals carry the greatest amount of body weight. Guarding of the patient's knees is also necessary.

Step 3. A second person should be positioned on the mat table or behind the patient to assist with moving the patient's posterior hips and trunk.

Step 4. On a specified count, the therapist positioned in front of the patient shifts the patient's weight forward and moves the patient's hips and buttocks to the transfer surface. The position of the patient's feet must also be monitored to avoid possible injury. Generally,

INTERVENTION 13.13 Two-Person Lift

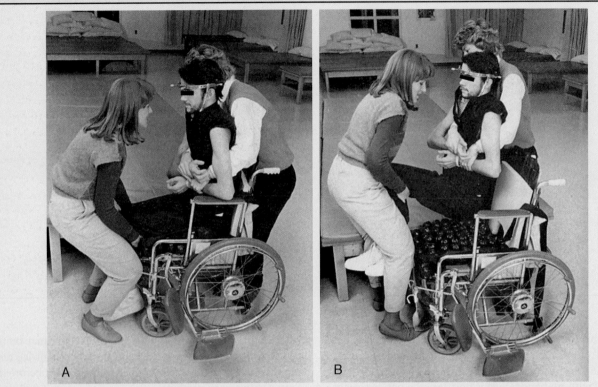

A. and B. Care must be taken so that the patient's buttocks clear the wheel during the two-person lift. Good body mechanics are equally important for the individuals assisting with this type of transfer.

(From Buchanan LE, Nawoczenski DA: *Spinal cord injury and management approaches*, Baltimore, 1987, Williams & Wilkins.)

prepositioning the feet in the direction that the patient will assume at the end of the transfer is beneficial.

Step 5. Once the patient is on the mat, the therapist in front of the patient aligns the patient to an upright position. The therapist does not, however, take her hands off the patient because of the patient's lack of trunk control. Without necessary physical assistance, a patient with tetraplegia could lose balance and fall. Intervention 13.14 demonstrates a sit-pivot transfer with a patient.

Modified stand-pivot transfer. A modified stand-pivot transfer can also be used with some patients who have incomplete injuries and lower extremity innervation. Additionally, patients with lower extremity extensor tone may be able to perform a modified stand-pivot transfer. The steps in completion of this transfer are similar to the ones described earlier and the techniques discussed in Chapter 12. Intervention 13.15 illustrates this type of transfer.

Airlift. The airlift transfer is depicted in Intervention 13.16 and may be the preferred type of transfer for patients with significant lower extremity extensor tone. The patient's legs are flexed and rest on the clinician's thighs. The patient is then rocked out of the wheelchair and moved to the transfer surface. The therapist must maintain proper body mechanics and initiate the patient lift with her legs to avoid possible injury to the therapist's low back. This type of transfer is often preferred because it prevents shear forces on the buttocks.

Sliding board transfers. A sliding board can also be used to assist with transfers. The chair should be prepositioned as close as possible to the transfer surface and at approximately a 30-degree angle. As the patient's trunk is flexed forward over her knees, the PT or PTA places the sliding board under the patient's hip that is closer to the mat table. The clinician may need to lift up the patient's buttocks to assist with board placement. Clinicians must be aware of the patient's active trunk control. Many individuals with SCIs are not able to maintain their trunks in an upright position. Once the board is in the proper position, it helps support the patient's body weight during the transfer. The board also provides the patient's skin some protection during the transfer. The patient's buttocks may be bumped or scraped on various wheelchair parts. This can be dangerous to the patient and can lead to skin breakdown. Intervention 13.17 illustrates a patient who is performing a sliding board transfer with the help of the therapist.

> **SPECIAL NOTE** Although patients with high cervical injuries are not physically able to assist in the transfer, the patient must be verbally able to direct caregivers in the completion of the task.

INTERVENTION 13.14 **Sit-Pivot Transfer**

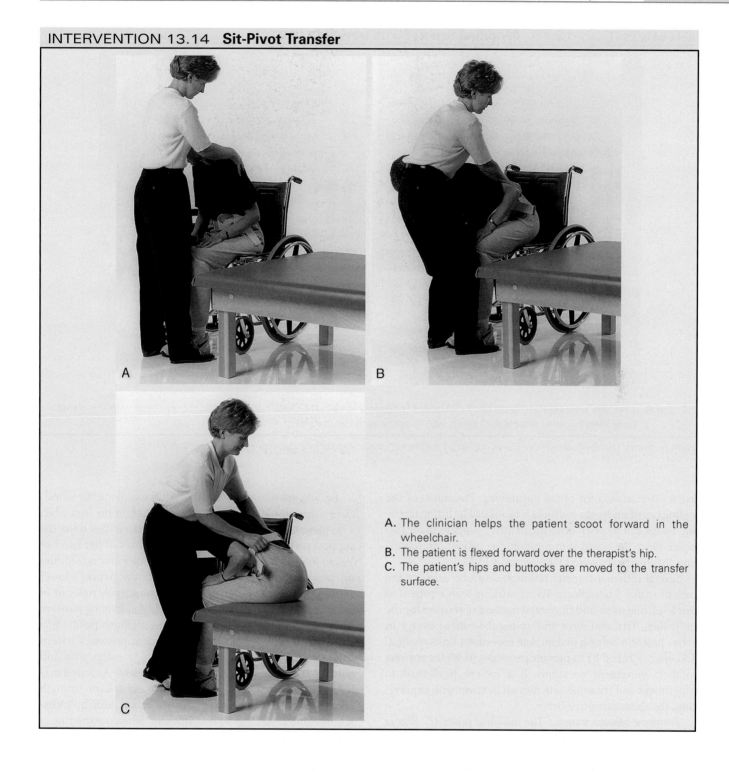

A. The clinician helps the patient scoot forward in the wheelchair.
B. The patient is flexed forward over the therapist's hip.
C. The patient's hips and buttocks are moved to the transfer surface.

A patient with C6 tetraplegia has the potential to transfer independently using a sliding board. Although the patient has the potential for this type of independence, patients with C6 tetraplegia often use the assistance of a caregiver or a family member because of the time and energy involved with transfers. To be independent with sliding board transfers from the wheelchair, the patient must be able to manipulate the wheelchair parts and position the sliding board. Extensions applied to the wheelchair's brakes are common and allow the patient to use wrist movements to maneuver these wheelchair parts. Leg rests and armrests may also be equipped with these extensions to provide the patient with a mechanism to negotiate the wheelchair parts independently. In an effort to prevent the development of upper extremity overuse injuries, patients should be instructed to limit the numbers of transfers they perform each day and avoid extremes of joint range (Somers, 2010).

To position the board, the patient can use tightness in the finger flexors to move the board to the proper location. The patient can also place her wrist at the end of the board and

INTERVENTION 13.15   Modified Stand-Pivot Transfer

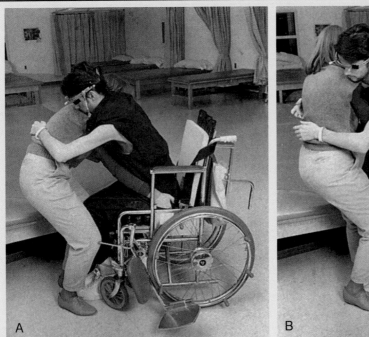 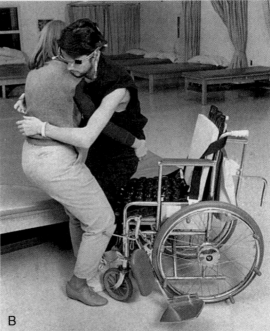

A. and **B.** Leverage principles and good body mechanics facilitate this stand-pivot transfer. The patient may assist with this transfer by holding his arms around the person who is completing the transfer.

(From Buchanan LE, Nawoczenski DA: *Spinal cord injury and management approaches*, Baltimore, 1987, Williams & Wilkins.)

use wrist extension for board positioning. Placement of the sliding board under the buttocks is facilitated by lifting up the leg. Loops can be sewn onto the patient's pants to make this easier. Once the board is in position, the patient can reposition the lower extremities (Intervention 13.18).

Several different transfer techniques can be used for the patient with C6 tetraplegia. When working with a patient at this level, one must find the easiest method of transfer for the individual. Trial and error and having the patient engage in active problem solving to complete movement tasks are best. Too often, PTs and PTAs provide patients with all the answers to their movement questions. If a patient is allowed to experiment and try some activities on her own with supervision, the results are often better.

Prone-on-elbows transfer. The modified prone-on-elbows transfer is one transfer method the patient may employ. The patient with C6 tetraplegia rotates her head and trunk to the opposite direction of the transfer while still in the wheelchair. Once the patient is in this position, she flexes both elbows and places them on the wheelchair armrest. The patient then flexes her trunk forward and pushes down on the upper extremities, thus scooting over onto the mat or bed. Some patients may also use the head to assist with the transfer. The patient can place her forehead on the armrest to provide additional trunk stability while attempting to move from the wheelchair. Once the patient is on the mat table, the patient hooks her arm under her knee and uses the sternal fibers of the pectoralis major to extend her trunk.

Rolling out of the wheelchair. After removing the wheelchair armrest, the patient rotates the trunk to the mat table. The patient then positions the lower extremities onto the support surface. The patient can use the back of her hand or Velcro loops attached to her pants to lift the lower extremities up and onto the support surface. Once the patient's lower extremities are up on the bed, the patient actually rolls out of the wheelchair. The patient can move to a side-lying position or can roll all the way over to a prone-on-elbows position.

Lateral push-up transfer. If the patient possesses triceps function, the potential for independent transfers with and without the sliding board is greatly enhanced. As stated earlier, a patient with a C7 injury and good triceps strength should eventually be able to perform a lateral push-up transfer without a sliding board. Initially, when instructing a patient in this type of transfer, the therapist should use a sliding board. The patient positions the board under the posterior thigh. With both upper extremities in a relatively extended position, the patient pushes down with her arms and lifts the buttocks up off the sliding board. The patient's feet and lower extremities should be prepositioned before the start of the transfer. Both feet should be placed on the floor and rotated away from the direction of the transfer. The patient moves slowly, using the board as a place to rest if necessary. As the strength in the patient's upper extremities improves, the patient will be able to complete the transfer faster and will not need to use the sliding board. Patients with high-level paraplegia also perform lateral push-up

INTERVENTION 13.16 Airlift Transfer

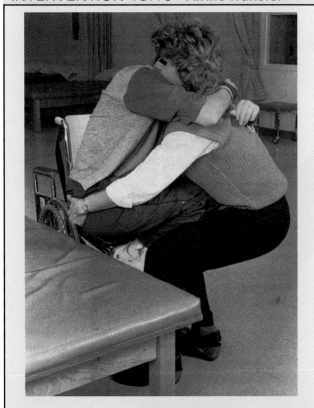

In the airlift transfer, the patient's flexed legs rest on or between the therapist's thighs. The patient can be "rocked" out of the chair and lifted onto the bed or mat. The patient's weight is carried through the therapist's legs and not the back.

(From Buchanan LE, Nawoczenski DA: *Spinal cord injury and management approaches*, Baltimore, 1987, Williams & Wilkins.)

transfers. Not until a patient possesses fair strength in the lower extremities are stand-pivot transfers possible.

Intermediate Treatment Interventions

Mat Activities

A major component of the patient's plan of care at this stage of rehabilitation includes mat activities. Mat activities are chosen to assist the patient in increasing strength and in improving functional mobility skills. The functional mobility activities previously described, including rolling, supine to prone, supine to long sitting, and prone to supine, continue to be practiced until the patient masters those tasks. Other, more advanced mat activities are now discussed in more detail.

Independent Self-Range of Motion

A patient with C7 tetraplegia should also be instructed in self-range of motion to the lower extremities. Assuming long sitting without upper extremity support is a prerequisite for becoming independent in self-range of motion. The first exercise that should be addressed is hamstring stretching. Two methods can be employed. The patient can assume a long-sitting position and then can lean forward toward the toes. The patient may rest the elbows on her knees to assist in

keeping the lower extremities extended. The maintenance of lumbar lordosis is important in preventing overstretching of the low-back musculature (Intervention 13.19).

The second method requires the patient to place her hands under the knee and pull the knee back as she leans backward into a supine position. With one hand at the anterior knee and the other at the ankle, the patient raises the leg while trying to keep the knee as straight as possible. The patient can then pull the lower extremity closer to the chest to achieve a better stretch. If the patient does not possess adequate hand function to grasp, she can use the back of the wrist or forearm to complete the activity. Intervention 13.19 shows a patient who is performing hamstring stretching.

The gluteus maximus should also be stretched. In a long-sitting position with one upper extremity used for balance, the patient places her free hand under the knee on the same side. The patient then pulls the knee up toward her chest and holds the position. Once the lower extremity is in the desired position, the patient can bring the volar surface of the forearm to the anterior shin and pull the leg closer. This maneuver gives an added stretch to the gluteus maximus (Intervention 13.20).

Patients must also spend a portion of each day stretching their hip flexors. This is especially important for individuals who spend a majority of their day sitting. The most effective way to stretch the hip flexors is for patients to assume a prone position. Patients should be advised to lie prone for at least 20 to 30 minutes every day. Patients can do this in their beds or on the floor if they are able to transfer into and out of their wheelchairs.

To stretch the hip abductors, adductors, and internal and external rotators, the patient should assume a long-sitting position as described earlier. The knee is brought up into a flexed position. With the nonsupporting hand, the patient should slowly move the lower extremity medially and laterally. The patient can maintain the arm under the knee or can place her hand on the medial or lateral surface of the knee to support the lower extremity (Intervention 13.21).

Stretching of the ankle plantar flexors is also necessary. The patient supports herself with the same upper extremity as the foot she is stretching. With the knee flexed approximately 90 degrees, the patient places either the dorsal or volar surface of the opposite hand on the plantar surface of the foot. Placement of the hand depends on the amount of hand function the patient possesses. Patients with strong wrist extensors can use motion at the wrist to stretch the ankle into dorsiflexion slowly (Intervention 13.22). Patients with paraplegia who possess wrist and finger function are able to complete this activity without difficulty. Stretching the ankle plantar flexors with the knee flexed stretches only the soleus muscle. The patient can stretch the gastrocnemius in a long-sitting position with a folded towel placed along the plantar surface of the foot. The ends of the towel are pulled to provide a prolonged stretch.

Advanced Treatment Interventions

Advanced Mat Activities

For the patient with paraplegia, practicing more advanced mat exercises is also appropriate. In a short- or long-sitting position, the patient can practice maintaining her sitting

INTERVENTION 13.17   Sliding Board Transfer

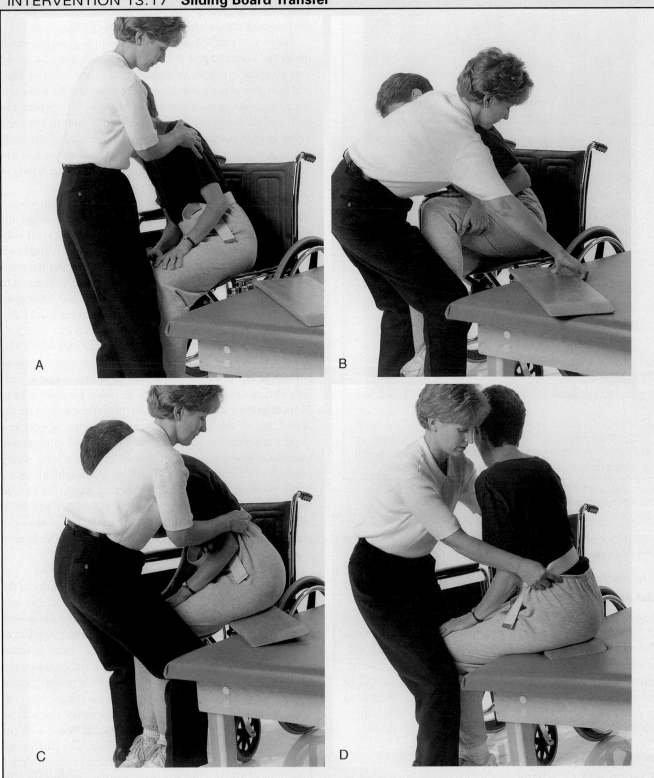

A. The patient's weight is shifted to the side farther away from the transfer surface.
B. The patient's thigh is lifted to position the board. The therapist remains in front of the patient, blocking the patient's lower extremities and trunk.
C. and D. The patient is transferred over to the support surface.

INTERVENTION 13.18   **Independent Sliding Board Transfer**

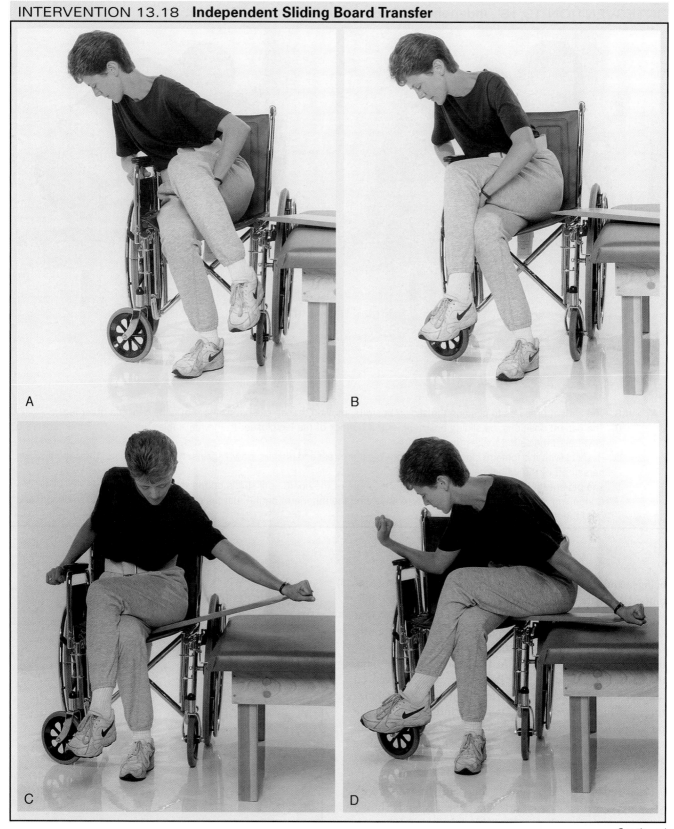

A

B

C

D

Continued

INTERVENTION 13.18 Independent Sliding Board Transfer—cont'd

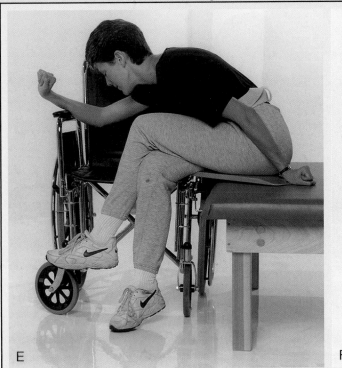
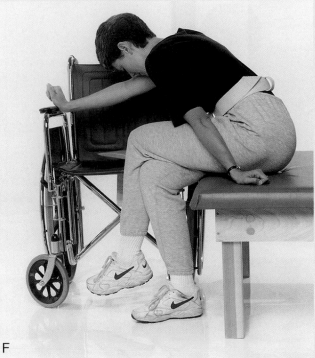

E   F

A. and **B.** The patient prepares to position the sliding board by moving the leg closest to the mat table over the other leg.

C. The patient positions the sliding board under the buttock of the leg closest to the mat table. The patient can uncross the lower extremities if it makes the transfer easier.

D. Pushing with the forearm closest to the wheelchair armrest and pushing down against the sliding board, the patient slides herself off of the wheelchair seat.

E. The patient then slides her buttocks down the length of the board until she is on the table.

F. Continuing to push off the wheelchair arm and using the other arm on the mat table, the patient scoots off the board and onto the table itself.

balance and finding her center of balance and limits of stability. Use of the upper extremities to maintain sitting balance will be dependent on the patient's motor level. Weight shifting, reaching, and other functional upper extremity tasks can be performed while the patient attempts to maintain her posture and balance. As the patient progresses, the therapist may choose to alter the surface. Other advanced mat activities that can be performed include sitting swing-through, hip swayers, trunk twisting and raising, prone push-ups, forward reaching in quadruped, creeping, and tall kneeling. The techniques used to execute each of these activities are as follows:

Sitting Swing-Through:

Step 1. The patient assumes a long-sitting position with upper extremity support. The patient's hands should be approximately 6 inches behind the patient's hips.

Step 2. The patient depresses the shoulders and extends the elbows. The buttocks should be lifted off the support surface.

Step 3. The patient swings the hips back between her hands.

INTERVENTION 13.19 Hamstring Stretching

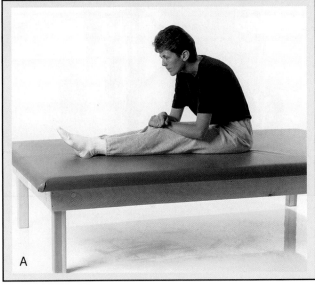

A

INTERVENTION 13.19 Hamstring Stretching—cont'd

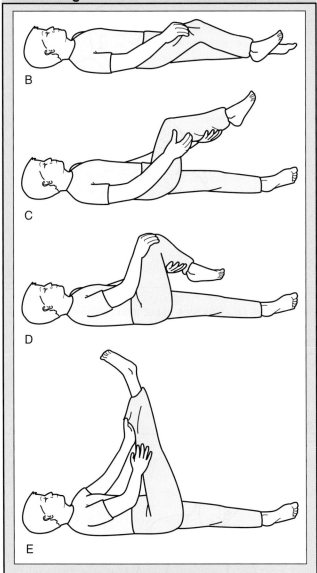

A. When stretching the hamstrings in the long-sitting position, the patient may rest her elbows on her knees to assist in keeping the lower extremities straight.

B. to E. Stretching the hamstrings in the supine position.

Hip Swayer:

Step 1. The patient assumes a long-sitting position with upper extremity support.

Step 2. The patient places one hand as close to her hip as possible; the other hand should be placed approximately 6 inches away from the other hip.

Step 3. The patient raises her buttocks and moves the hips toward the hand that is farther away.

Step 4. The patient travels sideways across the mat.

Step 5. The patient should practice moving in both directions.

Trunk Twisting and Raising:

Step 1. The patient assumes a side-sitting position.

Step 2. The patient places both hands near the hip that is closer to the support surface.

Step 3. The patient straightens her elbows to raise the hips to a semi-quadruped position and then lowers herself to the mat.

Step 4. The activity should also be practiced on the opposite side.

Prone Push-Ups:

In a prone position with the hands positioned next to the shoulders, the patient extends the elbows and lifts the upper body off of the support surface.

Forward Reaching:

Step 1. The patient assumes a four-point position. Some patients may need assistance achieving the position. The four-point position is achieved by having the patient assume a prone position. The therapist facilitates a posterior weight shift at the patient's pelvis while the patient extends her elbows. With a gait belt around the patient's low waist or hips, the clinician straddles the patient and pulls the patient's hips up and back as the patient pushes down with the upper extremities.

Step 2. If the patient is having difficulty maintaining the four-point position, a bolster or other object can be placed under the patient's abdomen to maintain the position. Care must be taken with patients who have increased lower extremity extensor tone; if the patient is unable to flex the hips and knees, the patient's lower extremities can spasm into extension.

Step 3. Once the patient can maintain the quadruped position, the patient can practice anterior, posterior, medial, and lateral weight shifts, as well as alternating isometrics and rhythmic stabilization.

Step 4. The patient can also practice forward reaching with one upper extremity while maintaining balance.

Step 5. If the patient possesses innervation of the trunk musculature, the patient can practice arching the back and letting it sag.

Creeping:

A patient's ability to creep depends on lower extremity muscle innervation. Strength in the hip flexors is needed to perform this activity.

Step 1. The patient assumes a quadruped position.

Step 2. The patient alternately advances one upper extremity followed by the opposite lower extremity.

Tall Kneeling:

Step 1. The patient assumes a quadruped position.

Step 2. Using a chair, bench, or bolster, the patient pulls up into a tall-kneeling position. The hips must remain forward while the patient rests on the Y ligaments in the hips.

Step 3. Initially, the patient works on maintaining balance in the position.

Step 4. Once the patient is able to maintain balance, the patient can work on alternating isometrics, rhythmic stabilization, and reaching activities.

INTERVENTION 13.20   Gluteus Maximus Stretching

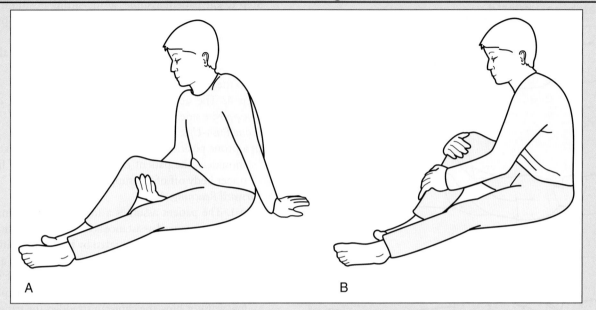

A | B

A. In the long-sitting position, the patient uses one upper extremity for support and his free hand to pull the knee on the same side up toward his chest.
B. Once the lower extremity is in position, the patient grasps the knee and shin with both hands and pulls the leg toward his trunk.

INTERVENTION 13.21   Stretching the Hip Rotators

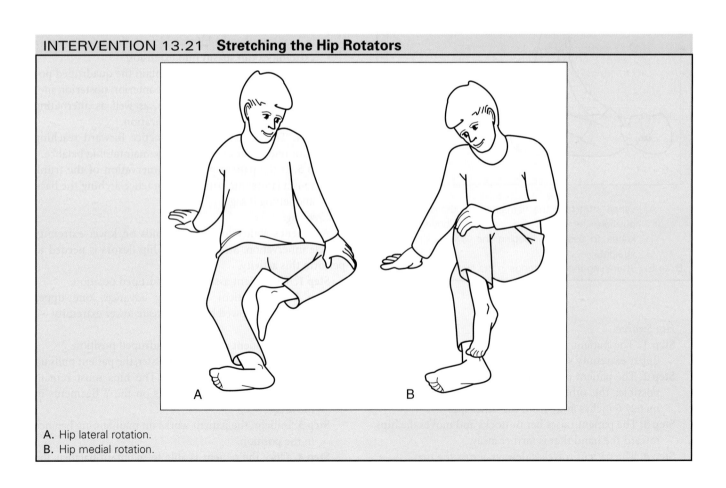

A | B

A. Hip lateral rotation.
B. Hip medial rotation.

INTERVENTION 13.22 Ankle Dorsiflexion

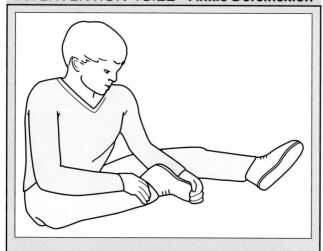

Ankle dorsiflexion. When completing this stretch, patients with C7 innervation will need to maintain one upper extremity in extension for trunk support.

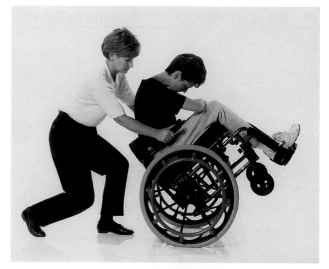

Fig. 13.14 The therapist lowers the wheelchair to the floor.

Step 5. The patient can advance to kneeling-height crutches. The patient can balance in the position with the crutches, lift one crutch, advance both crutches forward, or pull both crutches back.

The functional significance of these activities is widespread. The sitting swing-through, hip swayer, and prone push-up exercises work to improve upper extremity strength necessary for transfers and assisted ambulation. The trunk twisting exercise helps improve the patient's trunk control for transfers, including those from the wheelchair to the floor. Unilateral reaching in the quadruped position assists the patient in developing upper extremity strength and coordination and improves the patient's ability to transfer from the floor into the wheelchair. Creeping on all fours helps develop the patient's trunk and lower extremity muscle control. It is also a useful position for the patient to be able to assume while on the floor. Tall kneeling promotes the development of trunk control. It can be used as a position of transition for patients as they transfer from the floor back into their wheelchairs, and it serves as a preambulation activity. Stages of motor control (mobility, stability, controlled mobility, and skill) must also be considered when implementing these interventions.

Transfers

Wheelchair-to-floor transfers. Patients with paraplegia should be instructed how to fall while in their wheelchairs and how to transfer back into the chair if, for some reason, they are displaced. In addition, the floor is a good place to perform hip-flexor stretching. In the clinic, the PT or PTA will initiate practice of this skill by lowering the patient to the floor as shown in Fig. 13.14. The patient should be instructed to tuck her head and to keep her arms in the wheelchair. The patient must be cautioned against trying to soften the fall by using her arms. Extension of the upper extremities can result in wrist fractures. The patient will also want to place one of her upper extremities over the knees to prevent the lower extremities from coming up and hitting her in the face.

Once the patient is on the floor, she has several options for transferring back into the wheelchair. It may be easiest for the patient to right the wheelchair and then to transfer back into it. If the patient can position herself in a supported kneeling position in front of the wheelchair, she can pull herself back into the wheelchair, as depicted in Intervention 13.23. If the patient possesses adequate upper extremity strength and range of motion, she can back up to the wheelchair in a long-sitting position, depress her shoulders, and lift her buttocks back into the wheelchair. The patient's hands are positioned near the buttocks. Flexion of the neck while attempting this maneuver aids in elevating the buttocks through the head-hips relationship. Although this type of transfer is possible, many patients do not have adequate strength to complete the transition successfully. In the clinic, one can practice this by using a small step stool or several mats. In a long-sitting position, the patient transfers first to the step stool and then back up into the wheelchair. Intervention 13.24 illustrates a patient who is performing a transfer from the floor back into the wheelchair. The patient rotates the wheelchair casters forward and places one hand on the caster and the other on the wheelchair seat and pushes upward.

Righting the wheelchair. Individuals with good upper body strength may be able to right a tipped chair while remaining in it. To be successful with this activity, the individual must be able to push down with the arm in contact with the floor, use the head and upper trunk to shift weight forward, and remember to push down on the hand in contact with the wheelchair instead of pulling on it. Intervention 13.25 shows an individual who is completing this activity.

INTERVENTION 13.23   Transfer to Wheelchair From Tall Kneeling

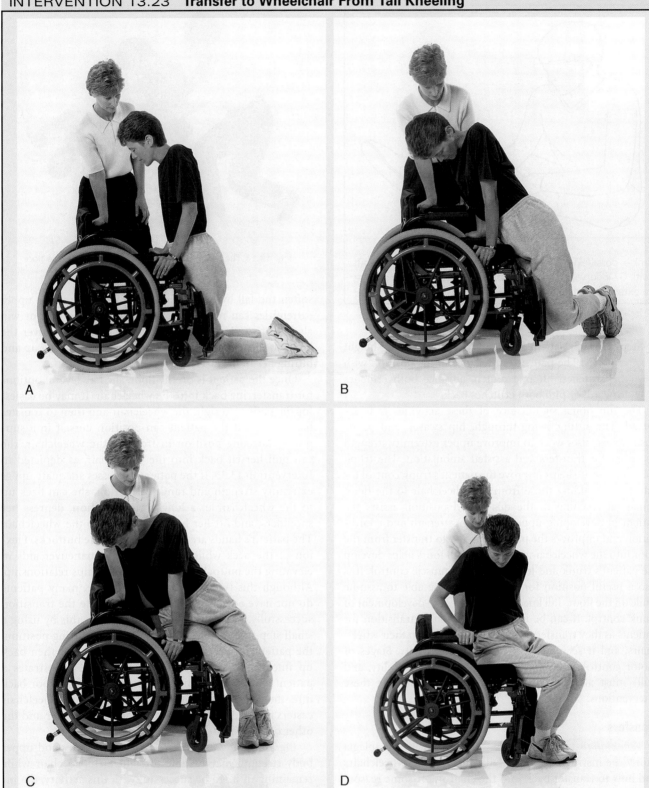

A

B

C

D

A. The patient assumes a tall-kneeling position and pulls herself into the wheelchair.

B. to D. The patient must rotate over her hips to assume a sitting position. The sequence can be reversed to transfer out of the wheelchair.

INTERVENTION 13.24 Transfer to Wheelchair From Long-Sitting Position

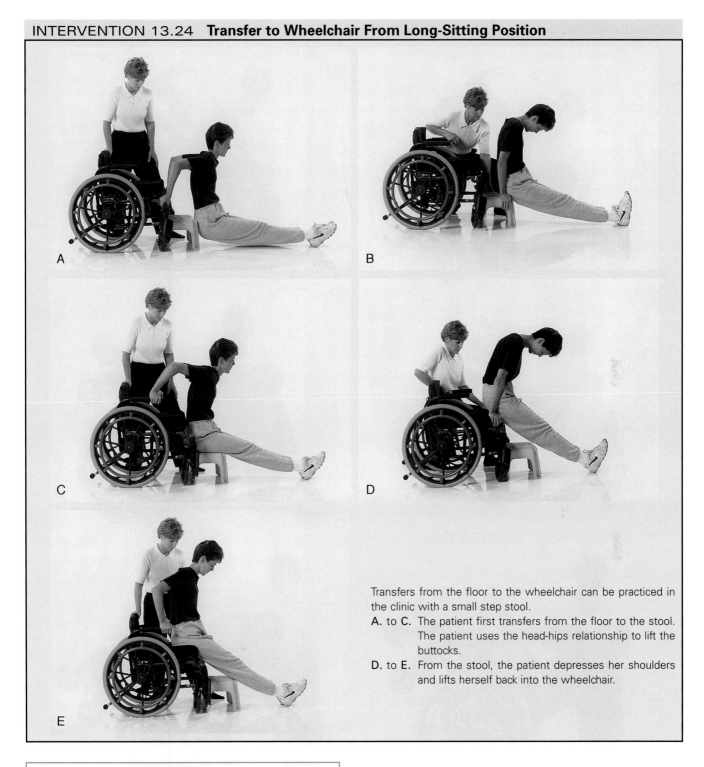

Transfers from the floor to the wheelchair can be practiced in the clinic with a small step stool.

A. to C. The patient first transfers from the floor to the stool. The patient uses the head-hips relationship to lift the buttocks.

D. to E. From the stool, the patient depresses her shoulders and lifts herself back into the wheelchair.

CAUTION A word of caution must be expressed during the performance of these activities. Patients who lack sensation in the lower extremities and buttocks must monitor the position of their lower extremities during activity performance. Patients can accidentally bump themselves on sharp wheelchair parts; these injuries can cause skin tears during these activities.

Although patients with tetraplegia cannot complete wheelchair to floor transfers independently, they should practice the task. These individuals must be able to instruct others in ways to assist should this situation occur in the home or community.

Advanced Wheelchair Skills

Patients with innervation and strength in the finger muscles should receive instruction in advanced wheelchair skills. Attaining wheelies and ascending and descending curbs should be taught so that the patient can be as independent in the community as possible.

Wheelies. Before the patient can learn to perform a wheelie independently, the patient must be able to find her balance point in a tipped wheelchair position (Fig. 13.15). The easiest way to do this is to tip the patient gently back onto

INTERVENTION 13.25   Righting the Wheelchair While Seated

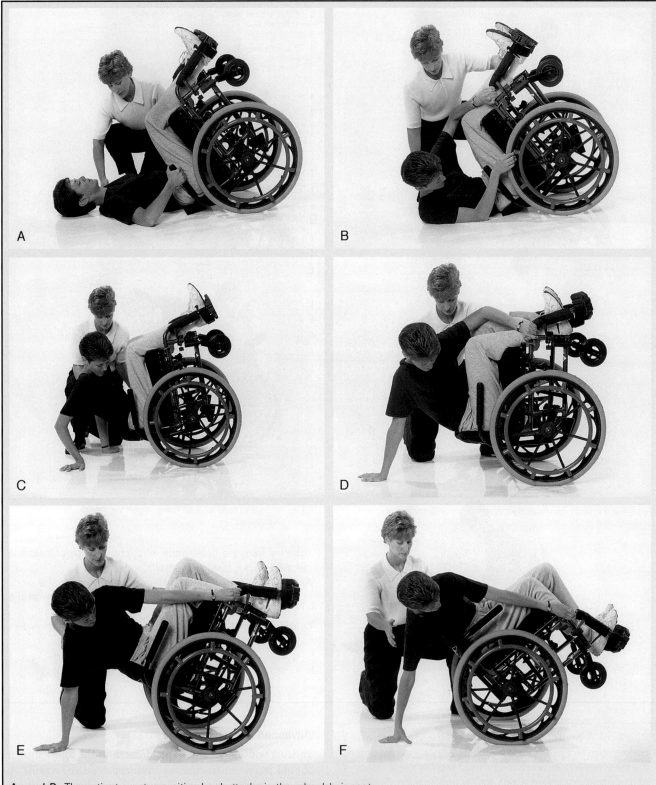

A. and B. The patient must reposition her buttocks in the wheelchair seat.

   C. The patient flexes her trunk forward and places both hands in contact with the floor to push herself up.

D. and E. The patient moves one arm to the opposite legrest and begins to push the legrest and front casters to the floor while she continues to push down and move the hand in contact with the floor closer to the wheelchair backrest.

   F. The patient flexes her head and trunk towards her legs.
   Patients should be carefully guarded while they practice this skill.

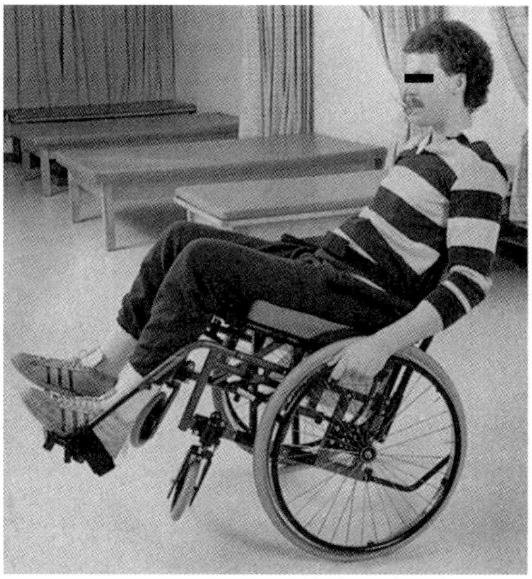

Fig. 13.15 Finding the balance point is a prerequisite to popping and maintaining a wheelie position. (From Buchanan LE, Nawoczenski DA: *Spinal cord injury and management approaches*, Baltimore, 1987, Williams & Wilkins.)

the rear wheels. The therapist should find the point at which the wheelchair is most perfectly balanced. The patient must keep her back against the wheelchair back. The patient then grasps the hand rims. If the wheelchair begins to tip backward, the patient should be instructed to pull back slightly on the hand rims. If the front casters begin to fall forward, the patient should push forward on the hand rims. Most patients initially overcompensate while learning to attain a balance point by leaning forward or pulling or pushing too much on the rims.

During these early stages of practice, you must guard the patient carefully. Standing behind the patient with your hands resting near the push handles of the wheelchair and standing near the backrest are the best places to guard the patient. Once the patient is able to maintain a wheelie with your assistance, the patient must learn to achieve the position independently. The patient must master this activity to negotiate curbs independently. To attain the wheelie position, have the patient lean forward in the wheelchair. The patient pulls back on the wheelchair rims and then quickly pushes forward at the same time she moves her shoulders posteriorly against the back of the wheelchair. The quick forward movement of the chair, combined with the shifting of the patient's weight backward, causes the front casters of the wheelchair to pop up. With practice, the patient learns how much force is needed to attain the position. Eventually, the patient is able to achieve the wheelie position from a stationary or rolling position.

Ascending ramps. A patient should ascend a ramp while in a forward position. The length and inclination must be considered before the patient attempts to negotiate any ramp. When the patient is going up a ramp, instruct her to lean forward in the wheelchair. If the ramp is long, the patient uses long, strong pushes on the hand rims. If the ramp is

relatively short and steep, the patient uses short, quick pushes to accelerate forward. A grade aid on the wheelchair may be needed to prevent the chair from rolling backward between pushes. The grade aid serves as a type of braking mechanism to assist the patient to change hand position for the next push without rolling backward.

Descending ramps. Patients should be encouraged to descend ramps with their wheelchairs facing forward. The patient is instructed to lean back in the wheelchair. The patient then places both hands on the hand rims or on the rims and wheels themselves. The movement of the wheelchair is controlled by friction applied to the hand rims and wheels by the patient. The patient must let the rims move equally between both hands to guarantee that the wheelchair will move in a straight path. Patients may also elect to apply the wheelchair brakes partially when descending ramps. Although this technique provides added friction to the wheels, it can cause mechanical failure to the braking mechanism of the wheelchair.

Ramps can also be descended with the patient in a backward position if the patient feels safer using this technique. The patient is instructed to line the wheelchair up evenly at the top of the ramp. The patient leans forward and grasps the hand rims near the brakes. The rims are then allowed to slide through the patient's hands during the descent. Patients must be careful at the bottom of the ramp because the casters and footrests can catch on the ramp and cause the chair to tip backward. Fig. 13.16 shows two methods for descending a ramp.

Ramps can also be ascended or descended in a diagonal or zigzag manner. Negotiating the ramp in a diagonal pattern decreases the tendency to roll down the ramp during ascent and decreases speed during descent.

SPECIAL NOTE During the performance of wheelchair skills, the patient may elect to wear gloves to protect the hands.

Ascending a curb. Going up a curb should always be performed with the patient in a forward direction. If the patient is going to be independent with this activity, she must be able to elevate the front casters of the wheelchair. As the patient approaches the curb, she pops the front casters up with a wheelie. Once the casters have cleared the curb, the patient leans forward and pushes on the hand rims. Patients require a great deal of practice to master this activity because the timing of the individual components is extremely important and the completion of the task takes considerable muscle strength. Intervention 13.26, *A* and *B*, illustrates this skill.

Descending a curb. It is often easiest to instruct patients to descend curbs backward; however, most clinicians agree that it presents more danger to the patient because of the risk from unseen traffic. In this technique, the patient backs the wheelchair down the curb. Again, the patient should lean forward and grasp the wheel rims near the brakes on the chair. The position of the footplates must also be observed during performance of this activity. The footplates may catch on the curb as the chair

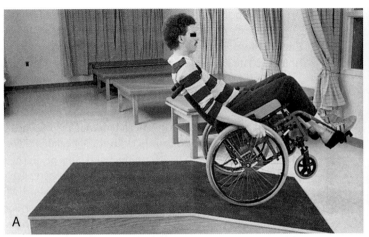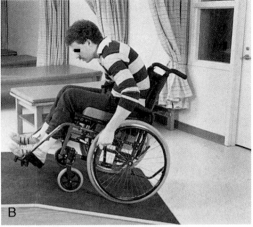

Fig. 13.16 A, A person with good wheelchair mobility skills may be able to descend a ramp in a wheelie position. **B,** The safest method to descend a ramp is backward. The person must remember to lean forward while controlling the rear wheels. Ascending a ramp is performed in a similar manner. (From Buchanan LE, Nawoczenski DA: *Spinal cord injury and management approaches*, Baltimore, 1987, Williams & Wilkins.)

descends. If this occurs, the patient will need to lean back into the chair to allow the casters to clear the curb (see Intervention 13.26, *C* and *D*).

A second method of descending a curb is for the patient to go down in a forward position. Before the patient attempts this maneuver, she must be able to achieve a wheelie and roll forward while in a tilted position. As the patient approaches the curb, she pops a wheelie. The rear wheels are allowed to roll or bounce off the curb. Once the rear wheels have cleared the curb, the patient leans forward so that the front casters once again are on the ground. Care must be taken when patients learn this task because incorrect shifting of the patient's weight either too far backward or too far forward can cause the patient to fall out of the wheelchair. It is often easiest to begin training using lower height curbs. A 1- to 2-inch curb should be used initially with patients as they try to perfect these skills.

Powered mobility. Patients with high-level tetraplegia need to master powered mobility. Often, equipment vendors will provide power chairs for individuals on a trial basis. A portion of your treatment session should be devoted to assisting the patient with the operation of the power chair. Descriptions of different types of power wheelchairs and the operation of these units are outside the scope of this text. Clinicians are encouraged to work with equipment vendors to become knowledgeable about the different wheelchairs and accessories that are available.

Wheelchair cushions. Individuals who will be spending a considerable amount of time each day sitting in a wheelchair should also have some type of wheelchair cushion. Specialized cushions are available that reduce some of the pressure applied to the individual's buttocks. Fig. 13.17 depicts various commercially available cushions. No cushion completely eliminates pressure, and individuals must continue to perform some method of pressure relief throughout the day in order to minimize the risk of pressure ulcers.

Cardiopulmonary Training/Aerobic Conditioning

Cardiopulmonary training should also be included in the patient's rehabilitation program and must be based on the patient's exercise capacity as determined by the motor level. Use of inspiratory muscle trainers and diaphragmatic strengthening should be continued to further maximize vital capacity. Endurance training should be incorporated into the patient's treatment plan and can include activities such as wheelchair propulsion for extended distances, upper extremity ergometry (arm bikes), swimming, and wheelchair aerobics. Although these activities improve the patient's endurance, the upper extremity muscles are smaller and, as such, are capable of performance at a higher intensity for a shorter duration of time than the muscles in the lower extremities. Therefore, muscles fatigue occurs more quickly (Decker and Hall, 1986; Morrison, 1994). Additionally, with muscle atrophy there is a shift in muscle fiber type from oxidative to nonoxidative "which leads to rapid onset fatigue and muscle intolerance" (Macko, 2016). Passive leg cycling has also been shown to provide cardiovascular, neuromuscular, and musculoskeletal benefits (Phadke et al., 2019). Unfortunately, this equipment is often only available in rehabilitation centers, making access difficult for patients.

Patients with SCIs lack normal cardiovascular responses to exercise. Individuals with injuries above T4 will generally exhibit maximal heart rates of 130 beats/min or less with exercise, whereas patients with lower level paraplegia will present with increased heart rate responses comparable to the general public (Jacobs and Nash, 2004). Blood pressure, heart rate, cardiac output, and sweating responses are altered secondary to autonomic sympathetic dysfunction and the resultant disturbed blood flow. Therefore, the use of target heart rate alone may not be an appropriate indicator of exercise intensity for patients with spinal cord injuries. Additional methods of monitoring the patient's exercise response, including blood pressure and the Borg Rating of Perceived Exertion (RPE) Scale (a subjective measure of individual

INTERVENTION 13.26 Ascending and Descending a Curb

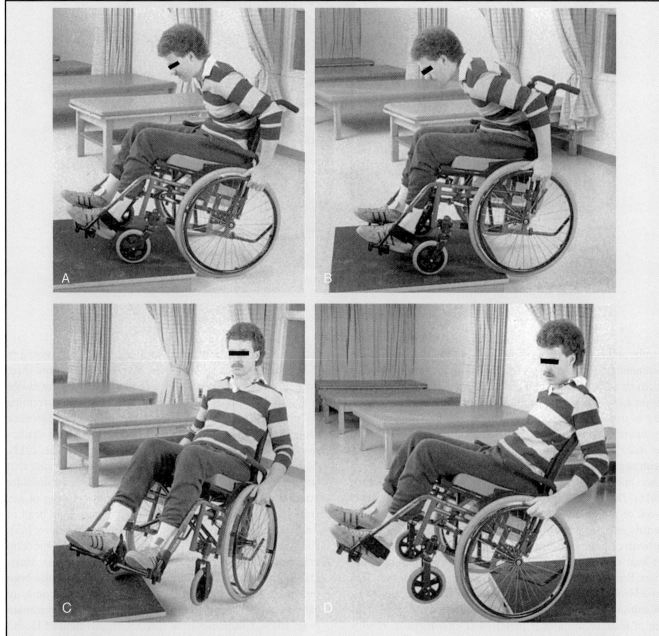

A. and B. A person ascends a curb by "popping a wheelie" to place the front casters onto the curb, then pulls the rear wheels upward. Timing and good upper extremity strength are important for this activity.

C. Descending a curb may be performed by lowering the rear wheels evenly off the curb and completing the activity by spinning the chair to clear the front casters.

D. A person may descend the curb forward in a controlled wheelie position.

(From Buchanan LE, Nawoczenski DA: *Spinal cord injury and management approaches*, Baltimore, 1987, Williams & Wilkins.)

exercise intensity), should be employed. A target RPE rating of 12 to 15/20 is recommended (Borello-France et al., 2000; Ferrara and Tappan, 2019).

Aerobic training effects are, however, still possible and patients can benefit from exercise programs to decrease the risk of secondary complications, including hypertension, diabetes mellitus, and elevated cholesterol. Improvements in body composition (increasing fat-free muscle mass and reducing intramuscular and abdominal fat), systemic and cardiac vasomotor function, bone health, skin integrity, bowel function, and an individual's psychological function (mood, anxiety, depression, and in older adults, cognition) can also be achieved with regular exercise (Department of Health & Human Services, 2018; Macko, 2016; Burr et al., 2012;

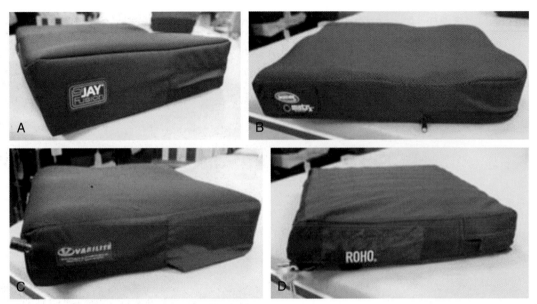

Fig. 13.17 Pressure-relieving wheelchair cushions. **A–D**, Immersion and envelopment-type cushions are made of foams, gel, air-based cells, or a hybrid or mixture of these mediums. (From Webster JB, Murphy DP, editors: *Atlas of orthoses and assistive* devices, ed 5, Philadelphia, 2019, Elsevier, p 388.)

Jacobs and Nash, 2004; Lewthwaite et al., 1994). Exercise recommendations for persons with SCIs do not vary drastically from those for the general public. If the individual plans to begin a low-intensity exercise program, formal exercise testing is usually not necessary because the intensity is likely comparable to that which is associated with physical therapy or daily activities. Individuals at higher risk or those who wish to exercise at a greater level should receive medical clearance and complete a formal graded exercise test (Macko, 2016). Duration of exercise should be 150 to 300 minutes a week of moderate intensity aerobic activity. If moderate intensity exercise is too difficult then 75 to 150 minutes of light intensity can be substituted. Individuals should also perform at least 2 days of flexibility and muscle strengthening exercises. Persons at risk for falls should also incorporate exercises to address balance. If a patient is unable to tolerate 20 to 60 minutes of continuous activity, aerobic activity performed for at least 10 minutes is preferred (Department of Health & Human Services, 2018; Macko, 2016; Gordon et al, 2016; Jacobs and Nash, 2004). Evidence suggests that cardiovascular fitness can be achieved through several shorter bouts of exercise instead of one longer session (Lewthwaite et al., 1994). Possible activities that may be performed include leg cycling with electric stimulation, body-weight-supported treadmill ambulation, upper extremity and wheelchair ergometry, circuit training, swimming, and wheelchair sports (Macko, 2016; Somers, 2010). If an individual is unable to meet the guidelines presented, it is recommended to engage in some type of regular physical activity and avoid inactivity.

Circuit Training

Researchers have also studied the effects of circuit training (weight training with exercise equipment and upper extremity ergometry) in individuals with paraplegia. Significant increases in shoulder strength and endurance were noted in individuals who participated in a training program three times a week for 12 weeks. The results of a study by Jacobs et al. (2001) support the beneficial effects of circuit training on fitness levels in individuals with paraplegia. These exercise programs have the potential to decrease the risk for cardiovascular disease in this population (Sasso and Backus, 2013). Additionally, upper extremity strengthening programs that target the serratus, middle and lower trapezius, and shoulder external rotators combined with selective stretching of key areas (the pectoralis muscles, upper trapezius, long head of the biceps, and posterior capsule of the shoulder) have been effective in reducing shoulder pain and improving function in patients with paraplegia (Nawoczenski et al., 2006). Maximal-intensity lower extremity strength training has also been shown to improve strength, gait, and balance outcomes in patients with chronic motor incomplete SCIs (Jayaraman et al., 2013). Guidelines from the U.S. Department of Health and Human Services (2018) recommend 8 to 10 repetitions (progressing to three sets) of general whole body muscle-strengthening exercises for 2 or more days a week to achieve maximal health benefits.

Aquatic (Pool) Therapy

Pool therapy can be a valuable addition to the patient's overall treatment plan. Water offers an excellent medium for exercising without the effects of gravity and friction and for practicing ambulation skills. Many facilities have warm-water (92° to 96° F) therapeutic pools for their patients. The warm water provides physiologic effects, including increased circulation, heart rate, and respiration rate and decreased blood pressure. In addition, general relaxation is usually accomplished with warm-water immersion. These effects must be kept in mind as the PT develops a pool program for the patient.

When designing a therapeutic pool program for a patient with SCI, the PT should consider the following as therapeutic benefits of this type of treatment intervention. Activities performed in the water will help to:

1. Decrease abnormal muscle tone
2. Increase muscle strength
3. Increase range of motion
4. Improve pulmonary function
5. Provide opportunities for standing and weight bearing
6. Exercise muscles with fair-minus strength more easily
7. Improve cardiovascular fitness

Although most patients can exercise safely in the water, several situations have been identified as contraindications to aquatic programs. A patient with any of the following medical conditions should not be allowed to participate in the program: fever, infectious diseases, tracheostomy, uncontrolled blood pressure, vital capacities less than 1 liter, urinary or bowel incontinence, and an open wound or sore that cannot be covered by a waterproof dressing. Patients with halo traction devices can be taken into the pool as long as their heads are kept out of the water and components of the device that retain water are replaced. Individuals with catheters may participate in pool programs if the drain tubes are clamped and storage bags are attached to the lower extremity (Giesecke, 1997).

Pool program. Several logistic factors must be considered before taking the patient in the water for a treatment session. As stated previously, warm water is desirable. However, to accommodate the many patients who may need to use a therapeutic pool at a given facility, the temperature of water may be cooler. This factor must be considered when one works with patients with SCIs because their temperature regulation is often impaired. Different facilities have specific requirements regarding safety procedures that must be followed when working with the patient in the water. Previous water safety experience is beneficial. A minimal number of people may also be needed in the pool area to ensure safety. To prepare the patient for the treatment session, the PT or PTA must discuss the benefits of the program and describe a typical session. The patient's previous affinity for water must also be determined. Many individuals profoundly dislike water and may be apprehensive about the experience. Reassuring the patient should help. The patient should arrive for the treatment session in a swimsuit. Catheters should be clamped to avoid the potential for leakage. The patient should also be instructed to wear socks, and elbow and knee pads, depending on the treatment activities to be performed. Because sensory impairments are common, areas that could become scraped during the session must be protected.

Transfers into and out of the pool can occur in a number of different ways and depend on the type of equipment and facilities present. Frequently, a lift transfers the patient into the pool, or the pool may have a ramp and entrance is in some type of wheelchair or shower chair. Once the patient is in the water, the therapist must guard the patient carefully. Patients with tetraplegia and paraplegia have decreased movement, proprioception, and light touch sensation. The patient may have difficulty maintaining her position in the water. At times, the lower extremities may float toward the surface of the water, and the clinician may have a difficult time keeping the patient's feet and lower extremities on the bottom of the pool in a weight-bearing position. Gentle pressure applied to the top of the patient's foot by the therapist's foot can help alleviate this problem. Flotation vests are helpful and can be reassuring to the patient. Once the patient is more confident in the water, the vest can be removed if allowed by facility policy.

Pool exercises. Many pools have steps into them or an area where the clinician and the patient can sit down. This feature provides an excellent environment to work on upper extremity strengthening. With the upper extremity supported, the patient moves the arm in the water and uses the buoyancy of the water to complete range-of-motion exercises. The patient can also work on lifting the extremity out of the water to provide more challenge to the activity. The anterior, middle, and posterior deltoids, as well as the pectoralis major and rhomboids, can be exercised in this position. Triceps strengthening can also occur in a gravity-neutralized or supported position. In addition to working on upper extremity strengthening, use of the sitting position serves to challenge the patient's sitting balance and trunk muscles that remain innervated. Alternating isometrics and rhythmic stabilization can be applied at the shoulder region to work on trunk strengthening.

Exercises to increase pulmonary function can be practiced while the patient is in the water. Having the patient hold her breath or blow bubbles while in the water assists in improving pulmonary capacity.

The patient can practice standing at the side of the pool while in the water. The PT or PTA may need to guard the patient at the trunk and to use the lower extremities to maintain proper alignment of the patient's legs. Approximation can be applied down through the hips to assist with lower extremity weight bearing. Some therapeutic pools possess parallel bars within the water to assist with standing and ambulation activities. If the patient has an incomplete injury with adequate lower extremity innervation, assisted walking can be performed. As stated previously, this is an excellent way to strengthen weak lower extremity muscles and to improve the patient's endurance. Kickboards can also be used to assist with lower extremity strengthening.

Floating and swimming. Patients with tetraplegia or paraplegia can be taught to float on their backs. Floating assists with breathing, as well as general body relaxation. Patients can also be instructed in modified or adaptive swimming strokes. Patients with tetraplegia can be taught a modified backstroke and breaststroke. Performance of these swimming strokes assists the patient with upper extremity strengthening and also improves the patient's cardiovascular fitness. Patients with paraplegia can be instructed in the front crawl or butterfly stroke, which can also increase upper extremity strength and improve the patient's cardiovascular endurance.

Other Advanced Rehabilitation Interventions

Other treatment activities may be performed as part of the patient's treatment plan. *Neuromuscular stimulation (NMS)/Functional Electrical Stimulation (FES)* may be used in patients with muscle weakness to increase strength and to decrease muscle fatigue. NMS is often suggested when a patient has muscle innervation and weakness as a consequence of an incomplete injury. Other benefits of NMS include decreasing range-of-motion limitations, decreasing spasticity, minimizing muscle imbalances, and providing positioning support for patients who are attempting ambulation. Electrical stimulation can be used to improve hand and upper extremity function in patients with SCI (Ho et al., 2014). In a study conducted by Hoffman and Field-Fote (2010), improved hand function in individuals with chronic tetraplegia was recorded with unilateral massed practice and electrical stimulation. Increases in the size of the corticomotor map for the thenar muscles were also noted, suggesting changes in cortical organization following the interventions. Clinicians can also apply NMS to the upper or lower extremity musculature to assist with arm and leg ergometry. Previous research with lower extremity cycling and FES has shown decreases in muscle atrophy and an increase in muscle mass as well as improvements in endurance, pulmonary function, and lower extremity circulation (Ferrara and Tappan, 2019).

As stated previously, patients with incomplete injuries often have increased muscle tone that interferes with function. Therefore, a component of the patient's treatment plan is the management of this problem. Stretching, ice, pool therapy, and functional electrical stimulation may be appropriate forms of intervention. Electrical stimulation can be applied either to the antagonist muscle to promote increased strength or to the agonist muscle to induce fatigue. Patients with excessive amounts of abnormal tone may also be receiving pharmacologic interventions, as mentioned previously in this chapter.

Ambulation Training (Compensatory Approach)

One of the first questions that patients with SCIs often ask is whether they will be able to walk again. This question is frequently posed in the acute-care center immediately following the injury. Early on, it may be difficult to determine the patient's ambulation potential secondary to spinal shock and the depression of reflex activity; however, once this condition resolves, many patients expect an answer to this question. In a study by van Middendorp et al. (2011), the researchers developed a clinical prediction rule for ambulation based on a patient's age and her results on four neurologic tests (motor scores for the quadriceps and gastrocsoleus and light touch sensation in dermatomes L3 and SI). A patient's motor scores, sensory status, and age can provide health care providers with an early prognosis regarding the patient's ability to walk independently after injury (van Middendorp et al., 2011).

Different philosophies regarding gait training are recognized, and much depends on the rehabilitation team with which you work. Some health care professionals believe that it is best to give patients with the potential to ambulate every opportunity to do so. These individuals believe that most patients, given the opportunity to try walking with orthoses and an assistive device, will not continue to do so after they realize the difficulty encountered. It may be best to allow the patient to come to her decision on ambulation independent of the PT or health care team. Other health care professionals believe that a patient should possess strength in the hip-flexor musculature before ambulation is attempted because of the high-energy costs, time, and financial resources associated with gait training. Most patients with higher-level injuries choose wheelchair mobility as their preferred method of locomotion after trying ambulation with orthoses and assistive devices because of the energy expenditure and decreased speed associated with the activity (Lavis and Codamon, 2019; Cerny et al., 1980; Decker and Hall, 1986; Somers, 2010).

The *compensatory versus recovery* approaches to the treatment of the patient with SCI are best illustrated in the therapist's approach to gait training. The use of orthoses, assistive devices, functional electrical stimulation, and robotic exoskeletons are examples of *compensatory strategies* that can be employed to assist patients with ambulation on level surfaces. Locomotor training through partial body-weight-supported treadmill ambulation provides an excellent example of the *recovery approach* to patient care.

Benefits of Standing and Walking

Although functional ambulation may not be possible for all of our patients with SCIs, therapeutic standing has documented benefits. Standing prevents the development of osteoporosis and also helps decrease the patient's risk for bladder and kidney stones. Self-reported improvements in spasticity, bladder and bowel management, and psychological benefits have been noted in individuals who are able to participate in standing and walking programs (Lavis and Codamon, 2019; Eng et al., 2001; Nixon, 1985).

Guidelines have been established regarding assessment of the patient's likelihood for success with ambulation. Factors to consider include the following: (1) the patient's motivation to walk and to continue with ambulation once discharged from rehabilitation (given the opportunity to try assisted ambulation with orthoses, some patients decide it is too difficult a task and prefer not to continue with the training); (2) the patient's weight and body build (the heavier the patient is, the more difficult it will be for the patient to walk, and taller patients usually find it more challenging to ambulate with orthoses); (3) the passive range of motion present at the hips, knees, and ankles (hip, knee, or ankle plantar flexion contractures limit the patient's ability to ambulate with orthoses and crutches; in addition, patients need approximately 110 degrees of passive hamstring range of motion to be able to don their orthoses and transfer from the floor if they fall); (4) the amount of spasticity present (lower extremity or trunk spasticity can make wearing orthoses difficult); (5) the cardiopulmonary status of the patient (patients with better pulmonary function have an easier time meeting the energy demands of walking); and (6) status of the integumentary system. The rehabilitation team must consider all of these factors when discussing ambulation goals with the patient (Atrice et al., 2013; Basso et al., 2000).

Depending on the patient's motor level, different types of ambulation potential have been described. The literature varies on the specific motor level and the potential for ambulation. For patients with T2 through T11 injuries, therapeutic standing or ambulation may be possible. This means that the patient is able to stand or ambulate in the physical therapy department with assistance. However, functional ambulation is not possible. Therapeutic ambulators require assistance to transfer from sitting to standing and to walk on level surfaces. These patients ambulate for the physiologic and therapeutic benefits it offers. Patients with injuries at the T12 through L2 level have the potential to be household ambulators, whereas patients with innervation at L3 can achieve functional community ambulation (Atrice et al., 2013).

Individuals who achieve *household or community ambulation* are able to ambulate in their homes with orthoses and assistive devices. Patients at this level are able to transfer independently, to ambulate on level surfaces of varying textures, and to negotiate doorways and other minor architectural barriers.

Community ambulation is possible for patients with injuries at L3 or lower. These patients are able to ambulate with or without orthoses and assistive devices. Community ambulators are able to ambulate independently in the community and can negotiate all environmental barriers (Atrice et al., 2013; Decker and Hall, 1986).

The energy cost for ambulation in patients with complete injuries above T12 is above the anaerobic threshold and cannot be maintained for an extended period (Atrice et al., 2013). Cerny et al. (1980) reported that gait velocities for patients with paraplegia were significantly slower than normal walking, and gait required a 50% increase in oxygen consumption and a 28% increase in heart rate. Consequently, individuals with paraplegia discontinue ambulation with their orthoses and assistive devices and use their wheelchairs for environmental negotiation (Cerny et al., 1980).

Orthoses

Patients with paraplegia who decide to pursue ambulation training need some type of orthosis. Fig. 13.18 depicts the most common lower extremity orthoses prescribed. Knee-ankle-foot orthoses may be recommended for patients with paraplegia. These orthoses typically have a thigh cuff and an external knee joint with a locking mechanism (drop locks or bail locks are the most common). They have a calf band and an adjustable locked ankle joint. Scott-Craig knee-ankle-foot orthoses are frequently prescribed for patients with paraplegia. These orthoses consist of a single thigh and pretibial band, a bail lock at the knee joint, and modified footplates. The design of this orthosis provides built-in stability at the knee and ankle while passively positioning the hip in extension. "An extension moment is created at the hips that prevents the individual from folding forward" while the Y ligaments in the hip

maintain the hip in extension (Lavis and Codamon, 2019). This provides the patient with inherent stability while standing.

The reciprocating gait orthosis is a hip-knee-ankle-foot orthosis (HKAFO) that may be prescribed for patients with SCIs. This device is used with patients with limited trunk control. The reciprocating gait orthosis has an external hip joint that is operated by a cable mechanism. When the patient shifts weight forward and laterally onto one lower extremity, the cable system advances the opposite leg. Individuals using reciprocating gait orthoses often use a walker instead of Lofstrand crutches as their preferred assistive device. Other orthoses are available that have expanded on the basic principles of the reciprocating gait orthosis (RGO). Therapists are advised to consult with an orthotist to determine the most effective bracing system for a given patient.

New orthotic systems are also being developed that utilize robotic exoskeletons and electric stimulation. These systems may decrease some of the physiologic demands of ambulation with orthotics; however, barriers to use include cost, donning and doffing, and the ability to use the device when in one's wheelchair. Additional research is necessary to determine the long-term benefits of these systems (Lavis and Codamon, 2019).

Ambulation Outcomes

The decision to attempt gait training is made by the patient and the rehabilitation team. Realistic goals and expectations must be conveyed during the decision-making process. As stated previously, the patient's motor level and other factors must be considered. Patients with motor complete, AIS A, have very limited abilities to achieve functional ambulation. Individuals who do achieve some level of walking function are those who have lower thoracic and lumbar injuries (Lavis and Codamon, 2019). For patients with a diagnosis of AIS B, motor complete and sensory incomplete, the ability to ambulate is approximately 33%, whereas in patients with AIS C the recovery of walking is about 75%. Age does appear to be a prognostic factor in patients with AIS C because individuals younger than 50 have a significantly improved chance of walking (80% to 90%) as compared with older adults (30% to 40%). Independent ambulation is possible for all patients who are classified as AIS D (Lavis and Codamon, 2019).

SPECIAL NOTE In general, the patient should be independent in mat mobility, wheelchair-to-mat transfers, and wheelchair mobility on level surfaces before beginning gait training. Many clinics possess training orthoses that allow the patient to practice standing before permanent orthoses are prescribed and manufactured. An orthotist should work with the patient to assist in identifying and fabricating the best orthosis for the patient. Depending on the patient's length of stay in the rehabilitation facility, gait training may begin at the end of the patient's inpatient hospitalization, or it may begin in earnest in the outpatient setting.

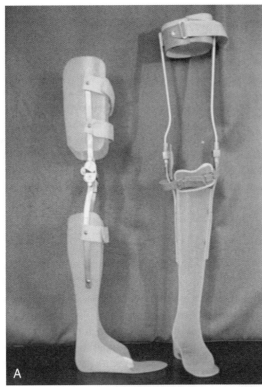
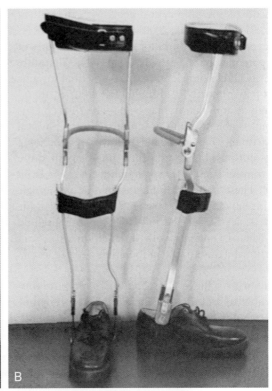
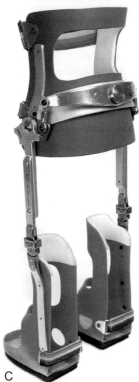
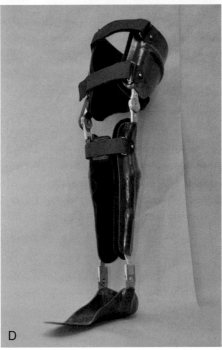

Fig. 13.18 A, Combination plastic and metal knee-ankle-foot orthoses. **B,** The Scott-Craig knee-ankle-foot orthosis is a special design for spinal cord injury. The orthosis consists of double uprights, offset knee joints with locks and bail control, one posterior thigh band, a hinged anterior tibial band, an ankle joint with anterior and posterior adjustable pin stops, a cushion heel, and specially designed footplates made of steel. **C,** The reciprocating gait orthosis, although generally used with children, is also used with adults. Its main components are a molded pelvic band, thoracic extensions, bilateral hip and knee joints, polypropylene posterior thigh shells, ankle-foot orthosis sections, and cables connecting the two hip joint mechanisms. **D,** Electronic knee-ankle-foot orthosis. (**A–C,** From Umphred DA, editor: *Umphred's neurological rehabilitation*, ed 6, St. Louis, 2013, Elsevier; **D,** From Webster JB, Murphy DP, editors: *Atlas of orthoses and assistive devices*, ed 5, St. Louis, 2019, Elsevier, p 253.)

Once the permanent orthoses have been delivered, it is time to begin the first gait training session. If possible, the orthotist should be present for this session. Having the patient don the orthoses is the first step. It is often easiest for the patient to do this on the mat in a long-sitting position. The patient should be encouraged to do as much as possible on this first attempt. She should start by placing one foot into the shoe and then locking the knee joint. During the performance of this activity, one realizes the necessity of possessing 110 degrees of hamstring range. Once the knee is in the orthosis, the patient can tighten the thigh pad. From there, the patient should start to put the other foot in the orthosis. Once both orthoses are on, the therapist and the orthotist, if present, will inspect the orthoses and check the fit. The orthoses must not rub the patient's skin. This situation can cause areas of redness and can lead to skin breakdown. If everything looks satisfactory, the patient should then be instructed to transfer back to the wheelchair to begin standing activities in the parallel bars. Upon completion of the gait training session and removal of the orthoses, the patient's skin should be inspected once again to ensure that there are no areas of pressure or skin breakdown.

Standing in the Parallel Bars

The first thing the patient needs to do is to transfer to standing. The therapist should initially demonstrate this maneuver for the patient. It is easiest to have the patient hold on to the parallel bars and pull forward. In preparation for this transition, the patient needs to move forward in the wheelchair. Having the patient push up and lift the buttocks forward is best to prevent shearing of the patient's skin. Once the patient is forward in the chair, the therapist will want to make sure the patient's orthoses are locked. If this is the patient's first time to stand up, it will be safest to have two individuals assist. While the patient is wearing the safety belt, one person is positioned in front of the patient and the other person is at the side or the back of the patient. On the count of three, the patient pulls herself forward on the bars. The individuals assisting the patient also provide the patient with the needed strength and momentum to complete the transfer.

Once upright, the patient must work to find her *balance point.* The patient's lower extremities should be slightly apart; the low back should be in hyperextension; the shoulders are toward the back; and the hands must be forward of the hips and holding on to the parallel bars. Essentially, the patient is resting on the Y ligaments in the hip and pelvic region. The lower extremity orthoses and positioning allow the patient to move her center of gravity behind the hip joints. Once the patient is able to find her balance point, she will eventually be able to stand and maintain balance without the use of the upper extremities. To guard the patient during this activity, the therapist will be behind the patient or off to the side. The therapist holds on to the gait belt and should avoid holding on to the patient's upper arms. The therapist may place a supporting hand on the patient's anterior shoulder as long as the therapist does not provide a counterbalancing or rotational force.

During practice of achievement of the balance point, the patient should initially have both hands on the parallel bars. The patient should be encouraged to hold the bars lightly and should avoid grabbing or pulling on them. Often, just having the patient rest the hands on the bars may be best. Eventually, you will want the patient to balance with one hand, and finally with no hands. The patient should ultimately be able to stand in the orthoses without any upper extremity support.

After the patient feels comfortable finding and maintaining the balance point, she can begin to practice push-ups in the bars. With the hands in a forward position, the patient pushes down on the bars by depressing the shoulders and tucking the head. Depending on the type of lower extremity orthosis and the presence or absence of a spreader bar, the therapist will want to note what happens to the patient's lower extremities during the push-up. Most often, the legs dangle free. If a spreader bar is attached to the orthoses, the legs will move as one unit. Performing a push-up is a prerequisite activity for the patient to ambulate in a forward direction.

After the patient practices maintaining the balance point, she should also practice jack-knifing. *Jack-knife* can be described as movement of the patient's upper body and head forward of the pelvis. Although jack-knifing is an undesirable occurrence, the activity should be practiced in the parallel bars during early gait training sessions. With the hands forward, the patient bends forward at the waist and lowers the trunk down toward the parallel bars. The patient then pushes back up to an upright position by extending her elbows. Once the patient feels comfortable with this activity, she can practice falling into a jack-knife position. The patient can initiate this fall either by moving the hands posterior to the hips or by flexing the head forward. The therapist can also assist the patient with the achievement of the jack-knife position by gently pulling the patient's hips and pelvis in a posterior direction.

To review, the jack-knife position is the position the patient will likely assume if she loses her balance during ambulation activities. The patient should recognize this position and needs to know what to do if it occurs during gait activities. If this position should occur during gait, the patient will want to straighten her elbows while extending the head and trunk.

Gait Progression

Once the patient can maintain her balance point and can perform a push-up to clear her feet from the floor, she is ready to begin forward ambulation in the parallel bars. You may be wondering how long this typically takes. Normally, you will want to progress the patient to taking a few steps on the first standing and ambulation attempt. However, the clinician has to monitor the patient's responses closely during standing and ambulation. The effects of fatigue, orthostatic hypotension, decreased cardiopulmonary endurance, and the anxiety associated with standing and walking can easily overwhelm the patient. To monitor physiologic responses during the treatment, the clinician should take baseline pulse, respiration, and blood pressure readings before the patient is standing. Careful monitoring of vital signs during the gait training portion of the treatment session is also indicated. In addition, the patient must be instructed to report any feelings of light-headedness or dizziness immediately.

The therapist should instruct the patient to find her balance point before advancing forward in the parallel bars. The patient's head should be held upright, looking forward. The patient then flexes her head, pushes down on the hands, depresses the shoulders, and lifts the lower extremities off the ground. As the patient depresses her shoulders and straightens the elbows, she must extend the head and neck and return them to a neutral position. To maintain balance, the patient needs to move her hands forward of the hips immediately. If the patient were to maintain her hands in the same place after completing the lift, she would jack-knife. After the patient's feet make contact with the floor, she must retract the scapula and move the upper trunk and head posteriorly. This type of gait pattern is known as a swing-to pattern because the patient is moving the feet the same distance as her hands. The patient should repeat the steps just described until she progresses to the end of the parallel bars. Using the verbal instructions "Lean, lift, and land" is helpful. At this point, someone can pull the wheelchair up behind the patient, or the patient can be instructed in performing a quarter-turn. If the patient is not too tired, she should continue and learn the turning technique at this time. Intervention 13.27 illustrates the correct head and trunk positions for gait-training activities.

Quarter-Turns

To complete a quarter-turn, the patient depresses her shoulders and lifts the legs while rotating the trunk and changing her hand position on the parallel bars. In essence, she is completing two quarter-turns to turn around. The patient must practice turning in both directions.

Sitting

Before transferring back to sitting, the patient should be instructed in the proper technique. The wheelchair should not be pulled up to the back of the patient's legs. Remember, the patient transfers from standing to sitting with the lower-extremity orthoses locked in extension. For this reason, the chair should be at least 12 inches from the patient so she will be able to land in the wheelchair seat. If the chair is too close to the patient, she might tip the chair over backward. The PT or PTA should have the patient keep both of her hands on the parallel bars during the descent. In time, the patient will be instructed in other methods to perform transfers from sitting to standing and from standing to sitting without the use of the parallel bars.

Swing-Through Gait Pattern

Once the patient feels comfortable with the swing-to gait pattern, the patient can progress to a swing-through pattern. The technique is the same as the swing-to pattern, except the patient advances her legs a little farther forward instead of stopping between steps. This gait pattern allows the patient to move forward a little faster and is more energy-efficient.

Other Gait Patterns

If the patient possesses lower extremity innervation, specifically hip flexion, the patient may have the potential to use a four-point or two-point gait pattern. Both patterns more closely resemble normal reciprocal gait patterns with upper and lower extremity movement. These patterns are described in standard texts and are not discussed here.

Backing Up

Patients should also be instructed in backing up. This is important when the patient begins to use her crutches on level surfaces within the physical therapy department. Initially, backing up should be practiced in the parallel bars. The patient tucks the head, depresses the shoulders, and extends the elbows. This position causes the patient to perform a mini–jack-knife and allows the patient's legs to move backward by virtue of the head-hips relationship. The patient repeats this sequence several times to move the desired distance backward.

Progressing the Patient

After the patient has practiced ambulation in the parallel bars several times, it is time to progress to ambulation outside of them. It is advisable to progress out of the bars without delay because patients can become reliant on them and may find it difficult to make the transition to overground ambulation in a less secure environment. To assist with this transition, the clinician may elect to introduce Lofstrand (Canadian or forearm) crutches while the patient is still ambulating in the parallel bars.

Care must be exercised when practicing transitions into and out of the wheelchair. These techniques are best practiced with the back of the wheelchair positioned next to a wall for greater safety. In addition, the patient should check to make sure the wheelchair brakes are locked.

Standing from the Wheelchair

If the patient is to become independent in ambulation activities, she must learn to transfer from sitting to standing independently. Several methods are possible for the patient. The first method described is probably the easiest.

Step 1. The patient places the wheelchair against the wall and locks the brakes.

Step 2. The patient places her crutches behind the wheelchair to rest on the push handles.

Step 3. The patient moves to the edge of the wheelchair. The patient needs to complete mini–push-ups as she does this. Scooting forward can cause unnecessary shearing to the patient's skin.

Step 4. With the orthoses locked, the patient crosses one leg over the other.

Step 5. The patient then pivots over the fixed foot and pushes up to standing.

INTERVENTION 13.27 Gait Progression

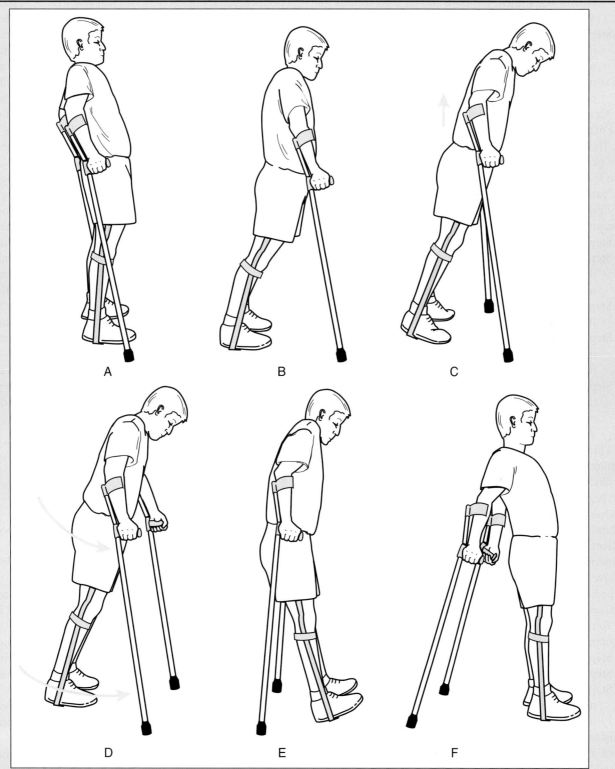

A. The patient finds his balance point.
B. He advances the crutches forward.
C. The patient tucks his head and pushes down on the crutches.
D. His pelvis and lower extremities swing forward.
E. His feet strike the floor.
F. The patient lifts his head and resumes a lordotic posture.

Step 6. Holding on to the wheelchair armrest, the patient secures one crutch, positions it, and then secures the second crutch.

Step 7. Once the crutches are in place, the patient backs up from the wheelchair, taking two or three steps backward. Intervention 13.28 shows the steps needed to transfer from sitting to standing with lower extremity orthoses and Lofstrand crutches.

An alternative way of completing this transfer is to unlock one of the orthoses and pivot over the unlocked lower extremity. This technique can be less stressful to the hip joint than the one previously described. The patient completes the transition to upright in the same way as noted earlier, except that the patient needs to lock the knee joint of the bent knee once an upright position has been achieved. The patient can also assume standing from the wheelchair by transferring forward.

Step 1. The patient moves forward to the edge of the chair.

Step 2. With the arms in the crutches, the patient places the crutches flat on the floor, slightly behind the front wheels.

Step 3. The patient flexes his head and pushes down on the crutches to propel out of the wheelchair.

Step 4. Once standing, the patient must quickly extend the head and trunk to regain the lumbar lordosis necessary for standing stability.

Step 5. The patient's upper extremities remain behind until the patient feels he has regained balance. Then he can move the arms and crutches forward. Intervention 13.29 shows a patient completing this activity.

This method is difficult for many patients because it requires a great deal of strength, balance, and coordination.

Once the patient is standing and has regained balance, he can begin to ambulate using a swing-through gait pattern, as described previously. The clinician guards the patient from behind, with one hand on the gait belt and the other on the patient's posterior shoulder, as depicted in Fig. 13.19. The clinician must be careful to avoid the tendency to apply excessive tactile cues to the patient. Pulling on the gait belt or impeding the movement of the patient's upper trunk may, in fact, cause the patient to experience balance disturbances.

To regain a sitting position after walking, the following is recommended:

Step 1. The patient faces the wheelchair initially.

Step 2. The patient places the crutches behind the chair.

Step 3. The patient unlocks one of the knee joints and rotates over that knee to assume a sitting position.

Patients can return to sitting using a straight-back method. This technique is difficult, however, and may best be used when a second person is present to assist with the transition to stabilize the wheelchair.

Gait Training With Crutches

As the patient begins ambulation training on level surfaces with the crutches, she once again needs to find her balance point. The patient must maintain the hands forward of the hips to prevent jack-knifing. Initially, the clinician may elect to perform a swing-to gait pattern with the patient. The clinician

should guard the patient from behind by holding on to the gait belt as necessary. Some clinicians may find it easier to guard the patient from the side initially by holding on to the gait belt and placing the other hand on the patient's shoulder. Verbal and tactile cueing may be necessary to assist the patient with head positioning and the hyperlordotic posture. Should the patient lose her balance and begin to jack-knife, the clinician will push the patient's pelvis forward and bring the shoulders back to resume the hyperextended posture. Because the patient will be moving relatively quickly, the clinician will need to take bigger steps. As the patient becomes more proficient, the patient can begin a swing-through gait pattern.

Falling. All patients who attempt gait training with crutches should also be instructed in proper falling techniques to avoid injury. The first attempts at falling should be completed in a controlled manner. You will want to have the patient fall onto a floor mat. The patient is instructed to let go of the crutches and remove the hands from the handgrips. The patient then reaches toward the ground and flexes the elbows to avoid trauma to the wrist. Holding onto the gait belt, the therapist slowly helps to lower the patient to the floor. If the facility has a crash mat (these mats are higher and softer), having the patient fall onto it is an easier starting point for the patient.

Getting up from the floor. Once the patient has practiced falling to the floor, the patient must also learn how to get up from the floor. The following steps should be used to assist the patient with this activity.

> **CAUTION** This transfer should be practiced close to a wall so the patient has something to lean against as he transitions to upright.

Step 1. The patient is instructed to assume a prone position on the floor.

Step 2. The patient positions the crutches with the tips pointing toward the head and the hand gripping at the hips.

Step 3. The patient pushes up to a plantigrade position. (The patient ensures that both orthoses are locked before attempting this maneuver.)

Step 4. The patient reaches for one of his crutches and puts the crutch tip on the floor to assist in the transition to an upright position. The patient's hand is on the crutch handle, and the crutch rests against the shoulder.

Step 5. The patient uses the crutch on the floor as a point of stability as he reaches for the other crutch and positions it on the forearm.

Step 6. The patient turns the opposite crutch around and places the forearm cuff at his elbow region.

Step 7. The patient regains balance with the crutches. Intervention 13.30 depicts this sequence.

Negotiating Environmental Barriers

If the patient is to be independent with ambulation in the community, she must be able to negotiate ramps, curbs, and stairs with orthoses and braces.

INTERVENTION 13.28 Sit-to-Stand Transfer With Orthoses

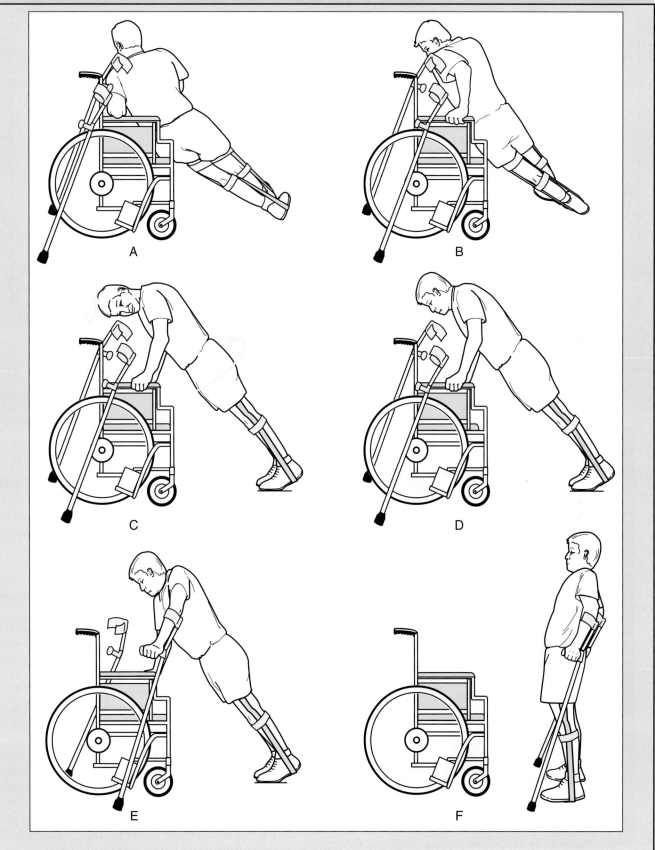

The sequence for transferring from sit to stand with lower extremity orthoses. (See text description on steps 1 through 7.)

INTERVENTION 13.29   Coming to Stand From the Wheelchair

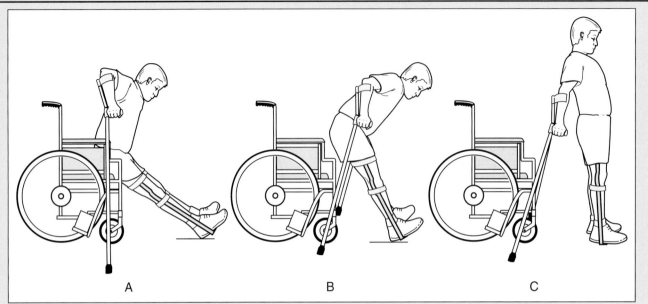

A   B   C

A. The patient flexes his head and upper trunk.
B. The patient uses the head-hips relationship and muscle action from the latissimus dorsi and triceps to push himself upright.
C. Upright standing.

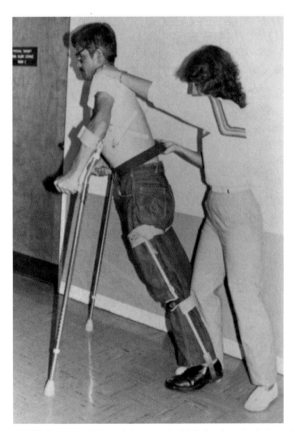

Fig. 13.19 Patient with an injury at the T12 level ambulating with crutches and bilateral knee-ankle-foot orthoses for balance and lower extremity advancement. (From Adkins HV, editor: *Spinal cord injury,* New York, 1985, Churchill Livingstone.)

Ascending a ramp.

Step 1. The patient uses a swing-to gait pattern to move forward up the ramp.

Step 2. To maintain balance, the patient keeps her crutches several inches in front of her feet.

Step 3. To increase hip stability, the patient's pelvis must be forward in a lordotic posture.

Descending a ramp. The same technique used for ambulation on level surfaces can be employed. A swing-through gait pattern is recommended.

Ascending a curb.

Step 1. The individual approaches the curb head-on.

Step 2. In a balanced position near the edge of the curb, the patient places the crutch tips on the curb.

Step 3. The patient leans forward, tucks the head, extends the elbows, and depresses the scapulae (jack-knifes) to elevate her lower extremities onto the curb. (The patient's toes drag up the elevation of the curb.)

Step 4. The patient can step to or past the crutches.

Step 5. Once the patient's feet land on the curb, she will need to regain the balance point.

Descending a curb.

Step 1. The individual approaches the curb head-on.

Step 2. In a balanced position near the edge of the curb, the patient steps off the curb, tucking the head, straightening the elbows, and depressing the scapulae.

Step 3. Once the patient's lower extremities have swung past the edge of the curb, she lowers her legs by eccentrically contracting the elbow and shoulder musculature.

Step 4. When the patient's feet come in contact with the ground, she needs to regain the balance point.

INTERVENTION 13.30 Getting Up From the Floor

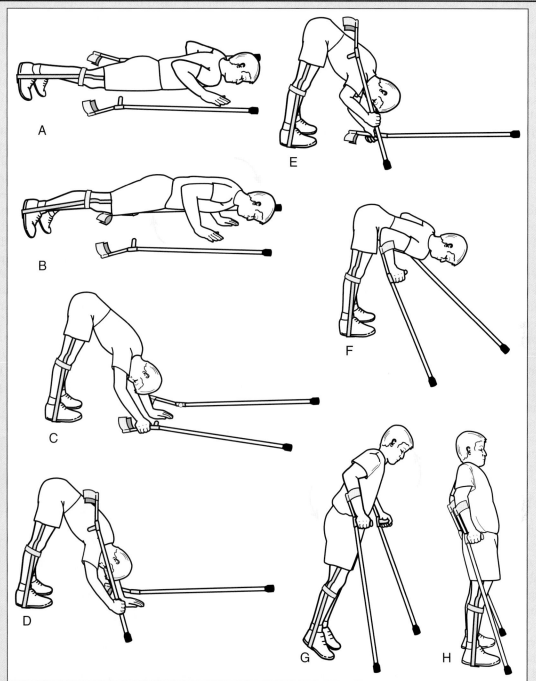

A. Instruct the patient to assume a prone position on the floor. Have the patient position the crutches with the tips pointing toward his head and the handgrips at the patient's hips.

B. The patient pushes up to a plantigrade position. (The patient will want to make sure that both orthoses are locked before attempting this.)

C. and D. The patient reaches for one of his crutches, using it for balance. The crutch rests against his shoulder.

E. and F. The patient uses the crutch on the floor as a point of stability as he reaches for the other crutch and positions it on his forearm.

G. and H. The patient regains his balance with the crutches.

Although the Americans with Disabilities Act increased the accessibility of many public and private buildings, many homes and community buildings are not accessible to certain individuals. For this reason, we review the techniques for instructing the patient in stair negotiation.

Ascending stairs. Patients can ascend stairs using the same techniques described to go up a single curb. In addition, patients can be instructed in an alternative approach to ascend the stairs backward.

Step 1. The patient stands with the back to the stairs and in a balanced position.

Step 2. With the crutches on the step above, the patient leans into the crutches, straightens the elbows, and depresses the scapulae. This maneuver causes the lower extremities to be lifted onto the step.

Step 3. Once the patient's feet have landed, she extends the neck and retracts the scapulae to regain a forward pelvis position.

The patient repeats these steps until she has successfully ascended all the required steps.

Descending stairs. The patient who must descend a series of steps can use the techniques described for going down a curb. However, the patient must be careful because the space in which she can land is limited. The patient must accurately gauge the length of her step so that she will not miss a step.

SPECIAL NOTE When teaching a patient any new skill (a transfer, wheelie, gait), it is important for the therapist to demonstrate the skill first and the steps necessary to achieve the outcome.

LOCOMOTOR TRAINING

Research in the basic sciences has been conducted in an effort to attenuate the deficits caused by SCI. Animal research suggests that cats with complete spinal cord transections can regain the ability to walk on a treadmill after training. This research "suggests that the spinal cord is able to integrate and adapt to sensory information during locomotion" (de Leon et al., 2001). Of particular interest to researchers and clinicians alike is the existence of central pattern generators (CPGs), a network of nerve cells in the spinal cord. CPGs produce locomotion and are facilitated by supraspinal input; however, CPGs can be activated by external stimuli in the absence of cortical influence (Hultborn and Nielsen, 2007; Basso, 2000). Key to our understanding of the recovery of locomotion abilities is the role that sensory feedback plays in stepping (Hultborn and Nielsen, 2007). Neuronal reorganization that occurs after locomotor training reinforces sensory feedback from plantar mechanoreceptors and proprioceptors in the hip and thus can modify the function of the CPG. This coincides with improvements in patient motor function and a decrease in spasticity (Smith and Knikou, 2016).

Recent research suggests that the central state of excitability of the spinal cord is a critical component in the recovery of locomotion and voluntary movement (Behrman et al., 2017).

Locomotor training for patients with incomplete spinal cord injury is based on the principles of activity-dependent plasticity, repetition, and automatic movement patterns. Activity-based, task-specific interventions focusing on limiting compensation while activating the nervous system below the injury level are important components of this training (Behrman et al., 2017: Basso, 2000). Locomotor training provides the nervous system with "appropriate sensory input to stimulate the remaining spinal cord injury networks to facilitate their continued involvement even when supraspinal input is compromised" (Harkema et al., 2012a).

The use of body-weight-supported treadmill training (BWSTT) with manual cues, electric stimulation, or robotic assistance has provided patients with improved outcomes relative to distance and walking speed (Behrman et al., 2017; Field-Fote and Roach, 2011; Harkema et al., 2012a, 2012b). Significant gains in muscle strength, walking distance, and speed have been reported in people with incomplete injuries (AIS C and D) (Basso and Lang, 2017; Harkema et al., 2012b). During BWSTT the patient is suspended by a harness, over a treadmill, which provides for upright posturing and decreased loading of the lower extremities. Approximately 35% to 40% of the patient's weight is supported. Trainers can assist with movement of the patient's lower extremities while the treadmill is moving. Intervention 13.31 illustrates this type of locomotor training. The movement of the treadmill pulls the hip

---

INTERVENTION 13.31 Locomotor Training

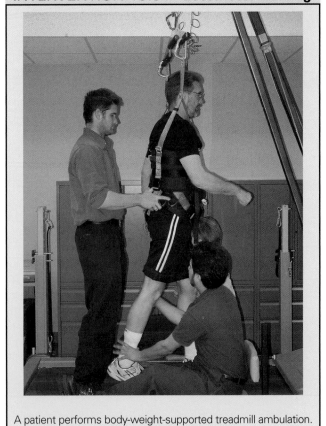

A patient performs body-weight-supported treadmill ambulation.

(From Sisto SA, Druin E, Sliwinski MM: *Spinal cord injury: management and rehabilitation,* St. Louis, 2009, Mosby.)

into extension and facilitates the swing phase of the gait cycle, thus providing patients with the sensory experience of walking. Treadmill speeds of 0.8 to 1.0 m/sec are recommended for training. As the patient progresses, treadmill speed, amount of body weight supported, and length of time the patient spends walking can be increased. In addition, the patient must participate in a significant number of sessions, greater than 60, and sessions must be at least 1.5 hours per day (Behrman et al., 2017). It is important to remember that overground ambulation and ambulation in the community are required in addition to the treadmill training in order to produce motor learning. (Refer to Chapter 11 for a review of BWSTT.)

Another important patient consideration is the loss of eccentric motor control, which is common in many neurologic conditions. "Eccentric control requires a precise gradation of descending drive from the brain to match peripheral muscle actions among a changing environment" (Basso and Lang, 2017). Owing to the patient impairments that develop with a loss of this control (maintenance of the lower extremity in extension or limb collapse), task-specific eccentric treadmill training should be considered and may provide improved outcomes (Basso and Lang, 2017).

In some research studies, BWSTT and overground ambulation is combined with electrical stimulation. The electrical stimulation elicits reflex-based movements (a flexor-withdrawal response) in the lower extremities to promote stepping and can be used as an orthosis. This approach is thought to facilitate the spinal circuitry underlying locomotion (Field-Fote and Roach, 2011; Field-Fote and Tepavac, 2002; Somers, 2010).

Robotic-assisted BWSTT is also available, providing the patient with kinematically appropriate lower extremity movements. Proprioceptive input is therefore precise and is thought to improve motor learning as it promotes development of an internal reference of correctness (Field-Fote and Roach, 2011). Although less physically demanding for the therapist, there are some concerns with robotic-assisted gait relative to the passive nature of the lower extremity movement and the fact that movement occurs only in the sagittal plane. Additionally, robotic-assisted locomotor training has not been found superior to other forms of gait training and it has been suggested that it should not replace overground walking training (Shumway-Cook and Woollacott, 2017). Intervention 13.32 illustrates robotic-assisted ambulation (Somers, 2010).

Robotic exoskeleton systems are also utilized for overground ambulation and are gaining popularity (Fig. 13.20). Exoskeletons provide intense stepping opportunities and allow patients to ambulate in hospital and community settings. Heinemann et al. (2018) found that robotic exoskeletons were often used in outpatient and wellness centers. Benefits of exoskeleton use include "improved posture and reduced spasticity and reduced complications affecting cardiovascular, gastrointestinal, and renal systems" (Heinemann, et al., 2018). Additional benefits can be derived from the patient's ability to increase levels of physical activity (Gorey et al., 2019). Patient reports of improved self-confidence and self-image have also been noted, although there are risks associated with use,

INTERVENTION 13.32 Robotic-Assisted Locomotor Training

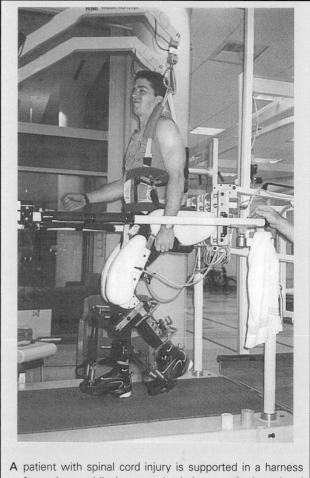

A patient with spinal cord injury is supported in a harness from above while he uses the Lokomat robotic-assisted gait training device.

(From Sisto SA, Druin E, Sliwinski MM: *Spinal cord injury: management and rehabilitation*, St. Louis, 2009, Mosby.)

including falls, skin irritation, and unrealistic patient expectations. As therapists and patients consider the use of robotic exoskeletons, it is important to remember that this technology is still in the early days of its development and that additional research is needed to guide practice and to assist patients in the development of realistic goals and expectations of device usage (Heinemann et al., 2018). Cost and accessibility are other concerns with exoskeleton usage and must be considered when discussing ambulation goals with our patients (Gorey et al., 2019).

An important issue for patients with SCIs and for PTs is the timing of the intervention, the specificity of the task, and the inflammatory process within the cellular environment. Animal studies have shown that treadmill-based rehabilitation delivered during the inflammatory process produced lasting locomotor deficits. Additionally, in rats it has been found that "high inflammation early after moderate or complete SCI contributes to maladaptive changes in neuroplasticity, hyperreflexia, and loss of segmental learning in the

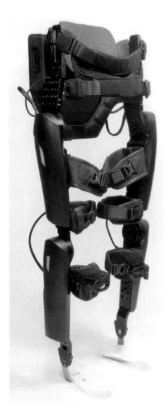

Fig. 13.20 ReWalk Exoskeleton (Robotic/Powered Exoskeleton). (From Webster JB, Murphy DP, editors: *Atlas of orthoses and assistive devices*, ed 5, Philadelphia, 2019, Elsevier, p 442.)

lumbar cord" (Basso and Lang, 2017). Thus, timing when task-specific interventions are administered to correspond with a conducive cellular environment may provide patients with SCI and other neurologic conditions greater opportunities for functional recovery (Basso and Lang, 2017).

High-intensity locomotor training

As discussed in Chapter 12, data from patients with stroke indicate that gait training programs delivered at high aerobic intensities and in variable environments can improve walking to a greater degree than gains made with conventional therapy (Holleran et al., 2018). Few studies have evaluated the feasibility and efficacy of this intervention in patients with motor incomplete injuries. The challenges for initiating a high-intensity stepping program for patients with SCIs present a unique set of challenges including bilateral impairments, more limited access to residual neural pathways, and the risk of adverse events, such as autonomic dysreflexia, may be greater at higher exercise intensities (Holleran et al., 2018). In a case series conducted by Holleran et al., (2018), high-intensity step training in individuals with chronic incomplete SCI was evaluated. Modest improvements in walking function, balance, and metabolic function were recorded in the four participants. Participants averaged 2200 steps during the one-hour session, although this number is lower than average stepping amounts recorded in individuals with chronic stroke who participated in a similar protocol (2500 to 3000 steps). Additionally, participants were not able consistently to achieve a heart rate range of 70% of predicted heart rate maximum, despite the therapist's efforts to reach 85%. Decreased heart rate responses may be owing to reduced afferent feedback or "decreased central drive to thoracic level sympathetic neural circuits that innervate the heart" (Holleran et al., 2018). With consideration of these challenges, the effectiveness of this intervention for patients may be limited (Holleran et al., 2018). However, in a study conducted by Leech et al. (2016), subjects who participated in a graded intensity locomotor training program (45 minutes of high-intensity gait training, with assistance, at RPE intensities of 14 or greater) demonstrated significant increases in gait speed and increased muscle activity and gait kinematics. Reinforcement of abnormal movement patterns was not evident after training. The ability to generalize these results to overground ambulation or to assess the efficacy of this intervention as compared with others was not possible as a control group was not a part of the research design (Leech et al., 2016).

Locomotor training principles

Harkema et al. (2012b) described four guiding principles for locomotor training: (1) maximize weight bearing on the lower extremities while limiting upper extremity weight bearing; (2) optimize the sensory experience associated with the activity; (3) promote proper limb kinematics; and (4) maximize independence and limit compensations. To improve the patient's functional abilities, locomotor training must also be performed overground and in the community. For motor learning to occur, the patient must be able to translate skills from one environment to the next. Patients must be able to adapt their gait to changing task and environmental conditions to allow for participation in the community (Shumway-Cook and Woollacott, 2017). In studies conducted by Field-Fote and Roach (2011) and Harkema et al. (2012b), outcome measures, including the 10-meter walk, Berg Balance Scores, and walking speed, were improved in patients with incomplete injuries who participated in intensive activity-based locomotor programs.

Discharge planning

As stated previously, lengths of stay for inpatient rehabilitation continue to decrease. As a consequence, one must begin discharge planning during the patient's first visit to physical therapy. All members of the patient's rehabilitation team, including the patient, family members, significant others, and caregivers, must be included in the process. The combined efforts of all involved parties help the patient make a successful transition from the hospital to her previous home and work environments.

The discharge planning process ideally includes a number of different activities aimed at improving the patient's functional outcome and providing an easy transition from health care facility to home. Activities that should be a part of the discharge planning process include (1) a discharge planning conference; (2) a trial home pass; (3) an assessment of the home environment to ensure accessibility; (4) development of a vocational plan; (5) procurement of all necessary adaptive equipment and supplies; (6) driver's training (if appropriate) or transportation; (7) education regarding community resource availability; and (8) recommendations regarding additional rehabilitation services and the need for long-term health and wellness services.

Discharge Planning Conference

The discharge planning conference should be held approximately 1 to 2 weeks before the patient's anticipated discharge date. At this time, continued medical and rehabilitation follow-up should be addressed, and a review of resources available to both patient and family should be provided. Ideally, patients will have access to comprehensive follow-up services. Spinal cord clinics that offer routine reassessments at predetermined times are beneficial. At these follow-up appointments, many potential long-term complications are discovered and are successfully managed. Unfortunately, many patients are discharged to areas where medical specialists trained in providing long-term care to this patient population are not available. For this reason, patients must be educated regarding their injuries, possible secondary complications, and potential outcomes for their recovery.

During the discharge planning conference, certain issues must be addressed. Areas of concern include the following:

1. The patient's attitude and discharge plans must be discussed. Is the patient realistic regarding what it will be like at home? Is discharge to home possible?
2. The knowledge base and understanding exhibited by the patient's primary caregivers regarding SCIs and their management should be assessed. Do caregivers understand the patient's condition and the level of care required?
3. The availability of a physician who can deal with the medical problems and secondary complications encountered by patients with SCIs should be discussed.
4. The amount and degree of professional and attendant care required by the patient must be determined. Does the patient possess the financial means (insurance or income) to pay for personal care? Has the patient received all of the adaptive and ADL equipment necessary to function at home? Equipment, including wheelchairs and seat cushions, should be received before the patient's discharge, so any necessary training or modifications can be performed in the facility. In addition, a relationship with a durable medical provider is suggested.
5. Transportation issues associated with school, work, leisure activities, and doctors' appointments must be confirmed. Patients with power wheelchairs need access to vans with hydraulic chair lift capabilities. Patients who want to resume driving need to have adaptive hand controls installed in their automobiles. The timetable to receive these items can be long. Therefore, one is advised to begin this planning process early.
6. The accessibility of the patient's home, school, or workplace must be addressed. Architectural modifications should be completed in advance of the patient's discharge.
7. Other issues related to accessibility of community resources and support for the patient and her family members must be discussed. Support groups for patients and their family members are available in many communities. These groups can often provide the patient with both emotional support and a social outlet.

Therapeutic passes are often given to patients prior to an impending discharge and are extremely beneficial to the discharge planning process. When a patient is given a pass, the patient is released from the health care facility for several hours or, in some cases, overnight in the care of a family member. The pass is used to determine how the patient will function once she is discharged from the rehabilitation unit. During the pass, the patient and the family can practice essential skills that will be needed once the patient is at home full time. These passes also offer opportunities for the patient to solve problems that may be encountered at home, such as inaccessibility of various rooms. The pass assists the patient in regaining the confidence needed to function outside the safe confines of the rehabilitation setting. Many patients are often anxious about their discharge from rehabilitation. The rehabilitation hospital or unit is considered a safe environment with 24-hour daily care and the comfort of individuals with similar problems and physical deficits.

After the pass, the patient returns to the rehabilitation unit for continued intervention and planning for discharge. The patient and family are expected to share their experiences regarding the pass so that additional training and problem solving can occur. Concomitantly, if additional environmental modifications to the dwelling must be made, the pass provides the information necessary to complete those changes.

As a component of discharge planning, the patient and the rehabilitation team need to discuss vocational planning. A referral to a vocational rehabilitation specialist or, in some instances, a psychologist can foster adjustment toward the patient's disability and can assist the patient in having an optimistic attitude toward the future. Many times, the patient is not ready at this particular point to think about the future, especially her place in the work world. However, beginning a vocational evaluation and discussing the patient's return to school or work is extremely positive and helps to foster the expectation that participation in these activities can be resumed. However, data show that only 32% of individuals with SCIs are employed 30 years after initial injury (The National Spinal Cord Injury Statistical Center, 2019).

Procurement of Equipment

A detailed discussion about securing equipment that the patient will need before discharge from the facility is beyond the scope of this text. Some of the common items that must be considered are presented here. The occupational therapist and the rehabilitation team should be consulted for more specific information.

Items frequently needed by the patient at discharge include the following:

1. *Wheelchair:* The type and specific requirements are determined by the rehabilitation team. The benefits of power versus manual wheelchairs must be considered. Cost and reimbursement issues may be concerns for some patients.
2. *Wheelchair cushion to assist with pressure relief:* Although pressure-relieving devices are beneficial, they do not take the place of regularly performed pressure-relief or weight-shifting activities. Selecting the proper wheelchair cushion depends on the patient's ability to transfer on and off the cushion and the degree of support needed.

3. *Hospital or pressure-relieving bed:* Patients with high tetraplegia who are to be discharged to home may require hospital beds, other specialized beds, or air mattresses.

4. *ADL adaptive equipment:* Examples of items that may be needed include dressing sticks to assist with donning clothing, loops attached to pants to assist with putting them on, button and zipper hooks to assist with securing these items, Velcro straps and elastic shoelaces to increase the ease of donning shoes, bath brushes, handheld shower attachments, and tub benches. Built-up utensils, toothbrushes, and handles may be needed for patients with tetraplegia. Dorsal wrist supports or universal cuffs may be necessary to assist the patient with feeding activities.

5. *Assistive technology/environmental control units:* Environmental control units interfaced with personal computers, a cell phone, and appliances within the home may be recommended. These electronic systems allow the patient with tetraplegia some control over the environment. By activating the environmental control unit, the patient can turn on the lights, television, or other appliances within the home. Referral to a rehabilitation engineer or other provider with expertise in this area is advisable.

Home Exercise Program

For some patients, discharge from your facility is the end of their rehabilitation. Not all patients receive follow-up services once they are discharged. Therefore, the supervising PT and PTA must design a home exercise program for the patient that will meet the patient's immediate and long-term needs. It is not reasonable to expect that once a patient is discharged, she will spend hours each day performing a home exercise program. The individual will spend a considerable amount of time each day completing ADLs. Thus, the physical therapy team should select only a few activities that will provide the patient with the greatest functional benefits.

Things to Consider When Developing a Home Exercise Program

Several factors must be considered when developing a home exercise program for your patient. Following is a list of questions you should ask yourself before you finalize the patient's home program:

1. What activities will the patient be able to perform when she is discharged? Will the patient be able to transfer independently? Is progress likely in other functional skills?

2. What motor and cardiopulmonary capacities will the patient need to possess to complete ADLs? Areas to consider include range of motion, strength, flexibility, balance, and vital capacity.

3. How will the patient maintain skin integrity and respiratory status and prevent possible secondary complications?

4. What skills and capacities can the patient maintain by completing her daily routine? For example, getting dressed and bathing assist in maintaining upper and lower extremity range of motion.

5. What areas will require extra attention because they are not addressed during routine performance of ADLs? Areas to consider include the maintenance of hip extension and ankle dorsiflexion and cardiopulmonary endurance.

In addition to asking these questions about the patient's motor and cardiopulmonary function, one should also consider the patient and the role of the family or caregivers in designing the home exercise program. As stated earlier, patients who have SCIs must become active problem solvers and must be able to direct and initiate their care. Patients who become reliant on others for making decisions relative to their care may have difficulty in directing a home exercise program. Failure to understand the possible complications of immobility and contractures may lead to lack of interest in a home exercise program. Stretching activities and active wheelchair propulsion each day will do a great deal to assist the patient in maintaining an optimal level of functional independence.

Family Teaching

As discussed throughout this chapter, family involvement and training are of the utmost importance. Family teaching should be initiated early during the patient's rehabilitation stay and should not be deferred until a few days before discharge. Family members or caregivers should assist PTs and PTAs with patient transfers, ADL tasks, skin inspection, wheelchair mobility, equipment usage and maintenance, and range-of-motion exercises. We should be patient with family members as they begin to learn these activities because they are often anxious and afraid of causing the patient pain or additional injury. Not only is it important to teach families how to assist patients physically, but families must also be educated about the injury, potential complications, precautions, safety factors, and probable functional outcome. This instruction is best if given over a period of time to give the family member or caregiver adequate time to digest and assimilate information. If the patient is to be discharged home, all individuals responsible for assisting with the care of the patient should demonstrate a level of competence with techniques before the patient is released from the facility.

Community Reentry

As the patient prepares for discharge, a final area that must be considered is the individual's reentry into the community. The patient should be encouraged to resume previously performed activities as her level of functional independence and interests warrant. Significant advances have been made in the areas of employment, recreational activities, sports, and hobbies for patients with disabilities. Approximately 32% of individuals with an SCI are employed 30 years after their injury (National Spinal Cord Injury Statistical Center, 2019). Factors that positively affect employment following injury include younger age and those with a college degree. Barriers to employment include transportation, a loss of health benefits, discrimination, and an individual's physical and overall health status (Fulk et al., 2019).

Quality of Life

Patients who have sustained a spinal cord injury often experience depression immediately after their injury. Estimated rates of depression in the population range from 11% to 37% (Model Systems Knowledge Translation Center, 2019). In general, patients do experience a decreased quality of life as compared with their healthy counterparts. Quality of life is not, however, related to the severity of the injury or to the patient's functional potential (Fulk et al., 2019).

Long-Term Health Care Needs

As the population in the United States ages, so do the survivors with SCIs. Investigators have estimated that 40% of individuals with SCIs are more than 45 years of age. Individuals with SCIs experience many of the same age-related changes that occur in the general population. Research studies are investigating how the normal aging process affects the preexisting musculoskeletal and cardiopulmonary deficits experienced by individuals who have had an SCI and how cumulative stresses sustained from years of wheelchair propulsion, repetitive upper extremity activities, and assisted ambulation may accelerate problems encountered with aging. Additionally, with advancing age, individuals with SCIs may present with contractures, decreased bone density, cardiovascular disease, diabetes, fecal incontinence, an increased prevalence of cardiovascular disease, sleep apnea, and other respiratory complications (Tappan and Tessiatore, 2019). As patients age, they can also experience declines in function and the need to use greater assistance. Fatigue, weakness, medical complications, shoulder pain, weight gain, and postural changes have been attributed to declines in function. Fortunately, many of these functional limitations are amenable to physical therapy intervention, including the procurement of adaptive equipment, seating systems, and power wheelchairs. An important point for health care providers working with individuals with SCIs is that many of the problems associated with aging and overuse may be preventable through education, training, health promotion, and wellness activities. Comprehensive follow-up services are extremely important to these individuals and may enhance fitness and decrease the incidence of secondary complications (Tappan and Tessiatore, 2019; Gerhart et al., 1993; Somers and Bruce, 2014).

CHAPTER SUMMARY

Patients with SCIs benefit from comprehensive rehabilitation services to optimize their functional independence. Physical therapy treatment sessions started shortly after the patient's injury can help improve the patient's strength, mobility, and cardiopulmonary function. Treatment should continue with admission to a comprehensive rehabilitation center where additional resources can be devoted to the patient's optimal recovery. Multiple therapeutic interventions and modalities are available to assist the patient in achieving the highest level of functional independence. Emphasizing the patient's active participation in the rehabilitation process and development of meaningful goals is essential. In addition, patient and family education must be included from the very start of rehabilitation to ensure a successful transition from the health care facility to home. Early discussions with the patient regarding returning to home and work or school assist the patient with reintegration into the community. Adequate long-term follow-up care remains absolutely essential in order to eliminate or minimize the potential secondary complications that often develop in this patient population. Changes in our approach to various physical therapy interventions have developed as our understanding of nervous system plasticity continues to evolve.

REVIEW QUESTIONS

1. List the four most common causes of SCIs.
2. Differentiate between a complete SCI and an incomplete SCI.
3. What are the characteristics of spinal shock?
4. What is autonomic dysreflexia? Describe the clinical manifestations of a patient experiencing this condition.
5. What is the functional potential of a patient with C7 tetraplegia?
6. List three physical therapy interventions that will improve pulmonary function.
7. List the three primary goals of physical therapy intervention during the acute care phase of rehabilitation.
8. Discuss a typical mat exercise program for a patient with C6 tetraplegia.
9. What is the most functional type of wheelchair-to-mat transfer for a patient with C7 tetraplegia?
10. List the benefits of a therapeutic pool program.
11. Discuss the gait training sequence for a patient with paraplegia who will be using orthoses.
12. Describe important areas for patient and family teaching for a patient with SCI.

CASE STUDIES INITIAL EXAMINATION AND EVALUATION

History

Chart Review

The patient is a 20-year-old man who was transferred to the University of Evansville Medical Center 1 week after diving into a shallow wave and hitting a sandbar while surfing. He sustained a teardrop fracture of C5 resulting in a medical diagnosis of C6 incomplete tetraplegia. He aspirated water and lost consciousness. He was initially taken to a local hospital for immobilization and treatment of aspiration pneumonia. On admission to the Medical Center the patient was conscious and alert. He had decreased breath sounds with crackles over the lateral bases. Light touch and pinprick were intact to T1 with intact perianal sensation. Proprioception was intact in all extremity joints. Computed tomography showed no blockage and surgery was not indicated. X-ray showed diaphragm movement of two intercostal spaces. Past medical history includes childhood asthma and is otherwise unremarkable. Medications: Tylenol for pain, as needed. A halo and vest are to be applied tomorrow to provide immobilization of the fracture and to allow for participation in the rehabilitation process.

Physical therapy has been ordered for examination and treatment with transfer to rehabilitation unit.

Subjective

The patient states that he is not in pain. He is a part-time college student and lives at home with his parents. The home is a one-story house with a one-step entry with a railing. At school, all of the buildings have elevators. The patient's goals are to return home to live with his parents and to learn to get around by himself. He gives consent to participate in examination.

Objective

Appearance, Rest Posture, Equipment: The patient is lying supine in bed in a rigid cervical collar. His arms are in extension at his sides, and his legs are also in extension. He has a Foley catheter in place. IV present in left forearm. He is resting on a pressure reducing mattress.

Systems Review

Communication/Cognition: The patient is alert and oriented × 3. Communication is intact. Yes-no responses are reliable. He is able to follow complex verbal commands with 100% accuracy.

Cardiovascular/Pulmonary: BP = 120/75 mm Hg, HR = 70 bpm, RR = 16 breaths/min.

Integumentary: Skin is intact. No redness is noted. He is dependent in pressure relief.

Musculoskeletal: Gross strength and range of motion (ROM) are impaired bilaterally. No postural asymmetries are noted.

Neuromuscular: Movement is impaired bilaterally.

Tests and Measures

Anthropometrics: Height 5'9", weight 160 lbs, Body Mass Index 24 (20–24 is normal).

Ventilation/Respiration: Vital capacity is 1000 mL taken with spirometer in supine. Breathing pattern is 4-diaphragm. Epigastric rise is 1". Cough is nonfunctional. Oxygen saturation is 96%.

Range of Motion: Passive ROM: Upper extremity (UE) passive ROM limited bilaterally at shoulders to 90 degrees flexion and abduction owing to cervical instability. Shoulder internal and external passive ROM within functional limits (WFL).

Elbow, wrist, and hand passive ROM WFL. Lower extremity (LE) passive ROM WFL except passive straight leg raise limited to 60 degrees bilaterally.

Active ROM: UE active ROM limited bilaterally at shoulders to 90 degrees flexion and abduction owing to cervical instability. No active ROM of neck, trunk, and shoulders past 90 degrees owing to cervical instability. Bilateral elbow flexion WFL. Bilateral wrist extension WFL. All other joints: no active ROM noted.

Reflex Integrity: Deep tendon reflexes: biceps: 2 + bilaterally. Triceps, patellar, and Achilles: 0 bilaterally. Babinski present bilaterally. There is a mild increase in tone bilaterally in ankle plantar flexors and hamstrings.

Motor Function: The patient is dependent in log rolling and all other motor functions.

Neuromotor Development: Unable to assess postural reactions secondary to spinal instability.

Muscle Performance: All testing was done in the recumbent position. Neck, trunk, and shoulder girdle muscles limited to trace and humeral active motion only without resistance because of cervical instability.

Muscle Strength:

	Right	Left
Sternocleidomastoid	1/5	1/5
Upper trapezius	1/5	1/5
Deltoid	1/5	1/5
Pectoralis major	3/5	3/5
Teres major	3/5	3/5
Biceps	3/5	3/5
Wrist extensors	3/5	3/5
Triceps	0/5	0/5
Finger flexors	0/5	0/5
Finger abductors	0/5	0/5
Hip flexors	0/5	0/5
Knee extensors	0/5	0/5
Ankle dorsiflexors	0/5	0/5
Long toe extensors	0/5	0/5
Ankle plantar flexors	0/5	0/5

Mobility: The patient is dependent in gait and locomotion. He is limited to recumbent position because of cervical instability.

Sensory Integrity: Light touch and pinprick intact through T1, absent below; perianal sensation intact. Proprioception: intact in all UE and LE joints.

Self-Care: Patient is dependent in all self-care activities.

Assessment/Evaluation

The patient is a 20-year-old man. His status 1 week after C5 teardrop fracture shows a neurologic level at C5 with an incomplete lesion and anterior cord syndrome.

ASIA Impairment Scale: C Motor Incomplete

Functional Independence Measure: transfer—1, walk/wheelchair—1 (wheelchair), stairs—1

Problem List

1. Decreased respiratory function
2. Decreased tolerance to upright
3. Decreased strength all intact muscle groups
4. Decreased passive ROM of hamstrings
5. Dependent in pressure relief and skin inspection

CASE STUDIES INITIAL EXAMINATION AND EVALUATION—cont'd

6. Dependent in mobility and ADLs
7. Lack of patient and family education

Diagnosis

Incomplete neurologic injury AIS C

Prognosis

Patient will improve his level of functional independence and functional skills as muscle strength and stability of the cervical spine improve. Rehabilitation potential for stated goals is good. The patient is motivated and has good family support and financial resources. Physical therapy visits in acute care: up to 10 visits with continuation to rehabilitation up to 150 additional visits.

Short-Term Goals (to be Achieved by 2 Weeks)

1. Patient will tolerate being upright in wheelchair for 2 consecutive hours.
2. Patient will increase strength of innervated UE muscles by one muscle grade.
3. Patient will perform pressure relief and skin inspection with minimal assist of 1.
4. Patient will perform bed/mat mobility with moderate assist of 1.
5. Patient will perform a lateral transfer with a sliding board with maximal assist of 1.
6. Patient will propel wheelchair with rim projections 25 feet with minimal assist of 1.
7. Patient will maintain balance in short sitting with elbows biomechanically locked for 5 minutes independently.
8. Patient will require moderate assist of 1 to perform assisted cough.

Long-Term Goals (to be Achieved by 6 Weeks, the Anticipated Discharge to Home With Family)

1. Patient will be independent in diaphragm-strengthening exercises and assisted cough techniques.
2. Patient will tolerate being upright in his wheelchair for 8 consecutive hours.
3. Patient will increase strength of innervated UE muscles to 5/5.
4. Patient will increase passive ROM of hamstrings to at least 90 degrees to allow for long sitting.
5. Patient will be independent in pressure relief and skin inspection.
6. Patient will be independent in bed/mat mobility.
7. Patient will perform a modified prone-on-elbows transfer independently.
8. Patient will independently propel wheelchair with rim projections over level surfaces and ramps.
9. Patient will perform ADLs with minimal assist of 1.
10. Patient will be able to direct someone how to help him get back into the wheelchair in case of a fall.
11. Family will demonstrate how to assist patient with ADLs, transfers, home exercise program, and stretching.
12. Patient will participate in an aerobic training program for 30 minutes each day.

Plan of Care

Treatment Schedule: The PT and PTA will see the patient for 45-minute treatment sessions twice a day 5 days a week, and once on Saturday for the next 6 weeks. Treatment sessions will include improving tolerance to upright, respiratory training, strength training, stretching, pressure relief and skin inspection, functional mobility training, family education, and discharge planning. A home assessment will be recommended. The physical therapy team will reassess the patient weekly.

Coordination, Communication and Documentation: The PT and PTA will communicate with the patient and his family on a regular basis. The acute-care PT will communicate with the rehabilitation team on his discharge from this facility. Outcomes of physical therapy interventions will be documented on a daily basis.

Patient/Client Instruction: The patient and his family will be instructed in stretching exercises and pressure-relief techniques as his condition stabilizes. In rehabilitation, the patient's family will participate in family training to learn to assist him with ADLs, transfers, and functional mobility activities.

Interventions

1. *Motor Function Training:* Improve tolerance to upright:
   a. Elevate head of bed, monitoring vitals, and gradually increasing length of time in this position
   b. Sitting in a reclining wheelchair with footrests elevated, monitoring vitals, and gradually increasing length of time and decreasing amount of recline
   c. Standing on a tilt table, monitoring vitals, and gradually increasing incline and length of time
2. *Airway Clearance:*
   a. Manual chest wall stretching
   b. Teach huffing
   c. Assisted cough techniques in supine progressing to prone, short sitting, and then long sitting
   d. Inspiratory strengthening with manual resistance progressing to weights
3. *Therapeutic Exercise: Strengthening*
   a. Isometric strengthening of neck, trunk, and shoulder girdle muscles with halo in place after receiving approval from physician
   b. Active movements of humerus without resistance (limited to 90 degrees of flexion and abduction)
   c. Biceps strengthening against gravity progressing to using TheraBand or cuff weights
4. *Therapeutic Exercises: Stretching:*
   a. Passive stretching of hamstrings and other lower extremity muscles by therapist
   b. Prolonged stretching of hamstrings using overhead sling in bed
5. *Integumentary Repair and Protection Techniques:*
   a. Instruct on the importance of pressure relief and skin inspection
   b. Implement a turning schedule for when patient is in bed
   c. Implement prone-positioning program—at least 20 minutes in prone 3 times a day
   d. Teach weight-shifting techniques while in wheelchair—1 minute of pressure relief for every 15 to 20 minutes of sitting
   e. Teach skin inspection techniques using mirror
6. *Motor Function Training: Mat Mobility*
   a. Mat activities—gradually decreasing amount of assistance while rolling prone over a wedge
   b. Transition to prone on elbows

Continued

CASE STUDIES INITIAL EXAMINATION AND EVALUATION—cont'd

c. Rhythmic stabilization, alternating isometrics in developmental positions

d. Weight shifting in prone-on-elbows transition to supine

e. Pull-ups using therapist's hands

f. Transition to supine on elbows

g. Rhythmic stabilization, alternating isometrics, and weight shifting in supine on elbows

h. Transition to long sitting once hamstring range is sufficient

i. Teach elbow locking and rhythmic stabilization, alternating isometrics in long sitting

7. **Motor Function Training:** Transfers—gradually decreasing amount of assist:

a. Assisted sliding board transfer with elbow locking initially progressing to prone on elbows independently

b. Bed to wheelchair

c. Wheelchair to car

d. Toilet transfers

8. **Motor Function Training:** Wheelchair mobility—gradually decreasing amount of assistance:

a. Education about wheelchair parts (armrests, footrests, and so forth) and how to use them to propel wheelchair over level surfaces, gradually increasing distance

b. Consider use of a power wheelchair

c. Propel wheelchair up and down ramps

d. Educate on how to fall/tip over safely in wheelchair

e. Educate caregiver in how to assist the patient in getting back into wheelchair after a fall

9. **Patient and Family Instruction:**

a. Educate family members on appropriate ways to assist with transfers

b. Have family members assist with transfers

c. Educate family on how to assist with ADLs

d. Have family demonstrate assistance with ADLs

10. **Discharge Planning:**

a. Consult with other members of rehabilitation team, patient, and family regarding discharge to home with assistance of family

b. Perform home and school assessment

c. Secure equipment, such as universal cuff, sliding board, pressure-reducing bed

d. Obtain lightweight wheelchair with ROHO cushion, projection rims, push handles for pressure relief, swing-away desk arms, and swing-away leg rests with heel loops

e. Instruct patient in home exercise program and long-term fitness program to address cardiopulmonary fitness, flexibility, and strengthening

f. Refer patient to driver's training and vocational rehabilitation

Questions to Think About

- What type of specific upper extremity strengthening exercises should be included in the patient's plan of care?
- How can aerobic conditioning be included in the patient's treatment program?
- What types of activities or exercises would be included as part of the patient's home exercise program?
- What types of activities and patient/family instruction should be included to prevent the development of secondary complications?

REFERENCES

Alvarez SE: Functional assessment and training. In Adkins HV, editor: *Spinal cord injury*, New York, 1985, Churchill Livingstone, pp 131–154.

American Spinal Injury Association: *International standards for neurological classification of spinal cord injury*, Richmond, VA, 2019. Available at: www.asia-spinalinjury.org. Accessed June 23, 2019.

Atrice MB, Morrison SA, McDowell SL, et al.: Traumatic spinal cord injury. In Umphred DA, editor: *Umphred's neurological rehabilitation*, ed 6, St. Louis, 2013, Elsevier, pp 459–520.

Basso DM: Neuroanatomical substrates of functional recovery after experimental spinal cord injury: implications of basic science research for human spinal cord injury, *Phys Ther* 80:808–817, 2000.

Basso DM, Behrman AL, Harkema SJ: Recovery of walking after central nervous system insult: basic research in the control of locomotion as a foundation for developing rehabilitation strategies, *Neurol Rep* 24:47–54, 2000.

Basso DM, Lang CE: Consideration of dose and timing when applying interventions after stroke and spinal cord injury, *J Neurol Phys Ther* 41:S24–S31, 2017.

Behrman AL, Ardolino EM, Harkema SJ: Activity-based therapy: from basic science to clinical application for recovery after spinal cord injury, *J Neurol Phys Ther* 41:S39–S45, 2017.

Borello-France D, Rosen S, Young AB, et al.: The relationship between perceived exertion and heart rate during arm crank exercise in individuals with paraplegia, *Neurol Rep* 24(3):94–100, 2000.

Burns S, Biering-Sorensen F, Donovan W, et al.: International standards for neurological classification of spinal cord injury, revised 2011, *Top Spinal Cord Inj Rehabil* 18(1):85–99, 2012.

Burr JF, Shephard RJ, Zehr EP: Physical activity after stroke and spinal cord injury: evidence-based recommendations on clearance for physical activity and exercise, *Can Fam Physician* 58(11):1236–1239, 2012.

Cerny D, Waters R, Hislop H, et al.: Walking and wheelchair energetics in persons with paraplegia, *Phys Ther* 60:1133–1139, 1980.

Chang E, Ghosh N, Yanni D, et al.: A review of spasticity treatments: pharmacological and interventional approaches, *Crit Rev Phys Rehabil Med* 25(1-2):11–22, 2013.

Consortium for Spinal Cord Medicine: Prevention of venous thromboembolism in individuals with spinal cord injury: clinical practice guidelines for health care providers, ed 3, *Top Spinal Cord Inj Rehabil* 22(3):209–240, 2016.

Craik RL: Abnormalities of motor behavior. In *Contemporary management of motor control problems: proceedings of the II STEP Conference*, Alexandria, VA, 1991, Foundation for Physical Therapy, pp 155–164.

Cromwell SJ, Paquette VL: The effect of botulinum toxin A on the function if a person with poststroke quadriplegia, *Phys Ther* 76:395–402, 1996.

de Leon RD, Roy RR, Edgerton VR: Is the recovery of stepping following spinal cord injury mediated by modifying existing neural pathways or by generating new pathways? A perspective, *Phys Ther* 81:1904–1911, 2001.

Decker M, Hall A: Physical therapy in spinal cord injury. In Bloch RF, Basbaum M, editors: *Management of spinal cord injuries*, Baltimore, 1986, Williams & Wilkins, pp 320–334.

Eng JJ, Levins SM, Townson AF, et al.: Use of prolonged standing for individuals with spinal cord injuries, *Phys Ther* 81:1392–1399, 2001.

Ferrara J, Tappan R: *Academy of Neurologic Physical Therapy: physical activity interventions for cardiovascular health after SCI*, Minneapolis, MN, 2019. Available at: www.neuropt.org/docs/default-source/sci-sig/fact-sheets/scisig_factsheet_physicalactivityinterventionsforcardiovascularhealthaftersci.pdf?sfvrsn=7cc15343_2. Accessed June 9, 2019.

Field-Fote EC, Roach KE: Influence of a locomotor training approach on walking speed and distance in people with chronic spinal cord injury: a randomized clinical trial, *Phys Ther* 91(1):48–60, 2011.

Field-Fote EC, Tepavac D: Improved intralimb coordination in people with incomplete spinal cord injury following training with body weight support and electrical stimulation, *Phys Ther* 82:707–715, 2002.

Finkbeiner K, Russo SG, editors: *Physical therapy management of spinal cord injury: accent on independence*, Fishersville, VA, 1990, Woodrow Wilson Rehabilitation Center, through Project Scientia, a grant from the Paralyzed Veterans of America, pp 51–58.

Fulk GT, Bowden M, Behrman AL: Traumatic spinal cord injury. In O'Sullivan SB, Schmitz TJ, Fulk GD, editors: *Physical rehabilitation*, ed 7, Philadelphia, 2019, FA Davis, pp 855–917.

Gerhart KA, Bergstrom E, Charlifue SW, et al.: Long-term spinal cord injury: functional changes over time, *Arch Phys Med Rehabil* 74:1030–1034, 1993.

Giesecke C: Aquatic rehabilitation of clients with spinal cord injury. In Ruoti RG, Morris DM, Cole AJ, editors: *Aquatic rehabilitation*, Philadelphia, 1997, JB Lippincott, pp 134–150.

Gordon, BT, Durstine GL, Painter PL, Moore GE: Basic physical activity and exercise recommendations for persons with chronic conditions. In Moore GE, Durstine JL, Painter PL, editors: *ACSM's exercise management for persons with chronic diseases and disabilities*, ed 4, Champaign, IL, 2016, Human Kinetics, pp 15–32.

Gorey AS, Sumrell R, Goetz LL: Exoskeleton assisted rehabilitation after spinal cord injury. In Webster JB, Murphy DP, editors: *Atlas of orthoses and assistive devices*, ed 5, Philadelphia, 2019, Elsevier, pp 440–447.

Harkema SJ, Hillyer J, Schmidt-Read M, et al.: Locomotor training: as a treatment of spinal cord injury and in the progression of neurologic rehabilitation, *Arch Phys Med Rehabil* 93(9):1588–1597, 2012a.

Harkema SJ, Schmidt-Read M, Lorenz DJ, et al.: Balance and ambulation improvements in individuals with chronic incomplete spinal cord injury using locomotor training-based rehabilitation, *Arch Phys Med Rehabil* 93(9):1508–1517, 2012b.

Heinemann AW, Jayaraman A, Mummidisetty CK, et al.: Experience of robotic exoskeleton use at four spinal cord injury model systems centers, *J Neurol Phys Ther* 42:256–267, 2018.

Ho CH, Triolo RJ, Elias AL, et al.: Functional electrical stimulation and spinal cord injury, *Phys Med Rehabil Clin N Am* 25(3):631–654, 2014.

Hoffman LR, Field-Fote EC: Functional and corticomotor changes in individuals with tetraplegia following unimanual or bimanual massed practice training with somatosensory stimulation: a pilot study, *J Neurol Phys Ther* 34(4):193–201, 2010.

Holleran CL, Hennessey PW, Leddy AL, et al.: High-intensity variable stepping training in patients with motor incomplete spinal cord injury: a case series, *J Neurol Phys Ther* 42:94–101, 2018.

Hultborn H, Nielsen JB: Spinal control of locomotion: from cat to man, *Acta Physiol (Oxf)* 189:111–121, 2007.

Jacobs PL, Nash MS: Exercise recommendations for individuals with spinal cord injury, *Sports Med* 34(11):727–751, 2004.

Jacobs PL, Nash MS, Rusinowski JW: Circuit training provides cardiorespiratory and strength benefits in persons with paraplegia, *Med Sci Sports Exerc* 33(5):711–717, 2001.

Jayaraman A, Thompson CK, Rymer WZ, Hornby GT: Short-term maximal intensity resistance training increases volitional function and strength in chronic incomplete spinal cord injury: a pilot study, *J Neurol Phys Ther* 37(3):112–117, 2013.

Katz RT: Management of spasticity, *Am J Phys Med Rehabil* 67:108–115, 1988.

Katz RT: Management of spastic hypertonia after spinal cord injury. In Yarkony GM, editor: *Spinal cord injury medical management and rehabilitation*, Gaithersburg, MD, 1994, Aspen Publishers, pp 97–107.

Lavis TD, Codamon L: Lower limb orthoses for persons with spinal cord injury. In Webster JB, Murphy DP, editors: *Atlas of orthoses and assistive devices*, ed 5, Philadelphia, 2019, Elsevier, pp 247–255.

Leech KA, Kinnaird CR, Holleran CL, et al.: Effects of locomotor exercise intensity on gait performance in individuals with incomplete spinal cord injury, *Phys Ther* 96(12):1919–1929, 2016.

Łęgosz P, Drela K, Pulik Ł, et al.: Challenges of heterotopic ossification-molecular background and current treatment strategies, *Clin Exp Pharmacol Physiol* 45:1229–1235, 2018.

Lewthwaite R, Thompson L, Boyd LA, et al.: Reconceptualizing physical therapy for spinal cord injury rehabilitation: physical activity for long-term health and function, *Infusions Res Pract* 1:1–9, 1994.

Lundy-Ekman L: *Neuroscience: fundamentals for rehabilitation*, ed 5, St. Louis, 2018, Elsevier, pp 284–285, 372–378.

Macko R: Stroke, brain trauma, and spinal cord injury. In Moore GE, Durstine JL, Painter PL, editors: *ACSM's exercise management for persons with chronic diseases and disabilities*, ed 4, Champaign, IL, 2016, Human Kinetics, pp 237–247.

Reyes MR, Chiodo A, Model Systems Translation Center: *Spasticity and spinal cord injury*, Washington, DC, 2019. Available at: www.msktc.org/sci/factsheets/Spasticity. Accessed January 26, 2020.

Monroy E: *Integumentary changes and considerations impacting people with spinal cord injury*, Minneapolis, MN, 2017, Academy of Neurologic Physical Therapy. Available at: www.neuropt.org/docs/default-source/sci-sig/fact-sheets/scisig_factsheet_integumentary-considerations_11_25_17.pdf. Accessed April 24, 2019.

Moore JL, Potter K, Blankshain K, et al.: A core set of outcome measures for adults with neurologic conditions undergoing rehabilitation: a clinical practice guideline, *J Neurol Phys Ther* 42:174–220, 2018.

Morrison S: Fitness for the spinal cord population: establishing a program in your facility, *Neurol Rep* 18:22–27, 1994.

National Spinal Cord Injury Statistical Center: *Spinal cord injury facts and figures at a glance*, Birmingham, AL, March 2019, University of Alabama. Available at: www.msktc.org/lib/docs/Data_Sheets_/SCIMS_Facts_and_Figures_2017_August_FINAL.pdf. Accessed March 13, 2019.

Nawoczenski DA, Ritter-Soronen JM, Wilson CM, et al.: Clinical trial of exercise for shoulder pain in chronic spinal cord injury, *Phys Ther* 86(12):1604–1618, 2006.

Neurology Section: *SCI EDGE outcome measures for entry-level educa-tion*, 2013. Available at: http://www.neuropt.org/docs/sci-edge-/sci-edge-entry-level-recommendations.pdf?sfvrsn=71546a8F_2. Accessed June 20, 2019.

Nixon V: *Spinal cord injury: a guide to functional outcomes in physi-cal therapy management*, Rockville, MD, 1985, Aspen Systems, pp 41–66, 177–188.

Phadke CP, Vierira L, Mathur S, et al.: Impact of passive leg cycling in persons with spinal cord injury: a systematic review, *Top Spinal Cord Inj Rehabil* 25(1):83–96, 2019.

Sasso E, Backus D: Home-based circuit resistance training to over-come barriers to exercise for people with spinal cord injury: a case study, *J Neurol Phys Ther* 37:65–71, 2013.

Scelza W, Shatzer M: Pharmacology of spinal cord injury: basic mechanism of action and side effects of commonly used drugs, *J Neurol Phys Ther* 27(3):101–108, 2003.

Shumway-Cook A, Woollacott MH: *Motor control: translating research into clinical practice*, ed 5, Philadelphia, 2017, Wolters Kluwer, pp 148–149, 435, 443–444.

Smith AC, Knikou M: A review on locomotor training after spinal cord injury: reorganization of spinal neuronal circuits and re-covery of motor function, *Neural Plast* 2016:1216258, 2016.

Somers MF: *Spinal cord injury functional rehabilitation*, ed 3, Boston, MA, 2010, Pearson, pp 527–551, 67, 130, 136–153, 194–198, 29–300, 345–346.

Somers MF, Bruce J: *Spinal cord injury, Clinical Summaries*, Alexan-dria, VA, 2014, American Physical Therapy Association. Available at: http://www.ptnow.org/ClinicalSummaries.aspx. Accessed September 15, 2014.

Tappan R, Tessiatore A: *Aging after spinal cord injury: an overview*, Minneapolis, MN, 2019, Academy of Neurologic Physical Ther-apy. Available at: www.neuropt.org/docs/default-source/sci-sig/fact-sheets/scisig_factsheet_aging.pdf. Accessed June 9, 2019.

Tefertiller C, Wehrli LS, Fuller KS: Traumatic spinal cord injury. In Goodman CC, Fuller KS, editors: *Pathology implications for physical therapy*, ed 4, St. Louis, 2015, Elsevier, pp 1556–1575.

United States Department of Health and Human Services: *Physical activity guidelines for Americans*, ed 2, Washington, DC, 2018. Available at: www.health.gov/paguidelines/second-edition/pdf/PhysicaL_Activity_Guidelines_2nd_edition.pdf. Accessed June 24, 2019.

van Middendorp JJ, Hosman AJ, Donders AR, et al.: A clinical pre-diction rule for ambulation outcomes after traumatic spinal cord injury: a longitudinal cohort study, *Lancet* 377:1004–1010, 2011.

Wetzel J: Respiratory evaluation and treatment. In Adkins HV, editor: *Spinal cord injury*, New York, 1985, Churchill Living-stone, pp 75–98.

Yarkony GM, Chen D: Rehabilitation of patients with spinal cord injuries. In Braddom RL, editor: *Physical medicine and rehabili-tation*, Philadelphia, 1996, WB Saunders, pp 1149–1179.

14

Other Neurologic Disorders

OBJECTIVES

After reading this chapter, the student will be able to:

1. Describe the incidence, etiology, and clinical manifestations of Parkinson disease (PD), multiple sclerosis (MS), amyotrophic lateral sclerosis (ALS), Guillain-Barré syndrome (GBS), and post-polio syndrome (PPS).
2. Understand the typical medical and surgical management of persons with PD, MS, ALS, GBS, and PPS.
3. Identify specific treatment interventions relative to the stage or degree of progression, activity limitations, and participation restrictions of persons with PD, MS, ALS, GBS, and PPS.
4. Discuss strategies for patient/family education to address functional limitations in persons with PD, MS, ALS, GBS, and PPS.

INTRODUCTION

Many neurologic disorders are chronic in nature such as Parkinson disease (PD) and multiple sclerosis (MS), and some are progressive in nature such as amyotrophic lateral sclerosis (ALS) and Guillain-Barré syndrome (GBS). ALS is a terminal degenerative disease of the upper motor neurons (UMNs) and lower motor neurons (LMNs). Individuals with post-polio syndrome (PPS) experience new symptoms 25 to 30 years after having overcome polio. Recovery is not expected in these neurologic disorders, except for individuals with GBS. GBS is a peripheral as opposed to a central nervous system (CNS) phenomenon, and remyelination of nerves can occur.

PD and MS are both progressive disorders. Despite that fact, life expectancy in all of the neurologic conditions discussed, except ALS, is not usually seriously diminished. There are a few exceptions such as when the cardiopulmonary system is involved or when there is rapid progression of the disease. ALS is a major exception as death usually occurs within 4 years of diagnosis. Regardless of whether the disease is acute or chronic, or whether recovery occurs as part of the pathologic process, physical therapy can assist these individuals and their families to function optimally and participate in their lives.

Intervention strategies must relate to the level of involvement and stage of disease progression or, in some cases, recovery of abilities. For example, a person diagnosed in the early stages of MS, PD, or even ALS may be able to participate in a moderately intense exercise program, whereas a person in the later stages of PD, MS, or ALS may not. Exercise and other physical therapy interventions must be specific to the type and severity of the movement system dysfunction. For example, in a patient with MS who exhibits ataxia (a condition of too much movement), stability is more important than mobility. However, in PD in which the

body, especially the trunk, exhibits rigidity, mobility is more important than stability. As muscle weakness progresses in ALS, the person is able to do less, and interventions move from being restorative or preventative in nature to compensatory and palliative. Fatigue is an ever-present finding or concern in all of the neurologic disorders discussed in this chapter, and its management must be an integral part of any plan of care. Each disorder will be presented with its clinical features, incidence and etiology, physical therapy goals, and sample interventions.

PARKINSON DISEASE

PD was first described in 1817 by James Parkinson in an essay on the shaking palsy. It is a chronic, progressive neurologic condition that affects the motor system. The four primary symptoms are bradykinesia (slowness of movement), rigidity, tremor, and postural instability. These symptoms are caused by a decrease in dopamine (DA), a neurotransmitter, stored in the substantia nigra. The substantia nigra is a component of the basal ganglia (see Chapter 2). The basal ganglia are primarily responsible for the regulation of posture and movement. Lesions in the basal ganglia change the character of movement rather than produce weakness or paralysis (Fuller et al., 2015).

In actuality, parkinsonism is a group of disorders involving dysfunction of the basal ganglia. The most common type of parkinsonism is primary parkinsonism or PD. It is also known as idiopathic PD because there is no apparent cause. Other types of parkinsonism include secondary parkinsonism and Parkinson-plus syndromes. Secondary parkinsonism occurs as a result of other conditions and can be associated with encephalitis, alcoholism, exposure to certain toxins, traumatic brain injuries, vascular insults, and use of psychotropic medications. Long-term use of medications used to control mood and behavior can produce Parkinson-like symptoms. Parkinson-plus syndromes include disorders such as multisystem atrophy, progressive supranuclear palsy, and Shy-Drager syndrome. These syndromes produce other neurologic signs of multiple system degeneration such as cerebellar dysfunction and autonomic system dysfunction (dysautonomia) in addition to the classic signs indicative of degeneration of the DA-producing neurons of the substantia nigra.

PD is the second most common age-related neurodegenerative disorder in the United States, with Alzheimer disease being the first. Prevalence of PD has more than doubled between 1990 and 2015 and is expected to double again by 2040 (Dorsey and Bloem, 2018). PD accounts for 85% of the cases of parkinsonism. Further description and discussion will be confined to primary or idiopathic PD, with only minimal references to the other types of parkinsonism. Incidence of PD rises with increasing age. Although the majority of individuals with PD are over age 60 when diagnosed, 4% are diagnosed before age 50 (https://parkinson.org/Understanding-Parkinsons/Statistics). Currently, over 10 million people are living with PD worldwide, with 60,000 individuals diagnosed annually in the United States. Prevalence of PD varies by region of the country (Marras et al., 2018). The average age of onset is 62.4 years, with the majority of cases occurring between 50 and 79 years. Men are 1.5 times more likely to have PD than women. The etiology of PD is multifactorial because many factors contribute to the clinical entity. Lifestyle factors associated with a reduced risk for PD include cigarette smoking, drinking coffee, and high levels of physical activity (Ascherio and Schwarzschild, 2016; Fang et al., 2018). There is a long prodromal stage in PD that can last 10 years before symptoms become sufficient for a diagnosis. Seven genes have been identified that are linked to familiar parkinsonism. Four of these genes are autosomal dominant, meaning only one copy is needed to produce parkinsonism. PD is a result of a complex interaction between many genetic and environmental factors, which are beginning to be understood (Reichmann, 2017).

Pathophysiology

PD is a disorder of the DA-producing neurons of the substantia nigra in the basal ganglia. The substantia nigra is subcortical gray matter that contains pigmented neurons. As these neurons degenerate, they lose their color. A 70% to 80% loss of neurons occurs before symptoms become apparent. The severity of loss of DA correlates well with the amount of movement slowness or bradykinesia exhibited by the patient. Loss of DA neurons and the production of Lewy bodies within the pigmented substantia nigra neurons are hallmarks of idiopathic PD. Lewy bodies contain neurofilaments and hyaline. They are part of the aging process and are seen in certain vulnerable neuronal populations. Lewy bodies are found in smaller numbers in other neurodegenerative disorders, such as Alzheimer disease, but in different brain areas.

DA is both an excitatory and inhibitory neurotransmitter. Because of the role of the basal ganglia in movement initiation and in releasing one movement sequence in order for another one to begin, basal ganglia circuitry is altered. As DA is depleted, some pathways are insufficiently activated, whereas other pathways become hyperactive. Insufficient activity slows movement and affects timing. The cholinergic system becomes more active because of the lack of inhibition from DA. Acetylcholine is used by the small interconnecting neurons in the basal ganglia. The increased cholinergic activity means more acetylcholine and causes an increase in muscle activity on both sides of a joint. This results in symptoms of rigidity and further slowing of movement or hypokinesia/bradykinesia.

Clinical Features

PD is a movement disorder that has considerable variation in its presentation. Clinically, a patient with PD exhibits bradykinesia, rigidity, tremor, and postural instability. Bradykinesia is particularly evident in the performance of activities of daily living (ADLs). Slowing of oral movements can result in poor speech intelligibility and inadequate breath support, often manifested as a soft monotone voice. Swallowing may become impaired. Handwriting can be cramped and small, an occurrence known as micrographia. Akinesia is an inability to initiate movement such as rising from a chair, turning in bed, or simply crossing the legs. As movement slows, the patient tends to adopt a fixed forward-flexed posture, and the ability to extend against gravity is lost.

Rigidity occurs in the trunk and the extremities. An early sign of this problem occurs when the individual loses the ability to swing the arms during walking. Rigidity is resistance to passive movement regardless of the speed of the movement. Two forms of rigidity, lead-pipe and cogwheel, can be demonstrated in a person with PD. In lead-pipe rigidity, there is constant resistance to passive limb movement in any direction regardless of speed. Cogwheel rigidity is the result of combining lead-pipe rigidity and tremor. The rigidity causes a catch, and the tremor allows the letting go. This type of rigidity results in a jerky, ratchet-like response to passive movement characterized by a tensing and letting go. Rigidity of the trunk impairs breathing and phonation by restricting chest wall motion. Rigidity can increase energy expenditure throughout the day, and its presence may be related to the postexercise fatigue experienced by these patients.

Tremor is often the first sign of PD. Because it manifests at rest and disappears on voluntary movement, it is classified as a resting tremor as opposed to an intention (on action) tremor. The tremor of the hand has a regular rhythm (4 to 7 beats per second) and is described as "pill-rolling." Tremors can also occur in the oral area or within postural muscles of the head, neck, and trunk. Tremors may begin unilaterally and progress over time to all four limbs and the neck. Tremors rarely interfere with ADLs.

Postural instability is a very serious problem for patients with PD and is a major reason for restriction in a person's activities and participation in life. Loss of postural extension and the inability to respond to expected and unexpected postural disturbances can cause falls. A person's fall potential increases the longer the person has the disease. People with PD also have lower confidence in being able to avoid a fall while performing ADLs than healthy controls (Adkins et al., 2003; Mak et al., 2012). An increased risk of falling and a fear of repeated falling are common problems in individuals with advanced PD (Grimbergen et al., 2013). Visuospatial deficits and slow processing of sensory information related to balance do contribute to postural instability (Peterson et al., 2016). The person with PD does not accurately perceive proprioceptive and kinesthetic input (Konczak et al., 2009). Patients with PD mix hip and ankle strategies, which produces maladaptive balance responses (Horak et al., 1996, 2005). Anticipatory postural responses were found to be poor or absent in several studies (Mancini et al., 2009; Rogers et al., 2011). Abnormal postural responses result from an inability to distinguish self-movement from movement of the environment. The person with PD is overdependent on vision for movement cues because of impaired proprioception (Vaugoyeau et al., 2007; Hwang et al., 2016). The proprioceptive impairment is an important factor in postural instability.

Other typical features of PD include a flexed posture, masked facies, dysphagia, festinating gait, freezing episodes, and fatigue. Postural deficits include flexion of the head, neck, and trunk, which create a forward displacement of the center of gravity (Fig. 14.1). However, exaggeration of flexion in the hips and knees may assist in bringing weight more posteriorly. Over time, these postural changes become fixed because of the rigidity of the trunk and have been described as flexion dystonia. Loss of trunk extension occurs early in the disease, followed by loss of rotation and subsequent loss of arm swing. The face becomes rigid and shows little or no facial expression. As oral structures lose their ability to move and become rigid, swallowing becomes more and more difficult, leading to concerns about the person's nutritional intake.

The gait of a person with PD is shuffling, punctuated by short steps and a progressive increase in speed as if trying to catch up. This is called *festination*. If festination occurs while walking forward, it is referred to as *propulsion*; if it occurs while walking backward, it is referred to as *retropulsion*. Foot clearance is decreased because of the short, slow shuffling, therefore increasing the person's risk for falling. Freezing occurs when the person becomes stuck in a posture. This usually occurs while walking and can be triggered by environmental situations, such as a doorway or change of floor surface. Freezing episodes can occur at any time, such as when making arm movements, speaking, or blinking. Festinating gait, postural dysfunction, and freezing of gait (FoG) are three contributing causes of the postural instability seen in patients with PD. The majority will eventually develop FoG as the disease progresses and gait becomes more impaired (Forsaa et al., 2015). The loss of automaticity of gait is most apparent when the person with PD performs a secondary task along with walking. Individuals with PD and FoG have more cognitive dysfunction than those with PD without FoG (Peterson et al., 2016). FoG is associated with problems with attention, shifting attention between tasks, and divided attention all of which are compounded by altered cognition.

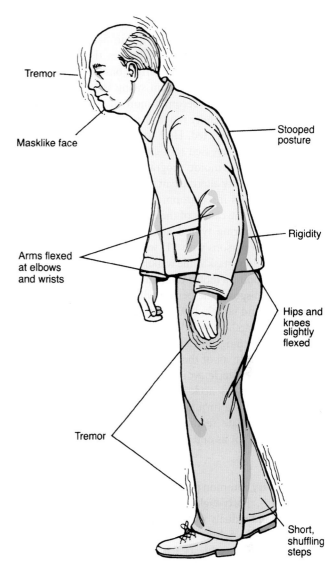

Fig. 14.1 Typical posture that results from Parkinson disease. (Modified from Monahan FD, Neighbors M: *Medical-surgical nursing: foundations for clinical practice,* ed 2, Philadelphia, 1998, WB Saunders. In Copstead LEC, Banasik JL: *Pathophysiology,* ed 3, St. Louis, 2005, Elsevier Saunders.)

Fatigue

Fatigue contributes to postural instability because of the difficulty the person with PD experiences while trying to sustain an activity. Fatigue affects 50% of this population and is often one of its most disabling effects (Friedman and Friedman, 2001; Miwa and Miwa, 2011). Fatigue is present even at the onset of the disease (Herlofson and Kluger, 2017). People with PD exhibit lethargy as the day progresses. A sedentary lifestyle with decreased activity contributes to general deconditioning. Fatigue is strongly correlated with high emotional distress and low quality of life (QOL) in patients with PD who are nondemented or depressed (Herlofson and Larsen, 2003). Patients with increased levels of fatigue are more likely to be sedentary and have poorer levels of physical function than those with lower levels of fatigue (Garber and Friedman, 2003). Fatigue is the most common symptom reported in disability claims in the United States (Zesiewicz et al., 2007)

Gait

Up to one-third of patients with PD initially present with postural instability and gait disturbances that constitute a group. Gait speed is slow with a narrow base and a characteristic festination or shuffling. Arm swing is lost early in the disease process. Posture becomes more and more forwardly flexed and lower extremity range of motion (ROM) becomes more and more restricted. Heel strike and toe-off are both lost, resulting in decreased foot clearance. Because of an inability to change a motor program once it has begun, the person has difficulty altering gait speed or stride length in response to changes in environmental demands. Bradykinesia and rigidity are the causes of the absent arm swing and trunk rotation seen during typical ambulation and turning. Gait dysfunction in persons with PD worsens when asked to perform an additional task while walking (Rochester et al., 2014). Difficulty stopping a motor program, such as when walking or running, predisposes the person with PD to slips, trips, and falls (Morris and Iansek, 1997). Smulders et al. (2016) recommend that research target additional components of gait such as initiation, turning, and adaptability as the person with PD has difficulty with all of these. For example, does the person with PD have obstacle avoidance skills? Speed of turning is related to increased neck tone (Franzén et al., 2009). Eye movement begins a turn and if the neck is stiff, the eyes are not able to initiate segmental turning and the individual moves "en bloc" or as one unit (eye-neck-trunk).

Falls

Falls are a very common problem in persons with PD (Morris et al., 2015). Forty-eight percent of early-stage optimally medicated individuals with PD reported a fall in a study by Kerr et al. (2010). Schrag et al. (2002) found that 64% of their community-based subjects with PD had experienced falls with postural instability. Self-selected gait speed can be used to predict fall risk in individuals with PD (Nemanich et al., 2013). A community-dwelling older adult with PD is twice as likely to experience a fall as is a community-dwelling older adult without PD (Wood et al., 2002). Additionally, it was found that previous falls, disease duration, dementia, and loss of arm swing were predictors of falling. Therefore people with PD who have fallen previously are more likely to fall again, and individuals with dementia or loss of arm swing are more likely to fall. FoG, impaired reactive and anticipatory balance, and impaired orientation were significantly associated with future falls (Paul et al., 2014). The longer a person has PD, the greater the risk for falling (Paul et al., 2018).

Systemic Manifestations/Nonmotor Symptoms

Half of the individuals with PD exhibit dementia and intellectual changes caused by the neurochemical changes in the basal ganglia (Fuller et al., 2015). Dementia along with bradyphrenia, dysautonomia, and depression are systemic manifestations of the disease. Bradyphrenia is a slowing of thought processes. It is usually accompanied by a lack of ability to attend and concentrate. Dysautonomia may result in orthostatic hypotension when changing position and lower than expected systolic blood pressure and heart changes with exercise. Low motivation and passivity can also be related to depression or to sensory deprivation from a lack of movement. Depression is common in patients with PD, but diagnosis may be delayed secondary to motor involvement that masks the underlying depression. Depression is also considered a nonmotor symptom of PD. Nonmotor symptoms in addition to depression include loss of sense of smell, constipation, pain, genitourinary problems, and sleep disturbances (Pfeiffer, 2016; Schapira et al., 2017). These nonmotor symptoms have been found 5 to 10 years before motor symptoms are present, and therefore may be able to be used to diagnose PD earlier (Reichmann, 2017).

Stages

The Hoehn and Yahr classification of disability (Hoehn and Yahr, 1967) (Table 14.1) is used to stage the severity of involvement of PD. New stages have been added to better describe the progression of the disease. Stage 0 indicates no signs of the disease. Stage 1 indicates minimal disease and stage 5 indicates that the person is in bed or using a wheelchair all of the time. In addition to stage 0, there are stages 1.5 and 2.5 (Goetz et al., 2004). The average patient shows slow, gradual progression of the disease over a period of 5 to 30 years. Therefore the life expectancy of someone with PD is only a little shorter than someone without PD of the same age.

Diagnosis

Up to now, diagnosis has been based on a person's clinical presentation of signs and symptoms and history. Presence of two of the four cardinal features and exclusion of the Parkinson-plus syndromes is usually employed to make the diagnosis (Bezkor et al., 2019). The presence of hyposmia (absence of smell) has been added as a cardinal feature of PD because over

TABLE 14.1 Hoehn and Yahr Staging Scale for Parkinson Disease

Stage	Progression of Symptoms
0	No signs of disease
1	Unilateral symptoms only
1.5	Unilateral and axial involvement
2	Bilateral symptoms, no impairment of balance
2.5	Mild bilateral disease with recovery on pull test
3	Balance impairment, mild to moderate disease, physically independent
4	Severe disability, but still able to walk or stand unassisted
5	Needing a wheelchair or bedridden unless assisted

The Hoehn and Yahr scale is commonly used to describe how the symptoms of Parkinson disease progress. The original scale included stages 1 to 5. Stage 0 has since been added, and stages 1.5 and 2.5 have been proposed to best indicate the relative level of disability in this population.
Modified from Goetz CG, Poewe W, Rascol O, et al.: Movement Disorder Society Task Force report of the Hoehn and Yahr staging scale: status and recommendations, *Mov Disord* 19:1020–1028, 2004.

90% of people with PD present with this problem (Berg et al., 2014; Haehner et al., 2009). Animal models have shown that the disease may be initiated by a substance originating in the environment that is inhaled or ingested. It causes the typical pathology (Lewy bodies, Lewy neurites) in the olfactory bulb, the submandibular gland, and the enteric nervous system (digestive tract). From there, it spreads via the vagal nerve to the brain. Theoretically, a diagnosis could be made by a biopsy of the submandibular gland or the gut (Reichmann, 2017). The Parkinson-plus syndromes do not respond typically to anti-Parkinson medication. Neuroimaging and laboratory tests are usually normal unless there are coexisting morbidities.

Medical Management

The mainstay of medical management of patients with PD is pharmacologic. Selegiline, also called deprenyl (Eldepryl), or rasagiline (Azilect) are often used as first medications after diagnosis because they delay the need for giving levodopa (L-dopa). These monoamine oxidase inhibitors block the breakdown of DA and are thought to slow the progression of PD and delay the need for replacement medication for up to 1 year (Sutton, 2009).

The major mainstay in treatment of PD remains L-dopa, which is used to replace the lost DA. It works best to decrease rigidity and make movement easier. DA cannot be given because it cannot cross the blood–brain barrier. L-dopa can cross the blood–brain barrier. However, because a lot of the L-dopa gets broken down before it reaches the brain, scientists add carbidopa to the L-dopa to delay its breakdown. This addition allows more L-dopa to reach the basal ganglia and smaller doses of medication can be given. Sinemet is the brand name of a commonly used combination of carbidopa and L-dopa. Anticholinergics are medications that block the increase in acetylcholine that results from the decrease in available DA. Smulders et al. (2016) present substantial evidence for the effectiveness of L-dopa and L-dopa-enhancing medications in improving simple, straight-ahead gait. Combining exercise and medication have produced greater effects on muscle force and mobility in persons with PD than either intervention alone (Dibble et al., 2015).

Anticholinergics are helpful in reducing the resting tremor but have little or no effect on the other symptoms including postural instability. A list of medications and their intended use is found in Table 14.2. The physical therapist should alert the physical therapist assistant to look for possible side effects of the patient's medications.

Unfortunately, with long-term use, L-dopa becomes less effective therapeutically. The medication usually works for only 4 to 6 years before its benefits are no longer evident. As the medication benefits decrease, other movement problems occur such as motor fluctuations, dyskinesias, and dystonia. Motor fluctuations are times when symptoms increase because the L-dopa is no longer able to cause a smooth and even effect. These times are also called "on/off" fluctuations or "on/off" phenomenon. Dyskinesias are involuntary movements involving the face, oral structures, head, trunk, or limbs. The timing of dyskinesias can vary. In some individuals,

TABLE 14.2 Medications Used for Neurologic Disorders

Brand Name of Medication	Usage
Artane	Moderate tremor and dystonia associated with wearing off in PD
Avonex	RRMS
Betaseron	RRMS, CIS
Copaxone	RRMS, CIS
Cogentin	End-of-dose "wearing off" in PD
Cortisone, corticosteroids, prednisone	Shorten acute attack in MS
Dantrium	Spasticity
Ditropan	Bladder urgency and frequency in MS
Eldepryl	Enhances levels of dopamine in early PD
Immunoglobulins	Duration and severity of GBS
Klonopin	Severe tremors in MS
Lioresal	Spasticity
Novantrone	SPMS, advanced RRMS, IV delivery
Parlodel	End-of-dose "wearing off" and dyskinesias in PD
Pro-Banthine	Bladder urgency and frequency in MS
Provigil	Fatigue in MS
Rebif	RRMS
Requip	Bradykinesia, rigidity, and motor fluctuations in PD
Sinemet IR or CR	Bradykinesia and rigidity in PD
Symmetrel	Bradykinesia and rigidity in PD Fatigue in MS, PPS
Tegretol	Tonic spasms in MS
Tysabri	RRMS not used initially, IV delivery
Urecholine	Urinary retention in MS
Valium	Night spasms in MS

CIS, Clinically isolated syndrome; *CR*, controlled release; *GBS*, Guillain-Barré syndrome; *IR*, immediate release; *IV*, intravenous; *MS*, multiple sclerosis; *PD*, Parkinson disease; *PPS*, post-polio syndrome; *RRMS*, relapsing-remitting multiple sclerosis; *SPMS*, secondary progressive multiple sclerosis.

they may occur at the peak effect of the medication. This is the most common pattern. For other individuals, they occur at the beginning or end of a dose. The medication-induced dyskinesias can be reversed by decreasing the dose of anti-Parkinson medication given; however, the tremors, slowness of movement, and gait difficulties worsen. Therefore some patients prefer to experience the dyskinesias rather than have more severe PD symptoms. Dystonia is a twisting or torsion of body parts caused by a prolonged involuntary contraction. Patients report toe clawing or cramping of back, neck, face, and calf muscles. Wearing-off phenomenon is the deterioration of movement often noted at the end of the time frame of medication. The therapist needs to be familiar with all of the medications a patient with PD is taking and their side effects.

Balancing medications is very challenging in this patient population.

Surgical Management

Deep brain stimulation (DBS) has emerged as a viable treatment option for patients with PD. Electrodes are implanted into the brain to stop nerve signals that produce symptoms. DBS is safer than formerly used surgical ablation or destruction of structures because it is reversible. Electrodes are implanted into the subthalamic nucleus with a stimulation box placed subcutaneously in the subclavicular area, much like an implantable cardiac pacemaker. The stimulation can be turned on and off by the patient. The amount of stimulation delivered is determined by the physician. Infection and hemorrhage are potential surgical risks. DBS reduces the need for medication, and therefore the dyskinesias that accompany long-term use of L-dopa. Benefits of subthalamic nucleus-DBS include improvement of bradykinesia, rigidity, and to a lesser degree tremor. L-dopa and DBS are not helpful for treating postural instability and FoG (Fasano et al., 2015; Nantel et al., 2012; Nutt et al., 2011).

Physical Therapy Management

Patients may be thought to present in three broad categories: tremor predominant, bradykinesia/akinesia, and postural instability/gait difficulty. Goals can be related to the type of presentation on examination, but there is considerable overlap. Physical therapy is a beneficial adjunct to medication for people with PD (Dibble et al., 2015; Ellis and Rochester, 2018; Silva-Batista et al., 2018). The primary physical therapy goal is to maximize function in the face of progressing pathology. Therefore the focus should be on early intervention. Gait bradykinesia or slowness affects almost everyone with PD. Stride length continues to shorten as the disorder progresses. Teaching the patient strategies to move more easily is of utmost importance. Table 14.3 shows activities that can be used as part of movement strategies training (Morris et al., 2011).

Progressive resistance training (RT) has been found to be effective in improving bradykinesia (David et al., 2016; Dibble et al., 2009) and postural control (Schlenstedt et al., 2015). Progressive resistance with instability (RTI) was found to improve mobility, balance, and cognition (Silva-Batista et al., 2016, 2017). RTI uses exercises with high motor complexity.

TABLE 14.3 Strategies to Enhance Daily Tasks

Task	Strategy
Walking	Instruct to walk with long steps Swing arms Place lines on the floor spaced at appropriate step lengths for person's age and height Incorporate starting and stopping
Turning around	Instruct patient to use a large arc of movement or clock pattern Practice different turn activities related to home and community environment
Sit to stand	Use mental rehearsal before moving Use gentle rocking back and forth before moving Ensure sufficient forward lean to get weight over the feet Increase height of seat or use armrests Use visual cues
Reaching in standing	Practice with objects of different sizes and weights at various heights within functional contexts (kitchen, shower, laundry room, grocery store, library)
Turning over and getting out of bed	Use a night light Use a lightweight bedcover Use mental rehearsal before moving Use momentum and normal timing Use verbal cues to trigger each part of the sequence or picture cards Sufficient bed height to stand easily
Protective stepping in standing	Practice large quick steps in different directions Use verbal or auditory cue to step Use a push or tug in a predictable or unpredictable direction
Complex walking tasks	Practice dual tasks Navigate an obstacle course Mentally rehearse before moving
Reaching, grasping, manipulating objects, and writing	Mentally rehearse before moving Use the object as a visual cue Break down the task into component parts Use verbal cues for each part of the sequence Avoid distractions or secondary tasks at the same time

From Morris ME, et al.: Falls and mobility in Parkinson's disease: protocol for a randomized controlled clinical trial, *BMC Neurol* 11:93, 2011; and Morris ME: Movement disorders in people with Parkinson disease: a model for physical therapy, *Phys Ther* 80:578–597, 2000.

Resistance exercises are performed on unstable surfaces such as a balance disc or BOSU (Hedstrom, Ashland, OH). Silva-Batista et al. (2018) compared the effects of RTI and RT on balance and fear of falling in patients with moderate PD. They also explored the association between cognitive function and changes in balance and fear of falling. RTI resulted in significantly better scores on the Balance Evaluation Systems Test than RT. Cognitive scores on the Montreal Cognitive Assessment were also significantly improved along with a decline in scores on the Falls Efficacy Scale–International.

A second goal is to prevent secondary sequelae, such as deconditioning, musculoskeletal changes related to stiffness, and loss of extension and rotation. Twelve weeks of strength and aerobic training improved fitness in patients with mild to moderate PD (Demonceau et al., 2017). A systematic review on strength training in PD found that using external resistance was well tolerated and resulted in improved QOL and physical function (Ramazzina et al., 2017). Because most individuals with PD succumb to respiratory infections, the longer a person with PD is physically active and mobile, the less likely he or she is to develop pneumonia. Physical therapy interventions should focus on slowing the onset of predictable changes in posture, locomotion, and general activity level. Changes in gait characteristics such as postural control, pace, and variability predicted decline in cognition in a group of newly diagnosed individuals with PD (Morris et al., 2017). Gait may be a clinical biomarker for cognitive decline.

Gait Interventions/Fall Prevention

The physical therapist needs to ascertain the cause of the gait disturbance to pick the correct strategy for intervention. The physical therapist assistant should also understand the rationale behind the selected gait intervention. One of the assistant's major roles with this population is to educate the patient and the family members about the importance of good posture and daily walking and the benefits of sustained activity. All components of daily mobility need to be addressed: gait initiation, straight walking, turning, and gait adaptability (obstacles). Using visual auditory and somatosensory cues to improve attention and optimize timing during a movement task are strategies that appear to be helpful in treating the gait hypokinesia (Frazzitta et al., 2009; Morris et al., 2011; Nieuwboer et al., 2009). Walking while holding onto poles can vary the motor program enough to elicit a faster gait. Markers can be placed on the floor and the person directed to step on or over them. Walking toward a mirror allows use of visual feedback to maintain an upright trunk. This strategy can be helpful in the early and middle stages. Attentional strategies can also be used to enhance walking including having the person think about taking long strides, mentally rehearsing the path to be taken before walking (Morris et al., 2011). In general, regardless of the task, breaking down the task into its component parts so the person can focus attention on each part separately is a very useful strategy. Practicing dual tasking to promote motor learning is a good intervention for people with mild to moderate involvement. Step hesitation is often the beginning of gait problems for the patient with PD.

Anticipatory postural adjustments (APAs) depend on proprioceptive awareness of the changes in weight displacement during step initiation (Mancini et al., 2009). People with PD produce less push-off force resulting in a delay in stepping and a shorter first step (Vallabhajosula et al., 2013). RTI has been shown to improve force production of the plantarflexors and knee extensors along with APAs (Silva-Batista et al., 2018). An accelerometer on the trunk can be used to measure APA. Proprioceptive deficits may appear before motor deficits in PD (Konczak et al., 2009). Slow gait in PD is characterized by a short stride so a way to document change in response to practice is to measure stride length before and after intervention. A measurable goal could be that the person would increase stride length by a certain amount or take fewer steps for a given distance.

Practice alternative walking patterns, such as side stepping, walking backward, braiding, and marching to various rhythms. Giving the person a mark on the floor to work toward or footprints to try and match or step on can also be helpful. Peripheral movement cues to walk are useful. The assistant would stand slightly to the side of the patient so that the patient could see his or her move as the request to walk is given. Freezing strategies that are often employed include having the person kick a box or pick up a penny. Freezing tends to happen in more confined spaces, such as going through a doorway. However, it can happen in an open environment, so several strategies need to be kept in mind.

There are no definitive guidelines regarding the use of assistive devices in persons with gait difficulty secondary to PD. The physical therapist will determine the efficacy of using an assistive device. Bryant et al. (2014) studied use of walking devices in PD. Those individuals who took more than 13 seconds to complete a 5-meter Timed Up and Go test used a device, and 78% of those who scored less than a 75 on the Activities-Specific Balance Confidence Scale used a walking device. Use of a cane or a walker will depend on the degree of coordination present in the upper and lower extremities. A rolling wheeled walker with pushdown brakes can be helpful for some people, whereas a reverse-facing walker may assist the person who loses balance in a backward direction. Regardless of the device, it should be adjusted to promote trunk extension not flexion. A U-step walker projects a laser line for the person with PD to step over. Research is ongoing to develop glasses that would project lines in the same manner (Zhao et al., 2016). Kegelmeyer et al. (2013) found that a four-wheeled walker provided the most consistent improvement in gait. Additionally, the laser on the U-step walker did not improve gait or safety compared with other devices in the study. A cane may be useful during a freezing episode. The person can turn it upside down and use it as a cue to continue walking. To date, no one assistive device has been found to be correct for everyone nor is everyone going to be able to benefit from using a device all of the time.

Interventions

Because trunk extension and rotation are lost early in the disease process, exercises to strengthen postural extensors are important to emphasize soon after diagnosis. Additionally, stretching exercises for tight pectorals are indicated if these muscles are shortened, thus preventing thoracic trunk extension. Stretching heel cords is indicated to maintain a plantigrade foot and normal weight transfer during gait. Rotational exercises of the trunk and limbs, such as those depicted in Interventions 14.1 and 14.2, have routinely been recommended. Rotational exercises were used to decrease the incidence of freezing in a small group of patients with advanced stage PD (Van Vaerenbergh et al., 2003). Stożek et al. (2016) showed an increase in trunk rotation after a 4 week rehabilitation program consisting of trunk mobility exercises, posture correction, simple dances, and distance walking. Improvements were also

seen in gait and balance, which were maintained for at least 1 month. They also included relaxation, breathing exercises, voice power, and a home exercise program. Rhythmic initiation, a proprioceptive neuromuscular facilitation (PNF) technique, can be used to assist the person to begin a movement or increase the ROM through which the movement occurs (see Chapter 10). This technique is most helpful when the patient is performing functional patterns of movement such as rolling and coming to sit or stand.

Relaxation techniques are used to treat rigidity and fatigue (O'Sullivan and Bezkor, 2014). Gentle, slow rocking of the trunk and rotation of the extremities can decrease rigidity. These techniques are best used while the person is sitting

---

INTERVENTION 14.1 **Rotational Activities in Supine**

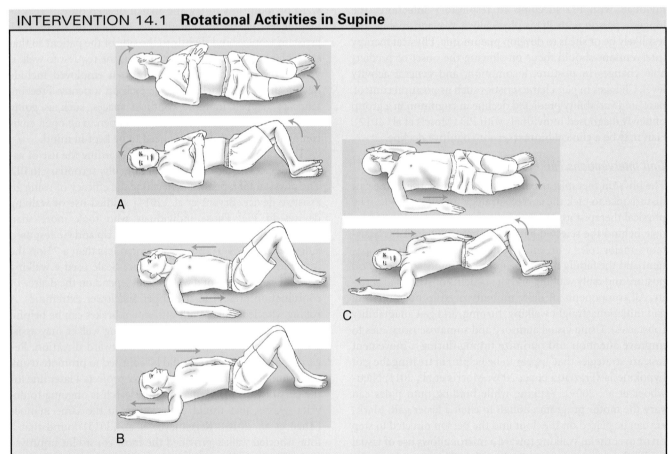

Rotational exercise sequence in supine can be used to increase range of motion of the neck and trunk. Any combination of motions can be used.

A. The head is rotated slowly side to side within the available range of motion while lower extremities are rotated side to side in the opposite direction.

B. The upper extremities are positioned in 45 degrees of shoulder abduction with 90 degrees of elbow flexion. One shoulder is externally rotated while the other shoulder is internally rotated. From this initial position, the shoulders are slowly rotated back and forth from an internally to an externally rotated position.

C. Advanced exercise: The head, shoulders, and lower extremities are rotated simultaneously from one position to the other. The head rotates opposite to the hips providing for counterrotation within the trunk. The upper extremity on the face side is externally rotated while the other arm is internally rotated.

Modified from Turnbull GI, editor: *Physical therapy management of Parkinson's disease*, New York, 1992, Churchill Livingstone, Fig. 9-11, p. 177.

INTERVENTION 14.2 Rotational Activities in Side-Lying

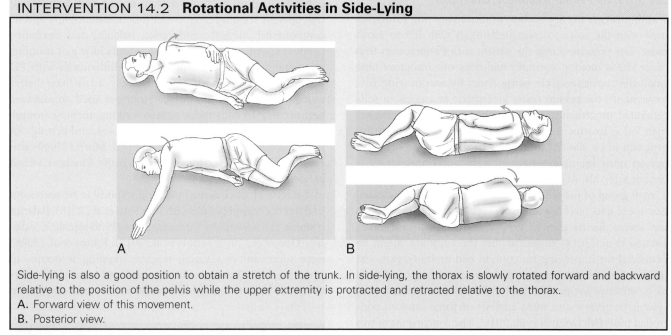

Side-lying is also a good position to obtain a stretch of the trunk. In side-lying, the thorax is slowly rotated forward and backward relative to the position of the pelvis while the upper extremity is protracted and retracted relative to the thorax.
A. Forward view of this movement.
B. Posterior view.

Modified from Turnbull GI, editor: *Physical therapy management of Parkinson's disease*, New York, 1992, Churchill Livingstone, Fig. 9-11, p. 178.

because in a supine position rigidity may be increased. Also, rhythmic rotation should be started proximally and then applied distally as proximal muscles are often stiffer than distal ones. After a decrease in rigidity, movement is often easier and less fatiguing. Large movements are especially helpful and need to encompass the entire range and should emphasize extension. Bilateral symmetrical movements are easier than reciprocal ones. The person can then be progressed to the use of diagonal patterns of movement, such as chops and lifts (see Chapter 10).

Deep breathing can be done to promote relaxation. The person can be in a comfortable supported position in supine and be taught to take slow deep breaths using the diaphragm. Progress the patient to sitting and standing while still concentrating on using the diaphragm and lateral chest expansion. Complete chest wall expansion is difficult for the patient to obtain because the trunk is often rigid. Therefore chest wall stiffness and any postural malalignment need to be addressed using visual feedback, stretching, and strengthening exercises. For example, the individual can perform bilateral D_2 flexion PNF patterns while taking a deep breath, and expiration can be carried out during D_2 extension (see Chapter 10). Stretching and flexibility exercises should be performed daily if possible but at a minimum of 2 to 3 days per week. Holding each stretch for 15 to 60 seconds for at least 4 repetitions is recommended (Protas et al., 2009). As the loss of extension is predictable, stretching of cervical, shoulder, trunk, hip, knee, and ankle joints is a must. If the person can lie flat in supine or get into a prone position for any amount of time, it can be beneficial. When implementing a stretching program, it is important to recognize when a deformity is fixed versus flexible. Some patients with PD require multiple pillows to support a permanently kyphotic spinal deformity. Such persons will not be able to regain normal postural alignment, and compensations in sitting and lying need to be made. Before the development of fixed contractures, wall and corner stretches for the pectorals and lying over a bolster or towel roll placed along the length of the spine to stretch the axial skeleton are all appropriate interventions.

Make automatic postural adjustments throughout the day to perform movement transitions of sit to stand, changing directions while walking, turning, talking and walking, carrying books, and going through a cafeteria line. Postural instability may be a major problem for someone who is moving slowly or for someone with advanced disease who is rigid. People with PD lose the ability to perform simple automatic postural adjustments like standing up straight and rising from a chair. Cognitive coaching can be a powerful tool to give the person with PD to think about a way of performing an activity that used to be done automatically. Telling a person to move his head forward and upward may be all that is necessary to help him rise to standing after many unsuccessful attempts. The exact cognitive strategy may differ from person to person, depending on the movement task and where the sequence is breaking down. Motor learning theory would indicate that practice of specific task is needed in an appropriate environmental context. It is very important to teach family members or caregivers the cognitive strategies that have been successful in therapy.

Lee Silverman Voice Treatment (LSVT) BIG

Training BIG is the application of motor training principles used with the voice to train individuals with PD to move more. The premise is that the person with PD perceives that he or she is moving normally and does not recognize how small the movements are being done. By encouraging BIG movements, the person resets kinesthetic awareness of self-generated movements. The individual who uses Lee Silverman Voice Treatment (LSVT) BIG undergoes a certification program to be allowed to use this treatment approach. The person must maintain certification by retaking courses at certain intervals. A study by Farley et al. (2008) showed that a small group of people with mild to moderate PD increased gait speed and reaching after a 4 week program. Those with less severe disease showed greater change. In a case series, Janssen et al. (2014) suggested that the approach might be beneficial for improving function in bed mobility, gait, and balance. LSVT BIG or amplitude-oriented training was found to be effective for persons with mild PD based on a recent systematic review and meta-analysis of three random controlled trials (McDonnell et al., 2018). The conclusions of this review have been questioned (Braun et al., 2018).

As the tremors usually do not interfere with ADLs function, those individuals are not as likely to be seen in physical therapy unless they also have problems with slowness of movement, postural instability, and gait difficulties. The patient and family can be taught strategies to deal with freezing episodes and the slowness in movement transitions, such as coming to stand, turning over in bed, or changing directions while walking. Dyskinesias are the least amenable to therapeutic intervention (Morris et al., 2001).

Fatigue is an important determinant of the physical function of persons with PD (Garber and Friedman, 2003). Fatigue can be the cause or result of inactivity; therefore aerobic conditioning should be begun as soon as the diagnosis of PD is made. The greater the level of fatigue, the less a person with PD participates in leisure activities and in moving around during the day. Additionally, people with PD show a greater decline in activity than age-matched peers (Fertl et al., 1993). However, Canning et al. (1997) thought that with regular aerobic exercise, people with mild to moderate PD have the potential to maintain normal exercise capacity. Recently Ahlskog (2018) provided evidence to support the use of long-term aerobic exercise and cardiovascular fitness training to slow disease progression in PD. Therefore incorporating an aerobic element into movement interventions is strongly suggested. Not only does aerobic exercise provide musculoskeletal benefits but it also can keep airway secretions mobilized while maximizing ventilation.

Exercise Strategies and Results

Exercise is a cornerstone of the intervention strategies used for people with PD. Exercise promotes physical activity, maintains flexibility, improves initiation and fluidity of movement, and decreases postural instability and fatigue. Exercise must be designed within the context of ADLs and should represent the range from practicing writing on lined paper to turning over and getting out of bed. Functional/task-specific training must target functional mobility and its components: strength, endurance, balance, and flexibility. Context-specific tasks/exercises should include gait training, sit to stand, and fine motor dexterity. Individuals with PD who exercise and/or who are physically active have better outcomes (Oguh et al., 2014). Strategies used to enhance performance of daily tasks, such as walking, turning around, standing up and sitting down, turning over, and getting out of bed, are clearly described in Table 14.3. Morris (2000) also recommends exercises for upper extremity function, which are depicted in Table 14.4.

Exercise must challenge postural stability to be successful in reducing falls in people with PD (Paul et al., 2018). Balance training can take many forms from tai chi to slackline training (Gao et al., 2014; Santos et al., 2017). Protas et al. (2005) were successful in training reactive stepping responses in persons with PD using an intense and well-supervised intervention. The intervention resulted in a short term decrease in

TABLE 14.4 Exercises for Upper Extremity Function

Task	Exercises
Buttoning	Button clothing, practicing with buttons of different sizes and shapes.
Handwriting	Practice handwriting by doing crossword puzzles, writing on lined paper, signing name, and filling in forms with multiple boxes.
Reaching/grasping	Reach, grasp, and drink from cups of different sizes, shapes, and weights.
Pouring	Pour water from one cup to another.
Opening/closing	Open and close food jars of different sizes.
Lifting	Lift jars and boxes of different weights onto and off of pantry shelves of different heights.
Fine-motor skills	Pick up grains of rice with the thumb and forefinger and place them in a teacup.
	Pick up a straw between the thumb and forefinger and place it in a soda can.
Dressing	Practice dressing, such as putting on a coat or sweater using verbal cues, such as "left arm," "right arm," and "pull."
Pressing/pushing	Practice pushing the correct sequence of telephone buttons to call family, friends, and local businesses while sitting or standing.
Folding	Fold napkins and place folded paper into envelopes.

Modified from Morris ME: Movement disorders in people with Parkinson disease: a model for physical therapy, *Phys Ther* 80:578–597, 2000, p. 588.

falls. Morris et al. (2015) found that both a movement strategy intervention and an LE strengthening intervention resulted in a similar reduction in falls. Both groups worked at a high rate of perceived exertion. Tai chi can allow a person with PD to explore limits of stability. Slackline training has a low fatigue impact while being safe and challenging. In summary, balance training is effective in reducing fall risk for those with lower levels of disease severity.

Treadmill exercise testing is safe in persons with PD (Bryant et al., 2016). Treadmill training with and without virtual reality is often used as an intervention in rehabilitation. Mirelman et al. (2016) studied individuals with a positive fall history, which included persons with PD. Their intensive treadmill training intervention uses a multimodal intervention to reduce fall risk (Fig. 14.2). V-TIME addresses both motor and cognitive deficits that contribute to fall risk. Using virtual reality, the environment can be altered to present different challenges, obstacles, and provide feedback. The treadmill also affords the motor benefits from walking and actual obstacle negotiation. The group that received treadmill training + virtual reality showed a greater reduction in fall risk than the group that received only treadmill training. Both interventions resulted in decreases in fall risk. In the PD subgroup, treadmill training + virtual reality decreased fall risk by almost 60%. Virtual reality imposes a high cognitive demand for attention, planning, response selection, and sensory processing. Intervention studies that provide larger amounts of exercise practice and supervision show the largest benefits in fall reduction (Paul et al., 2018). Based on their synthesis of studies they recommend a dose of greater than 30 hours over 3 months. Because the tasks used are challenging, high levels of supervision are needed. Individuals with high disease severity appear to only benefit from high-intensity training with complete supervision to reduce falls (Gao et al., 2014; Mirelman et al., 2016; Smania et al., 2010).

Cognitive dysfunction can create challenges to rehabilitation of persons with PD (Peterson et al., 2016). For people with PD who have FoG, the likelihood of having impaired cognitive function is greater than those with PD but without FoG. The potential for developing FoG increases with disease severity and with it the risk for falling. Peterson et al. (2016) outlined the cognitive contributions to FoG and implications for rehabilitation. They recommend combining cognitive and exercise training for those individuals with PD and FoG. Intervention 14.3A depicts examples of agility training with prioritization of the task based on either the motor component or the cognitive component. Agility courses can incorporate tight spaces, doorways, and other potential environments that can typically trigger FoG. Plotnik et al. (2014) improved FoG by using narrow passages. Intervention 14.3B is an example of providing conflicting visual and verbal cues during boxing. Rock steady boxing is an exercise program that has been modified for people with PD. It is often available at local YMCAs. Such a program may or may not include the cognitive component as described by Peterson et al. (2016). Research is needed to determine the effectiveness of integrating cognitive and motor training for people with PD + FoG.

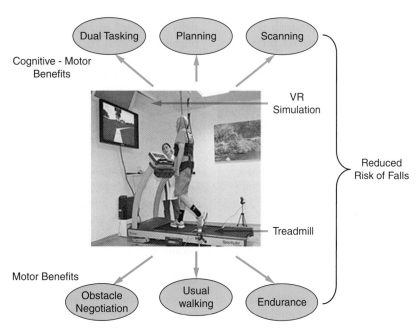

Effects of TT + VR on Fall Risk Mediators

Fig. 14.2. V-TIME: A treadmill training *(TT)* program that uses virtual reality *(VR)*. A patient trains on a treadmill while viewing a virtual environment that presents obstacles, different types of challenges, and feedback. (From Mirelman A, et al.: V-TIME: a treadmill training program augmented by virtual reality to decrease fall risk in older adults: study design of a randomized controlled trial, *BMC Neurol* 13:15, 2013.)

INTERVENTION 14.3   Integration of Cognitive and Mobility Training

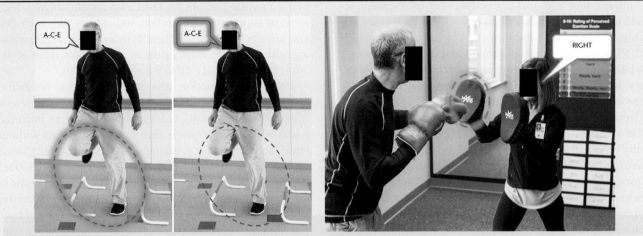

A. The patient completes a secondary cognitive task during agility training and is instructed to switch giving priority to the mobility/stepping component (shown on the left) and the cognitive component (shown on the right).

B. Conflicting visual-auditory cues are given while boxing. The instructor simultaneously visually cues for a left punch and verbally cues for a right punch. For this trial the patient is instructed to respond to the visual cue and ignore the auditory cue.

From Peterson DS, King LA, Cohen RG, Horak FB: Cognitive contributions to freezing of gait in Parkinson disease: implications for physical rehabilitation, *Phys Ther* 96:659–670, 2016.

MULTIPLE SCLEROSIS

MS is a chronic debilitating demyelinating disease of the CNS. It is a disease of young adults between the ages of 20 and 40. The incidence for women is two times higher than for men. The disease is aptly named because sclerotic plaques form throughout the brain and spinal cord. Charcot's triad of intention tremor, scanning speech, and nystagmus were described as early as 1869. Today, visual problems, such as optic neuritis, are often part of the initial event. However, presentation of symptoms is not always consistent within an individual or from one attack to another. Before the availability of magnetic resonance imaging (MRI), it was more difficult to diagnose a person with MS because the person might present with only one symptom, or symptoms might be mild or remit after a time.

MS affects more than 450,000 people in the United States (Fuller et al., 2015). The incidence has been reported to be 4.2 per 100,000 (Hirtz et al., 2007). Rates are higher in the United States, Canada, and northern Europe, possibly because people of northern European heritage are more likely to be affected than other racial groups. Incidence is very low in Asians, Eskimos, and North- and South-American Indians (Sutton, 2009). A US study found that black women have a higher risk for MS than black men, whose risk is similar to whites (Langer-Gould et al., 2013). MS does, however, have a worldwide distribution. More cases of MS are found in temperate climates with fewer cases closer to the equator. Although the etiology is still as yet unknown, viral infections and autoimmune dysfunction have been implicated. Viral infections can trigger an MS attack, and immune cells are present in acute MS lesions (Fuller et al., 2015). Susceptibility

to immune system dysfunction may be inherited but not the disease of MS.

Pathophysiology

Patches of demyelination occur in the white matter of the brain and spinal cord. Areas of the nervous system with a high concentration of myelin appear white because it is partially composed of fat. In the CNS, myelin is produced by oligodendrocytes. Their destruction leaves the axon unprotected and vulnerable to possible damage. Inflammation accompanies the destruction of the myelin sheath and can lead to axon damage and plaque formation. Plaques are replaced by scar tissue produced by glial cells, and the trapped axons degenerate (Fuller et al., 2015). Glial cells constitute the connective tissue of the nervous system. Because the immune system response in the brain of a patient with MS is more robust than normal, it may also play a role in plaque formation. Plaques are part of acute or chronic lesions that may be evident on MRI. The areas of the nervous system more likely to be involved include the optic nerve, periventricular white matter, corticospinal tracts, posterior columns, and cerebellar peduncles.

Clinical Features

Sensory symptoms are often the first signs of MS. The person may complain of "pins and needles" (paresthesias) or abnormal burning or aching (dysesthesias). Visual symptoms occur in 80% of individuals with the disease and can present as decreased visual acuity, inflammation of the optic nerve (neuritis) that causes graying or blurring of the vision, or double vision (diplopia). Nystagmus, also a common symptom, is caused by a lesion of the cerebellum or central vestibular pathways. Nystagmus is an oscillating movement of an eye at rest. The type of nystagmus depends on the direction the eye is moving. Horizontal nystagmus is the most common type although the person may exhibit vertical or rotatory eye movements. Nystagmus is named for the direction of the fast component of the oscillating movement.

Motor pathways are involved, as well as sensory pathways in MS. Motor weakness, typically in one or both legs, indicates involvement of the corticospinal tract. Clumsiness in reaching is often seen with the person overshooting the target. Coordination of alternating movements like flexion and extension is impaired, resulting in walking difficulty. Gait is often characterized by poor balance and lurching. Ataxia or general incoordination is evident when there is involvement of the white matter of the cerebellum. A postural tremor of an extremity or the trunk may be evident in sitting or standing. Difficulty coordinating oral movements may interfere with speaking and swallowing. Scanning speech is slow with long pauses and lacks fluidity. There is an increased risk for aspiration in a person who cannot adequately coordinate breathing and eating.

Fatigue

Fatigue is a major problem in people with MS. It is the most frequently reported symptom, slightly ahead of walking difficulty. Over 80% of individuals with MS have fatigue (Yang et al., 2017). Although fatigue is a major symptom of the disease, its relationship to disease severity is weak. In other words, someone does not need to have a severe case of the disease to be severely fatigued. In fact, the fatigue is often out of proportion to the extent of the disease. Despite a decade of research, the underlying pathophysiologic process of fatigue in MS remains obscure. There is no laboratory or physiologic marker of fatigue in patients with MS. Fatigue is worsened by heat. This fact distinguishes it from fatigue seen in healthy individuals or those with other progressive neurologic diseases. Uhthoff phenomenon is the heat-related onset of blurred vision, increased paresthesias, or overwhelming fatigue. It is considered a pseudoattack that is resolved when the body temperature returns to normal.

Fatigue has a profound effect on the individual's ability to complete ADLs and to continue to be employed. It is very important to understand the patient's perception of fatigue because MS fatigue is closely linked to how the person perceives his QOL and general and mental health (Bakshi, 2003). In a meta-analysis, exercise was found to modify behavior and positively affect the QOL in individuals with MS (Motl and Gosney, 2008). Cakit et al. (2010) found that exercise decreased depression, and Dalgas et al. (2010) saw an improvement in mood, fatigue, and QOL. There is evidence to support Amantadine (Symmetrel) and modafinil (Provigil) to treat MS fatigue (Yang et al., 2017; Shangyan et al., 2018).

Cognitive Impairment

Prevalence of cognitive impairment in patients with MS can be as high as 70% (Chiaravalloti et al., 2015). These deficits range from mild to moderate in severity and may involve problem solving, short-term memory, visual-spatial perception, and conceptual reasoning. Information processing speed is most commonly affected, as evidenced by bradyphrenia or slow thinking (Bergendal et al., 2007). General intellectual ability, conversational ability, long-term memory, and reading comprehension are usually preserved. Cognitive impairment is related to location of brain regions, not disease severity or disability status (McIsaac et al., 2019). Lesions in the frontal lobe can affect executive brain functions such as judgment and reasoning, making the patient cognitively inflexible. Global deterioration of intelligence or dementia is rare but may occur if the disease is the rapidly progressive type.

People who have chronic diseases are more prone to depression, and individuals with MS have more bouts of depression than the general population (Boeschoten et al., 2017; Patten et al., 2017). The rates reported in these reviews range from 30% to 50%. Higher levels of helplessness were associated with more fatigue and depressive mood (Van der Werf et al., 2003). The experience of fatigue and depression may be mediated by similar factors. Greeke et al. (2017) assessed depression and fatigue in patients with MS longitudinally and found that depression scores declined over time and were moderately correlated to fatigue. Subjects with low depression and high fatigue scores at baseline were more likely to develop high depression scores at follow-up than subjects with low fatigue and depression scores at baseline. Depression is also related to emotional stability. Patients with MS can demonstrate emotional lability, being euphoric one minute and crying uncontrollably the next.

Autonomic Dysfunction

Bowel and bladder problems in patients with MS are indicative of involvement of the autonomic nervous system. The bladder can fail to empty completely, leading to urinary retention, and thus setting up a perfect culture medium for bacterial growth. The reflex control of the bowel and bladder can be impaired and lead to constipation or inadequate emptying, urinary frequency, and nocturia (frequency at night). Complete loss of bowel and bladder control, as well as sexual dysfunction, are possible in the later stages of the disease. Some medications used to treat these bladder problems can be found in Table 14.2.

Disease Course

The course of the disease is unpredictable because its presentation is highly variable. The first demyelinating attack that may indicate MS has been termed the *clinically isolated syndrome*. It often presents as optic neuritis. It can be an isolated occurrence and be deemed inactive if no other episode occurs. If it is active the person goes on to develop *relapsing-remitting multiple sclerosis* (RRMS). RRMS constitutes 85% of cases of MS in which there are definable periods of exacerbations and remissions. Exacerbations occur when symptoms worsen acutely and then remit or recover with a time of symptom stability. Symptoms may completely resolve or there may be residual neurologic deficits. The amount of time that passes between attacks or relapses can be as long as 1 year at the beginning of the disease. The time between attacks may shorten as the disease progresses. Despite the relapsing-remitting course, there is evidence that the disease is active even when symptoms appear stable, considering that 60% go on to develop secondary progressive MS within 2 decades of being diagnosed (Fuller et al., 2015).

Secondary progressive MS begins with relapses and remissions but then becomes progressive with only occasional relapses and minor remissions. This type has also been further divided into subtypes that will not be discussed. The last type of MS is the least common type, affecting about 15% of individuals with MS. Primary progressive MS is characterized by a relentless progression from the onset without distinct attacks. It too is also divided into subtypes that will not be discussed. The progressive-relapsing subtype has been eliminated (Lublin et al., 2013).

The Kurtzke Expanded Disability Status Scale is used to provide an overall rating of disability in MS (Kurtzke, 1983). It is a standard in MS research and describes neurologic function and impairment with a focus on ambulation and need for assistive devices. Scores range from 0 (normal neurologic function) to 10.0 (death from MS) and increase by 0.5 points. Scores less than 4.0 are considered indicative of mild MS, scores between 4 and 5.5 are moderate MS, and 6.0 or above is severe MS. Patients with scores of 7 or above are unable to walk. Most participants in research studies are usually within the mild to moderate categories. The form is available at: https://www.nationalmssociety.org/NationalMSSociety/media/MSNationalFiles/Brochures/10-2-3-29-EDSS_Form.pdf.

Diagnosis

The diagnosis of MS continues to be based on clinical evidence of multiple lesions in the CNS white matter, distinct time (temporal) intervals, and occurrence in an individual between the ages of 10 and 50 years old. The cerebrospinal fluid is usually examined for the presence of higher amounts of myelin protein and oligoclonal bands. The former would be elevated during an acute episode and be indicative of immune system involvement. If sensory pathways are involved, recording evoked sensory potentials may provide further evidence of demyelination. As vision is often affected, assessing visual-evoked potentials can be a helpful part of the diagnostic process. MRI is the best tool to assist in confirming the diagnosis of MS. An MRI can visualize small and large lesions. With the proper enhancement, it is possible to tell if the lesions are new and active. McDonald criteria for MS are used to make the diagnosis easier (Polman et al., 2011). These criteria have been updated recently (Thompson et al., 2018) and the presence of oligoclonal bands in the cerebrospinal fluid is now recognized as specific to MS.

Medical Management

Medications are the mainstay in the management of MS. The majority of these disease-modifying drugs are synthetic immune system modulators developed for the most common form of MS, which is relapsing-remitting. They are approved by the US Food and Drug Administration for that form but are used off-label for other forms of MS. The purpose of a disease modifying agent is to modify the disease and reduce the frequency and severity of attacks. Avonex, Betaseron, and Copaxone modify the disease. Copaxone has been shown to reduce the frequency of attacks. All of the drugs are injected. Avonex is taken weekly, Betaseron every other day, and Copaxone daily. These medications are currently recognized as standard treatment for patients with RRMS. Newer medications such as Tysabri and Novantrone have to be delivered intravenously while the person is in a medical center because constant monitoring is indicated. Individuals may need to try several disease-modifying drugs to find one that is best tolerated.

A person with MS may exhibit myriad symptoms that reflect the diverse areas of the nervous system that are involved. Common symptoms that are treated pharmacologically include muscle spasms, spasticity, weakness, fatigue, visual symptoms, urinary symptoms, pain, and depression. Refer to Table 14.2 for a partial list of medications that might be prescribed for a patient with MS. Symptoms related to muscle spasms or spasticity can be managed by using physical therapy interventions in addition to medication.

Physical Therapy Management

The goals of rehabilitation in the patient with MS are to:
1. minimize progression;
2. maintain an optimum level of functional independence;
3. prevent or decrease secondary complications;
4. maintain respiratory function;
5. conserve energy/manage fatigue; and
6. educate the patient and their family.

These goals are met by managing the symptoms that the patient presents with in such a way that the impact on function is minimized.

Weakness

The most common neurologic symptoms of MS are weakness, spasticity, and ataxia. Weakness can result directly from lesions involving the corticospinal tract or cerebellum. Weakness also develops secondary to inactivity and generalized deconditioning. Therefore strengthening is an important goal of physical therapy, and exercise should be initiated early before secondary impairments develop (McIsaac et al., 2019). Many types of exercise training can be used.

People with MS require comprehensive rehabilitation that includes exercise training, aerobic conditioning, fatigue management, and gait training. In a study by Hameau et al. (2017), walking performance was predicted by the strength of the weakest limb and the Expanded Disability Status Scale score. There is credible evidence that physical therapy improves activity and participation of people with MS (Khan and Amatya, 2017). Exercise and physical activity increases mobility, strength, and aerobic capacity (Amatya et al., 2019), which in turn improves QOL. High-intensity exercise has been shown to be safe if well-controlled and supervised (Wens et al., 2015). In two recent systematic reviews, aerobic high-intensity exercise was found to be safe and effective for those with mild disability due to MS (Campbell et al., 2018), and exercise training demonstrated positive benefits in adults with severe mobility problems and MS (Edwards and Pilutti, 2017). Most exercise programs previously in the literature have targeted those individuals with mild to moderate disability and have utilized low to moderate intensity exercise (Cakit et al., 2010; Dalgas et al., 2010). Short-term exercise programs have had a positive effect on aerobic fitness, health perception, fatigue, and activity level in individuals with MS (Mostert and Kesselring, 2002).

It is possible to increase strength and endurance in patients with MS. RT can use isokinetic or progressive resistive modes or water. A recent pilot study found that combining high-intensity interval training with RT improved not only physical capacity but QOL in men and women with MS (Zaenker et al., 2018). Exercises can be made more functional by having the person perform PNF patterns because functional movements almost always have some rotational component (see Chapter 10). Additionally, the rotation may help to reduce tone. Resistance within the PNF diagonals should be graded to match the patient's abilities. Energy consumption can be decreased during functional activities by placing an emphasis on strengthening proximal muscle groups. Exercise for this population should also have an aerobic component as a means of preventing or treating deconditioning.

Individuals with MS have been shown to have a normal cardiovascular response to exercise.

Aerobic capacity is severely reduced in those with MS fatigue (Driehuis et al., 2018). Aerobic capacity was significantly related to participation in indoor and outdoor activities, social life, and physical functioning. Physical activity in people with MS appears to be more related to demographic characteristics and MS severity than behavioral-cognitive status (Beckerman et al., 2010). People with MS are at greater risk for developing impaired glucose tolerance. Wens et al. (2017) studied the effect of a 12-week high-intensity aerobic and resistance exercise program on glucose tolerance in three groups: a control group, a high-intensity interval plus resistance group, and a high-intensity continuous aerobic training plus resistance group. Glucose tolerance was improved in both of the intervention groups. In an earlier study by Wens et al. (2015), interval training showed greater improvements in endurance than continuous training.

Intensity of exercise is being recognized more and more as an important factor to improve fitness, decrease hypertension, and improve glucose tolerance.

An exercise test is indicated before having the person take part in an aerobic training program because as the disease progresses, the potential for autonomic cardiovascular dysfunction increases. Use of established protocols, as in cardiac rehabilitation, is indicated to assess a person's ability to respond to increasing working loads by using either a treadmill or a cycle ergometer. Based on recent literature, the exercise protocol used to assess initial exercise tolerance may not need to be limited to low-level ones.

Increases in core body temperature in patients with MS can result in a temporary increase in clinical symptoms.

Precooling (lowering the body temperature) was found to be effective in preventing increases in core temperature during exercise (White et al., 2000). A recent systematic review concluded that precooling can prevent an increase in symptoms related to exercise-induced overheating (Kaltsatou and Flouris, 2019). To avoid any adverse effects of heat, exercise should be performed in cool environments. Additional cooling sources, such as fans and even personal cooling suits, can be used. Heat sensitivity is related to MS fatigue. Exercise in a cool pool that is between 80°F and 85°F is recommended for patients with MS. Exercise testing has been used to guide aquatic therapy with individuals with MS that resulted in improved cardiovascular fitness (Pariser et al., 2006). Water provides challenges and support to balance and can be an effective medium for exercise. A recent systematic review found good evidence that aquatic therapy improved QOL in 8 out of 10 studies (Corvillo et al., 2017).

Patients with MS can experience fatigue related to the disease process. Secondarily, fatigue is related to deconditioning and respiratory muscle weakness and overuse. Training of respiratory muscles is indicated for patients with MS as dysfunction of respiratory muscles will decrease exercise tolerance (Martin-Valero et al., 2014). There is some evidence that resistive inspiratory muscle strengthening is effective in those with mild to moderate MS (Rietberg et al., 2017). Exercising to fatigue is contraindicated. Submaximal levels of exercise appear to be the safest with a discontinuous schedule of training. Submaximal levels are less than 85% of the person's age-predicted heart rate (220 minus age), or less than 85% of the maximum heart rate achieved on a graded exercise test. For deconditioned patients, starting at 50% to 60% of their maximum heart rate may produce aerobic conditioning. A discontinuous schedule builds in sufficient rest times to prevent or lessen fatigue. The person's heart rate, blood pressure, and perceived exertion using the Borg scale should be used as a way to monitor exercise response. Nonfatiguing exercise protocols are discussed under Post-Polio Syndrome.

Spasticity

Stretching can be preparation for exercise, especially in muscles that exhibit increased tone. Individuals with MS have spasticity secondary to the UMN lesions and decreased flexibility secondary to decreased movement and activity. Slow static stretching is indicated with no bouncing. The patient and family should be taught self-stretching with particular attention to stretching the cervical region, hamstrings, and heel cords. Self-stretching combined with slow rhythmic rotation can be an effective means to gain range. The new stretched position should be held for 30 to 60 seconds to allow the muscle to adjust to the new length. PNF techniques, such as hold relax and contract relax, can be used to gain ROM. Refer to Chapter 10 for more information on PNF techniques.

The muscle groups exhibiting spasticity vary from patient to patient. However, the plantar flexors, adductors, and quadriceps are often involved in the lower extremity. Stretching the hamstrings can be accomplished several different ways, as seen in Intervention 14.4. Methods include static stretching

INTERVENTION 14.4   **Stretching Activities**

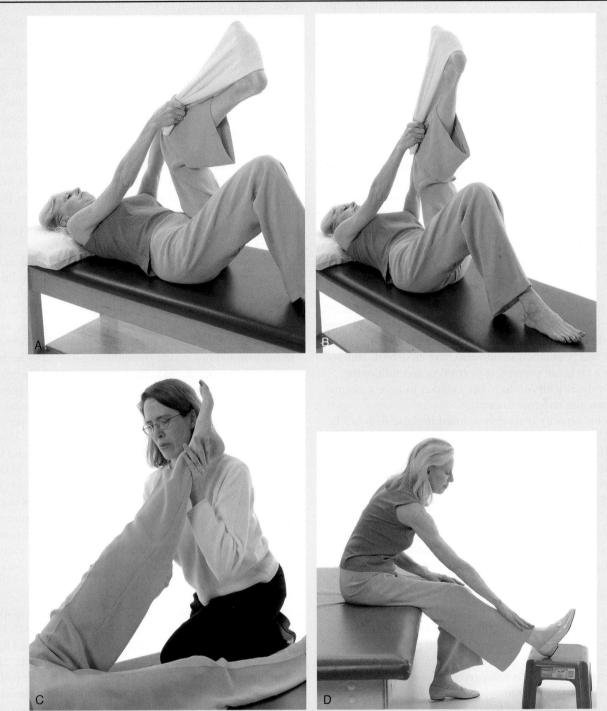

Supine static stretch of the heel cords and hamstrings using a towel:

A. The patient lies on a firm surface in the hook-lying position. Then while one leg is bent, the other leg is raised. A towel is placed around the foot. The free ends are grasped and pulled gently to stretch the ankle into dorsiflexion. The stretch is held for 30 to 60 seconds.

B. To stretch the hamstrings, the patient slowly straightens the raised leg as far as possible and holds the stretch for 30 to 60 seconds. The stretch is repeated with the other leg.

Supine static stretch of the hamstrings using another person:

C. The patient lies on a firm surface. The clinician raises one leg keeping the knee straight as in a straight-leg raise. The end position is held for 30 to 60 seconds. The other leg may be bent or straight, as pictured. If a pull is felt in the low back, the patient should bend the leg that is not being stretched to avoid lumbar strain. The clinician may use the proprioceptive neuromuscular facilitation technique hold relax in this position to gain additional range of motion (see Chapter 10 for an explanation of the technique).

INTERVENTION 14.4 Stretching Activities—cont'd

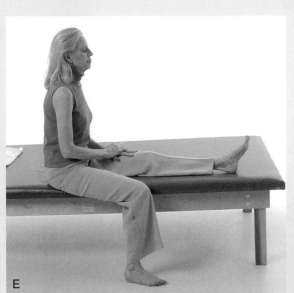
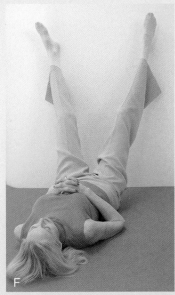
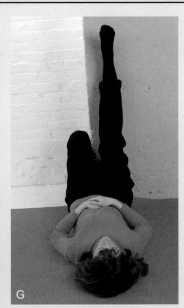

E F G

Sitting stretch of the hamstrings using a stool:

D. The patient sits with the heel of one leg resting on a stool or other stable raised object. The trunk is kept erect and the patient leans forward while maintaining a lumbar lordosis as much as possible. The patient reaches with one or both hands toward the ankle of the raised leg and tries to keep the knee as straight as possible to maximize the stretch of the hamstrings. The stretch is held for 30 to 60 seconds and repeated several times. The stretch is then repeated with the other leg. When stretching the heel cords in this position, the patient uses a towel around the foot as in Intervention 14.3A and pulls the foot gently into dorsiflexion while keeping the knee as straight as possible.

Sitting stretch of the hamstrings on a low mat:

E. The patient sits on a low mat with one leg on the floor and one leg on the mat table. The trunk is kept erect and the patient leans forward at the hips to ensure that the stretch occurs in the hamstrings and not the low back. The patient may reach with one or both hands toward the ankle. Again, the heel cord can be stretched by using a towel (as in Intervention 14.4A) in this position. The stretch is held for 30 to 60 seconds and then repeated with the other leg.

Wall stretch of the hamstrings and hip adductors:

F. The patient lies on the floor on her back with the legs supported by the wall. The hips should be as close to the wall as possible to obtain the greatest stretch of the hamstrings. The patient may need assistance to get into and out of this position. The patient should not lift the pelvis or arch the back. When the patient slides the legs out to either side, the hip adductors are stretched. Depending on the patient's ability, the legs can be moved one at a time or together. The legs are slowly separated and the stretched position held for 30 to 60 seconds.

Hamstring stretch against a wall:

G. The patient lies on the floor on her back (preferably in a doorway). One of the patient's legs protrudes through the doorway; it can be bent at the knee, as pictured, or straight. The leg to be stretched is propped up against the wall or door frame with its knee straight. The patient brings her hips as close to the wall/door frame as possible to obtain the best possible stretch.

in supine and in sitting. Hip flexors and hamstrings can also be kept flexible by using a program that consists of lying in a prone position on a firm surface several times a day for at least 20 to 30 minutes. A tilt table can be used if the person is unable to get into a prone position, but straps are necessary to maintain hips and knees in extension. Some benefit is derived from weight-bearing in an upright position for tone management. Heel cords can be stretched passively using the tilt table. If the ankles are plantar flexed, a wedge may be used to ensure weight is borne through the entire foot. Over time, the size of the wedge may be decreased.

Lower trunk rotation is quite effective in reducing tone in the trunk and proximal pelvic girdle muscles. Use of a ball in modified hook lying is shown in Intervention 14.5. The ball supports the weight of the legs, keeping them in flexion as the assistant guides the ball and the patient's limbs to either side, producing trunk rotation. A person can also practice trunk rotation when moving from a hands-and-knees position to side sitting, as seen in Intervention 14.6. The person may need assistance to attain the four-point position and may need to be guarded while moving through the available range. If the person cannot get all the way to side sitting, pillows or a wedge can be used to allow the person to go through as much range as possible. Hand position can be varied. Hands can be on the support surface or on a raised bench. In the case of the latter, the person can move from kneeling to side sitting.

INTERVENTION 14.5   Rhythmical Rotation of the Lower Trunk

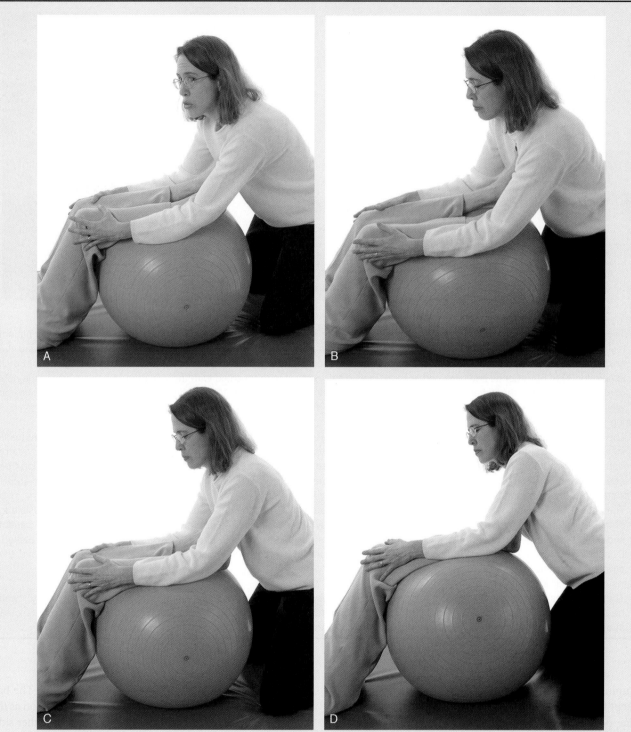

The patient lies supine on a firm surface. A therapy ball is used to support the lower extremities. The ball should be large enough to support the lower legs but small enough to keep the hips and knees in a flexed position. This technique is used as a preparation for functional movements, such as rolling and coming to sit.

A. The clinician places the patient's knees and lower legs on the ball and uses manual hand contact on the outside of the patient's knees.

B. The clinician gently rotates the patient's lower extremities, supported by the ball to one side.

C. The clinician moves the patient's lower extremities back to center.

D. Then the clinician gently rotates the patient's lower extremities, which are still supported by the ball to the other side. Trunk rotation will occur with greater amounts of rotation.

INTERVENTION 14.6   Movement Transition From Four-Point to Side Sitting

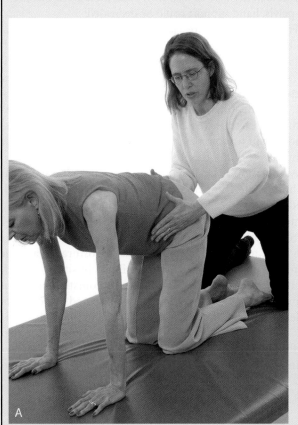

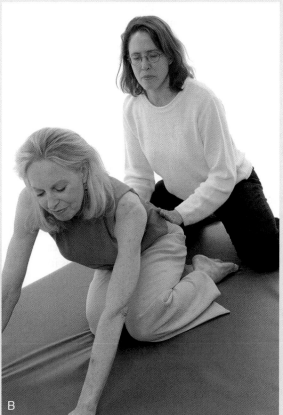

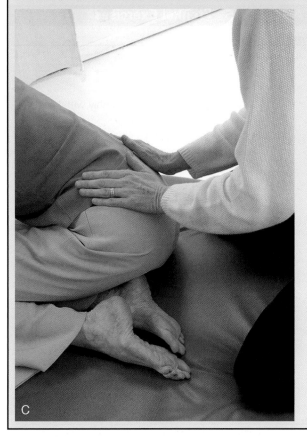

Movement transitions, such as from four-point to side sitting, can be used to practice trunk rotation. The clinician's hand placement provides manual cues for either moving into side sitting or back into four-point.

A. The patient begins in a hands-and-knees or four-point position. The clinician uses manual hand contacts on the sides of the hips to guide the patient.

B. The clinician guides the patient to rotate diagonally backward from four-point into a side-sitting position.

C. The clinician then guides the patient's return from side sitting to the four-point position. The movements can be assisted at first and then resisted.

Ataxia

Control of static postures or postural stability is difficult for the patient with MS exhibiting ataxia. Postures that enable the person to load the trunk and other extremities not involved in movement are helpful in providing stability. Unilateral limb holding in mid ranges and weight-bearing, especially in antigravity postures, with slow-controlled weight shifting can be beneficial. The limits of stability of these individuals can be quite precarious. The developmental sequence, especially the prone progression, can provide a wealth of treatment ideas. PNF techniques that are helpful with this problem include alternating isometrics, rhythmic stabilization, and slow reversal hold in an ever-decreasing range.

Functional movement transitions are very important to focus on for the patient with MS to ensure safety. Should the patient have the upper extremities loaded when moving from sit to stand to give more stability to the upper trunk? Does the person reach more smoothly if the nonreaching arm is in weight-bearing (loaded)? Does the person have more distal control if the elbow is loaded? Can the person benefit from the use of weights around the waist or trunk? Weight belts and vests are available that may increase proprioceptive awareness and enhance stability in sitting, standing, and walking. Light distal weights have been used to improve coordination of the upper extremities during reaching, and of the lower extremities during walking. Although such weights can provide some improved awareness, they can also produce a rebound phenomenon when removed. Dysmetric movements (overshooting) may appear to worsen after weights are removed, so caution must be practiced when deciding to weight a limb distally. Using the least amount of weight to achieve the desired effect and loading the axial skeleton (trunk) rather than the extremities is preferable. TheraBand (Performance Health, Akron, OH) wrapped around a limb can provide resistance to movement in both directions, such as reaching out and returning the arm to the lap. Of course, graded manual resistance can do the same thing but that requires having an assistant or caregiver available any time the person wants to reach, which is not practical.

Balance training incorporates dynamic as well as static interventions. However, movable surfaces are more challenging for the patient and the assistant. The patient must be safe at all times, which may necessitate the need of additional support staff. Use of a tilt board, a biomechanical ankle platform system (BAPS) board (BAPS Spectrum Therapy, Adrian, MI), a ball, or a balance master may all be indicated, but safety must always be the first consideration. If the person is not safe when trying to control movement on a movable surface, a nonmovable surface may be indicated. Another modification that can be used would be to have the person seated while an extremity or extremities are placed on a movable surface. For example, the person could be seated on a low mat table with hand support and the feet could be placed on a tilt board or a BAPS board. Another modification would be to use a DynaDisc (Exertools, Petaluma, CA) or an inflatable disc for the person to sit on while the feet are supported on

the floor and the hands are on the support surface. As the person is better able to deal with a disturbance of balance at the pelvis, hand support could be decreased.

Frenkel exercises are classic coordination exercises that can be done in four standard positions: lying, sitting, standing, and walking. Although described for the lower extremities, similar ones can be developed for the upper extremities. These exercises are intended to be done slowly with even timing. The patient may initially need to have a limb supported so that the exercises can be progressed from assisted to independent and from unilateral to bilateral. See Table 14.5 for a complete list of these exercises.

Ambulation is challenging for a person with ataxia. As an immediate compensation, the base of support is widened, and the knees are often stiffened to increase stability. Some individuals may compensate by bending the knees, thereby lowering the body's center of gravity. The arms are also used to counteract the increased postural sway. The increased postural sway is also exhibited in sitting and often necessitates that the person leans on outstretched arms to provide stability. A recent study compared the effect of different exercise interventions on ataxia in MS (Salci et al., 2017). The researchers found that by combining either lumbar stabilization or task-specific training with balance training was more successful than balance training alone.

TABLE 14.5	**Frenkel Exercises**
Position	**Movements**
Supine	
	1. Flex and extend one leg, heel sliding down a straight line on a table.
	2. Abduct and adduct hip smoothly with knee bent, heel on a table.
	3. Abduct and adduct leg with knee and hip extended, leg sliding on a table.
	4. Flex and extend hip and knee with heel off a table.
	5. Place one heel on knee of opposite leg and slide heel smoothly down shin toward ankle and back to knee.
	6. Flex and extend both legs together, heels sliding on table.
	7. Flex one leg while extending other leg.
	8. Flex and extend one leg while abducting and adducting other leg.
Sitting	
	1. Place foot in therapist's hand, which will change position on each trial.
	2. Raise leg and put foot on traced footprint on floor.
	3. Sit steady for a few minutes.

Modified from Umphred DA: *Neurological rehabilitation*, ed 5, St. Louis, 2001, Mosby, p. 735.

Despite difficulties, a majority of patients with MS are still able to walk after 20 years (Schapiro, 2003).

Mobility options are many and varied. For persons with ataxia, a weighted walker may be the best option as it affords stability and mobility. A wheeled walker with hand brakes and a seat can provide for frequent rest periods. A motorized scooter or other forms of power mobility may be indicated when fatigue is the overriding problem or tremors and weakness make propulsion of a standard wheelchair difficult. Wheelchairs should be prescribed using typical seating guidelines with a seatbelt for safety. A cushion should always be used to provide extra protection from pressure when an individual becomes wheelchair-dependent. Using a three-wheeled scooter may have less social stigma than using a wheelchair.

There are also many types of orthotic options. Probably the most typical type of orthosis used by someone with MS is an ankle-foot orthosis (AFO). Indications for use of an AFO include saving energy, improving foot/toe clearance, providing greater ankle stability, controlling knee hyperextension, and improving overall gait pattern. Guidelines for use of an AFO can be found in Table 14.6. The rehabilitation team consisting of the physical therapist and the orthotist will make a final recommendation. Rocker clogs have also been found to be helpful in accommodating for loss of ankle mobility (Perry et al., 1981). Some have reported use of a reciprocal gait orthosis, a type of hip-knee-ankle-foot orthosis, for patients with MS.

Additional Concerns

Some patients with MS exhibit emotional lability. They can demonstrate rather volatile swings in mood, ranging from euphoria to crying. These abrupt changes in behavior need to be managed with calmness and firm direction in order for them to not totally disrupt a treatment session. In some cases, the patient can benefit from psychologic intervention. Another challenging situation occurs when a patient continuously exhibits nystagmus. The patient extends the head to minimize the amount of movement of the eyes. The tilted head posture should not be corrected, as that will remove the compensation and may negatively affect the patient's balance. Other patients may experience vertigo with sudden head movements. In this situation, the person needs to move the head more slowly or actually fix the head in a position before attempting a movement so as to not produce a loss of balance.

Summary

Exercise is a crucial part of the physical therapy intervention for a person with MS. Exercise balanced with rest can improve the QOL of an individual dealing with this chronic disease. Although symptoms vary depending on the sites in the nervous system that are involved, fatigue is a pervasive problem. Whether the fatigue is stress-related or heat-related, it can produce immobility, which may all too quickly become

TABLE 14.6 Guidelines for Use of Ankle-Foot Orthoses

Type of AFO	Advantages	Disadvantages	Relative Contraindications
Standard polypropylene	Saves energy Improves toe and foot clearance Improves safety Improved knee control during midstance Avoids knee hyperextension Greater ankle stability	Impedes tibial advancement during sit to stand	Moderate or severe spasticity Severe edema in the foot Severe weakness (2/5 or less) at the hips
Polypropylene with articulating ankle joint	All of the above Tibial advancement during sit to stand More normal ankle movement during gait Able to squat May have a plantar flexion stop or a dorsiflexion assist		Same as above
Double upright metal with articulating ankle joint	All of the above May have straps to correct valgus or varus May accommodate significant fluctuations in limb volume		Weight Poor cosmesis

AFO, Ankle-foot orthoses.
Data from Schapiro R: *Multiple sclerosis: a rehabilitation approach to management,* New York, 1991, Demos Publications; Edelstein JE, Wong CK: Orthotics. In O'Sullivan SB, Schmitz TJ, Fulk GD, editors: *Physical rehabilitation,* ed 6, Philadelphia, 2014, FA Davis, pp. 1325–1363; and Lusardi MM, Bowers DM: Orthotic decision making in neurological and neuromuscular disorders. In Lusardi MM, Jorge M, Nielsen CC, editors: *Orthotics and prosthetics in rehabilitation,* ed 3, Philadelphia, 2013, Saunders, pp. 266–307.

part of a cycle of disuse and deconditioning. Therefore regular exercise at an appropriate intensity is essential to preserving function in this population.

AMYOTROPHIC LATERAL SCLEROSIS

ALS is a terminal progressive disease involving both UMNs and LMNs. It is commonly known as Lou Gehrig disease. UMNs degenerate in the cortex and corticospinal tract, LMNs degenerate in the brainstem (cranial nerve nuclei) and anterior horn cells in the spinal cord. Therefore signs of both UMN and LMN involvement will be evident. The loss of LMNs results in muscle atrophy and weakness (amyotrophy) and the destruction of the corticospinal and corticobulbar tracts, which results in the lateral sclerosis (UMN symptoms) (Fuller et al., 2015). Muscle weakness is the cardinal sign of ALS (Dal Bello-Haas, 2014). ALS is a rare adult-onset progressive motor neuron disease that can also demonstrate multisystem involvement. Life expectancy is usually 2 to 5 years after the onset of symptoms. The only approved medication, riluzole, appears to have a modest effect on survival (Miller et al., 2012).

Incidence and Etiology

ALS is the most common motor neuron disease in adults, with an incidence of 2 per 100,000 individuals. There are an estimated 30,000 people with ALS in the United States, with a prevalence of 5 per 100,000 people (Mehta et al., 2018). ALS usually occurs between the middle and late sixth decade of age. Men are slightly more likely to be affected than women. The cause of ALS is unknown, with the exception of the inherited form, which is an autosomal trait. In about 20% of inherited cases, the person has a mutation of a gene involved in producing enzymes that eliminate free radicals. The majority of people with ALS have no prior family history. There is as yet no clear cause of ALS (Fuller et al., 2015).

Clinical Presentation

ALS can present with limb loss onset or bulbar loss onset. The majority of people with ALS (70% to 80%) present asymmetric weakness in an arm or a leg. A smaller percentage (20% to 30%) present difficulty swallowing or speaking. Fasciculation (twitching of muscle fibers) may be seen in the tongue. Earliest signs of ALS include muscle cramps, weakness, atrophy, and fatigue. Involvement spreads regionally with distal symptoms occurring before proximal ones. Bulbar signs commonly occur later in the disease progression, unless the initial presentation of loss is in the cranial nerves, which are responsible for tongue movements, chewing, and swallowing.

There is no one definitive laboratory test for ALS. Diagnosis is based on the combination of signs and symptoms in the UMNs and LMNs, supplemented by electromyography (EMG), nerve conduction velocity tests, neuroimaging, and nerve and muscle biopsies. According to the revised El Escorial criteria, a "definite" diagnosis of ALS requires LMN + UMN findings in three regions (Brooks et al., 2000;

Fuller et al., 2015). Regions include bulbar, cervical, thoracic, or lumbosacral.

In "pure" ALS, there is no sensory involvement or eye muscle involvement. Spinocerebellar and sensory systems are sparred. Previously, the presence of cognitive deficits would exclude a diagnosis of ALS. However, up to half of patients with ALS have cognitive impairments (Phukan et al., 2012; Montuschi et al., 2015). Fifteen percent meet the criteria for frontotemporal dementia (FTD). FTD is characterized by behavioral and personality changes, as well as decline in executive function. FTD can present before the ALS or with the ALS or develop after the ALS. Previously, the presence of cognitive deficits would exclude a diagnosis of ALS. A therapist should be suspicious of cognitive involvement in a patient with ALS who exhibits delays in executive function, such as not following through on exercise or medication recommendations and verbal fluency (Abrahams et al., 2000). Research has shown shared genetic, clinical, and neuropathologic features of ALS and FTD (Beeldman et al., 2016; Majounie et al., 2012). Scientists now recognize a continuum in which "pure" ALS with no cognitive involvement is at one end, and "pure" FTD is at the other end with no motor involvement. The diagnosis of FTD, along with ALS, decreases median survival time (Elamin et al., 2011; Olney et al., 2005). Multisystem involvement in ALS is further reinforced by data that shows cerebellar involvement (Prell and Grosskreutz, 2013).

Because of the relentless progression of ALS, staging is best thought of as early, middle, and late. More in-depth staging has been devised for drug research, but to provide a framework for intervention, three stages works well. Early on, the person has mild to moderate weakness in specific muscle groups. Realize that a person may have lost 80% of motor neurons before reporting weakness (Hallum and Allen, 2013), so there may not be an extreme impact on gait, ADLs, or speech. By the end of the early stage, the person is experiencing difficulty with ADLs and mobility. During the middle stage, mobility continues to decrease with a wheelchair needed for long distances. People with ALS are at a high risk for falls, owing to a decreased ability to use vestibular input (Sanjak et al., 2014). ADLs continue to decline. Pain is manifested because of decreased ROM, faulty posture, or spasticity. Late stage is marked by total dependence in mobility and ADLs, dysarthria and dysphagia, respiratory compromise, and pain. The patient may be restricted to bed. Death results from respiratory failure as muscles of ventilation, the diaphragm, intercostals, and accessory muscles, become weak.

Medical Management

There is no cure for ALS, and medical management focuses on symptom management. A multidisciplinary clinic is best equipped to provide the most optimal and comprehensive care for individuals with ALS and their families. Riluzole (Rilutek, Sanofi-Aventis, Paris, France) is the only disease-modifying medication presently approved for the treatment of ALS. Other medications may be prescribed for muscle cramping, spasticity, sialorrhea, and depression. With bulbar involvement, swallowing and nutrition issues are best addressed by a speech-language pathologist and a nutritionist or registered dietitian. The need for augmented feeding via a percutaneous endoscopic gastrostomy tube may be considered in the middle stage of the disease. Some individuals choose invasive mechanical ventilation during the later stage of the disease.

Physical Therapy Management

During the early stages of the disease, individuals may participate in preventive exercise programs to forestall activity limitations. Exercise involving moderate loads and moderate resistance was found to improve function in a group of patients with early-stage ALS compared with a matched control group doing stretching (Dal Bello-Haas et al., 2007). Research from other patients with progressive neuromuscular disorders has resulted in several suggestions or guidelines for exercise in the ALS population. These general suggestions include: (1) avoid heavy eccentric exercise; (2) moderate resistance can increase strength in muscles with a manual muscle testing grade of 3 or higher out of 5; (3) overuse is not an issue if the muscles exhibit a manual muscle testing grade of 3 or better out of 5. As the disease progresses, mobility concomitantly decreases so the strategy becomes one of support for weak muscles and modification of the home and workplace. Some individuals are helped by a custom orthosis to support the neck and upper thoracic spine. It is appropriate to assess the person's need for pressure-relieving devices, such as a mattress or a wheelchair cushion. As with all the diseases discussed so far, the balance between rest and activity is essential. Pulmonary care in the patient with ALS must be geared to prevention and education regarding potential for aspiration and difficulty with airway clearance as the respiratory muscles weaken. The physical therapist can play a very important role in assisting the patient with ALS and the family to cope with this devastating disease. The reader is referred to a recent review by Dal Bello-Haas (2018) on physical therapy for people with ALS.

GUILLAIN-BARRÉ SYNDROME

GBS is the most frequent cause of acute generalized weakness now that polio is all but eradicated. It is referred to as a syndrome because it represents a broad group of demyelinating inflammatory polyradiculoneuropathies. There are two major subtypes of GBS, which can be distinguished based on pathologic and electrophysiologic findings: acquired inflammatory demyelinating polyneuropathy (AIDP) and acute motor axonal neuropathy (AMAN) (Van Doorn, 2013). Cranial nerves, which are a part of the peripheral nervous system, may also be involved. Seventy percent of patients with GBS exhibit facial nerve palsy (Van Doorn et al., 2008). Another common variant of GBS involving cranial nerves is Miller-Fisher syndrome, consisting of ophthalmoplegia, ataxia, and areflexia. GBS is a classic LMN disorder that involves peripheral nerves (polyneuropathy) and results in flaccid paralysis.

Incidence and Etiology

GBS is rare with an incidence of about 1.2 to 2.3 cases per 100,000 people (Hughes and Cornblath, 2005). About 100,000 people develop the disorder every year worldwide (Willison et al., 2016). It occurs in all age groups, both children and adults. The majority of individuals who acquire GBS experience a respiratory or gastrointestinal illness before the onset of weakness and sensory changes. GBS is an autoimmune disorder triggered by a preceding viral or bacterial infection. *Campylobacter jejuni*, a common bacterial cause of gastroenteritis, is the most frequent infectious agent. Cytomegalovirus, Epstein-Barr virus, and mycoplasma pneumonia have also been identified as common antecedent pathogens. There is no one causal agent. It is a reactive, self-limited autoimmune disease with a good overall prognosis.

Pathophysiology

The pathophysiology of GBS is complex because it involves autoimmune reactions. The infection-induced immune responses cause a cross-reaction with neural tissue. When myelin is destroyed, destruction is accompanied by inflammation. These acute inflammatory lesions are present within several days of the onset of symptoms. Nerve conduction is slowed and may be blocked completely. Even though the Schwann cells, which produce myelin in the peripheral nervous system, are destroyed, the axons are left intact in all but the most severe cases. Two to three weeks after the original demyelination, the Schwann cells begin to proliferate, inflammation subsides, and remyelination begins.

GBS is the most common cause of severe acute flaccid paralysis. AIDP is more common in Europe and North America, whereas AMAN is most frequent in Japan and Asia (Kuwabara, 2004). In the AMAN form, the infecting organism mimics a component of the peripheral nerves and the immune response cross-reacts causing axonal degeneration (Kuwabara, 2007). The target molecule has not been identified in AIDP. Variants such as Miller-Fisher are poorly understood (Jacobs et al., 2017). The progression of the demyelination appears to be different in the AMAN type of GBS versus the AIDP type. Patients with the AMAN GBS have a more rapid progression and reach nadir earlier. Nadir is the point of greatest severity. The only way to classify a patient with GBS as having axonal (i.e., AMAN) or nonaxonal type (i.e., AIDP) is electrodiagnostically.

Clinical Features

GBS is characterized by a rapid, symmetrical ascending progressive loss of motor function that begins distally and progresses proximally. Distal sensory impairments often present as paresthesias (burning and tingling) of the toes or hypesthesia (an abnormal sensitivity to touch). The sensory involvement varies and is usually not as significant as the motor involvement. The progression of motor and sensory changes may be limited to the limbs, or the progression of weakness can impair the diaphragm and cranial nerves. The diaphragm is the major muscle of ventilation. Weakness of shoulder elevators and neck flexion parallels diaphragmatic weakness.

The diaphragm is innervated by cervical nerve roots 3, 4, and 5. If the diaphragm becomes involved, ventilatory failure occurs. About 25% of patients require mechanical ventilation for days to months (Van Doorn, 2013). Additionally, 50% of the people with GBS experience changes in the autonomic nervous system, which can result in fluctuations of blood pressure, pooling of blood with poor venous return, tachycardia, and arrhythmias.

Pain is reported by patients as being muscular in nature, which is myalgia. Pain can be an early symptom and requires constant intervention. Hypesthesia may make using a bed sheet uncomfortable. Pain can be difficult to manage and can add to the person's fear and anxiety. The cause of pain is often unclear, but it may come from spontaneous transmissions from demyelinated nerves (Sulton, 2002).

Half of the patients with GBS have oral-motor involvement in the form of weakness that causes difficulty speaking (dysarthria) and swallowing (dysphagia). Alternative means of communication may need to be explored, as well as measures taken to prevent aspiration. The facial nerve (cranial nerve VII) is frequently involved and bilateral facial weakness is common. Double vision (diplopia) can result from eye muscle weakness secondary to cranial nerves III, IV, and VI involvement. Paralysis of cranial nerves is termed bulbar palsy. Cranial nerve involvement is referred to as bulbar because the majority of cranial nerves exit the bulb or brainstem. Deep tendon reflexes are absent because of the demyelination of the peripheral nerves, therefore making areflexia a core feature of this LMN disorder.

Medical Management

Plasmapheresis, or plasma exchange, or infusion of intravenous immunoglobulins (IVIGs) have been found to be equally effective in treating GBS (Van Doorn et al., 2008; Van Koningsveld et al., 2007; Willison et al., 2016). However, IVIG is the preferred treatment because of availability and greater convenience (Hughes et al., 2006). Either of these interventions needs to be initiated within the first or second week of symptom onset to shorten the course of the disease (Van Doorn et al., 2008). IVIG may need to be repeated depending on patient response. Despite the use of either plasma exchange or IVIG treatment, about 20% of affected patients are unable to ambulate after 6 months (Hughes et al., 2007; Van Doorn, 2013) and 3% to 10% die (Van Doorn, 2013). GBS is a severe disease despite current treatment.

There are three phases of GBS: acute, plateau, and recovery. The first stage lasts up to 4 weeks. During this time, symptoms appear; 80% of individuals present with paresthesias, 70% with areflexia, and 60% with weakness in all limbs. In time, the percentages of patients exhibiting the core symptoms increase to close to 100%. The plateau phase is defined by the stabilization of symptoms. Although symptoms are present, they are not progressing or worsening. This phase can also last up to 4 weeks. Finally, the recovery phase is evident when the patient begins to improve. Eighty percent of patients recover within 1 year but may have some neurologic sequela or residual deficits. The recovery phase can last a few

months to a couple of years. Patients who tend to have a poorer outcome are those who needed ventilatory support, had a rapid progression of demyelination, and demonstrated low distal motor amplitudes on EMG (Ropper et al., 1991). The latter finding is reflective of the amount of axonal damage incurred.

Physical Therapy Management

Acute Phase

Supportive care during the acute stage is a necessity. Because of the possibility of respiratory involvement, people with GBS are hospitalized and may spend a long time in intensive care. During the acute phase, it is most appropriate for the physical therapist to treat the patient as symptoms are usually progressing. If a patient's respiratory musculature becomes involved, he or she will likely require ventilatory support and be in an intensive care unit. Physical therapy goals during the acute stage include minimizing the acute signs and symptoms; supporting pulmonary function, preventing skin breakdown, and contracture formation; and managing pain. Exercise is limited to those movements that can be made without pain or excessive fatigue (Van Doorn, 2013).

If the physical therapist assistant is providing passive ROM and positioning under the supervision of the physical therapist, the therapist needs to provide information about oxygen saturation and vital capacity parameters in order for the assistant to be alert to the changes in the patient's respiratory status. The physical therapist assistant may also provide postural drainage with percussion to maintain airway clearance. Gentle stretching of the chest wall and trunk rotation may be done while the patient is still on a ventilator. The person is positioned to decrease potential contractures with hand and foot splints. Extra care should be taken when performing ROM as denervated muscles can easily be damaged. The assistant should be careful to support the limb to prevent overstretching. Always ensure that the ankle is in a subtalar neutral position before stretching the heel cord. Subtalar neutral is the position in which the talus is equally prominent when palpated anteriorly, as seen in Fig. 14.3. ROM should be performed at least twice a day. The schedule of positioning, splinting, and the ROM program should be posted at the patient's bedside.

Pain is one of the most difficult symptoms to treat in patients with GBS. Medications are not always effective. Passive ROM, massage, and transcutaneous electrical nerve stimulation may be helpful. If the patient demonstrates an increased sensitivity to light touch, a cradle can be used to keep the bed sheet away from the skin. Low-pressure wrapping or a snug-fitting garment may provide a way to avoid light moving touch on the limbs. Pain may be heightened by the patient's fear as to what has happened. Reassurance and an explanation about what to expect may help alleviate anxiety that could compound the pain.

Plateau Phase

When respiratory and autonomic functions stabilize, a program to increase tolerance to upright can be begun. This

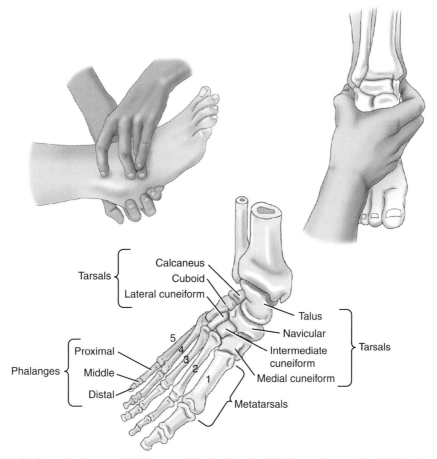

Fig. 14.3. Finding subtalar neutral before stretching heel cords. With the patient supine, hold the heel of the foot with one hand. Grasp the foot over the fourth and fifth metatarsal heads using the thumb, index, and ring fingers of the other hand. Palpate both sides of the talus on the dorsum of the foot (refer to the frontal view and skeletal structure). Passively dorsiflex the foot until resistance is felt. In this position, supinate and pronate the foot; the talus will bulge laterally and medially, respectively. Positioning the foot so that there is no bulge is subtalar neutral.

must be initiated gradually as the patient may still be on a ventilator. Physical therapy goals during the plateau phase include acclimation to upright posture, maintenance of ROM, improvement in pulmonary function, and avoidance of fatigue and overexertion. The patient is acclimated to sitting upright with appropriate postural alignment and truncal support because the trunk may still have minimal innervation. Pressure relief is still provided by changing positions on a regular basis. If the patient continues to experience pain, it may lead to holding limbs in potentially contracture-prone positions. Heat may be used before stretching if there is no sensory loss. Return of oral musculature may signal the need for additional team members to work on the movement patterns needed for swallowing, eating, and speaking. The physical therapist assistant may provide postural support for the patient during these sessions. At the very least, the assistant needs to be aware of any precautions regarding potential aspiration and any requirement for maintaining an upright upper body posture after any oral intake of food or fluids.

Recovery Phase

Muscle strength is gradually recovered 2 to 4 weeks after the condition has reached a plateau. The muscles return in the reverse order or descending pattern. This is opposite from the ascending order of loss. As the neck and trunk muscles recover, the patient may begin to use a tilt table for continued acclimation to upright and weight-bearing on the lower extremities. Positioning splints may be needed for the lower extremities, as well as thromboembolic deterrent stockings to decrease venous pooling. Muscles of respiration can be weak if the person required ventilatory assistance, and this weakness may limit tolerance to upright.

Physical therapy goals at this time now encompass strengthening and maximizing functional abilities in addition to carrying over any goals from the previous phases. Strengthening activities and exercise prescription for these individuals is challenging. Depending on the number of intact motor units present in any given muscle, the same amount of exercise can be harmful or beneficial. If there are too few motor units, working the muscle may be detrimental to its recovery.

Unfortunately, there is no easy way to ascertain how many motor units are present in a patient recovering from GBS.

Once the patient has stabilized or reached a plateau, active exercise can begin. Each patient must be progressed individually based on the response to exercise. Rehabilitation should begin as soon as improvement starts (Van Doorn et al., 2008). Gupta et al. (2010) found that patients continued to improve over a 1-year period following initial hospitalization. Patients were transferred from the hospital to a neurorehabilitation unit on average of 29.5 days after initial hospital admission. The mean length of stay in the unit was 32.9 days. Longer stays were associated with autonomic dysfunction, but not with cranial nerve involvement or need for ventilator assistance. Khan and Amatya (2012) found "satisfactory" evidence that both inpatient rehabilitation and physical therapy/exercise produced positive functional gains in patients with GBS. There was "good" evidence for outpatient high-intensity rehabilitation to produce long-term gains even 6.5 years after initial diagnosis with GBS. Their call for more high-quality randomized controlled trials to determine effectiveness of timing, intensity, and progression of rehabilitation programs for this very challenging and complex condition has not been heeded. Arsenault et al. (2016) attempted to evaluate the effectiveness of exercise interventions in patients with GBS. Their systematic review included only one randomized controlled trial that showed a high-intensity exercise program was better than a low-intensity exercise program at reducing disability in patients with GBS based on changes in Functional Independence Measure scores (Khan et al., 2011). In summary, cycling seems to be a beneficial type of training with programs lasting three times a week for 12 weeks (Arsenault et al., 2016). Exercise bouts lasted from 30 to 60 minutes at 70% to 90% of maximum heart rate. A two stage rehabilitation program was recommended by Khan et al. (2011). Early in recovery the goal is to decrease disability burden, and later in recovery the goal is to support reconditioning. Exercise intensity must be monitored closely.

Bensman's recommendations in 1970 are still useful guidelines for exercise in this population:

1. Use short periods of nonfatiguing exercise matched to the patient's strength.
2. Increase the difficulty of an activity or level of exercise only if the patient improves or if there is no deterioration in status after 1 week.
3. Return the patient to bed rest if a decrease in strength or function occurs.
4. Direct the strengthening exercises at improving function, not merely at improving strength.

Overworking a partially denervated muscle produces a profound decrease in that muscle's ability to demonstrate strength and endurance. Exercise of partially denervated muscles can interfere with axon regrowth (Lundy-Ekman, 2018; Van Doorn, 2013). Signs of overuse weakness are delayed onset of muscle soreness, which gets worse 1 to 5 days after exercising, and a reduction in the maximum amount of force the muscle is able to generate (Faulkner et al., 1993). Bassile (1996) recommends training muscles that are

at a 2/5 muscle strength in a gravity-eliminated plane using only the weight of the limb. Once the person can move the limb against a resistance equal to the mass of the limb, the person can perform antigravity exercise. Exercise progression in this population must be taken slowly. Care must be taken to avoid straining weaker muscles while increasing resistance to those showing good recovery. The distal muscles of the hands and feet are often the ones most likely to not recover fully. Use of lightweight orthoses can be helpful to support muscles around the ankle from overuse.

Regardless of the terminology, most everyone agrees that it is best to start with low repetitions and short, frequent bouts of exercise matched to the patient's muscular abilities, that is, muscle strength. For example, someone who has poor (2/5) deltoid muscle strength could exercise in a pool, or with an overhead sling apparatus or a powder board. All of these situations are gravity-eliminated. Facilitation techniques, such as stroking, brushing, vibration, and tapping of the muscle, can be combined with gravity-eliminated exercise. The patient is restricted from moving against gravity until the deltoid muscles' strength is a 3/5. The lower extremities are going to recover after the upper extremities. Most people walk within 6 months of the onset of symptoms (Van Doorn et al., 2008), but 20% do not achieve this milestone. The dilemma comes as to whether to attempt ambulation with a patient before the muscles of the lower extremities have at least a fair grade (3/5) (Bassile, 1996). No one outcome measure was consistently used in the studies reviewed by Arsenault et al. (2016). At present, physical exercise is positively associated with improved health outcomes.

Adaptive equipment needs change as the patient recovers. Once acclimated to upright, mobility may initially be limited to a wheelchair. When ambulation is achieved, a walker, forearm crutches, or a cane may be needed as an assistive device. Orthotic assistance needs to be lightweight. A plastic AFO or even an air stirrup splint can provide support for weak ankles. Residual weakness is most often apparent in the distal muscles of the hands and feet, such as the wrist extensors, finger intrinsics, ankle dorsiflexors, and foot intrinsics. The gluteal and quadriceps may also remain weak. Endurance is often lacking and may be a major obstacle even if the person is strong enough to return to work. Endurance training should be included in the patient's home exercise program; otherwise, the patient may continue to be minimally active despite adequate strength. Pitetti et al. (1993) studied a 54-year-old man who had been 3 years post-GBS. He was able to improve leg strength and total work capacity after a three-times-a-week aerobic exercise program using a bike ergometer. He was even able to return to gardening. A highly trained athlete with GBS (Fisher and Stevens, 2008) was reported in the literature. The individual recovered within 3 weeks using a combined treatment with IVIG, plasma exchange, and corticosteroids.

Summary

The prognosis for a person with GBS is usually very good. Fortunately, the muscle weakness is reversed as the peripheral nervous system recovers. However, patients with GBS are often immobilized for lengthy periods of time because of the slow nature of the recovery process. The health care team's role during that time is to safeguard the musculoskeletal and cardiopulmonary systems so that when recovery occurs, the patient is able to make the most of the changes. The role of exercise in this neuromuscular disease is to improve function without causing overuse damage. The use of nonfatiguing exercise protocols is indicated in persons with GBS. These protocols will be further discussed in the next section. There is some evidence that high-intensity exercise may lead to improved function (Khan et al., 2011), but this finding needs to be further supported by more research.

POST-POLIO SYNDROME

PPS is the name given to the late effects of poliomyelitis. Polio is a viral infection that attacks some of the anterior horn cells in the spinal cord and causes muscular paralysis. Polio was epidemic in the United States from 1910 to 1959. Decades after having survived polio, 25% to 40% of these individuals experience fatigue, new muscle weakness, and loss of functional abilities. PPS was first described and recognized as a clinical entity in 1972 when Mulder et al. published criteria for its diagnosis. The universal criteria consist of: (1) having had polio based on history, signs of residual weakness and muscle atrophy on neurologic examination, and signs of denervation on EMG; (2) period of partial or complete functional recovery followed by relative stability lasting at least 15 years; (3) development of new neurologic weakness and abnormal fatigue, with or without other symptoms; (4) symptoms persist for at least 1 year; and (5) exclusion of other neurologic, medical, or orthopedic problems as reasons for the symptoms (March of Dimes, 2000).

Because records are not as accurate as one might expect, we only have an estimate of the number of people who actually had polio. According to Post-Polio Health International, there are 640,000 survivors in the United States. Twenty to forty percent of those or 128,000 to 256,000 individuals may be expected to have PPS in the United States. The severity of PPS is related to the severity of the original polio infection. If a person had a mild case of polio, the PPS is also going to be mild. Conversely, if a person had a severe case, which required the use of an iron lung, the PPS was likely to be severe. Although PPS slowly progresses over a long period of time and is rarely life-threatening, it substantially affects QOL.

Etiology

Despite being incompletely understood, most sources accept the theory that PPS is caused by decades of increased metabolic demand made on the body by giant motor units (Gonzalez et al., 2010; Lo and Robinson, 2018a; Trojan and Cashman, 2005). These giant motor units were formed during the recovery process from the original viral infection. After the poliovirus destroys anterior horn cells, muscle fibers innervated by those anterior horn cells are orphaned. During recovery, the anterior horn cells not destroyed by the virus reinnervate some of the orphaned fibers, creating giant motor units. The repair process involves branching and cutting back of neural processes. Repair continues for a while after the original infection and is the basis for recovery and return of function. Stress and overuse of the enlarged motor units over a lifetime lead to distal degeneration of axons and new weakness (Wiechers and Hubbell, 1981). The body's response is probably compounded by age-related changes that typically occur in the nervous system. Because there is a loss of motor units during normal aging, a person who had polio may lose some giant motor units. The end result is a subsequent loss of function by the person with PPS.

Clinical Features

Fatigue

One of the most commonly reported and debilitating problems in patients with PPS is fatigue (Gonzalez et al., 2010). In fact, fatigue is one of a triad of symptoms, which include pain and a decline in strength. This fatigue goes beyond the typical fatigue everyone has felt after working hard. This fatigue is described as an overwhelming tiredness or exhaustion occurring with only minimal effort. It can be so severe that the person's ability to concentrate is affected. The fatigue can occur at the same time of day and be accompanied by signs of autonomic distress such as sweating or headaches. Some people have described the feeling of fatigue as "hitting the wall." Defects in neuromuscular transmission caused by the degeneration of the distal motor unit in PPS may contribute to this fatigue (Trojan and Cashman, 2005). Fatigue is multidimensional. Muscular factors, such as overuse, high-energy cost of even submaximal workloads, and decreased cardiovascular and pulmonary deconditioning, can contribute to fatigue. Mental fatigue may impact psychosocial function and lead to a decreased QOL. Modifiable risk factors for fatigue such as stress and physical exertion must be considered in the management of patients with PPS (Trojan et al., 2009). Regardless of the source of fatigue it most definitely impacts QOL and overall functional status (Young et al., 2018b). Researchers are working to develop a disease-specific QOL questionnaire for PPS (Young et al., 2018a, 2018b).

New Weakness

New weakness is a hallmark of PPS. It occurs in muscles already involved and in muscles that did not clinically show any effects of the original polio infection. There is evidence that these "new" muscles may actually have been involved at a subclinical level based on EMG results. The weakness is asymmetric, usually proximal, and slowly progressive in nature.

As mentioned previously, overuse has been associated with the new muscle weakness seen in individuals with PPS. If fatigue is a contributing factor, the weakness may be transient. Motor units normally break down with increasing age, and in the case of individuals with PPS, these may be giant motor units. After years of increased metabolic effort, these giant motor units degrade and cause new weakness, which is permanent. Because of increased muscle weakness, patients with PPS may experience impaired balance, and therefore be at greater risk for falls. Assistive devices for ambulation including a wheelchair may need to be considered.

Pain

Pain is a major symptom in individuals with motor neuron disease such as PPS. It is owing to overuse of muscles and increased ligamentous stress secondary to weakness. Muscle and joint pain are common manifestations of PPS. The pain and fatigue in weak muscles occurs 1 to 2 days after an activity. It lessens with rest and responds well to pacing of activities to avoid excessive fatigue. Muscle pain is diffuse and takes a long time to recover from, as evidenced by research on patients' adherence to recommendations regarding pacing and lifestyle changes (Peach and Olejnik, 1991). Those subjects that followed the recommendations had a higher percentage of resolution or improvements in muscular pain.

Joints can become unstable when muscles are weak or when excessive daily physical activity overstresses these muscles and their surrounding soft tissues. Mobility is often curtailed in the presence of joint or muscle pain, which then leads to muscular atrophy. Pain is usually the result of repetitive microtrauma from years of moving joints that are misaligned or malaligned, owing to weakness or frank postural deformity. Joint pain is a result of wear and tear on joints, poor posture, and of deterioration of soft tissue or orthopedic surgical procedures done to treat the residual effects of polio. Patients with muscle pain had higher levels of fatigue and lower QOL (Jensen et al., 2011; Werhagen and Borg, 2013). Pain severity has also been associated with poorer physical function and greater levels of depression (Stoelb et al., 2008; Werhagen and Borg, 2013). Psychosocial factors also need to be considered in the pain management of people with PPS (Lo and Robinson, 2018a, 2018b).

Other Symptoms

Cold Intolerance

Because of sympathetic involvement, the person with PPS is intolerant of cold. The limbs are often cold and require extra clothing to minimize heat loss. Use of cold as a modality is usually met with resistance because of this intolerance. If the person has difficulty with edema, heat is often not the modality of choice. Therefore extensive patient education may be required to convince a person with PPS to use local cold to treat swelling.

Decreased Function

Fatigue, pain, and weakness conspire to produce a cycle of inactivity in the person with PPS. When inquiring about what the person does on a daily basis, it is not unusual to hear "not much" as a reply. With probing you may realize that the person used to be very active and do a lot but has curtailed her activity level because of a combination of pain, fatigue, and weakness. Less activity results in deconditioning of the cardiopulmonary systems. Deconditioning further exacerbates fatigue and weakness, leading to less activity and even lower levels of social engagement. Any one of the triad of symptoms, fatigue, pain, or weakness, can trigger the cycle that results in activity restrictions and participation limitation.

Vital functions, such as eating and breathing, can be affected if the person with PPS had bulbar involvement. Cranial nerves exiting from the brainstem or bulb support oral motor and cardiorespiratory function. If the polio virus attacked the brainstem, the central control of breathing could have been compromised in addition to the muscles of ventilation, such as the diaphragm and intercostals. Subsequently, after years of working, the person with PPS may be so exhausted at the end of the day she collapses at night. Shortness of breath is a common complaint. Sleep may be disrupted by periods of apnea or pain, and thus further compound the fatigue, pain, and weakness problems encountered during waking hours. The individual with oral motor or significant pulmonary involvement or sleep disturbances will be more appropriately treated by a team member with expertise in that area, such as an occupational or speech therapist. A pulmonologist may recommend use of a positive-pressure breathing device at night to ensure adequate oxygenation.

Having walked for years with significant gait deviations, people with PPS are at risk for falls and loss of bone density. People with PPS have a greater chance for having osteoarthritis than the general population. They may also exhibit postural abnormalities secondary to polio or aging such as a forward head, absent lumbar curve, forward-leaning trunk, uneven pelvic base, or scoliosis. Individuals with PPS have prided themselves on using assistive devices only when absolutely necessary, although others have walked with knee-ankle-foot orthoses and forearm crutches. Many have established compensatory movements with or without orthoses and assistive devices that allowed them functional movement. General orthotic recommendations for common postpolio presentations can be found in Lovegreen et al., 2019. With the onset of PPS, these compensations may no longer be adequate and put them at high fall risk. One study of polio survivors reported a four times higher rate of falling than of other older adults (Bickerstaffe et al., 2010). Brogårdh and Lexell (2014) found that 50% to 84% of individuals with PPS reported at least one fall in the previous year. Brogårdh et al. (2017) identified knee muscle strength, dynamic balance, and decreased gait performance as determinants of falling and fear of falling in people with late effects of polio. A recent survey found that depression predicted falls in people living with late effects of polio (Da Silva et al., 2017). The results predicted falls in those with and without PPS. Screening for depression is recommended for polio survivors.

Medical Management

Medications for fatigue have not been proven effective. High doses of prednisone and amantadine do not improve strength or treat fatigue. Management of patients with PPS is based on physical activity levels and an individualized muscle training program. Ostlund et al. (2012, 2015) have used IVIG treatments to decrease pain in responding individuals with PPS. However, the consensus is that IVIG cannot be recommended at this time (Huang et al., 2015; Lo and Robinson, 2018b).

Physical Therapy Management

Goals for physical therapy management of the individual with PPS are to:

1. ambulate safely;
2. achieve optimal functional independence;
3. avoid fatigue;
4. avoid muscular overuse; and
5. educate the patient and family.

Physical Activity/Exercise

Individuals with PPS benefit from physical activity, which includes exercise and an active lifestyle. People with PPS that engage in regular physical activity reported a higher level of function and fewer symptoms than those who are not as active (Fillyaw et al., 1991; Willen et al., 2001). Every exercise program needs to be tailored to the person's presentation, as most people with PPS exhibit asymmetrical muscle weakness. General guidelines include avoiding overuse and disuse and modifying the level of physical activity to decrease pain. Heart rate, blood pressure, and rate of perceived exertion should be monitored. Trojan and Finch (1997) recommended a Borg rating of 14, which equates to "hard." The original scale is preferred over the 10-point one. Later studies recommend a Borg rating of 12 "somewhat hard," which is a moderate level of intensity (Voorn et al., 2014, 2016). In keeping with a nonfatiguing protocol, the duration of the exercise should be short and use a submax workload. Capacity to perform even at a submax workload is reduced in people with PPS, therefore workload needs to be adequately assessed (Nollet et al., 2001).

Customized strengthening exercises have been shown to be effective in multiple studies (Agre et al., 1996; Bertelson et al., 2009; Chan et al., 2003; Farbu et al., 2006; Jubelt and Agre, 2000; Spector et al., 1996). Short intervals of exercise are recommended with rest in-between to recover. Nonfatiguing protocols consist of submaximal and maximal strengthening exercises combined with short duration repetitions. An every-other-day schedule of exercise avoids overuse and provides for full recovery. Exercise should be supervised by a physical therapist or physical therapist assistant to ensure that correct techniques are being used, and to monitor that the patient avoids increasing muscle or joint pain and producing excessive muscle fatigue. Studies have found exercise and lifestyle modification to positively contribute to reducing signs of overuse, improving fatigue and function (Cup et al., 2007; Klein et al., 2002; Oncu et al., 2009). For examples of nonfatiguing protocols see Table 14.7.

Stretching

Stretching overworked muscles may not be indicated because of the potential for increasing joint instability. The person with PPS may have already achieved a delicate balance of ligamentous and muscular tightness that has substituted for

TABLE 14.7 Nonfatiguing Exercise Protocols

	Nonfatiguing Aerobic Interval Training	Nonfatiguing Strengthening Exercise
Resistance	Target heart rate—low range, 60%-70%	60%-80% of one repetition maximum
Frequency	3 times per week	3-5 times per week
Repetitions	NA	Goal of 5-10
Duration	15-30 minutes	NA
Contract time/rest time	NA	5 seconds/10 seconds
Intervals	Start with 2- or 3-minute exercise bouts interspersed with 1-minute rests for a session of 15 minutes; when able to do this comfortably for a total of 20 minutes for 2 weeks, increase each exercise bout by 1 minute. Goal: 4 minutes each exercise bout, 1-minute rest interval, total session: 30 minutes total of exercise bouts.	NA
Kinds of exercise	Walking, swimming, pool walking, stationary bicycling, arm ergometer—selection is based on strongest muscle group to achieve heart rate goals and avoid joint trauma.	Concentric
Measurable and reproducible testing	Pretest, then 2 and 4 months.	Pretest, then at 1, 3, 6 months, and yearly intervals.

NA, Not available.
Data from Owen RP: Postpolio syndrome and cardiopulmonary conditioning, in rehabilitation medicine—adding life to years, special issue, *West J Med* 154:557–558, 1991; McNelis A: Physical therapy management of post-polio syndrome, *Rehab Manag* 38–43, 1989; Dean E, Ross J: Modified aerobic walking program: effect on patients with postpolio syndrome, *Arch Phys Med Rehabil* 69:1033–1038, 1988; and Jones DR, Speier J, Canine K, Owen R, Stull GA: Cardiorespiratory responses to aerobic training by patients with postpoliomyelitis sequelae, *JAMA* 261:3255–3258, 1989.

weak or absent musculature. A mild shortening of the plantar flexors may increase knee stability when there is quadriceps weakness. In such case, stretching the heel cord could impair function. Any increase in ROM must be able to be supported by adequate muscle strength, which may not be possible in this population. Gentle stretching may be indicated as a strategy to combat pain or cramping from occasional overuse. Use of rehabilitation principles similar to those used in other neuromuscular disorders is appropriate (Skalsky and McDonald, 2012).

Pain Management

Pain management depends on the type of pain that the person with PPS is experiencing. Three types of pain have been described in the literature: cramping, musculoskeletal, and biomechanical (Lo and Robinson, 2018a). Gentle stretching after application of heat is indicated in the presence of cramping. This is very similar to the way people with polio were treated. As musculoskeletal pain often results from overuse, the structure involved, such as the tendon, bursa, fascia, or muscle, must be identified before an appropriate treatment can be determined. Treatment of inflammation or strains should incorporate use of antiinflammatory medication and appropriate modalities, as well as changes in patterns of use of the involved extremities. By far, the most frequent type of pain comes from biomechanical changes, resulting from degenerative joint disease, low-back pain, and nerve compression. Strategies should include posture education and/or use of an appropriate assistive device.

Orthoses may be indicated to provide better biomechanical alignment of the feet and lower extremities. In PPS, the individual usually has a combination of biomechanical malalignment and muscle imbalance. An orthosis may only be able to support better joint alignment, not accomplish a complete correction. The most frequently prescribed orthoses include shoe lifts, AFOs, and knee-ankle-foot orthoses. Use of lightweight carbon fiber orthoses, while more expensive, can improve gait efficiency (Brehm et al., 2007; Lo and Robinson, 2018b). Energy efficiency and improved gait were demonstrated using a stance control knee joint (Kim et al., 2016). See Lovegreen et al. (2019) for a discussion of orthotic management of polio and PPS. When orthotic interventions are being considered, the person should be assessed by an interdisciplinary team (a physician, orthotist, and a physical therapist) and should include a gait assessment.

Lifestyle Modification

People with PPS must change their lifestyle. Although this is easy to say, it is very difficult for them to do. Having survived polio and not let it get the best of them, these individuals often resist seeing the need for and implementing lifestyle changes. Mobility is freedom and independence that is something they fought for and achieved a long time ago. Change is going to come slowly. The adage of working through pain was used successfully before and so they might think that this strategy will work again. Slowing down seems a poor option when it is equated, in their mind, to giving in. A recent two part review suggests activity pacing, reducing physical and emotional stress, joint protection, modification of work and home environments, and use of mobility aids to reduce fatigue and preserver function (Lo and Robinson, 2018a, 2018b). Others recommend energy conservation and weight loss. Changes in lifestyle do not mean that the person with PPS is not active. Life satisfaction and perceived well-being appears to be less related to physical impairment and more related to engaging in an active lifestyle (Lexell and Brogårdh, 2012; Winberg et al., 2014).

Energy Conservation

Because of the far-reaching effects of fatigue and the danger of overuse, energy conservation must be an integral part of the management of a person with PPS, and may be the most important aspect of management. Energy conservation is a means of modifying a person's lifestyle to conserve energy. It can incorporate changes in the environment, the task, or the way the mover performs the task. One, two, or all three components can be changed. One person with PPS may need to use an assistive device when none was used before to conserve energy during ambulation. Someone else may require the use of an electric scooter. When performing ADLs, the person has to ask if the task can be done in one trip rather than three. For example, can all the dishes be unloaded from the dishwasher onto a cart, and the cart moved to a location where all the dishes can be put away rather than making multiple trips to and from the dishwasher to various locations? Can the person sit rather than stand to perform filing (if that is part of the person's job)? Analysis of daily routines can be helpful in determining where changes can be easily made.

Activity pacing is part of energy conservation, and therefore of lifestyle modification. Pacing requires a balance between rest and activity. Does the person have more energy in the morning or afternoon? Taking advantage of planning activities according to when energy is available makes good sense. Taking more frequent rest breaks may allow someone to continue to work, as well as perform daily household activities. The amount of rest that is adequate may be different for every individual with PPS. Daytime naps may be needed. Continuing to do our "jobs," whatever that entails, leads to having a better, more positive sense of self and QOL. The physical therapist assistant should empower the person with PPS to figure out ways to increase rest while reducing stress.

Balance Between Activity and Rest

Physical therapy management of the person with PPS is aimed at decreasing the workload of muscles used on a daily basis. Nonfatiguing exercise protocols, energy conservation activity pacing, breathing exercises, and coordination of breathing with activity are all strategies that are used at some point with the person experiencing PPS. The biggest challenge comes not in identifying intervention strategies but in helping the person find the most beneficial balance between rest and activity. How much exercise can the person do while conserving energy throughout the day? This is a real balancing act. More is not better in this case, less is best.

CHAPTER SUMMARY

The neurologic disorders reviewed in this chapter have several things in common. They all significantly impact the ability of a person to function. Mobility, daily living activities, job performance, and participation in leisure activities may all be seriously compromised as a result of these disorders. All of these disorders produce fatigue and create the potential for deconditioning regardless of the underlying pathologic process involved. Exercise is beneficial for the individual with any of these neurologic disorders, even in the case of an individual with ALS. Exercise is the central strategy and the most crucial part of the overall therapeutic management plan. Precautions regarding overuse are applicable to all patients with these types of neurologic disorders. Regardless of specific

disorder, interventions require all individuals to find a balance between the amount of rest and activity that can be tolerated while continuing to optimize function. Early intervention, which in this context means "soon after diagnosis," provides the person the best possible plan of care. This initial plan of care may contain many episodes and allows for continual modification of the intervention strategies based on disease progression or recovery. The plan is instituted and carried out by a team of health care practitioners. Exercise intensity is an essential component of the plan of care. The physical therapist and physical therapist assistant are part of the team that play an important role in managing individuals with PD, MS, ALS, GBS, and PPS.

REVIEW QUESTIONS

1. What is the most common cause of acute paralysis in adults?
2. What is one of the three most common movement disorders seen in the United States?
3. What is the most pervasive symptom seen in all the neurologic disorders discussed?
4. Give several interventions that could be used to improve lower extremity extensibility in a person with MS who exhibits increased lower extremity tone.
5. Identify three factors that could lead to inactivity and deconditioning in a person with PPS.
6. List signs and symptoms of overuse weakness.
7. What is the most prevalent type of MS?
8. How long can a person with PD usually benefit from taking L-dopa?
9. Describe strategies to use when a person with PD freezes.
10. When is a nonfatiguing exercise protocol warranted?
11. What are three exercise guidelines for a patient with GBS?

CASE STUDIES: REHABILITATION UNIT INITIAL EVALUATION: JB

History

Chart Review

JB was transferred to a regional medical center from a rural county hospital for severe progressive weakness 3 weeks ago. The patient was admitted through the emergency room on the day before the transfer, complaining of weakness in all extremities. He had a viral infection a few days earlier, with diarrhea, fever, and chills. No previous history of diabetes, chronic obstructive pulmonary disease, heart disease, or hypertension. Patient had previous hospitalization via the emergency room for kidney stones. He has no allergies and is on no medications. He recently completed a course of intravenous immunoglobulins. Physical therapist order for examination and treatment received on transfer to the rehabilitation unit.

Subjective

JB states that he is married and is a high school math teacher. He reports having a viral illness lasting 3 days from which he fully recovered. Three weeks ago, he noticed that he had difficulty writing because of arm weakness. On admission to the rural hospital, he had partial paralysis of his arms and total paralysis of his legs. He had no pain. He and his wife were anxious about the reason for his transfer to a regional medical center but following diagnosis and treatment of Guillain-Barré syndrome (GBS), they are looking forward to his recovery. He

grows tomatoes as a hobby. He lives in a one-story house with two steps to enter. He gives consent for the examination.

Objective

Appearance/Equipment: Patient is supine in bed on an egg-crate mattress. A Foley catheter is in place.

Systems Review

Communication/Cognition: Speech is normal. He understands multiple step directions, is alert and cooperative.

Cardiovascular/Pulmonary: Heart rate 82 beats per minute; blood pressure 130/90 mm Hg; respiratory rate 20 breaths per minute.

Integumentary: Skin intact, no redness or edema.

Musculoskeletal: Passive range of motion (ROM) intact; active ROM impaired.

Neuromuscular: Gait, locomotion, and balance are impaired. Upper extremity and lower extremity paralysis are present; sensation intact proximally, impaired distally.

Psychosocial: Wife is at bedside.

Tests and Measures

Anthropometric: Height, 6' 3", weight, 190 lbs.

Arousal, Attention, and Cognition: Oriented × 3, mental status intact.

Continued

CASE STUDIES: REHABILITATION UNIT INITIAL EVALUATION: JB—cont'd

Circulation: Skin is warm to touch, pedal pulses present bilaterally, strong radial pulse.

Ventilation/Respiration: Breathing pattern is 2-neck, 2-diaphragm. No chest wall expansion noted. Epigastric rise is 1.5". Vital capacity is 3 L, 50% of normal.

Cranial Nerve Integrity: Cranial nerves intact.

Reflex Integrity: Biceps 2 +, patellar, Achilles 0 bilaterally; Babinski absent bilaterally; muscle tone is flaccid in the lower extremities, trunk, and below the elbows; tone in the arms, shoulders, and neck appears normal.

Range of Motion: Passive ROM within functional limits; active shoulder flexion/abduction in sitting to 60 degrees bilaterally, active elbow flexion to 90 degrees bilaterally, elbow extension lacks 15 degrees from complete extension, neck motion within functional limits, no other active movement.

Motor Function: Patient requires max assist 1 for rolling and coming to sit. Patient can sit up supported in bed for 20 minutes at a time. He is dependent in sitting and standing. Patient requires max assist of 2 for bed ← → wheelchair transfer.

Muscle Performance: Tested per Berryman Reese manual muscle testing procedures. Patient is in supported sitting with appropriate stabilization. Muscles of facial expression are intact bilaterally.

	R	L
Upper trapezius	3	3
Deltoid	3−	3−
Biceps	3−	3−
Triceps	0	0
Wrist extensors	0	0
Finger flexors	0	0
Hip flexors	0	0
Quadriceps	0	0
Anterior tibialis	0	0
Gastrocsoleus	0	0

Sensory Integrity: Pinprick intact throughout the upper extremities, except diminished below the wrists; intact on the trunk and lower extremities to the knees, absent below.

Pain: 0 on a scale of 0 to 10.

Posture: At rest, the patient is in supine on an egg-crate mattress with a Foley catheter in place. His upper limbs are flexed across his lower trunk. His lower limbs are externally rotated at the hips, extended at the knees, and plantar flexed at the feet.

Gait, Locomotion, and Balance: Dependent in gait and locomotion. Patient is unable to take any challenges in a supported sitting position.

Self-Care: Dependent in feeding, dressing, personal hygiene.

Assessment/Evaluation

JB is a 53-year-old married, male teacher who, after experiencing a viral illness, was hospitalized with paralysis of his arms and legs. On day 2, he was transferred from a local hospital to a regional medical center for continued evaluation and treatment. The diagnosis of GBS was made and he underwent infusion with intravenous immunoglobulins. He is dependent in transfers and locomotion. Functional Independence Measure: transfers 1, locomotion 1. He is being transferred to the rehabilitation unit at the medical center.

Problem List

1. Dependent in mobility.
2. Dependent in activities of daily living (ADLs) and transfers.
3. Decreased strength and endurance.
4. Dependent in pressure relief.
5. Lacks knowledge of disease course and rehabilitation.

Diagnosis: JB exhibits impaired force production and diminished sensory integrity associated with an acute polyneuropathy, Guillain-Barré syndrome.

Prognosis: Over the course of 2 months, JB will improve his level of functional independence and functional skills. Changes will be limited by the degree and rapidity of recovery of muscle function and strength and any residual musculoskeletal or neuromuscular deficits.

Short-term Goals (2 Weeks)

1. JB will maintain passive ROM of all joints within functional limits for ADLs.
2. JB will increase vital capacity to 100% to improve cough effectiveness.
3. JB will demonstrate a 2-chest, 2-diaphragm breathing pattern to increase tolerance to upright.
4. JB will increase strength in all innervated muscles to 3 + to improve sitting and standing balance.
5. JB will increase tolerance to upright sitting in a wheelchair to 4 hours a day with no loss of skin integrity.
6. JB will roll supine → prone and back with min assist of 1 for pressure relief.
7. JB will transfer from bed to wheelchair with min assist of 1 using stand pivot.

Long Term Goals (6 Weeks at Discharge from Rehabilitation Unit)

1. JB will ambulate 150 feet × 3 independently, with or without an assistive device.
2. JB will negotiate a set of 4 stairs with handrails.
3. JB will stand for 45 consecutive minutes (class period) without a break.
4. JB will drive his car from home to school.
5. JB will plant 5 tomato plants without a rest break.

Plan

Patient will be seen twice a day 5 days a week and once on Saturday and Sunday for 45-minute treatment sessions. Treatment sessions are to include positioning, ROM, pulmonary rehabilitation, functional mobility training, patient/family education, and discharge planning. Patient will be reassessed weekly.

Coordination, Communication, and Documentation: The physical therapist and physical therapist assistant will be in constant contact. The physical therapist will also be communicating with the occupational therapist, the respiratory therapist, the physician, the nursing staff, and the nutritionist.

Patient/Client Instruction: JB and his wife will be educated regarding the pathologic process involved in GBS, the importance of ROM, monitoring for changes in muscle function, and avoiding overuse.

Interventions

1. Passive ROM to all extremities that lack voluntary movement.
2. Positioning program to prevent contractures including low top tennis shoes.

CASE STUDIES: REHABILITATION UNIT INITIAL EVALUATION: JB—cont'd

3. Turning schedule for pressure relief.
4. Chest wall stretching.
5. Diaphragm strengthening and incentive spirometry.
6. Transfer training progressing from sit pivot → stand pivot to and from the bed to commode, bed to wheelchair; wheelchair to car.
7. Tilt table for standing.
8. Strengthening exercises as muscle function returns.
9. Endurance training using a nonfatiguing protocol.
10. Wheelchair mobility training.
11. Gait training progressing from parallel bars to level ground to elevations.
12. ADLs training with upper extremity support and hand-over-hand progressing to independent feeding, dressing, and toileting.
13. Monitor muscle and sensory return.

Discharge Planning
JB will be discharged to home with spouse. A home and school assessment will be performed if needed and equipment secured as necessary. Vocational rehabilitation will be contacted.

Questions to Think About
- What procedural interventions are appropriate for the physical therapist assistant to perform?
- When would transfers to sitting and standing be initiated?
- What signs and symptoms should the physical therapist assistant use to indicate a negative change in status?

REFERENCES

Abrahams S, Leigh PN, Harvey A, et al.: Verbal fluency and executive dysfunction in amyotrophic lateral sclerosis, *Neuropsychologia* 38:734–747, 2000.

Adkins AL, Frank JS, Jog MS: Fear of falling and postural control in Parkinson's disease, *Mov Disord* 18:496–502, 2003.

Agre JC, Rodriquez AA, Franke TM, et al.: Low-intensity, alternate-day exercise improves muscle performance without apparent adverse effect in postpolio patients, *Am J Phys Med Rehabil* 75:50–58, 1996.

Ahlskog JE: Aerobic exercise: evidence for a direct brain effect to slow Parkinson disease progression, *Mayo Clin Proc* 93(3):360–372, 2018.

Amatya B, Khan F, Galea M: Rehabilitation for people with multiple sclerosis: an overview of Cochrane Reviews, *Cochrane Database Syst Rev* 1:CD012732, 2019. doi:10.1002/14651858.CD012732.pub2.

Arsenault NS, Vincent PO, Yu BH, Bastien R, Sweeney A: Influence of exercise on patients with Guillain-Barré syndrome: a systematic review, *Physiother Can* 68(4):367–376, 2016.

Ascherio A, Schwarzschild MA: The epidemiology of Parkinson's disease: risk factors and prevention, *Lancet Neurol* 15(12):1257–1272, 2016. doi:10.1016/S1474-442(916)30230-7.

Bakshi R: Fatigue associated with multiple sclerosis: diagnosis, impact, and management, *Mult Scler* 9:219–227, 2003.

Bassile CC: Guillain-Barré syndrome and exercise guidelines, *Neurol Rep* 20:31–36, 1996.

Beckerman H, de Groot V, Scholten MA, Kempen JC, Lankhorst GJ: Physical activity behavior of people with multiple sclerosis: understanding how they can become more physically active, *Phys Ther* 90:1001–1013, 2010.

Beeldman E, Raaphorst J, Klein Twennaar M, et al.: The cognitive profile of ALS: a systematic review and meta-analysis update, *J Neurol Neurosurg Psychiatry* 87(6):611–619, 2016.

Bensman A: Strenuous exercise may impair muscle function in Guillain-Barré patients, *JAMA* 214:468–469, 1970.

Berg D, Postuma RB, Bloem B, et al.: Time to redefine PD? Introductory statement of the MDS task force on the definition of Parkinson's disease, *Mov Disord* 29:454–462, 2014.

Bergendal G, Fredrikson S, Almkvist O: Selective decline in information processing in subgroups of multiple sclerosis: an 8-year longitudinal study, *Eur Neurol* 57(4):193–202, 2007.

Bertelson M, Broberg S, Madsen E: Outcome of physiotherapy as part of a multidisciplinary rehabilitation in an unselected polio population with one-year follow-up: an uncontrolled study, *J Rehabil Med* 41:85–87, 2009.

Bezkor EW, McIsaac TL, O'Sullivan SB: Parkinson's disease. In O'Sullivan SB, Schmitz TJ, Fulk GD, editors: *Physical rehabilitation*, ed 7, Philadelphia, 2019, FA Davis, pp 760–816.

Bickerstaffe A, Beelen A, Nollet F: Circumstances and consequences of falls in polio survivors, *J Rehabil Med* 42:908–915, 2010.

Boeschoten RE, Braamse AMJ, Beekman ATF, et al.: Prevalence of depression and anxiety in multiple sclerosis: a systematic review and meta-analysis, *J Neurol Sci* 372:331–341, 2017.

Braun T, Marks D, Thiel C: Comment on 'Lee Silverman Voice Treatment (LSVT)-BIG to improve motor function in people with Parkinson's disease: a systematic review and meta-analysis', *Clin Rehabil* 32(9):1284–1285, 2018. doi:10.1177/0269215518769436.

Brehm MA, Beelen A, Doorenbosch CA, Harlaar J, Nollet F: Effect of carbon-composite knee-ankle-foot-orthoses on walking efficiency and gait in former polio patients, *J Rehabil Med* 39:651–657, 2007.

Brogårdh C, Flansbjer UB, Lexell J: Determinants of falls and fear of falling in ambulatory persons with late effects of polio, *PM R* 9:455–463, 2017. doi:10.1016/j.pmrj.2016.08.006.

Brogårdh C, Lexell J: Falls, fear of falling, self-reported impairments and walking limitations in persons with late effects of polio. *PM R* 6:900–907, 2014.

Brooks BR, Miller RG, Swash M, et al.: El Escorial revisited: revised criteria for the diagnosis of amyotrophic lateral sclerosis, *Amyotroph Lateral Scler Other Motor Neuron Disord* 1:293–299, 2000.

Bryant MS, Jackson GR, Hou JG, Protas EJ: Treadmill exercise tests in persons with Parkinson's disease: responses and disease severity, *Aging Clin Exp Res* 28(5):1009–1014, 2016.

Bryant MS, Rintala DH, Graham JE, et al.: Determinants of use of a walking device in persons with Parkinson's disease, *Arch Phys Med Rehabil* 95:1940–1945, 2014.

Cakit BD, Nacir B, Gene H, et al.: Cycling progressive resistance training for people with multiple sclerosis: a randomized controlled study, *Am J Phys Med Rehabil* 89:446–457, 2010.

Campbell E, Coulter EH, Paul L: High intensity interval training for people with multiple sclerosis: a systematic review, *Mult Scler Relat Disord* 24:55–63, 2018.

Canning CG, Alison JA, Allen NE, Groeller H: Parkinson's disease: an investigation of exercise capacity, respiratory function, and gait, *Arch Phys Med Rehabil* 78:199–207, 1997.

Chan KM, Amirjani N, Sumrain M, Clarke A, Strohschein FJ: Randomized controlled trial of strength training in post-polio patients, *Muscle Nerve* 27:332–338, 2003.

Chiaravalloti ND, Genova HM, DeLuca J: Cognitive rehabilitation in multiple sclerosis: the role of plasticity, *Front Neurol* 6:67, 2015.

Corvillo I, Varela E, Armijo F, et al.: Efficacy of aquatic therapy for multiple sclerosis: a systematic review, *Eur J Phys Rehabil Med* 53:944–952, 2017.

Cup EH, Pieterse AJ, Ten Broed-Pastoor JM, et al.: Exercise therapy and other types of physical therapy for patients with neuromuscular disease: a systematic review, *Arch Phys Med Rehabil* 88:1452–1464, 2007.

Da Silva CP, Zuckerman B, Olkin R: Relationship of depression and medications on incidence of falls among people with late effects of polio, *Physiother Theory Pract* 33(5):370–375, 2017.

Dal Bello-Haas V: Physical therapy for individuals with amyotrophic lateral sclerosis: current insights, *Degener Neurol Neuromuscul Dis* 8:45–54, 2018.

Dal Bello-Haas V, Florence JM, Kloos AD, et al.: A randomized controlled trial of resistance exercise in individuals with ALS, *Neurology* 68:2003–2007, 2007.

Dal Bello-Haas V: Amyotrophic lateral sclerosis. In O'Sullivan SS, Schmitz TJ, Fulk GD, editors: *Physical rehabilitation*, ed 6, Philadelphia, 2014, FA Davis, pp 769–806.

Dalgas U, Stenager E, Jakobsen J, et al.: Fatigue, mood, and quality of life improve in MS patients after progressive resistance training, *Mult Scler* 16:480–490, 2010.

David FJ, Robichaud JA, Vaillancourt DE, et al.: Progressive resistance exercise restores some properties of the triphasic EMG pattern and improves bradykinesia: the PREt-PD randomized clinical trial, *J Neurophysiol* 116:2298–2311, 2016.

Demonceau M, Maquet D, Jidovtseff B, et al.: Effects of twelve weeks of aerobic or strength training in addition to standard care in Parkinson's disease: a controlled study, *Eur J Phys Med Rehabil Med* 53(2):184–200, 2017.

Dibble LE, Foreman KB, Addison O, Marcus RL, LaStayo PC: Exercise and medication effects on persons with Parkinson disease across the domains of disability: a randomized clinical trial, *J Neurol Phys Ther* 39(2):85–92, 2015.

Dibble LE, Hale TF, Marcus RL, Gerber JP, LaSrayo PC: High intensity eccentric resistance training decreases bradykinesia and improves quality of life in persons with Parkinson's disease: a preliminary study, *Parkinsonism Relat Disord* 15:752–757, 2009.

Dorsey ER, Bloem BR: The Parkinson pandemic: a call to action, *JAMA Neurol* 75(1):9–10, 2018. doi:10.1001/jamaneurol.2017.3299.

Driehuis ER, Van Den Akker LE, De Groot V, Bekerman H: Aerobic capacity explains physical functioning and participation in patients with multiple-sclerosis fatigue, *J Rehabil Med* 50:185–192, 2018.

Edwards T, Pilutti LA: The effect of exercise training in adults with multiple sclerosis with severe mobility disability: a systematic review and future directions, *Mult Scler Relat Disord* 16:31–39, 2017.

Elamin M, Phukan J, Bede P, et al.: Executive dysfunction is a negative prognostic indicator in patients with ALS without dementia, *Neurology* 76:1263–1269, 2011.

Ellis T, Rochester L: Mobilizing Parkinson's disease: the future of exercise, *J Parkinsons Dis* 8:S95–S100, 2018.

Fang X, Han D, Cheng Q, et al.: Association of levels of physical activity with risk of Parkinson disease: a systematic review and meta-analysis, *JAMA Netw Open* 1(5):e182421, 2018. doi:10.1001/jamanetworkopen.2018.2421.

Farbu E, Gilhus NE, Barnes MP, et al.: EFNS guideline on diagnosis and management of postpolio syndrome: report of an EFNS task force, *Eur J Neurol* 13:795–801, 2006.

Farley BG, Fox CM, Ramig LO, McFarland DH: Intensive amplitude-specific therapeutic approaches for Parkinson's disease: toward a neuroplasticity-principled rehabilitation model, *Top Geriatr Rehabil* 24:99–114, 2008.

Fasano A, Aquino CC, Krauss JK, et al.: Axial disability and deep brain stimulation in patients with Parkinson disease, *Nat Rev Neurol* 11:98–110, 2015.

Faulkner JA, Brooks SV, Opiteck JA: Injury to skeletal muscle fibers during contractions: conditions of occurrence and prevention, *Phys Ther* 73:911–921, 1993.

Fertl E, Doppelbauer A, Auff E: Physical activity and sports in patients suffering from Parkinson's disease in comparison with healthy seniors, *J Neural Transm Park Dis Dement Sect* 5:157–161, 1993.

Fillyaw M, Badger G, Goodwin G, et al.: The effects of long-term non-fatiguing resistance exercise in subjects with post-polio syndrome, *Orthopedics* 14:1253–1256, 1991.

Fisher TB, Stevens JE: Rehabilitation of a marathon runner with Guillain-Barré syndrome, *J Neurol Phys Ther* 32:203–209, 2008.

Forsaa EB, Larsen JP, Wentzel-Larsen R, Alves G: A twelve-year populations-based study of freezing of gait in Parkinson's disease, *Parkinsonism Relat Disord* 21(3):254–258, 2015.

Franzén E, Paquette C, Gurfinkel VS, et al.: Reduced performance in balance, walking and turning tasks is associated with increased neck tone in Parkinson's disease, *Exp Neurol* 219(2):430–438, 2009.

Frazzitta G, Maestri R, Uccellini D, Bertoti G, Abelli P: Rehabilitation treatment of gait in patients with Parkinson's disease with freezing: a comparison between two physical therapy protocols using visual and auditory cues with and without treadmill training, *Mov Disord* 24:1139–1143, 2009.

Friedman JH, Friedman H: Fatigue in Parkinson's disease: a nine-year follow-up, *Mov Disord* 16:1120–1122, 2001.

Fuller KS, Demarche, Winkler PS: Degenerative diseases of the central nervous system. In Goodman CC, Fuller KS, editors: *Pathology: implications for the physical therapist*, ed 4, Philadelphia, 2015, Elsevier, pp 1455–1506.

Gao Q, Leung A, Yang Y, et al.: Effects of tai chi on balance and fall prevention in Parkinson's disease: a randomized controlled trial, *Clin Rehabil* 28:748–753, 2014.

Garber CE, Friedman JH: Effects of fatigue on physical activity and function in patients with Parkinson's disease, *Neurology* 60:1119–1124, 2003.

Goetz CG, Poewe W, Rascol O, et al.: Movement Disorder Society Task Force report of the Hoehn and Yahr staging scale: status and recommendations, *Mov Disord* 19:1020–1028, 2004.

Gonzalez H, Olsson T, Borg K: Management of postpolio syndrome, *Lancet Neurol* 9(6):634–642, 2010.

Greeke EE, Chua AS, Healy BC, et al.: Depression and fatigue in patients with multiple sclerosis, *J Neurol Sci* 380:236–241, 2017.

Grimbergen YA, Schrag A, Mazibrada G, Borm GF, Bloem BR: Impact of falls and fear of falling on health-related quality of life in patients with Parkinson's disease, *J Parkinsons Dis* 3(3):409–413, 2013. doi:10.3233/JPD-120113.

Gupta A, Taly AB, Srivastava A, Murali T: Guillain-Barré syndrome: rehabilitation outcome, residual deficits, and requirement of lower-limb orthosis for locomotion at 1-year follow up, *Dis Rehabil* 32:1897–1902, 2010.

Haehner A, Boesveldt S, Berendse HW, et al.: Prevalence of smell loss in Parkinson's disease – a multicenter study, *Parkinsonism Relat Disord* 15:490–494, 2009.

Hallum A, Allen DD: Neuromuscular diseases. In: Umphred DA, Lazaro RT, Roller ML, Burton GU, editors: *Umphred's neurological rehabilitation*, ed 6, St. Louis, 2013, Elsevier, pp 521–570.

Hameau S, Zory R, Latrile C, Roche N, Bensmail D: Relationship between neuromuscular and perceived fatigue and locomotor performance in patients with multiple sclerosis, *Eur J Phys Rehabil Med* 53(6):833–840, 2017.

Herlofson K, Kluger BM: Fatigue in Parkinson's disease, *J Neurol Sci* 374:38–41, 2017.

Herlofson K, Larsen JP: The influence of fatigue on health-related quality of life in patients with Parkinson's disease, *Acta Neurol Scand* 107:1–6, 2003.

Hirtz D, Thurman D, Gwinn-Hardy K, et al.: How common are the "common" neurologic disorders? *Neurology* 68:326–327, 2007.

Hoehn MM, Yahr MD: Parkinsonism: onset, progression, and mortality, *Neurology* 17:427, 1967.

Horak FB, Frank J, Nutt J: Effects of dopamine on postural control in parkinsonian subjects: scaling, set, tone, *J Neurophysiol* 75:2380–2396, 1996.

Horak FB, Dimitrova D, Nutt JG: Direction-specific postural instability in subjects with Parkinson's disease, *Exp Neurol* 193:504–521, 2005.

Huang YH, Chen HC, Huang KW, et al.: Intravenous immunoglobulin for postpolio syndrome: a systematic review and meta-analysis, *BMC Neurol* 15:39, 2015.

Hughes RA, Cornblath DR: Guillian-Barré syndrome, *Lancet* 366:1653–1666, 2005.

Hughes RA, Raphael JC, Swan AV, van Doorn PA: Intravenous immunoglobulin for Guillain-Barré syndrome, *Cochrane Database Syst Rev* (1):CD002063, 2006.

Hughes RA, Swan AV, Raphael JC, et al.: Immunotherapy for Guillain-Barré syndrome: a systematic review, *Brain* 130:2245–2257, 2007.

Hwang S, Agada P, Grill S, et al.: A central sensory processing deficit with Parkinson's disease, *Exp Brain Res* 234(8):2369–2379, 2016. doi:10.1007/s00221-016-4642-4.

Jacobs BC, van den Berg B, Verboon C, et al.: International Guillain-Barré syndrome outcome study: protocol of a prospective observational cohort study on clinical and biological predictors of disease course and outcome in Guillain-Barré syndrome, *J Peripher Nerv Syst* 22:68–76, 2017.

Janssens J, Malfroid K, Nyffeler T, Bohlhalter S, Vanbellingen T: Application of LSVT BIG intervention to address gait, balance, bed mobility, and dexterity in people with Parkinson disease: a case series, *Phys Ther* 94:1014–1023, 2014.

Jensen MP, Alschuler KN, Smith AE, et al.: Pain and fatigue in persons with postpolio syndrome: independent effects on functioning, *Arch Phys Med Rehabil* 92:1796–1801, 2011.

Jubelt B, Agre JC: Characteristics and management of postpolio syndrome, *JAMA* 284:412–414, 2000.

Kaltsatou A, Flouris AD: Impact of pre-cooling therapy on the physical performance and functional capacity of multiple sclerosis patients: a systematic review, *Mult Scler Relat Disord* 27:419–423, 2019.

Kegelmeyer DA, Parthasarathy S, Kostyk SK, White SE, Kloos AD: Assistive devices alter gait patterns in Parkinson disease: advantages of the four-wheeled walker, *Gait Posture* 38:20–24, 2013.

Kerr GK, Worringham DJ, Cole MH, et al.: Predictors of future falls in Parkinson disease, *Neurology* 75:116–124, 2010.

Khan F, Amatya B: Rehabilitation in multiple sclerosis: a systematic review of systematic reviews, *Arch Phys Med Rehabil* 98:353–367, 2017.

Khan F, Amatya B: Rehabilitation interventions in patients with acute demyelinating inflammatory polyneuropathy: a systematic review, *Eur J Phys Rehabil Med* 48:507–522, 2012.

Khan F, Pallant JF, Amatya B, et al.: Outcomes of high- and low-intensity rehabilitation programme for persons in chronic phase after Guillain-Barré syndrome: a randomized controlled trial, *J Rehabil Med* 43:638–646, 2011.

Kim JH, Ji SG, Jung KJ: Therapeutic experience on stance control knee-ankle-foot orthosis with electromagnetically controlled knee joint system in poliomyelitis, *Ann Phys Med Rehabil* 40:356–361, 2016.

Klein MG, Whyte J, Esquenazi A, et al.: A comparison of the effects of exercise and lifestyle modification on the resolution of overuse symptoms of the shoulder in polio survivors: a preliminary study, *Arch Phys Med Rehabil* 83:708–713, 2002.

Konczak J, Corcos DM, Horak F, et al.: Proprioception and motor control in Parkinson's disease, *J Mot Beh* 41:543–552, 2009.

Kurtzke JF: Rating neurologic impairment in multiple sclerosis: an expanded disability status scale (EDSS), *Neurology* 33:1444–1452, 1983.

Kuwabara S: Guillain-Barré syndrome: epidemiology, pathophysiology and management, *Drugs* 64:597–610, 2004.

Kuwabara S: Guillain-Barré syndrome, *Curr Neurol Neurosci Rep* 7:57–62, 2007.

Langer-Gould A, Brara SM, Beaber BE, Zhang JL: Incidence of multiple sclerosis in multiple racial and ethnic groups, *Neurology* 80:1734–1739, 2013.

Lexell J, Brogårdh C: Life satisfaction and self-reported impairments in persons with late effects of polio, *Ann Phys Rehabil Med* 55:577–589, 2012.

Lo JK, Robinson LR: Postpolio syndrome and the late effects of poliomyelitis. Part 1. Pathogenesis, biomechanical considerations, diagnosis, and investigations, *Muscle Nerve* 58:751–759, 2018a.

Lo JK, Robinson LR: Postpolio syndrome and the late effects of poliomyelitis. Part 2. Treatment, management, and prognosis, *Muscle Nerve* 58:760–769, 2018b.

Lovegreen W, Kwasnieski M, Panchang P, Smith MJ: Orthotic management of polio and postpolio syndrome. In Webster JB, Murphy DP, editors: *Atlas of orthoses and assistive devices*, ed 5, Philadelphia, 2019, Elsevier, pp 277–288.

Lublin FD, Reingold SC, Cohen JA, et al.: Defining the clinical course of multiple sclerosis: the 2013 revisions, *Neurology* 83(3):278–286, 2013.

Lundy-Ekman L: *Neuroscience: fundamentals for rehabilitation*, ed 5, St. Louis, 2018, Elsevier, pp 115–117, 255–256.

Majounie E, Renton AE, Mok K, et al.: Frequency of the C9orf72 hexanucleotide repeat expansion in patients with amyotrophic lateral sclerosis and frontotemporal dementia: a cross-sectional study, *Lancet Neurol* 11(4):323–330, 2012.

Mak MK, Pang MY, Mok V: Gait difficulty, postural instability, and muscle weakness are associated with fear of falling in people with Parkinson's disease, *Parkinsons Dis* 2012:901721, 2012. doi:10.1155/2012/901721.

Mancini M, Zampieri C, Carlson-Kuhta P, et al.: Anticipatory postural adjustments prior to step initiation are hypometric in untreated Parkinson's disease: an accelerometer-based approach, *Eur J Neurol* 16:1028–1034, 2009.

March of Dimes. *Identifying best practices in diagnosis and care. International Conference on Post-Polio Syndrome*, Warm Springs, GA, May 19-20, 2000. Available at: http://www.polioplace.org/sites/default/files/files/MOD-%20Identifying.pdf. Accessed May 8, 2019.

Marras C, Beck JC, Bower JH, et al.: Prevalence of Parkinson's disease across North America, *NPJ Parkinson's Disease* 4(1):1–7, 2018.

Martin-Valero R, Zamora-Pascual N, Armenta-Peiado JA: Training of respiratory muscles in patients with multiple sclerosis: a systematic review, *Resp Care* 59(11):1764–1772, 2014.

McDonnell MN, Rischbieth B, Schammer TT, et al.: Lee Silverman Voice Treatment (LSVT)-BIG to improve motor function in people with Parkinson's disease: a systematic review and meta-analysis, *Clin Rehabil* 32(5):607–618, 2018. doi:10.1177/0269215517734385.

McIsaac TL, Frtiz NE, O'Sullivan SB: Multiple sclerosis. In O'Sullivan SB, Schmitz TJ, Fulk GD, editors: *Physical rehabilitation*, ed 7, Philadelphia, 2019, FA Davis, pp 662–711.

Mehta P, Kaze W, Ramond J, et al.: Prevalence of amyotrophic lateral sclerosis - United States, 2015, *MMWR Morb Mortal Wkly Rep* 67(46):1285–1289, 2018.

Miller RG, Mitchell JD, Moore DH: Riluzole for amyotrophic lateral sclerosis (ALS)/motor neuron disease (MND), *Cochrane Database Syst Rev* (3):CD001447, 2012.

Mirelman A, Rochester L, Maidan I, et al.: Addition of a non-immersive virtual reality component to treadmill training to reduce fall risk in older adults (V-TIME): a randomised controlled trial, *Lancet* 388:1170–1182, 2016.

Miwa H, Miwa T: Fatigue in patients with Parkinson's disease: impact on quality of life, *Intern Med* 50(15):1553–1558, 2011.

Montuschi A, Iazzolino B, Calvo A, et al.: Cognitive correlates in amyotrophic lateral sclerosis: a population-based study in Italy, *J Neurol Neurosurg Psychiatry* 86(2):168–173, 2015.

Morris ME: Movement disorders in people with Parkinson disease: a model for physical therapy, *Phys Ther* 80:578–597, 2000.

Morris ME, Iansek R: Gait disorders in Parkinson's disease: a framework for physical therapy practice, *Neurol Rep* 21:125–131, 1997.

Morris ME, Huxham FE, McGinley J, Iansek R: Gait disorders and gait rehabilitation in Parkinson's disease, *Adv Neurol* 87:347–361, 2001.

Morris ME, Menz HB, McGinley JL, et al.: Falls and mobility in Parkinson's disease: protocol for a randomized controlled clinical trial, *BMC Neurol* 11:93, 2011.

Morris ME, Menz HB, McGinley JL, et al.: A randomized clinical trial to reduce falls in people with Parkinson's disease, *Neurohabil Neural Repair* 29(8):777–785, 2015.

Morris R, Lord S, Lawson RA, et al.: Gait rather than cognition predicts decline in specific cognitive domains in early Parkinson's disease, *J Gerontol A Biol Sci Med Sci* 72(12):1656–1662, 2017.

Mostert S, Kesselring J: Effects of a short-term exercise training program on aerobic fitness, fatigue, health perception, and activity level of subjects with multiple sclerosis, *Mult Scler* 8:161–168, 2002.

Motl RS, Gosney JL: Effect of exercise training on quality of life in multiple sclerosis: a meta-analysis, *Mult Scler* 14:129–135, 2008.

Mulder DW, Rosenbaum RA, Layton DD Jr: Later progression of poliomyelitis or forme fruste amyotrophic lateral sclerosis?, *Mayo Clin Proc* 47:756–761, 1972.

Nantel J, McDonald JC, Bonte-Stewart H: Effect of medication and STN-DBS on postural control in subjects with Parkinson's disease, *Parkinsonism Relat Disord* 18:285–289, 2012.

Nemanich ST, Duncan RP, Dibble LE, et al.: Predictors of gait speeds and the relationship of gait speeds to falls in men and women with Parkinson disease, *Parkinsons Dis* 2013:141720, 2013. doi:10.1155/2013/141720.

Nieuwboer A, Baker K, Willems AM, et al.: The short-term effects of different cueing modalities on turn speed in people with Parkinson's disease, *Neurorehabil Neural Repair* 23:831–836, 2009.

Nollet F, Beelen A, Sargeant AJ, et al.: Submaximal exercise capacity and maximal power output in polio subjects, *Arch Phys Med Rehabil* 82:1678–1685, 2001.

Nutt JG, Horak FB, Bloem BR: Milestones in gait, balance, and falling, *Mov Disord* 26:1166–1174, 2011.

Oguh O, Eisenstein A, Kwasny M, Simuni T: Back to the basics: regular exercise matters in Parkinson's disease: results from the National Parkinson foundation QII registry study, *Parkinsonism Relat Disord* 21:1221–1225, 2014.

O'Sullivan SB, Bezkor EW: Parkinson's disease. In O'Sullivan SB, Schmitz TJ, Fulk GD, editors: *Physical rehabilitation: assessment and treatment*, ed 6, Philadelphia, 2014, FA Davis, pp 807–858.

Olney RK, Murphy J, Forshew D, et al.: The effects of executive and behavioral dysfunction on the course of ALS, *Neurology* 65:1774–1777, 2005.

Oncu J, Durmaz B, Karapolat H: Short-term effects of aerobic exercise on functional capacity, fatigue, and, quality of life in patients with post-polio syndrome, *Clin Rehabil* 23:155–163, 2009.

Ostlund G, Broman L, Werhagen L, Borg K: IVIG treatment in post-polio patients: evaluation of responders, *J Neurol* 259:2571–2578, 2012.

Ostlund G, Broman L, Werhagen L, Borg K: Immunoglobulin treatment in post-polio syndrome: identification of responders and non-responders, *J Rehabil Med* 47:727–733, 2015.

Pariser G, Madras D, Weiss E: Outcomes of an aquatic exercise program including aerobic capacity, lactate threshold, and fatigue in two individuals with multiple sclerosis, *J Neurol Phys Ther* 30:82–90, 2006.

Patten SB, Marrie RA, Carta MG: Depression in multiple sclerosis, *Int Rev Psychiatry* 29(5):463–472, 2017.

Paul SS, Dibble LE, Peterson DS: Motor learning in people with Parkinson's disease: implications for fall prevention across the disease spectrum, *Gait Posture* 61:311–319, 2018.

Paul SS, Sherrington C, Canning CG, et al.: The relative contribution of physical and cognitive fall risk factors in people with Parkinson's disease: a large prospective cohort study, *Neurorehabil Neural Repair* 28(3):282–290, 2014.

Peach PE, Olejnik S: Effect of treatment and noncompliance on post-polio sequelae, *Orthopedics* 14:1199–1203, 1991.

Perry J, Gronley JK, Lunsford T: Rocker shoe as walking aid in multiple sclerosis, *Arch Phys Med Rehabil* 62:59–65, 1981.

Peterson DS, King LA, Cohen RG, Horak FB: Cognitive contributions to freezing of gait in Parkinson disease: implications for physical rehabilitation, *Phys Ther* 96:659–670, 2016.

Pfeiffer RF: Non-motor symptoms in Parkinson's disease, *Parkinsonism Relat Disord* 22(Suppl 1):S119–S122, 2016. doi:10.1016/j.parkreldis.2015.09.004.

Phukan J, Elamin M, Bede P, et al.: The syndrome of cognitive impairment in amyotrophic lateral sclerosis: a population-based study, *J Neurol Neurosurg Psychiatry* 83(1):102–108, 2012.

Pitetti KH, Barrett PJ, Abbas D: Endurance exercise training in Guillain-Barré syndrome, *Arch Phys Med Rehabil* 74:761–765, 1993.

Plotnik M, Shema S, Dofman M, et al.: A motor learning-based intervention to ameliorate freezing of gait in subjects with Parkinson's disease, *J Neurol* 261:1329–1339, 2014.

Polman CH, Reingold SC, Banwell B, et al.: Diagnostic criteria for multiple sclerosis: 2010 revisions to the McDonald criteria, *Ann Neurol* 69:292–302, 2011.

Prell T, Grosskreutz J: The involvement of the cerebellum in amyotrophic lateral sclerosis, *Amyotroph Lateral Scler Frontotemporal Degener* 14(7-8):507–515, 2013.

Protas EJ, Mitchell K, Williams A, et al.: Gait and step training to reduce falls in Parkinson's disease, *NeuroRehabilitation* 20:183–190, 2005.

Protas E, Stanley R, Jankovic J: Parkinson's disease. In Durstine JL, Moore G, Painter P, Roberts S, editors: *ACSM's exercise management for persons with chronic diseases and disabilities*, ed 3, Champaign, IL, 2009, Human Kinetics, pp 350–356.

Ramazzina I, Bernazzoli B, Costantino C: Systematic review on strength training in Parkinson's disease: an unsolved question, *Clin Interv Aging* 12:619–628, 2017.

Reichmann, H: Premotor diagnosis of Parkinson's disease, *Neurosci Bull* 33(5):526–534, 2017.

Rietberg MB, Veerbeek JM, Gosselink R, Kwakkel G, van Wegen EE: Respiratory muscle training for multiple sclerosis, *Cochrane Database Syst Rev* 12:CD009424, 2017.

Rochester L, Galna B, Lord S, Burn D: The nature of dual-task interference during gait in incident Parkinson's disease, *Neuroscience* 265:83–94, 2014.

Rogers MW, Kennedy R, Palmer S, et al.: Postural preparation prior to stepping in patients with Parkinson's disease, *J Neurophysiol* 106(2):915–924, 2011.

Ropper AH, Wijdicks E, Truax BT: *Guillain-Barre syndrome, contemporary neurology series* (vol 34), Philadelphia, 1991, FA Davis.

Salci Y, Fil A, Armutlu K, et al.: Effects of different exercise modalities on ataxia in multiple sclerosis patients: a randomized controlled study, *Disabil Rehabil* 39(26):2626–2632, 2017.

Sanjak M, Hirsch MA, Bravver EK, et al.: Vestibular deficits leading to disequilibrium and falls in ambulatory amyotrophic lateral sclerosis, *Arch Phys Med Rehabil* 95:1933–1939, 2014.

Santos L, Fernandez-Rio J, Winge K, et al.: Effects of supervised slackline training on postural instability, freezing of gait, and falls efficacy in people with Parkinson's disease, *Disabil Rehabil* 39:1573–1580, 2017.

Schapira AHV, Chaudhuri KR, Jenner P: Non-motor features of Parkinson disease, *Nat Rev Neurosci* 18(7):435–450, 2017. doi:10.1038/nrn.2017.62.

Schapiro RT: *Managing the symptoms of multiple sclerosis*, ed 4, New York, 2003, Demos Publications.

Schlenstedt C, Paschen S, Kruse A, et al.: Resistance versus balance training to improve postural control in Parkinson's disease: a randomized rater blinded controlled study, *PLoS One* 10:e0140584, 2015.

Schrag A, Ben-Shlomo Y, Quinn N: How common are complications of Parkinson's disease? *J Neurol* 249:419–423, 2002.

Shangyan H, Kuiqing L, Yumin X, Jie C, Weixiong L: Meta-analysis of the efficacy of modafinil versus placebo in the treatment of multiple sclerosis fatigue, *Mult Scler Relat Disord* 19:85–89, 2018. doi:10.1016/j.msard.2017.10.011.

Silva-Batista C, Corcos DM, Roschel H, et al.: Resistance training with instability for patients with Parkinson's disease, *Med Sci Sports Exerc* 48:1678–1687, 2016.

Silva-Batista C, Corcos DM, Barroso R, et al.: Instability resistance training improves neuromuscular outcome in Parkinson's disease, *Med Sci Sports Exerc* 49:652–660, 2017.

Silva-Batista C, Corcos DM, Kanegusuku H, et al.: Balance and fear of falling in subjects with Parkinson's disease is improved after exercise with motor complexity, *Gait Posture* 61:90–97, 2018.

Skalsky AJ, McDonald CM: Prevention and management of limb contractures in neuromuscular diseases, *Phys Med Rehabil Clin N Am* 23:675–687, 2012.

Smania N, Corato E, Tinazzi C, et al.: Effect of balance training on postural instability in patients with idiopathic Parkinson's disease, *Neurorehabil Neural Repair* 24:826–834, 2010.

Smulders K, Dale ML, Carson-Kuhta P, Nutt JG, Horak FB: Pharmacological treatment in Parkinson's disease: effects on gait, *Parkisonism Relat Disord* 31:3–13, 2016.

Spector SA, Gordon PL, Feuerstein IM, et al.: Strength gains without muscle injury after strength training in patients with post-polio muscular atrophy, *Muscle Nerve* 19:1282, 1996.

Stoelb BL, Carter GT, Abresch RT, et al.: Pain in persons with post-polio syndrome: frequency, intensity and impact, *Arch Phys Med Rehabil* 89:1933–1940, 2008.

Stożek J, Rudzińska M, Pustułka-Piwnik U, Szczudlik A: The effect of the rehabilitation program on balance, gait, physical performance and trunk rotation in Parkinson's disease, *Aging Clin Exp Res* 28:1169–1177, 2016.

Sulton LL: Meeting the challenge of Guillain-Barré syndrome, *Nursing Manage* 33:25–31, 2002.

Sutton AL, editor: *Movement disorders source book*, ed 2, Detroit, 2009, Omnigraphics.

Thompson AJ, Banwell BL, Barkhof F, et al.: Diagnosis of multiple sclerosis: 2017 revisions of the McDonald criteria, *Lancet Neurol* 17(2):162–173, 2018.

Trojan DA, Cashman NR: Post-poliomyelitis syndrome, *Muscle Nerve* 31:6–19, 2005.

Trojan DA, Finch L: Management of post-polio syndrome, *NeuroRehabilitation* 8:93–105, 1997.

Trojan DA, Arnold DL, Shapiro S, et al.: Fatigue in post-poliomyelitis syndrome: association with disease-related, behavioral, and psychosocial factors, *PM R* 1:442–449, 2009.

Vallabhajosula S, Buckley TA, Tillman MD, Hass CJ: Age and Parkinson's disease related kinematic alterations during multi-directional gait initiation, *Gait Posture* 37(2):280–286, 2013.

Van der Werf SP, Evers A, Jongen PJH, Bleijenberg G: The role of helplessness as mediator between neurological disability, emotional instability, experienced fatigue and depression in patients with multiple sclerosis, *Mult Scler* 9:89–94, 2003.

Van Doorn PA: Diagnosis, treatment and prognosis of Guillain-Barré syndrome (GBS), *Presse Med* 42:193–201, 2013.

Van Doorn PA, Ruts L, Jacobs BC: Clinical features, pathogenesis, and treatment of Guillain-Barré syndrome, *Lancet Neurol* 7:939–950, 2008.

Van Koningsveld R, Steyerberg EW, Hughes RA, et al.: A clinical prognostic scoring system for Guillain-Barré syndrome, *Lancet Neurol* 6:589–594, 2007.

Van Vaerenbergh J, Vranken R, Baro F: The influence of rotational exercises on freezing in Parkinson's disease, *Funct Neurol* 18:11–16, 2003.

Vaugoyeau M, Viel S, Assaiante C, et al.: Impaired vertical postural control and proprioceptive integration deficits in Parkinson's disease, *Neuroscience* 146(2):852–863, 2007.

Voorn EI, Gerrits KH, Koopman FS, Nollet F, Beelen A: Determining the anaerobic threshold in postpolio syndrome: comparison with current guidelines for training intensity prescription, *Arch Phys Med Rehabil* 95:935–940, 2014.

Voorn EI, Koopman FS, Brehm MA, et al.: Aerobic exercise training in post-polio syndrome: process evaluation of a randomized controlled trial, *PLoS One* 11:e0159280, 2016.

Wens I, Dalgas U, Vandenabeele F, et al.: High intensity exercise in multiple sclerosis: effects on muscle contractile characteristics and exercise capacity, a randomized controlled trial, *PLOS One* 10(9):e0133697, 2015. doi:10.1371/journal.pone.0133697.

Wens I, Dalgas U, Vandenabeele F, et al.: High intensity aerobic and resistance exercise can improve glucose tolerance in person with multiple sclerosis: a randomized controlled trial, *Am J Phys Med Rehabil* 96(3):161–166, 2017.

Werhagen L, Borg K: Impact of pain on quality of life in patients with post-polio syndrome, *J Rehabil Med* 45:161–163, 2013.

White AT, Wilson TE, Davis SL, Petajan JH: Effect of precooling on physical performance in multiple sclerosis, *Mult Scler* 6:176–180, 2000.

Wiechers DO, Hubbell SL: Late changes in the motor unit after acute poliomyelitis, *Muscle Nerve* 4:524–528, 1981.

Willen C, Sunnerhagen KS, Grimby G: Dynamic water exercise in individuals with late poliomyelitis, *Arch Phys Med Rehabil* 82:66–72, 2001.

Willison HJ, Jacobs BC, Van Doorn PA: Guillain-Barré syndrome, *Lancet* 388:717–727, 2016.

Winberg C, Flansbjer UB, Carlsson G, Rimmer J, Lexell J: Physical activity in persons with late effects of polio: a descriptive study, *Disabil Health* 7:302–308, 2014.

Wood BH, Bilclough JA, Bowron A, Walker RW: Incidence and prediction falls in Parkinson's disease: a prospective multidisciplinary study, *J Neurol Neurosurg Psychiatry* 72:721–725, 2002.

Yang TT, Wang L, Deng XY, Yu G: Pharmacological treatments for fatigue in patients with multiple sclerosis: a systematic review and meta-analysis, *Neurol Sci* 380:256–261, 2017.

Young CA, Quincey AC, Wong SM, Tennant A: Quality of life for post-polio syndrome: a patient derived, Rasch standard scale, *Disabil Rehabil* 40(5):597–602, 2018a. doi:10.1080/09638288.2016.1260650.

Young CA, Wong SM, Quincey AC, Tennant A: Measuring physical and cognitive fatigue in people with post-polio syndrome: development of the Neurological Fatigue Index for Post-Polio Syndrome (NFI-PP), *PM R* 10(2):129–136, 2018b. doi:10.1016/j.pmrj.2017.06.014.

Zaenker P, Favret F, Lonsdorfer E: High-intensity interval training combined with resistance training improves physiological capacities, strength and quality of life in multiple sclerosis patients: a pilot study, *Eur J Phys Rehabil Med* 54(1):58–67, 2018.

Zesiewicz TA, Patel-Larson A, Hauser RA, Sullivan KL: Social security disability insurance (SSDI) in Parkinson's disease, *Disabil Rehabil* 29(24):1934–1936, 2007.

Zhao Y, Nonnekes J, Storcken EJ, et al.: Feasibility of external rhythmic cueing with the Google Glass for improving gait in people with Parkinson's disease, *J Neurol* 263:1156–1165, 2016.